The Encyclopedia of

NEUROPSYCHOLOGICAL DISORDERS

CHAD A. NOGGLE, PhD, is Assistant Professor of Clinical Psychiatry and Chief of the Division of Behavioral and Psychosocial Oncology at Southern Illinois University-School of Medicine. He previously served as an Assistant Professor at both Ball State University and Middle Tennessee State University. Dr. Noggle holds a BA in Psychology from the University of Illinois at Springfield and completed his MA and PhD at Ball State University in School Psychology with specialization in Clinical Neuropsychology. He completed a 2-year post-doctoral residency at the Indiana Neuroscience Institute at St. Vincent's Hospital with specialization in Pediatric and Adult/Geriatric Neuropsychology. To date, Dr. Noggle has published more than 250 articles, book chapters, encyclopedia entries, and research abstracts, and has made over 80 presentations at national and international conferences in neuropsychology. He currently serves as a reviewer for a number of neuropsychology journals. Dr. Noggle is a member of the American Psychological Association (Divisions 5, 16, 22, 38, 40), National Academy of Neuropsychology, and International Neuropsychological Society. He is a licensed Psychologist in both Illinois and Indiana. His research interests focus on both adult and pediatric populations, spanning psychiatric illnesses, dementia, PDDs, and neuromedical disorders. He has particular interest in the neuropsychological consequences of cancer and its treatment in both adults and children.

RAYMOND S. DEAN, PhD, ABPP, ABPN, holds a BA degree in Psychology (Magna cum laude) and an MS degree in Research and Psychometrics from the State University of New York at Albany. As a Parachek-Frazier Research Fellow, he completed a PhD in School/Child Clinical Psychology at Arizona State University in 1978. Dr. Dean completed an internship focused on neuropsychology at the Arizona Neurophychiatric Hospital and post-doctoral work at the University of Wisconsin at Madison. From 1978–1980, Dr. Dean was Assistant Professor and Director of the Child Clinic at the University of Wisconsin at Madison. During this time he was awarded the Lightner Witmer Award by the School Psychology Division of the American Psychological Association. From 1980–1981, he served as Assistant Professor of Psychological Services at the University of North Carolina at Chapel Hill. From 1981–1984, Dr. Dean served as Assistant Professor of Medical Psychology and Director of the Neuropsychology Internship at Washington University School of Medicine in St. Louis. During this time, Dr. Dean received both the Outstanding Contribution Award from the National Academy of Neuropsychology and the Early Contribution Award by Division 15 of the APA. He was named the George and Frances Ball Distinguished Professor of Neuropsychology and Director of the Neuropsychology Laboratory at Ball State University and has served in this position since 1984. In addition, Dr. Dean served as Distinguished Visiting Faculty at the Staff College of the NIMH. Dr. Dean is a Diplomate of the American Board of Professional Psychology, the American Board of Professional Neuropsychology, and the American Board of Pediatric Neuropsychology. He is a Fellow of the American Psychological Association (Divisions Clinical, Educational, School and Clinical Neuropsyhology), the National Academy of Neuropsychology, and the American Psychopathological Association. Dr. Dean is a past president of the Clinical Neuropsychology Division of the American Psychological Association and the National Academy of Neuropsychology. He also served as editor of the *Archives of Clinical Neuropsychology*, *Journal of School Psychology*, and the *Bulletin of the National Academy of Neuropsychology*. Dr. Dean has published some 600 research articles, books, chapters, and tests. For his work he has been recognized by awards from the National Academy of Neuropsychology, the *Journal of School Psychology*, and the Clinical Neuropsychology Division of the American Psychological Association.

ARTHUR MACNEILL HORTON JR., EdD, ABPP, ABPN, received his EdD degree in Counselor Education from the University of Virginia in 1976. He also holds Diplomates in Clinical Psychology and Behavioral Psychology from the American Board of Professional Psychology and in Neuropsychology from the American Board of Professional Neuropsychology. Dr. Horton is the author/editor of over 15 books, more than 30 book chapters, and over 150 journal articles. He also coauthored (with Cecil Reynolds, PhD) *The Test of Verbal Conceptualization and Fluency*, a measure of executive functioning in children, adults, and the elderly. He is past president of the American Board of Professional Neuropsychology, a doctoral-level certification board in neuropsychology, the Coalition of Clinical Practitioners in Neuropsychology, the National Academy of Neuropsychology, and the Maryland Psychological Association. In addition, Dr. Horton was a member of the State of Maryland Board of Examiners of Psychologists for two terms. Dr. Horton is a Fellow of the American Psychological Association (Divisions 6, 42, 50 and 56). Previously, Dr. Horton was a Program Officer with the National Institute of Drug Abuse and National Institutes of Health, with responsibilities for neuropsychology. He has taught at the University of Virginia, The Citadel, West Virginia University, Johns Hopkins University, The University of Baltimore, Loyola College in Maryland, the Department of Psychiatry of the University of Maryland School of Medicine, and the Fielding University Graduate Program in Neuropsychology. Currently, Dr. Horton is in independent practice as Director of the Neuropsychology Section at Psych Associates of Maryland and Editor-in-Chief of *Applied Neuropsychology*. Dr. Horton also consults on neuropsychology and drug abuse research issues.

The Encyclopedia of

NEUROPSYCHOLOGICAL DISORDERS

Edited by

Chad A. Noggle, PhD

Raymond S. Dean, PhD, ABPP, ABPN

Arthur MacNeill Horton Jr., EdD, ABPP, ABPN

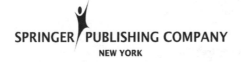

SPRINGER PUBLISHING COMPANY

NEW YORK

Springer Publishing Company, LLC
11 West 42nd Street
New York, NY 10036
www.springerpub.com

Acquisitions Editor: Nancy Hale
Composition: S4Carlisle Publishing Services

ISBN: 978-0-8261-9854-9
E-book ISBN: 9780826198556

11 12 13/ 5 4 3 2 1

The authors and the publisher of this Work have made every effort to use sources believed to be reliable to provide information that is accurate and compatible with the standards generally accepted at the time of publication. The authors and publisher shall not be liable for any special, consequential, or exemplary damages resulting, in whole or in part, from the readers' use of, or reliance on, the information contained in this book. The publisher has no responsibility for the persistence or accuracy of URLs for external or third-party Internet Web sites referred to in this publication and does not guarantee that any content on such Web sites is, or will remain, accurate or appropriate.

Cataloging-in-Publication Data is available from the Library of Congress.

Printed in the United States of America by Bang Printing.

To my wife and children for your love and support: You are my everything.
To my parents, for your encouragement and many life lessons,
among them the importance of hard work.
CAN

I dedicate this book to my three daughters,
Sarah, Whitney, and Heather.
RSD

To my wife Mary, with all of my love.
AMH

EDITORIAL BOARD

CONTENTS

PREFACE

The Encyclopedia of Neuropsychological Disorders was created as a reference manual of disorders that have a biological-psychological interaction. In many ways the title of this text can be seen as a misnomer. As professionals, we speak of neurological disorders and psychiatric disorders, but the concept of neuropsychological disorders is not readily used by the medical and psychological professions. The book makes this distinction in the discussion of the potential neuropsychological sequelae for an array of recognized neurological, psychiatric, as well as other medical disorders. As such, the book provides firm bases for numerous health care professionals to better understand and treat neurological, psychiatric, and neuromedical patients. While the book offers a wide array of disorders, the crux of the discussion is directed toward the fields of neuropsychology, neuropsychiatry, and behavioral neurology. Indeed, what we know of the functioning of normal and diseased brains has grown more in the last four decades than any other time in history. And, because there is an increased appreciation of the potential impact on the central nervous system by various unsuspected disorders, the variety of presentations now seen by clinicians in the neurosciences is steadily expanding. Along with this knowledge comes vast improvements in the approaches to diagnosis and treatment by professionals across a wider band of specialties. As a consequence, there is need for a concise and synthesized discussion of the presenting features of recognized disorders. With this in mind specifically, we sought to create a reference work in which individual disorders are discussed with the fields of neuropsychology, neuropsychiatry, and neurology in mind, covering those domains of clinical relevance with emphasis placed on empirically based information.

The internet can be a powerful tool, but in many ways it can be difficult to determine the reliability of that information. Thus, empirical backing of the information shared was of greatest importance. The product is designed to be useful to both veteran clinicians as well students in training. In all, the text includes a structured coverage of the clinical and neuropsychological features, neuropathological/pathophysiological correlates, diagnostic considerations, and methods of treatment for nearly 300 recognized disorders and diseases across the lifespan.

CONTRIBUTORS

J. Aaron Albritton, BA
Research Assistant
Functional Neurosurgery Laboratory
Vanderbilt University
Nashville, TN

Ana Arenivas, MS
Doctoral Student
University of Texas Southwestern
Dallas, TX

Amanda Ballenger, MA
Doctoral Student
Department of Educational Psychology
Ball State University
Muncie, IN

Mark T. Barisa, PhD, ABPP-CN
Clinical Neuropsychologist
Department of Neuropsychology
Baylor Institute for Rehabilitation
Dallas, TX

Alyse Barker, MA
Doctoral Candidate
Department of Psychology
Louisiana State University
Baton Rouge, LA

Jeffrey T. Barth, PhD, ABPP-CN
John Edward Fowler Professor
Neurocognitive Assessment Laboratory
Department of Psychiatry and Neurobehavioral Sciences
University of Virginia School of Medicine
Charlottesville, VA

Audrey Baumeister, PhD
Clinical Psychologist
NeuroBehavioral Institute
Weston, Florida

Melanie Blahnik, PsyD
Clinical Psychologist
Department of Physical Medicine
  and Rehabilitation
Minneapolis Veterans Affairs
  Medical Center
Minneapolis, MN

Tonya M. Bennett, MS
Graduate Student
Department of Psychology
Fielding Gradute University
Santa Barbara, CA

Ryan Boddy, BA
Graduate Student
Center for Psychological Studies
Nova Southeastern University
Fort Lauderdale, FL

Josie Bolanos, BA
Graduate Student
Center for Psychological Studies
Nova Southeastern University
Fort Lauderdale, FL

Justin J. Boseck, MA
Doctoral Student
Department of Educational
  Psychology
Ball State University
Muncie, IN

W. Howard Buddin Jr., MS
Doctoral Student
Center for Psychological Studies
Nova Southeastern University
Fort Lauderdale, FL

Shane S. Bush, PhD, ABPP, ABN
Clinical Neuropsychologist
Long Island Neuropsychology, PC
Lake Ronkonkoma, NY
Department of Psychology
VA New York Harbor Healthcare System
St. Albans, NY

Mei Chang, MA
Doctoral Student
Department of Educational Psychology
Ball State University
Muncie, IN

Sarah C. Connolly, MA
Doctoral Student
Department of Educational Psychology
Ball State University
Muncie, IN

Christine Corsun-Ascher, PsyD
Center for Psychological Studies
Nova Southeastern University
Fort Lauderdale, FL

Nicole Cruz, PhD
Instructor of Clinical Neurology
Department of Neurology
Washington University School of Medicine
Department of Psychology
St. Louis Children's Hospital
St. Louis, MO

George M. Cuesta, PhD
Supervisory Psychologist and Team Leader
Department of Veterans Affairs
Veterans Health Administration
Readjustment Counseling Service
New York, NY
Clinical Assistant Professor of Neuropsychology
Department of Neurology and Neuroscience
Weill Medical College of Cornell University
New York, NY

Danielle S. Dance, MS
Doctoral Student
Center for Psychological Studies
Nova Southeastern University
Fort Lauderdale, FL

Andrew S. Davis, PhD, HSPP
Associate Professor of Psychology, Director of
    Doctoral Internships
Department of Educational Psychology
Ball State University
Muncie, IN

Jeremy Davis, PsyD
School of Psychological Sciences
University of Indianapolis
Indianapolis, IN

Raymond S. Dean, PhD, ABPP, ABN, ABPdN
George and Frances Ball Distinguished
    Professor of Neuropsychology
Department of Educational Psychology
Ball State University
Muncie, IN

Brenda Deliz-Roldán, MD
Neurologist-Neuromuscular Specialist
University of Puerto Rico Medical School
San Juan, Puerto Rico

Angela Dortch, BA, MA
Graduate Student
Department of Educational Psychology
Ball State University
Muncie, IN

Maryellen C. Dougherty, MA
Doctoral Student
Center for Psychological Studies
Nova Southeastern University
Fort Lauderdale, FL

Valeria Drago, MD, PhD
Neurologist
Services of Neurology and Rehabilitation
ASP Siracusa
Siracusa, Italy
Adjunct Assistant Professor
Department of Neurology
University of Florida
Gainesville, FL

Rebecca Durkin, MD
Department of Psychiatry
Rush University Medical Center
Chicago, IL

Jennifer N. Fiebig, PhD
Instructor
Department of Psychology
Loyola University
Chicago, IL

Glen R. Finney, MD
Assistant Professor
Department of Neurology University of Florida
Gainesville, FL

Jessica Foley, PhD
Center for Psychological Studies
Nova Southeastern University
Fort Lauderdale, FL

Paul S. Foster, PhD
Associate Professor
Department of Psychology
Middle Tennessee State University
Murfreesboro, TN
Adjunct Assistant Professor
Department of Neurology
University of Florida
Gainesville, FL

Jason R. Freeman, PhD
Associate Professor
Neurocognitive Assessment Laboratory
Department of Psychiatry and
   Neurobehavioral Sciences
University of Virginia School of Medicine
Charlottesville, VA

Daniel L. Frisch, BA
Graduate Student
Center for Psychological Studies
Nova Southeastern University
Fort Lauderdale, FL

Jessica Garcia, PhD
Paralegal Studies Coordinator
Nova Southeastern University
Fort Lauderdale, FL

Jacob M. Goings, BA
Doctoral Student
Educational Psychology and
   Counseling Department
University of Tennessee
Knoxville, TN

Charles Golden, PhD, ABPP, ABN
Professor and Director
Center for Psychological Studies
Nova Southeastern University
Fort Lauderdale, FL

Amy J. Goldman, PT, DPT
Physical Therapist-Stroke Program Manager
Department of Physical Therapy
Madonna Rehabilitation Hospital
Lincoln, NE

Gerald Goldstein, PhD
Senior Research Career Scientist,
Mental Illness Research, Education, and Clinical Center
VA Pittsburgh Healthcare System
Clinical Professor of Psychiatry
Department of Psychiatry
University of Pittsburgh
Pittsburgh, PA

Javier Gontier, MA
Department of Psychology
Universidad del Desarrollo
Concepcioen, Chile

William Drew Gouvier, PhD
Professor
Department of Psychology
Louisiana State University
Baton Rouge, LA

Peyton Groff, MA
Doctoral Student
Department of Educational Psychology
Ball State University
Muncie, IN

Mary E. Haines, PhD, ABPP-CN
Clinical Neuropsychologist
Clinical Associate Professor
Departments of Physical Medicine and Rehabilitation
   and Psychiatry
University of Toledo Medical Center
Toledo, OH

Vishnumurthy S. Hedna, MD
Resident
Department of Neurology
University of Florida
Gainesville, FL

Margie Hernandez, BA
Graduate Student
Department of Psychology
University of North Carolina-Wilmington
Wilmington, NC

Jeremy Hertza, PsyD
Director of Behavioral Medicine
Clinical Neuropsychologist
Walton Rehabilitation Hospital
Assistant Clinical Professor of Psychiatry and
   Health Behavior
Medical College of Georgia
Augusta, GA

Daniel J. Heyanka, MA
Doctoral Student
Center for Psychological Studies
Nova Southeastern University
Fort Lauderdale, FL

Lindsay J. Hines, MS
Doctoral Student
Center for Psychological Studies
Nova Southeastern University
Fort Lauderdale, FL

James B. Hoelzle, PhD
Assistant Professor
Department of Psychology
Marquette University
Milwaukee, WI

Matth Holcombe, MA
Doctoral Student
Department of Educational Psychology
Ball State University
Muncie, IN

Jessica Holster, BA
Graduate Student
Center for Psychological Studies
Nova Southeastern University
Fort Lauderdale, FL

Javan Horwitz, PsyD
Clinical Neuropsychologist
Department of Extended Care and Rehabilitation
VA Northern Indiana Healthcare System
Marion, IN

Natalie Horwitz, MA
Private Practice
Indianapolis, IN

Haojing Huang, MD, PHD
Assistant Professor of Clinical Psychiatry
Department of Psychiatry
Southern Illinois University - School of Medicine
Springfield, IL

Kelly N. Hutchins, MS
Private Practice
Bakersfield, CA

J. T. Hutton, MD, PhD
University of North Carolina
Wilmington, NC

Gaurav Jain, MD
Resident
Department of Psychiatry
Southern Illinois University-School of Medicine
Springfield, IL

Christina Weyer Jamora, PhD
San Francisco General Hospital/UCSF School of Medicine
San Francisco, CA

Nick P. Jenkins, MD
Internal Medicine
St.Vincent Hospital
Indianapolis, IN

Sarah C. Jenkins
Counseling and Guidance Services
Ball State University
Muncie, IN

Velisa M. Johnson, MA
Graduate Student
Department of Psychology
Fielding Graduate University
Santa Barbara, CA

Evan Koehn, MA
Doctoral Student
Department of Educational Psychology
Ball State University
Muncie, IN

Abhay Kumar, MD
Resident
Department of Neurology
University of Florida
Gainesville, FL

Darla J. Lawson, PhD
Pediatric Neuropsychology Department
Pediatric Neurobehavioral Diagnostics
Idaho Falls, ID

Gershom T. Lazarus, MA
University of North Carolina
Wilmington, NC

Hannah Lindsey, BA
Graduate Student
Department of Psychology
University of North Carolina-Wilmington
Wilmington, NC

Raquel Vilar López, PhD
Universidad de Granada
Granada, Spain

Shira Louria, PsyD
Resident
Neuroscience Institute
Long Island Jewish Medical Center
Long Island, NY

Courtney Lund, MA
Doctoral Student
Department of Educational Psychology
Ball State University
Muncie, IN

Jacob T. Lutz, MA
Doctoral Student
Department of Educational Psychology
Ball State University
Muncie, IN

Jennifer Mariner, PsyD, HSPP
Clinical Psychologist
Geriatrics and Extended Care
Department of Psychiatry
Richard L. Roudebush VA Medical Center
Assistant Professor of Clinical Psychology
Department of Clinical Psychiatry
Indiana University School of Medicine
Indianapolis, IN

Alyssa M. Maulucci, PhD
VA Medical Center
Washington, DC

Anya Mazur-Mosiewicz, MA
Doctoral Student
Department of Educational Psychology
Ball State University
Muncie, IN

Kathryn McGuire, PhD
Clinical Psychologist
Department of Physical Medicine and Rehabilitation
Minneapolis Veterans Affairs Medical Center
Assistant Professor
Department of Psychiatry
University of Minnesota
Minneapolis, MN

Teri J. McHale, PhD
Psychological Assistant
Developmental Neuropsychology Laboratory
Ventura, CA
Bay Psychiatric Medical Group
Torrance, CA

Katherine Meredith, MS
Doctoral Student
Center for Psychological Studies
Nova Southeastern University
Fort Lauderdale, FL
Department of Neuropsychology
Baylor Institute for Rehabilitation
Dallas, TX

Kynan Eugene Metoyer, BA
Graduate Student
Center for Psychological Studies
Nova Southeastern University
Fort Lauderdale, FL

Liza San Miguel-Montes, PsyD
Clinical Neuropsychologist
Neurology Section-Medicine
University of Puerto Rico Medical School
San Juan, Puerto Rico

Kathryn M. Lombardi Mirra, MA
Doctoral Student
Department of Psychology
Suffolk University
Boston, MA

Ashleigh R. Molz, BS
Doctoral Student
Temple University
Department of Psychology
Philadelphia, PA

Jessie L. Morrow, MS
Doctoral Student
Center for Psychological Studies
Nova Southeastern University
Fort Lauderdale, FL

Monica O. Murray, EdS
Graduate Student
School of Psychology
Fielding Graduate University
Santa Barbara, CA

Mandi Musso, BS
Doctoral Candidate
Department of Psychology
Louisiana State University
Baton Rouge, LA

Mónica Muzquiz, MA
University of North Carolina
Wilmington, NC

Thomas E. Myers, MS
Doctoral Student
Department of Psychology
The Graduate Center and Queens College
City University of New York
Flushing, NY

Chad A. Noggle, PhD
Assistant Professor of Clinical Psychiatry
Chief, Division of Behavioral and Psychosocial Oncology
Department of Psychiatry
Southern Illinois University-School of Medicine
Springfield, IL

Kyle Noll, MA
Doctoral Student
University of Texas Southwestern
Dallas, TX

Anthony P. Odland, BA
Graduate Student
Center for Psychological Studies
Nova Southeastern University
Fort Lauderdale, FL

Carlos Ojeda, MA
Graduate Student
Department of Psychology
University of Arkansas
Fayetteville, AR

Michelle R. Pagoria, PsyD
Clinical Neuropsychologist
Director of Neuropsychology
Benchmark Psychiatric Services, Ltd
Orland Park, IL

Lisa A. Pass, MA
Doctoral Student
Department of Educational Psychology
Ball State University
Muncie, IN

Kelly R. Pless, MS
Doctoral Student
Center for Psychological Studies
Nova Southeastern University
Fort Lauderdale, FL

Lena M. F. Prinzi, BA
Graduate Student
Center for Psychological Studies
Nova Southeastern University
Fort Lauderdale, FL

Stephen E. Prover, MD
Diplomate-American Board of Psychiatry and Neurology
Bay Psychiatric Medical Group
Torrance, CA

Antonio E. Puente, PhD
Clinical Neuropsychologist
Professor
Department of Psychology
University of North Carolina, Wilmington
Wilmington, NC

Antonio N. Puente, BA
Graduate Student
Department of Psychology
University of Georgia
Athens, GA

Sandra Santiago Ramajo, PhD
Universidad de Granada
Granada, Spain

Donna Rasin-Waters, PhD
VA New York Harbor Healthcare System
Brooklyn, NY

Luz M. Restrepo, BA
Graduate Student
Center for Pscyhological Studies
Nova Southeastern University
Fort Lauderdale, FL

Jamie Rice, BA
Graduate Student
Center for Psychological Studies
Nova Southeastern University
Fort Lauderdale, FL

Ann M. Richardson
Attorney at Law
California State Government
Sacramento, CA

David Ritchie, MA
Doctoral Student
Center for Psychological Studies
Nova Southeastern University
Fort Lauderdale, FL

Jessi H. Robbins, MS
Doctoral Student
Center for Psychological Studies
Nova Southeastern University
Fort Lauderdale, FL

Stephen Robinson, MD
Assistant Professor of Clinical Psychiatry
Director, Adult Inpatient Services
Assistant Chair, Department of Psychiatry
Southern Illinois University–School of Medicine
Springfield, IL

Rachel Rock, MA
Department of Psychology
The University of Alabama
Tuscaloosa, AL

Miriam Jocelyn Rodriguez, BA, MS
Doctoral Student
Center for Psychological Studies
Nova Southeastern University
Fort Lauderdale, FL

Ronald Ruff, PhD, ABPP
Clinical Neuropsychologist
Clinical Professor
Department of Psychiatry
University of California-San Francisco
San Francisco, CA

Saralyn Ruff, MEd
Doctoral Student
Department of Human Development and Family Studies
Purdue University
West Lafayette, IN

Daniela Rusovici, MD
Neurologist
Private Practice
Palm Beach, FL

Mark A. Sandberg, PhD
Clinical Neuropsychologist
Independent Practice
Smithtown, NY

J. Forrest Sanders, PsyD
Neurocognitive Assessment Laboratory
Department of Psychiatry and Neurobehavioral Sciences
University of Virginia Health System
Charlottesville, VA

Stephanie Lei Santiso, MS
Doctoral Student
Center for Psychological Studies
Nova Southeastern University
Fort Lauderdale, FL

David M. Scarisbrick, BA
Graduate Student
Center for Psychological Studies
Nova Southeastern University
Fort Lauderdale, FL

Mindy Scheithauer, MA
Doctoral Student
Department of Educational Psychology
Ball State University
Muncie, IN

Brian Schmitt, MA
Doctoral Student
Department of Educational Psychology
Ball State University
Muncie, IN

Eric Silk, MA, MS
Visiting Professor of Psychology
Farquhar College of Arts and Sciences
Nova Southeastern University
Fort Lauderdale, FL

Anita H. Sim, PhD
Clinical Neuropsychologist
Physical Medicine and Rehabilitation
Minneapolis VA Medical Center
Minneapolis, MN

Melissa Singh, MA
Doctoral Student
Department of Educational Psychology
Ball State University
Muncie, IN

Sarita Singhal, MD
Resident
Department of Pediatrics
Southern Illinois University-School of Medicine
Springfield, IL

Henry V. Soper, PhD
Professor
School of Psychology
Fielding Graduate University
Santa Barbara, CA

Tara V. Spevack, PhD, ABPP
Pediatric Neuropsychologist
St. Louis Children's Hospital
Washington University Medical Center
St. Louis, MO

Susan Spicer, MA
Doctoral Student
School of Psychology
Fielding Graduate University
Santa Barbara, CA

Amanda R. W. Steiner, PhD
University of Virginia
Department of Psychology
Charlottesville, VA

Amy R. Steiner, PsyD, LP
Clinical Neuropsychologist
HealthPartners Neurology
Center for Dementia and Alzheimer's Care
Minneapolis, MN

Andrea Stephen, MA
Doctoral Student
Department of Educational Psychology
Ball State University
Muncie, IN

Carol Swann, MA
Doctoral Student
School of Psychology
Fielding Graduate University
Santa Barbara, CA

Melissa Swanson, PhD
Clinical Neuropsychology Postdoctoral Fellow
Department of Physical Medicine
  and Rehabilitation
University of Toledo Medical Center
Toledo, OH

Lori S. Terryberry, SPOHR, PhD, ABPP
Clinical Neuropsychologist
Manager, Brain Injury Program
Department of Neuropsychology
Madonna Rehabilitation Hospital
Lincoln, NE

Jon C. Thompson, PsyD, HSPP
Department of Neuropsychology
St.Vincent Hospital
Indianapolis, IN

Erin L. Tireman, MS
Doctoral Student
Center for Psychological Studies
Nova Southeastern University
Fort Lauderdale, FL

Jeffrey B. Titus, PhD
Department of Psychology
St. Louis Children's Hospital
Assistant Professor of Clinical Neurology
Department of Neurology
Washington University School of Medicine
St. Louis, MO

Issac Tourgeman, BA
Graduate Student
Center for Psychological Studies
Nova Southeastern University
Fort Lauderdale, FL

Beth Trammell, MA
Doctoral Student
Department of Educational Psychology
Ball State University
Muncie, IN

Krista Puente Trefz, PsyD
Licensed Psychologist
Circles of Care
Melbourne, FL

Chriscelyn Tussey, PsyD
Clinical Neuropsychologist
Director of Psychological Assessment
Bellevue Hospital Center
New York University School of Medicine
New York, NY

Sarah M. Viamonte, PhD, MSPH
Clinical Neuropsychology Post-doctoral Fellow
Department of Psychology
Nebraska Medical Center
Omaha, NE

O. J. Vidal, MA
University of North Carolina, Wilmington
Wilmington, NC

Jacqueline Remondet Wall, PhD, HSPP, CRC
Director, Undergraduate Programs in Psychology
Associate Professor
School of Psychological Sciences
University of Indianapolis

Ashley Ware, BA
University of North Carolina, Wilmington
Wilmington, NC

Sarah E. West, BA
Graduate Student
Center for Psychological Studies
Nova Southeastern University
Fort Lauderdale, FL

Timothy F. Wynkoop, PhD, ABPP-CN
Clinical/Forensic Neuropsychologist
Private Practice, Maumee, OH
Clinical Assistant Professor
Department of Psychiatry
University of Toledo Medical Center
Toledo, OH

Maya Yutsis, PhD
Clinical Neuropsychology Post-Doctoral Fellow
Mayo Clinic, Rochester, MN

Amy E. Zimmerman, MA
Doctoral Student
Department of Educational Psychology
Ball State University, Muncie, IN

Sophia Zavrou, PsyD
Morrison Child and Family Services Center
Portland, OR

List of Entries

ACKNOWLEDGMENTS

Seeing this project through to publication has been very rewarding and has been made
possible by the many authors and by the support of our colleagues and
associated institutions (SIU School of Medicine, Middle Tennessee State University,
Ball State University, Psych Associates of Maryland),
as well as our editors (Nancy Hale and Phil Laughlin)
at Springer Publishing Company, LLC.

The Encyclopedia of
NEUROPSYCHOLOGICAL DISORDERS

ACUTE DISSEMINATED ENCEPHALOMYELITIS

DESCRIPTION

Acute disseminated encephalomyelitis (ADEM) is classified as a demyelinating disease of the central nervous system (CNS) and has onset in all age ranges, with more cases found in the pediatric population. Empirical studies suggest that ADEM is an immune-mediated inflammatory process that predominately involves the white matter of the brain. Onset may manifest spontaneously, or, in most cases, it is triggered by a systemic viral infection such as mumps, rubella, varicella-zoster, herpes simplex virus, hepatitis A virus, and coxsackie virus. There are rare cases in which vaccinations have triggered this disease.

Symptoms are characterized by rapid onset of encephalopathy with or without meningeal signs and focal/multifocal neurological signs (Alper, Heyman, & Wang, 2008; Marchioni et al., 2008; Sejvar, 2008; Tenembaum, 2007). Altered mental status, as minimal as lethargy or as severe as coma, may be present. Some focal neurologic deficits may be present, specifically extrapyramidal or pyramidal signs, which are shown in 60–90% of cases. Hemiplegia is present in 50–75% of cases, cranial nerve deficits in 7–45%, and concomitant spinal cord involvement in 25% (Sejvar, 2008). These symptoms are generally short lived with resolution over weeks or months. Complete recovery has been reported at 57–89% (Alper et al., 2008).

Although ADEM shares similar characteristics to other CNS disorders, it can be distinguished because of its rapid onset, progression of the illness, rapid remission, and the characteristic pattern and distribution of brain lesions on a MRI. However, none of these differences are pathognomic of ADEM making diagnosis unclear. Furthermore, symptoms of ADEM are most similar to first episodes of multiple sclerosis (MS), which makes it difficult to distinguish (Marchioni et al., 2008; Sejvar, 2008). ADEM can be classified into two types. The classic form is characterized by brain and spinal cord involvement, and there is a site-restricted form that is characterized by pure encephalitis, myelitis, cerebellitis, and optic neuritis. Peripheral nervous system (PNS) involvement is suggested in 5–43% of cases (Marchioni et al., 2008).

NEUROPATHOLOGY/PATHOPHYSIOLOGY

Neuroimaging studies have suggested that ADEM is a result of an inflammatory autoimmune response with resultant CNS inflammation and demyelination. A lack of biological markers make the pathophysiological basis of the condition unclear. Though the pathophysiological underpinnings of this response are unclear, one suggested explanation for ADEM, as well as other inflammatory CNS and PNS disorders, is that factors stimulate the immune system to produce antigen-specific humoral and/or cellular immunity (Sejvar, 2008; Tenembaum, 2007).

A few mechanisms have been offered to explain the process of immune stimulation induced by an infection or vaccination. "Molecular mimicry" is a term used to describe the involvement of epitopes of a virus, vaccine, or other antigenic stimulus in developing immune antibodies and/or T cells that cross-react with epitopes on myelin or axonal glycoproteins of nerves. Another mechanism describes the initial event as the binding of cross-reactive antibodies and subsequent damage to oligodendrocytes. Also, the introduction of sequestered myelin antigens into the circulation could damage myelin cells and therefore incite autoimmunity (Sejvar, 2008).

NEUROPSYCHOLOGICAL/CLINICAL PRESENTATION

In most cases, the clinical course of ADEM involves a rapid onset and resolution of the disorder while resulting deficits develop within days. Predominately spontaneous recovery (of neurological deficits) occurs over a period of weeks to months. Some cases result in persistent motor deficits, cognitive impairment, and recurrent seizures. In general, outcome is favorable in adult ADEM (Sejvar, 2008). One study of adult ADEM followed patients diagnosed with ADEM over a period of 30 months and found some residual mild cognitive impairment, as shown by problems with memory and concentration, and speech (Hollinger, Sturzenegger, Mathis, Schroth, & Hess, 2002). Therefore, the literature supports that in adult cases of ADEM, long-lasting neuropsychological and behavioral deficits are minimal or nonexistent.

Long-term neuropsychological or behavioral impairment in children with history of ADEM seems to be minimal or nonexistent as well. Although cognitive and motor deficits predominate in the initial stages of ADEM in adults, children may initially present with behavioral disturbances prior to diagnosis of ADEM. One study reported two cases where the child initially presented with symptoms of abnormal behavior such as irritability, violent tendencies, and behaviors mimicking delusions, suggestive of acute psychotic disorder. This suggests a different psychological manifestation of the disorder in some children. However, both these cases had positive outcomes and no residual cognitive, academic, or neuropsychological deficits were found (Krishnakumar, Jayakarishnan, Beegum, & Riyaz, 2008). This is consistent with the current literature that states serious complications are rare in childhood ADEM. However, some studies have found that the rate of relapse is considerable in this population (Anlar et al., 2003; Hollinger et al., 2002).

DIAGNOSIS

The major differential diagnosis of ADEM is MS. Interestingly, it has been suggested that 10–30% of patients initially diagnosed with ADEM end up developing MS (Sejvar, 2008). Two more differential diagnoses are also important: that is, infectious meningoencephalitis of possibly treatable etiology and acute brain swelling (Hollinger et al., 2002; Schwarz, Mohr, Knauth, Wildemann, & Storch-Hagenlocher, 2001).

MRIs generates similar results for MS. An MRI image of a case with ADEM would typically include widespread, bilateral, and asymmetric involvement of the white matter, deep gray nuclei, and spinal cord (Beleza et al., 2008). This is similar to MRI findings of 18% of children who are ultimately diagnosed with MS, making it indistinguishable (Alper et al., 2008; Callen et al., 2008). Several neuroimaging studies have made suggestions on how to distinguish between ADEM and first episodes of MS. Callen et al. (2008) proposed that the criteria for pediatric MS should include any two of the following: ≥ 2 periventricular legions, presence of black holes, or absence of diffuse bilateral legion distribution pattern. It has also been suggested that, in many cases, the presence of

encephalopathy is a strong indicator for the diagnosis of ADEM (Alper et al., 2008).

Recently, four patterns of MRI results in ADEM have been identified. These include ADEM with small (<5 mm) lesions, with large confluent lesions with edema and mass effect, with symmetric bilateral thalamic involvement, and acute hemorrhagic encephalomyelitis with features of hemorrhage within demyelinating lesions. However, correlation of the above to clinical outcome has not been found (Sejvar, 2008).

It is not sufficient to rely solely on one diagnostic procedure when diagnosing ADEM. Some minimal requirements have been identified that include a preceding infection, a monophasic disease course, neurological findings that indicate a disseminated CNS disease, and an absence of metabolic or infectious disorders (Hollinger et al., 2002). The classic definition of ADEM does not consider the PNS aspect of the disease. This type is found in 5–43% of cases and is associated with worse prognosis for functional recovery after the first episode and likelihood of relapse (Marchioni et al., 2008).

Relapse of ADEM is an issue of concern particularly in pediatric ADEM. Currently, relapse has been reported to occur in 5–25% of cases (Marchioni et al., 2008; Tenembaum, 2007). There are two categories of this relapsing form of ADEM. The disease can be classified as "recurrent" if it recurs at least 2 months after its onset, and the lesions affect the same area as in the first episode. ADEM can be classified as multiphasic, if the lesions present dissemination in space and time (Marchioni et al., 2008; Supplej et al., 2008).

TREATMENT

The treatment of choice for ADEM lies in different immunosuppressive or immunomodulatory strategies. These options are thought to be effective under the assumption that ADEM is the result of an autoimmune response against CNS structures. Some medical treatment examples of this nature are high-dose corticosteroids, plasmapheresis, or intravenous immunoglobulins. Corticosteroids are considered to be the first choice and most widely used treatment for ADEM. Treatment regimen, in most cases, includes intravenous methylprednisolone or dexamethasone for 3–5 days, followed by an oral taper for 3–6 weeks. Steroid treatment may be administered. However, this has been associated with relapse. These treatments combined with rehabilitation for any cognitive or neurological impairment or residual physical deficits, such as cognitive, occupational, and physical therapy, should result in full recovery of the disorder in a relatively short period of time (Hollinger et al., 2002; Sejvar, 2008).

Miriam Jocelyn Rodriguez
Charles Golden

Alper, G., Heyman, R., & Wang, L. (2008). Multiple Sclerosis and acute disseminated encephalomyelitis diagnosed in children after long-term follow-up: comparison of presenting features. *Developmental Medicine and Child Neurology.* Advance online publication. Retrieved December 22, 2008. doi: 10.1111/j.1469-8749.2008.03136.x

Anlar, B., Basaran, C., Kose, G., Guven, S., Haspolat, S., Yakut, A., et al. (2003). Acute disseminated encephalomyelitis in children: Outcome and prognosis. *Neuropediatrics, 34,* 194–199.

Beleza, P., Ribeiro, M., Pereira, J., Ferreira, C., Jordao, M. J., & Almeida, F. (2008). Probable acute disseminated encephalomyelitis due to *Haemophilus influenzae* meningitis. *Developmental Medicine & Child Neurology, 50,* 388–391.

Callen, D. J. A., Shroff, M. M., Branson, H. M., Li, D. K., Lotze, T., Stephens, D., et al. (2008). Role of MRI in the differentiation of ADEM from MS in children. *Neurology.* Retrieved December 22, 2008. doi: 10.1212/01.wnl.0000338630.20412.45

Hollinger, P., Sturzenegger, M., Mathis, J., Schroth, G., & Hess, C. W. (2002). Acute disseminated encephalomyelitis in adults: A reappraisal of clinical, CSF, EEG, and MRI findings. *Journal of Neurology, 249,* 320–329.

Krishnakumar, P., Jayakarishnan, M. P., Beegum, M. N., & Riyaz, A. (2008). Acute disseminated encephalomyelitis presenting as acute psychotic disorder. *Indian Pediatrics, 45,* 999–1001.

Marchioni, E., Tavazzi, E., Minoli, L., Del Bue, S., Ferrante, P., Piccolo, G., et al. (2008). Acute disseminated encephalomyelitis. *Neurological Sciences, 29,* 286–288.

Schwarz, S., Mohr, A., Knauth, M., Wildemann, B., & Storch-Hagenlocher, B. (2001). Acute disseminated encephalomyelitis: A follow up study of 40 adult patients. *Neurology, 56,* 1313–1318.

Sejvar, J. J. (2008). Acute disseminated encephalomyelitis. *Current Infectious Disease Reports, 10,* 307–314.

Supplej, A., Vittorini, R., Fontanin, M., De Grandis, D., Manara, R., Atzori, M., et al. (2008). Acute disseminated encephalomyelitis in children: Focus on relapsing patients. *Pediatric Neurology, 39,* 12–17.

Tenembaum, S. N. (2007). Disseminated encephalomyelitis in children. *Clinical Neurology and Neurosurgery, 110,* 928–938.

ADRENOLEUKODYSTROPHY

DESCRIPTION

Adrenoleukodystrophy, also referred to as ALD, is one of a group of genetic disorders referred to as leukodystrophies. These disorders are so named as they correspond with deterioration of myelin within the central nervous system (CNS). ALD specifically is characterized by the widespread demyelination of white matter throughout the CNS and atrophy in the adrenal gland secondary to a buildup of very long chain fatty acids (VLCFAs). Formerly classified along with other presentations under the umbrella of Schilder's disease (Beers, Porter, & Jones, 2006), it is now recognized as an independent metabolic encephalopathy (Ropper & Brown, 2005).

Two different subtypes fall under the umbrella of ALD. The most common is the X-linked form, which corresponds with a genetic abnormality on the sex chromosome, thus affecting young males rather than females. Onset is usually before age 7 (approximately 4–10 years of age) but may present in young adults in the early 20s as a more slowly developing disorder. The child cerebral form is the most common form and also the most severe. In some cases, it may occur in neonatal stages of development as an autosomal recessive type that represents the second subtype.

Symptoms present across cognitive, sensorimotor, academic, emotional, and behavioral domains as discussed under Neuropsychological/Clinical Presentation. As the disease progresses, neural impulses become further broken and thus greater functional impairments are seen. Given the progressive nature of the disease, prognosis for the childhood form is poor with individuals usually succumbing 1–10 years after initial symptom onset. In comparison, the adult form does not usually onset until the early to late 20s, sometimes early 30s, and is associated with a far slower and milder progressive course. Nevertheless, prominent cerebral deterioration can be seen. The disease is still noted far more in males compared with females, although an even milder form of adult-onset ALD has been noted in females who are carriers of the disease.

NEUROPATHOLOGY/PATHOPHYSIOLOGY

ALD most commonly presents as an X-linked recessive trait that corresponds with an inability to metabolize VLCFAs and subsequently their accumulation in the brain and adrenal glands. This leads to demyelination and progressive dysfunction of the adrenal gland, corresponding with the clinical presentation of ALD as discussed below. In the X-linked ALD, the genetic abnormality has been mapped to the Xq28 region resulting in the mutation of the *ALDP* gene, which encodes a peroxisomal membrane protein member of the ATP-binding cassette family (Maertens & Dyken, 2007).

Several pathological abnormalities in ALD patients have been noted. First, they have elevated levels of cerebrospinal fluid's protein content that corresponds with their inability to efficiently metabolize VLCFAs. The adrenal glands may be hard to identify as they are commonly severely atrophic and correspond with adrenal insufficiency. In addition, adrenal biopsies in the zona fasciculata and reticularis show microvacoules, striated cytoplasms, and many ballooned cytoplasmic cortical cells (Lake, 1997; Maertens & Dyken, 2007).

MRI scans reveal diffuse demyelination and CT scans may show hyperdense or hypodense regions in the parieto-occipital white matter, with the frontal lobes being less involved. As such, on the cortical surfaces, the brain and spinal cord are usually normal, but on slicing, the involved white matter is gray and firm, and in most cases, there is a caudorostral progression of the leukodystrophy (Lake, 1997). This white matter degradation presents bilaterally and generally symmetrically. Still, pathological review suggests particular susceptibility of the optic nerves, the fornix, hippocampal commissure, posterior cingulum, posterior limbs of the internal capsule, and the corpus callosum with characteristic contrast enhancement at the rim of the lesions (Lake, 1997; Maertens & Dyken, 2007; Powers, 1985).

NEUROPSYCHOLOGICAL/CLINICAL PRESENTATION

The disease is progressive in nature and is thus associated with a gradually expanding clinical picture in terms of functional compromise. Again, the childhood-onset form is not only the most common but also the most severe type. Beginning between the ages of 4 and 10, a gradual onset of behavioral and functional changes may be seen. Children may begin to act out more, appearing regressive in their behavioral regulation. Motoric deficits may also begin to be seen in the form of diminished coordination and eventually disturbance of gait and spasticity. Independent ambulation eventually becomes impossible, and in some instances, even quadriplegia is seen, and thus individuals become wheelchair bound (Maertens & Dyken,

2007). Increasing difficulties in memory and school performance are also seen early on. As the disease continues to progress, individuals often develop dysphagia, deafness, blindness (due to demyelination of the entire visual pathway), aphasia, and mental disorientation leading to dementia (Beers et al., 2006; Dox, Melloni, Eisner, & Melloni, 2002; Rowland, 2005). In addition, seizures may develop but do so in less than one-third of patients (Naidu & Moser, 1994). Other symptoms include characteristic signs of adrenal failure. This includes salt craving, hyperpigmentation in skin folds, vomiting, and fatigue. Eventually, deterioration culminates in a vegetative state (Maertens & Dyken, 2007).

There is also an adolescent-onset form, in which the signs and symptoms of cerebral involvement are the same as those seen in the childhood form but instead develop between the ages of 10 and 21 (i.e., the period between childhood onset and adult onset) (Lake, 1997).

In the adult-onset form, the disease is primarily characterized by motoric changes early on. Individuals will demonstrate progressive rigidity that leads to a decrease in gross motor magnitude, amplitude, and coordination. Preferential compromise of the lower extremities can at times be seen leading to paresis or paralysis, whereas the upper limbs are largely spared (Lake, 1997). Ataxia is also commonly noted. The array of motor anomalies is directly related to the disease's infiltration of spinocerebellar regions (Maertens & Dyken, 2007). Spastic paraparesis tends to occur later in life (i.e., 30s–40s), again with notation of a slow progression (Ropper & Brown, 2005). Psychiatric disturbances and seizures are also commonly seen (Maertens & Dyken, 2007). Finally, cognitive deterioration can occur in the adult-onset form, although the progression is far slower and tends not be of the same degree of severity. When presenting in women who are carriers of the disease, these features are milder; however, it is worth noting that neurological symptoms have been reported to occur in less than 50% of these women (Ropper & Brown, 2005).

DIAGNOSIS

Diagnosis of ALD is often multifaceted, although some methods are more favored and definitive than others. Specifically, identification of an excess of VLCFAs and than other biochemical abnormalities noted previously is the major method of making the diagnosis (Maertens & Dyken, 2007) and may be viewed as the definitive means of diagnosis. Low serum sodium and chloride levels and elevated potassium levels are also noted on laboratory workup corresponding with degradation of the adrenal glands (Ropper & Brown, 2005). In some instances, genetic testing can identify the abnormality as discussed previously and has been suggested in early identification and even prenatal diagnosis. Diagnosis during the first trimester can be accomplished by the measurement of VLCFA ester in chorionic villus samples and by restriction fragment length polymorphism using a DNA probe (Boué et al., 1985).

Although the above are considered definitive, it is noted that often these laboratory tests are only carried out after previous clinical workup including taking of a thorough history, neurological and/or neuropsychological workup, and neuroimaging suggest the potential of ALD. When considering ALD, both CT and MRI scans are viewed as helpful clinical tools (Lake, 1997). Commonly, MRI scans can demonstrate the diffuse white matter disease that is the hallmark of the presentation, which in combination with noted clinical features can lead to the aforementioned laboratory tests.

TREATMENT

Prognosis for patients with ALD is poor with those stricken with the disease succumbing to its effects within 1–10 years of symptom onset. Neurological deterioration progresses until patients finally enter a vegetative state; however, patients generally die from adrenal crisis or other causes soon after. Although the disease course cannot be halted, there is some evidence to support methods of slowing progression and addressing symptoms. Adrenal replacement therapy prolongs life and occasionally effects a partial neurological remission. Lorenzo's oil (glyceryl trierucate/glyceryl trioleate: 4/1) therapy can diminish the frequency and severity of neurological disability if started early, before any symptoms appear (Lake, 1997). Bone marrow transplantation has also demonstrated some benefit when done early, but the efficacy is limited (Krivit, Lockman, Watkins, Hirsch, & Shapiro, 1995). Specifically, although the bone marrow transplantation seems to cure the biochemical defects, it does not affect radiological or neurological defects. All cases show neurological progression regardless of transplantation (Beers et al., 2006). The procedure also carries risk of mortality and morbidity and is not recommended for those whose symptoms are already severe or who have the adult-onset or neonatal forms.

Oral administration of docosahexanoic acid may help infants and children with neonatal ALD. In addition, when administered before the age of 6, a diet enriched with monounsaturated fatty acids and devoid of long chain fatty acids has been said to slow the progress of the disease. Therapeutic plasma exchanges are successful in reducing VLCFA but without altering the clinical course.

Although the above are considered options for treatment, in many ways still therapy is primarily directed at supportive care and treatment including physical therapy, psychological support, and special education.

J. Aaron Albritton
Chad A. Noggle

Beers, M. H., Porter, R. S., & Jones, T. V. (2006). *The Merck manual of diagnosis and therapy* (18th ed.). Whitehouse Station, NJ: Merck.

Boué, J., Oberle, I., Heilig, R., Mandel, J. L., Moser, A., Moser, H., et al. (1985). First trimester prenatal diagnosis of adrenoleukodystrophy by determination of very long chain fatty acid levels and linkage analysis to a DNA probe. *Human Genetics, 69,* 272–274.

Dox, I. G., Melloni, B. J., Eisner, G. M., & Melloni, J. L. (2002). *Melloni's illustrated medical dictionary* (4th ed.). London: The Parthenon Publishing Group.

Krivit, W., Lockman, L. A., Watkins, P. A., Hirsch, J., & Shapiro, E. G. (1995). The future for treatment by bone marrow transplantation for adrenoleukodystrophy, metachromatic leukodystrophy, globoid cell leukodystrophy, and Hurler syndrome. *Journal of Inherited Metabolic Disorders, 18,* 398–412.

Lake, B. (1997). Lysosomal and peroxisomal disorders. In D. I. Graham & P. L. Lantos (Eds.), *Greenfield's neuropathology* (6th ed., pp. 657–753). New York: Oxford University Press.

Maertens, P., & Dyken, P. R. (2007). Storage diseases: Neuronal ceroid-lipofuscinoses, lipidoses, glycogenoses, and leukodystrophies. In C. G. Goetz (Ed.), *Textbook of clinical neurology* (3rd ed., pp. 613–639). Philadelphia: Saunders Elsevier.

Naidu, S., & Moser, H. (1994). Peroxisomal disorders. In K. Swaiman (Ed.), *Pediatric neurology: Principles and practices* (2nd ed., Vol. 2, pp. 1357–1383). St. Louis, MO: Mosby.

Powers, J. M. (1985). Adrenoleukodystrophy. *Clinical Neuropathology, 4,* 181–199.

Ropper, A. H., & Brown, R. H. (2005). *Adams and Victor's principles of neurology* (8th ed., pp. 797–849). New York: McGraw-Hill.

ADULT ANXIETY DISORDERS

DESCRIPTION

It may appear inappropriate to characterize psychopathology associated with anxiety as a neuropsychologically based condition, since traditionally the anxiety disorders have been thought to be the result of environmental stressors, and, particularly within a psychoanalytic framework, stressors occurring during early life. However, with recent developments in neuroscience, a literature has developed that has been supportive of the view that there are neurobiological aspects to at least some of these disorders. Anxiety is an affect characterized by unpleasant features involving physical and psychological experiences. Physically there may be disturbed breathing, increased heart activity, trembling, paralysis, and sweating. Psychologically there are unpleasant feelings and sensations, and a sense of apprehension. Traditionally, anxiety is distinguished from fear, in that fear is associated with objective real or threatened danger, whereas anxiety is more associated with unreal or imagined danger. Although anxiety itself is a commonly experienced and normal human emotion, some individuals experience anxiety or fear to such a degree that it interferes with their lives. At the point when anxiety becomes debilitating, it is likely that the person would be diagnosed with one of the anxiety disorders as a psychiatric diagnosis currently described and defined in the *Diagnostic and Statistical Manual of Mental Disorders*, Fourth Edition, Text Revision (*DSM-IV-TR;* American Psychiatric Association [APA], 2000).

The term Anxiety Disorders in the *DSM-IV* is actually an umbrella that covers all pathological disorders that are characterized by intense anxiety, fear, or stress. These include Panic Disorder With or Without Agoraphobia, Specific Phobia, Social Anxiety Disorder, Obsessive-Compulsive Disorder, Posttraumatic Stress Disorder, Acute Stress Disorder, and Generalized Anxiety Disorder. Anxiety disorders are often found to be comorbid with mood disorders or other anxiety disorders, but comorbid depression predicts a poorer outcome (van Balkom et al., 2008).

Panic Disorder (PD) is a mental illness characterized by frequent panic attacks and worry of impending attacks, which may or not be brought on by agoraphobia. Panic attacks are defined as a brief attack of extreme terror with feelings of imminent death, loss of control, confusion, and often dizziness and shortness of breath. These frightening attacks occur abruptly, peaking in 10 minutes or less, but can last for hours. People experiencing panic attacks often believe they are experiencing a heart attack, due to the very similar physiological symptoms. The constant worry about when the next attack will occur only adds to patients' tension and anxiety, as these attacks are perceived as occurring without cause or warning.

Agoraphobia is an intense fear of enclosed spaces where escape is difficult or impossible. PD is often complicated by agoraphobia, such that there is an agoraphobic specifier: Panic Disorder With Agoraphobia (PDA). Unfortunately, people with agoraphobia commonly reinforce these feelings of danger by avoiding places where they believe an attack will occur; the more they avoid such places, the more they believe that attacks will occur there, and the more the places are feared. People with PDA often do not seek treatment for long periods of time.

In Specific Phobias (SPs), anxiety is provoked by exposure to a specific object or situation, such as a certain animal, heights, or air travel. SPs generally have an early childhood onset with a very long course of illness and a 9.4% lifetime prevalence in the United States. Very few people that could be diagnosed with SP ever seek treatment (Stinson et al., 2007).

People who suffer from Social Anxiety Disorder (SAD) have an intense fear of being evaluated or criticized in social situations, or that he or she will do something horribly humiliating. Some have this fear in all social settings, which would require the specifier "Generalized," whereas others are anxious only in the context of certain situations, such as eating in front of others, speaking in class, and so forth. When put in a situation that is so feared, the person will experience extreme anxiety, which may or may not develop into a panic attack. SAD manifests early in life, as around 50% of those with the disorder report the onset before adolescence (Hayward, Killen, Kraemer, & Taylor, 1998). Unfortunately, this diagnosis is often complicated by related, comorbid conditions, most notably substance abuse disorders and major depression (Stein & Chavira, 1998). Obsessive-Compulsive Disorder (OCD) is characterized by obsessive thoughts that provoke anxiety and/or compulsions or repetitive behaviors that help to neutralize anxiety. People with OCD feel that their compulsive behaviors reduce the stress brought on by the obsessive thoughts, but these may or may not be logically related. In order to be considered OCD, the prevalence of these thoughts and actions must impair the person's life in social or occupational functioning.

Posttraumatic Stress Disorder (PTSD) is a condition that may arise after a severely traumatic event. Symptoms include reexperiencing the event, feeling great anxiety or tension when reminded of the event, increased arousal and avoidance of stimuli that may be associated with the traumatic event. PTSD may be significantly disabling and has been reported to cause significant work production losses in the United States (Zatzick et al., 2008). The symptoms of Acute Stress Disorder (ASD) are similar to those of PTSD but occur immediately following the traumatic event and typically have a shorter duration.

Generalized Anxiety Disorder (GAD) is characterized by a pervasive, excessive, and uncontrollable continuous worry about life events and activities.

It affects women twice as much as men. Patients may also suffer from physical ailments that manifest their worry, such as fatigue, restlessness, and muscle tension. GAD is the most common anxiety disorder and is also one of the most common comorbid disorders with other anxiety and mood disorders (Kessler, Chiu, Demler, Merikangas, & Walters, 2005). Patients with GAD tend to have a chronic course with early onset (Newman, 2000).

Anyone that presents with significant anxiety symptoms or phobic avoidance that does not fully meet *DSM-IV* criteria for any of the above-specified disorders can be classified as having Anxiety Disorder NOS (Not Otherwise Specified).

NEUROPATHOLOGY/PATHOPHYSIOLOGY

The neuropathology and pathophysiology of the anxiety disorders are inextricably associated with the area of the neurobiology of stress and fear, which have an enormous literature. There is extensive research evidence indicating that stress has consequences for brain function based both on animal model and human studies. A good example is the now classical work of Sapolsky on how autonomic changes, notably involving glucocorticoids, influence the functioning of the hippocampus (Rodrigues, LeDoux, and Sapolsky, 2009) and the extensive work of LeDoux on the amygdala and fear conditioning (e.g., Delgado, Jou, LeDoux, & Phelps, 2009).

Some of the neurobiology of anxiety disorders is genetic or developmental, and some relates to interaction with the environment (Stein, Jang, Taylor, Vernon, & Lively, 2002). A portion of the neurobiology of the anxiety disorders has to do with developmental vulnerabilities, whereas other aspects are considered to be the consequences of stress. Areas of the brain involved appear to be in the limbic system, with major emphasis on the amygdala and hippocampus. There are also neurochemical considerations. For example, many researchers believe that the glutamate receptor, the primary excitatory neurotransmitter in the brain, is a key contributor to mood and anxiety disorders (Sanacora, Kendell, Fenton, Coric, & Krystal, 2004; Zarate et al., 2004). To this effect, several studies have been conducted looking to find symptom relief in mood and anxiety disorders with a variety of glutamate modulators (Mathew et al., 2008; Sanacora et al., 2004; Zarate et al., 2004).

Neuropathologies and pathophysiologies may differ according to type of anxiety disorder. In PD, patients have been found to have anatomical changes in the form of decreased anterior cingulate cortex (ACC) volume (Asami et al., 2008). Childhood Separation Anxiety Disorder often predates PD, and it has been shown that both disorders predict heightened sensitivity to inhaled CO_2. Researchers have found that genetic predispositions are correlated with both this developmental trajectory and CO_2 sensitivity and interact with the environmental event of parental loss as a significant mediating factor in both disorders (Battaglia et al., 2009). Researchers have found correlations with PD diagnosis and certain chemicals in the brain, as well: For instance, serotonin receptor binding is significantly reduced in patients as compared with healthy controls, and this dysfunction improves in treated patients (Nash et al., 2008).

Individuals with SP have greater activation responses in the insula and ACC to pictures of phobic avoidance than controls (Straube, Glauer, Dilger, Mentzel, & Miltner, 2006). In SAD, there is significant neurological evidence for the precipitating brain areas in which symptoms occur. Functional magnetic resonance imaging (fMRI) studies have shown consistently that the ACC is involved in experiencing physical pain but more recently some researchers have found the same area to also be involved in pain or discomfort arising from social situations, such as perceiving group exclusion (Eisenberger, Lieberman, & Williams, 2003). These same researchers also showed that ACC activation during social exclusion was correlated with self-reports of distress.

There has been extensive neurobiological research regarding PTSD involving both human studies and animal models. Summarizing an enormous literature, there appears to be a consensus that the amygdala, insula, and ACC all play crucial roles in PTSD symptomatology (Damsa, Kosel, & Mousally, 2009). Neurobiological studies now implicate both developmental or genetic and acquired aspects.

Wakizono et al. (2007) found that there is reduction in inhibition of memory circuits for fear extinction in animals due to exaggerated amygdala response associated with hypofunctioning medial prefrontal cortex (PFC) and hippocampus, but strain differences were found. Thus, in animal models of PTSD it appears that individual characteristics that mediate responses to stress and therefore the onset of PTSD can be genetic or environmental or an interaction of these two factors. A twin study showed that both exposure to trauma such as violent crime and ensuing PTSD symptoms are mediated by genetics and environment, whereas exposure to trauma via accidents and natural disasters are influenced only by shared environmental factors (Stein et al., 2002).

Bremner et al. (2003) is among many others that have found that characteristic features of brain dysfunction in PTSD patients (see also Gurvits et al., 1996; Liberzon et al., 1999). For example, while remembering negatively emotionally valenced words in a memory test, women with PTSD show very different fear and emotion brain pathways than women without PTSD, in a network that has been implicated in PTSD problems in previous studies. Patients with PTSD have shown decreased response to reward receipt, which may underlie decreased motivation associated with the disorder, most notably in animals exposed to inescapable shock (Maier & Seligman, 1976; Sailer et al., 2008). These deficits have been shown in fMRI studies to be associated with the PFC, which is responsible for decision making, and the nucleus accumbens, which is important in the reward pathway (Krawcyzk, 2002; Sailer et al., 2008).

The severity of GAD symptoms are highly correlated with salivary cortisol levels (Mantella et al., 2008). This evidence points to hypothalamic-pituitary-adrenal (HPA) axis dysfunction, which is associated with constant stress and worry and theorized to cause continual activation of the HPA axis. It is also speculated that the amino acid N-acetylaspartate's (NAA) occurrence in the hippocampus is related to severe anxiety. A recent study measuring levels of hippocampal NAA while treating GAD patients with Riluzole (an approved treatment for amyotrophic lateral sclerosis) showed that these levels dropped significantly during and after the course of treatment as compared to non-anxious controls, and great symptom relief was also seen (Matthew et al., 2008).

NEUROPSYCHOLOGICAL/CLINICAL PRESENTATION

It is generally understood that individuals with anxiety disorders typically do not have apparent neuropsychological deficits and that cognitive changes, when present, tend to be subtle and mild. Indeed, individuals with OCD may be exceptionally bright. The major descriptive considerations for these individuals are associated with personality, lifestyle, and symptoms associated with anxiety. Apparent cognitive features of these individuals may relate to cognitive style, such as the preoccupation with detail seen in OCD or amnesia for traumatic events seen in ASD or PTSD. People with anxiety disorders typically have very low quality of life, as 20% to 59% of patients diagnosed on the spectrum of anxiety disorders score at least two standard deviations below the community norm on a Quality of Life Scale (Rapaport, Clary, Fayyard, & Endicott, 2005).

Not all anxiety disorders present in the same way. In a study using the startle blink reflex, Grillon, Ameli, Goddard, Woods, and Davis (1994) showed that patients with PD overgeneralize conditioned fear to stimuli providing a danger cue. That is, they respond with a fear response to stimuli more distant from a conditioned danger cue than is the case for normal controls. Decreased function of short-term memory and attention has also been reported in people with PD (Gordeev, 2008). Onset of situational phobias is much later in life than the other subtypes. Animal phobics, however, do not have a fear of being harmed so much as an intense disgust (Lipsitz, Barlow, Mannuzza, Hofmann, & Fyer, 2002).

A study performed by Rapee and Lim (1992) had observers rate the performances of people with SAD in social situations, and the subjects also rated their own performances. The observers rated the subjects much higher than the subjects rated themselves, showing that people with SAD have some cognitive distortions about their performance in social situations. Other studies have shown, however, that people with SAD actually do perform worse in social situations than people with an anxiety disorder (Thompson & Rapee, 2002; Voncken & Bögels, 2008), although these deficits are seen only in interactive social situations, not in solo actions such as speech giving (Voncken & Bögels, 2008). Voncken and Bögels (2008) showed one cognitive distortion that is characteristic of social anxiety sufferers—there is a great discrepancy between how patients perceive themselves and what they believe others want them to be. This theory provides logic as to why SAD patients are fearful in social situations—because they feel unable to live up to others' expectations, and are constantly failing others.

Clinicians have long seen a great deal of heterogeneity in OCD, but a recent meta-analytic study found that while obsessions and compulsions range quite widely, they can be reduced to symmetry in ordering, forbidden thoughts, cleaning, and hoarding (Bloch, Landeros-Weisenberger, Rosario, Pittenger, & Leckman, 2008). Research has shown that patients with OCD also respond more extremely and more quickly to startling images (Kumari, Kaviani, Raven, Gray, & Checkley, 2001). Unfortunately, OCD symptoms tend to be stable across time (Mataix-Cols et al., 2002).

There are numerous studies of cognitive function in OCD, particularly involving memory and executive function. Performance on the Wisconsin Card Sorting Test in those with OCD has shown worse perseveration than found in normal controls; visuospatial deficits have also been found (Bucci et al., 2007). Others have identified a cognitive profile characterized by weaknesses in motor function and processing speed and strengths in language, verbal memory, and reasoning/problem-solving (Burdick, Robinson, Malhotra, & Szeszko, 2008). A suggested basis for the deficits found is altered corticostriatal functional connectivity involving the dorsal striatum and lateral PFC.

Although the severity of PTSD symptoms has been shown to be negatively correlated with the strength of one's social support network (Scarpa, Haden, & Hurley, 2006), researchers have recently discovered that social support does not mediate time to remission of symptoms (Laffaye, Cavella, Drescher, & Rosen, 2008). Some of these symptoms are neuropsychological in nature. There has been substantially more research conducted in the neuropsychological aspects of PTSD than any other anxiety disorder. The general consensus appears to be that even when one accounts for intelligence, education, alcoholism, and depression (Bremner et al., 1995, 2004; Samuelson et al., 2006; Vasterling et al., 2002), there is impairment of verbal declarative memory and attention associated with PTSD itself. These deficits appear to coexist with the common traumatic and negative emotionally valenced memories generally found in PTSD and the preference for remembrance of trauma-related material (Elzinga & Bremner, 2002). PTSD sufferers also experience early amnesia immediately after trauma exposure, which is correlated with later severity of symptoms (Granja et al., 2008).

ASD is very similar to PTSD except that it remits much more quickly. A diagnosis of ASD following a traumatic event is a high-risk factor for developing PTSD, which has a much longer course (Brewin, Andrews, Rose, & Kirk, 1999; Fullerton, Ursano, & Wang, 2004). Symptoms of PTSD have been noted in elderly veterans who experienced the "Bataan Death March" during World War II (Goldstein, van Kammen, Shelly, Miller, & van Kammen, 1987). Unfortunately, although it is established in the literature that a diagnosis of ASD predicts later diagnosis of PTSD, much more research needs to be conducted to see if early, aggressive treatment of ASD can stave off a diagnosis of PTSD (McKibben, Bresnick, Wiechman, & Fauerbach, 2008). ASD is highly correlated with dissociative symptoms (Ginzburg, Solomon, Dekel, & Bleich, 2006), which are characterized by a disruption in a person's consciousness, memory, and/or identity (APA, 2000). Persons that experience some kind of trauma and then proceed to blame others for their suffering are much more likely to develop ASD (Lambert, Difede, & Contrada, 2004), although the reasoning behind this phenomenon has yet to be illuminated.

Patients with GAD have been found to negatively evaluate their internal experiences (such as thoughts, emotions, and sensations) and use worry as a means of escaping and avoiding these experiences (Roemer, Orsillo, & Salters-Pedneault, 2008). Researchers now believe that patients with GAD not only have problems with worrying, but worry about their worry (called meta-worry), as they view their worrisome thoughts as dangerous and uncontrollable (Wells & Carter, 2002). It is believed that the implications for treatment from this new theory are that patients must learn to view worrying as a negative strategy for dealing with threat and also learn new behavioral strategies for appraising threats in the environment (Well & Carter, 1999). As with most anxiety disorders, GAD has been found to be associated with very low quality of life (Pollack et al., 2008). Although patients with GAD report experiencing negative thoughts that are unpleasant and anxiety-provoking, they have been shown not to present with signs of hyperarousal measured by skin conductance and heart rate (Upatel & Gerlach, 2008). Although individuals with GAD often have difficulties concentrating, there does not appear to be a specific cognitive literature on this disorder separate from phobias, PTSD, and OCD. Apparently, the disorder is so heterogeneous, often including the symptoms of other anxiety disorders and other comorbidities, that there can be no specific neuropsychological profile.

DIAGNOSIS

The Anxiety Disorders are a class of mental disorders, and there is a general consensus in the professional community to accept the diagnostic criteria contained in the various editions of the *DSM I–IV-TR*. The latest version (*DSM-5*) is in preparation at this writing. Therefore, diagnoses are made by determining whether the client meets the required number of criteria contained in the manual. Most clinicians use an interview and history review to determine whether those criteria are met, but a more precise and scientifically acceptable method is to use one of the structured psychiatric interviews. The most commonly used procedure at present is the Structured Clinical Interview for *DSM-IV-TR* (SCID) (First, Spitzer, Gibbon, & Williams, 2005) that will shortly be replaced by the SCID for *DSM-5*. Use of the SCID generally is a requirement for publication of diagnoses in professional and scientific journals and may be used in general clinical practice at the discretion of the psychologist or psychiatrist in routine clinical practice. It may be useful to supplement the SCID with one of many anxiety scales available and with psychological personality testing. The most commonly used anxiety scales are the Beck Anxiety Inventory, the Hamilton Anxiety Rating Scale, and the Spielberger State-Trait Anxiety Inventory (STAI). Numerous scales have been developed for PTSD including the Trauma Symptom Inventory, two Mississippi Scales, one for civilians and the other for the military, the PTSD Checklist, and others. The diagnosis of an anxiety disorder is therefore ideally made using a structured interview to evaluate presence of *DSM-IV-TR* criteria, and special scales as indicated. These criteria are briefly reviewed in what follows.

As indicated by the *DSM IV-TR*, clients are diagnosed with PD if they have recurrent panic attacks with four or more of the following symptoms: palpitations or accelerated heart rate, sweating, shaking, shortness of breath, feeling of being choked, chest pain, nausea, feeling faint, derealization or depersonalization, fear of losing control or going crazy, fear of dying, numbness or tingling, and/or chills or hot flushes (APA, 2000). Also, at least one panic attack must have been succeeded by a month or more of one or more of the following symptoms: worry of additional attacks, what they may mean or signify, and/or a change in behavior due to the attack. These attacks cannot be related to agoraphobia or due to the effects of a medical condition or substance. PDA follows the same criteria as for PD, but panic attacks are often caused by agoraphobia. One could also be diagnosed as having agoraphobia without history of PD.

For SP, clinicians must specify whether the client suffers from Animal, Natural Environment, Blood-Injection-Injury, Situational, or Other type.

In SAD the person meets criteria for phobia and knows that the fear is excessive, but the social or performance situations are either avoided or endured with intense distress (*DSM IV-TR*). In order for this to be diagnosable, the avoidance of fearful situations must significantly interfere with the person's daily life, occupational or social functioning, or have great distress. These symptoms cannot be accounted for by substances or any other mental disorder. Some overlapping diagnoses are Panic Disorder With or Without Agoraphobia, Body Dysmorphic Disorder, or Schizoid Personality Disorder. The fear or criticism can also not be related to a different, medical disorder, such as abnormal eating behavior in the presence of an eating disorder. There is a Generalized specifier if the person fears almost all social situations, not simply a few stressful ones.

In order to be diagnosed with OCD, one must have either obsessions or compulsions, or both. Obsessions are recurrent thoughts, impulses, or images that are thought to be intrusive and inappropriate and cause distress, which are not just excessive worries about real problems. They cannot be suppressed, ignored, or distracted away, and the patient must know these thoughts are from his own mind, not from an outside source. Compulsions are defined repetitive behaviors or mental acts that one feels compelled to complete in response to an obsession, or according to extremely strict rules. Some common examples of compulsions are hand washing, checking, and repeating words silently. These behaviors are intended to reduce distress or prevent a terrible event, but they are not connected in a realistic way to the observer. Also, at some point the patient has been aware that these compulsions and obsessions are excessive or unreasonable, and they take up more than an hour of the patient's day, everyday, and cause marked stress or interference in domains of daily life, such as occupational and social functioning.

Some obsessions and compulsions are considered separate disorders, such as obsession with one's appearance seen in Body Dysmorphic Disorder and obsession with food seen in Eating Disorders. Clinicians can specify whether a patient has Poor Insight, if the patient does not see these problems as excessive for most of an episode.

Regarding PTSD, witnessing a traumatic event that made the patient feel that his life was threatened or an event that included serious injury or death of another is the first criteria that must be fulfilled for a diagnosis of PTSD. The patient's response must have involved intense fear and helplessness. Throughout the course of the disorder, a patient will reexperience this event recurrently in one or more ways, including intrusive memories, upsetting dreams, "flashbacks," or a reliving of the event, perhaps in hallucinatory form, with distress at the exposure to stimuli that remind him of the event, and experience physiological fear. Patients avoid any stimuli that is associated with the precipitating event, in three or more of the following ways: avoiding thoughts, feelings, or talking; avoid places, people, or activities; inability to remember a part of the event; anhedonia; asociality; blunted affect; sense of no future. Arousal is indicated by two or more of the following: insomnia, irritability, difficulty in attention, hypervigilance, exaggerated startle response. The various PTSD scales document these symptoms in detail. All of them must last for longer than 1 month, and the illness must cause significant impairments in some areas of functioning. PTSD is considered Acute if it lasts for less than 3 months and Chronic if it lasts for longer. Usually, trauma survivors show symptoms within 6 months of the event, but if not, they are considered to have

Delayed Onset. In ASDs the symptom picture is similar, but the condition should last no more than 1 month from experiencing the extreme stressor.

People diagnosed with GAD not only worry excessively, but they meet the criteria for worrying more days than not for at least 6 months about a multitude of events or activities. GAD patients find it difficult, if not impossible, to control their feelings of worry, and this anxiety is associated with at least three of the following symptoms: restlessness, fatigue, difficulty concentrating or "mind going blank," irritability, muscle tension, or significant sleep disturbance of any kind. This anxiety cannot be due to another physical or mental disorder, or to the effects of a substance. As always, this worry and anxiety must cause the client significant amounts of distress or impairment in domains of their life, such as social or occupational.

Formal neuropsychological testing is of particular interest in the cases of OCD and PTSD where there are extensive literatures regarding brain function. Emphasis is generally placed on memory and executive function, individuals with these diagnoses typically having normal language and usually average or above general intelligence. Even in these cases, referral for neuropsychological assessment is relatively infrequent, and is generally made because of suspicion of some other disorder, usually substance abuse or a general medical condition. The clinician should not be surprised to find normal neuropsychological results in many individuals with anxiety disorders. The neuropsychological deficits reported in the literature often involve functions that require specific tests to evaluate, many of which are not contained in standard neuropsychological batteries. The task of the clinical neuropsychologist is often that of identifying a disorder of brain function associated with some other illness in the context of an anxiety disorder. A typical question involves whether impaired function may be a product of disabling anxiety. In any event, the most useful clinical procedures appear to be tests of executive abilities and memory (Fenger et al., 2005; Kuelz, Hohagen, & Vodeholzer, 2004).

TREATMENT

Treatment for all anxiety disorders is mostly the same, as psychologists and psychiatrists tend to use cognitive behavioral therapy (CBT), medications, and sometimes psychotherapy.

Behavioral therapy methods have been commonly used. Behavioral methods were mainly used in combination with other treatments but not much alone (Goisman et al., 1993). Formal psychotherapy for PD, social phobia, and GAD has all decreased in the past decades, but cognitive and behavioral treatments are still far less used than psychodynamic therapies (Goisman, Warshaw, & Keller, 1999). However, the use of orthodox psychoanalysis, commonly used early in the 20th century, is rarely used today.

One popular and effective type of CBT is in vivo exposure, in which an anxious patient is put in a feared situation over and over, learning how to deal with their responses with the help of the therapist. This is much more effective than imaginative exposure therapy (Emmelkamp, 2002) yet now researchers are finding that exposure therapy given in the form of virtual reality is just as effective as in person in vivo exposure therapy (Parsons & Rizzo, 2008). Exercising as an adjunct to CBT in treating anxiety disorders, even walking, has been found to have a significant effect on relieving symptoms rather than treatment with CBT alone (Merom et al., 2008). Unfortunately, several studies have shown through prospective experiments that patients with any anxiety disorders are very likely to have a chronic course of the disease, and that sufferers of social phobia had the smallest chance of recovery (Bruce et al., 2005).

A new theoretical perspective on PTSD and phobias (including SAD) is that a neutral stimulus has been found to be associated with some great fear. Therefore, accelerating the cognitive process known as extinction, which replaces the fear associated with something neutral or positive over time, is a new way of looking at treatment for PTSD and phobias. An interesting study conducted by Marchand, Roberge, Primiano, and Germain (2009) found that there were no statistical differences in PD treatment outcome for CBT, exposure therapy, or supportive therapy. More recently, there has been a focus on patients' subjective views of what helps them recover.

Subjects with SPs showed great activation reduction in associated brain areas after only two sessions of exposure therapy (Straube, 2006), but not enough studies have been conducted to tease out the differences in therapy application to the different anxiety disorder subtypes (Choy, Fyer, & Lipsitz, 2006). In vivo exposure therapy has shown strong effects in ameliorating symptoms, but patients tend to drop out (Choy et al., 2006).

Exposure therapy for SAD often consists of therapist and client working together to make a ranked list of fearful situations, since each person's fear hierarchy is different. Then the client learns the nature of social anxiety, cognitive restructuring strategies, goes through in vivo exposure, and receives social skills training. There are standard protocols for therapists' use (Antony, Craske, & Barlow, 2006; Antony &

Swinson, 2000). Recently, several studies have examined the validity of the exposure hierarchy and have shown good treatment outcomes for persons with SAD and other anxiety problems through measures of symptomatology after treatment, as well as high test-retest reliability (Coldwell et al., 1998; Katerelos, Hawley, Antony, & McCabe, 2008).

Numerous pharmacological treatments have been developed over the years for anxiety disorders. Several different pharmacological treatments have been approved by the FDA for both acute and long-term treatment, such as duloxetine (Hartford et al., 2007; Koponen et al., 2007; Rynn et al., 2008). A recent study has shown that patients who respond well to duloxetine in acute (short-term) therapeutic use also have a greatly decreased likelihood of relapse in 6 months if they continue its use (Davidson et al., 2008). However, some clinicians and researchers believe that patients with GAD treated with CBT still exhibit residual symptoms after treatment.

Paroxetine, a selective serotonin reuptake inhibitor (SSRI) type of antidepressant often known by its commercial name Seroquel, has much promise for treating anxiety disorders, as Ballenger showed that the greatest rates of remission from anxiety disorders are found when treated with paroxetine (2004; also see Baldwin, Bobes, Stein, Scharwachter, & Faure, 1999). Another SSRI, escitalopram, has been found to be effective with SAD and other anxiety disorders.

The N-methyl-D-aspartate (NMDA) receptor within the amygdala is very important in learning and extinction, and new research findings show that exposure therapy along with the drug D-cycloserine, which enhances the NMDA receptor, seems to be more helpful than therapy alone (Davis, Myers, Ressler, & Rothbaum, 2005; Hoffman et al., 2006) There are numerous other pharmacological approaches to the anxiety disorders, with the above examples only providing a small sample of the ongoing work in this area.

A study by Huppert et al. (2004), which looked at placebo effects in anxiety disorders, found that the effect was much weaker for patients with OCD than in patients with SAD or PD. The authors hypothesize that placebos enable those with social anxiety to face their fears and perhaps in the process help learn new emotional associations for social situations, while as in OCD, compulsions interfere with this process. Fortunately, several studies have found SSRIs and serotonin–norepinephrine reuptake inhibitors (SNRIs), such as clomipramine and venlafaxine, to be quite successful in relieving symptoms of OCD (for meta-analytic reviews, see Dello'osso, Nestadt, Allen, & Hollander, 2006; Fineberg & Gale, 2005). Although transcranial magnetic stimulation has been showing promise as a treatment in other mental disorders, as of yet there is little evidence for its therapeutic use in OCD (Alsonso et al., 2001; Martin, Barbanoj, Pérez, & Sacristán, 2003). Psychosurgery is still considered controversial by many medical and lay parties (Moran, 2004), but cingulotomies are still performed as a last-resort surgical effort to alleviate OCD symptoms, and some studies show improvements with few side effects in patients several years afterward (Dougherty et al., 2002). Different forms of CBT have been found to be helpful: though stress management training sounds plausible, in vivo exposure and ritual prevention forms of CBT have been found to be much more successful (Simpson et al., 2008).

PTSD is often treated with CT or CBT, and several studies have empirically shown them to be effective (Rabe, Zoellner, Beauducel, Maercker, & Karl, 2008; Sibrandij et al., 2007). Rabe et al. actually documented changes in brain activity after a course of CT treatment, using electroencephalogram readings. Previous studies have shown heightened right hemisphere activity for feelings of anxiety, and in this study Rabe et al. showed a significant decrease in right anterior activity upon viewing a trauma-related image, whereas the same area brain activity did not decrease in wait-list controls (2008). Another study showed that if PTSD is treated with CBT within 3 months after trauma exposure, recovery is accelerated (Sibrandij et al., 2007). Although PTSD symptoms have been shown empirically to respond well to cognitive behavioral and trauma-focused therapies, patients do not respond well to psychodynamic, supportive, nondirective, or hypnotherapy (Bisson & Andrew, 2007). Interestingly, one experiment showed that acupuncture is significantly better at treating PTSD than group CBT (Hollifield, Sinclair-Lian, Warner, & Hammerschlag, 2007).

For GAD, individual acceptance-based behavior therapy (ABBT) that alters the intensity and/or frequency of internal experiences has arisen as a conglomerate of several other types of therapy, such as CBT for GAD, dialectical behavior therapy, and acceptance and commitment therapy. ABBT has shown promise (Roemer & Orsillo 2007; Roemer et al., 2008). The therapy involves heightening patients' awareness of their anxious response habits and why avoiding experiences that cause such feeling make their stress worse. Clients self-monitor their progress between sessions and are encouraged to practice mindfulness everyday as well as conduct written exercises toward the same end. Mindfulness meditation in the context of mindfulness-based CT has been shown to alleviate these residual symptoms (Evans et al., 2008).

In summary, an exceptionally wide variety of behavioral and pharmacological approaches have been taken to the treatment of the anxiety disorders. Treatments of both types used individually or combined have had some success, and, in general, one could conclude that the anxiety disorders are quite treatable, with good outcomes. As new treatments emerge, such as mindfulness meditation, they are certain to be applied and evaluated.

ACKNOWLEDGMENTS

This work was supported by the Medical Research Service, Department of Veterans Affairs and by the VISN-IV Mental Illness Research, Educational and Clinical Center (MIRECC), VA Pittsburgh Healthcare System.

Gerald Goldstein
Ashleigh R. Molz

Alsonso, P., Pujol, J., Cardoner, N., Benlloch, L., Deus, J., Menchon, J. M., et al. (2001). Right prefrontal repetitive transcranial magnetic stimulation in obsessive-compulsive disorder: A double-blind, placebo-controlled study. *American Journal of Psychiatry, 158,* 1143–1145.

American Psychiatric Association. (2000). *Diagnostic and statistical manual of mental disorders* (4th ed., text revision). Washington DC: American Psychiatric Association.

Antony, M. M., & Swinson, R. P. (2000). *Phobic disorders and panic in adults: A guide to assessment and treatment.* Washington, DC: American Psychological Association.

Antony, M. M., Craske, M. G., & Barlow, D. H. (2006). *Mastering your fears and phobias: Workbook.* London: Oxford University Press: Incorporated.

Asami, T., Hayano, F., Nakamura, M., Yamasue, H., Uehara, K., Otsuka, T., et al. (2008). Anterior cingulate cortex volume reduction in patients with panic disorder. *Psychiatry and Clinical Neurosciences, 62,* 322–330.

Baldwin, D., Bobes, J., Stein, D. J., Scharwachter, I., & Faure, M. (1999). Paroxetine in social phobia/social anxiety disorder. Randomised, double-blind, placebo-controlled study. *The British Journal of Psychiatry, 175,* 120–126.

Ballenger, J. C. (2004). Remission rates in patients with anxiety disorders treated with paroxetine. *Journal of Clinical Psychiatry, 65,* 1696–1707.

Battaglia, M., Pesenti-Gritti, P., Medland, S. E., Ogliari, A., Tambs, K., Spatola, C. A. M. (2009). A genetically informed study of the association between childhood separation anxiety, sensitivity to CO2, Panic Disorder, and the effect of childhood parental loss. *Archives of General Psychiatry, 66,* 64–71.

Bisson, J., & Andrew, M. (2007). Psychological treatment of posttraumatic stress disorder. *Cochrane Database of Systematic Reviews, 2,* CD003388.

Bloch, M. H., Landeros-Weisenberger, A., Rosario, M. C., Pittenger, C., & Leckman, J. F. (2008). Meta-analysis of the symptom structure of obsessive-compulsive disorder. *American Journal of Psychiatry, 165,* 1532–1542.

Bremner, J. D. et al. (1995). (10 authors) MRI-based measurement of hippocampal volume in patients with combat-related posttraumatic stress disorder. *American Journal of Psychiatry, 152,* 973-981.

Bremner, J. D., Vermetten, E., Afzal, N., & Vythilingam, M. (2004). Deficits in verbal declarative memory function in women with childhood sexual abuse-related posttraumatic stress disorder. *The Journal of Nervous and Mental Disease, 192,* 643–649.

Bremner, J. D., Vythilingam, M., Vermetten, E., Southwick, S. M., McGlashan, T., Staib, L. H., et al. (2003). Neural correlates of declarative memory for emotionally valenced words in women with posttraumatic stress disorder related to early childhood sexual abuse. *Biological Psychiatry, 53,* 879–889.

Brewin, C. R., Andrews, B., Rose, S., & Kirk, M. (1999). Acute stress disorder and posttraumatic stress disorder in victims of violent crime. *American Journal of Psychiatry, 156,* 360-366.

Bruce, S. E., Yonkers, K. A., Otto, M. W., Eisen, J. L., Weisberg, R. B., Pagano, M., et al. (2005). Influence of psychiatric comorbidity on recovery and recurrence in generalized anxiety disorder, social phobia, and panic disorder: A 12 year prospective study. *American Journal of Psychiatry, 162,* 1179–1187.

Bucci, P., Galdensi, S., Catapano, F., Di Benedetto, R., Piegari, G., Mucci, A., et al. (2007). Neurocognitive indices of executive hypercontrol in obsessive-compulsive disorder. *Acta Psychiatrica Scandinavica, 115,* 380–387.

Burdick, K. E., Robinson, D. G., Malhotra, A. K., & Szeszko, P. R. (2008). Neurocognitive profile analysis in obsessive-compulsive disorder. *Journal of the International Neuropsychological Society, 14,* 640–645.

Choy, Y., Fyer, A. J., & Lipsitz, J. D. (2006). Treatment of specific phobia in adults. *Clinical Psychology Review, 27,* 266–286.

Coldwell, S. E., Getz, T., Milgrom, P., Prall, C. W., Spadafora, A., & Ramsay, D. S. (1998). CARL: A LabVIEW 3 computer program for conducting exposure therapy for the treatment of dental injection fear. *Behavior Research and Therapy, 36,* 429–441.

Damsa, C., Kosel, M., & Moussally, J. (2009). Current status of brain imaging in anxiety disorders. *Current Opinions in Psychiatry, 22,* 96–110.

Davidson, J. R. T., Wittchen, H. U., Llorca, P. M., Erickson, J., Detke, M., Ball, S. G., et al. (2008). Duloxetine treatment for relapse prevention in adults with generalized anxiety disorder: A double-blind placebo-controlled trial. *European Neuropsychopharmacology, 18,* 673–681.

A

Davis, M., Myers, K. M., Ressler, K. J., & Rothbaum, B. O. (2005). Facilitation of extinction of conditioned fear by d-cycloserine: Implications for psychotherapy. *Current Directions in Psychological Science, 14*, 214–219.

Delgado, M. R., Jou, R. L., Ledoux, J. E., & Phelps, E. A. (2009). Avoiding negative outcomes: Tracking the mechanisms of avoidance learning in humans during fear conditioning. *Frontiers of Behavioral Neuroscience, 3*, 33.

Dello'osso, B., Nestadt, G., Allen, A., & Hollander, E. (2006). Serotonin-norepinephrine reuptake inhibitors in the treatment of obsessive-compulsive disorder: A critical review. *The Journal of Clinical Psychiatry, 67*, 600–610.

Dougherty, D. D., Baer, L., Cosgrove, G. R., Cassem, E. H., Price, B. H., Nierenberg, A. A., et al. (2002). Prospective long-term follow-up of 44 patients who received cingulotomy for treatment-refractory obsessive-compulsive disorder. *American Journal of Psychiatry, 159*, 269–275.

Eisenberger, N. I., Lieberman, M. D., & Williams, K. D. (2003). Does rejection hurt? An fMRI study of social exclusion. *Science, 3032*, 290–292.

Elzinga, B. M., & Bremner, J. D. (2002). Are the neural substrates of memory the final common pathway in posttraumatic stress disorder? *Journal of Affective Disorders, 70*, 1–17.

Emmelkamp, P. M. G., Krijn, M., Hulsbosch, A. M., de Vries, S., Schuemie, M. J., & van der Mast, C. A. P. G. (2002). Virtual reality treatment versus exposure in vivo: A comparative evaluation in acrophobia. *Behavior Research and Therapy, 40*, 509–516.

Evans, S., Ferrando, S., Findler, M., Stowell, C., Smart, C., & Haglin, D. (2008). Mindfulness-based cognitive therapy for generalized anxiety disorder. *Journal of Anxiety Disorders, 22*, 716–721.

Fenger, M. M., Gade, A., Adams, K. H., Hansen, E. S., Bolwig, T. G., & Knudsen, G. M. (2005). Cognitive deficits in obsessive-compulsive disorder on tests of frontal lobe functions. *Nordic Journal of Psychiatry, 59*, 39–44.

Fineberg, N. A., & Gale, T. M. (2005). Evidence-based pharmacotherapy of obsessive–compulsive disorder. *The International Journal of Neuropsychopharmacology, 8*, 107–129.

First, M. B., Spitzer, R. L., Gibbon, M., & Williams, B. W. (2005). *Structured clinical interview for DSM-IV-TR Axis 1 disorders-patient edition (SCID-1/P, 4/2005 revision*. New York: Biometrics Research Department.

Fullerton, C. S., Ursano, R. J., & Wang, L. (2004). Acute stress disorder, posttraumatic stress disorder, and depression in disaster or rescue workers. *American Journal of Psychiatry, 161*, 1370–1376.

Ginzburg, K., Solomon, Z., Dekel, R., & Bleich, A. (2006). Longitudinal study of acute stress disorder, posttraumatic stress disorder and dissociation following myocardial infarction. *Journal of Nervous and Mental Disorders, 194*, 945–950.

Goisman, R. M., Rogers, M. P., Steketee, G. S., Warshaw, M. G., Cuneo, P., & Keller, M. B. (1993). Utilization of behavioral methods in a multicenter anxiety disorders study. *The Journal of Clinical Psychiatry, 6*, 213–218.

Goisman, R. M., Warshaw, M. G., & Keller, M. B. (1999). Psychosocial treatment prescriptions for generalized anxiety disorder, panic disorder, and social phobia. *American Journal of Psychiatry, 156*, 1819–1821.

Goldstein, G., van Kammen W., Shelly, C., Miller, D. J., & van Kammen, D. P. (1987). Survivors of imprisonment in the Pacific theater during World War II. *American Journal of Psychiatry, 144*, 1210–1213.

Gordeev, S. A. (2008). Cognitive functions and the state of nonspecific brain systems in panic disorders. *Neuroscience and Behavior Physiology, 38*, 707–714.

Granja, C., Gomes, E., Amaro, A., Ribeiro, O., Jones, C., Carneiro, A., & Costa-Pereira, A. (2008). Understanding posttraumatic stress disorder-related symptoms after critical care: The early illness amnesia hypothesis. *Critical Care Medicine, 36*, 2801–2809.

Grillon, C., Ameli, R., Goddard, A., Woods, S. W., & Davis, M. (1994). Baseline and fear-potentiated startle in panic disorder patients. *Biological psychiatry, 35*, 431–439.

Gurvits, T. V., Shenton, M. E., Hokama, H., Ohta, H., Lasko, N. B., Gilbertson, M. W., et al. (1996). Magnetic resonance imaging study of hippocampal volume in chronic, combat-related posttraumatic stress disorder. *Biological Psychiatry, 40*, 1091–1099.

Hartford, J., Kornstein, S., Liebowitz, M., Pigott, T., Russell, J. M., Detke, M., et al. (2007). Duloxetine as an SNRI treatment for generalized anxiety disorder: Results from a placebo and active-controlled trial. *International Clinical Psychopharmacology, 22*, 167–174.

Hayward, C., Killen, J. D., Kraemer, H. C., & Taylor, C. B. (1998). Linking reported childhood behavioral inhibition to adolescent social phobia. *Journal of the American Academy of Child and Adolescent Psychiatry, 37*, 1308–1316.

Hoffman, S. G., Meuret, A. E., Smits, J. A., Simon, N. M., Pollack, M. H., Eisenmenger, K., et al. (2006). Augmentation of exposure therapy with D-cycloserine for social anxiety disorder. *Archives of General Psychiatry, 63*, 298–304.

Hollifield, M., Sinclair-Lian, N., Warner, T. D., & Hammerschlag, R. (2007). Acupuncture for posttraumatic stress disorder: A randomized controlled pilot trial. *The Journal of Nervous and Mental Disease, 195*, 504–513.

Huppert, J. D., Schultz, L. T., Foa, E. B., Barlow, D. H., Davidson, J. R. T., Gorman, J. M., et al. (2004). Differential response to placebo among patients with Social Phobia, Panic Disorder, and Obsessive-Compulsive Disorder. *American Journal of Psychiatry, 161*, 1485–1487.

Katerelos, M., Hawley, L. L., Antony, M. M., & McCabe, R. E. (2008). The exposure hierarchy as a measure of progress

A

A

and efficacy in the treatment of social anxiety disorder. *Behavior Modification, 32*, 504–518.

Kessler, R. C., Chiu, W. T., Demler, O., Merikangas, K., & Walters, E. E. 2005. Prevalence, severity, and comorbidity of 12 month DSM-IV in the National Comorbidity Survery Replication. *Archives of General Psychiatry, 62*, 617–627.

Koponen, H., Allgulander, C., Erickson, J., Dunayevich, E., Pritchett, Y., Detke, M. J., et al. (2007). Efficacy of duloxetine for treatment of generalized anxiety disorder: Implications for primary care physicians. *Primary Care Companion to the Journal of Clinical Psychiatry, 9*, 100–107.

Krawczyk, D. C. (2002). Contributions of the prefrontal cortex to the neural basis of human decision making. *Neuroscience & Biobehavioral Reviews, 26*, 631–664.

Kuelz, A. K., Hohagen, F., & Voderholzer, U. (2004). Neuropsychological performance in obsessive-compulsive disorder: A critical review. *Biological Psychiatry, 65*, 185–236.

Kumari, V., Kaviani, H., Raven, P. W., Gray, J. A., & Checkley, S. A. (2001). Enhanced startle reactions to acoustic stimuli in patients with obsessive-compulsive disorder. *American Journal of Psychiatry, 158*, 134–136.

Laffaye, C., Cavella, S., Drescher, K., & Rosen, C. (2008). Relationships among PTSD symptoms, social support, and support source in veterans with chronic PTSD. *Journal of Traumatic Stress, 21*, 394–401.

Lambert, J. F., Difede, J., & Contrada, R. J. (2004). The relationship of attribution of responsibility to acute stress disorder among hospitalized burn patients. *Journal of Nervous and Mental Disorders, 192*, 304–312.

Liberzon, I., Taylor, S. F., Amdur, R., Jung, T. D., Chamberlain, K. R., Minoshima, S., et al. (1999). Brain activation in PTSD in response to trauma-related stimuli. *Biological Psychiatry, 45*, 817–826.

Lipsitz, J. D., Barlow, D. H., Mannuzza, S., Hofmann, S. G., & Fyer, A. J. (2002). Clinical features of four DSM-IV specific phobia subtypes. *The Journal of Nervous and Mental Disease, 190*, 471–478.

Maier, S. F., & Seligman, M. E. (1976). Learned helplessness: Theory and evidence. *Journal of Experimental Psychology: General, 105*, 3–46.

Mantella, R. C., Butters, M. A., Amico, J. A., Mazumdar, S., Rollman, B. L., Begley, A. E., et al. (2008). Salivary cortisol is associated with diagnosis and severity of late-life generalized anxiety disorder. *Psychoneuroendocrinology, 33*, 773–781

Marchand, A., Roberge, P., Primiano, S., & Germain, V. (2009). A randomized, controlled clinical trial of standard, group and brief cognitive-behavioral therapy for panic disorder with agoraphobia: A two-year follow-up. *Journal of Anxiety Disorders, 23*, 1139–1147

Martin, J. L., Barbanoj, M. J., Pérez, V., & Sacristán, M. (2003). Transcranial magnetic stimulation for the treatment of obsessive-compulsive disorder. *Cochrane Database of Systematic Reviews, 2003*, (2), CD003387.

Mataix-Cols, D., Rauch, S. L., Baer, L., Eisen, J. L., Shera, D. M., Goodman, W. K., et al. (2002). Symptom stability in adult obsessive-compulsive disorder: Data from a naturalistic two-year follow-up study. *American Journal of Psychiatry, 159*, 263–268.

Mathew, S. J., Amiel, J. M., Coplan, J. D., Fitterling, H. A., Sackeim, H. A., & Gorman, J. M. (2005). Open-label trial of riluzole in generalized anxiety disorder. *American Journal of Psychiatry, 162*, 2379–2381.

Mathew, S. J., Price, R. B., Mao, X., Smith, E. L. P., Coplan, J. D., Charney, D. S., et al. (2008). Hippocampal N-acetylaspartate concentration and response to riluzole in generalized anxiety disorder. *Biological Psychiatry, 63*, 891–898.

McKibben, J. B. A., Bresnick, M. G., Wiechman Askay, S. A., & Fauerbach, J. A. (2008). Acute stress disorder and posttraumatic stress disorder: A prospective study of prevalence, course, and predictors in a sample with major burn injuries. *Journal of Burn Care & Research, 29*, 22–35.

Merom, D., Phongsavan, P., Wagner, R., Chey, T., Marnane, C., Steel, Z., et al. (2008). Promoting walking as an adjunct intervention to group cognitive behavioral therapy for anxiety disorders: A pilot group randomized trial. *Journal of Anxiety Disorders, 22*, 959–968

Moran, M. (2004). Psychosurgery evolves into new neurosurgery approaches. *Psychiatry News, 39*, 28.

Nash, J. R., Sargent, P. A., Rabiner, E. A., Hood, S. D., Argyropoulos, S. V., Potokar, J. P., et al. (2008). Serotonin 5-HT1A receptor binding in people with panic disorder: Positron emission tomography study. *The British Journal of Psychiatry, 193*, 229–234.

Newman, M. G. (2000). Recommendations for a cost-offset model of psychotherapy allocation using generalized anxiety disorder as an example. *Journal of Consulting and Clinical Psychology, 68*, 549–555.

Parsons, T. D., & Rizzo, A. A. (2008). Affective outcomes of virtual reality exposure therapy for anxiety and specific phobias: A meta-analysis. *Journal of Behavior Therapy and Experimental Psychiatry, 39*, 250–261.

Rabe, S., Zoellner, T., Beauducel, A., Maercker, A., & Karl, A. (2008). Changes in brain electrical activity after cognitive behavioral therapy for posttraumatic stress disorder in patients injured in motor vehicle accidents. *Psychosomatic Medicine, 70*, 13–19.

Rapaport, M. H., Clary, C., Fayyard, R., & Endicott, J. (2005). Quality of life impairment in depressive and anxiety disorders. *American Journal of Psychiatry, 162*, 1171–1178.

Rapee, R. M., & Lim, L. (1992). Discrepancy between self- and observer ratings of performance in social phobics. *Journal of Abnormal Psychology, 101*, 729–731.

Rodrigues, S. M., LeDoux, J. E., & Sapolsky, R. M. (2009). The influence of stress hormones on fear circuitry. *Annual Review of Neuroscience, 32*, 289–313.

Roemer, L., & Orsillo, S. M. (2007). An open trial of an acceptance-based behavior therapy for generalized anxiety disorder. *Behavior Therapy, 38,* 72–85.

Roemer, L., Orsillo, S. M., & Salters-Pedneault, K. (2008). Efficacy of an acceptance-based behavior therapy for generalized anxiety disorder: Evaluation in a randomized controlled trial. *Journal of Consulting and Clinical Psychology, 76,* 1083–1089.

Rynn, M., Russell, J. M., Erickson, J., Detke, M. J., Ball, S., Dinkel, J., et al. (2008). Efficacy and safety of duloxetine in treatment of generalized anxiety disorder: A flexible-dose, progressive-titration, placebo-controlled trial. *Depression and Anxiety, 25,* 182–189.

Sailer, U., Robinson, S., Fischmeister, F. P., König, D., Oppenauer, C., Lueger-Schuster, B., et al. (2008). Altered reward processing in the nucleus accumbens and mesial prefrontal cortex of patients with posttraumatic stress disorder. *Neuropsychologia, 46,* 2836–2844.

Samuelson, K. W., Neylan, T. C., Lenoci, M., Metzler, T. J., Cardenas V., Weiner, M. W., et al. (2006). Longitudinal effects of PTSD on memory functioning. *Journal of the International Neuropsychological Society, 15,* 853–861.

Sanacora, G., Kendell, S. F., Fenton, L., Coric, V., & Krystal, J. H. (2004). Riluzole augmentation for treatment-resistant depression. *American Journal of Psychiatry, 161,* 2132.

Scarpa, A., Haden, S. C., & Hurley, J. (2006). Community violence victimization and symptoms of posttraumatic stress disorder. *Journal of Interpersonal Violence, 21,* 446–469.

Sibrandij, M., Olff, M., Reitsma, J. B., Carlier, I. V., de Vries, M. H., & Gersons, B. P. (2007). Treatment of acute posttraumatic stress disorder with brief cognitive behavioral therapy: A randomized controlled trial. *American Journal of Psychiatry, 164,* 82–90.

Simpson, H. B., Foa, E. B., Liebowitz, M. R., Ledley, D. R., Huppert, J. D., Cahill, S., et al. (2008). A randomized, controlled trial of cognitive-behavioral therapy for augmenting pharmacotherapy in obsessive-compulsive disorder. *American Journal of Psychiatry, 165,* 621–630.

Stein, M. B., & Chavira, D. A. (1998). Subtypes of social phobia and comorbidity with depression and other anxiety disorders. *Journal of Affective Disorder, 50,* S11–S16.

Stein, M. B., Jang, K. L., Taylor, S., Vernon, P. A., & Livesley, W. J. (2002). Genetic and environmental influences on trauma exposure and posttraumatic stress disorder symptoms: A twin study. *American Journal of Psychiatry, 159,* 1675–1681.

Stinson, F. S., Dawson, D. A., Chou, S. P., Smith, S., Goldstein, R. B., Ruan, W. J., et al. (2007). The epidemiology of DSM-IV specific phobia in the USA: Results from the National Epidemiologic Survey on alcohol and related conditions. *Psychological Medicine, 37,* 1047–1059.

Straube, T., Glauer, M., Dilger, S., Mentzel, H., & Miltner, W. H. R. (2006). Effects of cognitive-behavioral therapy on brain activation in specific phobia. *NeuroImage, 29,* 125–135.

Thompson, S., & Rapee, R. M. (2002). The effect of situational structure on the social performance of socially anxious and non-anxious participants. *Journal of Behavioral Therapy and Experimental Psychiatry, 33,* 91–102.

Upatel, T., & Gerlach, A. L. (2008). Appraisal of activating thoughts in generalized anxiety disorder. *Journal of Behavior Therapy and Experimental Psychiatry, 39,* 234–249.

van Balkom, A. J., Boeijen, C. A., Boeke, A. J., van Oppen, P., Kempe, P. T., & van Dyck, R., (2008). Comorbid depression, but not comorbid anxiety disorders, predicts poor outcome in anxiety disorders. *Depression and Anxiety, 25,* 408–415.

Vasterling, J. J., Duke, L. M., Brailey, K., Constants, J. I., Allain, A. N., Jr., & Sutker, P. B. (2002). Attention, learning, and memory performance and intellectual resources in Vietnam veterans: PTSD and no disorder comparisons. *Neuropsychology, 16,* 5–14.

Voncken, M. J., & Bögels, S. M. (2008). Social performance deficits in social anxiety disorder: Reality during conversation and biased perception during speech. *Journal of Anxiety Disorders, 22,* 1384–1392.

Wakizono, T., Sawamura, T., Shimizu, K., Nibuya, M., Suzuki, G., Toda, H., et al. (2007). Stress vulnerabilities in an animal model of Posttraumatic Stress Disorder. *Physiology & Behavior, 90,* 687–695.

Watson, D. (2005). Rethinking the mood and anxiety disorders: A quantitative hierarchical model for DSM-V. *Journal of Abnormal Psychology, 114,* 522–536.

Wells, A., & Carter, K. (1999). Preliminary tests of a cognitive model of generalized anxiety disorder. *Behaviour Research and Therapy, 37,* 585–594.

Zarate, C. A., Payne, J. L., Quiroz, J., Sporn, J., Denicoff, K. K., Luckenbaugh, D., et al. (2004). An open-label trial of riluzole in patients with treatment resistant major depression. *American Journal of Psychiatry, 161,* 171–174.

Zatzick, D., Jurkovich, G. J., Rivara, F. P., Wang, J., Fan, M. Y., Joesch, J., et al. (2008). A national US study of posttraumatic stress disorder, depression, and work and functional outcome after hospitalization for traumatic injury. *Annals of Surgery, 248,* 429–437.

Adult Criminality

DESCRIPTION

Adult criminality refers to the commission of illegal behaviors by adults. It is not a diagnostic entity in the *Diagnostic and Statistical Manual of Mental Disorders, Fourth Edition, Text Revision* (*DSM-IV-TR*; American

Psychiatric Association [APA], 2000), nor is it a neurocognitive disorder. However, it is a behavioral pattern not entirely foreign to patients seen by neuropsychologists. One potential cause is behavioral disinhibition consequent to neurodevelopmental disorder or acquired neuropathology. Conversely, acquired brain injury can be a consequence of a risk-taking pattern of behavior often associated with adult criminality.

In 2008, 3.2% of U.S. adults were in prison or under community supervision (Sabol, West, & Cooper, 2009). In 2006, 1,331,100 of these persons were incarcerated in state prisons (Sabol et al., 2009). Of those prisoners, 50% were sentenced for violent offenses, 21% for property offenses, 20% for drug offenses, and 9% for other offenses (Sabol et al., 2009). One-half of state and one-third of federal prisoners reportedly committed their current offense under the influence of alcohol or drugs, with roughly three-quarters of all prisoners reporting some type of alcohol or drug use in the time leading up to their instant offense (Mumola, 1999).

NEUROPATHOLOGY/PATHOPHYSIOLOGY

Associations have been observed between prefrontal dysfunction and aggressive and violent behavior in neuroimaging studies using adults (Bufkin & Luttrell, 2005) and in studies using neuropsychological testing, neurological examination, and EEG (Brower & Price, 2001). Impulsive aggression has been associated with overactivation of right hemispheric subcortical regions (Raine et al., 1998) and/or underactivation of prefrontal regions (Raine et al., 1998). Predatory violence does not show the same prefrontal underactivation as does affective violence (Raine et al., 1998). Left temporal activity is also associated with acts of violence (Bufkin & Luttrell, 2005). A study by Gatze-Kopp, Raine, Buchsbaum, and LaCasse (2001) found functional deficits in both the frontal and temporal regions in persons convicted of murder.

Criminals diagnosed with antisocial personality disorder (APD) are known to have a substantially decreased volume of prefrontal gray matter, but not white matter, compared with controls (Raine, Lencz, Bihrle, LaCasse, & Colletti, 2000), and to demonstrate reduced autonomic activity via lower mean skin conductance under conditions of stress (Patrick, 2008; Raine et al., 2000), as well as lower heart rates (Raine et al., 2000) and startle reflex potentiation (Patrick, 2008). Psychopathy has also been associated with late frontocentral event-related potential negativities for a variety of stimuli (Kiehl, 2006) and is associated with paralimbic system dysfunction,

including the orbital frontal cortex, insula, amygdala, parahippocampal regions, anterior superior temporal gyrus, and rostral, caudal, and posterior cingulate (Kiehl, 2006).

Readers can also reference the articles entitled Conduct Disorder and Oppositional Defiant Disorder by Wynkoop, Haines, and Swanson, and Juvenile Delinquency by Wynkoop in this text for developmental information related to criminality.

NEUROPSYCHOLOGICAL/CLINICAL PRESENTATION

Although not definitive, a number of studies have demonstrated that adult criminals experience deficits in executive function, verbal abilities, and impulsivity compared with controls. This is despite research demonstrating that convicted violent and nonviolent felons can reason morally as well as noncriminals (Priest, Kordinak, & Wynkoop, 1991). A meta-analysis by Morgan and Lilienfeld (2000) supported the finding of executive dysfunction in groups defined by high levels of antisocial behavior. Violent index offenders including batterers are known to experience increased executive dysfunction compared with non-offenders and nonbatterers (Baker & Ireland, 2007; Cohen et al., 2003). Batterers are also known to fare less well on measures of impulsivity than are nonbatterers (Cohen et al., 2003). Similarly, impulsivity and aggression correlate inversely with performance on tests of concept formation and abstract reasoning (Dolan & Anderson, 2002).

Convicted criminals generally perform weakly on most neuropsychological tests including verbal tests when compared with noncriminal controls (Barratt, Stanford, Kent, & Felthous, 1997). Poor verbal performance has been associated with early age of onset of behavioral problems, involvement in violent and nonviolent offending, and chronic offending (Piquero, 2001). In addition, a study by Rasmussen, Almvik, and Levander (2001) found that verbal deficits (poor vocabulary, slow decoding of verbal stimuli) were associated with a history of crimes of violence. The study by Cohen et al. (2003) found that batterers had a weaker vocabulary score than nonbatterers but did not differ from the nonbatterers with respect to education level or general intelligence as measured by the Wechsler Adult Intelligence Scale-Revised.

However, research has not always demonstrated consistent differences between criminal and noncriminal groups. For example, a study by Hare (1984) found that the neurocognitive test performances of psychopaths and other inmates were similar to that of noncriminal controls and not at all like that of

A

frontal lobe patients. In addition, a study by Hart, Forth, and Hare (1990) found that the test scores and global impairment ratings of psychopaths and other criminals were not appreciably different from those typically obtained with noncriminals of approximately the same age and education.

DIAGNOSIS

Adult criminality is not a diagnosis per se but characterizes illicit behaviors committed by adults. The typical associated *DSM-IV-TR* (APA, 2000) diagnoses include APD and adult antisocial behavior, but can also include conduct disorder that persists into adulthood (not converted to APD), and even impulse control disorders (among others). The prevalence of personality disorders in forensic settings is about three times that of nonforensic settings (Rotter, Way, Steinbacher, Sawyer, & Smith, 2002). For example, the prevalence of APD (APA, 2000) among male inmates ranges from 40% to 60%, whereas in the community it ranges between 2% and 3% (Fazel & Dunseh, 2002; Moran, 1999).

TREATMENT

Treatment/intervention for criminal offenders is demonstrably effective in reducing recidivism (Hollin, 1999), including lower rates of reconviction for those who complete programing versus noncompleters and comparison groups (Palmer et al., 2007; see also Hollin et al., 2008; McGuire et al., 2008). Women have also responded to programmed intervention with significantly greater reductions in arrests for new crimes (Sacks et al., 2008).

Given the rampant abuse of substances among offender populations, with its known contribution to poor judgment and behavioral disinhibition, it makes sense to consider the beneficial effects of substance abuse treatment in corrections. Research by Passey, Bolitho, Scantleton, and Flaherty (2007) suggested that such treatment is an effective crime prevention strategy. In addition, Sullivan et al. (2007) demonstrated that reduced crime is related more so to preventing drug and alcohol relapse than to improving mental health symptoms.

Research also demonstrates that reduced recidivism is enhanced by structured behavioral and multimodal approaches compared with less-focused approaches (Bourgon & Armstrong, 2005; Hollin, 1999), with cognitive-behavioral interventions being among the most efficacious (Hollin, 1999; Hollin & Palmer, 2009; Lowenkamp, Latessa, & Holsinger, 2006), including Enhanced Thinking Skills

(Friendship, Blud, Erikson, Travers, & Thornton, 2003; Mullin & Simpson, 2007) and Reasoning and Rehabilitation programs (Friendship et al., 2003; Tong & Farrington, 2006). However, the efficacy of these approaches is not without conflicting results (see Howells et al., 2005, for nonsignificant group differences).

Matching multimodal interventions to multiple offender needs has produced favorable results. For example, matching the amount of intervention with degree of risk to reoffend and targeting specific offending risk needs (e.g., family structure and processes, criminal associates, antisocial cognitions, deficits in self-control) matched with the intellectual capacities and learning styles of the offender demonstrably reduces recidivism (meta-analysis by Dowden & Andrews, 1999; see also Hollin & Palmer, 2009; Lowenkamp et al., 2006). Research also demonstrates that the amount of clinically and psychologically appropriate treatment in relation to the degree of recidivism risk is much stronger for female offenders and young offenders than are other approaches (Andrews & Dowden, 2006). Other studies demonstrate that there may be minimum levels of treatment required to reduce recidivism that is dependent on the level of an offender's risk and need (Bourgon & Armstrong, 2005; Lowenkamp et al., 2006).

Program integrity (e.g., structure, highly trained and supported staff) appears to provide an independent source of enhanced effectiveness (Andrews & Dowden, 2005; see also Hollin, 1999; Hollin & Palmer, 2009). Results have been mixed, however, regarding the relative effectiveness of residential (Lowenkamp et al., 2006) versus community (Hollin, 1999) interventions.

Melissa M. Swanson
Timothy F. Wynkoop

American Psychiatric Association. (2000). *Diagnostic and statistical manual of mental disorders* (4th ed., with text revision). Washington, DC: Author.

Andrews, D. A., & Dowden, C. (2005). Managing correctional treatment for reduced recidivism: A meta-analytic review of programme integrity. *Legal and Criminological Psychology, 10,* 173–187.

Andrews, D. A., & Dowden, C. (2006). Risk principle of case classification in correctional treatment: A meta-analytic investigation. *International Journal of Offender Therapy and Comparative Criminology, 50,* 88–100.

Baker, S. F., & Ireland, J. L. (2007). The link between dyslexic traits, executive functioning, impulsivity, and social self-esteem among an offender and non-offender sample. *International Journal of Law and Psychiatry, 30,* 492–503.

A

Barratt, E. S., Stanford, M. S., Kent, T. A., & Felthous, A. (1997). Neuropsychological and cognitive psychophysiological substrates of impulsive aggression. *Biological Psychiatry, 41,* 1045–1051.

Bourgon, G., & Armstrong, B. (2005). Transferring the principles of effective treatment into a "real world" prison setting. *Criminal Justice and Behavior, 32,* 3–25.

Brower, M. C., & Price, B. H. (2001). Neuropsychiatry and frontal lobe dysfunction in violent and criminal behavior: A critical review. *Journal of Neurology, Neurosurgery, and Psychiatry, 71,* 720–726.

Bufkin, J. L., & Luttrell, V. R. (2005). Neuroimaging studies of aggressive and violent behavior. Current findings and implications for criminology and criminal justice. *Trauma, Violence, Abuse, 6,* 176–191.

Cohen, R. A., Brumm, V., Zawacki, T. M., Paul, R., Sweet, L., & Rosenbaum, A. (2003). Impulsivity and verbal deficits associated with domestic violence. *Journal of the International Neuropsychological Society, 9,* 760–770.

Dolan, M., & Anderson, I. M. (2002). Executive and memory function and its relationship to trait impulsivity and aggression in personality disordered offenders. *The Journal of Forensic Psychiatry, 13,* 503–526.

Dowden, C., & Andrews, D. A. (1999). What works for female offenders: A meta-analytic review. *Crime & Delinquency, 45*(4), 438–452.

Fazel, S., & Danesh, J. (2002). Serious mental disorder among 23,000 prisoners: Systematic review of 62 surveys. *Lancet, 16,* 545–550.

Friendship, C., Blud, L., Erikson, M., Travers, R., & Thornton, D. (2003). Cognitive-behavioural treatment for imprisoned offenders: An evaluation of HM Prison Service's cognitive skills programmes. *Legal and Criminological Psychology, 8,* 103–114.

Gatze-Kopp, L. M., Raine, A., Buchsbaum, M., & LaCasse, L. (2001). Temporal lobe deficits in murderers: EEG finding undetected by PET. *The Journal of Neuropsychiatry and Clinical Neurosciences, 13,* 486–491.

Hare, R. D. (1984). Performance of psychopaths on cognitive tasks related to frontal lobe function. *Journal of Abnormal Psychology, 93,* 133–140.

Hart, S. D., Forth, A. E., & Hare, R. D. (1990). Performance of criminal psychopaths on selected neuropsychological tests. *Journal of Abnormal Psychology, 99,* 374–379.

Hollin, C. R. (1999). Treatment programs for offenders: Meta-analysis, "what works," and beyond. *International Journal of Law and Psychiatry, 22,* 361–372.

Hollin, C. R., McGuire, J., Hounsome, J. C., Hatcher, R. M., Bilby, C. A. L., & Palmer, E. J. (2008). Cognitive skills behavior programs for offenders in the community. *Criminal Justice and Behavior, 35,* 269–283.

Hollin, C. R., & Palmer, E. J. (2009). Cognitive skills programmes for offenders. *Psychology, Crime, & Law, 15,* 147–164.

Howells, K., Day, A., Williamson, P., Bubner, S., Jauncey, S., & Parker, A. (2005). Brief anger management programs with offenders: Outcomes and predictors of change. *The Journal of Forensic Psychiatry & Psychology, 16,* 296–311.

Kiehl, K. A. (2006). A cognitive neuroscience perspective on psychopathy: Evidence for paralimbic dysfunction. *Psychiatry Research, 142,* 107–128.

Lowenkamp, C. T., Latessa, E. J., & Holsinger, A. M. (2006). The risk principle in action: What have we learned from 13,676 offenders and 97 correctional programs? *Crime & Delinquency, 52,* 77–93.

McGuire, J., Bilby, C. A. L., Hatcher, R. M., Hollin, C. R., Hounsome, J., & Palmer, E. J. (2008). Evaluation of structured cognitive-behavioural treatment programmes in reducing recidivism. *Journal of Experimental Criminology, 4,* 21–40.

Moran, P. (1999). The epidemiology of antisocial personality disorder. *Social Psychiatry and Psychiatric Epidemiology, 34,* 231–242.

Morgan, A. B., & Lilienfeld, S. O. (2000). A meta-analytic review of the relation between antisocial behavior and neuropsychological measures of executive function. *Clinical Psychology Review, 20,* 113–136.

Mullin, S., & Simpson, J. (2007). Does executive functioning predict improvement in offenders' behavior following enhanced thinking skills training? An exploratory study with implications for rehabilitation. *Legal and Criminological Psychology, 12,* 117–131.

Mumola, C. J. (1999). *Substance abuse and treatment, state and federal prisoners, 1997.* Retrieved February 18, 2010, from The Bureau of Justice Statistics.

Palmer, E. J., McGuire, J., Hounsome, J. C., Hatcher, R. M., Bilby, C. A. L., & Hollin, C. R. (2007). Offending behaviour programmes in the community: The effects on reconviction of three programmes with adult male offenders. *Legal and Criminological Psychology, 12,* 251–264.

Passey, M., Bolitho, J., Scantleton, J., & Flaherty, B. (2007). The magistrate's early referral into treatment (MERIT) pilot program: Court outcomes and recidivism. *The Australian and New Zealand Journal of Criminology, 40,* 199–217.

Patrick, C. J. (2008). Psychophysiological correlates of aggression and violence: An integrative review. *Philosophical Transactions of the Royal Society B, 363,* 2543–2555.

Piquero, A. (2001). Testing Moffitt's neuropsychological variation hypothesis for the prediction of life-course persistent offending. *Psychology, Crime & Law, 7,* 193–215.

Priest, B. J., Kordinak, S. T., & Wynkoop, T. F. (1991). Type of offense and level of moral development among adult male inmates. *Journal of Addictions and Offender Counseling, 12,* 2–11.

Raine, A., Lencz, T., Bihrle, S., LaCasse, L., & Colletti, P. (2000). Reduced prefrontal gray matter volume and reduced autonomic activity in antisocial personality disorder. *Archives of General Psychiatry, 57,* 119–127.

Raine, A., Meloy, J. R., Bihrle, S., Stoddard, J., LaCasse, L., & Buchsbaum, M. S. (1998). Reduced prefrontal and increased subcortical brain functioning assessed using positron emission tomography in predatory and affective murderers. *Behavioral Sciences and the Law, 16,* 319–332.

Rasmussen, K., Almvik, R., & Levander, S. (2001). Performance and strategy indices of neuropsychological tests: Relations with personality, criminality, and violence. *Journal of Forensic Neuropsychology, 2,* 29–43.

Rotter, M., Way, B., Steinbacher, M., Sawyer, D., & Smith, H. (2002). Personality disorders in prison: Aren't they all antisocial? *Psychiatric Quarterly, 73,* 337–349.

Sabol, W. J., West, H. C., & Cooper, M. (2009). *Prisoners in 2008.* Retrieved February 18, 2010, from The Bureau of Justice Statistics.

Sacks, J. Y., Sacks, S., McKendrick, K., Banks, S., Scheoneberger, M., Hamilton, Z., et al. (2008). Prison therapeutic community treatment for female offenders: Profiles and preliminary findings for mental health and other variables (crime, substance use, and HIV risk). In D. Phillips (Ed.), *Probation and parole: Current Issues* (pp. 233–261). New York: Taylor & Francis.

Sullivan, C. J., Sacks, S., McKendrick, K., Banks, S., Sacks, J. Y., & Stommel, J. (2007). Modified therapeutic community treatment for offenders with co-occurring disorders: Mental health outcomes. *Mental Health Issues in the Criminal Justice System,* 227–247.

Tong, L. S. J., & Farrington, D. P. (2006). How effective is the "Reasoning and Rehabilitation" programme in reducing reoffending? A meta-analysis of evaluations in four countries. *Psychology, Crime & Law, 12,* 3–24.

ADULT MOOD DISORDERS

DESCRIPTION

Mood disorders encompass an array of presentations. Major depressive disorder (MDD) is characterized by the presence of at least one major depressive episode in a person's life. The manifestation of this disorder is wildly heterogeneous. In order to meet diagnostic criteria (American Psychiatric Association [APA], 2000), one must experience a significant loss of interest or pleasure in usually enjoyed activities, and/or a depressed mood. Aside from exhibiting one of these required symptoms, people diagnosed with MDD must have four other symptoms, which are varied: weight or appetite loss or gain, insomnia or hypersomnia, psychomotor agitation or retardation, fatigue or loss of energy, feelings of worthlessness or excessive guilt, lack of ability to concentrate, and/or recurrent thoughts of death or suicidal ideation or plan (APA, 2000). These symptoms must be present nearly everyday, most of the day for at least 1 week to qualify as meeting criteria for an episode. These symptoms also must be severe enough to interfere with the patient's life in the way of social, occupational, or other functioning. Major depressive episodes can last as short as 1 week or as long as several months or even years. Two people diagnosed with MDD can have very different characteristics. One person may have a lifetime history of many episodes, each one lasting several months, with many symptoms including depressed mood, significant weight gain, hypersomnia, fatigue, and trouble concentrating. Another may have one episode lasting a week, characterized by loss of interest, appetite loss, insomnia, psychomotor agitation, and suicidality. Because of this variability MDD is sometimes difficult to diagnose.

Some people with MDD experience differential amounts of episodes in different seasons of the year. When this is the case, the diagnosis is augmented by the qualifier Seasonal Pattern. Most often, it happens that patients experience more major depressive episodes in the winter rather than other seasons of the year. This disorder is also called Seasonal Affective Disorder.

There are numerous other qualifiers including mild, moderate, severe with and without psychotic features, chronic, or with catatonic, melancholic or atypical features, and postpartum onset. Some individuals have only a single major depressive episode, whereas others have recurrent depression. A recurrent depression is diagnosed when there is an interval of at least 2 months between episodes. An important specific feature that sometimes occurs is melancholia in which there is loss of interest or pleasure in all activities. Individuals with melancholia do not improve their mood even when something good happens; their depression is worse in the morning, and they may have abnormal motor behavior in the form of agitation or retardation.

Dysthymic Disorder is a less severe but more chronic manifestation of depressed mood. In adults, this mood must be present for most of the day, most days of the week, for at least 2 years (APA, 2000). Two of the above-listed symptoms must also be present, and there must be no relapse in symptoms for greater than 2 months. There is also a diagnosis colloquially called Double Depression, to indicate that one has a history of Dysthymia punctuated by major depressive episodes.

The spectrum of Bipolar Disorders (BDs) is at the other end of mood disorders. They are characterized by the presence of manic and/or hypomanic episodes. A manic episode is a period of at least 1 week of abnormally and persistently high, grandiose, or irritable mood. If the patient is hospitalized for such a mood, there is no duration cutoff. Three more of the following symptoms are required (four if the mood criterion is irritability): high self-esteem or grandiosity, less need for sleep, more talkative than usual or a pressure to keep talking, flight of ideas, distractibility, increase in goal-directed activity or psychomotor agitation, and overinvolvement in enjoyable activities with high potential for negative consequences. Episodes must cause impairment in social or occupational functioning. A mixed episode is one that meets criteria for a manic and depressive episode for at least 1 week. Hypomania is a lesser version of mania which lasts at least 4 days rather than a week. The same symptoms are required, and the change should be visible to others, but impaired functioning is not a problem in hypomania. Rather, many people that have experienced hypomanic episodes enjoy them, as they feel better about themselves and are more productive or social.

A distinction is now made between Bipolar I Disorder (BD I) and Bipolar II Disorder (BD II). BD I is characterized by the presence of at least one manic episode. No history of major depressive episodes is required, but they are commonly seen. There are several diagnostic qualifiers for BD I, mostly detailing the type and severity of the most recent episode. A person who has only had one manic episode in the past will be diagnosed with BD I, as well as a person who has a recurring history of several manic, hypomanic, and major depressive episodes. BD II is a less severe version of BD, characterized by the presence of at least one major depressive episode and the presence of at least one hypomanic episode. Again, the symptoms must cause significant impairment in social or occupational functioning. If someone diagnosed with BD II ever has a manic episode, their diagnosis is immediately raised to that of BD I. Cyclothymia is an even less severe form in terms of the symptomatology, but patients experience many more episodes each year than most of those with BD I or II. Receiving a diagnosis requires the presence of both and many hypomanic and depressive episodes that do not meet criteria for a major depressive episode, for at least 2 years without any relapse longer than 2 months. Some people with any of the bipolar spectrum disorders may meet criteria for the qualifier Rapid Cycling, indicating the presence of 4 mood episodes within 12 months that meet criteria for a major depressive, manic, mixed, or hypomanic episode.

Certain life events have been found to predict to the onset of mood episodes. One theory is that a biobehavioral system called the behavioral activation system (BAS), which is theorized to regulate actions toward goal attainment, is dysregulated in people at risk for bipolar spectrum disorders. When confronted with a stimulus that activates the BAS, the system overcompensates and the ensuing cascade causes manic or hypomanic symptoms rather than just optimism, as in healthy people (Uroševic, Abramson, Harmon-Jones, & Alloy, 2008). Keeping with this, many investigators have found that life events involving goal attainment and/or anger predict manic symptoms and episodes (Alloy et al., 2006; Hammen & Gitlin, 1997). Conversely, negative life events have been shown to predict depressive symptoms and episodes (Alloy et al., 2006; Hammen & Gitlin, 1997).

Several studies have implicated dysregulation of the circadian rhythm as one predictor of mood episodes (Azorin & Kaladjian, 2009). One study that involved forcing a dysregulation of the circadian pacemaker in human adults found evidence that even small differences in sleep schedules can affect mood (Boivin et al., 1997). Recent research has shown that daily routines, especially sleep times, can affect the circadian rhythm (Boivin, 2000). Conversely, other studies have shown that depriving those with depressive disorders of sleep actually improves their symptoms (Graw, Huag, Leaonhardt, Wirz-Justice, 1998), although it is not known how sleep deprivation works (Giedke & Schwärzler, 2002). However, reduction in rapid eye movement sleep and slow wave sleep may be involved (Boivin, 2000).

NEUROPATHOLOGY/PATHOPHYSIOLOGY

The original conceptions of depression viewed it as an acquired disorder thought to be produced by life stresses. It was not always clearly distinguished from bereavement in which the depression is clearly associated with mourning for a recent death or other catastrophic event. Subsequently, it was recognized that some depressions are endogenous and cannot be directly associated with some unfortunate life experience. This form is now often characterized as "biological" depression and is distinguished from "reactive" depression, which can be associated with an identifiable life experience, such as losing a job or becoming ill.

There is now a very substantial literature in the area of depression involving anatomical studies based largely on various neuroimaging procedures or direct examination of brain tissue at autopsy and neurochemical studies. We borrow from an informative review of this research provided in Langenecker, Lee, and Bieliauskas (2009), who distinguish among neuroanatomy, structural imaging, functional imaging, and affective neuroscience research. The neuroanatomic studies have implicated limbic, frontal, and subcortical systems in depression. Various abnormalities have been noted in these systems based on direct observation with MRI or CT scan procedures. There is particular involvement of the hippocampus marked by atrophy, and there have been numerous studies relating volume loss to behavioral variables including cognition and functional status. The amygdala has also received substantial attention with some studies showing increased volume. The possibility has been raised that there is increased volume at the onset of the depression and smaller or normal volume with recurrence. The major focus of investigation has involved functional neuroimaging including functional magnetic resonance imaging (fMRI), cerebral blood flow studies, and positron emission tomography (PET). Numerous studies of BD have identified gray matter decreases in the insula bilaterally, the perigenual anterior cingulate, and the subgenual anterior cingulate (Ellison-Wright & Bullmore, 2010). It was pointed out by the authors of the meta-analytic study that produced these findings that these areas are structures involved in functional systems for pain, reward, punishment, and emotional processing.

The use of these neurobiological procedures has become associated with the relatively new field of affective neuroscience that deals with the neurobiology of mood and affect. Neurochemistry is also involved with major attention being paid to the status of dopamine and serotonin. These new procedures typically study relationships between findings derived from them and cognitive variables such as attention, working memory, and social cognition. There is clear evidence that individuals with depression have a different pattern of physiological reactivity to emotional stimuli, typically demonstrated with fMRI. Evidence also comes from electroencephalographic (EEG) research. Siegle, Condray, Thase, Keshavan, and Steinhauer (2010) showed that individuals with depression have increased gamma-band EEG particularly in the seconds following hearing negative words indicating sustained elaboration following emotional stimuli. Summarizing a substantial literature very briefly, depression appears to be associated with limbic, frontal, and subcortical system dysfunction that mediates neurochemical changes associated with mood and cognitive alterations. Some of these changes are better characterized in terms of different ways of processing information than as an abnormality of the type that may be demonstrated by atrophy of other signs of neuropathology.

NEUROPSYCHOLOGICAL/CLINICAL PRESENTATION

Consistent with the heterogeneity of the mood disorders noted, cognitive status is quite variable. Some depressed individuals are quite bright or at least cognitively intact. Others have performance difficulties when depressive symptoms interfere with taking cognitive tests, such as an inability to maintain concentration or slowness in action. Still others may be affected by side effect of antidepressive treatment. Some years ago, the use of electroconvulsive therapy in treatment of depression appeared to have resulted in memory dysfunction (e.g., Squire & Zouzounis, 1986). In some cases, however, certain forms of cognitive dysfunction appear to be a part of the disorder itself and can be demonstrated not only by test performance but also by corresponding positive findings on neuroimaging procedures, notably fMRI. Sometimes serial testing can resolve these matters. The patient can be tested when the course of medication has been completed or when the depressive episode is over. Improvement at these time points suggests that previously observed deficits were not the result of permanent, irreversible brain dysfunction.

It should be recognized that neuropsychological studies of depression are very frequently done with patients with other illnesses. There are numerous studies of patients who are HIV-positive or who have epilepsy, cancer, traumatic brain injury, substance-use disorders, heart disease, and numerous other illnesses which themselves may serve to alter neuropsychological functioning. Depression in the elderly is a field of research unto itself. The cognitive status of this group of individuals is of great interest, but studies involving them cannot resolve the matter of identifying neurocognitive aspects of depression itself. In addition, depression can vary greatly in severity consequently altering the degree of neurocognitive impairment. The status of neurocognitive function in depression remains an unsettled area with inconsistent research findings, and extensive heterogeneity. A comprehensive, recent review by McClintock, Husain, Greer, and Cullum (2010) has made this point forcefully. These investigators concur with the view that some patients with MDD show cognitive difficulties whereas others do not. They also identify the areas of executive function, attention and concentration, processing speed and memory as the domains of most concern, and the prefrontal cortex and hippocampus as the most involved brain regions. However, the pertinent literature is characterized by studies in which deficits were identified relative to normal controls and studies in which normal cognitive function was found.

It would appear that the best conceptual model for neuropsychological aspects of depression is that it is a heterogeneous disorder, although clear cognitively based subtypes have not been developed. Factors contributing to the heterogeneity may be severity of the depression, age, and presence of co-occurring illnesses that may independently produce cognitive deficits. Thus, the depressed patient with diabetes may have cognitive deficits because of the diabetes and not specifically because of the depression.

Neuropsychological testing for depression is not usually a routine procedure but can be productively used to help answer several questions. In its typical role, it can be used to determine whether the patient has a neurobehavioral disorder aside from the depression and to describe its behavioral consequences. It can be used to determine the presence, extent, and pattern of possible cognitive disorders associated with the depression itself. Sometimes this procedure is used productively in association with online neuroimaging. It is often used to resolve the so-called pseudodementia matter in which usually elderly individuals show signs of apparent dementia when in fact they are depressed, and the dementia signs disappear once the depression has been resolved (Raskind, 1998). The understanding of this condition has become complicated by the considerations that in some cases it is thought that depression is the first manifestation of actual Alzheimer's disease or other form of dementia and that individuals, generally in the early course of the illness, become depressed in the face of learning that they have Alzheimer's disease. Individuals in the later course of the disease tend to become less depressed because of increasing failure to be able to comprehend the cognitive consequences of the disorder (Lopez et al., 2003).

In performing a neuropsychological assessment, tests of attention probably are most important to administer, but speed of processing, memory, and executive function are typically given. Thus, a typical battery may include such procedures as the Wisconsin Card Sorting Test, the Stroop Test, the Trail-Making Test, and a memory test such as the Wechsler Memory Scale or the California or Hopkins Verbal Learning Test. The "Freedom from Distractibility" tests from the Wechsler intelligence scales are often quite helpful as well. Less-emphasized areas such as sensory-motor function have also been found to be useful in some research (Davis, Horwitz, Noggle, Dean, & Davis, 2010).

It is clear that unlike some other disorders, one cannot characterize a prototype neuropsychological profile for depression. Therefore, one cannot recommend particular tests or a particular test battery to be used with depressed patients. There is not only heterogeneity among depressed patients but within the

patient. Cognitive function may be quite different in an individual during an episode of depression or mania from when the episode is resolved. Thus retesting at appropriate times is of great importance in evaluating the stability of neuropsychological deficits. The psychologist should not be surprised at finding completely intact performance in some patients and substantial impairment in others.

DIAGNOSIS

The mood disorders are a class of mental disorders and, as pointed out in our entry on anxiety disorders in this book, there is a general consensus in the professional community to accept the diagnostic criteria contained in the various editions of the *Diagnostic and Statistical Manual of the American Psychiatric Association* (*DSM I* through *IV-TR*) and will be contained in the forthcoming *DSM-5*. Therefore, diagnoses are made by determining whether the client meets the required number of criteria contained in the manual. We have recommended, if a precise and scientifically acceptable diagnosis is to be made, the use of structured interviews. The most commonly used procedure at present is the structured clinical interview for *DSM-IV-TR* (SCID) (First & Spitzer, 1997). Use of the SCID generally is a requirement for publication of diagnoses in professional and scientific journals and may be used in general clinical practice at the discretion of the psychologist or psychiatrist in routine clinical practice. The currently proposed changes for *DSM-5* are relatively minor involving the addition of a Mixed Anxiety Depression diagnosis, and removal of the BD I – Most Recent Episode Mixed diagnosis and will be included in the anticipated forthcoming edition of the SCID.

It may be useful to supplement the SCID with one of the many depression scales available and with psychological personality testing. The most commonly used depression scales are the Beck Depression Inventory and the Hamilton Depression Rating Scale. The Zung Depression Scale is also commonly used. Because some changes associated with normal aging may resemble depression, scales have been developed for the elderly. The Geriatric Depression Scale created by Yeasavage et al. (1982–1983) is commonly used, and the Zung Scale is also often appropriate for elderly individuals. Clinicians often find it useful to use a more comprehensive personality assessment, such as the Minnesota Multiphasic Personality Inventory to understand the context in which the depression occurs. The diagnosis of a mood disorder as in the case of other psychiatric disorders is therefore ideally made using a structured interview to evaluate presence

A

of *DSM-IV* criteria, and special tests and scales as indicated. In diagnostic assessment of the mood disorders, it is important to describe the patient's current state. That is, the patient may be presently in a depressive episode or has a history, or lifetime diagnosis of a mood disorder, but is not currently depressed. It is often important to make an assessment as to whether further episodes of depression may be anticipated. In the case of BD, patients may be in manic or depressed states or euthymic: that is, neither manic nor depressed. Scales for mania are also available, the most popular of which is the Young Mania Rating Scale (Young, Biggs, Ziegler, & Meyer, 1978).

TREATMENT

Major efforts have been made to develop effective treatments for depression in general and more specific forms of it such as suicidality or seasonal affective disorder. The choice is usually between pharmacological and behavioral therapy. But some studies have found that there are benefits to be gained when both forms of treatment are combined. Evaluating the effectiveness of treatment is beset by numerous methodological problems prominent among them being placebo effects and the fact that depression is often a self-limiting disorder, and recovery may occur with or without active treatment. Patients in both the United States and the United Kingdom have shown an interest in augmenting their treatment of pharmacotherapy and psychotherapy with self-help techniques as reported in an extensive literature (e.g., Osgood-Hynes et al., 1998; Richardson, Richards, & Barkham, 2010). Research into the risk factors for relapse has provided impetus for research into whether training patients to be aware of these warning signs are helpful in long-term treatment. A review of six randomized controlled trials showed that interventions with this form of psychoeducation were more helpful than psychotherapy and medication (Morriss et al., 2007). This training lengthened the amount of time to the next episode relapse and resulted in better functioning and less hospitalization of patients overall. Therefore, there is probably a common tendency to underevaluate the successful efforts patients sometime make to conquer depression on their own.

Based upon extensive studies involving large sample randomized trials sponsored by the NIMH (Klerman) there is widespread acceptance of the view that behavioral therapy, usually in the form of cognitive behavioral or interpersonal therapy, and pharmacotherapy with antidepressant medications are equally efficacious and that combined treatment is better than any treatment by itself. Guided by this general principle, there has been extensive study of different forms of psychotherapy and of different medications.

Behavioral Approaches

Most of the more recent literature in the area of psychotherapy for depression involves the application of three methods: cognitive behavioral therapy, interpersonal therapy, and social rhythm therapy. These are all evidence-based, manualized treatments that are behaviorally oriented. Cognitive behavioral therapy (Beck, 1993) includes a number of methods of systematic treatment aimed at problem-solving in the areas of the emotions, cognition, and behavior. It may take the form of different techniques including diary keeping, dealing with the patient's cognitions, assumptions, evaluations and beliefs and specific methods such as cognitive therapy, rational emotive behavior therapy, relaxation, mindfulness, and distraction. In the case of mood disorders, it is oriented toward Beck cognitive theory of depression based upon thinking biased toward negative interpretations. Depressed people make negative evaluations of themselves, and it is the aim of the treatment to correct the negative schema these individuals develop. Interpersonal therapy addresses itself to the relationship between mood and interpersonal events. It deals with interpersonal problems related to grief and interpersonal deficits. When combined with social rhythm therapy, it involves stabilization of daily routines and sleep/wake cycles.

Pharmacological Approaches

There are several options for treating mood disorders with medications. For depressive disorders, selective serotonin reuptake inhibitors (SSRIs) are one of the most common choices of medication, as they are the most effective of the drugs available and have less severe side effects. Atypical antidepressants are drugs that exert effects on the norepinephrine as well as serotonin systems in the brain, and they may be helpful to people that do not improve on SSRIs. One of the oldest kinds of drugs are monoamine oxidase inhibitors, which have dangerous interactions with foods and other drugs. They are still used but very rarely. Unfortunately, about 30% of patients treated with antidepressant medications do not significantly improve on any of these drugs. Furthermore, meta-analyses of clinical trials have shown that though these drugs are more effective than placebo, the effect is low to moderate (Kirsch et al., 2008). However, the effects on treating severe depression are considered clinically significant. It has therefore been suggested that the medications are more effective with severely depressed patients than with patients with mild or moderate depression. An extensive meta-analytic study has supported the view that combined approaches are the best. This study found that though medication may have a rapid and robust effect it does little to reduce risk of recurrence of the depression once its use is discontinued. Cognitive behavior therapy and interpersonal therapy are as effective as medications, with cognitive behavior therapy showing enduring benefits. Combined therapy provides the advantages of both methods. The treatment of choice particularly for severely depressed patients appears to be combined therapy.

Seasonal Affective Disorder

Highly specialized techniques have been developed for seasonal affective disorder, largely involving circadian rhythm abnormalities. These methods include 20-h days (Koorengevel, Beersma, den Boer, & Hoofdakker, 2003), sleep deprivation (Boivin, 2000), a medication called duloxetine (Pirek et al., 2008), and phototherapy or light therapy involving prolonged exposure to bright light (Rastad, Ulfberg, & Lindberg, 2008). Successful results have generally been reported.

Suicidal Ideation

Treatment of depressed patients with suicidal behaviors involving ideation or attempts has stressed use of a variety of medications as well as employment of cognitive or interpersonal therapy. The use of antidepressant medication has been criticized on the basis of reports of increased suicidal behavior, particularly in depressed adolescents. An FDA advisory committee recommended a black box warning on antidepressants providing this information for adolescents with a recommended extension to young adults. Subsequent research confirmed the absence of such a risk in adults and recommended continued use of these medications. Lithium has been described as a particularly effective medication for reduction of suicidal behavior (Müller-Oerlinghausen & Lewitzka, 2010).

Bipolar Disorder

As suggested by Gershon, Chengappa, and Malhi (2009) lithium is the classic, gold standard treatment for BD. They indicate that in 2009, lithium had been used for that purpose for a half century and continues to be used as the treatment of choice. Other medications and their combination have also been used

successfully, particularly with individuals who are not lithium responders, but lithium remains the generally most efficacious and universally used treatment. Behavioral treatments may be used with BD patients but typically in conjunction with lithium or other medication (Gonzalez-Isasi et al., 2010). It is noted that patients with BD frequently have comorbid substance use and chronic medical illnesses that need to be considered in treatment planning (McIntyre, 2009).

ACKNOWLEDGMENTS

This work was supported by the Medical Research Service, Department of Veterans Affairs and the Mental Illness Research, Education, and Clinical Center (MIRECC) VA Pittsburgh Healthcare System.

Ashleigh R. Molz
Gerald Goldstein

Alloy, L. B., Abramson, L. Y., Walshaw, P. D., Cogswell, A., Smith, J. M., Neeren, A. M., et al. (2006). Behavioral approach system (BAS) sensitivity and bipolar spectrum disorders: A retrospective and concurrent behavioral high-risk design. *Motivation and Emotion, 30,* 143–155.

American Psychiatric Association. (2000). *Diagnostic and statistical manual of mental disorders* (4th ed., text revision). Washington, DC: Author.

Azorin, J. M., & Kaladjian, A. (2009). Depression and circadian rhythm. *Encephale, 35* (Suppl. 2), S68–S71.

Beck, A. (1993). *Cognitive behavior therapy and the emotional disorders.* New York: Penguin.

Boivin, D. B. (2000). Influence of sleep-wake and circadian rhythm disturbances in psychiatric disorders. *Journal of Psychiatry and Neuroscience, 25,* 446–458.

Boivin, D. B., Czeisler, C. A., Dijk, D., Duffy, J. F., Folkard, S., Minors, D. S., et al. (1997). Complex interaction of the sleep-wake cycle and circadian phase modulates mood in healthy subjects. *Archives of General Psychiatry, 54,* 145–152.

Davis, A. S., Horwitz, J. L., Noggle, C. A., Dean, R. S., & Davis, K. M. (2010). Cortical and subcortical sensory-motor impairment in patients with major depression: A preliminary analysis. *International Journal of Neuroscience, 120,* 352–354.

Ellison-Wright, I., & Bullmore, E. (2010). Anatomy of bipolar disorder and schizophrenia: A meta-analysis. *Schizophrenia Research,* doi:10.1016/j.schres.2009.12.22

First, M., & Spitzer, R. (Eds.). (1997). *Structured clinical interview for DSM-IV Axis I disorders (clinician version) SCID-I administration booklet.* Washington, DC: American Psychiatric Association.

A

Gershon, S., Chengappa, K. N., & Malhi, G. S. (2009). Lithium specificity in bipolar illness: A classic agent for the classic disorder. *Bipolar Disorders*, (Suppl. 2), 34–44.

Giedke, H., & Schwärzler, F. (2002). Therapeutic use of sleep deprivation in depression. *Sleep Medicine Review, 6*, 361–377.

González-Isasi, A., Echeburúa, E., Mosquera, F., Ibáñez, B., Aizpuru, F., & González-Pinto, A. (2010). Long-term efficacy of a psychological intervention program for patients with refractory bipolar disorder: A pilot study. *Psychiatry Research, 176*, 161–165.

Graw, P., Haug, H. J., Leaonhardt, G., & Wirz-Justic, A. (1998). Sleep deprivation response in seasonal affective disorder during a 40-h constant routine. *Journal of Affective Disorders, 48*, 69–74.

Hammen, C., & Gitlin, M. (1997). Stress reactivity in bipolar patients and its relation to prior history of disorder. *American Journal of Psychiatry, 154*, 856–857.

Kirsch, I., Deacon, B. J., Huedo-Medina, T. B., Scoboria, A., Moore, T. J., & Johnson, B. T. (2008). Initial severity and antidepressant benefits: A meta-analysis of data submitted to the food and drug administration. *PLoS Medicine, 5*, e45.

Koorengevel, K. M., Beersma, D. G., den Boer, J. A., & Hoofdakker, R. H. (2003). Mood regulation in seasonal affective disorder patients and healthy controls studied in forced desynchrony. *Psychiatry Research, 25*, 57–74.

Langenecker, S. A., Lee, H. J., & Bieliauskas, L. A. (2009). Neuropsychology of depression and related mood disorders. In I. Grant & K. A. Adams (Eds.), *Neuropsychological assessment of neuropsychiatric and neuromedical disorders* (3rd ed., pp. 523–559). New York: Oxford University Press.

Lopez, O. L., Becker, J. T., Sweet, R. A., Klunk, W., Kaufer, D. I., Saxton, J., et al. (2003). Psychiatric symptoms vary with the severity of dementia in probable Alzheimer's disease. *Journal of Neuropsychiatry and Clinical Neuroscience, 15*, 346–353.

McClintock, S. M., Husain, M. M., Greer, T. L., & Cullum, C. M. (2010). Association between depression severity and neurocognitive function in major depressive disorder: A review and synthesis. *Neuropsychology, 24*, 9–34.

McIntyre, R. S. (2009). Overview of managing medical comorbidities in patient with severe mental illness. *Journal of Clinical Psychiatry, 70*, e17.

Morriss, R., Faizal, M. A., Jones, A. P., Williamson, P. R., Bolton, C. A., & McCarthy, J. P. (2007). Interventions for helping people recognise early signs of recurrence in bipolar disorder (Review). *Cochrane Database System Review*, 1, CD004854.

Müller-Oerlinghausen, B., & Lewitzka, U. (2010). Lithium reduces pathological aggression and suicidality: A mini-review. *Neuropsychology, 62*, 43–49.

Osgood-Hynes, D. J., Greist, J. H., Marks, I. M., Baer, L., Heneman, S. W., Wenzel, K. W., et al. (1998). Self-administered psychotherapy for depression using a telephone-accessed computer system plus booklets: An open U.S.-U.K. study. *Journal of Clinical Psychiatry, 59*, 358–365.

Pirek, E., Willeit, M., Praschak-Rieder, N., Konstantinidis, A., Semlitsch, H. V., Kasper, S., et al. (2008). Treatment of seasonal affective disorder with duloxetine: An open-label study. *Pharmacopsychiatry, 41*, 100–105.

Raskind, M. A. (1998). The clinical interface of depression and dementia. *Journal of Clinical Psychiatry, 59* (Suppl. 10), 9–12.

Rastad, C., Ulfberg, J., & Lindberg, P. (2008). Light room therapy effective in mild forms of seasonal affective disorder-a randomised controlled study. *Journal of Affective Disorders, 108*, 291–296.

Richardson, R., Richards, D. A., & Barkham, M. (2010). Self-help books for people with depression: The role of the therapeutic relationship. *Behavioral and Cognitive Psychotherapy, 38*, 67–81.

Siegle, G. J., Condray, R., Thase, M. E., Keshavan, M., & Steinhauer, S. R. (2010). Sustained gamma-band EEG following negative words in depression and schizophrenia. *International Journal of Psychophysiology, 75*, 107–118.

Squire, L. R., & Zouzounis, J. A. (1986). ECT and memory: Brief pulse versus sine wave. *American Journal of Psychiatry, 143*, 586–601.

Urošević, S., Abramson, L. Y., Harmon-Jones, E., & Alloy, L. B. (2008). Dysregulation of the behavioral approach system (BAS) in bipolar spectrum disorders: Review of theory and evidence. *Clinical Psychology Review, 28*, 1188–1205.

Yeasavage, J. A., Brink, T. L., Rose, T. L., Lum, O., Huang, V., Adey, M., et al. (1982–1983). Development and validation of a geriatric depression screening scale: A preliminary report. *Journal of Psychiatric Research, 17*, 37–49.

Young, R. C., Biggs, J. T., Ziegler, V. E., & Meyer, D. A. (1978). A rating scale for mania: Reliability, validity and sensitivity. *British Journal of Psychiatry, 133*, 429–435.

ADULT REFSUM DISEASE

DESCRIPTION

Adult Refsum disease (ARD), also known as hereditary sensory motor neuropathy Type IV and heredopathia atactica polyneuritiformis, is an autosomal recessive disorder whose symptoms were first described in 1946 by Norwegian neurologist Sigvald Bernhard Refsum, after whom the disease is named (Wierzbicki, Lloyd, Schofield, Feher, & Gibberd, 2002; Zalewska & Schwartz, 2007). ARD belongs to a group of genetic diseases called leukodystrophies, which damage the white matter of the brain and cause motor impairments.

The disease is characterized by flawed peroxisomal alpha-oxidation of phytanic acid. ARD was originally thought to be caused by a mutation in the gene phytanoyl-CoA hydroxylase (*PAHX*); however, Wierzbicki et al. (2002) found the disease to have multiple causes, with 55% of cases likely to be attributed to mutations in other genes. Van den Brink et al. (2003) discovered that mutations of the peroxisomal biogenesis factor 7 gene (*PEX7*) are also associated with patients clinically diagnosed with ARD. ARD usually begins in late childhood presenting the clinical features retinitis pigmentosa (deterioration of the retina causing progressive night blindness) and anosmia (loss of smell). As the disease progresses, other symptoms may appear such as ataxia (loss of the ability to coordinate muscular movement), deafness, peripheral neuropathy (muscle weakness), cardiac arrhythmias (irregular heart rhythm), ichthyosis (dry and scaly skin), and the buildup of phytanic acid in plasma-containing and lipid-containing tissues.

NEUROPATHOLOGY/PATHOPHYSIOLOGY

ARD is characterized by flawed peroxisomal alpha-oxidation of phytanic acid. Phytanic acid levels are elevated in the blood of patients with ARD. This exogenous C20-branched-chain fatty acid, which is introduced into the body by ingesting dietary plant chlorophyll and animal products, builds up in the brain, blood, and tissues. Other essential fatty acids such as linoleic and arachidonic acids in lipid moieties are replaced by excessive phytanic acid, which is linked to ichthyosis due to the essential fatty acid deficiency. The normal level of phytanic acid increases by 50 times or more (Zalewska & Schwartz, 2007). ARD is genetically heterogeneous with mutations in the *PAHX* and *PEX7* genes both being linked to cases.

NEUROPSYCHOLOGICAL/CLINICAL PRESENTATION

The only emotional impairment that is documented is the development of depression when ARD goes untreated or is diagnosed late (Zalewska & Schwartz, 2007). Numerous sensory-motor impairments occur such as retinitis pigmentosa, anosmia, deafness, ataxia, and peripheral neuropathy. Retinitis pigmentosa and anosmia usually appear during late childhood, whereas ataxia, peripheral neuropathy, and deafness may appear as the disease advances. Cognitive functions have not been examined independent of these sensory and motor losses.

DIAGNOSIS

The diagnosis of ARD is based on clinical observations of introductory symptoms (retinitis pigmentosa and anosmia) and biochemical analysis detecting elevated levels of phytanic acid in the bloodstream. ARD can be differentiated from Zellweger's syndrome, infantile Refsum disease, neonatal adrenoleukodystrophy, and rhizomelic chondrodysplasia because ARD presents in late childhood with introductory features being progressively worsening night vision, retinitis pigmentosa, and anosmia (Wierzbicki et al., 2002). ARD is the only one of the leukodystrophies that has an elevated phytanic acid level in the bloodstream.

TREATMENT

ARD is the most treatable of the leukodystrophies because phytanic acid is only produced in food and not in the body (National Institute of Neurological Disorders and Stroke [NINDS], 2007). The main method of treating ARD is to cut down or eliminate foods containing phytanic acid from the diet. Phytanic acid is made from phytol, which is a part of chlorophyll. Animals such as cows, sheep, and rabbits eat grass, which is then broken down to make phytanic acid. Phytanic acid is then bound into their fatty tissues and into the milk they produce.

Therefore, grass eating animals and their milk should be avoided. Certain fatty fish and shellfish such as tuna, cod, and haddock should also be avoided since part of their diet is algae which contain chlorophyll (NINDS, 2007). Fruits and vegetables are allowed in the diet because recent research has shown that phytol is bound to chlorophyll in green foods; therefore, it is not broken down to phytanic acid and absorbed by the body. Fermented vegetable products are an exception as they appear to contain phytanic acid.

Certain individuals may need plasmapheresis, which is the removal, filtration, and return of blood plasma into the body to manage the buildup of phytanic acid in the bloodstream. Even if treated, there may still be hearing and vision problems. The sense of smell may never return either. Muscle weakness and numbness normally goes away, and dry and scaly skin normally clears up with successful treatment (NINDS, 2007). Death from cardiac arrhythmias is a possibility if the disorder is left untreated.

Kynan Eugene Metoyer
Charles Golden

National Institute of Neurological Disorders and Stroke. (2007). *NINDS Refsum Disease Information Page.* Retrieved December 25, 2008, from http://www.ninds.nih.gov/disorders/refsum/refsum.htm

Van den Brink, D. M., Brites, P., Haasjes, J., Wierzbicki, A. S., Mitchell, J., Lambert-Hamill, M., et al. (2003). Identification of PEX7 as the second gene involved in Refsum disease. *American Journal of Human Genetics, 72,* 471–477.

Wierzbicki, A. S., Lloyd, M. D., Schofield, C. J., Feher, M. D., & Gibberd, F. B. Refsum's disease: A peroxisomal disorder affecting phytanic acid alpha-oxidation. *Journal of Neurochemistry, 80* (2002), 727–735.

Zalewska, A., & Schwartz, R. (2007). *Refsum's Disease.* Retrieved December 25, 2008, from http://emedicine.medscape.com/article/1114720-overview

Agenesis of the Corpus Callosum

DESCRIPTION

Agenesis of the corpus callosum (ACC) represents a rare birth defect in which the corpus callosum, the bundle of fibers that connect the two hemispheres of the brain, is completely or partially absent. This typically occurs during intrauterine development and results in the hemispheres being disconnected. Although it can occur in isolation, it may also be seen in conjunction with other cerebral anomalies or neurological presentations such as Aicardi's syndrome, holoprosencephaly, Arnold–Chiari's malformation, Dandy–Walker's syndrome, Andermann's syndrome, and/or schizencephaly (Van Allen et al., 1993).

Clinically, symptoms vary and are largely dependent upon the degree of disconnection and whether it presents in isolation or in conjunction with other cerebral anomalies. Individuals may present as entirely asymptomatic or exhibiting severe deficits. As such, no unitary profile is indicative of the presentation, and diagnosis is only made and confirmed through radiological investigation utilizing CT or MRI (Kingsley, 1991) or through fetal ultrasound (Lynn, Buchanan, Fenichel, & Freeman, 1980). However, symptoms resembling disconnection syndromes have been noted as have higher risks of mental retardation and seizures (Golden & Bonnemann, 2007). Furthermore, given that the deficits coincide with cerebral defects, treatment is symptom based.

NEUROPATHOLOGY/PATHOPHYSIOLOGY

ACC has been primarily linked with disruption of prenatal brain development between the mid-first trimester and the early portion of the second trimester. This corresponds roughly with the 5th through 15th weeks of development. Research has long demonstrated that it may be sporadic or familial (Golden & Bonnemann, 2007; Naiman & Frazer, 1955), but, in general, it is impossible to accurately identify the underlying etiology. Some theories have centered around genetic contributions, whereas others have suggested chromosomal errors as the root cause. Metabolic disorders and prenatal teratogens (i.e., intrauterine toxins, infections, etc.) or injury have also been indicted.

ACC is often part of more extensive cerebral malformations/anomalies or a feature of specific physiological syndromes. For example, it has been noted in association with holoprosencephaly, Arnold–Chiari's malformation, Dandy–Walker's syndrome, Andermann's syndrome, schizencephaly, X-linked dominant Aicardi's syndrome (Aicardi, Lefebvre, & Lerique-Koechlin, 1965; Hoyt, Billson, Ouvrier, & Wise, 1978; Renier, Gabreels, Mol, & Korten, 1973), acrocallosal syndrome (Nelson & Thompson, 1982), Meckel's syndrome (Paetau, Salonen, & Haltia, 1985), and hydrolethalus syndrome (Salonen, Herva, & Norio, 1981). It has also been noted in association with midline cerebral masses including meningiomas, cysts, hamartomas, and/or lipomas, although it is noted that this is rare (Golden & Bonnemann, 2007; Nelson & Thompson, 1982).

The corpus callosum may be partially or entirely absent. When absent, in lieu of connecting the hemispheres, the bundle of fibers that would form the corpus callosum align longitudinally in each hemisphere and are called Probst bundles. At the same time the cingulated gyrus is absent, the remaining gyri have a radiating pattern extending perpendicularly to the roof of the third ventricle, and there is no structural separation of the lateral ventricles (Harding & Copp, 1997). Partial agenesis is most commonly associated with an absence of the posterior portion of the structure.

NEUROPSYCHOLOGICAL/CLINICAL PRESENTATION

The signs and symptoms of ACC vary based on the extent of the structure defect and whether it presents in conjunction with other cerebral anomalies or physiological syndromes. When ACC presents in conjunction with infantile spasms, chorioretinopathy and depigmented lacunae, mental retardation, and vertebral anomalies, Aicardi's syndrome is probable (Aicardi et al., 1965; Hoyt et al., 1978; Renier et al., 1973). Acrocallosal syndrome includes polydactyly, macrocephaly, and mental retardation in conjunction with ACC (Nelson & Thompson, 1982). Arnold–

Chiari's malformation, Dandy–Walker's syndrome, Andermann's syndrome, schizencephaly (clefts or deep divisions in brain tissue), and holoprosencephaly may all also present with ACC in addition to their commonly associated clinical features. Still, it is feasible that ACC will present as asymptomatic on the behavioral surface with only minor deficits being detected on neuropsychological/psychological testing (Golden & Bonnemann, 2007; Jeeves, 1990). In severe cases, mental retardation becomes more probable. In addition, individuals may present with seizures, prominent sensory and motor deficits, and potential hydrocephalus due to alterations in the structural composition of the ventricles as discussed above (Golden & Bonnemann, 2007).

DIAGNOSIS

The clinical presentation of ACC may vary from individuals being asymptomatic to severely impaired. This is most effectively determined through comprehensive neuropsychological evaluation and potentially physical and occupational workup. Speech therapy may also be indicated to determine the nature and extent of any deficits along these lines. Optometry examination may help to diagnose any visual impairments. However, when it comes to the actual diagnosis of ACC, this can only be done through neuroimaging, preferably MRI although CT may also be used. Electroencephalography may also be necessary to evaluate for seizures. With the advancement of fetal ultrasound (Lynn et al., 1970), identification intrauterine is also feasible.

TREATMENT

Given there is no unitary profile of ACC, no standard treatment course is suggested. Treatment is symptom based and may require a multidisciplinary approach based on severity. In general, neuropsychological assessment can prove quite useful in identifying neurocognitive strengths and weaknesses that may be used to develop appropriate cognitive and/or educational interventions. Even in instances where individuals appear asymptomatic, such assessment commonly reveals subtle deficits that may suggest directions for intervention. Physical and occupational therapies may be utilized as needed. Similarly, speech therapy may be indicated on a case-by-case basis. If seizures are present, antiepileptic drugs may be indicated following consultation with a neurologist.

Chad A. Noggle
Javan Horwitz

Aicardi, J., Lefebvre, J., & Lerique-Koechlin, A. (1965). A new syndrome: Spasms in flexion, callosal agenesis, ocular abnormalities. *Electroencephalography and Clinical Neurophysiology, 19,* 609–610.

Golden, J. A., & Bonnemann, C. G. (2007). Developmental structural disorders. In C. G. Goetz (Ed.), *Textbook of clinical neurology* (3rd ed., pp. 561–591). Philadelphia: Saunders Elsevier.

Harding, B., & Copp, A. J. (1997). Malformations. In D. I. Graham & P. L. Lantos (Eds.), *Greenfield's neuropathology* (6th ed., pp. 397–533). New York: Oxford University Press.

Hoyt, C. S., Billson, F., Ouvrier, R., & Wise, G. (1978). Ocular features of Aicardi's syndrome. *Archives of Ophthalmology, 96,* 291–295.

Jeeves, M. (1990). Agenesis of the corpus callosum. In F. Boller & J. Grafman (Eds.), *Handbook of neuropsychology* (4th ed., pp. 99–114). New York: Elsevier.

Kingsley, D. P. E. (1991). Neuroimaging. In E. M. Brett (Ed.), *Pediatric neurology* (pp. 836–837). London: Churchill Livingston.

Lynn, R. B., Buchanan, D. G., Fenichel, G. M., & Freeman, F. R. (1980). Agenesis of the corpus callosum. *Archives of Neurology, 37,* 444–445.

Naiman, J., & Frazer, F. C. (1955). Agenesis of the corpus callosum. *Archives of Neurology and Psychiatry, 74,* 182–185.

Nelson, M. M., & Thompson, A. J. (1982). The acrocallosal syndrome. *American Journal of Medical Genetics, 12,* 195–199.

Paetau, A., Salonen, R., & Haltia, M. (1985). Brain pathology in the Meckel syndrome: A study of 59 cases. *Clinical Neuropathology, 4,* 56–62.

Renier, W., Gabreels, F. J. M., Mol, L., & Korten, J. (1973). Agenesis of the corpus callosum, chorioretinopathy and infantile spasms (Aicardi syndrome). *Psychiatria Neurologia Neurochirurgia, 76,* 39–45.

Salonen, R., Herva, R., & Norio, R. (1981). The hydrolethalus syndrome: Delineation of a "new" lethal malformation syndrome based on 28 patients. *Clinical Genetics, 19,* 321–330.

Van Allen, M. I., Kalousek, D. K., Chernoff, G. F., Juriloff, D., Harris, M., McGillivray, B. C., et al. (1993). Evidence for multisite closure of the neural tube in humans. *American Journal of Medical Genetics, 47,* 723–743.

AGNOSIAS

DESCRIPTION

Agnosia is a relatively rare disorder (Zihl & Kennard, 1996) and has been defined as a failure of recognition that cannot be attributed to elementary sensory defects,

A

mental deterioration, attentional disturbances, aphasic misnaming, or unfamiliarity with sensorially presented stimuli (Benson, 1989; De Renzi, 2000; Frederiks, 1969; Schnider, 1994). Although neuroradiology might be useful in detecting the focal lesions that may account for the appearance of these symptoms, the best way to recognize the symptoms of agnosia is through behavior. Visiting patients and studying the behavioral implications of the disorder are the best methods that allow clinicians to detect and recognize the symptoms associated with agnosia. Further, there are no pathognomonic signs based either on neuroradiological or neurochemical procedures that indicate the presence of agnosia. Given the importance of behavioral and neuropsychological assessment in determining this disorder, we will discuss the neuropsychological aspects of agnosia and the associated behavioral impairments.

Agnosia may be modality specific. For example, the patient may fail to recognize objects such as a fork or a watch when presented through a particular sensory channel (e.g., vision). However, the patient might successfully identify the same object if presented under a different sensory modality, such as through tactile manipulation of the item or hearing characteristic sounds associated with the item. Additionally, the patient might be able to describe the objects. Visual, auditory, and tactile agnosias have been widely described, but many other kinds of agnosias have been identified (Bauer, 1993).

Lissauer (1890) was perhaps the first to provide a detailed description of a recognition disturbance in a patient. Since then, significant debates have arisen regarding the functional mechanisms responsible for agnosia. Among the first of the models that have been suggested to explain the brain mechanisms behind disorders of object recognition has been the "stage" model. This model proposes that the cortex first constructs a percept from elementary sensory impressions and then recognition occurs when the resulting percept is matched or compared with information that is stored about the object. The model proposed by Lissauer is such a stage model and has been widely used in conceptualizing agnosia and the different subtypes of agnosia. Essentially, Lissauer argued that recognition proceeds in two stages, apperception and association. Apperception is the conscious perception of a sensory impression and then putting together or combining these different sensory impressions, such as visual attributes, to construct a meaningful whole. Association refers to matching this whole or gestalt to a previous experience. This model allows researchers and clinicians to distinguish between apperceptive and associative agnosias, or between a failure in the ability to perceive stimuli consciously and a failure to give meaning to what is perceived. Patients with apperceptive agnosia will have problems with perceiving the object and with their ability to construct the whole, meaning that they will not only be unable to recognize the object but also to copy the object or match the object. A different deficit will characterize individuals with associative agnosia. Patients with associative agnosia might still be able to copy or match the given object or picture, but they lose the ability to recognize it because of the disruption in the association between the visual representation of the object and the knowledge of the object. Hence, patients may be able to copy or draw a given object but later not be able to recognize the object that they drew and deny any familiarity to the drawing (De Renzi, Scotti, & Spinnler, 1969). In summary, patients with apperceptive disorders would be unable to copy or to match the object, whereas patients with associative disorders would not be able to identify the object although they will be able to copy the given object or picture.

Another model of visual recognition was proposed by Ellis and Young (1988). In this model, the initial, viewer, and object-centered representations are matched to stored descriptions of known objects or object recognition units. When the object matches a structure in the object recognition unit, the object recognition unit becomes active and access to the stored semantic information about the object becomes possible (Zoltan, 1996). Name retrieval occurs in the final stage of the model. A deficit prior to the object recognition unit corresponds to Lissauer's apperceptive agnosia and a deficit after this point is associative.

The most common cause of agnosia is a cerebrovascular event, but cases of agnosia have also been reported after severe traumatic brain injury (McKenna, Cooke, Fleming, Jefferson, & Ogden, 2006). Often this syndrome follows occipitotemporal lesions that extend into the underlying white matter (Shelton, Bowers, Duara, & Heilman, 1994). Recently, a great deal of research has been conducted using neuroimaging techniques and cognitive models to better understand the processing networks that are damaged in individuals with agnosia (Damasio, Tranel, & Rizzo, 2000; Mesulam, 2000; Riddoch & Humphreys, 2001). Tractography has also been used as a tool with which to explore the neuroanatomy of occipitotemporal connections and has provided evidence in support of a direct connection from the extrastriate occipital cortex to the anterior temporal structures, compatible with the classical anatomical description of the inferior longitudinal fasciculus (Catani, Jones, Donato, & Ffytche, 2003). A lesion of this white matter tract might contribute to the development of agnosia.

PRIMARY TYPES OF AGNOSIA

Visual Agnosia

Visual agnosia refers to a class of disorders characterized by impairment in visual object recognition, but with intact elementary visual functioning, memory, language, and general intellectual functioning. The impairment in recognition is also modality specific in that stimuli may be recognized through some other sensory modality. Hence, patients with visual agnosia are not able to recognize stimuli presented visually but they often will be able to recognize the stimuli through touch or sound, or if the examiner verbally describes the object (Banich, 2004; Bauer, 1993). Visual agnosia may be distinguished from anomia because patients with anomia will often use circumlocution when attempting to describe a stimulus that they cannot name. Also, patients with anomia will not benefit from presenting objects through a different sensory modality. Hence, the examiner may determine whether patients have no knowledge of visually presented objects (visual agnosia) or whether they are merely unable to name the object (anomia). Patients with anomia will be unable to name stimuli regardless of the sensory modality used (Goodglass, Barton, & Kaplan, 1968). Visual agnosia is typically associated with lesions to the visual association areas of the occipital lobes (Benson, 1989), either bilaterally (Albert, Soffer, Silverberg, & Reches, 1979) or at the left hemisphere (Giovagnoli et al., 2009; Schnider, Benson, & Scharre, 1994). Visual agnosia has also been reported in neurodegenerative diseases, including Alzheimer's disease (Helmes & Ostbye, 2002; Mendez, Mendez, Martin, Smyth, & Whitehouse, 1990), Lewy body dementia (Mori et al., 2000), and posterior cortical atrophy (McMonagle, Deering, Berliner, & Kertesz, 2006).

Visual agnosia may be rather selective, with category-specific deficits (Farah, McMullen, & Meyer, 1991). Some have reported discrepancies between living and nonliving things (Riddoch & Humphreys, 2003; Warrington & Shallice, 1984). Indeed, within the category of visual agnosias, there are several subcategories or types that differ in regard to the nature of the material that the patients are unable to recognize. Types of agnosia that have been described include orientation agnosia (Turnbull, Beschin, & Della Sala, 1997), topographic or landmark agnosia (Farah, 2003b; Mendez & Cherrier, 2003), and even a brightness agnosia (Nijboer, Nys, van der Smagt, & de Haan, 2009; Nijboer, te Pas, & van der Smagt, 2011). Additionally, many other subtypes have received much attention in the research literature and include simultanagnosia

(a deficit in attending to more than one stimulus at a time), color agnosia (a deficit in recognizing colors), and prosopagnosia (a deficit in recognizing faces). Additional forms of visual agnosia include apperceptive visual agnosia (a deficit in forming a percept) and associative agnosia (a deficit in associating a percept with its meaning). Many of the individual types of agnosias, including those agnosias from other sensory modalities, may have apperceptive and associative types. Also, these additional forms of agnosia may be present separately or in various combinations in the same patient.

Apperceptive Visual Agnosia

Patients affected by apperceptive visual agnosia have difficulty at the perceptual level but with intact elementary sensory functions, such as acuity, discrimination, and color vision (Banich, 2004; Farah & Feinberg, 2003). Patients with apperceptive visual agnosia will demonstrate normal acuity on testing and will be able to navigate their environment while avoiding obstacles (Bauer, 1993). Despite the fact that elementary sensory functions appear to be relatively intact, these patients cannot synthesize what they see (Grossman, Galetta, & D'Esposito, 1997) or combine visual information into a percept or meaningful whole (Banich, 2004). They exhibit distortion in higher-order visual perception and severe impairment in describing the features of visual objects, copying objects, and matching the object to similar objects or pointing to an object named by the examiner (Bauer, 1993; Jankowiak & Albert, 1994). The drawings produced by these patients are often incomplete and fragmented, with different pieces or individual elements drawn but not put together, or may be so distorted as to be rendered unidentifiable. Furthermore, patients with apperceptive visual agnosia have difficulties in recognizing objects from different, atypical, or unusual perspectives (Davidoff & Warrington, 1999; Warrington & Taylor, 1973). When given incomplete line drawings with missing contour information, patients with apperceptive agnosia will have difficulty in identifying the object. They will also exhibit problems in tasks requiring them to disembed objects that have been superimposed, such as with the Poppelreuter–Ghent's overlapping figures (Banich, 2004). These patients often complain that they cannot see well, that the lighting of the room is poor, or that they have little experience with the stimuli that they are being asked to identify (Bauer, 1993).

The etiology of apperceptive agnosia is often associated with carbon monoxide poisoning, although bilateral posterior cerebral dysfunction is also often seen (Jankowiak & Albert, 1994). Shelton et al. (1994) reported the case of an individual with apperceptive visual agnosia who had a bilateral inferior temporal and occipital lobe infarction. The occipital lobe involvement was in the association areas and spared the primary visual cortex. Apperceptive visual agnosia has also been described in patients with posterior cortical atrophy (Gardini et al., 2011; Mendez, Ghajarania, & Perryman, 2002).

Associative Visual Agnosia

In contrast to patients with apperceptive visual agnosia, patients with associative visual agnosia exhibit relatively intact visual perception but yet are still unable to recognize objects presented visually. Even though visual information may be integrated into a meaningful percept, the ability to connect the percept to meaning and stored knowledge is impaired (Banich, 2004; Farah & Feinberg, 2003). Some have proposed that associative agnosia is characterized by a disconnection between a visual memory store and the semantic system (Carlesimo, Casadio, Sabbadini, & Caltagirone, 1998) or a deficit in visual access to stored semantic knowledge (Riddoch & Humphreys, 2003). Patients with associative visual agnosia will be able to identify objects through other sensory modalities and will also be able to produce a drawn copy of the objects (Banich, 2004; Bauer, 1993; Farah & Feinberg, 2003). Pointing to objects is often impaired but might be better than naming the objects spontaneously. The reason pointing to objects is not as impaired as spontaneously naming may be that pointing takes place within the context of a limited number of objects, whereas naming involves choosing from a myriad of potential names (Bauer, 1993). Further, identification of objects presented in photographs or line drawings is often worse than identification of real objects (Kertesz, 1979; Sparr, Jay, Drislane, & Venna, 1991; Wilson & Davidoff, 1993), which is likely related to the inability of these patients to derive 3D information from 2D pictorial cues (Turnbull, Driver, & McCarthy, 2004). Visual associative agnosia may be found together with various combinations of alexia, prosopagnosia, and/or color agnosia (Freedman & Costa, 1992; Kawahata & Nagata, 1989; Kertesz, 1979; Sparr et al., 1991; for a review, see also Jankowiak & Albert, 1994). These patients are also impaired in demonstrating the semantic meaning and functional properties of the object. They often fail when asked to sort objects and pictures into categories and to match different representations of the same object (Bauer, 1993).

A number of different etiologies have been reported to give rise to associative visual agnosia, but most of these seem to involve bilateral temporo-occipital and parietal dysfunction (Jankowiak & Albert, 1994). However, there have been several reports of associative visual agnosia following left hemisphere lesions (Benke, 1988; Ferro & Santos, 1984; Goldberg, 1990; McCarthy & Warrington, 1986). Associative visual agnosia has also been reported in patients with Alzheimer's disease (Giannakopoulos et al., 1999) and in a patient with progressive multifocal leukoencephalopathy (Butter & Trobe, 1994).

Simultanagnosia

Simultanagnosia has been considered a type of apperceptive agnosia (Bauer, 1993; Farah & Feinberg, 2003) and has two subtypes, dorsal simultanagnosia and ventral simultanagnosia. Dorsal simultanagnosia refers to the inability to attend to more than one object at the same time (Luria, 1959), a definition that is consistent with that of Damasio (1985). Hence, the disorder may be conceptualized as a bias for processing local elements and/or a deficit in processing more global elements. However, the deficit in global processing may be modulated by stimulus density (Dalrymple, Kingstone, & Barton, 2007) and spatial distance between local elements (Huberle & Karnath, 2006). Differences in identifying animate versus inanimate objects have also been reported (Riddoch & Humphreys, 2004). Dorsal simultanagnosia is typically associated with bilateral parietal lobe lesions (Berti, Papagno, & Vallar, 1986; Coslett & Lie, 2008a, 2008b; Duncan et al., 2003; Michel & Henaff, 2004), although bilateral superior occipital lesions (Rizzo & Hurtig, 1987) and inferior parietal damage (Kase, Troncoso, Court, Tapia, & Mohr, 1977) have also been reported. Given the involvement of the bilateral parietal lobes in dorsal simultanagnosia, it is not surprising that this disorder is often seen in patients with posterior cortical atrophy (Delamont, Harrison, Field, & Boyle, 1989; Kirshner & Lavin, 2006; Mendez & Cherrier, 1998; Yoon, Park, & Na, 2002). Dorsal simultanagnosia has also been described in patients with corticobasal degeneration (Mendez, 2000) and Huntington's disease (Finke et al., 2007).

Ventral simultanagnosia is associated with relatively spared ability to recognize whole objects, but limitations in how many objects may be recognized within a specific period of time (Farah & Feinberg, 2003). This form may be distinguished from the dorsal variant in that patients with ventral simultanagnosia are more successful on dot-counting tasks and seem to be less impaired in navigating their environment

(Bauer, 1993). Additionally, patients with ventral simultanagnosia are able to read using a letter-by-letter approach (Kinsbourne & Warrington, 1962; Levine & Calvanio, 1978). Ventral simultanagnosia is associated with left occipital (Trivelli, Turnbull, & Sala, 1996) and left occipitotemporal (Duncan et al., 2003) dysfunction.

Color Agnosia

Several different disorders of color processing have been described in the literature but they are not related to problems with gnosis (Bauer, 1993; Tranel, 2003). Central achromatopsia is a disorder characterized by the loss of color vision due to CNS disease (Bauer, 1993) and is associated with lesions to the occipital lobes and neighboring regions (Damasio, Yamada, Damasio, Corbett, & McKee, 1980; Tranel, 2003). Color anomia refers to the inability to name colors, either when presented with colored stimuli or when asked to point to colors when provided with the names (Tranel, 2003), but they can match and sort colors and answer questions about the colors of objects that are not presented; e.g., what is the color of the sky? (Bauer, 1993). It is associated with left mesial occipitotemporal lesions (Damasio, Tranel, & Rizzo, 2000). Specific color aphasia is also characterized by deficits with naming the colors of items presented visually and pointing to colors when provided the names, but these patients also have problems when answering questions about colors of stimuli (Bauer, 1993). Kinsbourne and Warrington (1964) described a patient with color aphasia who had a left posterior parietal subdural hematoma due to a head injury.

Color agnosia has been defined as the inability to retrieve color knowledge that is pertinent to a given stimulus and that is not due to problems with perception or naming (Tranel, 2003). Patients affected by color agnosia are unable to name colors or point to colors named by the examiner, although they are able to recognize colors on nonverbal tasks (Bauer, 1993). For example, if an examiner asks a patient with color agnosia to name the color of the grass, the patient will likely not be able to name the color. Patients with color agnosia will also have problems retrieving basic information about colors and choosing the correct color for some object or entity (Tranel, 2003). Some have found that patients with color agnosia maintain an ability to implicitly process color information (Nijboer, van Zandvoort, & de Haan, 2006). Differences in color processing of natural and nonnatural scenes have also been reported (Nijboer, van der Smagt, van Zandvoort, & de Haan, 2007). Color agnosia has been reported to result from lesions at the left

posterior regions (Goldenberg, 1992) and in particular the left temporo-occipital area (Luzzatti & Davidoff, 1994; Schnider, Landis, Regard, & Benson, 1992). However, van Zandvoort, Nijboer, and de Haan (2007) reported the case of an individual with color agnosia who had a right cerebellar stroke.

Prosopagnosia

Prosopagnosia refers to the inability to recognize faces and may include the faces of friends, family, and even the patient's own face (Farah, 2003a), even in the presence of intact object recognition (Riddoch, Johnston, Bracewell, Boutsen, & Humphreys, 2008). Patients with prosopagnosia may be unable to haptically recognize faces as well (Kilgour, de Gelder, & Lederman, 2004). Patients with prosopagnosia may be able to recognize the sex, relative age, and emotional expression of faces (Tranel, Damasio, & Damasio, 1988) and be able to recognize that the stimulus is a face (Banich, 2004; Bauer, 1993; Farah, 2003a), but they are not able to identify to whom the face belongs. Deficits identifying facial emotional expressions have been termed as prosopaffective agnosia by some (Vuilleumier, Ghika-Schmid, Bogousslavsky, Assal, & Regli, 1998). Patients with prosopagnosia may attempt to use different cues to assist in recognizing faces, such as the presence of glasses, the tone of the voice, hair style, etc. (Bauer, 1993; Damasio, Damasio, & Van Hoesen, 1982). The inability of patients with prosopagnosia to identify friends and family may lead to the belief that they are experiencing a memory deficit or dementia (Bauer, 1993). Prosopagnosia has been described together with achromatopsia, topographical disorientation, and object agnosia in various combinations (Green & Lessell, 1977; Nardelli et al., 1982; see also Jankowiak & Albert, 1994). Reports on prosopagnosia in the literature indicate that it is about four times more common in men than in women, a finding that might reflect sex difference in cerebral organization (Mazzucchi & Biber, 1983). As with visual agnosia, both apperceptive and associative forms of prosopagnosia have been proposed (De Renzi, Faglioni, Grossi, & Nichelli, 1991). Apperceptive prosopagnosia results from faulty perceptual processes, and associative prosopagnosia refers to the inability to recognize faces that is not due to a disruption in perceptual processing or a loss of semantic knowledge (De Renzi, 2000).

The lesions causing prosopagnosia often involve the ventral or inferior occipitotemporal regions bilaterally (Damasio et al., 1982; Green & Lessell, 1977; Nardelli et al., 1982). However, there is also evidence

A

A

that lesions restricted to the right hemisphere may be sufficient to cause prosopagnosia (Benton, 1990; Cals, Devuyst, Afsar, Karapanayiotides, & Bogousslavsky, 2002; De Renzi, Perani, Carlesimo, Silveri, & Fazio, 1994). Research has indicated that characteristic hemisphere processing differences appear in face recognition performances of patients with unilateral occipital lobe lesions (Damasio, Tranel, & Rizzo, 2000). It is thought by some that damage to the occipitotemporal region may disconnect visual input from the association cortex in which visual representation of faces is located (Damasio et al., 1982). Also, occipitotemporal lesions that involve the inferior longitudinal fasciculus may be posterior enough to affect portions of inferotemporal cortex that are important in recognizing, categorizing, and discriminating visual forms (Gross, Rocha-Miranda, & Bender, 1972).

Auditory Agnosia

Auditory agnosia refers to an impaired ability to recognize sounds despite the presence of otherwise adequate hearing as measured by standard audiometry (Bauer & McDonald, 2003). The disorder represents an inability to associate auditory sensory information to meaning (Banich, 2004). A generalized form of the disorder is associated with impaired ability to recognize both verbal and nonverbal sounds (Bauer, 1993). Auditory agnosia may be differentiated from cortical deafness in that individuals with cortical deafness possess a lack of awareness of auditory stimuli of any type and whose audiometric pure tone thresholds are markedly abnormal. Receptive amusia may be distinguished from auditory deafness in that receptive amusia refers to the inability to appreciate various characteristics of heard music (Bauer, 1993). Auditory agnosia is often associated with bilateral temporal lobe lesions (Oppenheimer & Newcombe, 1978; Parving, Salomon, Elberling, Larsen, & Lassen, 1980; Rosati et al., 1982; Satoh, Takeda, & Kuzuhara, 2007) and may be subcortical (Kazui, Naritomi, Sawada, Inoue, & Okuda, 1990). Auditory agnosia has also been described in individuals with mitochondrial encephalomyopathy with lactic acidosis and stroke (Miceli et al., 2008), Landau–Kleffner's syndrome (Baynes, Kegl, Brentari, Kussmaul, & Poizner, 1998; Kaga, 1999), and with neurodegeneration (Matthews, Chang, De May, Engstrom, & Miller, 2009). Specific or selective auditory agnosias have been described, including auditory verbal agnosia (pure word deafness), auditory sound agnosia (agnosia for nonspeech sounds), and paralinguistic agnosia (auditory affective agnosia).

Auditory Verbal Agnosia

Auditory verbal agnosia (pure word deafness or auditory agnosia for speech) refers to the inability to comprehend spoken language, although the ability to read, write, and speak is relatively preserved (Buchman, Garron, Trost-Cardamone, Wichter, & Schwartz, 1986; Coslett, Brashear, & Heilman, 1984). Comprehension of nonverbal sounds is relatively spared (Buchman et al., 1986), which distinguishes this disorder from auditory sound agnosia (Coslett et al., 1984). The syndrome is "pure" in the sense that it is relatively free of the aphasic symptoms found with posterior aphasia syndromes (Bauer & McDonald, 2003). Many patients with pure words deafness complain that speech sounds like a foreign language and their speech might contain occasional word-finding pauses and paraphasias and is often slightly louder than normal (Bauer, 1993). Pure word deafness has been associated with a bilateral disconnection of Wernike's area from auditory input (Bauer & McDonald, 2003; Takahashi et al., 1992). Pure word deafness is rather uncommon because the associated lesion is typically very circumscribed within the superior temporal gyrus, specific enough to involve Heschl's gyrus but sparing Wernike's area (Bauer & McDonald, 2003). In addition to left superior temporal lobe lesions (Stefanatos, Gershkoff, & Madigan, 2005), pure word deafness has been associated with bilateral temporal lobe lesions (Coslett et al., 1984; Di Giovanni, D'Alessandro, Baldini, Cantalupi, & Bottacchi, 1992), a tumor within the third ventricle (Shivashankar, Shashikala, Nagaraja, Jayakumar, & Ratnavalli, 2001), left subcortical temporal hemorrhage (Hayashi & Hayashi, 2007), left thalamic hemorrhage (Takahashi et al., 1992), and frontotemporal dementia (Iizuka, Suzuki, Endo, Fujii, & Mori, 2007).

Auditory Sound Agnosia

Auditory sound agnosia (or agnosia for nonspeech sounds) is associated with a selective deficit in identifying and recognizing nonverbal sounds (Bauer & McDonald, 2003). It is relatively rare, possibly because these patients are less inclined to seek medical advice because they are able to understand spoken language and their audiometry is often normal (Bauer, 1993; Bauer & McDonald, 2003). As with visual agnosia, two different forms of auditory sound agnosia have been proposed. The perceptual-discriminative type is associated with right hemisphere lesions and disruption of processing melody. The semantic-associative type is associated with left hemisphere lesions and disruption of processing rhythm (Buchtel & Stewart, 1989; Vignolo, 1982, 2003). Whereas the former group is more prone to error when detecting sounds and matching the sounds to the correct source, the latter group produces more semantic errors (Bauer, 1993; Bauer & McDonald, 2003). This subdivision between perceptual and semantic types has also been found in patients with Alzheimer's disease (Rapcsak, Kentros, & Rubens, 1989). Many investigators have reported that generalized auditory agnosia eventually progresses to an auditory sound agnosia for environmental or nonverbal sounds (Lambert, Eustache, Lechevalier, Rossa, & Viader, 1989; Motomura, Yamadori, Mori, & Tamaru, 1986; Taniwaki, Tagawa, Sato, & Iino, 2000). Auditory sound agnosia has been associated with a right temporal lobe lesion (Fujii et al., 1990) and also a lesion to the left temporal and parietal regions (Saygin, Leech, & Dick, 2010).

Paralingusitic Agnosia

Paralinguistic agnosias include auditory affective agnosia and phonagnosia. Heilman, Scholes, and Watson (1975) reported that patients with right temporoparietal lesions and neglect were impaired in comprehending the affective qualities of speech (nonpropositional speech), although they were relatively capable of comprehending the content of speech (propositional speech). This finding raises the possibility that auditory affective agnosia is a variant of auditory sound agnosia and represents a category-specific auditory agnosia (Bauer, 1993). Van Lancker and colleagues reported another type of paralinguistic deficit that follows right hemisphere dysfunction and termed this disorder "phonagnosia." Specifically, patients with unilateral right hemisphere damage exhibited deficits in discriminating and recognizing familiar voices. However, patients with left hemisphere damage were impaired in discriminating between famous voices. Right parietal lobe damage has been associated with impairment in voice recognition, whereas damage to either hemisphere was related to a deficit in voice discrimination between two famous voices (Van Lancker, Cummings, Kreiman, & Dobkin, 1988; Van Lancker & Kreiman, 1988; Van Lancker, Kreiman, & Cummings, 1989). A progressive form of phonagnosia has also been described in patients with frontotemporal dementia (Hailstone, Crutch, Vestergaard, Patterson, & Warren, 2010).

Somatosensory Agnosia

The terms somatosensory agnosia, tactile agnosia, and astereognosia have been used interchangeably

(Banich, 2004, Bauer, 1993). However, some distinctions between these terms have been proposed. Tactile agnosia refers to the impairment of tactile object recognition but in the presence of relatively intact elementary somatosensory, attentional, intellectual, and linguistic functioning (Bauer, 1993; Caselli, 2003). Some have proposed that astereognosis refers to impaired tactile spatial perception and tactile agnosia refers to a selective disturbance in tactile object recognition (Caselli, 1991, 2003). Bauer (1993) views astereognosis as an apperceptive form of tactile agnosia. Other forms of somatosensory agnosia have also been identified, including anosognosia, autotopagnosia, and finger agnosia. It is felt that these disorders represent forms of somatosensory agnosia in as much as somatosensation is involved.

Astereognosis

Patients with astereognosis experience sensory defects at some point in the clinical course of the disorder, though they do not necessarily have a defect in identifying the objects (Bauer, 1993; Caselli, 2003). The deficit in these patients is often limited to one hand, usually the left, due to unilateral lesions (Roland, 1976). For instance, an early case was described by Harris and Fearnsides (1915) who had astereognosis at the left hand. However, cases of astereognosis affecting the right hand have also been reported, such as the patient described by Stewart (1908). Additionally, in some cases the asymbolic hand recognizes the object but only after an extensive linguistic exam of all the separate features that comprise the object (Bauer, 1993). The fact that these patients often do not manipulate the objects placed in their hand has led to the suggestion that elementary sensory function is not actively brought to bear and this information is not adequately integrated with motor information in the perceptual processing of the stimulus that is placed in the hand (Bauer, 1993). Research has implicated the parietal lobes in astereognosis (Mauguiere, Desmedt, & Courjon, 1982; Stewart, 1908) and, in particular, damage to the anterior portion of the middle third of the postcentral gyrus causes astereognosis (Roland, 1976). Astereognosis has also been associated with tumors (Feinsod, Bentin, Moscovitch, & Wald, 1980; Rubinstein, 1938), cerebral commissurotomy (Zaidel, 1998), and Alzheimer's disease (Davis, Mazur-Mosiewicz, & Dean, 2010).

Tactile Agnosia

Disorders of tactile object recognition (tactile agnosia) without sensory or perceptual deficits have been

A

rarely reported (Bauer, 1993). Tactile agnosia typically affects one hand and results from a unilateral lesion (Balsamo, Trojano, Giamundo, Grossi, 2008; Caselli, 1991, 1993b; Endo, Miyasaka, Makishita, Yanagisawa, & Sugishita, 1992; Reed & Caselli, 1994; Reed, Caselli, & Farah, 1996). The patients are often able to match or draw tactually presented stimuli (Caselli, 1993a, 2003). The types of errors committed by patients with tactile agnosia have been described as misidentifications in spatial approximation, confusion with spatially similar objects, and generic descriptions of the object (Caselli, 2003). Tactile agnosia is distinguished from astereognosis in that astereognosis may be considered a more specific deficit that represents an apperceptive tactile agnosia. Further, astereognosis is often caused by a lesion in the region of the middle third of the postcentral gyrus, where the hand is represented, and the cortical and subcortical connections to this region (Bauer, 1993). However, tactile agnosia seems to result from parietotemporal lesions (Caselli, 1991, 1993b; Reed & Caselli, 1994). However, the case reported by Endo et al. (1992) had a left parietal lesion as well as lesions at the right parietal, temporal, and occipital lobes. Also, the case reported by Balsamo et al. (2008) had a hemorrhagic lesion involving the posterior regions of the corpus callosum.

Anosognosia

The term anosognosia was originally used by Babinski (1914) to refer to patients who did not recognize their hemiplegia (Heilman, Watson, & Valenstein, 1993; Starkstein, Fedoroff, Price, Leiguarda, & Robinson, 1992). Currently, though, anosognosia more generally refers to the lack of awareness or denial of illness (Banich, 2004; Caselli, 2003; Heilman et al., 1993). Anosognosia has been described together with hemiplegia (Pia, Neppi-Modona, Ricci, & Berti, 2004; Vocat, Staub, Stroppini, & Vuilleumier, 2010), neglect (Heilman et al., 1993; Jehkonen, Laihosalo, & Kettunen, 2006; Starkstein et al., 1992), emotional changes following stroke (Biran & Chatterjee, 2003; Spalletta et al., 2007), deficits in recognizing emotions (Starkstein et al., 1992), and achromatopsia (von Arx, Muri, Heinemann, Hess, & Nyffeler, 2010). Anosognosia has also been described in patients with degenerative diseases (Rosen, 2011), including Alzheimer's disease (Galeone, Pappalardo, Chieffi, Iavarone, & Carlomagno, 2011; Orfei et al., 2010; Starkstein, Brockman, Bruce, & Petracca, 2010), frontotemporal dementia (Rosen, 2011; Zamboni, Grafman, Krueger, Knutson, & Huey, 2010), and even mild cognitive impairment (Galeone et al., 2011; Orfei et al.,

2010). Anosognosia is differentiated from a similar disorder called anosodiaphoria. Unlike anosognosia, anosodiaphoria is associated with intact awareness of deficits, but the patients express little or no concern about their deficits (Critchley, 1966). Anosodiaphoria is often associated with right hemisphere damage (Stone, Halligan, & Greenwood, 1993; Takayama, Sugishita, Hirose, & Akiguchi, 1994) and has been noted in patients with frontotemporal dementia (Mendez & Shapira, 2005).

Anosognosia is typically associated with lesions to the right hemisphere (Heilman et al., 1993; Jehkonen et al., 2006; Pia et al., 2004; Stone et al., 1993; Vocat et al., 2010), and in particular the right temporal-parietal region (Starkstein, Brockman, et al., 2010; Starkstein et al., 1992). However, the lesion location has been found to vary (Appelros, Karlsson, & Hennerdal, 2007). Specifically, anosognosia has been associated with lesions in the subcortical regions (Pia et al., 2004), including the thalamus (De Witte et al., 2011) and left internal capsule (Biran & Chatterjee, 2003), as well as left hemisphere lesions (Stone et al., 1993).

Autotopagnosia

Autotopagnosia refers to a disorder involving the inability of patients to localize the parts of their body, on the body of someone else, or on the body of a model (Goldenberg, 2003). Patients with autotopagnosia are unable to point to specified body parts, with many of the errors being within the vicinity of the designated body part. However, many patients are able to name the body parts when pointed at by an examiner (Buxbaum & Coslett, 2001; De Renzi & Scotti, 1970; Ogden, 1985; Sirigu, Grafman, Bressler, & Sunderland, 1991). The disorder may be seen independent of aphasia and dementia and these patients may still be able to point to individual parts of objects, animals, and plants when requested to do so (Benton & Sivan, 1993). Awareness of their body and the ability to orient themselves on their body may be intact (Semenza, 1988; Sirigu et al., 1991); hence, the disorder seems to result from an inability to associate spatial orientation of their body with stored conceptual knowledge about the human body (Goldenberg, 2003). Thus, autotopagnosia may be conceptualized as a form of associative agnosia. Additionally, intact localization of the individual fingers has been reported in patients with autotopagnosia (De Renzi & Scotti, 1970). Autotopagnosia has been described in patients with left parietal dysfunction (Buxbaum & Coslett, 2001; De Renzi & Scotti, 1970; Ogden, 1985; Semenza, 1988).

Finger Agnosia

Finger agnosia was originally described as part of a syndrome that also included agraphia, left-right disorientation, and acalculia and that has since been referred to as Gerstmann's syndrome (Gerstmann, 1940). Finger agnosia refers to a disorder involving the inability of patients to localize or recognize the fingers of their hands (Banich, 2004). Finger agnosia may be considered by some as a specific form of autotopagnosia. However, as mentioned earlier, there are cases where patients with autotopagnosia remain able to identify individual fingers (De Renzi, 1982; De Renzi & Scotti, 1970). Gerstmann (1940) thought the disorder resulted from a disturbance in body schema from left parietal lobe dysfunction. Finger agnosia has also been described in patients with Alzheimer's disease, who exhibit particular difficulty in identifying the index finger (Shenal, Jackson, Crucian, & Heilman, 2006).

Paul S. Foster
Valeria Drago

Albert, M. L., Soffer, D., Silverberg, R., & Reches, A. (1979). The anatomic basis of visual agnosia. *Neurology, 29,* 876–879.

Appelros, P., Karlsson, G. M., & Hennerdal, S. (2007). Anosognosia versus unilateral neglect: Coexistence and their relations to age, stroke severity, lesion site and cognition. *European Journal of Neurology, 14,* 54–59.

Balsamo, M., Trojano, L., Giamundo, A., & Grossi, D. (2008). Left hand tactile agnosia after posterior callosal lesion. *Cortex, 44,* 1030–1036.

Banich, M. T. (2004). *Cognitive neuroscience and neuropsychology* (2nd ed.). Boston: Houghton Mifflin Company.

Bauer, R. M. (1993). Agnosia. In K. M. Heilman & E. Valenstein (Eds.), *Clinical neuropsychology* (3rd ed., pp. 215–278). New York: Oxford University Press.

Bauer, R. M., & McDonald, C. R. (2003). Auditory agnosia and amusia. In T. E. Feinberg & M. J. Farah (Eds.), *Behavioral neurology and neuropsychology* (2nd ed., pp. 257–270). New York: McGraw Hill.

Baynes, K., Kegl, J. A., Brentari, D., Kussmaul, C., & Poizner, H. (1998). Chronic auditory agnosia following Landau-Kleffner syndrome: A 23 year outcome study. *Brain and Language, 63,* 381–425.

Benke, T. (1988). Visual agnosia and amnesia from a left unilateral lesion. *European Neurology, 28,* 236–239.

Benson, D. F. (1989). Disorders of visual gnosis. In J. W. Brown (Ed.), *Neuropsychology of visual perception*. New York: IRBN Press.

Benton, A. L. (1990). Face recognition. *Cortex, 26,* 491–499.

Benton, A. L., & Sivan, A. B. (1993). Disturbances of the body schema. In K. M. Heilman & E. Valenstein (Eds.), *Clinical neuropsychology* (3rd ed., pp. 123–140). New York: Oxford University Press.

Berti, A., Papagno, C., & Vallar, G. (1986). Balint syndrome: A case of simultanagnosia. *Italian Journal of the Neurological Sciences, 7,* 261–264.

Biran, I., & Chatterjee, A. (2003). Depression with anosognosia following a left subcortical stroke. *Clinical Neurology and Neurosurgery, 105,* 99–101.

Buchman, A. S., Garron, D. C., Trost-Cardamone, J. E., Wichter, M. D., & Schwartz, M. (1986). Word deafness: One hundred years later. *Journal of Neurology, Neurosurgery, and Psychiatry, 49,* 489–499.

Buchtel, H. A., & Stewart, J. D. (1989). Auditory agnosia: Apperceptive or associative disorder? *Brain and Language, 37,* 12–25.

Butter, C. M., & Trobe, J. D. (1994). Integrative agnosia following progressive multifocal leukoencephalopathy. *Cortex, 30,* 145–158.

Buxbaum, L. J., & Coslett, H. B. (2001). Specialized structural descriptions for human body parts: Evidence from autotopagnosia. *Cognitive Neuropsychology, 18,* 289–306.

Cals, N., Devuyst, G., Afsar, N., Karapanayiotides, T., & Bogousslavsky, J. (2002). Pure superficial posterior cerebral artery territory infarction in The Lausanne Stroke Registry. *Journal of Neurology, 249,* 855–861.

Carlesimo, G. A., Casadio, P., Sabbadini, M., & Caltagirone, C. (1998). Associative visual agnosia resulting from a disconnection between intact visual memory and semantic systems. *Cortex, 34,* 563–576.

Caselli, R. J. (1991). Rediscovering tactile agnosia. *Mayo Clinic Proceedings, 66,* 129–142.

Caselli, R. J. (1993a). Somesthetic syndrome. *Neurology, 43,* 2423–2424.

Caselli, R. J. (1993b). Ventrolateral and dorsomedial somatosensory association cortex infarctions produce distinct somesthetic syndromes. *Neurology, 43,* 762–771.

Caselli, R. J. (2003). Tactile agnosia and disorders of tactile perception. In T. E. Feinberg & M. J. Farah (Eds.), *Behavioral neurology and neuropsychology* (2nd ed., pp. 271–283). New York: McGraw-Hill.

Catani, M., Jones, D. K., Donato, R., & Ffytche, D. H. (2003). Occipito-temporal connections in the human brain. *Brain, 126,* 1–15.

Coslett, H. B., Brashear, H. R., & Heilman, K. M. (1984). Pure word deafness after bilateral primary auditory cortex infarcts. *Neurology, 34,* 347–352.

Coslett, H. B., & Lie, E. (2008a). Simultanagnosia: Effects of semantic category and repetition blindness. *Neuropsychologia, 46,* 1853–1863.

Coslett, H. B., & Lie, E. (2008b). Simultanagnosia: When a rose is not red. *Journal of Cognitive Neuroscience, 20,* 36–48.

Critchley, M. (1966). *The parietal lobes.* New York: Hafner.

A

A

Dalrymple, K. A., Kingstone, A., & Barton, J. J. (2007). Seeing trees OR seeing forests in simultanagnosia: Attentional capture can be local or global. *Neuropsychologia, 45,* 871–875.

Damasio, A. R. (1985). Disorders of complex visual processing: Agnosia, achromatopsia, Balint's syndrome, and related difficulties of orientation and construction. In M. M. Mesulam (Ed.), *Principles of behavioral neurology* (pp. 259–288). Philadelphia: F. A. Davis.

Damasio, A. R., Damasio, H., & Van Hoesen, G. W. (1982). Prosopagnosia: Anatomic basis and behavioral mechanisms. *Neurology, 32,* 331–341.

Damasio, A. R., Tranel, D., & Rizzo, M. (2000). Disorders of complex visual processing. In M. M. Mesulam (Ed.), *Principles of behavioral and cognitive neurology* (pp. 332–372). Philadelphia: F. A. Davis.

Damasio, A. R., Yamada, T., Damasio, H., Corbett, J., & McKee, J. (1980). Central achromatopsia: Behavioral, anatomic, and physiologic aspects. *Neurology, 30,* 1064–1071.

Davidoff, J., & Warrington, E. K. (1999). The bare bones of object recognition: Implications from a case of object recognition impairment. *Neuropsychologia, 37,* 279–292.

Davis, A. S., Mazur-Mosiewicz, A., & Dean, R. S. (2010). The presence and predictive value of astereognosis and agraphesthesia in patients with Alzheimer's disease. *Applied Neuropsychology, 17,* 262–266.

De Renzi, E. (1982). Memory disorders following focal neocortical damage. *Philosophical Transactions of the Royal Society of London. Series B, Biological Sciences, 298,* 73–83.

De Renzi, E. (2000). Disorders of visual recognition. *Seminars in Neurology, 20,* 479–485.

De Renzi, E., Faglioni, P., Grossi, D., & Nichelli, P. (1991). Apperceptive and associative forms of proso-pagnosia. *Cortex, 27,* 213–221.

De Renzi, E., Perani, D., Carlesimo, G. A., Silveri, M. C., & Fazio, F. (1994). Prosopagnosia can be associated with damage confined to the right hemisphere—An MRI and PET study and a review of the literature. *Neuropsychologia, 32,* 893–902.

De Renzi, E., & Scotti, G. (1970). Autotopagnosia: Fiction or reality? *Archives of Neurology, 23,* 221–227.

De Renzi, E., Scotti, G., & Spinnler, H. (1969). Perceptive and associative disorders of visual recognition: Relationship to the side of the cerebral lesion. *Neurology, 19,* 634–642.

De Witte, L., Brouns, R., Kavadias, D., Engelborghs, S., De Deyn, P. P., & Marien, P. (2011). Cognitive, affective and behavioural disturbances following vascular thalamic lesions: A review. *Cortex, 47,* 273–319.

Delamont, R. S., Harrison, J., Field, M., & Boyle, R. S. (1989). Posterior cortical atrophy. *Clinical and Experimental Neurology, 26,* 225–227.

Di Giovanni, M., D'Alessandro, G., Baldini, S., Cantalupi, D., & Bottacchi, E. (1992). Clinical and neuroradiological findings in a case of pure word deafness. *Italian Journal of the Neurological Sciences, 13,* 507–510.

Duncan, J., Bundesen, C., Olson, A., Humphreys, G., Ward, R., Kyllingsbaek, S., et al. (2003). Attentional functions in dorsal and ventral simultanagnosia. *Cognitive Neuropsychology, 20,* 675–701.

Ellis, A. W., & Young, A. W. (1988). *Human cognitive neuropsychology.* Hillsdale, NJ: Lawrence Erlbaum.

Endo, K., Miyasaka, M., Makishita, H., Yanagisawa, N., & Sugishita, M. (1992). Tactile agnosia and tactile aphasia: Symptomatological and anatomical differences. *Cortex, 28,* 445–469.

Farah, M. J. (2003a). Prosopagnosia. In T. E. Feinberg & M. J. Farah (Eds.), *Behavioral neurology and neuropsychology* (2nd ed., pp. 239–241). New York: McGraw Hill.

Farah, M. J. (2003b). Visuospatial function. In T. E. Feinberg & M. J. Farah (Eds.), *Behavioral neurology and neuropsychology* (2nd ed., pp. 295–300). New York: McGraw Hill.

Farah, M. J., & Feinberg, T. E. (2003). Visual object agnosia. In T. E. Feinberg & M. J. Farah (Eds.), *Behavioral neurology and neuropsychology* (2nd ed., pp. 233–238). New York: McGraw Hill.

Farah, M. J., McMullen, P. A., & Meyer, M. M. (1991). Can recognition of living things be selectively impaired? *Neuropsychologia, 29,* 185–193.

Feinsod, M., Bentin, S., Moscovitch, M., & Wald, U. (1980). Brainstem tumor presenting with unilateral astereognosis. *Annals of Neurology, 8,* 191–192.

Ferro, J. M., & Santos, M. E. (1984). Associative visual agnosia: A case study. *Cortex, 20,* 121–134.

Finke, K., Schneider, W. X., Redel, P., Dose, M., Kerkhoff, G., Muller, H. J., et al. (2007). The capacity of attention and simultaneous perception of objects: A group study of Huntington's disease patients. *Neuropsychologia, 45,* 3272–3284.

Frederiks, J. A. M. (1969). The agnosias. In P. J. Vinken & G. W. Bruyn (Eds.), *Handbook of clinical neurology* (Vol. 4). Amsterdam: North-Holland.

Freedman, L., & Costa, L. (1992). Pure alexia and right hemi-achromatopsia in posterior dementia. *Journal of Neurology, Neurosurgery, and Psychiatry, 55,* 500–502.

Fujii, T., Fukatsu, R., Watabe, S., Ohnuma, A., Teramura, K., Kimura, I., et al. (1990). Auditory sound agnosia without aphasia following a right temporal lobe lesion. *Cortex, 26,* 263–268.

Galeone, F., Pappalardo, S., Chieffi, S., Iavarone, A., & Carlomagno, S. (2011). Anosognosia for memory deficit in amnestic mild cognitive impairment and Alzheimer's disease. *International Journal of Geriatric Psychiatry, 26,* 695–701.

Gardini, S., Concari, L., Paliara, S., Ghetti, C., Venneri, A., & Caffarra, P. (2011). Visuo-spatial imagery impairment in posterior cortical atrophy: A cognitive and SPECT study. *Behavioral Neurology, 24,* 123–132.

Gerstmann, J. (1940). Syndrome of finger agnosia, disorientation for right and left, agraphia and acalculia. *Archives of Neurology and Psychiatry, 44*, 398–408.

Giannakopoulos, P., Gold, G., Duc, M., Michel, J. P., Hof, P. R., & Bouras, C. (1999). Neuroanatomic correlates of visual agnosia in Alzheimer's disease: A clinicopathologic study. *Neurology, 52*, 71–77.

Giovagnoli, A. R., Aresi, A., Reati, F., Riva, A., Gobbo, C., & Bizzi, A. (2009). The neuropsychological and neuroradiological correlates of slowly progressive visual agnosia. *Neurological Sciences, 30*, 123–131.

Goldberg, E. (1990). Associative agnosias and the functions of the left hemisphere. *Journal of Clinical and Experimental Neuropsychology, 12*, 467–484.

Goldenberg, G. (1992). Loss of visual imagery and loss of visual knowledge — A case study. *Neuropsychologia, 30*, 1081–1099.

Goldenberg, G. (2003). Disorders of body perception and representation. In T. E. Feinberg & M. J. Farah (Eds.), *Behavioral neurology and neuropsychology* (2nd ed., pp. 285–294). New York: McGraw Hill.

Goodglass, H., Barton, M. I., & Kaplan, E. F. (1968). Sensory modality and object-naming in aphasia. *Journal of Speech and Hearing Research, 11*, 488–496.

Green, G. J., & Lessell, S. (1977). Acquired cerebral dyschromatopsia. *Archives of Ophthalmology, 95*, 121–128.

Gross, C. G., Rocha-Miranda, C. E., & Bender, D. B. (1972). Visual properties of neurons in inferotemporal cortex of the macaque. *Journal of Neurophysiology, 35*, 96–111.

Grossman, M., Galetta, S., & D'Esposito, M. (1997). Object recognition difficulty in visual apperceptive agnosia. *Brain and Cognition, 33*, 306–342.

Hailstone, J. C., Crutch, S. J., Vestergaard, M. D., Patterson, R. D., & Warren, J. D. (2010). Progressive associative phonagnosia: A neuropsychological analysis. *Neuropsychologia, 48*, 1104–1114.

Harris, W., & Fearnsides, E. G. (1915). Case of astereognosis of the left hand. *Proceedings of the Royal Society of Medicine, 8*, 79–83.

Hayashi, K., & Hayashi, R. (2007). Pure word deafness due to left subcortical lesion: Neurophysiological studies of two patients. *Clinical Neurophysiology, 118*, 863–868.

Heilman, K. M., Scholes, R., & Watson, R. T. (1975). Auditory affective agnosia: Disturbed comprehension of affective speech. *Journal of Neurology, Neurosurgery, and Psychiatry, 38*, 69–72.

Heilman, K. M., Watson, R. T., & Valenstein, E. (1993). Neglect and related disorders. In K. M. Heilman & E. Valenstein (Eds.), *Clinical neuropsychology* (3rd ed., pp. 279–336). New York: Oxford University Press.

Helmes, E., & Ostbye, T. (2002). Beyond memory impairment: Cognitive changes in Alzheimer's disease. *Archives of Clinical Neuropsychology, 17*, 179–193.

Huberle, E., & Karnath, H. O. (2006). Global shape recognition is modulated by the spatial distance of local elements — Evidence from simultanagnosia. *Neuropsychologia, 44*, 905–911.

Iizuka, O., Suzuki, K., Endo, K., Fujii, T., & Mori, E. (2007). Pure word deafness and pure anarthria in a patient with frontotemporal dementia. *European Journal of Neurology, 14*, 473–475.

Jankowiak, J., & Albert, M. L. (1994). Lesion localization in visual agnosia. In A. Kertesz (Ed.), *Localization and neuroimaging in neuropsychology* (pp. 429–471). San Diego, CA: Academic Press.

Jehkonen, M., Laihosalo, M., & Kettunen, J. (2006). Anosognosia after stroke: Assessment, occurrence, subtypes and impact on functional outcome reviewed. *Acta Neurologica Scandinavica, 114*, 293–306.

Kaga, M. (1999). Language disorders in Landau-Kleffner syndrome. *Journal of Child Neurology, 14*, 118–122.

Kase, C. S., Troncoso, J. F., Court, J. E., Tapia, F. J., & Mohr, J. P. (1977). Global spatial disorientation. *Journal of the Neurological Sciences, 34*, 267–278.

Kawahata, N., & Nagata, K. (1989). A case of associative visual agnosia: Neuropsychological findings and theoretical considerations. *Journal of Clinical and Experimental Neuropsychology, 11*, 645–664.

Kazui, S., Naritomi, H., Sawada, T., Inoue, N., & Okuda, J. (1990). Subcortical auditory agnosia. *Brain and Language, 38*, 476–487.

Kertesz, A. (1979). Visual agnosia: The dual deficit of perception and recognition. *Cortex, 15*, 403–419.

Kilgour, A. R., de Gelder, B., & Lederman, S. J. (2004). Haptic face recognition and prosopagnosia. *Neuropsychologia, 42*, 707–712.

Kinsbourne, M., & Warrington, E. K. (1962). A disorder of simultaneous form perception. *Brain, 85*, 461–486.

Kinsbourne, M., & Warrington, E. K. (1964). Observations on colour agnosia. *Journal of Neurology, Neurosurgery, and Psychiatry, 27*, 296.

Kirshner, H. S., & Lavin, P. J. (2006). Posterior cortical atrophy: A brief review. *Current Neurology and Neuroscience Reports, 6*, 477–480.

Lambert, J., Eustache, F., Lechevalier, B., Rossa, Y., & Viader, F. (1989). Auditory agnosia with relative sparing of speech perception. *Cortex, 25*, 71–82.

Levine, D. N., & Calvanio, R. (1978). A study of the visual defect in verbal alexia-simultanagnosia. *Brain, 101*, 65–81.

Lissauer, H. (1890). Ein Fall von seelenblindheit nebst conem Beitrage zur Theorie derselben. *Archiv für Psychiatrie und Nervenkrankheiten, 21*, 222–270.

Luria, A. R. (1959). Disorders of "simultaneous perception" in a case of bilateral occipitoparietal brain injury. *Brain, 83*, 437–449.

A

Luzzatti, C., & Davidoff, J. (1994). Impaired retrieval of object-colour knowledge with preserved colour naming. *Neuropsychologia, 32,* 933–950.

Matthews, B. R., Chang, C. C., De May, M., Engstrom, J., & Miller, B. L. (2009). Pleasurable emotional response to music: A case of neurodegenerative generalized auditory agnosia. *Neurocase, 15,* 248–259.

Mauguiere, F., Desmedt, J. E., & Courjon, J. (1982). Astereognosis and dissociated loss of frontal or parietal components of somatosensory evoked potentials in hemispheric lesions: Detailed correlations with clinical signs and computerized tomographic scanning. *Brain, 106,* 271–311.

Mazzucchi, A., & Biber, C. (1983). Is prosopagnosia more frequent in males than in females? *Cortex, 19,* 509–516.

McCarthy, R. A., & Warrington, E. K. (1986). Visual associative agnosia: A clinico-anatomical study of a single case. *Journal of Neurology, Neurosurgery, and Psychiatry, 49,* 1233–1240.

McKenna, K., Cooke, D. M., Fleming, J., Jefferson, A., & Ogden S. (2006). The incidence of visual perceptual impairment in patients with severe traumatic brain injury. *Brain Injury, 20,* 507–518.

McMonagle, P., Deering, F., Berliner, Y., & Kertesz, A. (2006). The cognitive profile of posterior cortical atrophy. *Neurology, 66,* 331–338.

Mendez, M. F. (2000). Corticobasal ganglionic degeneration with Balint's syndrome. *Journal of Neuropsychiatry and Clinical Neurosciences, 12,* 273–275.

Mendez, M. F., & Cherrier, M. M. (1998). The evolution of alexia and simultanagnosia in posterior cortical atrophy. *Neuropsychiatry, Neuropsychology, and Behavioral Neurology, 11,* 76–82.

Mendez, M. F., & Cherrier, M. M. (2003). Agnosia for scenes in topographagnosia. *Neuropsychologia, 41,* 1387–1395.

Mendez, M. F., Ghajarania, M., & Perryman, K. M. (2002). Posterior cortical atrophy: Clinical characteristics and differences compared to Alzheimer's disease. *Dementia and Geriatric Cognitive Disorders, 14,* 33–40.

Mendez, M. F., Mendez, M. A., Martin, R., Smyth, K. A., & Whitehouse, P. J. (1990). Complex visual disturbances in Alzheimer's disease. *Neurology, 40,* 439–443.

Mendez, M. F., & Shapira, J. S. (2005). Loss of insight and functional neuroimaging in frontotemporal dementia. *Journal of Neuropsychiatry and Clinical Neurosciences, 17,* 413–416.

Mesulam, M. (2000). Behavioral neuroanatomy. In M. M. Mesulam (Ed.), *Principles of Behavioral and Cognitive Neurology* (2nd ed., pp. 1–120). New York: Oxford University Press.

Miceli, G., Conti, G., Cianfoni, A., Di Giacopo, R., Zampetti, P., & Servidei, S. (2008). Acute auditory agnosia as the presenting hearing disorder in MELAS. *Neurological Sciences, 29,* 459–462.

Michel, F., & Henaff, M. A. (2004). Seeing without the occipito-parietal cortex: Simultanagnosia as a shrinkage of the attentional visual field. *Behavioral Neurology, 15,* 3–13.

Mori, E., Shimomura, T., Fujimori, M., Hirono, N., Imamura, T., Hashimoto, M., et al. (2000). Visuoperceptual impairment in dementia with Lewy bodies. *Archives of Neurology, 57,* 489–493.

Motomura, N., Yamadori, A., Mori, E., & Tamaru, F. (1986). Auditory agnosia: Analysis of a case with bilateral subcortical lesions. *Brain, 109,* 379–391.

Nardelli, E., Buonanno, F., Coccia, G., Fiaschi, A., Terzian, H., & Rizzuto, N. (1982). Prosopagnosia: Report of four cases. *European Neurology, 21,* 289–297.

Nijboer, T. C., Nys, G. M., van der Smagt, M. J., & de Haan, E. H. (2009). A selective deficit in the appreciation and recognition of brightness: Brightness agnosia? *Cortex, 45,* 816–824.

Nijboer, T. C., te Pas, S. F., & van der Smagt, M. J. (2011). Detecting gradual visual changes in colour and brightness agnosia: A double dissociation. *Neuroreport, 22,* 175–180.

Nijboer, T. C., van der Smagt, M. J., van Zandvoort, M. J., & De Haan, E. H. (2007). Colour agnosia impairs the recognition of natural but not of non-natural scenes. *Cognitive Neuropsychology, 24,* 152–161.

Nijboer, T. C., van Zandvoort, M. J., & de Haan, E. H. (2006). Covert colour processing in colour agnosia. *Neuropsychologia, 44,* 1437–1443.

Ogden, J. A. (1985). Autotopagnosia: Occurrence in patients without nominal aphasia and with an intact ability to point to parts of animals and objects. *Brain, 108,* 1009–1022.

Oppenheimer, D. R., & Newcombe, F. (1978). Clinical and anatomic findings in a case of auditory agnosia. *Archives of Neurology, 35,* 712–729.

Orfei, M. D., Varsi, A. E., Blundo, C., Celia, E., Casini, A. R., Caltagirone, C., et al. (2010). Anosognosia in mild cognitive impairment and mild Alzheimer's disease: Frequency and neuropsychological correlates. *American Journal of Geriatric Psychiatry, 18,* 1133–1140.

Parving, A., Salomon, G., Elberling, C., Larsen, B., & Lassen, N. A. (1980). Middle components of the auditory evoked response in bilateral temporal lobe lesions: Report on a patient with auditory agnosia. *Scandinavian Audiology, 9,* 161–167.

Pia, L., Neppi-Modona, M., Ricci, R., & Berti, A. (2004). The anatomy of anosognosia for hemiplegia: A meta-analysis. *Cortex, 40,* 367–377.

Rapcsak, S. Z., Kentros, M., & Rubens, A. B. (1989). Impaired recognition of meaningful sounds in Alzheimer's disease. *Archives of Neurology, 46,* 1298–1300.

Reed, C. L., & Caselli, R. J. (1994). The nature of tactile agnosia: A case study. *Neuropsychologia, 32,* 527–539.

A

A

Reed, C. L., Caselli, R. J., & Farah, M. J. (1996). Tactile agnosia: Underlying impairment and implication for normal tactile object recognition. *Brain, 119*, 875–888.

Riddoch, M. J., & Humphreys, G. W. (2001). Object recognition. In B. Rapp (Ed.), *The hand book of cognitive neuropsychology: What deficits reveal about the human mind* (pp. 45–74). Philadelphia: Psychology Press.

Riddoch, M. J., & Humphreys, G. W. (2003). Visual agnosia. *Neurologic Clinics of North America, 21*, 501–520.

Riddoch, M. J., & Humphreys, G. W. (2004). Object identification in simultanagnosia: When wholes are not the sum of their parts. *Cognitive Neuropsychology, 21*, 423–441.

Riddoch, M. J., Johnston, R. A., Bracewell, R. M., Boutsen, L., & Humphreys, G. W. (2008). Are faces special? A case of pure prosopagnosia. *Cognitive Neuropsychology, 25*, 3–26.

Rizzo, M., & Hurtig, R. (1987). Looking but not seeing: Attention, perception, and eye movements in simultanagnosia. *Neurology, 37*, 1642–1648.

Roland, P. E. (1976). Astereognosis: Tactile discrimination after localized hemispheric lesions in man. *Archives of Neurology, 33*, 543–550.

Rosati, G., De Bastiani, P., Paolino, E., Prosser, S., Arslan, E., & Artioli, M. (1982). Clinical and audiological findings in a case of auditory agnosia. *Journal of Neurology, 227*, 21–27.

Rosen, H. J. (2011). Anosognosia in neurodegenerative disease. *Neurocase, 17*, 231–241.

Rubinstein, J. E. (1938). Astereognosis associated with tumors in the region of the foramen magnum. *Archives of Neurology and Psychiatry, 39*, 1016–1032.

Satoh, M., Takeda, K., & Kuzuhara, S. (2007). A case of auditory agnosia with impairment of perception and expression of music: Cognitive processing of tonality. *European Neurology, 58*, 70–77.

Saygin, A. P., Leech, R., & Dick, F. (2010). Nonverbal auditory agnosia with lesion to Wernicke's area. *Neuropsychologia, 48*, 107–113.

Schnider, A., Benson, D. F., & Scharre, D. W. (1994). Visual agnosia and optic aphasia: Are they anatomically distinct? *Cortex, 30*, 445–457.

Schnider, A., Landis, T., Regard, M., & Benson, D. F. (1992). Dissociation of color from object in amnesia. *Archives of Neurology, 49*, 982–985.

Semenza, C. (1988). Impairment of localization of body parts following brain damage. *Cortex, 24*, 443–450.

Shelton, P. A., Bowers, D., Duara, R., & Heilman, K. M. (1994). Apperceptive visual agnosia: A case study. *Brain and Cognition, 25*, 1–23.

Shenal, B. V., Jackson, M. D., Crucian, G. P., & Heilman, K. M. (2006). Finger agnosia in Alzheimer disease. *Cognitive and Behavioral Neurology, 19*, 202–203.

Shivashankar, N., Shashikala, H. R., Nagaraja, D., Jayakumar, P. N., & Ratnavalli, E. (2001). Pure word deafness in two patients with subcortical lesions. *Clinical Neurology and Neurosurgery, 103*, 201–205.

Sirigu, A., Grafman, J., Bressler, K., & Sunderland, T. (1991). Multiple representations contribute to body knowledge processing. *Brain, 114*, 629–642.

Spalletta, G., Serra, L., Fadda, L., Ripa, A., Bria, P., & Caltagirone, C. (2007). Unawareness of motor impairment and emotions in right hemispheric stroke: A preliminary investigation. *International Journal of Geriatric Psychiatry, 22*, 1241–1246.

Sparr, S. A., Jay, M., Drislane, F. W., & Venna, N. (1991). A historic case of visual agnosia revisited after 40 years. *Brain, 114*, 789–800.

Starkstein, S. E., Brockman, S., Bruce, D., & Petracca, G. (2010). Anosognosia is a significant predictor of apathy in Alzheimer's disease. *Journal of Neuropsychiatry and Clinical Neurosciences, 22*, 378–383.

Starkstein, S. E., Fedoroff, P., Price, T. R., Leiguarda, R., & Robinson, R. G. (1992). Anosognosia in patients with cerebrovascular lesions: A study of causative factors. *Stroke, 23*, 1446–1453.

Starkstein, S. E., Jorge, R. E., & Robinson, R. G. (2010). The frequency, clinical correlates, and mechanism of anosognosia after stroke. *Canadian Journal of Psychiatry, 55*, 355–361.

Stefanatos, G. A., Gershkoff, A., & Madigan, S. (2005). On pure word deafness, temporal processing, and the left hemisphere. *Journal of the International Neuropsychological Society, 11*, 456–470.

Stewart, P. (1908). Gross lesion of post-central gyrus associated with astereognosis. *Proceedings of the Royal Society of Medicine, 1*, 220–223.

Stone, S. P., Halligan, P. W., & Greenwood, R. J. (1993). The incidence of neglect phenomena and related disorders in patients with an acute right or left hemisphere stroke. *Age and Ageing, 22*, 46–52.

Takahashi, N., Kawamura, M., Shinotou, H., Hirayama, K., Kaga, K., & Shindo, M. (1992). Pure word deafness due to left hemisphere damage. *Cortex, 28*, 295–303.

Takayama, Y., Sugishita, M., Hirose, S., & Akiguchi, I. (1994). Anosodiaphoria for dressing apraxia: Contributory factor to dressing apraxia. *Clinical Neurology and Neurosurgery, 96*, 254–256.

Taniwaki, T., Tagawa, K., Sato, F., & Iino, K. (2000). Auditory agnosia restricted to environmental sounds following cortical deafness and generalized auditory agnosia. *Clinical Neurology and Neurosurgery, 102*, 156–162.

Tranel, D. (2003). Disorders of color processing. In T. E. Feinberg & M. J. Farah (Eds.), *Behavioral neurology and neuropsychology* (2nd ed., pp. 243–256). New York: McGraw Hill.

Tranel, D., Damasio, A., & Damasio, H. (1988). Intact recognition of facial expression, gender, and age in patient with impaired recognition of face identity. *Neurology, 38*, 690–696.

Trivelli, C., Turnbull, O. H., & Sala, S. D. (1996). Recovery of object recognition in a case of simultanagnosia. *Applied Neuropsychology, 3*, 166–173.

Turnbull, O. H., Beschin, N., & Della Sala, S. (1997). Agnosia for object orientation: Implications for theories of object recognition. *Neuropsychologia, 35*, 153–163.

Turnbull, O. H., Driver, J., & McCarthy, R. A. (2004). 2D but not 3D: Pictorial-depth deficits in a case of visual agnosia. *Cortex, 40*, 723–738.

Van Lancker, D. R., Cummings, J. L., Kreiman, J., & Dobkin, B. H. (1988). Phonagnosia: A dissociation between familiar and unfamiliar voices. *Cortex, 24*, 195–209.

Van Lancker, D. R, & Kreiman, J. (1988). Unfamiliar voice discrimination and familiar voice recognition are independent and unordered abilities. *Neuropsychologia, 25*, 829–834.

Van Lancker, D. R., Kreiman, J., & Cummings, J. (1989). Voice perception deficits: Neuroanatomical correlates of phonagnosia. *Journal of Clinical and Experimental Neuropsychology, 11*, 665–674.

Van Zandvoort, M. J., Nijboer, T. C., & de Haan, E. (2007). Developmental colour agnosia. *Cortex, 43*, 750–757.

Vignolo, L. A. (1982). Auditory agnosia. *Philosophical Transactions of the Royal Society of London. Series B, Biological Sciences, 298*, 49–57.

Vignolo, L. A. (2003). Music agnosia and auditory agnosia: Dissociations in stroke patients. *Annals of the New York Academy of Science, 999*, 50–57.

Vocat, R., Staub, F., Stroppini, T., & Vuilleumier, P. (2010). Anosognosia for hemiplegia: A clinical-anatomical prospective study. *Brain, 133*, 3578–3597.

Von Arx, S. W., Muri, R. M., Heinemann, D., Hess, C. W., & Nyffeler, T. (2010). Anosognosia for cerebral achromatopsia — A longitudinal case study. *Neuropsychologia, 48*, 970–977.

Vuilleumier, P., Ghika-Schmid, R., Bogousslavsky, J., Assal, G., & Regli, F. (1998). Persistent recurrence of hypomania and prosopaffective agnosia in a patient with right thalamic infarct. *Neuropsychiatry, Neuropsychology, and Behavioral Neurology, 11*, 40–44.

Warrington, E. K., & Shallice, T. (1984). Category specific semantic impairments. *Brain, 107*, 829–854.

Warrington, E. K., & Taylor, A. M. (1973). The contribution of the right parietal lobe to object recognition. *Cortex, 9*, 152–164.

Wilson, B. A., & Davidoff, J. (1993). Partial recovery from visual object agnosia: A 10 year follow-up study. *Cortex, 29*, 529–542.

Yoon, S. J., Park, J. M., & Na, D. L. (2002). Simultanagnosia in posterior cortical atrophy. *Journal of Neurology, Neurosurgery, and Psychiatry, 72*, 269.

Zaidel, E. (1998). Stereognosis in the chronic split brain: Hemispheric differences, ipsilateral control and sensory integration across the midline. *Neuropsychologia, 36*, 1033–1047.

Zamboni, G., Grafman, J., Krueger, F., Knutson, K. M., & Huey, E. D. (2010). Anosognosia for behavioral disturbances in frontotemporal dementia and corticobasal syndrome: A voxel-based morphometry study. *Dementia and Geriatric Cognitive Disorders, 29*, 88–96.

Zihl, J., & Kennard, C. (1996). Disorders of higher visual functions. In T. Brandt, L. R. Caplan, J. Dichgans, H. C. Diener, & C. Kennard (Eds.), *Neurological disorders, course and treatment* (pp. 201–212). San Diego, CA: Academic Press.

Zoltan, B. (1996). Vision, perception, and cognition: A model for the evaluation and treatment of the neurologically impaired adult. New Jersey: Slack Incorporated.

AGRAPHIAS

DESCRIPTION

Agraphia is a disorder of writing first described by Benedikt in 1865 (see Roeltgen, 1993). Nielson in 1946 classified different types of agraphias with some forms associated with aphasia and others not. Specifically, Nielson (1946) described an apraxic aphasia, which is often seen in patients affected by other kind of apraxias, an aphasic agraphia that can be seen in patients affected by different kinds of aphasia, motor, sensitive, or transcortical, and an isolated agraphia, when agraphia was not associated with any other neuropsychological disturbance. The isolated form of agraphia was thought to result from a lesion located at the foot of the second frontal convolution, an area called Exner's area, or from a lesion of the angular gyrus. Nielson (1946) hypothesized a connection between the angular gyrus and Exner's area, along with Broca's area, and these anatomical and functional connections would explain why agraphia is often seen in aphasic patients.

Goldstein (1948) classified agraphias as either primary or secondary. Primary agraphia is associated with a disorder of the *motor act of writing*, whereas secondary agraphia is associated with an *impairment of speech*. Primary agraphias were subsequently subdivided into several forms, including those with poor impulse for writing; impairment in abstract words with better production of concrete words; ideatoric agraphia, which is associated with a loss of the idea of the letter form; pure or motor agraphia that is characterized by production of incorrect letters; and agraphia associated with apraxia of the minor hand. The secondary forms of agraphia are then parallel to the various types of aphasia (e.g., transcortical, motor, sensory, etc.)

To test for agraphia, the motor and linguistic components of this disorder must be examined. The usual approach to accomplish this is to ask the patient to write spontaneously and to dictation, and to copy writing (Beeson & Rapcsak, 2010; Roeltgen, 1993). During the spontaneous writing task it is possible to identify the content as well as the form of the words, thereby providing information about the motoric and conceptual aspects of writing. The writing under dictation condition is a very important task that allows the examiner to have more control over the stimuli as well as using words that differ in class (regular or irregular), abstractness, and even using words versus nonwords. Another important aspect to examine is copying. By having the patient provide a copy of written work, the examiner can detect if the patient experiences difficulty with the motoric act of writing. Problems with the motoric aspect of writing is often noticeable when the patient begins copying letter by letter or even stroke by stroke instead of reading or retaining the sentence and then writing the sentence autonomously by memory. Furthermore, it is important to examine the patient for potential neurological disorders that may present as confounds by interfering with writing, oral spelling, or copying. The neurological evaluation may include disorders of speech, reading, ideomotor apraxia, visuoperceptual deficits, visuospatial neglect, constructional abilities, and elementary motor and sensory functions (Roeltgen, 1993).

PRIMARY TYPES OF AGRAPHIA

Recently, several different classifications of agraphia have been proposed (Lorch, 1995). One possible classification is dividing agraphia into those with "central" and "peripheral" causes (Beeson & Rapcsak, 2010). The central agraphias result from disorders of central language processing. These types of agraphia might affect lexical processing (the ability to choose the right word), semantic processing (word meaning), and phonological processing (the ability to generate the correct grapheme). The "peripheral" agraphias result from disorders of the motor aspect of writing, such as those involving the selection of the right letter string and the motor output required to write it. Based on the associated cognitive deficits and clinical evaluations, five different classifications of agraphia have been proposed. These classifications include pure agraphia, aphasic agraphia, agraphia with alexia, apraxic agraphia, and spatial agraphia (Roeltgen, 1993).

Pure Agraphia

Pure agraphia is when agraphia is presented without any other significant language disturbance, such as oral language or reading ability (Croisile, Laurent, Michel, & Trillet, 1990; Roeltgen, 1993). It might result from a focal lesion (Maeshima, Shigeno, Dohi, Kajiwara, & Komai, 1992; Roeltgen, 1994), a neurodegenerative process (Fukui & Lee, 2008; Ishihara et al., 2010; Kirshner & Lavin, 2006; LaBarge, Smith, Dick, & Storandt, 1992), or an acute confusional state (Chedru & Geschwind, 1972). Focal lesions leading to pure agraphia may involve a number of regions, including Exner's area (second frontal circonvolution; Aimard, Devick, Lebel, Trouillas, & Boisson, 1975; Kaplan & Goodglass, 1981), Broca's area and surrounding regions (Hillis, Chang, Breese, & Heidler, 2004), the posterior perisilvian regions (Auerbach & Alexander, 1981), posterior parasagittal parieto-occipital region (Levine, Mani, & Calvanio, 1988; Schomer et al., 1998), superior parietal lobe (Basso, Taborelli, & Vignolo, 1978; Paolino, De Bastiani, Monetti, Boldrini, & Rosati, 1983), the left temporal lobe (Rosati & De Bastiani, 1979), as well as the region of the left caudate and internal capsule (Laine & Marttila, 1981) and other subcortical structures (Croisile et al., 1990; Nagaratnam, Plew, & Cooper, 1998; Toyokura, Kobayashi, & Aono, 2010). Patients with pure agraphia are often capable of writing the characters correctly, but they misspell the words. However, pure agraphia that results from an acute confusional state is characterized by graphemic errors in addition to problems writing on the lines of the pages (Chedru & Geschwind, 1972).

Aphasic Agraphia

Disorders of speaking and writing are often comorbid. Basso and colleagues (1978) examined 500 cases of individuals with language disturbances following left hemisphere damage and found only seven patients with selective impairment is speech and another seven patients with selective impairment in writing. Aphasic agraphia has been described together with Broca's or nonfluent aphasia (Davous & Boller, 1994; Sgaramella, Ellis, & Semenza, 1991; Tanridag & Kirshner, 1985), conduction aphasia (Balasubramanian, 2005; Sgaramella et al., 1991), Wernike's or fluent aphasia

A

(Kirshner & Webb, 1982; Sgaramella et al., 1991; Tanridag & Kirshner, 1985), sensory transcortical aphasia (Clark & Grossfeld, 1983), anomic aphasia (Krishnan, Rao, & Rajashekar, 2009), primary progressive aphasia (Graham, Patterson, & Hodges, 2004; Rohrer, Rossor, & Warren, 2009), and aphemia (Kaminski, Adams, Burnstine, Civil, & Ruff, 1992). Patients with Broca's, Wernicke's, and conduction aphasia have all been reported to make relatively more selection errors in writing as opposed to movement errors (Sgaramella et al., 1991). Patients with Broca's or nonfluent aphasia may present with agraphia characterized by problems writing spontaneously with relatively intact ability to copy material. Writing to dictation is better for words than for nonwords in many patients. Also, these patients may exhibit correct graphemic production but with their writing characterized by omissions, distortions, additions, and substitutions of graphemes. They often also exhibit severe spelling deficits. Other patients will exhibit an agrammatical sentence structure and their writing will resemble speech, and therefore will be brief, effortful, and lacking in syntax (Marcie & Hecaen, 1979). Patients with conduction aphasia often have difficulty with crossing out words, overwriting, and stopping (Marcie & Hacaen, 1979). Patients with Wernicke's aphasia often write how they speak, with writing that is abundant but unintelligible with occasional jargon agraphia (Marcie & Hacaen, 1979). However, some have reported severe telegraphic writing, limited to a single or just a few words (Kirshner & Webb, 1982). Coping is relatively preserved, but spelling is impaired (Kirshner & Webb, 1982; Marcie & Hacaen, 1979; see also Lorch, 1995). The agraphia reported in primary progressive aphasia has been described as having neologistic jargon (Rohrer et al., 2009) and telegraphic production (Graham et al., 2004).

Agraphia With Alexia

Agraphia with alexia is the inability to write and read. This type of agraphia is also called parietal agraphia (Marcie & Hacaen, 1979) as lesions of the parietal lobe often cause agraphia and alexia in absence of aphasia. Patients who have agraphia with alexia make poorly formed graphemes when writing, such as distortions and inversions, and when spelling aloud they pronounce letters correctly but have difficulties in spelling. However, some have reported preserved spelling in these patients (Rothi & Hielman, 1981). Copying is relatively preserved in these patients, as is the syntactic structure of sentences (Marcie & Hacaen, 1979; Roeltgen, 1993). Lesions to the posterior parietal lobe, and in particular the angular gyrus, are typically associated with agraphia with alexia (Davous & Boller, 1994; Greenblatt, 1977; Marcie & Hacaen, 1979; Sheldon, Malcolm, & Barton, 2008), although some have reported lesions to left temporal lobe (Sakurai, Mimura, & Mannen, 2008).

Apraxic Apgaphia

Apraxic agraphia is characterized by severe difficulties in forming graphemes when writing spontaneously, writing to dictation, or copying, but often with intact spelling (Heilman, Coenen, & Kluger, 2008; Marcie & Hacaen, 1979; Roeltgen, 1993). Copying and oral spelling may be disturbed, although writing generally improves with the use of anagram letters (Roeltgen, 1993). The disorder may also be asymmetrical, which potentially signifies the onset of cortical basal degeneration (Heilman et al., 2008). Moreover, apraxic agraphia may be present in even in the absence of ideomotor apraxia (Coslett, Gonzales Rothi, Valenstein, & Heilman, 1986; Roeltgen & Heilman, 1983). The lesions causing apraxic agraphia in right-handed subjects are often located within the left parietal lobe (Alexander, Fischer, & Friedman, 1992; Otsuki, Soma, Arai, Otsuka, & Tsuji, 1999). However, subcortical lesions (Assmus, Buss, Milkereit, Meyer, & Fink, 2007) and thalamic infarction (Ohno, Bando, Nagura, Ishii, & Yamanouchi, 2000) have also been reported in association with apraxic agraphia.

Spatial Agraphia

Spatial agraphia is usually seen in patients with right parietal lesions, and it is often associated with visuospatial neglect (Ardila & Rosselli, 1993; Marcie & Hacaen, 1979). However, spatial agraphia may be seen in the absence of spatial neglect (Auclair, Sieroff, & Kocer, 2008) and has been reported in association with cerebellar atrophy (Silveri, Misciagna, Leggio, & Molinari, 1997). This type of agraphia is characterized by the tendency to write just in the right side of the page, failure to write one side of the word, trouble writing on horizontal lines, duplicate strokes, and intrusions of blank spaces between graphemes (Guerrero, Kumar, Khaku, & Heilman, 2010; Marcie & Hacaen, 1979; Roeltgen, 1993).

As noted by Roeltgen (1993), the aforementioned classification system is based on clinical observations and hampered by the fact that many agraphias do not seem to fit into these categories. For instance, Guerrero et al. (2010) reported the case of a patient whose agraphia was characterized by perseveration of the first letter of the word he was attempting to write.

Furthermore, the lesion presumably causing this form of agraphia was located in the right parietal lobe. The patients reported by Kirshner and Webb (1982) had agraphia with Wernicke's aphasia but exhibited very short sentences or could only write one word as opposed to writing abundantly but unintelligibly. Hence, Roeltgen (1993) proposed classifying the agraphias according to the underlying neuropsychological mechanisms responsible for the writing disturbances. This classification system includes agraphia arising from problems within linguistic components (including central mechanisms) and from problems within motor components (including peripheral mechanisms). This different classification system includes many of the aforementioned types of agraphia but also introduces new forms. Others have also used this type of classification system, or something similar (Beeson & Rapcsak 2010; Lorch, 1995).

DISORDERS OF LINGUISTIC COMPONENTS

A dysfunction of the linguistic component refers to difficulty in spelling words and with the lexical–semantic system. There are two strategies by which individuals spell words. Words may be spelled through access to the semantic system, referred to as the lexical–semantic spelling route, and is associated with whole-word processing. Access to the semantic system may occur directly or with input from the phonological lexicon. Alternatively, or in combination, spelling may also be achieved through the sublexical route, which is based on sound-to-letter correspondence strategies (phoneme–grapheme strategy; Beeson & Rapcsak, 2010; Roeltgen, Gonzalez Rothi, & Heilman, 1986). When spelling irregular words, individuals typically use a whole-word approach (such as yacht). In contrast, words with regular spellings may be spelled using a sound-to-letter approach (such as animal).

Lexical Agraphia

Agraphia associated with a dysfunction of the lexical system is called lexical agraphia. This disorder is characterized by the inability to spell irregular and ambiguous words, with a relatively preserved ability to spell regular or nonwords using a grapheme–phoneme approach to spell words as they sound. Lexical agraphic patients typically make errors in which words are misspelled but are phonologically plausible, such as "spaid" for "spade." The sound of the words is the same but the spelling is different. Patients with lexical agraphia lose the ability to spell the word by access to word meaning; instead, words are accessed by the

knowledge of sound and spelling is phonetic (spelling based on a sublexical strategy; Beeson & Rapcsak, 2010; Roeltgen, 1993). However, the patient's native language might influence pure agraphia. Italian, for example, is entirely regular in spelling, whereas English has many irregular spelled words. Lexical agraphia would be easier to detect in an English speaker than those who speak Italian.

The anatomy underlying lexical agraphia often involves lesions of the junction of the left posterior angular gyrus and the parieto-occipital lobule, but sparing the supramarginal gyrus (Roeltgen & Heilman, 1984). Other areas have also been implicated in lexical agraphia, including the right posterior parietal-occipital region (Gonzalez Rothi, Roeltgen, & Kooistra, 1987), the left posterior-inferior temporal cortex (Rapcsak & Beeson, 2004), and the left precentral gyrus (Rapcsak, Arthur, & Rubens, 1988). Lexical agraphia has also been reported in patients with Alzheimer's disease (Lambert et al., 1996; Rapcsak, Arthur, Bliklen, & Rubens, 1989), with some indication that problems within the lexical–semantic route may predominate at an earlier stage in the disease (Platel et al., 1993).

Phonological Agraphia

The phoneme-to-grapheme strategy involves the ability to parse the phonemic string into separate phonemes and then convert single phonemes into letters. This system is often used to spell unfamiliar orthographically regular words and nonwords that are pronounceable (Roeltgen, 1993) or when the lexical-semantic route (whole-word approach) system is dysfunctional (Beeson & Rapcsak, 2010; Roeltgen, 1993). A dysfunction of this phonological (sublexical) system causes phonological agraphia, and patients must rely on the lexical–semantic system for spelling. Phonological agraphia is characterized by problems spelling in nonwords, but with relatively preserved spelling for both regular and irregular familiar words (Alexander, Friedman, Loverso, & Fischer, 1992; Beeson & Rapcsak, 2010; Roeltgen, 1993).

The lesions responsible for phonological agraphia may involve a number of different perisylvian regions (Alexander et al., 1992). Roeltgen, Sevush, and Heilman (1983) reported four patients with phonological agraphia who had lesions involving the supramarginal gyrus. Similarly, Roeltgen and Heilman (1984) reported involvement of the left supramarginal gyrus, sparing the angular gyrus in patients with phonological agraphia. Other reported lesion locations have included the left temporo-parietal area (Iribarren, Jarema, & Leours, 2001), left anterior insula

(Marien, Pickut, Engelborghs, Martin, & De Deyn, 2001), left perisylvian region (Henry, Beeson, Stark, & Rapcsak, 2007), left posterior-superior temporal gyrus (Kim, Chu, Lee, Kim, & Park, 2002), and even the right supramarginal gyrus (Bolla-Wilson, Speedie, & Robinson, 1985).

Semantic Agraphia

The inability to write and spell with meaning is called semantic agraphia. However, patients affected by semantic agraphia may be able to spell irregular and nonwords correctly. Patients with semantic agraphia will typically make semantic-homophone substitutions with words that are phonetically similar, that is, they write and spell semantically incorrect but nevertheless correctly spelled homophones (Lorch, 1995; Roeltgen, 1993). For example, when asked to write the sentence "Tie a knot in your shoe," the patient may write "Tie a not in your shoe." In contrast, a healthy individual will realize the correct spelling from the context in which the word is used. Patients with semantic agraphia are often not able to understand the meaning of the word even if they hear it or read it. These patients can spell irregular words and nonwords.

Research concerning the functional neuroanatomy of semantic agraphia has been sparse. Roeltgen et al. (1986) reported five cases of individuals with semantic agraphia but whose lesion locations were rather varied. However, all patients had subcortical involvement. Semantic agraphia has also been described in patient with Alzheimer's disease (Forbes, Shanks, & Venneri, 2004; see also Neils-Strunjas, Groves-Wright, Mashima, & Harnish, 2006).

Deep Agraphia

As in phonological agraphia, patients have difficulty spelling nonwords. However, patients with deep agraphia have the added deficit of problems spelling certain classes of words and they make semantic paragraphic errors. Typically, these patients will exhibit greater difficulty spelling functor words than nouns, will spell nouns with high imageability better than those with low imageability, and will spell words with concrete meanings better than those with abstract meanings (Lorch, 1995; Roeltgen, 1993). A typical semantic paragraphic error may involve semantically related words, such as writing the word "chair" for "desk." Some have also described segmental spelling errors in patients with deep agraphia, where letters are deleted from the words, often toward the end of the word (Bormann, Wallesch, & Blanken, 2008). Some have suggested that deep agraphia and phonological agraphia are endpoints on a single continuum of severity in phonological and lexical–semantic spelling deficits (Rapcsak & Beeson, 2000).

Some have proposed that deep agraphia reflects writing contributions from the right hemisphere when large portions of the left hemisphere are lesioned (Rapcsak, Beeson, & Rubens, 1991). Bub and Kertesz (1982) reported a case of deep agraphia in a patient with a large left hemisphere lesion involving the left pre- and postcentral gyri, superior temporal gyrus, temporal operculum, and portions of the supramarginal and angular gyri.

DISORDERS OF MOTOR COMPONENTS

Writing necessarily involves the use of not only memory for graphemes but also motor and visuospatial skills. Peripheral writing involves several processes (Beeson & Rapcsak, 2010), including allographic conversion (converting orthographic representations into physical letter shapes), graphic motor programs (spatial and temporal codes for the movements necessary for writing and producing different letters), and graphic innervatory patterns (the motor commands for specific muscles needed for writing). Peripheral causes of agraphia may arise from dysfunction within these processes.

Apraxic Agraphia

Motor functions are necessary to be able to write including both the pyramidal and the extrapyramidal motor systems that are needed to perform fine motor movements as well as praxis. Regarding praxis, this involves the ability to hold the pen or pencil in the necessary position and the ability to perform the fine finger movements necessary for forming written letters or graphemes (Roeltgen, 1993). Apraxia is defined as a disorder of skilled movement and typically follows lesions to the left hemisphere (Heilman & Gonzalez Rothi, 1993). Given that the left hemisphere is dominant for language, apraxia is often accompanied by aphasia (Joshi, Roy, Black, & Barbour, 2003; Papagno, Della Sala, & Basso, 1993; Rohrer, Rossor, & Warren, 2010) and as a result it may be difficult to separate the aphasic from the apraxic contributions of agraphia (Roeltgen, 1993). Apraxic agraphia may be defined as a disorder arising from dysfunction from graphic motor programs (Beeson & Rapcsak, 2010) and patients with this type of agraphia will exhibit illegible writing, both spontaneously and to dictation (Roeltgen, 1993). As mentioned earlier, the critical lesion is often within the left parietal lobe or the parietal lobe contralateral to the preferred hand (Roeltgen, 1993).

Spatial Agraphia

Although intact motor skills are critical for writing, visuospatial skills are also required in that the individual must place the letters and words in the correct location on the page and maintain a line when writing. Moreover, visuospatial skills are required for the formation of letters and words. Hence, motor programs must interact with visuospatial skills in order to write successfully. As mentioned earlier, spatial agraphia is characterized by the tendency to write just in the right side of the page, failure to write one side of the word, trouble writing on horizontal lines, duplicated strokes, and intrusions of blank spaces between graphemes (Guerrero et al., 2010; Marcie & Hacaen, 1979; Roeltgen, 1993). Patients with spatial agraphia also often have difficulty copying, but oral spelling may be preserved (Roeltgen, 1993). Although the left half of the word is often omitted, consistent with unilateral spatial neglect, it has been reported that a patient committed errors on the right half of words (Caramazza & Hillis, 1990). This form of agraphia has also been referred to as visuospatial or constructional agraphia (Ellis, Young, & Flude, 1987) and afferent agraphia (Lebrun, 1980). Spatial agraphia is seen following lesions to the right hemisphere (Ardila & Rosselli, 1993; Baxter & Warrington, 1983; Cubelli, Guiducci, & Consolmagno, 2000) and in particular the right parietal region (Roeltgen, 1993).

Allographic Agraphia

As mentioned earlier, allographic conversion is the process of converting orthographic representations into the appropriate letter shapes (Beeson & Rapcsak, 2010). This allographic store is involved in selecting and producing the correct case and style of writing (Roeltgen, 1993). Hence, patients with impairment in the allographic store exhibit errors in case (such as writing aLlogRaphiC) and the style of writing (print or cursive). Oral spelling is generally better than written spelling and these patients exhibit normal praxis and visuospatial abilities as well as normal letter form (Beeson & Rapcsak, 2010; Roeltgen, 1993). Allograpic agraphia has been associated with bilateral parietal-occipital lobe dysfunction (Popescu & Vaidya, 2007), relative left parietal-occipital and frontal dysfunction (Grossman et al., 2001), left fronto-subcortical stroke (Catala, Fontaine, & Rancurel,

1994), frontotemporal dementia (Menichelli, Rapp, & Semenza, 2008), and vascular dementia (Forbes & Venneri, 2003).

TREATMENT

Given the central and peripheral causes of agraphia, different treatment approaches should be used for the various types of agraphia. McNeil and Tseng (1990) suggested that one of three strategies is typically employed, including retraining the behavior directly or indirectly, compensating for the behavior by strengthening a system that is capable of assuming the same function, or the behavior is conveyed and practiced through some alternative system or modality. Furthermore, one of these strategies is selected following a consideration of the cause of the disorder and the underlying theoretical model. Beeson and Rapcsak (2010) provide an excellent review of different treatment approaches for many of the aforementioned types of agraphia. Specifically, treatment for lexical agraphia may involve strengthening the interactive use of sublexical and lexical knowledge by training patients to detect and correct spelling errors. Alternatively, treatment may involve strengthening lexical–semantic spelling abilities by using tasks of increasing difficulty that address spelling knowledge, including the use of anagrams as well as direct or delayed copying of words. Treatment for apraxic agraphia may also involve repeated direct and delayed copying of words with increasing difficulty, when the patient is capable of copying. Beeson and Rapcsak (2010) also provided treatment approaches for phonological agraphia and allographic agraphia, among others.

Empirical treatment studies for agraphia are relatively sparse (see McNeil & Tseng, 1990). Raymer and colleagues treated a group of agraphia patients using both errorless and effortful procedures and found that both strategies were effective, although the effect sizes were greater for the effortful procedure. Moreover, they reported little generalization to untrained control words (Raymer, Strobel, Prokup, Thomason, & Reff, 2010). Other researchers have also reported successful treatment with agraphia patients (Beeson, Rising, Kim, & Rapcsak, 2008; Beeson, Rising, Kim, & Rapcsak, 2010).

Valeria Drago
Paul S. Foster

Aimard, G., Devick, M., Lebel, M., Trouillas, P., & Boisson, D. (1975). Agraphie pure (Dynamique?) d'origine frontale. *Revue Neurologique (Paris)*, 7: 505–512.

Alexander, M. P., Fischer, R. S., & Friedman, R. (1992). Lesion localization in apractic agraphia. *Archives of Neurology, 49,* 246–251.

Alexander, M. P., Friedman, R. B., Loverso, F., & Fischer, R. S. (1992). Lesion localization of phonological agraphia. *Brain and Language, 43,* 83–95.

Ardila, A., & Rosselli, M. (1993). Spatial agraphia. *Brain and Cognition, 22,* 137–147.

Assmus, A., Buss, A., Milkereit, E. L., Meyer, J., & Fink, G. R. (2007). Pure apraxic agraphia: A disconnection syndrome after left subcortical stroke. *European Journal of Neurology, 14,* e30–e31.

Auclair, L., Sieroff, E., & Kocer, S. (2008). A case of spatial neglect dysgraphia in Wilson's disease. *Archives of Clinical Neuropsychology, 23,* 47–62.

Auerbach, S. H., & Alexander, M. P. (1981). Pure agraphia and unilateral optic ataxia associated with a left superior lobule lesion. *Journal of Neurology, Neurosurgery, & Psychiatry, 44,* 430–432.

Balasubramanian, V. (2005). Dysgraphia in two forms of conduction aphasia. *Brain and Cognition, 57,* 8–15.

Basso, A., Taborelli, A., & Vignolo, L. A. (1978). Dissociated disorders of speaking and writing in aphasia. *Journal of Neurology, Neurosurgery, and Psychiatry, 41,* 556–563.

Baxter, D. M., & Warrington, E. K. (1983). Neglect dysgraphia. *Journal of Neurology, Neurosurgery, and Psychiatry, 46,* 1073–1078.

Beeson, P. M., & Rapcsak, S. Z. (2010). Neuropsychological assessment and rehabilitation of writing disorders. In J. M. Gurd, U. Kischka, & J. C. Marshall (Eds.), Handbook of clinical neuropsychology (pp. 323–348). New York: Oxford University Press.

Beeson, P. M., Rising, K., Kim, E. S., & Rapcsak, S. Z. (2008). A novel method for examining response to spelling treatment. *Aphasiology, 22,* 707–717.

Beeson, P. M., Rising, K., Kim, E. S., & Rapcsak, S. Z. (2010). A treatment sequence for phonological alexia/agraphia. *Journal of Speech, Language, and Hearing Research, 53,* 450–468.

Benedikt, M. (1865). *Uber Aphasie, Agraphie und verwandte pathologische Zustande.* Wiener Medizische Presse, 6.

Bolla-Wilson, K., Speedie, L. J., & Robinson, R. G. (1985). Phonologic agraphia in a left-handed patient after a right-hemisphere lesion. *Neurology, 35,* 1778–1781.

Bormann, T., Wallesch, C. W., & Blanken, G. (2008). "Fragment errors" in deep dysgraphia: Further support for a lexical hypothesis. *Cognitive Neuropsychology, 25,* 745–764.

Bub, D., & Kertesz, A. (1982). Deep agraphia. *Brain and Language, 17,* 146–165.

Caramazza, A., & Hillis, A. E. (1990). Spatial representation of words in the brain implied by studies of a unilateral neglect patient. *Nature, 346,* 267–269.

Catala, M., Fontaine, B., & Rancurel, G. (1994). Alphabetical paragraphia in a limited middle cerebral artery stroke.

Journal of Neurology, Neurosurgery, and Psychiatry, 57, 649–651.

Chedru, F., & Geschwind, N. (1972). Writing disturbance in acute confusional states. *Neuropsychologia, 10,* 343–353.

Clark, L. W., & Grossfeld, M. L. (1983). Nature of spelling errors in transcortical sensory aphasia: A case study. *Brain and Language, 18,* 47–56.

Coslett, H. B., Gonzales Rothi, L. J., Valenstein, E., & Heilman, K. M. (1986). Dissociations of writing and praxis: Two cases in point. *Brain and Language, 28,* 357–369.

Croisile, B., Laurent, B., Michel, D., & Trillet, M. (1990). Pure agraphia after deep left hemisphere haematoma. *Journal of Neurology, Neurosurgery, and Psychiatry, 53,* 263–265.

Cubelli, R., Guiducci, A., & Consolmagno, P. (2000). Afferent dysgraphia after right cerebral stroke: An autonomous syndrome? *Brain and Cognition, 44,* 629–644.

Davous, P., & Boller, F. (1994). Transcortical alexia with agraphia following a right temporo-occipital hematoma in a right-handed patient. *Neuropsychologia, 32,* 1263–1272.

Ellis, A. W., Young, A. W., & Flude, B. M. (1987). "Afferent dysgraphia" in a patient and in normal subjects. *Cognitive Neuropsychology, 4,* 465–486.

Forbes, K. E., Shanks, M. F., & Venneri, A. (2004). The evolution of dysgraphia in Alzheimer's disease. *Brain Research Bulletin, 63,* 19–24.

Forbes, K. E., & Venneri, A. (2003). A case for case: Handling letter case selection in written spelling. *Neuropsychologia, 41,* 16–24.

Fukui, T., & Lee, E. (2008). Progressive agraphia can be a harbinger of degenerative dementia. *Brain and Language, 104,* 201–210.

Gonzalez Rothi, L. J., Roeltgen, D. P., & Kooistra, C. A. (1987). Isolated lexical agraphia in a right-handed patient with a posterior lesion of the right cerebral hemisphere. *Brain and Language, 30,* 181–190.

Graham, N. L., Patterson, K., & Hodges, J. R. (2004). When more yields less: Speaking and writing deficits in nonfluent progressive aphasia. *Neurocase, 10,* 141–155.

Grossman, M., Libon, D. J., Ding, X. S., Cloud, B., Jaggi, J., Morrison, D., et al. (2001). Progressive peripheral agraphia. *Neurocase, 7,* 339–349.

Guerrero, W. R., Kumar, A., Khaku, A., & Heilman, K. M. (2010). Spatially adherent graphemic perseveration. *Cognitive and Behavioral Neurology, 23,* 269–273.

Heilman, K. M., Coenen, A., & Kluger, B. (2008). Progressive asymmetric apraxic agraphia. *Cognitive and Behavioral Neurology, 21,* 14–17.

Heilman, K. M., & Gonzalez Rothi, L. J. (1993). Apraxia. In K. M. Heilman & E. Valenstein (Eds.), *Clinical neuropsychology* (pp. 141–163). New York: Oxford University Press.

Henry, M. L., Beeson, P. M., Stark, A. J., & Rapcsak, S. Z. (2007). The role of left perisylvian cortical regions in spelling. *Brain and Language, 100*, 44–52.

Hillis, A. E., Chang, S., Breese, E., & Heidler, J. (2004). The crucial role of posterior frontal regions in modality specific components of the spelling process. *Neurocase, 10*, 175–187.

Iribarren, I. C., Jarema, G., & Lecours, A. R. (2001). Two different dysgraphic syndromes in a regular orthography, Spanish. *Brain and Language, 77*, 166–175.

Ishihara, K., Ichikawa, H., Suzuki, Y., Shiota, J., Nakano, I., & Kawamura, M. (2010). Is lesion of Exner's area linked to progressive agraphia in amyotrophic lateral sclerosis with dementia? An autopsy case report. *Behavioral Neurology, 23*, 153–158.

Joshi, A., Roy, E. A., Black, S. E., & Barbour, K. (2003). Patterns of limb apraxia in primary progressive aphasia. *Brain and Cognition, 53*, 403–407.

Kaminski, H. J., Adams, N., Burnstine, T. H., Civil, R. H., & Ruff, R. L. (1992). Relation of aphemia and agraphia. *European Neurology, 32*, 302–204.

Kim, H. J., Chu, K., Lee, K. M., Kim, D. W., & Park, S. H. (2002). Phonological agraphia after superior temporal gyrus infarction. *Archives of Neurology, 59*, 1314–1316.

Kirshner, H. S., & Lavin, P. J. (2006). Posterior cortical atrophy: A brief review. *Current Neurology and Neuroscience Reports, 6*, 477–480.

Kirshner, H., & Webb, W. G. (1982). Alexia and agraphia in Wernicke's aphasia. *Journal of Neurology, Neurosurgery, and Psychiatry, 45*, 719–724.

Krishnan, G., Rao, S. N., & Rajashekar, B. (2009). Apraxic agraphia: An insight into the writing disturbances of posterior aphasias. *Annals of Indian Academy of Neurology, 12*, 120–123.

LaBarge, E., Smith, D. S., Dick, L., & Storandt, M. (1992). Agraphia in dementia of the Alzheimer type. *Archives of Neurology, 49*, 1151–1156.

Laine, T., & Marttila, R. J. (1981). Pure agraphia: A case study. *Neuropsychologia, 19*, 311–316.

Lambert, J., Eustache, F., Viader, F., Dary, M., Rioux, P., Lechevalier, B., et al. (1996). Agraphia in Alzheimer's disease: An independent lexical impairment. *Brain and Language, 53*, 222–233.

Lebrun, I. (1980). Reading, writing and drawing disorder due to right brain damage. *Acta Neurologica Latinoamericana, 26*, 223–227.

Levine, D. N., Mani, R. B., & Calvanio, R. (1988). Pure agraphia and Gerstmann's syndrome as a visuospatial-language dissociation: An experimental case study. *Brain and Language, 35*, 172–196.

Lorch, M. P. (1995). Disorders of writing and spelling. In H. S. Kirshner (Ed.), *Handbook of neurological speech and language disorders* (pp. 295–324). New York: Marcel Dekker, Inc.

Maeshima, S., Shigeno, K., Dohi, N., Kajiwara, T., & Komai, N. (1992). A study of right unilateral spatial neglect in left hemispheric lesions: The difference between right-handed and non-right-handed post-stroke patients. *Acta Neurologica Scandinavica, 85*, 418–424.

Marcie, P., & Hacaen, H. (1979). Agraphia: Writing disorders associated with unilateral cortical lesions. In K. M. Heilman & E. Valenstein (Eds.), *Clinical neuropsychology* (pp. 92–127). New York: Oxford University Press.

Marien, P., Pickut, B. A., Engelborghs, S., Martin, J. J., & De Deyn, P. P. (2001). Phonological agraphia following a focal anterior insulo-opercular infarction. *Neuropsychologia, 39*, 845–855.

McNeil, M. R., & Tseng, C. H. (1990). Acquired neurogenic dysgraphias. In L. L. LaPointe (Ed.), *Aphasia and related neurogenic language disorders* (pp. 147–176). New York: Thieme Medical Publishers.

Menichelli, A., Rapp, B., & Semenza, C. (2008). Allographic agraphia: A case study. *Cortex, 44*, 861–868.

Nagaratnam, N., Plew, J., & Cooper, S. (1998). Pura agraphia following periendarterectomy stroke. *International Journal of Clinical Practice, 52*, 203–204.

Nielson, J. M. (1946). *Agnosia, apraxia, aphasia: Their value in cerebral localization.* New York: Paul B. Hoeber.

Neils-Strunjas, J., Groves-Wright, K., Mashima, P., & Harnish, S. (2006). Dysgraphia in Alzheimer's disease: A review for clinical and research purposes. *Journal of Speech, Language, and Hearing Research, 49*, 1313–130.

Ohno, T., Bando, M., Nagura, H., Ishii, K., & Yamanouchi, H. (2000). Apraxic agraphia due to thalamic lesion. *Neurology, 54*, 2336–2339.

Otsuki, M., Soma, Y., Arai, T., Otsuka, A., & Tsuji, S. (1999). Pure apraxic agraphia with abnormal writing stroke sequences: Report of a Japanese patient with a left superior parietal haemorrhage. *Journal of Neurology, Neurosurgery, and Psychiatry, 66*, 233–237.

Paolino, E., Bastiani, P., Monetti, V. C., Boldrini, P., & Rosati, G. (1983). Pure "aphasic" agraphia due to damage of the left superior parietal lobule. *Italian Journal of the Neurological Sciences, 4*, 233–237.

Papagno, C., Della Sala, S., & Basso, A. (1993). Ideomotor apraxia without aphasia and aphasia without apraxia: The anatomical support for a double dissociation. *Journal of Neurology, Neurosurgery, and Psychiatry, 56*, 286–289.

Platel, H., Lambert, J., Eustache, F., Cadet, B., Dary, M., Viader, F., et al. (1993). Characteristics and evolution of writing impairment in Alzheimer's disease. *Neuropsychologia, 31*, 1147–1158.

Popescu, I. M., & Vaidya, N. A. (2007). Isolated inability to write cursively after transient is chemic attack (TIA). *Cognitive and Behavioral Neurology, 20*, 131–135.

A

A

Rapcsak, S. Z., Arthur, S. A., Bliklen, D. A., & Rubens, A. B. (1989). Lexical agraphia in Alzheimer's disease. *Archives of Neurology, 46,* 65–68.

Rapcsak, S. Z., Arthur, S. A., & Rubens, A. B. (1988). Lexical agraphia from focal lesion of the left precentral gyrus. *Neurology, 38,* 1119–1123.

Rapcsak, S. Z., & Beeson, P. M. (2004). The role of left posterior inferior temporal cortex in spelling. *Neurology, 62,* 2221–2229.

Rapcsak, S. Z., Beeson, P. M., & Rubens, A. B. (1991). Writing with the right hemisphere. *Brain and Language, 41,* 510–530.

Raymer, A., Strobel, J., Prokup, T., Thomason, B., & Reff, K. L. (2010). Errorless versus errorful training of spelling in individuals with acquired dysgraphia. *Neuropsychological Rehabilitation, 20,* 1–15.

Roeltgen, D. P. (1993). Agraphia. In K. M. Heilman & E. Valenstein (Eds.), *Clinical neuropsychology* (pp. 63–89). New York: Oxford University Press.

Roeltgen, D. P. (1994). Localization of lesions in agraphia. In A. Kertesz (Ed.), *Localization and neuroimaging in neuropsychology* (pp. 377–405). San Diego: Academic Press.

Roeltgen, D. P., Gonzalez Rothi, L., & Heilman, K. M. (1986). Linguistic semantic agraphia: A dissociation of the lexical spelling system from semantics. *Brain and Language, 27,* 257–280.

Roeltgen, D. P., & Heilman, K. M. (1983). Apractic agraphia in a patient with normal praxis. *Brain and Language, 18,* 35–46.

Roeltgen, D. P., & Heilman, K. M. (1984). Lexical agraphia: Further support for the two-system hypothesis of linguistic agraphia. *Brain, 107,* 811–827.

Roeltgen, D. P., Sevush, S., & Heilman, K. M. (1983). Phonological agraphia: Writing by the lexical-semantic route. *Neurology, 33,* 755–765.

Rohrer, J. D., Rossor, M. N., & Warren, J. D. (2009). Neologistic jargon aphasia and agraphia in primary progressive aphasia. *Journal of the Neurological Sciences, 277,* 155–159.

Rohrer, J. D., Rossor, M. N., & Warren, J. D. (2010). Apraxia in progressive nonfluent aphasia. *Journal of Neurology, 257,* 569–574.

Rosati, G., & De Bastiani, P. (1979). Pure agraphia: A discrete form of aphasia. *Journal of Neurology, Neurosurgery, and Psychiatry, 42,* 266–269.

Rothi, L. J., & Heilman, K. M. (1981). Alexia and agraphia with spared spelling and letter recognition abilities. *Brain and Language, 12,* 1–13.

Sakurai, Y., Mimura, I., & Mannen, T. (2008). Agraphia for kanji resulting from a left posterior middle temporal gyrus lesion. *Behavioral Neurology, 19,* 93–106.

Schomer, D. L., Pegna, A., Matton, B., Seeck, M., Bidaut, L., Slossman. D., et al. (1998). Ictal agraphia: A patient study. *Neurology, 50*(2), 542–545.

Sgaramella, T. M., Ellis, A. W., & Semenza, C. (1991). Analysis of the spontaneous writing errors of normal and aphasic writers. *Cortex, 27,* 29–39.

Silveri, M. C., Misciagna, S., Leggio, M. G., & Molinari, M. (1997). Spatial dysgraphia and cerebellar lesion: A case report. *Neurology, 48,* 1529–1532.

Tanridag, O., & Kirshner, H. S. (1985). Aphasia and agraphia in lesions of the posterior internal capsule and putamen. *Neurology, 35,* 1797–1801.

Toyokura, M., Kobayashi, R., & Aono, K. (2010). A case of pure agraphia due to left thalamic hemorrhage. *Tokai Journal of Experimental and Clinical Medicine, 35,* 89–94.

AICARDI'S SYNDROME

DESCRIPTION

Aicardi's syndrome refers to a rare syndrome consisting of agenesis of the corpus callosum, chorioretinal lacunae, and infantile spasms. Other commonly seen features associated with Aicardi's syndrome are choroid plexus papillomas, ependymal cysts, cortical migration abnormalities, and optic disc coloboma (Aicardi, 1999). The prevalence of Aicardi's syndrome is not known; however, approximately 1% to 4% of referred infantile spasm cases may be due to it (Aicardi, 1999).

Aicardi's syndrome often results in severe cognitive and motor deficits. Most people with this syndrome are unable to walk or speak in complete sentences. About 76% of those with Aicardi's syndrome survive until age 6 and about 40% survive until age 14 (Menezes, MacGregor, & Buncic, 1994). A large variability of outcomes exists. Some infants with callosal agenesis have been known to have a normal development from 2 to 8 years of age, although prognosis is worse for those with other associated symptoms and chromosomal abnormalities (Aicardi, 2005).

NEUROPATHOLOGY/PATHOPHYSIOLOGY

One of the earliest signs of Aicardi's syndrome that can be detected is a partial or complete agenesis of the corpus callosum. Complete callosal agenesis can be detected via ultrasonography, MRI, or CT scan. MRI represents one of the best options for detecting partial callosal agenesis. Prenatal diagnosis based on agenesis of the corpus callosum is possible as early as 20 weeks gestation (Kligensmith & Cioffi-Ragan, 1986). Holoprosencephaly, which refers to an undivided anterior brain, may also be present in Aicardi's syndrome.

Infantile spasms are commonly reported with Aicardi's syndrome. Infantile spasms may precede or be triggered by clonic or tonic seizures. Often, these spasms and seizures are asymmetrical and only impact one side (Aicardi, 1999, 2005). According to Shah, Narendran, and Kalpana (2009), the most reliable feature of Aicardi's syndrome is chorioretinal lacunae.

Aicardi's syndrome does not appear to be hereditary. Instead, it is likely due to an X-linked dominant mutation (Aicardi, 1992). Only females are affected by this syndrome. Previously it was believed that the only males to have this syndrome have an XXY chromosomal configuration (Hopkins et al., 1979); however, there are very rare cases of XY males with the classic triad of Aicardi's syndrome characteristics (Chappelow, Reid, Parikh, & Traboulsi, 2008).

NEUROPSYCHOLOGICAL/CLINICAL PRESENTATION

Infantile spasms are a commonly reported feature of Aicardi's syndrome and may be asymmetrical. Next to infantile spasms, gastrointestinal dysfunction is the most commonly reported complication with Aicardi's syndrome (Glasmacher et al., 2007). Motor and cognitive deficits vary from case to case, but these deficits tend to be severe. Disconnection syndrome-like features may be seen in relation to partial or complete agenesis of the corpus callosum. Individuals may not acquire the ability to walk, or smile, or self-feed, but some cases show more subtle deficits in motor and cognitive functioning (Aicardi, 2005). Accurate assessment of vision can be confounded by motor and cognitive deficits, but reasonable visual functioning has been reported if chorioretinal lacunae do not impact the fovea (Shah et al., 2009).

DIAGNOSIS

Aicardi's syndrome was traditionally defined as having a triad of characteristics including agenesis of the corpus callosum, infantile spasms, and chorioretinal lacunae. Aicardi (1999) later defined other frequent features that could be considered for diagnosis. These frequently associated features are cortical malformations, periventricular and subcortical heterotopia, cysts around the choroid plexuses or third ventricle, papillomas of choroid plexuses, and optic disc or nerve coloboma. Some or most of these features may be absent in certain cases. The most commonly present features are cortical malformations and periventricular heterotopias. There are no completely consistent biological or genetic characteristics that have been deemed crucial for diagnosis. Due to variability in callosal agenesis and certain other features, Hopkins, Sutton, Lewis, Van den Veyver, and Clark (2008) proposed that diagnosis should be made upon some of the most frequently observed features detected via MRI. The most frequently detected features are frontal-dominant and perisylvian polymicrogyria, intracranial cysts, periventricular nodular heterotopias, and posterior fossa abnormalities.

TREATMENT

Varying manifestations and severity of Aicardi's syndrome features suggest that strategies for treatment or management of the conditions will also vary. Varying levels of cognitive and motor deficits may require different levels of care. Some individuals with Aicardi's syndrome may require intensive care and tube feeding. Infantile spasms are often found to be frequent and problematic but can be managed with therapy or medication. Saito et al. (2009) found zonisamide, clobazam, and a ketogenic diet to be partially effective in managing epileptic spasms and tonic seizures of those with this syndrome. Functional hemispherectomies may prove effective for managing seizures in some cases of Aicardi's syndrome (Saito et al., 2009). Convulsions associated with the syndrome may be successfully treated with adrenocorticotropic hormone therapy (Abe, Mitsudome, Ogata, Ohfu, & Takakusaki, 1990) or vigabatrin (Cossette, Riviello, & Carmant, 1999).

Evan Koehn
Beth Trammell
Raymond S. Dean

Abe, K., Mitsudome, A., Ogata, H., Ohfu, M., & Takakusaki, M. (1990). A case of Aicardi syndrome with moderate psychomotor retardation. *No To Hattatsu. Brain and Development, 22*, 4, 376–380.

Aicardi, J. (1992). *Diseases of the nervous system in childhood.* London: Mac Keith Press.

Aicardi, J. (1999). Aicardi syndrome: Old and new findings. *International Pediatrics, 14*, 1.

Aicardi, J. (2005). Aicardi syndrome. *Brain and Development, 27*, 164–171.

Chappelow, A., Reid, J., Parikh, S., & Traboulsi, E. (2008). Aicardi syndrome in a genotypic male. *Ophthalmic Genetics, 29*, 4, 181–183.

Cossette, P., Riviello, J. J., & Carmant, L. (1999). ACTH versus vigabatrin therapy in infantile spasms: A retrospective study. *Neurology, 52*, 8, 1691–1694.

Glasmacher, M., Sutton, V., Hopkins, B., Eble, T., Lewis, R., Parsons, D., et al. (2007). Phenotype and management of Aicardi syndrome: New findings from a survey of 69 children. *Journal of Child Neurology, 22*, 2, 176–184.

Hopkins, B., Sutton, V., Lewis, R., Van den Veyver, I., & Clark, G. (2008). Neuroimaging aspects of Aicardi syndrome. *American Journal of Medical Genetics. Part A, 146A*, 22, 2871–2878.

Hopkins, I. J., Humphrey, J., Keith, C. G., Sussman, M., Webb, G. C., & Turner, E. K. (1979). The Aicardi syndrome in a 47, XXY male. *Australian Pediatric Journal, 15*, 278–280.

Klingensmith, W.C., & Cioffi-Ragan, D.T. (1986). Schizencephaly: Diagnosis and progression in utero. *Radiology, 59*, 617–618.

Menezes, A. V., MacGregor, D. L., & Buncic, J. R. (1994). Aicardi syndrome: Natural history and possible predictors of severity. *Pediatric Neurology, 11*, 313–318.

Saito, Y., Sugai, K., Nakagawa, E., Sakuma, H., Komaki, H., Sasaki, M., et al. (2009). Treatment of epilepsy in severely disabled children with bilateral brain malformations. *Journal of the Neurological Sciences, 277*, 1/2, 37–49.

Shah, P. K., Narendran, V., & Kalpana, N. (2009). Aicardi syndrome: The importance of an ophthalmologist in its diagnosis. *Indian Journal of Ophthalmology, 57*, 3, 234–236.

ALEXANDER'S DISEASE

DESCRIPTION

Alexander's disease (AD) was first described by W.S. Alexander (Alexander, 1949), an Australian pathologist on a fellowship in England. Resulting from a progressive white matter deficiency of the brain (Nielsen, Jorgensen, & Jorgensen, 2002), AD is a rare genetic disorder that affects the astrocytes of the central nervous system (Alexander, 1949; Johnson, 1996). There are three main variants of AD: infantile, which is diagnosed between the ages of 0 and 2, juvenile, diagnosed between the ages of 2 and 12, and adult-onset, diagnosed after 12 years of age.

The infantile form of AD usually has an onset within the first 2 years of life. It is the most common subtype and is usually fatal within the first decade of life. Megalencephaly, seizures, psychomotor retardation, and progressive spastic quadriparesis are typical manifestations (Balbi et al., 2008). The infantile type can also include irritability, muscle weakness, and pyramidal tract signs (Franzoni, 2006). The juvenile form usually is first evident in children around the age of 4 years into the early teens. It tends to have more prominent brainstem

changes with speech and eating problems, has greater involvement of the lower limbs, and progresses more slowly (Johnson, 2002). Patients with the juvenile form of AD often do not have megalencephaly, are mentally intact, and show less white matter involvement at MRI compared with infantile forms (Balbi et al., 2008). The mean age at onset of the juvenile form of AD is 9 years, and the average survival is 8 years (Franzoni, 2006).

Both the infantile and juvenile forms generally appear to be caused by sporadic de novo and dominant genetic mutations (Suzuki et al., 2004). In contrast, adult-onset AD (AOAD) is often familial, meaning those with AOAD are carriers of a novel glial fibrillary acidic protein (GFAP) complex molecular defect composed of two mutations in one allele (Balbi et al., 2008). According to Quinlan, Brenner, Goldman, and Messing (2007), the genetic basis for AD is now firmly established. Pareyson et al. (2008) found that, in AOAD, there was evidence of autosomal dominant inheritance. AOAD has a different clinical and neuroradiological presentation with respect to early-onset AD, as abnormalities are mainly concentrated in the brainstem–spinal cord junction (Pareyson et al., 2008). In patients with AOAD, there are a number of clinical features that frequently present which include palatal tremors, dysphagia, and other bulbar and pseudobulbar signs (Quinlan et al., 2007).

NEUROPATHOLOGY/PATHOPHYSIOLOGY

Rosenthal fibers are a particular indicator of AD, but they can also sometimes be found in other conditions (fibrillary astrocytomas and prolonged debilitating systemic illnesses such as AIDS; van der Knaap et al., 2001). Balbi et al. (2008) found that a common neuropathological feature of AD is the diffuse presence of Rosenthal fibers, intracytoplasmic aggregates within astrocytes containing GFAP, the principal intermediate filament of astrocytes. GFAP contributes, when polymerized, to the stability of the cytoskeleton (Nielsen et al., 2002).

AD has also been associated with mutations in the GFAP gene (Brenner et al., 2001). Work by a number of investigators supports the idea that AD is a genetically homogenous disorder, with greater than 95% of patients who meet recognized MRI criteria for diagnosis having GFAP mutations (Quinlan et al., 2007). The most characteristic MRI findings are diffuse, symmetric, bifrontal white-matter signal abnormalities, with an intense enhancement in the infantile type (van der Knaap et al., 2001).

NEUROPSYCHOLOGICAL/CLINICAL PRESENTATION

The infantile form is characterized clinically by megalencephaly, developmental delay, psychomotor retardation, seizures, and a progressive course (Johnson & Brenner, 2003). The juvenile form is characterized by pseudobulbar and bulbar signs, such as problems with speech and swallowing. There may also be ataxia, spasticity of the lower extremities, and kyphoscoliosis.

AOAD is the least common type and may include features such as palatal myoclonus, ataxia, and dysautonomia (Johnson & Brenner, 2003). Seizures, cognitive delays, and/or regression are common symptoms (Quinlan et al., 2007) as are pyramidal involvement, cerebellar ataxia, and urinary disturbances. Less frequent findings include sleep disorders and dysautonomia (Pareyson et al., 2008). As such, AOAD must be considered in patients of any age with lower brain stem signs. When present, palatal myoclonus is strongly suggestive of the disease.

DIAGNOSIS

Prior to the development of GFAP, gene sequencing analysis diagnostic criteria was based on MRI findings. Criteria proposed by van der Knaap et al. (2001) included four of five of these criteria: (1) Extensive cerebral white matter abnormalities with a frontal predominance, (2) A periventricular rim of decreased signal intensity on T_2-weighted images and elevated signal intensity on T_1-weighted images, (3) Abnormalities of the basal ganglia and thalami, (4) Abnormalities of the brainstem, especially the medulla and midbrain, (5) Contrast enhancement of one or more of these structures: ventricular lining, periventricular tissue, frontal lobe white matter, optic chiasm, fornix, basal ganglia, thalamus, dentate nucleus, or brainstem.

Rosenthal fibers are the classical histopathological feature of AD. Given this, MRI is an extremely important diagnostic tool, but genotyping is the most secure method for confirming AD (Quinlan et al., 2007). In patients who do not meet previously established MRI criteria for AD, DNA diagnostics are warranted for the diagnosis (Franzoni et al., 2006).

TREATMENT

With GFAP mutations providing a firm genetic foundation for AD, attention is naturally turning to gene and replacement therapy. Since astrocyte dysfunction appears to depend in part upon elevation of GFAP above a toxic threshold, any damping of the elevation that occurs during the natural course of the disease is likely to be beneficial (Quinlan et al., 2007). An alternative approach to therapy currently under investigation is a systematic screening of existing drugs that are already approved by the FDA for previously unknown activities that may reduce expression of GFAP (Quinlan et al., 2007). Gorospe et al. (2002) suggested that quercetin or other compounds known to reduce GFAP expression in cultured astrocytes might be useful as therapeutics. Finally, modest success was found using thyrotropin releasing hormone in treating a juvenile AD patient (Quinlan et al., 2007).

Justin J. Boseck
Andrew S. Davis

Alexander, W. S. (1949). Progressive fibrinoid degeneration of fibrillary astrocytes associated with mental retardation in a hydrocephalic infant. *Brain, 72,* 373–381.

Balbi, P., Seri, M., Ceccherini, I., Uggetti, C., Casale, R., Fundarò, C., et al. (2008). Adult-onset Alexander disease. *Journal of Neurology, 255,* 24–30.

Brenner, M., Johnson, A. B., Boespflug-Tanguy, O., Rodriguez, D., Goldman, J., & Messing, A. (2001). Mutations in GFAP, encoding glial fibrillary acidic protein, are associated with Alexander's disease. *Nature Genetics, 27,* 117–120.

Franzoni, E., Van der Knaap, M. S., Errani, A., Colonnelli, M. C., Bracceschi, R., Malaspina, E., et al. (2006). Unusual diagnosis in a child suffering from juvenile Alexander disease: Clinical imaging report. *Journal of Child Neurology, 21*(12), 1075–1080.

Gorospe, J. R., Naidu, S., Johnson, A. B., Puri, V., Raymond, G. V., Jenkins, S. D., et al. (2002). Molecular findings in symptomatic and pre-symptomatic Alexander Disease patients. *Neurology, 58,* 1494–1500.

Johnson, A. B. (1996). In H. G. Moser (Ed.), *Handbook of clinical neurology: Neurodystrophies and neurolipidoses* (pp. 701–710). Amsterdam: Elsevier.

Johnson, A. B. (2002). Alexander disease: A review and the gene. *Journal of Developmental Neuroscience, 20,* 391–394.

Johnson, A. B., & Brenner, M. (2003). Alexander's disease: Clinical, pathologic, and genetic features. *Journal of Child Neurology, 18,* 625–632.

Nielsen, A. L., Jorgensen, P., & Jorgensen, A. L. (2002). Mutations associated with a childhood leukodystrophy, Alexander disease, cause deficiency in dimerization of the cytoskeletal protein GFAP. *Journal of Neurogenetics, 16,* 175–179.

Pareyson, D., Fancellu, R., Mariotti, C., Romano, S., Salmaggi, A., Carella, F., et al. (2008). Adult-onset Alexander disease: A series of eleven unrelated cases with review of the literature. *Brain, 131,* 2321–2331.

Quinlan, R. A., Brenner, M., Goldman, J. E., & Messing, A. (2007). GFAP and its role in Alexander disease. *Experimental Cell Research, 313*, 2077–2087.

Suzuki, Y., Kanazava, N., Takenaka, J., Okumura, A., Negoro, T., & Tsujino, S. (2004). A case of infantile Alexander disease with a milder phenotype and a novel GFAP mutation, L90P. *Brain and Development, 26*(3), 206–208.

van der Knaap, M. S., Naidu, S., Breitner, S. N., Blaser, S., Stroink, H., Springer, S., et al. (2001). Alexander disease: Diagnosis with MR imaging. *American Journal of Neurodialogy, 22*, 541–552.

ALEXIAS

DESCRIPTION

Alexia is an acquired disorder characterized by the loss of the ability to read. Alexia typically occurs following damage to the left hemisphere or to the areas that are responsible for processing visual aspects of language or visual access to the language system (De Renzi, Zambolin, & Crisi, 1987; Johansson & Fahlgren, 1979; Pyun, Sohn, Jung, & Nam, 2007; Sakurai et al., 2000; Sevush & Heilman, 1984; Weisberg & Wall, 1987). However, different types of alexia may be associated with different lesion locations in the brain. In contrast to alexia, which denotes reading defects in persons who could read before the onset of brain damage or disease, dyslexia typically refers to developmental disorders in otherwise competent children who do not make normal progress in reading (Coltheart, Patterson, & Marshall, 1987; Lovett, 2003).

PRIMARY TYPES OF ALEXIA

Attentional Alexia

Shallice and Warrington (1977) described a patient who could read single words but had difficulty with reading multiple words. When presented with a complete sentence, the patient reported that the letters tended to migrate, one word moving over the others. The underlying problem in attentional alexia seems to be related to a deficit of attention that is not limited to orthographic material (Friedman, Ween, & Albert, 1993).

Neglect Alexia

Neglect alexia refers to those groups of reading disturbances often associated with hemispatial neglect. Individuals affected by hemispatial neglect may have a variety of reading problems. Among the most common

of these disorders are right parietal stroke and left-sided neglect in patients. These patients neglect the left side of the page with subsequent omission of the words placed on the left side (subject-centered neglect) or omission of the left side of the words (object-centered neglect), result in characteristic substitution errors (Arduino, Burani, & Vallar, 2002; Lee et al., 2009; Martelli, Arduino, & Daini, 2011; Vallar, Burani, & Arduino, 2010). This effect disappears if the orientation of the words on the page is changed. Other patients may exhibit substitution errors without any of the features of neglect (Haywood & Coltheart, 2001). Also, some patients may omit the last segment of the printed word (the portion of the word appearing on the right side) and these errors may not be sensitive to the spatial orientation of the word (Friedman et al., 1993; Petrich, Greenwald, & Berndt, 2007). Overall, the majority of the errors seen in patients with neglect alexia are substitutions; thus, the length of the words is generally intact. Deletions and additions may also be seen but are rarer.

Neglect alexia has been considered a feature of visuospatial neglect (Ellis, Flude, & Young, 1987), although recent reports indicate cases of pure alexia without neglect (Riddoch, Humphreys, Cleton, & Fery, 1990), or left neglect alexia with a right hemispatial neglect (Costello & Warrington, 1987). Whether or not neglect alexia is dissociable from visuospatial neglect, it is highly probable that neglect alexia is related to an attentional deficit of that part of the reading system responsible for coding abstract letters and position information (Friedman et al., 1993). The majority of patients with neglect alexia produce orthography-related errors that are not restricted to one side, such as substitutions. This finding has led to the notion that information about letter position is retained in neglect alexia, while information about letter identity is lost (Ellis et al., 1987).

Pure Alexia

Pure alexia is a condition in which all aspects of the orthographic lexicon and semantic processing remain intact. Hence, agraphia and aphasia are typically not present. However, visual input is not able to activate the orthographic unit and thus the patients cannot read, although they can recognize single letters. To compensate for these dysfunctions, patients with pure alexia may read letter by letter aloud so that their auditory system may assist in recognizing the words (Friedman et al., 1993). Patients with pure alexia will have greater difficulty with long words (Behrmann, Shomstein, Black, & Barton, 2001; Cumming, Patterson, Verfaellie, & Graham, 2006; Henderson, Friedman, Teng, & Weiner, 1985), but will likely have no problems in recognizing words when they are orally spelled out by the examiner (Buxbaum & Coslett, 1996; Greenwald & Gonzalez Rothi, 1998). The syndrome of letter-by-letter reading has been described as equivalent to the syndrome of pure alexia (Friedman et al., 1993).

To read, the images entering the eyes must be translated into neural impulses, which must then travel from the retina to the calcarine or striate cortex of the occipital lobe. From the striate cortex the impulses travel to the visual association cortex and the angular gyrus, which is part of the fronto-temporo-parital language system. Damage to the connections between the angular gyrus and its input, without damaging the angular gyrus itself, will result in alexia without agraphia (Damasio & Damasio, 1983; Friedman et al., 1993; Johansson & Fahlgren, 1979; Naranjo, Espada, Torrella, Donderis, & De las Peñas, 1989; Quint & Gilmore, 1992; Weisberg & Wall, 1987). Patients with alexia without agraphia will be able to write (both spontaneously and to dictation) but will have difficulty reading even what he or she has written. Thus, it is thought that the angular gyrus is a central area involved in the processing of orthographic word forms (Friedman et al., 1993). Lesions to the angular gyrus itself result in alexia with agraphia, in which both reading and writing are affected (Davous & Boller, 1994; Greenblatt, 1977; Sheldon, Malcolm, & Barton, 2008). The typical event that causes a disconnection to the angular gyrus is an infarct in the territory of the posterior cerebral artery that simultaneously affects the mesial left occipital lobe and the splenium of the corpus callosum. A lesion in this area results in a right visual field defect but preservation of vision in the left hemifield because the right calcarine cortex is not affected. However, the patient will be alexic in both hemifields. The reason for alexia in both visual fields is related to the fact that the visual input from the left hemisphere travels to the right primary and secondary visual cortex. From here the visual input should access the left angular gyrus involved in the orthographic wordform. However, to access the left angular gyrus the right visual cortex must connect first with the left visual cortex as there are no direct callosal fibers between the right visual cortex and the left angular gyrus. The left angular gyrus is connected to the left secondary visual cortex through the vertical occipital fasciculus. A lesion of the vertical occipital fasciculus will result in alexia for both hemifields (Friedman et al., 1993; Greenblatt, 1990).

Surface Alexia

Written words activate an established pattern of orthographic units in lexical memory. An impairment in the orthographic lexicon appears when the appropriate word is not activated, which may result in a "regularity effect" (Friedman et al., 1993; Hanley & Kay, 2010). Languages such as English have both regular and irregular words. Regular words possess correspondence between the pronunciation of the word and the spelling. Irregular words, in contrast, do not have perfect correspondence between spelling and sound. Some individuals have no difficulty reading regular words, but they have more problems in reading irregular words. This type of disturbance is called surface alexia (or orthographic alexia; Coslett, 2003; Friedman et al., 1993; Hanley & Kay, 2010). The errors committed by these patients are referred to as "regularization" errors because irregular words are often pronounced with a regular pronunciation, according to the spelling of the word (Friedman et al., 1993; Hanley & Kay, 2010).

The semantic system in surface alexia must rely upon input from the phonological system as the word is typically comprehended according to how it is pronounced. If semantic information were obtained strictly on the basis of the sound of the word, then words with homophones would often be interpreted incorrectly, such as "would" being mistaken for "wood" (Coltheart, Masterson, Byng, Prior, & Riddoch, 1983). Thus, the diagnosis of orthographic (surface) alexia is made when regular and pseudowords are read significantly better than irregular words (Banich, 2004; Friedman, 1988; Friedman et al., 1993). If comprehension depends upon the phonological code assigned to the word, homophone confusions are common and pseudohomophone words are often accepted as real words. These instances result in surface alexia from impairment of orthographic lexicon (Friedman et al., 1993).

The neuroanatomy of surface alexia is difficult to ascertain because the lesion location and source may vary substantially. The left temporal lobe and surrounding areas seem to be involved in many cases (Deloche & Andreewsky, 1982; Gold et al., 2005; Vanier & Caplan, 1985). Based on their review of the literature, Friedman et al. (1993) found that the lesions typically involved the temporoparietal cortex and deep white and gray matter of the left hemisphere. The occipital cortex and white matter (areas involved in pure alexia) and frontal association cortex and Broca's areas (areas involved in deep alexia) are typically spared. Also, the right hemisphere was involved in some cases but never in isolation.

Phonological Alexia

Phonological alexia is characterized by a disconnection between orthographical units and phonological units, whereas all other connections remain intact.

Patients affected by phonological alexia are still able to read because the orthographic units access the semantic units and thus the phonological ones. For this reason, reading and comprehension will be preserved. However, some problems might be expected when the patients are asked to read pseudowords (Hanley & Kay, 2010). The pronunciation of pseudowords, unlike real words, cannot be attained through this alternate route and pseudoword reading should therefore be greatly impaired relative to words (Friedman et al., 1993). Several patients have been reported with this type of phonological alexia (Beauvois & Derouesnè, 1979; Cuetos, Valle-Arroyo, & Suarez, 1996; Friedman & Kohn, 1990; Glosser & Friedman, 1990; Rapcsak, Gonzalez Rothi, & Heilman, 1987). Phonological alexia is often associated with a stroke in the territory of the middle cerebral artery, typically involving the temporal lobe and surrounding regions (Lambon Ralph & Graham, 2000; Rapcsak et al., 1987), and damage to the angular and supramarginal gyri may also be involved (Friedman & Kohn, 1990).

Semantic Alexia

Semantic alexia is characterized by a preserved ability to read aloud either words or pseudowords but with a profound impairment in comprehension. This is often seen in people affected by Alzheimer's disease and semantic dementia who present difficulties understanding either spoken or written language (Friedman et al., 1993; Hanley & Kay, 2010).

Deep Alexia

Deep alexia is a syndrome characterized by the production of semantic paralexias. Semantic paralexias are reading errors in which the response has the same meaning, but the word is phonologically and orthographically different. Semantic paralexias can be opposite (e.g., soft–hard), superordinates (e.g., gun–weapon), subordinates (e.g., vegetable–broccoli), coordinates (e.g., arm–leg), synonyms (e.g., doctor–physician), or associate (e.g., sleep–dream). Patients are said to have deep alexia when more than 5% of all their reading errors are semantic paralexias (Friedman et al., 1993). Patients with deep alexia almost always have some other symptom of alexia (Coltheart, 1980), such as a part-of-speech effect (nouns and adjectives are read better than verbs, verbs are then read better then functors), a concreteness/imageability effect (concrete and imageable nouns are read better than abstract and nonimageable nouns), functor word substitutions, and deficits reading pseudowords

(Friedman et al., 1993; Hanley & Kay, 2010). The production of these errors indicates a disturbance within semantic and phonological reading routes. Thus, deep alexia is the result of the inability to use the direct orthography to phonology route for oral reading, in combination with a deficit within the semantic reading route (Friedman, 1991). The deficit in the semantic route may occur just within the semantic system or within the semantic and phonological routes. These two possibilities can be distinguished by having the patients first read a word aloud and then have them point to the corresponding picture from an array of several semantically related choices (Friedman & Perlman, 1982). If the patient chooses the incorrect picture, a semantic processing deficit may then be suggested. If the patient produces a semantic paralexia but then chooses the correct picture (even when the picture corresponding to the paralexia is among the choices), it is likely that the problem occurs subsequent to semantic processing. Friedman and Perlman (1982) patient evidenced both of these types of errors. However, the patients reported by Caramazza and Hillis (1990) fit the second pattern as they not only performed well on word–picture matching tasks but they also provided correct definitions of the words to which they had produced semantic paralexias.

TREATMENT

A successful treatment program described by de Partz (1986) consisted of the goal to retrain the patient to read through using the phonological route. Specifically, each letter was paired with a common word that begins with that letter, and by doing this the subject is forced to produce a phoneme corresponding to each letter. Success using this phoneme-blending technique has been reported by others as well (Nickels, 1992; Stadie & Rillig, 2006). However, patients with surface alexia have problems reading irregular words. One way to treat this patient group is to teach them the use of a whole-word approach. For instance, Coltheart and Byng (1989) paired written words with a mnemonic device. Friedman and Robinson (1991) grouped words according to pronunciation rather than using a mnemonic device. For example, all "ow" words pronounced /o/ such as "mow" and "grow" were grouped together. Patients with pure alexia typically learn that spelling the words letter by letter aloud helps them to recognize the words through their auditory system. There are pure alexia patients who have difficulty recognizing individual letters, and thus, they may use a kinesthetic approach (Goldstein, 1948; Kashiwagi & Kashiwagi, 1989). The kinesthetic approach involves the patient being taught to trace the presented letters either with the finger or with the head or eyes and the feedback provided from the body movement allows the patients to recognize the letters.

Valeria Drago
Paul S. Foster

Arduino, L. S., Burani, C., & Vallar, G. (2002). Lexical effects in left neglect dyslexia: A study in Italian patients. *Cognitive Neuropsychology, 19*, 421–444.

Beauvois, M. F., & Derouesnè, J. (1979). Phonological alexia: Three dissociations. *Journal of Neurology, Neurosurgery, and Psychiatry, 42*, 1115–1124.

Behrmann, M., Shomstein, S. S., Black, S. E., & Barton, J. J. (2001). The eye movements of pure alexic patients during reading and nonreading tasks. *Neuropsychologia, 39*, 983–1002.

Buxbaum, L. J., & Coslett, H. B. (1996). Deep dyslexic phenomena in a letter-by-letter reader. *Brain and Language, 54*, 136–167.

Caramazza, A., & Hillis, A. E. (1990). Where do semantic errors come from? *Cortex, 26*, 95–122.

Coltheart, M., & Byng, S. (1989). A treatment for surface dyslexia. In X. Seron & G. Deloche (Eds.), *Cognitive approaches in neuropsychological rehabilitation*. Hillsdale, NJ: Erlbaum.

Coltheart, M., Masterson, J., Byng, S., Prior, M., & Riddoch, J. (1983). Surface dyslexia. *Quarterly Journal of Experimental Psychology, 35A*, 469–495.

Coltheart, M., Patterson, K. E., & Marshall, J. C. (1987). Deep dyslexia since 1980. In M. Coltheart, K. E. Patterson, & J. Marshall (Eds.), *Deep dyslexia* (2nd ed.). London: Routledge and Kegan Paul.

Coslett, H. B. (2003). Acquired disorders of reading. In T. E. Feinberg & M. J. Farah (Eds.), *Behavioral neurology and neuropsychology* (2nd ed., pp. 195–205). New York: McGraw-Hill.

Costello, A. D. L., & Warrington, E. K. (1987). The dissociation of visuospatial neglect and neglect dyslexia. *Journal of Neurology, Neurosurgery, and Psychiatry, 50*, 1110–1116.

Cuetos, F., Valle-Arroyo, F., & Suarez, M. P. (1996). A case of phonological dyslexia in Spanish. *Cognitive Neuropsychology, 13*, 1–24.

Cumming, T. B., Patterson, K., Verfaellie, M., & Graham, K. S. (2006). One bird with two stones: Abnormal word length effects in pure alexia and semantic dementia. *Cognitive Neuropsychology, 23*, 1130–1161.

Damasio, A. R., & Damasio, H. (1983). The anatomic basis of pure alexia. *Neurology, 33*, 1573–1583.

Davous, P., & Boller, F. (1994). Transcortical alexia with agraphia following a right temporo-occipital hematoma in a right-handed patient. *Neuropsychologia, 32*, 1263–1272.

Deloche, G., & Andreewsky, E. (1982). Surface dyslexia: A case report and some theoretical implications to reading models. *Brain and Language, 15*, 12–31.

De Renzi, E., Zambolin, A., & Crisi, G. (1987). The pattern of neuropsychological impairment associated with left posterior cerebral artery infarcts. *Brain, 110*, 1099–1116.

Ellis, A. W., Flude, B. M., & Young, A. W. (1987). "Neglect dyslexia" and the early visual processing of letters in words and nonwords. *Cognitive Neuropsychology, 4*, 439–464.

Friedman, R. B. (1991). *Is there a continuum of phonological/deep dyslexia?* Paper presented at DD12 Conference, London.

Friedman, R. B., & Kohn, S. E. (1990). Impaired activation of the phonological lexicon: Effects upon oral reading. *Brain and Language, 38*, 278–297.

Friedman, R. B., & Perlman, M. B. (1982). On the underlying causes of semantic paralexias in a patient with deep dyslexia. *Neuropsychologia, 20*, 559–568.

Friedman, R. B., & Robinson, S. R. (1991). Whole-word training therapy in a stable surface alexic patient: It works. *Aphasiology, 5*, 1–7.

Friedman, R. F., Ween, J. E., & Albert, M. L. (1993). Alexia. In K. M. Heilman & E. Valenstein (Eds.), *Clinical neuropsychology* (3rd ed., pp. 37–62). New York: Oxford University Press.

Glosser, G., & Friedman, R. B. (1990). The continuum of deep/phonological alexia. *Cortex, 26*, 343–359.

Gold, B. T., Balota, D. A., Cortese, M. J., Sergent-Marshall, S. D., Snyder, A. Z., Salat, D. H., et al. (2005). Differing neuropsychological and neuroanatomical correlates of abnormal reading in early-stage semantic dementia and dementia of the Alzheimer type. *Neuropsychologia, 43*, 833–846.

Goldstein, K. (1948). *Language and language disturbances*. New York: Grune and Stratton.

Greenblatt, S. H. (1977). Neurosurgery and the anatomy of reading: A practical review. *Neurosurgery, 1*, 6–15.

Greenblatt, S. H. (1990). Left occipital lobectomy and the preangular anatomy of reading. *Brain and Language, 38*, 576–595.

Greenwald, M. L., & Gonzalez Rothi, L. J. (1998). Lexical access via letter naming in a profoundly alexic and anomic patient: A treatment study. *Journal of the International Neuropsychological Society, 4*, 595–607.

Hanley, J. R., & Kay, J. (2010). Neuropsychological assessment and treatment of disorders of reading. In J. M. Gurd, U. Kischka, & J. C. Marshall (Eds.), *Handbook of clinical neuropsychology* (2nd ed., pp. 296–322). New York: Oxford University Press.

Haywood, M., & Coltheart, M. (2001). Neglect dyslexia with a stimulus-centered deficit and without visuospatial neglect. *Cognitive Neuropsychology, 18*, 577–615.

Henderson, V. W., Friedman, R. B., Teng, E. L., & Weiner, J. M. (1985). Left hemisphere pathways in reading:

A

Inferences from pure alexia without hemianopia. *Neurology, 35*, 962–968.

Johansson, T., & Fahlgren, H. (1979). Alexia without agraphia: Lateral and medial infarction of left occipital lobe. *Neurology, 29*, 390–393.

Kashiwagi, T., & Kashiwagi, A. (1989). Recovery process of a Japanese alexic without agraphia. *Aphasiology, 3*, 75–91.

Lambon Ralph, M. A., & Graham, N. L. (2000). Acquired phonological and deep dyslexia. *Neurocase, 6*, 141–143.

Lee, B. H., Suh, M. K., Kim, E. J., Seo, S. W., Choi, K. M., Kim, G. M., et al. (2009). Neglect dyslexia: Frequency, association with other hemispatial neglects, and lesion localization. *Neuropsychologia, 47*, 704–710.

Lovett, M. M. (2003). Developmental reading disorders. In T. E. Feinberg & M. J. Farah (Eds.), *Behavioral neurology and neuropsychology* (2nd ed.). New York: McGraw-Hill.

Martelli, M., Arduino, L. S., & Daini, R. (2011). Two different mechanisms for omission and substitution errors in neglect dyslexia. *Neurocase, 17*, 122–132.

Naranjo, I. C., Espada, J. L., Torrella, J. E., Donderis, M. A., & De las Peñas, R. (1989). Alexia without agraphia: A new case studied by CT-scan. *Neuroradiology, 31*, 199.

Nickels, L. (1992). The autocue? Self-generated phonemic cues in the treatment of a disorder of reading and naming. *Cognitive Neuropsychology, 9*, 155–182.

dePartz, M. P. (1986). Re-education of a deep dyslexic patient: Rationale of the method and results. *Cognitive Neuropsychology, 3*, 149–177.

Petrich, J. A., Greenwald, M. L., & Berndt, R. S. (2007). An investigation of attentional contributions to visual errors in right "neglect dyslexia." *Cortex, 43*, 1036–1046.

Pyun, S. B., Sohn, H. J., Jung, J. B., & Nam, K. (2007). Differential reorganization of fusiform gyrus in two types of alexia after stroke. *Neurocase, 13*, 417–425.

Quint, D. J., & Gilmore, J. L. (1992). Alexia without agraphia. *Neuroradiology, 34*, 210–214.

Rapcsak, S. Z., Gonzalez Rothi, L. J., & Heilman, K. M. (1987). Phonological alexia with optic and tactile anomia: A neuropsychological and anatomical study. *Brain and Language, 31*, 109–121.

Riddoch, J., Humphreys, G., Cleton, P., & Fery, P. (1990). Interaction of attentional and lexical processes in neglect dyslexia. *Cognitive Neuropsychology, 7*, 479–517.

Sakurai, Y., Takeuchi, S., Takada, T., Horiuchi, E., Nakase, H., & Sakuta, M. (2000). Alexia caused by a fusiform or posterior inferior temporal lesion. *Journal of the Neurological Sciences, 178*, 442–451.

Sevush, S., & Heilman, K. M. (1984). A case of literal alexia: Evidence for a disconnection syndrome. *Brain and Language, 22*, 92–108.

Shallice, T., & Warrington, E. K. (1977). The possible role of selective attention in acquired dyslexia. *Neuropsychologia, 15*, 31–41.

Sheldon, C. A., Malcolm, G. L., & Barton, J. J. (2008). Alexia with and without agraphia: An assessment of two classical syndromes. *Canadian Journal of Neurological Sciences, 35*, 616–624.

Stadie, N., & Rilling, E. (2006). Evaluation of lexically and nonlexically based reading treatment in a deep dyslexic. *Cognitive Neuropsychology, 23*, 643–672.

Vallar, G., Burani, C., & Arduino, L. S. (2010). Neglect dyslexia: A review of the neuropsychological literature. *Experimental Brain Research, 206*, 219–235.

Vanier, M., & Caplan, D. (1985). CT scan correlates of surface dyslexia. In K. Patterson, J. Marshall, & M. Coltheart (Eds.), *Surface dyslexia: Neuropsychological and cognitive studies of phonological reading*. Hove, UK: Erlbaum.

Weisberg, L. A., & Wall, M. (1987). Alexia without agraphia: Clinical-computed tomographic correlations. *Neuroradiology, 29*, 283–286.

ALIEN HAND SYNDROME

DESCRIPTION

Alien hand syndrome is a phenomenon in which an upper limb engages in simple and complex motor actions against the individual's will or volitional control (Scepkowski & Cronin-Golomb, 2003). Dating back to the 19th century, descriptions have been found of hands acting involuntarily and seemingly not under the individual's control (Mark, 2007). The first case to characterize the limb as foreign to the patient was described in 1908 by Kurt Goldstein (Goldstein, 1908; Mark, 2007; Scepkowski & Cronin-Golomb, 2003). In the 1940s, Akelaitis described a series of patients who experienced the alien hand symptoms following severing of the corpus callosum, and he termed the phenomena "diagnostic dyspraxia" (Akelaitis, 1945; Biran & Chatterjee, 2004; Scepkowski & Cronin-Golomb, 2003). Brion and Jedynak applied the term alien hand syndrome (*la main étrangère*) in 1972 after describing several similar cases of individuals with brain tumors who experienced lack of control of a limb (Brion & Jedynak, 1972; Scepkowski & Cronin-Golomb, 2003).

NEUROPATHOLOGY/PATHOPHYSIOLOGY

There has been some difficulty in establishing a complete understanding of the syndrome because of the rarity of the phenomenon and lack of uniformity in assessment techniques (e.g., neuropsychological tests, imaging) in case reports. In addition, most of the available literature has been descriptive in nature, based on an individual's personal experiences rather than based on sound experimental design (Assal, Schwartz, & Vuilleumier, 2007; Biran & Chatterjee, 2004; Scepkowski & Cronin-Golomb, 2003).

Historically, the alien hand syndrome has been associated with disconnection of the corpus callosum, which limits the amount of communication between the two cerebral hemispheres. Surgical disconnection of the corpus callosum is used as a treatment to alleviate symptoms in severe cases of epilepsy. However, alien hand phenomenon has also been documented in individuals with brain tumors, neurodegeneration, infectious processes, and even following strokes.

The presentation of alien hand syndrome can differ greatly based on the nature of the involuntary movements, which is in part due to the localization of damage (Mark, 2007). There are distinct subtypes based on location of structural damage in the brain that is believed to trigger the phenomena. Three identified variants are frontal, callosal, and posterior alien hand syndromes (Scepkowski & Cronin-Golomb, 2003). The most common form, that being the *frontal variant* of the syndrome, is observed in individuals with lesions in the supplemental motor areas, anterior cingulate gyrus, medial prefrontal cortex, and anterior portions of the corpus callosum (Brazdil, Kuba, & Rektar, 2006). The traditional description of alien hand syndrome involves the *callosal variant* and is associated with damage that leads to a lack of communication between cerebral hemispheres. In the original documented case by Goldstein (1908), he examined the patient's brain upon death and described lesions in the right hemisphere and the corpus callosum (Scepkowski & Cronin-Golomb, 2003). *Posterior alien hand syndrome* involves damages to the posterior brain regions, but it is believed to be associated with much more global damage than is the case with the frontal or callosal types in which damage is rather focal.

NEUROPSYCHOLOGICAL/CLINICAL PRESENTATION

Alien hand syndrome is an intermittent involuntary movement disorder. It is present when one of the hands, typically the left, begins to act autonomously and engages in purposeful behaviors against what the individual intends to do, as if the alien hand "has a mind of its own" (Bundick & Spinella, 2000; Mark, 2007). The movements of the alien hand must appear to be purposeful and goal-directed despite being inconsistent with the individual's intended goal (Mark, 2007). The appearance of purposeful movement distinguishes alien hand syndrome from involuntary muscle contractions, such as clonus or tremors. Furthermore, the patient must be aware of the lack of control of the alien hand.

The nature of alien hand activity can vary greatly across patients, depending on the specific type of alien hand syndrome (Scepkowski & Cronin-Golomb, 2003). *Intermanual conflict* is present when the alien hand acts to counter the action of the other hand, such as when an individual is buttoning a shirt with the right hand and the left hand follows and unbuttons. *Mirror movements* occur when the alien hand imitates the actions of the other hand precisely. *Enabling synkinesis* is the term used to describe when the controlled hand can only perform a task in unison with the alien hand. *Grasp reflex* is the tendency of the alien hand to grab at objects involuntarily and the desire to have something in hand. *Magnetic apraxia* describes when the alien hand reaches toward or grasps objects involuntarily, as if pulled by a magnetic force. *Utilization behavior* involves compulsive activity and manipulation of objects and tools (Scepkowski & Cronin-Golomb, 2003).

All of these signs of alien hand syndrome are not evident in each case; the specific presentation is associated with the location of the cerebral lesion or damage (Scepkowski & Cronin-Golomb, 2003). For instance, frontal alien hand syndrome is often associated with exploratory behaviors, groping, compulsivity, and grasp reflex (Bundick & Spinella, 2000), whereas cases of intermanual conflict are more often associated with callosal damage (Bundick & Spinella, 2000). In comparison, the posterior type is often characterized by hand levitations and abnormal postures (Biran & Chatterjee, 2004).

DIAGNOSIS

The diagnosis of alien hand syndrome is initially based on descriptive accounts of the patient's unique experience, as well as behavioral observations by the examiner. Following the initial observations, neurological examination and neuroimaging may be used to determine the site of damage and gain an understanding of the etiology. A thorough understanding of the cause is an important factor to help inform proper treatment procedures. Differential diagnosis is important to eliminate other potential causes of the phenomena, such as an underlying psychiatric problem or dementia (Mark, 2007).

TREATMENT

Gradual recovery within a year of onset usually occurs in individuals that manifest alien hand syndrome caused by a focal injury (Mark, 2007). In instances associated with more global damage, the phenomena

A

may persist. Neither formal treatment protocols nor rehabilitation techniques have been developed to specifically treat alien hand syndrome (Mark, 2007). Instead, treatment involves (1) identifying and treating the cause when possible, (2) behavior modification, and (3) making changes in the individual's home environment to maximize safety. It is also vital to treat the specific symptoms of each case. For some individuals, occupying the hand with an action, such as by having the alien hand grasp an object, may be helpful to limit involuntary actions.

Shane S. Bush
Kathryn M. Lombardi Mirra

Akelaitis, A. I. (1945). Studies on the corpus callosum. IV. Diagnostic dyspraxia in epileptics following partial and complete section of the corpus callosum. *American Journal of Psychiatry, 101*, 594–599.

Assal, F., Schwartz, S., & Vuilleumier P. (2007). Moving with or without will: Functional neural correlates of alien hand syndrome. *Annals of Neurology, 62*, 301–306.

Biran, I., & Chatterjee, A. (2004). Alien hand syndrome. *Archives of Neurology, 61*, 292–294.

Brazdil, M., Kuba, R., & Rektar, I. (2006). Rostral cingulate motor area and paroxysmal alien hand syndrome. *Journal of Neurology, Neurosurgery, and Psychiatry, 77*, 992–993.

Brion, S., & Jedynak, C. P. (1972). Troubles du transfer interhemispherique. A propos de trios observations de tumeurs du corps calleux. Le signe de la main etrangere. *Revue Neurologique (Paris), 126*, 257–266.

Bundick, T., & Spinella, M. (2000). Subjective experience, involuntary movement, and posterior alien hand syndrome. *Journal of Neurology, Neurosurgery, and Psychiatry, 68*, 83–85.

Goldstein, K. (1908). Zur Lehre der motorischen Apraxie. *Journal fur Psychologie und Neurologie, 11*, 169–187.

Mark, V. A. (2007). Alien hand syndrome. In S. Gilman (Ed.), *MedLink Neurology*. San Diego, CA: MedLink Corporation. Retrieved January 24, 2009, from www.jsmf.org/meetings/2008/may/Mark%20VW%202008%20Alien%20hand%20syndrome.pdf

Scepkowski, L. A., & Cronin-Golomb, A. (2003). The alien hand: Cases, categorizations, and anatomical correlates. *Behavioral and Cognitive Neuroscience Reviews, 2*, 261–277.

ALPERS'S DISEASE

DESCRIPTION

Alpers's disease, also referred to as progressive sclerosing poliodystrophy, spongy glioneuronal dystrophy, progressive cerebral poliodystrophy, and/or progressive neuronal degeneration of childhood, is an autosomal-recessive disease characterized by refractory seizures, neurological deterioration with poliodystrophy, and terminal hepatopathy as a result of a respiratory chain deficiency in mitochondria (Wiltshire et al., 2008). Onset typically occurs between the ages of 1 and 3 years, although cases have been seen in late adolescence (Harding et al., 1995; Wiltshire et al., 2008). Treatment consists of palliative care as there is no known cure with the disease typically resulting in death by age 10.

NEUROPATHOLOGY/PATHOPHYSIOLOGY

Naviaux and Nguyen (2004) attributed Alpers's disease to mutations in mitochondrial DNA (mtDNA) and subsequent research has shown at least nine genetic mutations in the polymerase gene polymerase gamma (POLG1) resulting in the disease (Ferrari et al., 2005; Nguyen et al., 2005; Wiltshire et al., 2008). As such deficiency of polymerase gamma is the most common cause of Alpers's disease in children (Naviaux and Nguyen, 2004).

NEUROPSYCHOLOGICAL/CLINICAL PRESENTATION

Electroencephalography (EEG) results in patients with Alpers's disease typically show a distinctive pattern of slow high amplitude (delta) wave activity with polyspikes (Gordon, 2006; Harding et al., 1995; Rasmussen, Sanengen, Skullerud, Kvittingen, & Skjeldal, 2000). MRI may reveal lesions, most frequently in the occipital lobes, with lesions also seen in the thalamus, basal ganglia, and deep cerebellar nuclei (Tzoulis et al., 2006). CT scans may reveal cerebral atrophy, especially in the occipital lobe and posterior temporal lobes. In addition, both cerebrospinal fluid and blood may show elevated levels of lactic acid in patients with Alpers's disease (Gordon, 2006).

Hepatic symptoms may include bile-duct proliferation, steatosis (the abnormal retention of lipids), focal inflammation, fibrosis (formation of excessive connective tissue), and multifocal necrosis (Gordon, 2006; Rasmussen et al., 2000). Depletion of mtDNA in the liver is also associated with Alpers's disease.

Muscle biopsy may show an increase in raggedred fibers, which is an accumulation of diseased mitochondria, suggesting respiratory chain enzyme and mitochondrial involvement. Biopsy may also reveal Cytochrome C oxidase (CCO) negative fibers (Gordon, 2006; Rasmussen et al., 2000). Due to the lack of control data for liver, skin, and muscle biopsies, the most appropriate method of determining the presence of Alpers's disease currently is genetic testing (Horvath et al., 2006).

Neuropathological symptoms include intractable seizures and inconsistent neuronal degeneration of gray matter, especially in the striate cortex, which can result in blindness (Rasmussen et al., 2000). Seizures may be generalized, focal, or myoclonic, and epilepsia partialis continua may be seen (Gordon, 2006). Epilepsia partialis continua is a rare form of seizure disorder involving frequent focal seizures over a period of days or years. Developmental delays, progressive mental deterioration, cortical blindness, hypotonia (low muscle tone), psychomotor regression, ataxia, and spasticity may also be seen (Gordon, 2006; Longley, Graziewicz, Bienstock, & Copeland, 2005).

DIAGNOSIS

Biopsies of the liver and muscle tissue, EEG showing brain patterns distinctive to Alpers's disease, and/or an MRI may help in differential diagnosis, which should include Rasmussen's, lipofuscinosis, mitochondrial myopathy, encephalopathy, and lactic acidosis. Genetic screening from a blood sample showing one of nine known genetic mutations in the POLG1 can conclusively determine the presence of Alpers's disease. However, postmortem brain biopsies may be necessary.

Differential diagnosis should include other neuronal degenerative disorders and mitochondrial dysfunction disorders, including Rasmusson's encephalitis, lipofuscinosis, mitochondrial myopathy, encephalopathy, and lactic acidosis (Gordon, 2006). The presence of epilepsia partialis continua can narrow the differential diagnosis, as it is extremely rare. Although EEG should be used, as Alpers's disease presents with a very specific pattern discussed previously, genetic testing can conclusively determine Alpers's disease if one of the nine known POLG1 mutations are present. However, as unidentified mutations causing Alpers's disease may exist, genetic testing should not be used to conclusively exclude the possibility of the disease (Nguyen et al., 2005).

TREATMENT

Due to liver dysfunction endemic to Alpers's disease and its detrimental effect on hepatic function, valproic acid should be used with extreme caution. Treatment with valproic acid has resulted in fatal liver failure in several patients (Gordon, 2006). Genetic counseling, advice and support may be recommended for the patient's parents. Again, as there are no known ways to slow progression and no cure, treatment primarily consists of palliative care, including supportive counseling for the patient and family.

Further research regarding effective treatment is needed.

Maryellen C. Dougherty
Charles Golden

A

Ferrari, G., Lamantea, E., Donati, A., Filosto, M., Briem, E., Carrara, F., et al. (2005). Infantile hepatocerebral syndromes associated with mutations in the mitochondrial DNA polymerase-γA. *Brain, 128,* 723–731.

Gordon, N. (2006). Alpers syndrome: Progressive neuronal degeneration of children with liver disease. *Developmental Medicine and Child Neurology, 48,* 1001–1003.

Harding, B. N., Alsanjari, N., Smith, S. J., Wiles, C. M., Thrush, D., Miller, D. H., et al. (1995). Progressive neuronal degeneration of childhood with liver disease (Alpers' disease) presenting in young adults. *Journal of Neurology, Neurosurgery, and Psychiatry, 58,* 320–325.

Horvath, R., Hudson, G., Ferrari, G., Fütterer, N., Ahola, S., Lamantea, E., et al. (2006). Phenotypic spectrum associated with mutations of the mitochondrial polymerase γ gene. *Brain, 129,* 1674–1684.

Longley, M. J., Graziewicz, M. A., Bienstock, R. J., & Copeland, W. C. (2005). Consequences of mutations in human DNA polymerase. γ *Gene, 354,* 125–131.

Naviaux, R. K., & Nguyen, K. V. (2004). POLG mutations associated with Alpers' syndrome and mitochondrial DNA depletion. *Annals of Neurology, 55,* 706–712.

Nguyen, K. V., Østergaard, E., Ravn, S. H., Balslev, T., Danielsen, E. R., Vardag, A., et al. (2005). POLG mutations in Alpers syndrome. *Neurology, 65,* 1493–1495.

Rasmussen, M., Sanengen, T., Skullerud, K., Kvittingen, E. A., & Skjeldal, O. H. (2000). Evidence that Alpers-Huttenlocher syndrome could be a mitochondrial disease. *Journal of Child Neurology, 15,* 473–477.

Tzoulis, C., Engelsen, B. A., Telstad, W., Aasly, J., Zeviani, M., Winterthun, S., et al. (2006). The spectrum of clinical disease caused by the A467T and W748S POLG mutations: A study of 26 cases. *Brain, 129,* 1685–1692.

Wiltshire, E., Davidzon, G., DiMauro, S., Akman, H. O., Sadleir, L., Haas, L., et al. (2008). Juvenile Alpers disease. *Archives of Neurology, 65,* 121–124.

ALTERNATING HEMIPLEGIA IN CHILDHOOD

DESCRIPTION

Alternating hemiplegia in childhood (AHC) is a rare disorder that occurs in childhood. This disorder was first described in 1971 by Verret and Steele who reported eight clinical cases in infancy (Bourgeois,

Aicardi, & Goutieres, 1993). Currently, no more than 100 cases have been reported in the literature, and, subsequently, little is known about its etiology or pathophysiology. Onset of the disorder is predominately before 18 months of age.

Early symptoms are characterized by episodic hemi- or quadriplegia that lasts minutes to days and involve either side of the body or shift from one side to the other; other paroxysmal disturbances occur during the hemiplegic bouts or in isolation, and bilateral hemiplegia may be observed. The symptoms immediately abate with sleep and then reappear 10–20 minutes after the child awakens. The severity of the symptoms has preliminarily been shown to decrease with age. However, the child is left with evidence of developmental delay, mental retardation, and neurological abnormalities. (Bassi et al., 2008; Bourgeois et al., 1993; Mikati, Kramer, Zupanc, & Shanahan, 2000; Rinalduzzi, Valeriani, & Vigevano, 2006; Shafer, Mayfield, & McDonald, 2005).

NEUROPATHOLOGY/PATHOPHYSIOLOGY

A few studies have shown a familial component to AHC, but the etiology of the disorder is still unclear. It has been assumed that the pathophysiology of AHC involves an identifiable molecular basis. Therefore, some studies have been done using somatosensory evoked potentials (SEPs) and motor evoked potentials (MEPs) to try to pinpoint the mechanism that causes this disorder. Rinalduzzi et al. (2006) attempted to identify neurophysiological abnormalities at the cerebral cortex and the subcortical structure levels during the interictal phase using SEPs, MEPs, and blink reflex recording.

Their results showed blink reflex abnormalities that were indicative of impaired brainstem circuits and normal function of the motor pathways involved in both the upper and lower limb muscles. To explain their results, they inferred two hypotheses. The first suggests that AHC involves a basal ganglia dysfunction, and the second suggests a similarity between AHC, Huntington's disease, and hemiplegia. These neuropathological results are similar to those of a migraine attack, suggesting that there are similar mechanisms between these two disorders. Some genetic studies have attempted to pinpoint a genetic determination, though this remains unproven (Neville, 2007).

NEUROPSYCHOLOGICAL/CLINICAL PRESENTATION

Few studies have focused on the neuropsychological aspects of AHC. However, current findings have shown developmental delay of some kind in all cases, with significant relationship between age of onset and severity of deficits in intellectual functioning (Shafer et al., 2005). Residual deficits of AHC have been identified to result in ataxia, chorea, hypotonia, as well as delays in language and other psychomotor functioning. Shafer et al. (2005) reported a case study of an 11-year-old girl, first diagnosed with AHC at 18 months, and provided a closer look at typical neuropsychological manifestations in AHC. This child performed at the low-average to borderline range in all neuropsychological assessments. The patient's intellectual performance was in the deficient range, academic abilities significantly impaired, language skills were deficient, memory and manual dexterity were impaired.

Mikati et al. (2000) reported findings of developmental delay being present in 91% of their participants. In conclusion, empirical findings show that children with AHC show a range of intellectual deficit from borderline intelligence, to moderate to severe mental retardation. Furthermore, findings have indicated poorer developmental and neurological abnormalities with early onset (Mikati et al., 2000).

In the long term, there is a wide range of behavioral and psychiatric disorders associated with AHC as well. Common behavioral observations in children with this disorder include impulsivity, lack of attention control, problems with communication, obsession, and short-temperedness (Neville, 2007). There is also risk of mood disorder in these children due to difficulty in adjusting to school and social environments. They are often isolated and rejected by their peers due to frequent attacks. This is especially difficult for patients who have more mild attacks and borderline intelligence. As the child ages, and symptoms become less frequent, the risk of depression and other psychiatric disorders becomes greater (Neville, 2007; Shafer et al., 2005).

DIAGNOSIS

Seven criteria need to be met for diagnosis of AHC. These are (1) onset before 18 months of age; (2) repeated episodes of hemiplegia; (3) episodes of bilateral hemiplegia or quadriplegia (starting as generalization of hemiplegic episode or bilateral); (4) paroxysmal disturbance; (5) the disappearance of symptoms with sleep and recurrence 10–20 minutes after awakening in long-lasting attacks; (6) evidence of developmental delay, learning disability, neurological abnormalities, choreoathetosis, dystonia, or ataxia; and (7) no attribution to another disorder (Neville, 2007). Three distinct phases have been identified from the above-listed symptoms. The first is the presence of abnormal eye movements accompanied by dystonic episodes. The second phase includes the hemiplegic attacks and psychomotor regression. The final phase includes fixed neurologic deficits and persistent developmental delay (Auvin et al., 2005; Bourgeois et al., 1993).

The clinical manifestations of AHC are very similar to those of severe migraine disorder, and it is often misidentified. This strong link may allow for further investigation and understanding of AHC. This disorder has also been linked to other vascular disorders, epilepsy, seizures, movement disorders, and mitochondrial dysfunction. Epilepsy, in particular, coexists with AHC in about 50% of cases (Neville, 2007; Shafer et al., 2005).

AHC is often difficult to identify with neuroimaging at initial presentation. Initial evaluations include routine electroencephalography (EEG), video EEG to identify epileptiform activities during attacks, MRI to rule out lesions, magnetic resonance angiography (MRA) of the head, as well as several laboratory tests that can be done. However, all of the above result in normal or negative findings and no pathognomic lesions of the brain have been identified.

Single-photon emission computed tomography (SPECT) scans have shown promise in identifying AHC. (Bourgeois et al., 1993; Wong-Kisiel, Renaud, Kotagal, & Collins, 2008). SPECT scans performed in ictal and interictal phases show comparable results, with improvement in perfusion shown on the interictal scan. In one case, findings were most evident in the left frontal and parietal regions compared with the right (Wong-Kisiel et al., 2008). This asymmetric perfusion is what is most commonly found in previously reported cases of AHC, as well as familial hemiplegic migraine.

TREATMENT

The nature of AHC and variability of its symptoms make it a difficult disorder to treat and manage. Current clinical treatment trials for AHC have proven to reduce frequency and duration of the attacks, but few cases have successfully obtained complete control. Nevertheless, the treatment of behavioral and neuropsychological manifestations of the disorder has been insufficiently reported in the literature (Bourgeois et al., 1993; Mikati et al., 2000). Generally, treatment plans are made to target clinical manifestations, the cognitive impairments, motor impairments, as well as behavioral and psychiatric implications of the disorder. Successful management of AHC requires a multidisciplinary team and emergency availability as well as an efficient educational setting. Emergency care should be available and easily accessible during severe attacks with admission to a hospital when necessary, such as when the child shows difficulty breathing, maintaining hydration and feeding, risk for chest infection, or epileptic seizures (Neville, 2007).

Medical treatment focuses on avoiding triggers, long-term drug treatment, management of attacks, management of epilepsy, and the use of sleep as a management tactic. Previous studies have reported triggering events in about half of the cases, such as exposure to cold, emotional stress, fatigue, bathing, hyperthermia/hypothermia, and upper respiratory infection (Neville, 2007). Parents may try to avoid these factors, though it is advisable that this tactic be considered on an individual basis in order to avoid negative effect on the child's quality of life.

Cases with epilepsy may be treated with antiepileptic drugs (AEDs). Other common pharmacological treatments include the use of flunarizine. However, though this appears to reduce frequency and duration of attacks, it does not eliminate the attacks completely. In occasional cases, complete control of attacks has been obtained using this drug. Haloperidol has also been effective in some cases (Bourgeois et al., 1993). In the educational setting, it is important for sleeping facilities to be available. Overall, the best treatment for children with AHC would be in a multidisciplinary setting. If the child has epilepsy, a comprehensive epilepsy program would be the best place for managing this disorder. Here, a child can receive occupational and physical therapy for motor treatment, as well as be under the care of a neurologist and other specialists. Furthermore, this setting will allow for access to a psychologist or mental health professional to treat underlying psychiatric issues (Neville, 2007).

Miriam Jocelyn Rodriguez
Charles Golden

Auvin, S., Joriot-Chekaf, S., Cuvellier, J. C., Pandit, F., Cuisset, J. M., Ruchoux, M. M., et al. (2005). Small vessel abnormalities in alternating hemiplegia of childhood: Pathophysiologic implications. *Neurology, 66,* 499–504.

Bassi, M. T., Bresolin, N., Tonelli, A., Nazos, K., Crippa, F., Baschirotto, C., et al. (2008). A novel mutation in the ATP1A2 gene causes alternating hemiplegia of childhood. *Journal of Medical Genetics, 41,* 621–628.

Bourgeois, M., Aicardi, J., & Goutieres, F. (1993). Alternating hemiplegia in childhood. *The Journal of Pediatrics, 122,* 673–679.

Mikati, M. A., Kramer, U., Zupanc, M. L., & Shanahan, R. J. (2000). Alternating hemiplegia of childhood: Clinical manifestations and long-term outcome. *Pediatric Neurology, 23,* 134–141.

Neville, B. G. R. (2007). The treatment and management of alternating hemiplegia of childhood. *Developmental Medicine and Child Neurology, 49,* 777–780.

Rinalduzzi, S., Valeriani, M., & Vigevano, F. (2006). Brainstem dysfunction in alternating hemiplegia of childhood: A neurophysiological study. *Cephalagia, 26*, 511–519.

Shafer, M. E., Mayvield, J. W., & McDonald, F. (2005). Alternating hemiplegia of childhood: A study of neuropsychological functioning. *Applied Neuropsychology, 12*, 49–56.

Wong-Kisiel, L. C., Renaud, D. L., Kotagal, S., & Collins, D. A. (2008). Single-photon emission computed tomography in a child with recurrent alternating hemiplegia and quadriplegia. *Pediatric Neurology, 38*, 221–222.

ALZHEIMER'S DISEASE

DESCRIPTION

In 1907, a psychiatrist by the name of Alois Alzheimer published a brief abstract about a 51-year-old woman named Auguste D. whom he cared for as the attending physician at the Frankfurt Asylum. Modern science currently speculates that this particular case may have represented arteriosclerosis of the brain rather than the neurodegenerative effects of Alzheimer's disease (AD); however, this case provided novel intelligence in the study of neurodegenerative disease (O'Brien, 1996). Dr. Emil Kraeplin, Alzheimer's coworker, named the disease after Alzheimer in a brief report of the morphology of the disease in 1910. Speculation does, however, exist concerning the readiness of Kraeplin to adopt Alzheimer's description of the disease (Fischer, 1907). In 1911, Alzheimer published a more detailed report of Auguste D. and his second case Johann F., who was reported to have become forgetful, could not find his way, could not perform simple tasks, did not bother with food, and exhibited poor hygiene (Graeber et al., 1997). The histological findings from Graeber et al. (1997) yielded morphological results that were in complete agreement with Alzheimer's (1911) paper.

AD is a progressive neurodegenerative disease and is currently the seventh leading cause of death in the United States. It serves as the fifth leading cause of death for those aged 65 and older, and more than 5 million Americans are currently estimated to have AD (Alzheimer's Association, 2008). It is currently the most common in a group of disorders called dementias. AD involves the loss of intellectual, emotional, and social abilities. The most common symptoms apparent with AD include persistent short-term memory deficits, planning and problem-solving deficits, word finding difficulties, decreases in judgment, personality changes, impairments in new learning, and disorientation (Bruen, McGeown, Shanks, & Venneri, 2008; Galton, Patterson, Xuereb, & Hodges, 2000; Greene, Baddeley, & Hodges, 1996; Mckhann et al., 1984). Functional changes are also noticeable with AD and include difficulties with activities of daily living, such as dressing, counting, telling time, concentration, and short-term memory. These abilities may deteriorate markedly as the disease progresses (Weiner, Fields, Hynan, & Cullum, 2008). Other common symptoms of AD are associated with neurodegeneration of specific neural networks supporting personal memory, reality monitoring, processing of reward, interoceptive sensations, and subjective emotional experience (Breun et al., 2008). Research, however, shows that the most prominent and earliest reported neuropsychological impairment of AD is that of anterograde episodic memory (Greene et al., 1996; Welsh, Butters, Hughes, Mohs, & Heyman, 1991).

NEUROPATHOLOGY/PATHOPHYSIOLOGY

The exact cause of AD is not yet known; however, it is speculated to develop from a multitude of factors. The greatest risk factor is advancing age, and the majority of those suffering from AD are age 65 and older (Alzheimer's Association, 2009). AD progresses as healthy brain tissue begins to degenerate causing loss of cognition and mental ability. Neuropathological data suggests that cortical gray matter volume is reduced in Alzheimer's patients. Furthermore, elevated tau protein levels have been linked to the presence of AD, although they are not indicative of severity (Bruen et al., 2009; Haense et al., 2008; Zetterburg, 2008). A decrease in hippocampal volume was also related to AD pathology, along with hippocampal sclerosis (Jagust, Zheng, & Harvey, 2008). Of course, cortical atrophy, neurofibrillary tangles and neuritic plaques, and granulovacuolar degeneration are considered hallmark pathologies of AD. All of these neuropathological processes may converge on similar brain structures making the determination between other dementias and AD very complex.

Current research directed at identification of late-onset AD focuses on various risk factors and apolipoprotein E-e4 (APOE-e4). APOE-e4 found in the CSF is one of three common forms of the *APOE* gene, which provides the blueprint for a protein that carries cholesterol in the bloodstream. The presence of this protein has been shown to correlate with future development of AD (Alzheimer's Association, 2009). The inheritance of this gene does not guarantee that the person will acquire AD; however, those with one or two copies do have a higher risk. Genetic testing is available, but its use is controversial and raises complex ethical questions (Geldmacher & Whitehouse, 1997).

In one study completed by the Consortium to Establish a Registry for Alzheimer's Disease, 20 patients with a postmortem diagnosis based on neuropathological data of pure AD were found to have significant correlations between neuroimaging evidence of temporal horn enlargement and autopsy identified hippocampal atrophy. The same study also found a correlation between the severity of cerebral atrophy determined by neuroimaging and a lower Mini–Mental State Examination (MMSE) score (Fillenbaum et al., 2008). Furthermore, functional magnetic resonance imaging (fMRI) studies of mild cognitive impairment (MCI) and AD have revealed abnormalities in memory circuit function in patients suffering from memory disorders (Dickerson & Sperling, 2008). Current research shows that a reduction in temporoparietal metabolism has been correlated with AD by using PET and SPECT.

NEUROPSYCHOLOGICAL/CLINICAL PRESENTATION

AD is widely considered to be clinically consistent with a characteristic profile of neuropsychological deficits (Grossman, Bergman, & Parker, 2006; Locascio, Growdon, & Corkin, 1995; Morris et al., 1989). Episodic memory complaints were the primary feature, with subsequent involvement of attentional, language, semantic, and visuospatial abilities in most cases (Galton et al., 2000). Persons suffering from various stages of AD often present with decreased attention/concentration, learning, recall, and language (word finding) difficulties. They also exhibit problems with executive function (problem solving) and visuospatial abilities.

AD research has largely concentrated on the study of cognitive decline, but the associated behavioral and neuropsychiatric symptoms are of equal importance in the clinical profile of the disease (Bruen et al., 2009). Behavior and personality changes are prominent with Alzheimer's patients, most commonly with lapses of judgment. Recent research also suggests that a low conscientiousness (as measured by the NEO Five-Factor Inventory) may be correlated with an increased incidence in AD; however, research of this nature is limited and thus should be interpreted with caution (Wilson, Schneider, Arnold, Bienias, & Bennett, 2007). Dependency on caregivers, denial of illness, and motor agitation

are very common, whereas sexual disinhibition and self-destructive behaviors are rare. Behavioral disinhibition, apathy, and indifference tend to increase with greater severity of AD. Catastrophic reactions, aggression, and agitation were also associated with greater functional impairment (Devanand et al., 1992). Considering the behavioral correlates of AD, many clinicians find it tough to differentially diagnose AD, depression, and other dementias.

MCI, particularly of the amnestic type, is considered a prodromal stage of AD and is a condition defined by deficit in one domain (memory, language, or other essential cognitive function) that is severe enough to show up on cognitive tests but not severe enough to interfere with daily life (Alzheimer's Association, 2009). Furthermore, some, but not all of those diagnosed with MCI will progress to AD later in life. A diagnosis of AD carries a typical prognosis of 8–10 years from the diagnosis and not necessarily from when symptomatology is first observed. Stages post-diagnosis may assist clinicians in pinpointing the severity of the illness in a particular patient. Unfortunately, neuropathological studies also show that though this classic staging may fit the majority of cases, a significant percentage do not adhere to this orderly pattern (Gertz et al., 1998). Positively, a more recent study presented in 2008 by Fillenbaum et al. showed that clinical history and age-related neuritic plaque counts could indicate levels of certainty (definite, probable, possible, or no evidence) in the diagnosis of AD. Using histological diagnosis as the gold standard, current research criteria are accurate in up to 90% of cases (McKhann et al., 1984). The final diagnosis of AD must be made postmortem with a microscopic examination of brain tissue to check for plaques and tangles.

DIAGNOSIS

Due to atypical presentations, the diagnosis of AD is often complicated and definitive diagnosis is not usually made until postmortem. "An obvious point, but one that is frequently overlooked, is that it is the distribution of pathology rather than the nature of the disease that is reflected in the clinical syndrome" (Galton et al., 2000). Accurate diagnosis of dementia is essential to provide appropriate treatment as well as patient and family counseling. Routine diagnostic steps include a combination of history, mental status screening, blood work, imaging studies, and neuropsychological testing. Differential diagnosis of AD may be difficult between other types of dementia, delirium, depression, drug interactions, or other psychiatric disorders. Consequently, the diagnostic procedure often involves ruling out other causes of

A

memory loss such as stroke, metabolic changes, vitamin deficiencies, or anticholinergic medication. Blood and urine tests can be employed to rule out vitamin deficiencies or thyroid problems; however, the rest may be more difficult to tease apart. Unfortunately, the profiles of both typical and atypical presentations can appear focal in nature for many years before inevitable deterioration.

As suggested previously, neuroimaging can prove quite useful in diagnosing AD, although clinical determinations are usually limited to reporting "probable" AD in lieu of a definitive conclusion. However, when used in combination with a detailed history and neuropsychological data, diagnostic conclusions are quite accurate. Neuroradiological techniques utilize CT, MRI, fMRI, or PET and allow doctors to pinpoint visible abnormalities (Bozzao, Floris, Baviera, Apruzzese, & Simonetti, 2001; Dickerson & Sperling, 2008; Weiner et al., 2008). Functional neuroimaging has also been reported to be useful for the clinical assessment of cases with possible or probable AD. Furthermore, perfusion MRI studies have proven successful at differentiating patients with possible or probable AD (Bozzao et al., 2001).

Neuropsychological tests provide confirmatory evidence of the diagnosis of AD and help to assess the course and response to therapy (Jacova, Kertesz, Blair, Fisk, & Feldman, 2007; McKahnn et al., 1984). When neuropsychological testing is part of a comprehensive assessment, there is good evidence that it can be a key factor in decisions between MCI and dementia, including the determination of functional and vocational impact as well as cognitive abilities and opportunities for cognitive rehabilitation (Jacova et al., 2007). Primary screening measures such as the MMSE and the Montreal Cognitive Assessment are often used to obtain a baseline of functioning. These tests briefly measure memory, problem-solving abilities, attention, language, concentration, and drawing. Although a diagnosis cannot be made from these tasks, a score below the mean on either should prompt subsequent investigation.

Further neuropsychological assessment typically includes Clock Drawing, Verbal Fluency (FAS), California Verbal Learning Test-II, Cambridge Behavioral Inventory, Rey Auditory Verbal Learning Test, Boston Naming Test, Repeatable Battery for the Assessment of Neuropsychological Status, and Wechsler Memory Scale-III. These tests measure more specific abilities including semantic and categorical memory, visuospatial abilities, executive functions, language, attention, praxis, and psychomotor speed (Balthazar, Figueredo, Fernando, & Pereira, 2008; Duff et al., 2008; Gainotti, Ferraccioli, Vita, & Marra, 2008). Recent studies show that for AD patients, correlations range from 0.80 to 0.91 for measures of verbal fluency, The Boston Naming Test, MMSE, Word List Learning, and Constructional Praxis (Fillenbaum et al., 2008). Neuropsychological assessment should assist in diagnosing AD by further defining cognitive strengths and weaknesses in learning, memory, problem solving, executive function, visuospatial and language abilities as well as behavioral facets.

TREATMENT

To date, there is no cure for AD; however, the earlier the disease is discovered, the better the prognosis for treatment. The FDA-approved drugs — cholinesterase inhibitors (donepezil, rivastigmine, galantamine) and an N-methyl-D-aspartate receptor antagonist (memantine) — for the treatment of AD are symptomatically effective in some patients for short periods of time (Keowkase & Luo, 2008). Cholinesterase inhibitors exert additional pharmacological action beyond inhibition of cholinesterase that may maximize and prolong the effect of these drugs. The complexity of AD pathogenesis limits these drugs to correct every aspect of the disease (Keowkase & Luo, 2008). Medication can slow the progression of AD in most cases; therefore, caregivers and a comprehensive biopsychosocial interdisciplinary approach must be in place to maintain the health of an AD patient.

Aside from medication, interventions for the treatment of AD can include cognitive rehabilitation of memory problems and/or behavioral strategies. Cognitive rehabilitation involves activity planning, self-assertiveness training, relaxation techniques, stress management, use of external memory aids, memory training, and motor exercise (Kurz, Pohl, Ramsenthaler, & Sorg, 2009). Unfortunately, the existing literature is limited by a lack of consensus on what constitutes the most effective type of cognitive training, insufficient follow-up times, a lack of matched active controls, and few outcome measures showing changes in daily functioning, global cognitive skills, or progression to early AD (Papp, Walsh, & Snyder, 2009). There are also multiple behavioral strategies such as increased activity levels to reduce boredom and redirecting problem behavior without criticism that can assist in dealing with problems associated with AD.

Significant cost implications related to AD and other dementias include an estimated $148 billion in direct (Medicare/Medicaid) and indirect cost (caregiver lost wages and out-of-pocket expenses and decreased business productivity costs) not to mention the estimated $89 billion in unpaid services to those with AD by caregivers (Alzheimer's Association, 2008). The following are often involved in the care of an elder: physician consultation, monthly medical clinic visits, medication management, home health care, planned social activities, and psychiatric and neuropsychological services such as cognitive rehabilitation. Other variables must be considered including patients' enabling, need, predisposing characteristics, family considerations, and organization affiliation. Significant predictors for success include previous service use, patient functioning, family characteristics, and the specific center recommending the service (Ginther, Webber, Fox, & Miller, 1994).

Tiffany L. Cummings
Frank M. Webbe
Antonio E. Puente

Alzheimer, A. (1911). Uber eigenartige Krankheitsfalle des spateren Alters. *Zeitschrift fur die Gesamte Neurologie und Psychiatrie, 4*, 356–386.

Alzheimer's Association. (2008). 2008 Alzheimer's disease facts and figures. *Alzheimer's & Dementia, 4*, 110–133.

Alzheimer's Association. (2009). 2009 Alzheimer's disease facts and figures. *Alzheimer's & Dementia, 5*, 3, 234–270.

Balthazar, M., Figueredo, L., Fernando, C., & Pereira, D. P. (2008). Semantic error patterns on the Boston Naming Test in normal aging, amnestic mild cognitive impairment, and mild Alzheimer's disease: Is there semantic disruption? *Neuropsychology, 22*, 6, 703–709.

Bozzao, A., Floris, R., Baviera, M. E., Apruzzese, A., & Simonetti, G. (2001). Diffusion and Perfusion MR imaging in cases of Alzheimer's disease: Correlations with cortical atrophy and lesion load. *American Journal of Neuroradiology, 22*, 1030–1036.

Bruen, P., McGeown, W., Shanks, M., & Venneri, A. (2008). Neuroanatomical correlates of neuropsychiatric symptoms in Alzheimer's disease. *Brain: A Journal of Neurology, 131*, 9, 2455–2463.

Devanand, D. P., Brockington, C. D., Moody, B. J., Brown, R. P., Mayeux, R., Endicott, J., et al. (1992). Behavioral syndromes in Alzheimer's disease. *International Psychogeriatrics, 4*, 161–184.

Dickerson, B., & Sperling, R. (2008). Functional abnormalities of the medial temporal lobe memory system in mild cognitive impairment and Alzheimer's disease: Insights from functional MRI studies. *Neuropsychologia, 46*, 6, 1624–1635. Retrieved February 22, 2009, doi:10.1016/j.neuropsychologia.2007.11.030

Duff, K., Humphreys Clark, J., O'Bryant, S., Mold, J., Schiffer, R., & Sutker, P. (2008). Utility of the RBANS in detecting cognitive impairment associated with Alzheimer's disease: Sensitivity, specificity, and positive and negative predictive powers. *Archives of Clinical Neuropsychology, 23*, 5, 603–612. Retrieved February 22, 2009, doi:10.1016/j.acn.2008.06.004

Fillenbaum, G. G., Belle, G., Morris, J. C., Mohs, R. C., Mirra, S. S., Davis, P. C., et.al. (2008). Consortium to establish a registry for Alzheimer's disease (CERAD): The first twenty years. *Alzheimer's and Dementia, 4*, 96–109.

Fischer, O. (1907). Miliare Nekrosen mit drusigen Wucherungen de Neurofibrillen, eine regelmassige Veranderung der Hirnrinde bei senile Demenz. *Monatssachr Psychiatry Neurology, 22*, 361–372.

Gainotti, G., Ferraccioli, M., Vita, M. G., & Marra, C. (2008). Patterns of neuropsychological impairment in MCI patients with small subcortical infarcts or hippocampal atrophy. *Journal of the International Neuropsychological Society, 14*, 4, 611–619.

Galton, C. J., Patterson, K., Xuereb, J. H., & Hodges, J. H. (2000). Atypical and typical presentations of Alzheimer's disease: A clinical, neuropsychological, neuroimaging and pathological study of 13 cases. *Brain, 123*, 3, 484–498.

Geldmacher, D. S., & Whitehouse, P. J., Jr. (1997). Differential diagnosis of Alzheimer's disease. *Neurology, 48*, 5 and 6, 2–9.

Gertz, H. J., Xuereb, J., Huppert, F., Brayne, C., McGee, M. A., Paykel, E., et al. (1998). Examination of the validity of the hierarchical model of neuropathological staging in normal aging and Alzheimer's disease. *Neuropathology, 95*, 154–158.

Ginther, S. D., Webber, P., Fox, P., & Miller, L. (1994). A preliminary study of medical services for persons with Alzheimer's disease: Recommendations by California's Alzheimer's diagnostic and treatment program staff. *Journal of Gerontological Social Work, 21*, 3/4, 27–29.

Graeber, M. B., Kosel, S., Egensperger, R., Banati, R. B., Müller, U., Bise, K., et al. (1997). Rediscovery of the case described by Alois Alzheimer in 1911: Historical, histological and molecular genetic analysis. *Neurogenetics, 1*, 1, 73–80.

Greene, J. D., Baddeley, A. D., & Hodges, J. R. (1996). Analysis of the episodic memory deficit in early Alzheimer's disease: Evidence from the doors and people test. *Neuropsychologia, 34*, 537–551.

Grossman, H., Bergman, C., & Parker, S. (2006). Dementia: A brief review. *The Mount Sinai Journal of Medicine, 73*, 7, 985–992.

Haense, C., Buerger, K., Kalbe, E., Drzezga, A., Teipel, S. J., Markiewicz, P., et al. (2008). CSF total and phosphorylated tau protein, regional glucose metabolism and dementia severity in Alzheimer's disease. *European Journal of Neurology, 15*, 1155–1162.

Jacova, C., Kertesz, A., Blair, M., Fisk, J. D., & Feldman, H. H. (2007). Neuropsychological testing and assessment for dementia. *Alzheimer's & Dementia, 3*, 299–317.

Jagust, W. J., Zheng, L., & Harvey, D. J. (2008). Neuropsychological basis of magnetic resonance images in aging and dementia. *Annals of Neurology, 63*, 1, 72–80.

Keowkase, R., & Luo, Y. (2008). Mechanism of CNS drugs and their contributions for Alzheimer's disease: Central nervous system agents. *Medicinal Chemistry, 8*, 4, 241–248.

Kurz, A., Pohl, C., Ramsenthaler, M., & Sorg, C. (2009). Cognitive rehabilitation in patients with mild cognitive impairment. *International Journal of Geriatric Psychiatry, 24,* 2, 163–168. *MEDLINE*, EBSCOhost. Retrieved April 8, 2009.

Locascio, J. J., Growdon, J. H., & Corkin, J. (1995). Cognitive test performance in detecting, staging and tracking Alzheimer's disease. *Archives of Neurology, 52,* 1087–1099.

McKhann, G., Drachman, D., Folstein, M., Katzman, R., Price, D., & Stadlan, E. M. (1984). Clinical diagnosis of Alzheimer's disease: Report of the NINCDS-ADRDA Work Group under the auspices of the Department of Health and Human Services Task Force on Alzheimer's Disease. *Neurology, 34,* 939–944.

Morris, J. C., Heyman, A., Mohs, R. C., Hughes, J. P., van Belle, G., Fillenbaum, G., et al. (1989). The Consortium to Establish a Registry for Alzheimer's disease (CERAD). Part I. Clinical and neuropsychological assessment of Alzheimer's disease. *Neurology, 39,* 1159–1165.

O'Brien, C. (1996). Auguste D. and Alzheimer's disease. *Science, 273,* 28.

Papp, K. V., Walsh, S. J., & Snyder, P. J. (2009). Immediate and delayed effects of cognitive interventions in healthy elderly: A review of current literature and future directions. *Alzheimer's & Dementia: The Journal of the Alzheimer's Association, 5,* 1, 50–60. *MEDLINE*, EBSCOhost. Retrieved April 8, 2009.

Weiner, M., Fields, J., Hynan, L., & Cullum, C. M. (2008). Annualized functional change in Alzheimer's disease participants and normal controls. *Clinical Neuropsychology, 22,* 5, 801–806.

Welsh, K., Butters, N., Hughes, J., Mohs, R., & Heyman, A. (1991). Detection of abnormal memory decline in mild cases of Alzheimer's disease using CERAD neuropsychological measures. *Archives of Neurology, 48,* 278–281.

Wilson, R. S., Schneider, J. A., Arnold, S. E., Bienias, J. L., & Bennett, D. A. (2007). Conscientiousness and the incidence of Alzheimer's disease and MCI. *Archives of Gerontological Psychiatry, 64,* 10, 1204–1212.

Zetterberg, H. (2008). Biomarkers reflecting different facets of Alzheimer's disease. *European Journal of Neurology, 15,* 11, 1143–1144.

AMYOTROPHIC LATERAL SCLEROSIS

DESCRIPTION

Amyotrophic lateral sclerosis (ALS) is a fatal neurodegenerative disease that results in severe muscular atrophy and eventual paralysis (Cluskey & Ramsden, 2001; Irwin, Lippa, & Swearer, 2007; Lewis & Rushanan, 2007). The most common variant of adult-onset motor neuron disease, ALS presents with an annual incidence between 1 and 3 in 100,000 of the general population (Blumenfeld, 2002; Strong & Rosenfeld, 2003) and a prevalence of approximately 5 in 100,000 (Schefner, 2006). Comparatively, males are at slightly increased risk for the disease than females (Rowland, 2003; Shoesmith & Strong, 2006) with onset typically occurring in mid-to-late adulthood, with a mean age of onset in the 50s (Roman, 1996; Strong, Grace, Orange, & Leeper, 1996). The disease affects individuals of all races and ethnic backgrounds (Rowland & Schneider, 2001), with several isolated areas in the world demonstrating increased incidence, especially areas in the western Pacific, such as Guam (Galasko et al., 2007; Roman, 1996; Rowland & Schneider, 2001). Symptoms progress fairly rapidly and without remission, typically resulting in death within 3–5 years of diagnosis (Rowland & Schneider, 2001; Shoesmith & Strong, 2006) from respiratory failure (Mitsumoto & Rabkin, 2007; Newsom-Davis, Lyall, Leigh, Moxham, & Goldstein, 2001).

NEUROPATHOLOGY/PATHOPHYSIOLOGY

ALS involves complex pathology that targets upper motor neurons including the large pyramidal neurons and Betz cells in the motor cortex and associated corticospinal tracts, as well as the lower motor neurons originating in the brainstem and the anterior horn of the spinal cord that connect to the muscles (Bromberg, 2002; Wong, Rothstein, & Price, 1998). In comparison, motor neurons in the oculomotor, trochlear, and abducens cranial nerve nuclei are spared (Goetz, 2000; Kunst, 2004). Neurons in Onuf's nucleus, which controls urethral and sphincter function, are only slightly affected (Bergmann, Volpel & Kuchelmeister, 1995).

ALS can be divided into sporadic and familial forms with sporadic being the most common form, occurring in approximately 90% of affected individuals (Irwin et al., 2007; Mitsumoto & Rabkin, 2007; Roman, 1996). The causes of sporadic ALS are not clear. Case control studies have found increased risk among rural populations of lower socioeconomic level and in occupations involving manual labor and physical activity, such as agricultural and farm work and welding (Roman, 1996). It is thought that certain individuals may possess a genetic predisposition to developing motor neuron disease that is expressed under the right environmental conditions, such as exposure to excitotoxins or chemicals (Roman, 1996). Familial forms, which comprise 5% to 10% of individuals with ALS (Irwin et al., 2007; Phukan, Pender, & Hardiman 2007; Rowland & Schneider, 2001), tend to follow an autosomal dominant inheritance pattern, though there are recessive forms that are rarer. Mutations in the *SOD1* gene, which codes for Cu/Zn superoxide dismutase, are thought to affect approximately 20% of patients with familial ALS (Gaudette, Hirano, & Siddique, 2000). Research evidence indicates that the *SOD1* mutations result in a gain of cytotoxicity (Clusky & Ramsden, 2001). Cytotoxic mechanisms possibly associated with *SOD1* mutations include possible dysfunction in neuronal copper chelation, increased production of potentially damaging reactive oxygen species (e.g., O_2, OH, H_2O_2), increased glutamate concentration, impaired mitochondrial function, and aberrant protein aggregation (Cluskey & Ramsden, 2001; Wong et al., 1998). Associated cellular damage includes axonal swelling with neurofilamentous accumulations, Golgi apparatus fragmentation, mitochondrial degeneration, cytoplasmic neuronal inclusions, and Wallerian degeneration (Cluskey & Ramsden, 2001; Rowland & Schneider, 2001; Wong et al., 1998). Axonal swellings filled with neurofilaments observed in muscle biopsy specimens from early stage ALS suggest that neurofilament disarrangement may be an early pathological step (Bromberg, 2002). It is thought that ALS starts as a disease of upper motor neuron dysfunction that secondarily causes death of lower motor neurons (Eisen, Kim, & Pant, 1992). Dysfunction of cortical inhibitory neurons leads to excess glutamate at synaptic connections onto upper motor neurons and subsequent overactivity and excess glutamate at the synapse between upper and lower motor neurons (Enterzari-Taher, Eisen, Stewart, & Nakajima, 1997). It is important to note that no clinical or electrophysiological features distinguish sporadic from familial ALS (Bromberg, 2002).

Neuroimaging studies have yielded mixed results regarding the presence of cortical atrophy in ALS. Some studies have demonstrated no difference in total brain volume of gray or white matter, nor in gray matter volume in the precentral gyrus, in ALS patients in comparison with control participants (Ellis et al., 2001; Toft, Gredal, & Pakkenberg, 2005), as well as no difference in the average number of neurons in the neocortex or the motor cortex between ALS patients and control participants (Gredal, Pakkenberg, Karlsborg, & Pakkenberg, 2000; Toft et al., 2005). Conversely, other studies have demonstrated reduced gray matter volume in the pre and postcentral gyrus in ALS patients, as well as in extended areas, such as the frontal lobe (Chang et al., 2005; Grosskreutz et al., 2006). Several studies utilizing proton magnetic resonance spectroscopy looking at the motor cortex of ALS patients have shown a decrease in the absolute in vivo concentrations of a metabolite, N-acetyl aspartate, considered to be an indicator of neural integrity, which suggests either neuronal loss or dysfunction in the motor cortex (Giroud et al., 1996; Gredal et al., 1997; Pioro, Antel, Cashman, & Arnold, 1994; Pohl et al., 2001; Rooney et al., 1998). Some evidence suggests that a change in cell body shape rather than a loss of neurons occurs in ALS (Kiernan & Hudson, 1993). White matter reductions within motor and nonmotor areas have been found to be more extensive in cognitively impaired than unimpaired ALS patients (Abrahams et al., 2005). Regional cerebral glucose utilization studies using positron emission tomography have shown that glucose metabolism is significantly reduced in the frontal and entire cortex of ALS patients compared with controls, and that these patients also demonstrate mild frontal dysfunction on neuropsychological tests (Ludolph et al., 1992). Other studies also have demonstrated atrophy of the frontal lobe and hypometabolism in the frontotemporal regions of the cortex (Jeong et al., 2005; Talbot et al., 1995), as well as the dorsolateral prefrontal cortex (Kew et al., 1993a, 1993b), along with associated cognitive impairments in patients with ALS. Interestingly, other neuropathological correlates associated with cognitive decline are similar to what is found in frontotemporal dementia (FTD) and include neuronal loss in the frontal and temporal regions, as well as superficial linear spongiosis and ubiquitinated tau-negative and synuclein-negative intraneuronal inclusions (Gallassi et al., 1985; Yoshida, 2004).

NEUROPSYCHOLOGICAL/CLINICAL PRESENTATION

Until recently, it was widely believed that cognitive abilities were relatively preserved in ALS (Jokelainen, 1977a, 1977b; Strong et al., 1996). In the past few decades, a preponderance of evidence suggests that measureable cognitive impairments do exist in a relatively large percentage of individuals with ALS. Estimates vary widely, likely due to differing criteria used to define cognitive impairment and variability in selected samples and tests administered, as well as confounding variables such as motor slowing and dysarthria (Neumann & Kotchoubey, 2004) and reduced respiration (Kim et al., 2007; Newsom-Davis et al., 2001). Generally, rates of measurable cognitive impairment range from 36% (Massman et al., 1996) to 55% (Abe et al., 1997) of the ALS population, although estimates have varied as widely as 10% (Poloni, Capitani, Mazzini, & Ceroni, 1986) to 75% (Frank, Haas, Heinze, Stark, & Munte, 1997). A number of reviews exist summarizing the literature (Irwin et al., 2007;

A

Neary, Snowden, & Mann, 2000; Phukan et al., 2007; Strong et al., 1996; Woolley & Katz, 2008). The most frequently noted impairments appear consistent with frontal lobe dysfunction. Deficits in verbal fluency have been most commonly reported (Abe et al., 1997; Abrahams et al., 2005; Gallassi et al., 1985; Kew et al., 1993a; Ludolph et al., 1992; Massman et al., 1996; Strong et al., 1996). Deficits also have been reported in cognitive flexibility (Abe et al., 1997; Abrahams et al., 1997; Lomen-Hoerth et al., 2003; Massman et al., 1996), attention (Abe et al., 1997; Frank et al., 1997; Massman et al., 1996; Ringholz et al., 2005), naming (Abe et al., 1997; Abrahams et al., 2004; Ringholz et al., 2005), and, to a more variable degree, learning and memory (Frank et al., 1997; Kew et al., 1993a; Ringholz et al., 2005). Cognitive deficits often remain even when the need for motor or speeded responding is controlled (Abrahams et al., 1997, 2000; Neary et al., 2000; Ringholz et al., 2005). In reviewing the current literature, Woolley and Katz (2008) found that studies using more stringent criteria to define "cognitive impairment," namely requiring performance on two or more measures to fall below the fifth percentile, still demonstrated a rate of impairment around 50% in ALS populations.

In the majority of individuals with ALS demonstrating cognitive impairment, deficits are subtle (Gallassi et al., 1985; Phukan et al., 2007; Ringholz et al., 2005; Rottig et al., 2006; Strong et al., 1996). Estimates of those with ALS meeting criteria for frank dementia range from 15% to 41% (Woolley & Katz, 2008). Approximately 5% of individuals with ALS demonstrate more significant cognitive impairment consistent with FTD, a common manifestation of frontotemporal lobar degeneration characterized by changes in personality, apathy, poor insight, disturbance in eating and sleep, disinhibition and impulsivity, stereotyped behavior, poverty of speech, and pervasive impairments in executive functioning (Lomen-Hoerth et al., 2003; Neary et al., 1998; Phukan et al., 2007; Woolley & Katz, 2008). FTD is associated with focal degeneration of the frontal and temporal neocortex (Neary et al., 2000). Although longitudinal studies are sparse due to the rapid progression of the disease and significant limitations in communication in the later stages, several studies have found that cognitive decline progresses more slowly than decline in motor functioning (Abrahams, Leigh, & Goldstein, 2005; Schreiber et al., 2005).

Depression may be prevalent to varying degrees in the ALS population, although it does not account for cognitive deficits observed in some ALS patients (Irwin et al., 2007). Estimates of the percent of individuals with ALS experiencing depressive symptoms vary widely from study to study. In the few studies that have utilized structured clinical interviews, approximately 9% to 11% of individuals with ALS have met criteria for clinical depression (Kurt, Nijboer, Matuz, & Kubler, 2007; Rowland & Schneider, 2001). Anxiety in the ALS population is not well studied, and prevalence rates vary widely across studies, ranging from 0% to 30% (Kurt et al., 2007).

DIAGNOSIS

There is no clearly established test for diagnosing ALS (Mitsumoto & Rabkin, 2007). A diagnosis can only be determined with absolute certainty after death, with a pathologic examination (Irwin et al., 2007). The most viable diagnostic methods include physical examination by a neurologist and ruling out other potential conditions, such as other motor neuron diseases, structural disorders, metabolic and toxic disorders, immune and inflammatory disorders, hereditary neurologic disorders, infectious disorders, and other central nervous system (CNS) degenerative disorders (Shoesmith & Strong, 2006).

The El Escorial World Federation of Neurology (WFN) established criteria for the diagnosis of ALS in 1994 for the purpose of identifying individuals appropriate for clinical research inclusion and have since been adopted for clinical use (Brooks, 1994). These criteria were reviewed at a subsequent WFN meeting in 1998, resulting in a limited number of revisions (Brooks et al., 2000). Based on these criteria, the diagnosis of ALS requires the presence of (1) signs of lower motor neuron degeneration by clinical, electrophysiological, or neuropathologic examination, (2) signs of upper motor neuron degeneration by clinical examination, and (3) progressive spread of signs within a CNS region or to other regions, (4) along with no evidence of other disease processes that might explain the lower or upper motor neuron degeneration as suggested by electrophysiological or neuroimaging studies. The criteria are stratified into four levels of diagnostic certainty including definite, probable, possible, and suspected ALS. Clinical signs of upper motor neuron loss include labile emotional affect, forced yawning, exaggerated shout reflex, pathological jaw jerk, pathological gag reflex, spastic tone to passive limb movements, pathological tendon reflexes, preserved tendon reflexes in weak and atrophic limbs, clonus, Hoffmann responses, and extensor plantar responses. Clinical signs of lower motor neuron loss include muscle weakness, muscle atrophy, and fasciculations (Brooks et al., 2000).

In approximately 60% to 80% of affected individuals, initial symptoms may include muscle weakness and clumsiness, muscle cramping, spasticity, and fasciculations in the extremities (Mitsumoto & Rabkin, 2007; Rowland & Schneider, 2001), referred to as limb or spinal-onset ALS. A smaller percentage of individuals initially experience bulbar symptoms, such as dysarthria, dysphagia, or breathing difficulties (Blumenfeld, 2002), referred to as bulbar-onset ALS. Hyperreflexia, clonus, and Babinski and Hoffman signs may be noted on neurological examination, and symptoms tend to start locally and then progress to other regions (Rowland & Schneider, 2001). Most large motor muscles eventually become incapacitated, with the exception of oculomotor control and bladder and sphincter function (Mitsumoto & Rabkin, 2007; Shoesmith & Strong, 2006). Thus, patients often are able to communicate with eye movements when other methods of communication become compromised (Blumenfeld, 2002; Lakerveld, Kotchoubey, & Kubler, 2008; Kotchoubey, Lang, Winter, & Birbaumer, 2003). Phenotypic variants include progressive bulbar palsy, progressive muscular atrophy (lower motor syndrome), and primary lateral sclerosis (upper motor syndrome).

TREATMENT

There is no known cure for ALS. Given its rapid progression and fatal prognosis, end-of-life decisions should be made in the early stages (McCluskey, 2007a). Palliative care ultimately may be necessary, and a multidisciplinary or interdisciplinary approach often is recommended to provide comprehensive care, manage physical, spiritual, and emotional issues, and improve quality of life (McCluskey, 2007b; Mitsumoto & Rabkin, 2007; Shoesmith & Strong, 2006). Multidisciplinary clinics of care specializing in ALS exist throughout North America. Professionals contributing to care may include neurologists and/or physiatrists, nurses, occupational and physical therapists, speech language pathologists, dieticians, respiratory therapists, social workers, and mental health professionals, among others (Carter & Miller, 1998; Mitsumoto & Rabkin, 2007). Physical and occupational therapists can assist in maintaining an optimal level of independence for as long as possible. Treatment may include providing appropriate exercise plans, training/education, and equipment to assist with ambulation and mobility, transfers, dressing, showering, and support of weakened limbs and neck (Lewis & Rushanan, 2007). Speech language pathologists can assist with communication devices. Percutaneous endoscopic gastrostomy, nasogastric tube placement, or radiologically inserted gastrostomy may be necessary to ensure nutritional maintenance secondary to dysphagia (Radunovic, Mitsumoto, & Leigh, 2007). Once respiratory muscles weaken to the point where objective measures of forced vital capacity fall below 50% predicted, noninvasive ventilation is recommended (Miller et al., 1999). This can prolong a patient's life approximately 12–18 months (Bourke et al., 2006). Ultimately, long-term mechanical ventilation may need to be considered, although there is disagreement regarding this treatment, as patients may reach a "locked in" state and be unable to communicate their wishes (Lakerveld et al., 2008; Mitsumoto & Rabkin, 2007). Another consideration in long-term planning is the capacity of the individual to make medical and end-of-life decisions, secondary to cognitive deficits (McCluskey, 2007a; Phukan et al., 2007).

Regarding recommended medications, Riluzole is the only medication approved in the United States by the FDA for treatment of ALS. This medication can extend ALS patients' lives up to 2 months (Miller, Mitchell, Lyon, & Moore, 2007). In treating depressive symptoms, few standards exist, although selective serotonin reuptake inhibitors and tricyclic antidepressants tend to be the drugs of choice among treatment clinics (Kurt et al., 2007). Symptoms of anxiety tend to be treated with buspirone and benzodiazepines (Kurt et al., 2007). Efforts to better understand the mechanisms underlying this devastating disease are ongoing.

Melanie Blahnik
Kathryn McGuire

Abe, K., Fujimura, H., Toyooka, K., Sakoda, S., Yorifuji, S., & Yanagihara, T. (1997). Cognitive function in amyotrophic lateral sclerosis. *Journal of the Neurological Sciences, 148*(1), 95–100.

Abrahams, S., Goldstein, L. H., Al-Chalabi, A., Pickering, A., Morris, R. G., Passingham, R. E., et al. (1997). Relation between cognitive dysfunction and pseudobulbar palsy in amyotrophic lateral sclerosis. *Journal of Neurology, Neurosurgery, and Psychiatry, 62*(5), 464–472.

Abrahams, S., Goldstein, L. H., Simmons, A., Brammer, M., Williams, S. C., Giampietro, V., et al. (2004). Word retrieval in amyotrophic lateral sclerosis: A functional magnetic resonance imaging study. *Brain: A Journal of Neurology, 127*(7), 1507–1517.

Abrahams, S., Goldstein, L. H., Suckling, J., Ng, V., Simmons, A., Chitnis, X., et al (2005). Frontotemporal white matter changes in amyotrophic lateral sclerosis. *Journal of Neurology, 252,* 321–331.

Abrahams, S., Leigh, P. N., & Goldstein, L. H. (2005). Cognitive change in ALS: A prospective study. *Neurology, 64*(7), 1222–1226.

Abrahams, S., Leigh, P. N., Harvey, A., Vythelingum, G. N., Grise, D., & Goldstein, L. H. (2000). Verbal fluency and executive dysfunction in amyotrophic lateral sclerosis (ALS). *Neuropsychologia, 38*(6), 734–747.

Bergmann, M., Volpel, M. & Kuchelmeister, K. (1995). Onuf's nucleus is frequently involved in motor neuron disease/amyotrophic lateral sclerosis. *Journal of Neurological Science, 129,* 141–146.

Blumenfeld, H. (2002). Corticospinal tract and other motor pathways. *Neuroanatomy through clinical cases* (pp. 231–243). Sunderland, MA: Sinauer Associates.

Bourke, S. C., Tomlinson, M., Williams, T. L., Bullock, R. E., Shaw, P. J., & Gibson, G. J. (2006). Effects of non-invasive ventilation on survival and quality of life in patients with amyotrophic lateral sclerosis: A randomised controlled trial. *Lancet Neurology, 5*(2), 140–147.

Bromberg, M. (2002). Amyotrophic lateral sclerosis. In W. F. Brown, C. F. Bolton, & M. J. Aminoff (Eds.), *Neuromuscular function and disease: Basic, clinical, and electrodiagnostic aspects* (Vol. 2, pp. 1307–1325). Philadelphia: Saunders.

Brooks, B. R. (1994). El Escorial World Federation of Neurology criteria for the diagnosis of amyotrophic lateral sclerosis: Subcommittee on motor neuron diseases/amyotrophic lateral sclerosis of the World Federation of Neurology Research Group on neuromuscular diseases and the El Escorial "Clinical limits of amyotrophic lateral sclerosis" workshop contributors. *Journal of the Neurological Sciences, 124*(Suppl.), 96–107.

Brooks, B. R., Miller, R. G., Swash, M., Munsat, T. L., & World Federation of Neurology Research Group on Motor Neuron Diseases. (2000). El escorial revisited: Revised criteria for the diagnosis of amyotrophic lateral sclerosis. *Amyotrophic Lateral Sclerosis and Other Motor Neuron Disorders: Official Publication of the World Federation of Neurology, Research Group on Motor Neuron Diseases, 1*(5), 293–299.

Carter, G. T., & Miller, R. G. (1998). Comprehensive management of amyotrphic lateral sclerosis. *Physical medicine and rehabilitation clinics of North America, 9*(1), 271–284.

Chang, J. L., Lomen-Hoerth, C., Murphy, J., Henry, R. G., Kramer, J. H., Miller, B. L., et al (2005). A voxel-based morphometry study of patterns of brain atrophy in ALS and ALS/FTLD. *Neurology, 65,* 75–80.

Cluskey, S., & Ramsden, D. B. (2001). Mechanisms of neurodegeneration in amyotrophic lateral sclerosis. *Molecular Pathology, 54*(6), 386–392.

Eisen, A., Kim, S., & Pant, B. (1992). Amyotrophic lateral sclerosis (ALS): A phylogenetic disease of the corticomotoneuron? *Muscle & Nerve, 15*(2), 219–224.

Ellis, C. M., Suckling, J., Amaro E., Jr., Bullmore, E. T., Simmons, A., Williams, S. C. R., et al. (2001). Volumetric analysis reveals corticospinal tract degeneration and extramotor involvement in ALS. *Neurology, 57,* 1571–1578.

Enterzari-Taher, M., Eisen, A., Stewart, H., & Nakajima, M. (1997). Abnormalities of cortical inhibitory neurons in amyotrophic lateral sclerosis. *Muscle & Nerve, 20*(1), 65–71.

Frank, B., Haas, J., Heinze, H. J., Stark, E., & Munte, T. F. (1997). Relation of neuropsychological and magnetic resonance findings in amyotrophic lateral sclerosis: Evidence for subgroups. *Clinical Neurology and Neurosurgery, 99*(2), 79–86.

Galasko, D., Salmon, D., Gamst, A., Olichney, J., Thal, L. J., Silbert, L., et al. (2007). Prevalence of dementia in Chamorros on Guam: Relationship to age, gender, education, and APOE. *Neurology, 68*(21), 1772–1781.

Gallassi, R., Montagna, P., Ciardulli, C., Lorusso, S., Mussuto, V., & Stracciari, A. (1985). Cognitive impairment in motor neuron disease. *Acta Neurologica Scandinavica, 71*(6), 480–484.

Gaudette, M., Hirano, M., & Siddique, T. (2000). Current status of SOD1 mutations in familial amyotrophic lateral sclerosis. *Amyotrophic Lateral Sclerosis and Other Motor Neuron Disorders: Official Publication of the World Federation of Neurology, Research Group on Motor Neuron Diseases, 1*(2), 83–89.

Giroud, M., Walker P., Bernard D., Lemesle, M., Martin, D., Baudouin, N., et al. (1996). Reduced brain N-acetyl-aspartate in frontal lobes suggests neuronal loss in patients with amyotrophic lateral sclerosis. *Neurology Research, 18,* 241–243.

Goetz, C. G. (2000). Amyotrophic lateral sclerosis: Early contributions of Jean-Martin Charcot. *Muscle Nerve, 23,* 336–342.

Gredal, O., Pakkenberg, H., Karlsborg, M., & Pakkenberg, B. (2000). Unchanged total number of neurons in motor cortex and neocortex in amyotrophic lateral sclerosis: A stereological study. *Journal of Neuroscience Methodology, 95,* 171–176.

Gredal, O., Rosenbaum, S., Toop, S., Karlsborg, M., Stange, P., & Werdelin, L. (1997). Quantification of brain metabolites in amyotrophic lateral sclerosis by localized proton magnetic resonance spectroscopy. *Neurology, 48,* 878–881.

Grosskreutz, J., Kaufmann, J., Fradrich, J., Dengler, R., Heinze, H. J., & Peschel, T. (2006). Widespread sensorimotor and frontal cortical atrophy in Amyotrophic Lateral Sclerosis. *BMC Neurology, 6,* (17).

Irwin, D., Lippa, C. F., & Swearer, J. M. (2007). Cognition and amyotrophic lateral sclerosis (ALS). *American Journal of Alzheimer's Disease and Other Dementias, 22*(4), 300–312.

Jeong, Y., Park, K. C., Cho, S. S., Kim, E. J., Kang, S. J., Kim, S. E., et al. (2005). Pattern of glucose hypometabolism in frontotemporal dementia with motor neuron disease. *Neurology, 64*(4), 734–736.

Jokelainen, M. (1977a). Amyotrophic lateral sclerosis in Finland. I: An epidemiologic study. *Acta Neurologica Scandinavica, 56*(3), 185–193.

Jokelainen, M. (1977b). Amyotrophic lateral sclerosis in Finland. II: Clinical characteristics. *Acta Neurologica Scandinavica, 56*(3), 194–204.

Kew, J. J., Goldstein, L. H., Leigh, P. N., Abrahams, S., Cosgrave, N., Passingham, R. E., et al. (1993a). The relationship between abnormalities of cognitive function and cerebral activation in amyotrophic lateral sclerosis: A neuropsychological and positron emission tomography study. *Brain: A Journal of Neurology, 116*(6), 1399–1423.

Kew, J. J., Leigh, P. N., Playford, E. D., Passingham, R. E., Goldstein, L. H., Frackowiak, R. S., et al. (1993b). Cortical function in amyotrophic lateral sclerosis: A positron emission tomography study. *Brain: A Journal of Neurology, 116*(3), 655–680.

Kiernan, J. A., & Hudson, A. J. (1993). Changes in shapes of surviving motor neurons in amyotrophic lateral sclerosis. *Brain, 116*, 203–215.

Kim, S. M., Lee, K. M., Hong, Y. H., Park, K. S., Yang, J. H., Nam, H. W., et al. (2007). Relation between cognitive dysfunction and reduced vital capacity in amyotrophic lateral sclerosis. *Journal of Neurology, Neurosurgery, and Psychiatry, 78*(12), 1387–1389.

Kotchoubey, B., Lang, S., Winter, S., & Birbaumer, N. (2003). Cognitive processing in completely paralyzed patients with amyotrophic lateral sclerosis. *European Journal of Neurology: The Official Journal of the European Federation of Neurological Societies, 10*(5), 551–558.

Kunst, C. B. (2004). Complex genetics of amyotrophic lateral sclerosis. *American Journal of Human Genetics, 75*(6), 933–947.

Kurt, A., Nijboer, F., Matuz, T., & Kubler, A. (2007). Depression and anxiety in individuals with amyotrophic lateral sclerosis: Epidemiology and management. *CNS Drugs, 21*(4), 279–291.

Lakerveld, J., Kotchoubey, B., & Kubler, A. (2008). Cognitive function in patients with late stage amyotrophic lateral sclerosis. *Journal of Neurology, Neurosurgery, and Psychiatry, 79*(1), 25–29.

Lewis, M., & Rushanan, S. (2007). The role of physical therapy and occupational therapy in the treatment of amyotrophic lateral sclerosis. *NeuroRehabilitation, 22*(6), 451–461.

Lomen-Hoerth, C., Murphy, J., Langmore, S., Kramer, J. H., Olney, R. K., & Miller, B. (2003). Are amyotrophic lateral sclerosis patients cognitively normal? *Neurology, 60*(7), 1094–1097.

Ludolph, A. C., Langen, K. J., Regard, M., Herzog, H., Kemper, B., Kuwert, T., et al. (1992). Frontal lobe function in amyotrophic lateral sclerosis: A neuropsychologic and positron emission tomography study. *Acta Neurologica Scandinavica, 85*(2), 81–89.

Massman, P. J., Sims, J., Cooke, N., Haverkamp, L. J., Appel, V., & Appel, S. H. (1996). Prevalence and correlates of neuropsychological deficits in amyotrophic lateral sclerosis. *Journal of Neurology, Neurosurgery, and Psychiatry, 61*(5), 450–455.

McCluskey, L. (2007a). Amyotrophic lateral sclerosis: Ethical issues from diagnosis to end of life. *NeuroRehabilitation, 22*(6), 463–472.

McCluskey, L. (2007b). Palliative rehabilitation and amyotrophic lateral sclerosis: A perfect match. *NeuroRehabilitation, 22*(6), 407–408.

Miller, R. G., Mitchell, J. D., Lyon, M., & Moore, D. H. (2007). Riluzole for amyotrophic lateral sclerosis (ALS)/motor neuron disease (MND). *Cochrane Database System Review*, (1), CD001447.

Miller, R. G., Rosenberg, J. A., Gelinas, D. F., Mitsumoto, H., Newman, D., Sufit, R., et al. (1999). Practice parameter: The care of the patient with amyotrophic lateral sclerosis (an evidence-based review): Report of the quality standards subcommittee of the American Academy of Neurology. *Neurology, 52*(7), 1311–1323.

Mitsumoto, H., & Rabkin, J. G. (2007). Palliative care for patients with amyotrophic lateral sclerosis: Prepare for the worst and hope for the best. *The Journal of the American Medical Association, 298*(2), 207–216.

Neary, D., Snowden, J. S., Gustafson, L., Passant, U., Stuss, D., Black, S., et al. (1998). Frontotemporal lobar degeneration: A consensus on clinical diagnostic criteria. *Neurology, 51*(6), 1546–1554.

Neary, D., Snowden, J. S., & Mann, D. M. (2000). Cognitive change in motor neurone disease/amyotrophic lateral sclerosis (MND/ALS). *Journal of the Neurological Sciences, 180*, 15–20.

Neumann, N., & Kotchoubey, B. (2004). Assessment of cognitive functions in severely paralysed and severely brain-damaged patients: Neuropsychological and electrophysiological methods. *Brain Research Protocols, 14*(1), 25–36.

Newsom-Davis, I. C., Lyall, R. A., Leigh, P. N., Moxham, J., & Goldstein, L. H. (2001). The effect of non-invasive positive pressure ventilation (NIPPV) on cognitive function in amyotrophic lateral sclerosis (ALS): A prospective study. *Journal of Neurology, Neurosurgery, and Psychiatry, 71*(4), 482–487.

Phukan, J., Pender, N. P., & Hardiman, O. (2007). Cognitive impairment in amyotrophic lateral sclerosis. *Lancet Neurology, 6*(11), 994–1003.

Pioro, E. P., Antel, J. P., Cashman, N. R., & Arnold, D. L. (1994). Detection of cortical neuron loss in motor neuron disease by proton magnetic resonance spectroscopic imaging in vivo. *Neurology, 44*, 1933–1938.

Pohl, C., Block, W., Karitzky, J., Traber, F., Schmidt, S., Grothe, C., et al. (2001). Proton magnetic resonance spectroscopy

A

of the motor cortex in 70 patients with amyotrophic lateral sclerosis. *Archives of Neurology, 58,* 729–735.

Poloni, M., Capitani, E., Mazzini, L., & Ceroni, M. (1986). Neuropsychological measures in amyotrophic lateral sclerosis and their relationship with CT scan-assessed cerebral atrophy. *Acta Neurologica Scandinavica, 74*(4), 257–260.

Radunovic, A., Mitsumoto, H., & Leigh, P. N. (2007). Clinical care of patients with amyotrophic lateral sclerosis. *Lancet Neurology, 6,* 913–925.

Ringholz, G. M., Appel, S. H., Bradshaw, M., Cooke, N. A., Mosnik, D. M., & Schulz, P. E. (2005). Prevalence and patterns of cognitive impairment in sporadic ALS. *Neurology, 65*(4), 586–590.

Roman, G. C. (1996). Neuroepidemiology of amyotrophic lateral sclerosis: Clues to aetiology and pathogenesis. *Journal of Neurology, Neurosurgery, and Psychiatry, 61*(2), 131–137.

Rooney, W. D., Miller, R. G., Gelinas, D., Schuff, N., Maudsley, A. A., & Weiner, M. W. (1998). Decreased N-acetylaspartate in motor cortex and corticospinal tract in ALS. *Neurology, 50,* 1800–1805.

Rottig, D., Leplow, B., Eger, K., Ludolph, A. C., Graf, M., & Zierz, S. (2006). Only subtle cognitive deficits in non-bulbar amyotrophic lateral sclerosis patients. *Journal of Neurology, 253*(3), 333–339.

Rowland, L. P. (2003). Clinical aspects of sporadic amyotrophic lateral sclerosis/motor neuron disease. In P. J. Shaw & M. J. Strong (Eds.), *Motor neuron disorders* (pp. 111–143). Philadelphia: Butterworth-Heinemann.

Rowland, L. P., & Shneider, N. A. (2001). Amyotrophic lateral sclerosis. *The New England Journal of Medicine, 344*(22), 1688–1700.

Schreiber, H., Gaigalat, T., Wiedemuth-Catrinescu, U., Graf, M., Uttner, I., Muche, R., et al. (2005). Cognitive function in bulbar- and spinal-onset amyotrophic lateral sclerosis: A longitudinal study in 52 patients. *Journal of Neurology, 252*(7), 772–781.

Shefner, J. M. (2006). Creatine as a potential treatment for amyotrophic lateral sclerosis. *Progress in Neurotherapeutics and Neuropsychopharmocology, 1*(1), 79–90.

Shoesmith, C. L., & Strong, M. J. (2006). Amyotrophic lateral sclerosis: Update for family physicians. *Canadian Family Physician Medecin De Famille Canadien, 52*(12), 1563–1569.

Strong, M. J., Grace, G. M., Orange, J. B., & Leeper, H. A. (1996). Cognition, language, and speech in amyotrophic lateral sclerosis: A review. *Journal of Clinical and Experimental Neuropsychology, 18*(2), 291–303.

Strong, M., & Rosenfeld, J. (2003). Amyotrophic lateral sclerosis: A review of current concepts. *Amyotrophic Lateral Sclerosis and other motor neuron disorders: Official publication of the World Federation of Neurology, Research Group on Motor Neuron Diseases, 4*(3), 136–143.

Talbot, P. R., Goulding, P. J., Lloyd, J. J., Snowden, J. S., Neary, D., & Testa, H. J. (1995). Inter-relation between "classic" motor neuron disease and frontotemporal dementia: Neuropsychological and single photon emission computed tomography study. *Journal of Neurology, Neurosurgery, and Psychiatry, 58*(5), 541–547.

Toft, M. H., Gredal, O., & Pakkenberg, B. (2005). The size and distribution of neurons in the motor cortex in amyotrophic lateral sclerosis. *Journal of Anatomy, 207,* 399–407.

Wong, P. C., Rothstein, J. D., & Price, D. L. (1998). The genetic and molecular mechanisms of motor neuron disease. *Current Opinion in Neurobiology, 8*(6), 791–799.

Woolley, S. C., & Katz, J. S. (2008). Cognitive and behavioral impairment in amyotrophic lateral sclerosis. *Physical Medicine and Rehabilitation Clinics of North America, 19*(3), 607–617.

Yoshida, M. (2004). Amyotrophic lateral sclerosis: The clinicopathological spectrum. *Neuropathology, 24,* 87–102.

ANENCEPHALY

DESCRIPTION

Anencephaly is a neural tube defect that develops as a result of the rostral neuropore failing to close during the third and fourth weeks of gestation. Anencephaly corresponds with a broader spectrum of disorders called cephalic disorders, referring to improper development of the brain and head. At birth, infants present with an absence of a major portion of the brain, skull, and scalp (Beers, Porter, & Jones, 2006). This leads to the infant being born without a forebrain or cerebrum and often without bone and skin (Golden & Bonnemann, 2007).

Although a brainstem may be present, which may correspond with reflexive actions such as breathing and response to sound and touch, the absence of the forebrain and cerebrum eliminates the possibility of infants ever gaining consciousness. At most, infants are born unconscious and present as blind, deaf, and unable to feel pain. Although most fetuses succumb to spontaneous abortion or are stillborn, those who survive birth usually die within a few days (Dox, Melloni, Eisner, & Melloni, 2002) and none live past infancy (Judd, 2007). Consequently, there is no treatment for anencephaly. Rather, regulation of the mother's diet, particularly supplementation with folic acid, has been shown to significantly reduce the incidence of anencephaly as well as other neural tube defects.

NEUROPATHOLOGY/PATHOPHYSIOLOGY

Anencephaly occurs in 0.1–0.7 per 1,000 births, and females predominate in ratios ranging between 3:1 and 7:1 (Ropper & Brown, 2005). Although the cause of anencephaly is unknown, theories have emerged. As with many presentations, genetics has been suggested as a potential source of risk for the presentation. There is a 3% increased chance for anencephalic development if one prior pregnancy has presented with the defect, and there is as high as a 10% chance if this has occurred for more than two prior pregnancies. However, it is noted that 95% of anencephalic defects occur in families with no reported history of the disease (Beers et al., 2006).

Geographic location has also been associated with the presentation. For example, higher incidence of anencephaly has been noted in Ireland and Wales than in comparison to the United States and France. This has led some to postulate the role of population genetics and environmental toxins in the development of anencephaly. However, geographic location also influences dietary practices that themselves are linked to anencephaly and other neural tube defects. As a result, the true role of geographical location in the risk of anencephaly requires further investigation as it may be an indirect correlate.

Regarding diet, although its role in the manifestation of anencephaly is still being investigated and debated (Harding & Copp, 1997), compelling evidence exists suggesting the role of folic acid in the development of the presentation. Specifically, taking folic acid supplements during the first trimester has been shown to significantly reduce the incidence of anencephaly as well as various other neural tube defects.

Infants with anencephaly present without the cerebral cortex and white matter of the brain, as well as large portions of the scalp and cranial bones. The brainstem, cerebellum, and spinal cord are generally present, but may be malformed themselves. Specifically, aplasia of descending tracts is commonly noted in the medulla and spinal cord, and the spinal leptomeninges are excessively vascular and contain islands of heterotopic neurological tissue (Bell, Gordon, & Maloney, 1981). A hemorrhagic nubbin of nerve, glial, and connective tissue is often viewable (Ropper & Brown, 2005).

NEUROPSYCHOLOGICAL/CLINICAL PRESENTATION

Anencephaly always leads to death, with 65% of fetuses dying in utero (Ropper & Brown, 2005). Of those infants that make it to the full term, most die within a few days after birth or are stillborn (Dox et al., 2002). Surviving infants do not live past infancy (Judd, 2007). For those that survive for this short amount of time, they are unconscious, blind, deaf, and unable to feel pain. Nevertheless, they will many times respond reflexively to stimuli from touch and sound and also breathe reflexively (Judd, 2007). Spontaneous movements of limbs may be observed as can papillary light reactions, ocular movements, corneal reflexes, and, in a few, crying and feeding reflexes (Ropper & Brown, 2005).

DIAGNOSIS

Anencephaly is usually diagnosed in very specific ways. With refined imaging in ultrasound, neural tube defects, including anencephaly, are being identified earlier in the pregnancy (Cuckle, 1994). In addition, anencephaly can be anticipated if the mother's serum levels of α-fetoprotein (AFP) and acetylcholine esterase are elevated (Ropper & Brown, 2007). More accurate predictions can be obtained by analyzing the level of AFP in the amniotic fluid by way of an amniocentesis (Brock & Sutcliffe, 1972).

TREATMENT

There is no treatment for anencephaly, and the prognosis is extremely poor with the few infants that do not die in utero or present as stillborn dying a few hours to days after birth. Consequently, treatment is supportive in nature and directed at parents and family.

Although there is no intervention that may be implemented, as suggested, preventive measures can be taken in the form of dietary supplementation with folic acid at about 0.4 mg per day. This has been shown to decrease the likelihood of most neural tube defects by as much as 70% (Judd, 2007).

J. Aaron Albritton
Chad A. Noggle

Beers, M. H., Porter, R. S., & Jones, T. V. (2006). *The Merck manual of diagnosis and therapy* (18th ed.). Whitehouse Station, NJ: Merck.

Bell, J. E., Gordon, A., & Maloney, A. F. J. (1981). Abnormalities of the spinal meninges in anencephalic fetuses. *Journal of Pathology, 133,* 131–144.

Brock, D. J. H., & Sutcliffe, R. G. (1972). Alpha-fetoprotein in the antenatal diagnosis of anencephaly and spina bifida. *Developmental Medicine and Child Neurology, 23,* 155–159.

A

Cuckle, H. S. (1994). Screening for neural tube defects. In G. Bock & J. Marsh (Ed.), *Neural tube defects* (pp. 253–266). Chichester: John Wiley.

Dox, I. G., Melloni, B. J., Eisner, G. M., & Melloni, J. L. (2002). *Melloni's illustrated medical dictionary* (4th ed.). London: The Parthenon Publishing Group.

Golden, J. A., & Bonnemann, C. G. (2007). Developmental structural disorders. In C. G. Goetz (Ed.), *Textbook of clinical neurology* (3rd ed., pp. 561–591). Philadelphia: Saunders Elsevier.

Harding, B., & Copp, A. J. (1997). Malformations. In D. I. Graham & P. L. Lantos (Eds.), *Greenfield's neuropathology* (6th ed., pp. 397–533). New York: Oxford University Press.

Judd, S. (Ed.) (2007). *Congenital disorders sourcebook*. Detroit, MI: Omnigraphics.

Ropper, A.H. & Brown, R.H. (2005). Adams and Victor's Principles of Neurology (8th Ed.). New York: McGraw-Hill (pp. 850–894).

ANEURYSMS

DESCRIPTION

A cerebral aneurysm is a bulge in an artery in the brain. Saccular aneurysm is the most common type, and its shape appears like a round berry attached to the artery by a small neck, whereas fusiform aneurysms are less common and appear in the shape of a spindle around the artery (Goedee, Depauw, Zwam, & Temmink, 2009). Some aneurysms go undetected, producing no signs or symptoms, whereas others are large enough to place significant pressure on surrounding brain tissue. Between 2% and 5% (nearly 15 million people) of the U.S. population is afflicted with saccular brain aneurysm, and approximately 30,000 of these rupture each year. Ruptured aneurysms can quickly become life threatening, requiring prompt medical attention. The severity of the medical threat is dependent upon the size and location of the aneurysm as well as the patient's age and health. Aneurysms have been shown to present more commonly in males than in females with a ratio of 1.8:1 (Huang, McGirt, Gailloud, & Tamargo, 2005).

According to Goedee et al. (2009), aneurysms in children are very rare, with prevalence rates reported between 0.5% and 4.6%. Pediatric aneurysm cases have been attributed to congenital, connective tissue disorders (such as polycystic kidney disease, Marfan's syndrome, and Ehlers–Danlos syndrome), trauma, AIDS, and myotic and bacterial infection. Pediatric cases often present clinically with subarachnoidal hemorrhage or seizure (Allison et al., 1998; Buis, van Ouwerkerk, Takahata, & Vandertop, 2006; Norris & Wallace, 1998; Proust et al., 2001), and Goedee et al. noted that less frequent presenting symptoms include headaches, vomiting, lethargy, diplopia, irritability, facial nerve palsy, or other focal motor deficits.

Ruptured Aneurysms

Ruptured aneurysms lie within the category of nonprogressive brain disorders, along with afflictions such as traumatic brain injury, completely metabolic/toxic or infectious disorders, anoxia, and nutritional deficiencies. Nonprogressive brain disorders have direct, time-limited action on the brain (Howieson, Loring, & Hannay, 2004). Among individuals experiencing a ruptured aneurysm, approximately 40% do not survive after 24 hours, and a mortality rate of 25% occurs within 6 months due to complications.

NEUROPATHOLOGY/PATHOPHYSIOLOGY

Intracranial aneurysms typically occur due to the wear and tear of arteries as a person ages. They typically form at artery branches or forks as these areas of the blood vessel are weaker. Infection or a blow to the skull may also weaken an artery wall resulting in aneurysm, though this cause is rare.

The circle of Willis at the base of the brain is a typical location for aneurysm formation. Aneurysm appearance occurs almost exclusively in humans (Hashimoto, Handa, Nagata, & Hazama, 1984), and high blood pressure has been noted as a probable cause (Kim & Cervos-Navarro, 1991). Cerebral vasculature is particularly susceptible to aneurysm, and this is likely an effect of the thinness of cerebrovascular walls as well as the lack of support around these vessels (Ostergaard & Oxlund, 1987). Continuous turning over of collagen fibers is widely believed to be the driving mechanism of aneurysm development (Kroon & Holzapfel, 2008).

Risk for aneurysm is greater than twice as likely for individuals with close relatives who have developed aneurysms. Aneurysms with genetic links are more likely to rupture at a smaller size and at younger patient ages. Hypertension is a risk factor as readings greater than 160/95 have been linked to aneurysm development and rupture. Further, rapid and brief increases in blood pressure, such as those that occur when exerting energy to lift a heavy object, may be more closely linked to aneurysm than chronic hypertension.

Smoking has been cited as an intracranial aneurysm risk factor as risk of ruptured brain aneurysm increases as number of cigarettes smoked increases. Individuals with high blood pressure who smoke are 15 times as likely to experience brain aneurysm rupture versus nonsmokers without high blood pressure. Smokers are also at greater risk for unruptured aneurysms as well as multiple aneurysms.

Medical conditions associated with intracranial aneurysm include connective tissue disorders (such as pseudoxanthoma and Ehlers–Danlos syndrome), arteriovenous malformation (intracranial abnormal connections between arteries and veins), polycystic kidney disease, and narrowing of the aorta at birth.

Ruptured Aneurysm

According to Hannay, Howieson, Loring, Fischer, and Lezak (2004), intracranial arterial rupture occurs due to either pathological alternation caused by hypertension or ruptures associated with vascular abnormalities such as tumor, arteriovenus malformation, deficient coagulation (Qureshi et al., 2001; Walton, 1994), or aneurysm. Older patients and women have increased risk of aneurysm rupture, though great variation exists among patients (Rinkel, Djibuti, Alagra, & van Gijn, 1998).

Risk of aneurysm rupture is more closely related to aneurysm characteristics versus patient characteristics (Hannay et al., 2004). Of ruptured aneurysm cases, 90% are subarachnoid, and 41% of these cases occur in the anterior communicating/anterior cerebral artery, whereas 34% involve the middle cerebral artery. Both of these sites hold potential for profound neuropsychological damage (Morita, Puumala, & Meyer, 1998). Aneurysms larger than 10 mm are considered symptomatic, and these as well as basilar artery aneurysms, have significantly increased rupture likelihood.

Brain aneurysm rupture can result in stroke, permanent nerve damage, or death. Blood escaping from the rupture can damage nearby brain cells. A vasospasm is a delayed complication that involves the narrowing of blood vessels, which deprives the brain of nutrients and oxygen. Four days to 2 weeks is the typical time frame for vasospasm occurrence. Hydrocephalus can also develop as pressure can increase if the blood leaking from the ruptured aneurysm blocks CSF circulation.

Aneurysm rupture of the anterior communicating artery (ACoA) damages the basal forebrain, which results in memory impairment (Everitt & Robbins, 1997; von Cramon & Markowitsch, 2000). Further damage can affect the ventromedial prefrontal cortex, which can lead to personality change and attention deficits (DeLuca & Chiaravalloti, 2002; DeLuca & Diamond, 1995).

NEUROPSYCHOLOGICAL/CLINICAL PRESENTATION

Patients with large aneurysms may present with diplopia or vision loss due to mass effect. Also, many present with headache, pain above and behind the eye, numbness, weakness, and paralysis on one side of the face, and drooping of one eyelid (Hauck et al., 2009).

Ruptured Aneurysm

It is rare that warning signs precede subarachnoid hemorrhages (Ogden, 1996; van Gijn & Rinkel, 2001), and clinical manifestation of ruptured aneurysm is typically severe (Hannay et al., 2004). Patients typically suffer severe headache, vomiting, and nausea. Within the hour, patients exhibit focal neurological dysfunction, double vision, and stiff neck. Based on severity of bleeding and intensity and site of vasospasm, the patient may or may not lose consciousness (Hannay et al., 2004). Notably, vasospasm occurs in approximately 30% of cases, producing infarction and ischemia (Britz & Mayberg, 1997; Mohr, Spetzler, & Kistler 1986).

Ruptured aneurysms can be fatal if massive bleeding or extensive vasospasm occurs, as a 50% rate of mortality has been found within the month following stroke (Estol, 2001). Severity of impairment is based on the severity of bleeding following the rupture. If bleeding ceases in adequate time, the patient may experience minimal brain damage and little cognitive deficit, if at all (Ogden, Mee, & Henning, 1993). Those who survive aneurysm rupture but undergo significant damage experience behavioral changes attributable to focal damage. Lishman (1997) and Okawa, Maeda, Nukui, and Kawafuchi (1980) found that patients with ruptured aneurysms in the ACoA experience behavioral disturbances similar to individuals with frontal lobe lesions such as indifference, childishness, spontaneity, and memory retrieval problems. Anterograde amnesia has been observed among survivors of ACoA aneurysm rupture (DeLuca & Chiaravalloti, 2002; DeLuca & Diamond, 1995), and this involves impairment of declarative (event and fact) learning while relative cognitive functions are spared (Myers et al., 2008). Hannay et al. (2004) noted that compared with cognitive impairments following ischemic cerebrovascular accidents, impairments following ruptured aneurysms are more widespread, do not follow regular neuropsychological patterns, and are less anatomically well defined.

A

In a study by Myers, DeLuca, Hopkins, and Gluck (2006), feedback-based learning deficits were compared among amnesic hypoxic patients, amnesic ACoA patients, and controls. Both patient groups showed similar declarative memory impairment on tests of figural and prose recall. Patients were then tested on conditional discrimination and unsignaled reversal. The ACoA group could reverse as quickly as controls but demonstrated impairment on discrimination. Alternatively, the hypoxic group was impaired at reversal, but their acquired discrimination abilities were on par with the control group. Indeed ACoA aneurysm patients demonstrate a unique pattern of memory deficits.

Through the use of a feedback-based learning task, Myers et al. (2008) also examined the differences between amnesic hypoxic brain injury patients versus patients with memory impairments following ACoA aneurysm rupture. They found that hypoxic brain injury patients were unimpaired in learning but impaired in generalization phases containing new, irrelevant features. Alternatively, those with ACoA aneurysm rupture demonstrated impairments in learning but were unimpaired in generalization phases. This is in line with findings of Myers et al. (2006) who noted that ACoA amnesic patients needed approximately two times the number of trials to achieve simple conditional discrimination versus hypoxic patients and healthy controls.

Given that AcoA patients demonstrate similar scores on neuropsychological measures of executive function and attention versus hypoxic and control groups, the acquisition deficit demonstrated by ACoA patients cannot be easily attributed to frontal dysfunction, despite varying degrees of frontal damage (Myers et al., 2008). In a review by Myers, Ermita, Hasselmo, and Gluck (1998), it is noted that basal forebrain damage likely disrupts neuromodulatory systems, which slows simple stimulus–response associations, while sparing hippocampal-dependent contextual processing and generalization. Thus, current literature demonstrates that patients who develop anterograde amnesia following ACoA aneurysm rupture may demonstrate retarded learning; however, given the time to complete learning, generalization abilities are mostly intact. These findings provide implications for the development of rehabilitation therapies that may cater treatments to particular amnesic groups based on learning and generalization abilities (Meyers et al., 2008).

DIAGNOSIS

In assessing headaches, differential diagnosis is crucial in order to provide optimal treatment (Hannay et al., 2004). Initially, aneurysm as a headache source must be differentiated from migraines, cluster headaches, tension-type headaches, aneurysm, brain tumor, subdural hematoma, subarachnoid hemorrhage, or idiopathic intracranial hypertension (Mathew, 2000). Goedee et al. (2009) noted that unilateral, pulsating headaches lasting 4–72 hours, accompanied with nausea and the disabling of character, are likely symptomatic of migraine (Detsky et al., 2006). Alternatively, headaches involving aura or vomiting, undefined or cluster-type headaches, and headaches with aggravation upon Valsalva-like maneuvers or exertion, suggest nonmigraine origin, which may indicate the need for neuroimaging particularly when abnormalities in neurological examination are discovered (Detsky et al., 2006).

Diagnosing aneurysm involves multidisciplinary evaluation within specialized centers (Goedee et al., 2009). Current imaging modalities include CT and CT angiography or the preferred methods of MRI and MR angiography. According to Goedee et al. (2009), following aneurysm identification, balloon test occlusion (BTO) with angiography may be used for treatment option evaluation. This test determines whether collateral flow would be sufficient if the parent artery containing the aneurysm was occluded.

TREATMENT

When an unruptured aneurysm is discovered, clinicians must determine whether or not operation is necessary. Risk assessment must be made, and Kroon and Holzapfel (2008) suggested that it may be more effective to assess mechanical fields, such as the stress or strain on the aneurysm, as opposed to the current criteria of assessing risk based on the size of lesion (Austin, Fisher, Dickson, Anderson, & Richardson, 1993; Canham, Finlay, Dixon, & Ferguson, 1991).

Surgical clipping and coiling are well-supported treatments for saccular aneurysms, whereas fusiform aneurysms require a BTO test to determine whether collateral flow can support occlusion of the parent artery (Goedee et al., 2009). Goedee et al. noted that in 1995, the FDA approved the use of detachable coils for the endovascular treatment of intracranial aneurysms, and, subsequently, endovascular treatment has become the preferred treatment over surgical procedure (Guan & Want, 2008; Koebbe, Veznedaroglu, Jabbour, & Rosenwasser, 2006).

In small aneurysms, endovascular treatment often requires the use of balloon-assisted coiling, as the balloon can aid in aneurysm catheterization while stabilizing the microcatheter and decreasing risk in the event of perforation (Lubicz et al., 2009). Following this procedure, aneurysm obliteration is determined through angiography.

Treatment of giant aneurysms is difficult given the likely presence of a wide neck, calcification, and thrombosis. Giant aneurysms are aneurysms measuring 2 cm or greater (Hauck et al., 2009). If left untreated, the risk for rupture resulting in patient death or disability over a 5-year span ranges between 40% and 50% (Wiebers et al., 2003). Currently, Hauck et al. (2009) noted that the treatments of choice are clip ligation, complete exclusion from circulation, and aneurysm decompression. Further, they note the newer, less invasive treatment, endovascular management with optional stenting as a successful alternative.

Although surgery is typically the ideal treatment for giant aneurysms to reduce mass effects, some patients present with medical conditions that increase their risk during surgery; therefore, stent/coil treatment is a preferred alternative. A disadvantage of the stent/coil treatment is the high rate of incomplete occlusion upon the first treatment, and, therefore, there is a great need for multiple treatments along with follow-up angiography (Hauck et al., 2009). However, it is suggested by Hauck et al. that partial occlusion of giant aneurysm likely reduces the risk of rupture.

Audrey L. Baumeister
William Drew Gouvier

Allison, J. W., Davis, P. C., Sato, Y., James, C. A., Haque, S. S., Angtuaco, E. J., et al. (1998). Intracranial aneurysms in infants and children. *Pediatric Radiology, 28*, 223–229.

Austin, G., Fisher, S., Dickson, D., Anderson, D., & Richardson, S. (1993). The significance of the extracellular matrix in intracranial aneurysms. *Annals of Clinical and Laboratory Science, 23*, 97–105.

Britz, G. W., & Mayberg, M. R. (1997). Pathology of cerebral aneurysms and subarachnoid hemorrhage. In K. M. A. Welch et al. (Eds.), *Primer on cerebrovascular diseases.* San Diego, CA: Academic Press.

Buis, D. R., van Ouwerkerk, W. J., Takahata, H., Vandertop, W. P. (2006). Intracranial aneurysms in children under 1 year of age: A systematic review of the literature. *Child's Nervous System, 22*, 1395–1409.

Canham, P. B., Finlay, H. M., Dixon, J. G., & Ferguson, S. E. (1991). Layered collagen fabric of cerebral aneurysms quantitatively assessed by the universal stage and polarized light microscopy. *The Anatomical Record, 231*, 579–592.

DeLuca, J., & Chiaravalloti, N. (2002). Neuropsychological consequences of ruptured aneurysms of the anterior communicating artery. In J. Harrison & A. Owen (Eds.), *Cognitive deficits in brain disorders* (pp. 17–36). London: Duntz.

DeLuca, J., & Diamond, B. (1995). Aneurysm of the anterior communicating artery: A review of neuroanatomical and neurophysiological sequelae. *Journal of Clinical and Experimental Neuropsychology, 17*(1), 100–121.

Detsky, M. E., McDonald, D. R., Baerlocher, M. O., Tomlinson, G. A., McCroy, D. C., & Booth, C. M. (2006). Does this patient with headache have a migraine or need neuroimaging? *Journal of the American Medical Association, 296*, 1274–1283.

Estol, C. J. (2001). Headache: Stroke symptoms and signs. In J. Bogousslavsky & L. R. Caplan (Eds.), *Stroke syndromes* (2nd ed.). Cambridge, UK: Cambridge University Press.

Everitt, B., & Robbins, T. (1997). Central cholinergic systems and cognition. *Annual Review of Psychology, 48*, 649–684.

Goedee, H. S., Depauw, P. R., vd Zwam, B., & Temmink, A. H. (2009). Superficial temporal artery-middle cerebral artery bypass surgery in a pediatric giant intracranial aneurysm presenting as migraine-like episodes. *Child's Nervous System, 25*, 257–261.

Guan, Y. S., & Wang, M. Q. (2008). Endovascular embolization of intracranial aneurysms. *Angiology, 59*, 342–351.

Hannay, H. J., Howieson, D. B., Loring, D. W., Fischer, J. S., & Lezak, M. D. (2004). Neuropathology for neuropathologists. In M. D. Lezak, D. B. Howieson, & D. W. Loring (Eds.), *Neuropsychological assessment* (pp. 157–285). New York: Oxford.

Hashimoto, N., Handa, H., Nagata, I., & Hazama, F. (1984). Animal model of cerebral aneurysms: Pathology and pathogenesis of induced cerebral aneurysms in rats. *Neurological Research, 6*, 33–40.

Hauck, E. F., Welch, B. G., White, J. A., Replogle, R. E., Purdy, P. D., Pride, L. G., et al. (2009). Stent/coil treatment of very large and giant unruptured ophthalmic and cavernous aneurysms. *Surgical Neurology, 71*, 19–24.

Huang, J., McGirt, M. J., Gailloud, P., Tamargo, R. J. (2005). Intracranial aneurysms in the pediatric population: Case series and literature review. *Surgical Neurology, 63*, 424–432.

Howieson, D. B., Loring, D. W., & Hannay, H. J. (2004). Neurobehavioral variables and diagnostic issues. In M. D. Lezak, D. B. Howieson, & D. W. Loring (Eds.), *Neuropsychological assessment* (pp. 157–285). New York: Oxford.

Kim, C., & Cervos-Navarro, J. (1991). Spontaneous saccular cerebral aneurysm in a rat. *Neurological Research, 6*, 33–40.

Koebbe, C. J., Veznedaroglu, E., Jabbour, P., Rosenwasser, R. H. (2006). Endovascular management of intracranial aneurysms: Current experience and future advances. *Neurosurgery, 59*, 93–113.

Kroon, M., & Holzapfel, G. A. (2008). Modeling of saccular aneurysm growth in a human middle cerebral artery.

Journal of Biomechanical Engineering, 130(5), 51012-1–51012-10.

Lishman, W. A. (1997). *Organic psychiatry* (3rd ed.). Oxford, UK: Blackwell.

Lubicz, B., Bruneau, M., Dewindt, A., Lefranc, F., Baleriaux, D., & De Witte, O. (2009). Endovascular treatment of proximal anterior cerebral artery aneurysms. *Neuroradiology, 51*, 99–102.

Randolph W. Evans & Ninan T. Mathew, N. (2000). Migraine. In *Handbook of headache*. Philadelphia: Lippincott William & Wilkins.

Mohr, J. P., Spetzler, R. F., & Kistler, J. P. (1986). Intracranial aneurysms. In H. J. M. Bennett et al. (Eds.), *Stroke. Pathophysiology, diagnosis, and management*. New York: Churchill Livingstone.

Morita, A., Puumala, M. R., & Meyer, F. B. (1998). Intracranial aneurysms and subarachnoid hemorrhage. In M. Swash (Ed.), *Outcomes in neurological and neurosurgical disorders*. Cambridge, UK: Cambridge University Press.

Myers, C. E., Hopkins, R. O., DeLuca, J., Moore, N. B., Wolansky, L. J., Sumner, J. M., et al. (2008). Learning and generalization deficits in patients with memory impairments due to anterior communicating artery aneurysm rupture or hypoxic brain injury. *Neuropsychology, 22*(5), 681–686.

Myers, C., DeLuca, J., Hopkins, R., & Gluck, M. (2006). Conditional discrimination and reversal in amnesia subsequent to hypoxic brain injury or an anterior communicating artery aneurysm rupture. *Neuropsychologia, 44*, 130–139.

Myers, C., Ermita, B., Hasselmo, M., & Gluck, M. (1998). Further implications of a computational model of septohippocampal cholinergic modulation in eyeblink conditioning. *Psychobiology, 26*(1), 1–20.

Norris, J. S., & Wallace, M. C. (1998). Pediatric intracranial aneurysms. *Neurosurgery Clinics of North America, 9*, 557–563.

Ogden, J. A. (1996). *Fractured minds*. New York: Oxford University Press.

Ogden, J. A., Mee, E. W., & Henning, M. (1993). A prospective study of impairment of cognition and memory and recovery after subarachnoid hemorrhage. *Neurosurgery, 33*, 1–15.

Okawa, M., Maeda, S., Nukui, H., & Kawafuchi, J. (1980). Psychiatric symptoms in ruptured anterior communicating aneurysms: Social prognosis. *Acta Psychiatrica Scandinavica, 61*, 306–312.

Ostergaard, J. R., & Oxlund, H. (1987). Collagen type III deficiency in patients with rupture of intracranial saccular aneurysms. *Journal of Neurosurgery, 67*, 690–696.

Proust, F., Toussaint, P., Garnieri, J., Hannequin, D., Legars, D., Houtteville, J. P., et al. (2001). Pediatric cerebral aneurysms. *Journal of Neurosurgery, 94*, 733–739.

Qureshi, A. I., Tuhrim, S., Broderick, J. P., Batjer, H. H., Hondo, H., & Hanley, D. (2001). Spontaneous intracerebral hemorrhage. *New England Journal of Medicine, 344*, 1450–1460.

Rinkel, G. J., Djibuti, M., Algra, A., & van Gijn, J. (1998). Prevalence and risk of rupture of intracranial aneurysms: A systematic review. *Stroke, 29*, 251–256.

van Gijn, J., & Rinkel, G. J. E. (2001). Subarachnoid hemorrhage syndromes. In J. Bogousslavsky & L. Caplan (Eds.), *Stroke syndromes* (2nd ed.). Cambridge, UK: Cambridge University Press.

von Cramon, D., & Markowitsch, H. (2000). Human memory dysfunctions due to septal lesions. In R. Numan (Ed.), *The behavioral neuroscience of the septal region* (pp. 380–413). New York: Springer.

Walton, J. N. (1994). *Brain's diseases of the nervous system* (10th ed.). Oxford, UK: Oxford University Press.

Wiebers, D. O., Whisnant, J. P., Huston, J., Meissner, I., Brown, R. D., Piepgras, D. G., et al. (2003). Unruptured intracranial aneurysms: Natural history, clinical outcome, and risks of surgical and endovascular treatment. *The Lancet, 362*(9378), 103–110.

ANGELMAN SYNDROME

DESCRIPTION

Angelman syndrome (AS) is a genetic neurodevelopmental disorder that occurs as a result of chromosomal abnormality of the 15q11.2–15q13 region. It is primarily characterized by developmental delay, severe speech impairment, motor weakness, and behavioral abnormalities such as excessive laughter, inappropriate happiness, and hyperactivity. Frequent features include microcephaly, abnormal EEG, and seizures (Saadeh, Lisi, Batista, McIntosh, & Hoover-Fong, 2007). In addition, 20% to 80% of individuals with AS present with a protruding tongue, wide mouth, prominent mandible, depressed occiput, hypopigmented skin, sleep disturbances, abnormal feeding behaviors, hyperactive reflexes of the lower limbs, an attraction to water and sensitivity to heat (Horsler & Oliver, 2006).

Initially termed "happy puppet" syndrome, AS was first recognized in 1965 by Harry Angelman. However, it was not until 1987, with the development of the first diagnostic tests and criteria, that it became a prevalent condition (Clayton-Smith, 2001). It is now estimated to occur in 1 out of 12,000–20,000 births (Coppola et al., 2007) in both genders equally (Walz, 2007).

NEUROPATHOLOGY/PATHOPHYSIOLOGY

The behavioral and developmental phenotypes of AS are a result of particular genetic mechanisms, most commonly a dysfunction or deletion from maternal chromosome 15q11.2–15q13, deletion accounting for 70% of all cases (Jolleff, Emmerso, Ryan, & McConachie, 2006). Additional genetic mechanisms include paternal uniparental disomy (UPD; i.e., the father contributes two copies of chromosome), imprinting center defects, and gene mutation of *UBE3A*. The outcome of each mechanism is the lack of a functional copy of the *UBE3A* gene that is maternally derived (Walz, 2007). Each individual mechanism is indicative of particular phenotypes.

The deletion of the maternally contributed portion of chromosome 15 results in an abnormal expression of certain genes. AS is the result of a silenced paternal allele and maternal contribution that is not received or mutated (Lombroso, 2000). Typical presentation associated with this mechanism includes seizures, microcephaly, language impairments, and motor deficits (Jolleff et al., 2006).

In the case that both copies of the chromosome are paternally derived as with UPD, the gene remains silenced, and the functional protein is not produced. Compared with other forms, UPD tends to feature better physical growth, less motor difficulties and ataxia, fewer seizures, higher developmental level, language and ability to spontaneously demonstrate expressive skills (Jolleff et al., 2006).

A less common cause is a mutation of the imprinting center. This region is responsible for determining which portions of the DNA are imprinted, and with this abnormality normal functioning is disrupted (Lombroso, 2000). Single gene mutation of *UBE3A* is an additional mechanism involving maternal and paternal differences in imprinting. The gene from the maternal chromosome is limited to expression in the hippocampus and cerebellum (Walz, 2007). *UBE3A* functions in both ubiquitin ligase activity and as a transcriptional coactivator. The *UBE3A* gene, due to its direct interaction with hormone activity, has a role in growth and development. Mutations of this gene are associated with the neurodevelopmental abnormalities of AS, including cerebellar dysmyelination and Purkinje cell loss, ventricular enlargement, and cortical atrophy (Wilkinson, Davies, & Isles, 2007). Analysis of AS will reveal neuropathological abnormality of the cerebrum, including a decrease in arborization of dendritic spines. Impairment in dendritic development contributes to the seizures and mental retardation of AS (Volpe, 2008).

NEUROPSYCHOLOGICAL/CLINICAL PRESENTATION

Cognitive, social, behavioral, and communication deficits are essential aspects underlying AS presentation. Difficulties in social skills are characteristic and may contribute to the impaired development of expressive language. Severe developmental delay and failure to reach developmental milestones (i.e., imitation) is common (Walz, 2007). Cognitively, individuals present with severe intellectual retardation (Lombroso, 2000). Attention is limited, negatively impacting concentration and communication (Pelc, Cheron, & Dan, 2008).

Behavioral deficits are a dominant aspect of AS presentation. Individuals are described as being behaviorally hyperactive. They present with a happy disposition and engage in hypermotor activities, such as hand flapping, excessive laughter, and mouthing behaviors (Walz, 2007). The developmental delay characteristic of AS progressively becomes more apparent during infancy. Infants may demonstrate less crying behavior and decreased motor activity. Although social smiling develops at the appropriate age, it may be distinctive and an early indication of the happy demeanor of AS. Laughter occurs within a few weeks of life, which may appear as appropriate social development, sometimes causing the intellectual deficits to go undetected. Developmental delay is also apparent in the emergence of babbling and head control. The flattened back of the skull of AS is a result of delayed head control. (Pelc et al., 2008). In children with AS, cognitive and fine motor difficulties impede normal development of play. Ultimately, play appears to be repetitive, exploratory, and manipulative. Occasionally, movement is hindered by ataxia or tremor, but typically eye-hand coordination is good (Pelc et al., 2008).

DIAGNOSIS

Diagnosis is based on an established set of criteria that identify four clinical characteristics of AS, which are: developmental delay, movement disorder, behavioral uniqueness, and speech impairment (Horsler & Oliver, 2006). The final diagnosis is based on both clinical features and molecular genetic testing. Detection of AS includes identifying an unmethylated allele. A DNA methylation analysis (Southern Blot analysis, methylation specific PCR assay) may be used to detect the abnormal DNA methylation imprint. DNA methylation tests often require further investigation to determine the underlying genetic mechanism (Kubota et al., 1997). Fluorescent in situ hybridization or

A

array-based comparative genomic hybridization is used to identify deletions. UPD is identified with a DNA polymorphism test. Imprinting mutations are identified through an imprinting center analysis (Buiting et al., 2003). Lastly, sequence analysis is used when an individual presents with clinical features of AS, but methylation tests appear normal. The sequence analysis will identify any mutation of the *UBE3A* gene (Lossie and Drsicoll, 1999). Molecular genetic testing allows for the identification of AS, as well as the specific underlying genetic mechanism responsible.

Considerations surrounding a diagnosis of AS, should include its similarity to other diagnoses in clinical presentation. Chromosome 15 deletions that cause AS are also responsible for Prader–Willi syndrome. Prader–Willi syndrome reveals similarity in its presentation, including intellectual deficits, feeding difficulties, and developmental delay. The difference being that it is the result of the loss of the paternal contribution to the 15q11.2–15q13 region, as opposed to the maternal contribution loss of AS (Horsler & Oliver, 2006).

Autism spectrum disorders share similar pathophysiological abnormalities with AS. Repetitive behaviors, absence of speech and language development are characteristics of both autism and AS. However, there are behavioral differences that distinguish between the disorders. A preoccupation with order and moving objects is found in autism but not AS. Those with autism demonstrate impaired social interaction and disengagement. In contrast, those with AS demonstrate excessive hypersocial behaviors. The main distinction to consider for diagnosis is, the prominent social deficit characteristic of autism that is distinctly different from the social reciprocity and good social seeking behaviors of AS (Walz, 2007).

Due to the seizures and psychomotor delay characteristic of AS, a diagnosis of idiopathic epilepsy, static encephalopathy, and cerebral palsy must be ruled out. Hypotonia of AS introduces the possibility of a myopathic disorder. However, in AS a muscle biopsy and electromyography will appear normal, whereas a myopathic disorder will be abnormal. Abnormal speech and ataxia allows for the distinction between AS and cerebral palsy, as both present with jerky and tremulousness movements (Williams et al., 2006). Rett syndrome is one of the most common differentials. Seizures of infant girls are characteristic of both AS and Rett syndrome. However, in Rett syndrome the purposeful use of hands is lost, whereas in AS it is not. In addition, the happy disposition of AS is not present in Rett syndrome. Lastly, genetic testing can reveal a MECP2 mutation, which is the cause of Rett syndrome (Watson et al. 2001).

TREATMENT

There is no cure for this genetic condition; therefore, treatment is centered around symptom management. Through anticipation of clinical features of AS, complications can be treated effectively early in development. Mobility is a major concern, making the maintenance of a full range of movement, essential. Therefore, physiotherapy is recommended as a part of an active early intervention (Beckung, Steffenburg, & Kyllerman, 2004).

Treatment should include a form of language and speech therapy that compensate for communication and language deficits. Communication skills should include the use of gestures and signs, which ultimately can improve overall verbal comprehension. A multimethod approach should be taken by presenting several forms of communication in order to increase the chances of being able to communicate successfully. Augmentive communication strategies, such as the use of symbols and pictures, should be utilized to increase their expressive language and comprehension of the world through objects of reference (Jolleff et al., 2006). Seizures can be controlled through various types of anticonvulsants, such as sodium valproate and clonazepam (Valente et al., 2006).

Management of AS requires a multifocused form of intervention. Speech therapy, occupational therapy, music therapy, and hydrotherapy are additional forms of treatment that have proven to be helpful in the management of this condition. Individuals are more resistant to behavioral therapies. Intervention and treatment can help to make an individual with AS manageable. It can help them develop a form of communication allowing them to express themselves. Ultimately, individuals will grow to develop limited self-help skills (Pelc et al., 2008). It is likely that individuals will require constant supervision for the remainder of their lives.

Jamie Rice
Charles Golden

Beckung, E., Steffenburg, S., & Kyllerman, M. (2004). Motor impairments, neurological signs, and developmental level in individuals with Angelman syndrome. *Developmental Medicine & Child Neurology, 46*(4), 239–243.

Buiting, K., Gross, S., Lich, C., Gillessen-Kaesbach, G., el-Maarri, O., & Horsthemke, B. (2003). Epimutations in Prader-Willi and Angelman syndromes: A molecular study of 136 patients with an imprinting defect. *American Journal of Human Genetic, 72,* 571–577.

Clayton-Smith, J. (2001). Angelman syndrome: Evolution of the phenotype in adolescents and adults. *Developmental Medicine and Child Neurology, 43*(7), 476–480.

Coppola, G., Verrotti, A., Mainolfi, C., Auricchio, G., Fortunato, D., Operto, F. F., et al., (2007). Bone mineral density in Angelman syndrome. *Pediatric Neurology, 37*(6), 411–416.

Horsler, K., & Oliver, C. (2006). The behavioral phenotype of Angelman syndrome. *Journal of Intellectual Disability, 50*(1), 33–53.

Jolleff, N., Emmerson, F., Ryan, M., & McConachie, H. (2006). Communication skills in Angelman syndrome: Matching phenotype to genotype. *Advances in Speech-Language Pathology, 8*(1), 28–33.

Kubota, T., Das, S., Christian, S. L., Baylin, S. B., Herman, J. G., & Ledbetter, D. H. (1997). Methylation-specific PCR simplifies imprinting analysis. *Nature Genetics, 16*, 16–7.

Lombroso, P. J. (2000). Genetics of childhood disorders: XVI. Angelman syndrome: A failure to process. *Journal of the American Academy of Child and Adolescent Psychiatry, 39*(7), 931–933.

Lossie, A. C., & Driscoll, D. J., (1999). Transmission of Angelman syndrome by an affected mother. *Genetics in Medicine, 1*, 262–266.

Pelc, K., Cheron, G., & Dan, B. (2008). Behavior and neuropsychiatric manifestations in Angelman syndrome. *Neuropsychiatric Disease and Treatment, 4*(3), 577–584.

Saadeh, R., Lisi, E. C., Batista, D. A., McIntosh, I., & Hoover-Fong, J. E. (2007). Albinism and developmental delay: The need to test for 15q11-q13 deletion. *Pediatric Neurology, 37*(4), 299–302.

Valente, K. D., Koiffmann, C. P., Fridman, C., Varella, M., Kok, F., Andrade, J., et al. (2006). Epilepsy in patients with Angelman syndrome caused by deletion of the chromosome 15q11-13. *Archives of Neurology, 63*, 122–128.

Volpe, J. J. (2008). *Neurology of the newborn* (5th ed.). Philadelphia: Saunders Elsevier.

Walz, N. C. (2007). Parent report of stereotyped behaviors, social interaction, and developmental disturbances in individuals with Angelman syndrome. *Journal of Autism and Developmental Disorders, 37*, 940–947.

Watson, P., Black, G., Ramsden, S., Barrow, M., Super, M., Kerr, B., & Clayton-Smith, J. (2001). Angelman syndrome phenotype associated with mutations in MECP2, a gene encoding a methyl CpG binding protein. *American Journal of Medical Genetics, 38*, 224–228.

Wilkinson, L. S., Davies, W., & Isles, A. R. (2007). Genomic imprinting effects on brain development and function. *Neuroscience, 8*, 832–843.

Williams, C., Beaudet, A., Clayton-Smith, J., Knoll, J., Kyllerman, M., Laan, L. A., et al. (2006). Angelman syndrome 2005: Updated consensus for diagnostic criteria. *American Journal of Medical Genetics Part A, 140*, 413–418.

ANTIPHOSPHOLIPID ANTIBODY SYNDROME

A

DESCRIPTION

Antiphospholipid syndrome (APS) is an autoimmune disorder first identified in 1983 by Graham Hughes. Antiphospholipid antibodies (aPLs) are found in 1–2% of the general population, and in 25–50% of individuals with systemic lupus erythematosus (SLE); however, the mere presence of aPLs alone is not sufficient to warrant the diagnosis of this syndrome. An essential feature of APS is hypercoagulability of the blood, which leads to the presence of large vessel venous occlusions, and less commonly, arterial occlusions. These thrombotic events will commonly result in transient ischemic attacks, cerebral vascular attacks, and myocardial infarctions. Recurrent pregnancy loss is also not uncommon in individuals with APS (Diz-Küçükkaya, 2005).

APS has been classified into two categories, the first of which is primary APS, wherein no definitive etiology is identified. The second category is secondary APS, which is associated with an autoimmune disease, such as SLE. Other clinical associations, however, are malignancy, infections, and drug ingestion (Olmstead, 2001). A form of APS exists known as catastrophic APS (CAPS), which manifests as the presence of three or more thrombotic events in multiple organ systems over a period of several days or weeks (Diz-Küçükkaya, 2005; Frances & Piette, 2001; Sharma et al., 2005).

NEUROPATHOLOGY/PATHOPHYSIOLOGY

The exact causative mechanism in APS is uncertain. Hypotheses include elevated platelet activity, decreased antithrombin III plasma levels, inhibition of prostacyclin release, and inhibition of protein C–protein S thrombomodulin system. Antiphospholipid antibodies have been identified in patients with SLE, and have been posited as possible causative mechanisms in the syndrome and associated cognitive sequelae (Aharon-Peretz, Brenner, Amyel-Zvi, Metz, & Hemli, 1996).

Thrombotic events occur as a result of APS and are associated with secondary cognitive and physiological sequelae. These occlusions are the pathophysiological basis for hemorrhage, organ failure, and cognitive deficits such as impaired attention, verbal and visual memory, and executive functioning. Multiple occlusions and organ system failures are the most common pathophysiological findings in CAPS.

A

NEUROPSYCHOLOGICAL/CLINICAL PRESENTATION

Cognitive dysfunction is seen in individuals with aPLs. APS is associated with diffuse brain damage, leading to cognitive dysfunction in the domains of attention, verbal fluency, verbal learning, and executive functioning (Leritz, Brandt, Minor, Reis-Jensen, & Petri, 2002), as well as dementing processes (Mosek et al., 2000). Further neurobehavioral presentations may also include vascular dementia, movement disorders, suicidal ideation, choreiform movement, mood lability, slowed cognition, anorexia, hemihypesthesia, visual distortions, psychosis, derealization, and memory problems (Gorman & Cummings, 1993). In addition to the neurological and neuropsychological manifestations of APS, patients may present with mood and affective disorders and psychosis (Kurtz & Müller, 1994).

Cerebral ischemia may be present in individuals with APS, even when cognitive symptoms are not overt. A series of neuropsychological tests were administered to 20 patients diagnosed with APS in an attempt to quantify potential neuropsychological impairment (Aharon-Peretz et al., 1996). The groups were divided into neurologic symptomatic APS and neurologic asymptomatic APS. The tests employed were: digit span, logical memory (from the Wechsler Memory Scale), three words-three figures, and three trials for word list learning (eight words), the Rey–Osterrieth Complex Figure, Trails A and B, digit symbol substitution, and word fluency. The neurologic symptomatic APS group performed significantly worse on all measures, with the exception of Trail B. These findings potentially implicate subcortical and frontal systems. Other, similar definitive patterns of cognitive dysfunction have not been observed in individuals with aPLs (Leritz et al., 2002).

Some research (Whitelaw, Spangenberg, Rickman, Hugo, & Roberts, 1999) has indicated that the prolonged presence of APS negatively impacts cognition as measured by neuropsychological testing, in the domains of broad intelligence, and visual and verbal recall. Overall, patients with aPLs exhibit impairment in the areas of executive functioning, verbal memory, and visuospatial performance when compared with controls. There is also evidence to suggest that these cognitive impairments may present as prodromal markers for APS (Jacobson, Rapport, Keenan, Coleman, & Tietjen, 1999). MRI scans in that study also revealed a nonsignificant percentage of abnormalities in the brains of APS positive patients. Diffuse and focal ischemic changes were the most frequently noted.

The clinical presentation of APS may include pain in the leg and swelling, redness, loss of sensation in the limb (Olmstead, 2001). The syndrome may also present with a host of dermatologic abnormalities and lesions, including but not limited to: livedo reticularis, skin ulcerations, pseudovasculitis lesions, superficial skin necrosis, and anetoderma (Frances & Piette, 2001). Addison's disease may also present as part of APS. Adrenal insufficiency may be secondary to renal artery occlusions or as a result of anticoagulant therapy. The result is renal failure secondary to hemorrhage in either case. Adrenal hemorrhage is of particular concern, as the presence of aPLs increases the risk of hemorrhage in those receiving anticoagulants (Satta et al., 2000). The clinical presentation of CAPS may include the aforementioned and has been reported that hypertension occurs in approximately three-fourths of individuals with CAPS (Sharma et al., 2005).

DIAGNOSIS

Although the neuropsychological and clinical presentation of APS is somewhat heterogeneous, the diagnosis has been systematized and is thus relatively unambiguous. Clinical and laboratory diagnostic criteria were established in 1998 at the International Symposium on aPLs. The criteria include the presence of a vascular thrombosis with one or more episodes of arterial or venous occlusions, or history of pregnancy morbidity (one or more unexplained fetal deaths, premature births, or three or more spontaneous terminations). Serum tests will reveal the presence of anticardiolipin antibody of IgG and/or IgM inmunoglobin present in two separate tests spaced at 6-week intervals, or positive serum test for lupus anticoagulant. Meeting one each of clinical and lab criterion results in a positive diagnosis of APS. Blood analysis will reveal a low platelet count due to the inability of the marrow to keep up with the destruction of platelets in APS (Frances & Piette, 2001; Olmstead, 2001). Patients may also have a history of difficult pregnancies, silent retinal venous thrombosis, thrombocytopenia, and test positive for lupus anticoagulant and anticardiolipin antibody (Fukui, Kawamura, Hasegawa, Kato, & Kaga, 2000). Although it is not considered a primary differential of APS per se, clinicians should also include SLE as a rule out, as the two disorders are strongly linked (Diz-Küçükkaya, 2005; Frances & Piette, 2001; Whitelaw et al., 1999).

TREATMENT

Treatment of APS is disputed due to a dearth of long-term outcome studies on treatments. It is generally held, however, that medication treatment may include anticoagulants (typically wafarin), aspirin, and immunosuppressive drugs. It has been noted that successful treatment may result as a combination of the aforementioned, with the addition of prednisone and intravenous gamma globulin (Espinoza, 1996). The treatment of APS is aimed at preventing the presence or recurrence of thrombotic events (venous or arterial) (Lim, Crowther, & Eikelboom, 2006) and fetal loss (Espinoza, 1996). Also recommended are elimination of oral contraceptives, smoking cessation, and exercise (Olmstead, 2001). Long-term oral anticoagulant therapy with wafarin is also recommended, as thromboses have a tendency to recur. For individuals with no history of thrombosis, a lifetime regimen of aspirin should be used (Sarvis, 2005).

Treatment of CAPS has been recommended as intravenous heparin, plasmapheresis, and steroids. The greatest chance for successful treatment and prevention of recurring thromboses is early identification and aggressive treatment. The mortality rate, however, is greater than 50%, even with appropriate treatment (Diz-Küçükkaya, 2005; Sharma et al., 2005).

As previously noted, patients with primary or secondary APS and CAPS may present with a host of comorbid neuropsychological and psychiatric/psychological disorders. A review of individual and group cases for these comorbid conditions does not indicate an alteration in otherwise standard, best practice treatments (i.e., an antipsychotic regimen for treatment of psychosis, serotonin-specific reuptake inhibitors for major depressive disorder). It should be noted, however, that none of the studies reviewed pertained to the direct treatment of these disorders, per se; rather they were treated as secondary clinical conditions.

W. Howard Buddin
Charles Golden

Aharon-Peretz, J., Brenner, B., Amyel-Zvi, E., Metz, L., & Hemli, J. A. (1996). Neurocognitive dysfunction in the antiphospholipid antibody syndrome (APS). *Neuropsychiatry, Neuropsychology, and Behavioral Neuropsychology, 9*(2), 123–126.

Diz-Küçükkaya, R. (2005). Antiphospholipid antibody syndrome. *Hematology, 10*(4), 33–38.

Espinoza, L. R. (1996). Antiphospholipid antibody syndrome: Treatment. *Lupus, 5*(5), 456–457.

Frances, C., & Piette, J. (2001). Antiphospholipid antibody syndrome (Hughes' syndrome). *Dermatologic Therapy, 14*, 117–125.

Fukui, T., Kawamura, M., Hasegawa, Y., Kato, T., & Kaga, E. (2000). Multiple cognitive impairments associated with systemic lupus erythematosus and antiphospholipid antibody syndrome: A form of progressive vascular dementia? *European Neurology, 43*(2), 115–116.

Gorman, D. G., & Cummings, J. L. (1993). Neurobehavioral presentations of the antiphospholipid antibody syndrome. *The Journal of Neuropsychiatry and Clinical Neurosciences, 5*(1), 37–42.

Jacobson, M. W., Rapport, L. J., Keenan, P. A., Coleman, R. D., & Tietjen, G. E. (1999). Neuropsychological deficits associated with antiphospholipid antibodies. *Journal of Clinical and Experimental Neuropsychology, 21*(2), 251–264.

Kurtz, G., & Müller, N. (1994). The antiphospholipid syndrome and psychosis. *The American Journal of Psychiatry, 151*(12), 1841–1842.

Leritz, E., Brandt, J., Minor, M., Reis-Jensen, F., & Petri, M. (2002). Neuropsychological functioning and its relationship to antiphospholipid antibodies in patients with systemic lupus erythematosus. *Journal of Clinical and Experimental Neuropsychology, 24*(4), 527–533.

Lim, W., Crowther, M. A., & Eikelboom, J. W. (2006). Management of antiphospholipid antibody syndrome: A systematic review. *Journal of the American Medical Association, 295*(9), 1050–1057.

Mosek, A., Yust, I., Treves, T. A., Vardinon, N., Korczyn, A. D., & Chapman, J. (2000). Dementia and antiphospholipid antibodies. *Dementia and Geriatric Cognitive Disorders, 11*(1), 36–38.

Olmstead, J. (2001). A review of antiphospholipid antibody syndrome. *Journal of the American Academy of Nurse Practitioners, 13*(10), 460–463.

Sarvis, C. M. (2005). Antiphospholipid antibody syndrome: When wounds won't heal. *Nursing, 35*(9), 24.

Satta, M. A., Corsello, S. M., Della Casa, S., Rota, C. A., Pirozzi, B., Colasanti, S., et al. (2000). Adrenal insufficiency as the first clinical manifestation of the primary antiphospholipid antibody syndrome. *Clinical Endocrinology, 52*(1), 123–126.

Sharma, J., Karthik, S., Rao, S., Phadke, K., Crasta, J., & Garg, I. (2005). Catastrophic antiphospholipid antibody syndrome. *Pediatric Nephrology, 20*(7), 998–999.

Whitelaw, D. A., Spangenberg, J. J., Rickman, R., Hugo, F. H., & Roberts, M. (1999). The association between the antiphospholipid antibody syndrome and neuropsychological impairment in SLE. *Lupus, 8*(6), 444–448.

APHASIAS

DESCRIPTION

Aphasia refers to the loss or impairment of language due to brain dysfunction. Although there are many different aspects of language, such as gestures, prosody, and pragmatics, aphasia nearly always refers to disorders of the semantic and syntactic aspects of language. Both semantic (the meaning of the words) and syntactic (the grammatical aspects of words) functions rely on the left hemisphere functioning (Benson, 1985; Tyler et al., 2011).

The primary aphasia disorders may be divided into disorders of lexical output and disorders of comprehension. Based on conversational speech, Jackson (1868/1915) described two types of aphasias differentiated in terms of lexical output, including a nonfluent aphasia and a fluent aphasia. Nonfluent aphasia is characterized by poorly articulated speech and the use of short sentences (telegraphic). Also, there may be a lack of prosody (abnormal rhythm, melody, inflection, and timbre) and the preferential use of substantive, meaningful words but with poor syntax (agrammatism). Fluent aphasia, in contrast, is characterized by well-articulated speech with intact prosody, although there is often an excess of words. However, the sentences typically lack substantive meaning and there may be paraphasic errors, including both semantic and phonemic errors. The speech of patients with fluent aphasia is often described as empty due to the characteristic lack of meaning (Jackson, 1868/1915). Neuroanatomically, nonfluent aphasia is typically associated with dysfunction of the inferior left frontal cortex around the motor area (i.e., Broca's area) and fluent aphasia is seen with dysfunction of superior left temporal gyrus and regions posterior to the Rolandic fissure (i.e., Wernicke's area). The ability to repeat is often tested in patients with aphasia as this information yields important information regarding the localization of dysfunction. Repetition is impaired in patients with perisylvian lesions and not

in cases where the lesion spares this perisylvian region (Benson, 1993). Word-finding deficits (anomia) may also be seen in aphasia, although these deficits do not seem to provide reliable localizing information (Benson & Geschwind, 1985). Table 1 provides a list of common signs and symptoms associated with aphasia. Based on the location of dysfunction and the associated clinical presentation, aphasias have been divided into several different syndromes. The most common syndromes include those affecting the perisylvian region, such as Broca's aphasia, Wernicke's aphasia, conduction aphasia, and global aphasia.

NEUROPATHOLOGY/PATHOPHYSIOLOGY

Vascular lesions, especially from ischemic strokes but also from hemorrhagic strokes, are the most common cause of aphasia (Kirshner, 2004). Lesions that affect the basal ganglia may also yield aphasia (Bhatia & Marsden, 1994; Parkinson, Raymer, Chang, Fitzgerald, & Crosson, 2009). Language deficits arising from basal ganglia lesions tend to worsen over time and improve less with treatment, in contrast to the characteristic sudden onset from an ischemic cortical stroke (Parkinson et al., 2009). Furthermore, as hemorrhages compress cerebral tissue without necessarily destroying the tissue, recovery from hemorrhages is often easier. Other etiologies that might cause an intracerebral hemorrhage include arteriovenous malformations, anticoagulant therapy, head injury, infarctions, tumors, aneurysms, thrombocytopenia, and cerebral vasculitis (Kirshner, 2004).

Traumatic brain injury is another common cause of aphasia (Levin, Grossman, & Kelly, 1976; Pachalska, Macqueen, Jastrzebowska, & Pufal, 2004; Reeves & Panguluri, 2011; Safaz, Alaca, Yasar, Tok, & Yilmaz,

Table 1
APHASIA TERMS AND DEFINITIONS

Term	Definition
Adynamia	Difficulty initiating speech
Agrammatism	Absence of grammatical elements (verbs, articles, pronouns, and prepositions)
Anomia	Difficulty producing nouns
Circumlocution	Utterance of associated words related to the word that cannot be retrieved
Echolalia	Repetition of an utterance that does not require repetition
Jargon	Well-articulated but mostly incomprehensible language
Logorrhea	Excessively lengthy, often incomprehensible, but well-articulated language
Neologism	Substitution of contrived or invented words, well-articulated
Paragrammatism	Misuse of grammatical elements
Phonemic paraphasia	Substitution of one sound for another (for example, "fable" for "table")
Semantic paraphasia	Word substitution belonging to the same semantic class (such as "table" for "chair")
Stereotypes	Repetition of nonsensical syllables for all communicative attempts ("dee, dee, dee")
Telegraphic speech	Utterance of mostly nouns and verbs

2008). Recovery is better in patients with aphasia resulting from traumatic injury as compared with patients with aphasia from stroke (Vukovic, Vuksanovic, & Vukovic, 2008). Cerebral contusions, depressed skull fractures, and hematomas of the intracerebral, subdural, and epidural spaces may all cause aphasia when they disrupt or compress the language centers of the left hemisphere. However, trauma tends to be less localized than ischemic stroke. Thus, aphasia following traumatic brain injury is often present with the other symptoms of the trauma, such as loss of consciousness, delirium, and amnesia. Aphasia is occasionally associated with subdural hematomas overlying the left hemisphere and is often present with headache, memory loss, and drowsiness (Moster, Johnston, & Reinmuth, 1983; Rahimi & Poorkay, 2000).

A number of other conditions may cause aphasia. Tumors of the left hemisphere or temporal lobes may be associated with the gradual onset of aphasia and other cognitive problems (Gomori et al., 2009; Inskip et al., 2003; Nakamura, Roser, Bundschuh, Vorkapic, & Samii, 2003; Schramm & Aliashkevich, 2008) with more slowly progressing tumors being associated with the transfer of language functioning to the right hemisphere (Thiel et al., 2006). Chronic infections such as herpes simplex that have a predilection for the temporal lobe and orbitofrontal cortex may be associated with aphasia as well as a range of other symptoms such as seizures, confusion, headaches, and fever (Kennedy, Adams, Graham, & Clements, 1988; Khan & Ramsay, 2006; Ku, Lachmann, & Nagler, 1996). Aphasia has also been reported in patients with HIV/AIDS (Kure et al., 1989; Oelschlaeger et al., 2010; Udgirkar et al., 2003), which may cause focal lesions everywhere in the brain or multifocal leukoencephalopathy (Bowers, 1997; Singer et al., 1994). Aphasia has been reported in patients with multiple sclerosis (Devere, Trotter, & Cross, 2000; Lacour et al., 2004; Staff, Lucchinetti, & Keegan, 2009). Epileptic seizures may also cause aphasia (Sahaya, Dhand, Goyal, Soni, & Sahota, 2010; Smith Doody, Hrachovy, & Feher, 1992; Steinlein, 2009; Toledo et al., 2008; Wells et al., 1992), such as in the Landau–Kleffner syndrome's in children (Mouridsen, 1995; Steinlein, 2009) or in adults during the ictal phase or after the postictal phase (Devinsky et al., 1994; Profitlich, Hoppe, Reuber, Helmstaedter, & Bauer, 2008) and may be a feature of Todd's phenomenon (Rolak, Rutecki, Ashizawa, & Harati, 1992; Rosche et al., 2011).

Finally, neurodegenerative diseases such as Alzheimer's disease (Cummings, Benson, Hill, & Read, 1985; Greene, Patterson, Xeureb, & Hodges, 1996; Kertesz, Appell, & Fisman, 1986), semantic dementia (Fletcher & Warren, in press; Hodges, Patterson, Oxbury, & Funnell, 1992; Kertesz, Jesso, Harciarek, Blair, & McMonagle, 2010), primary progressive nonfluent aphasia (Mesulam, 1982), and primary progressive aphasia logopenic type (Gorno-Tempini et al., 2008; Henry & Gorno-Tempini, 2010) can also affect language functions and may be associated with aphasia. Primary progressive aphasia may be considered the neurodegenerative parallel of Broca's aphasia. Patients with primary progressive aphasia are nonfluent, almost mute, and exhibit problems with naming, syntax, and repetition (Amici, Gorno-Tempini, Ogar, Dronkers, & Miller, 2006; Gorno-Tempini et al., 2004; Mesulam, 2001; Neary et al., 1998). The atrophy is often greater in the left inferior frontal lobe (Gorno-Tempini et al., 2004; Mesulam, 2001). Patients with primary progressive aphasia logopenic type exhibit problems naming and have speech filled with phonemic paraphasic errors. Verbal output is slow and they have impaired repetition (Gorno-Tempini et al., 2004, 2008; Henry & Gorno-Tempini, 2010). The atrophy is often located at the posterior region of the temporoparietal lobe (Gorno-Tempini et al., 2004, 2008). Semantic dementia might be considered the neurodegenerative parallel of transcortical sensory aphasia in that these patients are often fluent but exhibit problems with comprehension (Mesulam, 2001; Neary et al., 1998). Also, they have problems with word and object meaning (Amici et al., 2006). The atrophy is usually greater at the left anterior temporal lobe (Gorno-Tempini et al., 2004, 2011).

NEUROPSYCHOLOGICAL/CLINICAL PRESENTATION

The syndromes of aphasia are differentiated in terms of the presence and/or absence of a number of signs, including language output, repetition, and comprehension. Research has generally supported the existence of these individual syndromes, in terms of both the clinical signs that comprise the syndromes and the associated neuroanatomy. Certainly, though, there are many exceptions. The syndromes described below have been generally accepted and might be considered the classic syndromes of aphasia.

PRIMARY TYPES OF PERISYLVIAN APHASIAS

Broca's Aphasia

Broca's aphasia (motor or nonfluent aphasia) is characterized by nonfluent lexical output, problems with repetition, and poor naming (Benson, 1993). Comprehension of verbal information is preserved (Benson,

1979; Goodglass & Berko, 1960; Wernicke, 1908). Sentences are often truncated and characterized by the presence of agrammatism. Also, hesitation and delays in speech production are often present. Speech quality is typically poor and the patients may exhibit hypophonia (Alexander, 2003). Many patients with Broca's aphasia also experience depression (Robinson, Kubos, Starr, Rao, & Price, 1984). Ideomotor apraxia may be seen at the left hemibody (Alexander, 2003; Benson & Geschwind, 1985). Hemi sensory loss or the loss of a visual field is less commonly observed (Alexander, 2003). Recovery of speech following stroke is related to the size and location of the lesion, with critical lesions being centered around the medial subcallosal fasciculus region and the middle third of the periventricular white matter area (Naeser, Palumbo, Helm-Estabrooks, Stiassny-Eder, & Albert, 1989). Furthermore, Knopman et al. (1983) found that lesions in the rolandic cortical region and underlying white matter were associated with persistent nonfluency.

The neuropathology of Broca's aphasia often involves the frontal opercular gyrus of the dominant hemisphere and for this reason right hemiplegia is often present (Damasio, 1991; Price & Crinion, 2005). A CT scan of the brain of Broca's patient, Leborgne, evidenced an extensive lesion involving the third frontal convolution, precentral gyrus, operculum, and insula (Signoret, Castaigne, Lhermitte, Abelanet, & Lavorel, 1984), with later analyses also indicating involvement of the medial subcallosal fasciculus (Naeser, 1994). The complete syndrome is associated with large lesions that involve Broca's area as well as the precentral gyrus, the anterior insula, the underlying white matter tracts, and sometimes the basal ganglia and the anterior temporal lobe (Mohr et al., 1978). Chronic Broca's aphasia typically involves lesions that extend into the subcortical white matter (Naeser et al., 1989).

Wernicke's Aphasia

Patient's with Wernicke's aphasia (sensory or fluent aphasia) have fluent lexical output but with many paraphasic errors (semantic and/or phonemic) and neologisms. Also, Wernicke's aphasia is characterized by problems with repetition and naming. Comprehension of speech is impaired (Benson, 1993), which is a key feature distinguishing Wernicke's aphasia from Broca's aphasia. Furthermore, as patients with Wernicke's aphasia are not aware of their deficits, their speech is often "empty" (without any meaning) and filled with jargon. Deficits may be seen in the right visual field, often a superior quadrantanopia (Alexander, 2003; Benson, 1993), particularly in cases where the lesion is deeper, extending into the optic radiations.

Patients with Wernicke's aphasia may also exhibit anosognosia (Lebrun, 1987). Wernicke's aphasia may be associated with relatively greater impairment in reading than in speech comprehension (Kirshner & Webb, 1982a), although others have reported poor speech comprehension with relatively preserved written comprehension (Heilman, Rothi, Campanella, & Wolfson, 1979; Kirshner, Webb, & Duncan, 1981).

Neuroanatomically, Wernicke's area has been defined as the region comprising the posterior two-thirds of the left superior temporal gyrus (Naeser, 1994). The neuropathology of Wernicke's aphasia involves the superior temporal lobe of the dominant hemisphere, often including the auditory association cortex and the posterior-superior temporal gyrus (Naeser & Hayward, 1978). More extensive damage involving the deep temporal white matter and/or the supramarginal gyrus will often result in more persistent deficits (Kertesz, Lau, & Polk, 1993; Naeser, Helm-Estabrooks, Haas, Auerbach, & Srinivasan, 1987; Selnes, Knopman, Niccum, Rubens, & Larson, 1983). The presence of word deafness suggests pathology involving Heschl's gyrus or its connections (Kirshner et al., 1981). Predominance of word blindness suggests greater involvement of the contiguous parietal cortex, primarily the angular gyrus (Swanberg, Nasreddine, Mendez, & Cummings, 2007).

Conduction Aphasia

Patients affected by conduction aphasia are fluent, but their language is characterized by many paraphasic errors such as substitutions of syllables or phonemes. Comprehension is also preserved in these patients (Benson, 1993). Hence, this syndrome differs from Broca's aphasia, in that language is fluent, and from Wernicke's aphasia as comprehension is intact. However, conduction aphasia shares a common feature with both Broca's and Wernicke's aphasias, namely impaired repetition (Alexander, 2003; Benson, 1993). Limb and/or buccofacial ideomotor apraxia may be seen in patients with conduction aphasia (Alexander, Baker, Naeser, & Kaplan, 1992; Benson et al., 1973; Poncet, Habib, & Robillard, 1987). Patients with conduction aphasia also exhibit problems with naming to confrontation (Axer, von Keyserlingk, Berks, & von Keyserlingk, 2001; Li & Williams, 1991) as well as short-term memory (Bartha & Benke, 2003; De Renzi & Nichelli, 1975; Shallice & Warrington, 1977).

The neuropathology often involves dysfunction within the supramarginal gyrus and the underlying white matter (Benson, 1993; Palumbo, Alexander, & Naeser, 1992), with involvement of the arcuate fasciculus (Benson et al., 1973). However, dysfunction in other regions may also result in conduction aphasia, such as the left temporal cortex, left parietal cortex, and both left and right subcortical white matter (Benson et al., 1973; Damasio & Damasio, 1980; Mendez & Benson, 1985). Lesions to the posterior portion of the left planum temporal have also been implicated in conduction aphasia (Buchsbaum et al., in press).

Global Aphasia

Global aphasia is characterized by impairment in all aspects of language affected by Broca's and Wernicke's aphasias. Thus, patients with global aphasia possess poor fluency, comprehension deficits, and an inability to repeat (Alexander, 2003; Benson, 1993). Naming and reading are also impaired (Kirshner & Webb, 1982b; Kumar, Masih, & Pardo, 1996). Patients also typically experience buccofacial and limb apraxia (Alexander et al., 1992). Patients with global aphasia typically experience weakness at the right side of the face and right hemiplegia, although many patients do not experience right-sided hemiplegia (Ferro, 1983; Legatt & Brust, 1992; Legatt, Rubin, Kaplan, Healton, & Brust, 1987; Tranel, Biller, Damasio, Adams, & Cornell, 1987). Three different forms of global aphasia without hemiparesis have been proposed, including those patients with persistent global aphasia over time, patients whose global aphasia evolves into a transcortical aphasia, and patients whose global aphasia evolves into a Wernicke's aphasia (Hanlon, Lux, & Dromerick, 1999). Also, the presence or absence of hemiplegia may have important implications in anatomical localization, with global aphasia and hemiplegia resulting from a large middle cerebral artery lesion and global aphasia without hemiplegia resulting from separate foci that individually affect the frontal and temporoparietal regions (Damasio, 1992).

This syndrome is typically associated with dysfunction in the territory of the middle cerebral artery that includes a significant portion of the perisylvian region (Benson, 1979). Both Broca's and Wernicke's areas are often involved, although variability exists and the lesions may include lesions that spare either area (Cappa & Vignolo, 1983; Vignolo, Boccardi, & Caverni, 1986). A case of global aphasia following a left thalamic stroke has also been reported (Kumar et al., 1996).

PRIMARY TYPES OF EXTRASYLVIAN APHASIAS

Another group of aphasias are referred to as the extrasylvian aphasias, or the "transcortical aphasia" (Benson, 1993). As with the perisylvian aphasias, this class of aphasias involves dysfunction within the dominant hemisphere. However, unlike the previous group of aphasias, the extrasylvian aphasias arise from dysfunction in regions outside the perisylvian areas. The extrasylvian aphasias are all characterized by the spared ability to repeat, which distinguishes them from the perisylvian aphasias. Several different forms exist that closely parallel the perisylvian aphasias, including transcortical motor aphasia, supplementary motor aphasia, transcortical sensory aphasia, and transcortical mixed aphasia (Benson, 1993).

Transcortical Motor Aphasia

Transcortical motor aphasia is characterized by difficulties in lexical output (nonfluent) and problems with names (anomia). Many patients with transcortical motor aphasia are initially mute (Alexander, 2003). However, comprehension is intact and the ability to repeat is preserved (Benson, 1993). A form of transcortical motor aphasia termed adynamic aphasia has also been identified and is characterized by sparse but normal spontaneous speech that improves when the patient is provided with external cues or prompting (Gold et al., 1997). Some patients with transcortical motor aphasia may also present with hemiparesis (Freedman, Alexander, & Naeser, 1984) and buccofacial apraxia (Alexander et al., 1992). Typically, pathology is located in the frontal/prefrontal regions of the dominant hemisphere, anterior or superior to Broca's area (Atkinson, 1971; Price & Crinion, 2005). However, a case of transcortical motor aphasia following a subdural hematoma has been reported (Liu, Moore, & Goldman, 1991).

Supplementary Motor Aphasia

The language pattern is basically identical to transcortical motor aphasia, with nonfluent lexical output, the presence of echolalia, good comprehension, and intact repetition. Patients with supplementary motor aphasia are often initially mute, which later progresses to a slow hypophonic output that improves with repetition. Unlike patients with transcortical motor aphasia, patients with supplemental motor aphasia often have other neurological signs such as weakness of the right lower extremities and shoulder but normal strength in the arms and face (Alexander, Benson, & Stuss, 1989; Swanberg et al., 2007).

The neuropathology of the syndrome involves the medial frontal structures of the dominant hemisphere, such as the cingulate cortex and supplementary motor area (Masdeu, Schoene, & Funkenstein, 1978; Pai, 1999; Ziegler, Kilian, & Deger, 1997). However, cases of transcortical motor aphasia

A

following lesions involving the supplementary motor area have also been reported (Freedman, Alexander, & Naeser, 1984; Iragui, 1990; Tijssen, Tavy, Hekster, Bots, & Endtz, 1984).

Transcortical Sensory Aphasia

Transcortical sensory aphasia is characterized by difficulties in comprehension but with fluent lexical output and preserved ability to repeat, including repetition of words that the patients cannot understand (Benson, 1993). Speech content is often empty and perseverative and filled with semantic paraphasic errors (Alexander, 2003). Additionally, naming, reading, and writing are impaired (Alexander, 2003; Benson, 1993; Chiacchio, Grossi, Stanzione, & Trojano, 1993). Different subtypes of transcortical sensory aphasia have been proposed based on the deficits underlying the repetition impairment in these patients. Specifically, one subtype is associated with a lexical process and another subtype is associated with a phonological process (Coslett, Roeltgen, Gonzalez-Rothi, & Heilman, 1987). Transcortical sensory aphasia has been described in patients with posterior cortical atrophy (Benson, Davis, & Snyder, 1988; Zakzanis & Boulos, 2001) and Alzheimer's disease (Cummings et al., 1985; Murdoch, Chenery, Wilks, & Boyle, 1987).

Transcortical sensory aphasia has been associated with lesions to the middle and inferior temporal gyri (Alexander, Hiltbrunner, & Fischer, 1989) and the occipitotemporal area (Servan, Verstichel, Catala, Yakovleff, & Rancurel, 1995). However, Kertesz, Sheppard, and MacKenzie (1982) found posterior parieto-occipital lesions in a sample of patients with transcortical sensory aphasia. An interesting investigation by Boatman and colleagues temporarily induced transcortical sensory aphasia in a group of seizure patients undergoing routine cortical mapping. The findings indicated that electrical stimulation of the posterior superior and middle temporal gyri induced transient transcortical sensory aphasia (Boatman et al., 2000). Numerous cases of transcortical sensory aphasia following left frontal lobe damage have also been reported (Kim et al., 2009; Maeshima et al., 1999; Maeshima, Osawa, Nakayama, & Miki, 2004; Sethi, Burke, Torgovnick, & Arsura, 2007).

Transcortical Mixed Aphasia

This form of aphasia is characterized by difficulties in spoken language (nonfluent) and an inability to comprehend, although, as with the other transcortical aphasias, repetition is intact (Alexander, 2003; Benson, 1993). As such, it may be considered a "transcortical" version of global aphasia. Naming is generally impaired

(Bogousslavsky, Regli, & Assal, 1988; Maeshima et al., 2002) but is sometimes preserved (Heilman, Tucker, & Valenstein, 1976; Silveri & Colosimo, 1995). Reading and writing may also be impaired (Maeshima et al., 2002). Also, patients with transcortical mixed aphasia may present with a hemianopia (Bogousslavsky, Bernasconi, & Kumral, 1996).

Some have proposed that transcortical mixed aphasia represents the isolation of the perisylvian speech areas (Maeshima et al., 2002). Bogousslavsky et al. (1988) reported involvement of the anterior pial territory and the watershed region between the middle and posterior cerebral artery in patients with transcortical mixed aphasia following left internal carotid occlusion. Maeshima et al. (1996) reported the case of a patient with transcortical mixed aphasia following a left frontoparietal infarct. Left thalamic lesions have also been associated with transcortical mixed aphasia (McFarling, Rothi, & Heilman, 1982).

OTHER TYPES OF APHASIAS

A number of additional aphasias have been identified that do not necessarily fit the perisylvian or extrasylvian classifications. These additional aphasias include anomic aphasia, aphemia, pure word deafness, and subcortical aphasia.

Anomic Aphasia

Patients with anomic aphasia possess intact fluency, comprehension, and repetition. However, they exhibit a deficit with word retrieval, although paraphasic errors are not common (Alexander, 2003; Benson, 1993). When unable to find the desired word, patients will often engage in circumlocution (Benson, 1993). Many aphasic patients will eventually progress or improve to an anomic aphasia (Kertesz & McCabe, 1977). Anomic aphasia has been described in patients with frontotemporal dementia (Short, Broderick, Patton, Arvanitakis, & Graff-Radford, 2005) and in particular primary progressive aphasia (Kertesz & Munoz, 2003).

Lesions involving the left basal ganglia (Sonobe, Yashima, Takahashi, Katayose, & Kumashiro, 1991) and the subcortical left temporal-parietal-occipital region (Takeda et al., 1999) have been reported. Krishnan, Rao, and Rajashekar (2009) reported the case of a patient with anomic aphasia with multiple lesions, including the left posterior parietal and frontal lobe, left caudate and lentiform nuclei, and anterior limb of the internal capsule. However, a case of crossed anomic aphasia following a right temporal lobe hematoma has been reported (Hadar, Ticehurst, & Wade, 1991).

Aphemia

Aphemia or anarthria typically begins with mutism and recovers to a hypophonic, slow and grammatically intact lexical output. Comprehension is preserved as well as the ability to write and read (Benson, 1993; Fox, Kasner, Chatterjee, & Chalela, 2001; Kaminski, Adams, Burnstine, Civil, & Ruff, 1992). Agrammatism and anomia are not present and it is the lack of agrammatism that makes aphemia distinct from Broca's aphasia (Benson, 1993). However, some patients may exhibit lexical errors and misspellings when writing (Kaminski et al., 1992). Buccofacial apraxia is also often present (Nathan, 1947; Sakurai et al., 1998). Occasionally with recovery there may remain a disorder of rhythm, prosody, inflection, and articulation called "foreign accent syndrome" (Benson, 1993). A progressive form of aphemia has been reported (Gallassi et al., in press) and the disorder has also been described in patients with Pick's disease (Sakurai et al., 1998) and primary progressive aphasia (Cohen, Benoit, Van Eeckhout, Ducarne, & Brunet, 1993). Herderschee, Stam, and Derix (1987) reported the case of a patient with multiple sclerosis who exhibited aphemia as an initial symptom, although whether the patient had multiple sclerosis has been called into question (Poser, 1987).

The pathology is located inferior to Broca's area in the dominant hemisphere (Lecours & Lhermitte, 1976; Schiff, Alexander, Naeser, & Galaburda, 1983). Many have reported left precentral lesions involving the motor and premotor areas leading to aphemia (Fox et al., 2001; Ojha, Nandavar, Pearson, & Demchuk, 2011; Ottomeyer et al., 2009; Rheims et al., 2006; Ruff & Arbit, 1981). However, Mendez (2004) reported the case of a patient with aphemia following a right supplementary motor lesion.

Pure Word Deafness

Patients affected by pure deafness cannot understand spoken language and exhibit an impaired ability to repeat, although their hearing is intact. However, the ability to identify nonverbal or environmental sounds remains intact (Benson, 1993; Buchman, Garron, Trost-Cardamone, Wichter, & Schwartz, 1986; Coslett, Brashear, & Heilman, 1984; Shivashankar, Shashikala, Nagaraja, Jayakumar, & Ratnavalli, 2001; Takahashi et al., 1992), which distinguishes pure word deafness from auditory agnosia. Comprehension of spoken language may be improved by lip reading and contextual cues (Buchman et al., 1986). Verbal output is often normal but may contain paraphasic errors (Buchman et al., 1986; Roberts, Sandercock, & Ghadiali, 1987). Reading comprehension is intact (Buchman et al., 1986; Roberts et al., 1987; Seliger et al., 1991; Slevc, Martin, Hamilton, & Joanisse, 2011) and many patients may hence use a writing tablet to communicate (Benson, 1993). However, some patients may exhibit impaired writing to dictation (Buchman et al., 1986). Naming is generally intact (Buchman et al., 1986), but may be mildly impaired (Roberts et al., 1987). Intact reading and writing are important factors that differentiate pure word deafness from Wernicke's aphasia (Benson, 1979; Hecaen & Albert, 1978). A progressive form of pure word deafness has been reported (Mesulam, 1982; Otsuki, Soma, Sato, Homma, & Tsuji, 1998) and the disorder has been described in frontotemporal dementia (Iizuka, Suzuki, Endo, Fujii, & Mori, 2007).

Cases of pure word deafness following head trauma have been reported (Seliger et al., 1991; Wirkowski, Echausse, Overby, Ortiz, & Radler, 2006). The pathological basis in most cases involves the bilateral temporal lobes (Buchman et al., 1986; Coslett et al., 1984; Di Giovanni, D'Alessandro, Baldini, Cantalupi, & Bottacchi, 1992; Szirmai, Farsang, & Csuri, 2003; Tanaka, Yamadori, & Mori, 1987; Wirkowski et al., 2006). However, pure word deafness has also been reported following a tumor in the third ventricle (Shivashankar et al., 2001), left thalamic lesion (Takahashi et al., 1992), a left temporoparietal lesion (Slevc et al., 2011), and a right temporoparietal lesion (Roberts et al., 1987).

Subcortical Aphasia

The specific language deficits that may arise from subcortical lesions often vary depending on the specific subcortical structures involved (Alexander & Benson, 1992). Subcortical aphasias are often characterized initially as the patient being mute, which eventually improves to a hypophonic, slow, poorly articulated speech output that contains paraphasic errors (Benson, 1993). Capsulostriatal lesions have been reported to cause subcortical aphasia (Mega & Alexander, 1994; Nadeau & Crosson, 1997) and are associated with poor speech fluency and paraphasic errors, but preserved comprehension and naming (Kuljic-Obradovic, 2003). Subcortical aphasia resulting from involvement of the thalamus generally consists of fluent speech, but impaired comprehension and naming as well as paraphasic errors (Karussis, Leker, & Abramsky, 2000; Kuljic-Obradovic, 2003). Left putaminal lesions cause a subcortical aphasia characterized by reduced fluency, impaired comprehension, and problems with repetition (D'Esposito & Alexander, 1995). Different forms of subcortical aphasia have been identified with capsular-putaminal lesions as well. Specifically, patients with capsular-putaminal

A

lesions extending into the anterior-superior white matter exhibit slow and dysarthric speech or a non-fluent aphasia, but with relatively intact comprehension. Capsular-putaminal lesions extending into the posterior white matter are associated with poor comprehension or a fluent aphasia. Finally, patients with both anterior and posterior capsular-putaminal lesions exhibit a global aphasia (Cappa, Cavallotti, Guidotti, Papagno, & Vignolo, 1983; Naeser et al., 1982). Most patients with capsular-putaminal lesions also exhibit a right hemiplegia (Naeser et al., 1982). Subcortical aphasia has also been reported following left caudate lesions (Hillis et al., 2004) and with atypical lacunar syndrome (Arboix et al., 2006).

DIAGNOSIS

The diagnosis of aphasia is based on the assessment of language functions and requires examining various aspects of language, such as conversational speech, simple naming, spelling, repetition, and comprehension as well as vocabulary and semantic reasoning. Among the first abilities that are usually evaluated is spontaneous speech or fluency. Fluency is often assessed in a bedside manner by asking patients various questions and engaging them in conversation during the clinical interview. Engaging patients in casual conversation may yield information regarding fluency, comprehension, correct use of syntax, prosody, naming, and accent. As mentioned earlier, patients with anterior lesions might evidence difficulties with fluency, agrammatic and dysprosodic speech, whereas patients with posterior lesions might possess very fluent but empty speech and have problems with comprehension. These characteristic symptoms are often readily observed during a clinical interview. Additionally, semantic and phonemic paraphasic errors are common and may be observed during conversation with patients who have a variety of different aphasias. More formal evaluation of fluency may be accomplished using tests such as the controlled oral word association test (lexical fluency) or the animal naming test (semantic fluency; see Strauss, Sherman, & Spreen, 2006). Repetition may also be assessed casually in the clinical interview by asking the patient to repeat a series of words and then progressively longer sentences. The sentence repetition test may also be used for more formal evaluation of repetition abilities (Strauss et al., 2006). Comprehension may be assessed by asking the patient to perform a series of actions of increasing difficulty. Examples may include asking simple questions requiring a "yes" or "no" response (i.e., "Are you at the store now?" or "Is your name Elizabeth?") or having the patient perform one-, two-, and three-step commands (i.e., "Close your

eyes"; "Before pointing to the door, point to the light"; or "Take this piece of paper with your right hand, fold it in half, and put it on the floor"). The Token test may be used to formally assess verbal comprehension (see Strauss et al., 2006). Naming is also often assessed in a casual manner by having the patient name objects that are present. However, it may be important to distinguish between naming impairment, visual/perceptual disturbance, and educational or cultural limitations. If the patient cannot recall the name of a given object, the examiner should provide a phonemic cue. Patients with true naming deficits may produce the target word when provided with a phonemic cue, whereas patients who are not familiar with the word will show no response to phonemic cueing. Formal evaluation of naming may be accomplished using tests such as the Boston Naming Test—2 (Kaplan, Goodglass, & Weintraub, 2001). Evaluation of reading, spelling, and written comprehension may also be important and may be accomplished using tests such as the Wide Range Achievement Test—4 (Wilkinson & Robertson, 2006).

Although informal, bedside evaluations and individual tests are often used to assess language functioning, many standardized batteries of tests are available to evaluate aphasia. These batteries are designed specifically to evaluate the patient's receptive and expressive language capacities by sampling various components, such as conversational speech, comprehension, repetition, naming, reading, and writing. The Minnesota Test for Differential Diagnosis of Aphasia (MTDDA; Schuell, 1965) is among the most comprehensive batteries to assess for language disturbance. The MTDDA can identify different aphasia types and contains several subtests to assess each major area of language. The Boston Diagnostic Aphasia Examination (BDAE; Goodglass & Kaplan, 1983) is one of the most commonly used; it can also assist in identifying different aphasia types and may be used to quantify the strengths and weaknesses in various areas of language. The Western Aphasia Battery (WAB; Kertesz, 1982) is another commonly used battery. The WAB is based on BDAE but can be completed in a much briefer period and may also be used to assist in classifying different aphasia syndromes and for providing an indication of the severity of impairment. The Porch Index of Communicative Ability (PICA; Porch, 1983) measures overall communication ability and uses 10 common objects (e.g., pen and comb) to elicit patient responses. The PICA may be used to predict and follow recovery. The Communication Effectiveness Index (CETI) assesses communication for basic needs, life skills, and health threats. The CETI is based on observations made by the patient's significant other. Finally, the Multilingual

Aphasia Examination (MAE; Benton, Hamsher, & Sivan, 1994) is another battery that is designed to assess the presence and severity of aphasic disorders. The MAE may be used to assess oral expression, oral and reading comprehension, speech articulation, writing, as well as oral, written, and block spelling. Following either casual or more formal examination of language functioning, it is also often useful to obtain either a CT or MRI of the brain to localize any lesion that might be affecting the patient's language ability.

TREATMENT

The symptoms of aphasia may be resolved by appropriate speech therapy techniques, although in some cases the disability remains permanent. There is strong evidence that aphasia therapy does produce worthwhile improvement in language function (Basso, Capitani, & Vignolo, 1979; Holland, Fromm, DeRuyter, & Stein, 1996; Robey, 1994, 1998; Wertz et al., 1981). Thus, most patients with aphasia deserve consideration for language therapy as many will experience benefits. That being said, it should be noted that considerable spontaneous recovery occurs, particularly in the first few months following the onset of aphasia. Generally, the greatest recovery occurs during the first 2-3 months, but improvement may continue over a prolonged period (Demeurisse et al., 1980; Lendrem & Lincoln, 1985; Sarno & Levita, 1979), especially in young patients (Kertesz & McCabe, 1977; Lendrem, McGuirk, & Lincoln, 1988) and in patients with global aphasia (Sarno & Levita, 1979). Many other factors can influence the degree and speed of recovery from aphasia, such as the type and size of lesion, initial severity, education, and intelligence (Demeurisse et al., 1980; Plowman, Hentz, & Ellis, in press). Additionally, the rates of recovery and prognosis vary for the different classes of aphasia (Demeurisse et al., 1980; Sarno & Levita, 1979). The type of aphasia often changes during recovery such that Broca's aphasia may evolve into a transcortical motor aphasia or anomic aphasia (Alexander, Naeser, & Palumbo, 1990; Mazzocchi & Vignolo, 1979) and global aphasia may evolve into a Broca's aphasia (Alexander, 2003). Anomic aphasia seems to be a common point of eventual evolution (Kertesz & McCabe, 1977). Although spontaneous recovery of some degree of language functioning is common and may be substantial, most clinicians now agree that language therapy is helpful for most aphasic patients (Basso, 1989). Further, patients with aphasia may benefit from treatment even well after the onset of aphasia (Moss & Nicholas, 2006). Studies of language activation using PET, SPECT, and functional imaging techniques are advancing our understanding of the neuroanatomy of language recovery (Crinion & Leff, 2007; Heiss, Kessler, Thiel, Ghaemi, & Karbe, 1999; Meinzer, Harnish, Conway, & Crosson, 2011).

Speech therapy, provided by a speech-language pathologist, attempts to facilitate language recovery by a variety of techniques and to help the patient compensate for lost functions. Repeated practice in articulation and comprehension tasks has traditionally been used to stimulate improvement. Melodic intonation therapy uses melody and rhythm to involve the right hemisphere in speech production as patients are often capable of singing words they cannot speak (Norton, Zipse, Marchina, & Schlaug, 2009; Sparks, Helm, & Albert, 1974). Melodic intonation therapy seems to be ideal for nonfluent aphasics (Albert, Sparks, & Helm, 1973; Schlaug, Marchina, & Norton, 2008; Sparks, Helm, & Albert, 1974). Visual action therapy is based on gestural expression and is essentially a nonvocal approach using pictures, drawings, and gestures to indicate objects (Helm-Estabrooks, Fitzpatrick, & Barresi, 1982). Visual action therapy ultimately trains patients to produce symbolic gestures for visually absent stimuli and may be indicated for patients affected by global aphasia. Additionally, promoting aphasics communication effectiveness (PACE) is a treatment that encourages patients to convey information through any available modality (e.g., speech, gestures, drawings, expressions, and mime) and may be of benefit to many different forms of aphasia (Davis & Wilcox, 1985). Computerized visual communication is a computer program that provides an alternative means of communication for patients with aphasia and is based on the premise that patients with aphasia may be able to learn a new system of symbols with which to communicate (Steele, Weinrich, Wertz, Kleczewska, & Carlson, 1989; Weinrich, 1991). However, patients with aphasia may benefit because they may be able to learn to produce simple sentences via a computer. Augmentation devices make language expression possible through the use of printers or voice simulators.

Speech therapy has remained controversial. Some studies have suggested that trained volunteers can produce as much improvement as speech language pathologists (Kelly, Brady, & Enderby, 2010; Marshall et al., 1989). However, meta-analyses of the literature have clearly indicated that patients who undergo formal speech therapy recover better than untreated patients (Holland et al., 1996; Robey, 1994, 1998). Another approach to language rehabilitation is the use of pharmacological agents to improve speech (Bakheit, 2004; Hillis, 2007). Albert, Bachman, Morgan, and Helm-Estabrooks (1988) were the first to report that the dopaminergic drug bromocriptine

A

improves speech fluency in a patient with transcortical motor aphasia. Others have also reported beneficial effects of bromocriptine (Raymer et al., 2001), especially when combined with speech therapy (Bragoni et al., 2000). However, not all studies have supported the use of bromocriptine, finding no difference between bromocriptine and placebo (Ashtary, Janghorbani, Chitsaz, Reisi, & Bahrami, 2006; Sabe, Salvarezza, Garcia Cuerva, Leiguarda, & Starkstein, 1995). Several studies have also shown that piracetam may be beneficial in treating patients with aphasia (Enderby, Broeckx, Hospers, Schildermans, & Deberdt, 1994; Greener, Enderby, & Whurr, 2001; Kessler, Thiel, Karbe, & Heiss, 2000). Other medications that may have beneficial effects in patients with aphasia include donepezil (Berthier et al., 2006; Berthier, Hinojosa, del Carmen Martin, & Fernandez, 2003) and amantadine (Barrett & Eslinger, 2007). However, further research must be conducted to examine the potential pharmacologic therapies in treating aphasic syndromes.

Research has supported the use of transcranial magnetic stimulation (TMS) as a treatment for aphasia (Galletta, Rao, & Barrett, 2011; Hamilton, Chrysikou, & Coslett, 2011; Naeser et al., 2010). Szaflarski et al. (2011) reported improved language skills following repetitive TMS (rTMS) targeted over Broca's area. A recent randomized, blinded study also found improvements following rTMS when applied to the right inferior frontal gyrus (Weiduschat et al., 2011). TMS has been reported to improve language skills in both nonfluent or motor aphasia (Barwood et al., 2011; Kakuda, Abo, Kaito, Watanabe, & Senoo, 2010) and global aphasia (Naeser et al., 2005). Finally, transcranial direct-current stimulation has also been reported to be of benefit to patients with aphasia (Baker, Rorden, & Fridriksson, 2010), including Wernicke's aphasia (You, Kim, Chun, Jung, & Park, 2011).

Valeria Drago
Paul S. Foster

Albert, M. L., Bachman, D. L., Morgan, A., & Helm-Estabrooks, N. (1988). Pharmacotherapy for aphasia. *Neurology, 38*, 877–879.

Albert, M. L., Sparks, R. W., & Helm, N. A. (1973). Melodic intonation therapy for aphasia. *Archives of Neurology, 29*, 130–131.

Alexander, M. P. (2003). Aphasia: Clinical and anatomic issues. In T. E. Feinberg & M. J. Farah (Eds.), *Behavioral neurology and neuropsychology* (2nd ed., pp. 147–164). New York: McGraw Hill.

Alexander, M. P., Baker, E., Naeser, M. A., & Kaplan, E. (1992). Neuropsychological and neuroanatomical dimensions of ideomotor apraxia. *Brain, 118*, 87–107.

Alexander, M. P., & Benson, D. F. (1992). The aphasias and related disturbances. In R. J. Joynt (Ed.), *Clinical neurology* (Vol. I, pp. 1–58). Philadelphia: Lippincott Williams & Wilkins.

Alexander, M. P., Benson, D. F., & Stuss, D. T. (1989). Frontal lobe and language. *Brain and Language, 37*, 656.

Alexander, M. P., Hiltbrunner, B., & Fischer, R. F. (1989). The distributed anatomy of transcortical sensory aphasia. *Archives of Neurology, 46*, 885–892.

Alexander, M. P., Naeser, M. A., & Palumbo, C. (1990). Broca's area aphasias: Aphasia after lesions including the frontal operculum. *Neurology, 40*, 353–362.

Amici, S., Gorno-Tempini, M. L., Ogar, J. M., Dronkers, N. F., & Miller, B. L. (2006). An overview on primary progressive aphasia and its variants. *Behavioral Neurology, 17*, 77–87.

Arboix, A., Lopez-Grau, M., Casasnovas, C., Garcia-Eroles, L., Massons, J., & Balcells, M. (2006). Clinical study of 39 patients with atypical lacunar syndrome. *Journal of Neurology, Neurosurgery, and Psychiatry, 77*, 381–384.

Ashtary, F., Janghorbani, M., Chitsaz, A., Reisi, M., & Bahrami, A. (2006). A randomized, double-blind trial of bromocriptine efficacy in nonfluent aphasia after stroke. *Neurology, 66*, 914–916.

Atkinson, M. S. (1971). Transcortical motor aphasia associated with left frontal lobe infarction. *Transactions of the American Neurological Association, 96*, 136–140.

Axer, H., von Keyserlingk, A. G., Berks, G., & von Keyserlingk, D. G. (2001). Supra- and infrasylvian conduction aphasia. *Brain and Language, 76*, 317–331.

Baker, J. M., Rorden, C., & Fridriksson, J. (2010). Using transcranial direct-current stimulation to treat stroke patients with aphasia. *Stroke, 41*, 1229–1236.

Bakheit, A. M. (2004). Drug treatment of poststroke aphasia. *Expert Review of Neurotherapeutics, 4*, 211–217.

Barrett, A. M., & Eslinger, P. J. (2007). Amantadine for adynamic speech: Possible benefit for aphasia? *American Journal of Physical Medicine and Rehabilitation, 86*, 605–612.

Bartha, L., & Benke, T. (2003). Acute conduction aphasia: An analysis of 20 cases. *Brain and Language, 85*, 93–108.

Barwood, C. H., Murdoch, B. E., Whelan, B. M., Lloyd, D., Riek, S., O'sullivan, J., et al. (2011). The effects of low frequency repetitive transcranial magnetic stimulation (rTMS) and sham condition rTMS on behavioural language in chronic non-fluent aphasia: Short term outcomes. *NeuroRehabilitation, 28*, 113–128.

Basso, A. (1989). Therapy of aphasia. In F. Boller & J. Grafman (Eds.), *Handbook of neuropsychology* (Vol. 2, pp. 67–82). Amsterdam: Elsevier.

Basso, A., Capitani, E., & Vignolo, L. A. (1979). Influence of rehabilitation on language skills in aphasia patients. *Archives of Neurology, 36*, 190–195.

Benson, D. F. (1979). *Aphasia, alexia, and agraphia*. New York: Churchill Livingstone.

Benson, D. F. (1985). Language in the left hemisphere. In D. F. Benson & E. Zaidel (Eds.), *The dual brain* (pp. 193–203). New York: Guilford Press.

Benson, D. F. (1993). Aphasia. In K. M. Heilman & E. Valenstein (Eds.), *Clinical neuropsychology* (pp. 17–36). New York: Oxford University Press.

Benson, D. F., Davis, R. J., & Snyder, B. D. (1988). Posterior cortical atrophy. *Archives of Neurology, 45*, 789–793.

Benson, D. F., & Geschwind, N. (1985). The aphasias and related disturbances. In A. B. Baker & R. J. Joynt (Eds.), *Clinical neurology* (Vol. I). Philadelphia: Harper and Row.

Benson, D. F., Sheremata, W. A., Bouchard, R., Segarra, J. M., Price, D., & Geschwind, N. (1973). Conduction aphasia: A clinicopathological study. *Archives of Neurology, 28*, 339–346.

Benton, A. L., Hamsher, K. de S., & Sivan, A. B. (1994). *Multilingual aphasia examination* (3rd ed.). Lutz, FL: Psychological Assessment Resources.

Berthier, M. L., Green, C., Higueras, C., Fernandez, I., Hinojosa, J., & Martin, M. C. (2006). A randomized, placebo-controlled study of donepezil in poststroke aphasia. *Neurology, 67*, 1687–1689.

Berthier, M. L., Hinojosa, J., Martin, M. C., & Fernandez, I. (2003). Open-label study of donepezil in chronic poststroke aphasia. *Neurology, 60*, 1218–1219.

Bhatia, K. P., & Marsden, C. D. (1994). The behavioural and motor consequences of focal lesions of the basal ganglia in man. *Brain, 117*, 859–876.

Boatman, D., Gordon, B., Hart, J., Selnes, O., Miglioretti, D., & Lenz, F. (2000). Transcortical sensory aphasia: Revisited and revised. *Brain, 123*, 1634–1642.

Bogousslavsky, J., Bernasconi, A., & Kumral, E. (1996). Acute multiple infarction involving the anterior circulation. *Archives of Neurology, 53*, 50–57.

Bogousslavsky, J., Regli, F., & Assal, G. (1988). Acute transcortical mixed aphasia: A carotid occlusion syndrome with pial and watershed infarcts. *Brain, 111*, 631–641.

Bowers, M. (1997). Progressive multifocal leukoencephalopathy. *Bulletin of Experimental Treatments for AIDS, September*, 23–26.

Bragoni, M., Altieri, M., Di Piero, V., Padovani, A., Mostardini, C., & Lenzi, G. L. (2000). *Neurological Sciences, 21*, 19–22.

Buchman, A. S., Garron, D. C., Trost-Cardamone, J. E., Wichter, M. D., & Schwartz, M. (1986). Word deafness: One hundred years later. *Journal of Neurology, Neurosurgery, and Psychiatry, 49*, 489–499.

Buchsbaum, B. R., Baldo, J., Okada, K., Berman, K. F., Dronkers, N., D'Esposito, M., et al. (in press). Conduction aphasia, sensory-motor integration, and phonological short-term memory—An aggregate analysis of lesion and fMRI data. *Brain and Language*.

Cappa, S. F., Cavallotti, G., Guidotti, M., Papagno, C., & Vignolo, L. A. (1983). Subcortical aphasia: Two clinical-CT scan correlation studies. *Cortex, 19*, 227–241.

Cappa, S. F., & Vignolo, L. A. (1983). CT scan studies of aphasia. *Human Neurobiology, 2*, 129–134.

Chiacchio, L., Grossi, D., Stanzione, M., & Trojano, L. (1993). Slowly progressive aphasia associated with surface dyslexia. *Cortex, 29*, 145–152.

Cohen, L., Benoit, N., Van Eeckhout, P., Ducarne, B., & Brunet, P. (1993). Pure progressive aphemia. *Journal of Neurology, Neurosurgery, and Psychiatry, 56*, 923–924.

Coslett, H. B., Brashear, H. R., & Heilman, K. M. (1984). Pure word deafness after bilateral primary auditory cortex infarcts. *Neurology, 34*, 347–352.

Coslett, H. B., Roeltgen, D. P., Gonzalez-Rothi, L., & Heilman, K. M. (1987). Transcortical sensory aphasia: Evidence for subtypes. *Brain and Language, 32*, 362–378.

Crinion, J. T., & Leff, A. P. (2007). Recovery and treatment of aphasia after stroke: Functional imaging studies. *Current Opinion in Neurology, 20*, 667–673.

Cummings, J. L., Benson, F., Hill, M. A., & Read, S. (1985). Aphasia in dementia of the Alzheimer type. *Neurology, 35*, 394–397.

Damasio, A. R. (1992). Aphasia. *New England Journal of Medicine, 326*, 531–539.

Damasio, H. (1991). Cerebral localization of the aphasias. In M. T. Sarno (Ed.), *Acquired aphasia* (pp. 45–73). New York: Academic Press.

Damasio, H., & Damasio, A. R. (1980). The anatomical basis of conduction aphasia. *Brain, 103*, 337–350.

Davis, G. A., & Wilcox, M. J. (1985). *Adult aphasia rehabilitation: Applied pragmatics*. San Diego, CA: College Hill Press.

De Renzi, E., & Nichelli, P. (1975). Verbal and non-verbal short-term memory impairment following hemispheric damage. *Cortex, 11*, 341–354.

Demeurisse, G., Demol, O., Derouck, M., de Beuckelaer, R., Coekaerts, M. J., & Capon, A. (1980). Quantitative study of the rate of recovery from aphasia due to ischemic stroke. *Stroke, 11*, 455–458.

D'Esposito, M., & Alexander, M. P. (1995). Subcortical aphasia: Distinct profiles following left putaminal hemorrhage. *Neurology, 45*, 38–41.

Devere, T. R., Trotter, J. L., & Cross, A. H. (2000). Acute aphasia in multiple sclerosis. *Archives of Neurology, 57*, 1207–1209.

Devinsky, O., Kelley, K., Yacubian, E. M., Sato, S., Kufta, C. V., Theodore, W. H., et al. (1994). Postictal behavior: A clinical and subdural electroencephalographic study. *Archives of Neurology, 51*, 254–259.

Di Giovanni, M., D'Alessandro, G., Baldini, S., Cantalupi, D., & Bottacchi, E. (1992). Clinical and neuroradiological findings in a case of pure word deafness. *Italian Journal of Neurological Sciences, 13*, 507–510.

A

Enderby, P., Broeckx, J., Hospers, W., Schildermans, F., & Deberdt, W. (1994). Effect of piracetam on recovery and rehabilitation after stroke: A double-blind, placebo-controlled study. *Clinical Neuropharmacology, 17,* 320–331.

Ferro, J. M. (1983). Global aphasia without hemiparesis. *Neurology, 33,* 1106.

Fletcher, P. D., & Warren, J. D. (in press). Semantic dementia: A specific network-opathy. *Journal of Molecular Neuroscience.*

Fox, R. J., Kasner, S. E., Chatterjee, A., & Chalela, J. A. (2001). Aphemia: An isolated disorder of articulation. *Clinical Neurology and Neurosurgery, 103,* 123–126.

Freedman, M., Alexander, M. P., & Naeser, M. A. (1984). Anatomic basis of transcortical motor aphasia. *Neurology, 34,* 409–417.

Gallassi, R., Sambati, L., Poda, R., Oppi, F., Stanzani Maserati, M., Cevolani, D., et al. (in press). Slowly progressive aphemia: A neuropsychological, conventional, and functional MRI study. *Neurological Sciences.*

Galletta, E. E., Rao, P. R., & Barrett, A. M. (2011). Transcranial magnetic stimulation (TMS): Potential progress for language improvement in aphasia. *Topics in Stroke Rehabilitation, 18,* 87–91.

Gold, M., Nadeau, S. E., Jacobs, D. H., Adair, J. C., Rothi, L. J., & Heilman, K. M. (1997). Adynamic aphasia: A transcortical motor aphasia with defective semantic strategy formation. *Brain and Language, 57,* 374–393.

Gomori, E., Halbauer, J. D., Kasza, G., Varga, D., Horvath, Z., & Komoly, S. (2009). Glioblastoma multiforme with an unusual location and clinical course. *Clinical Neuropathology, 28,* 165–167.

Goodglass, H., & Berko, J. (1960). Agrammatism and inflectional morphology in English. *Journal of Speech and Hearing Research, 3,* 257–267.

Goodglass, H., & Kaplan, E. (1983). *Boston diagnostic aphasia examination (BDAE).* Philadelphia: Lea and Febiger.

Gorno-Tempini, M. L., Brambati, S. M., Ginex, V., Ogar, J., Dronkers, N. F., Marcone, A., et al. (2008). The logopenic/phonological variant of primary progressive aphasia. *Neurology, 71,* 1227–1234.

Gorno-Tempini, M. L., Dronkers, N. F., Rankin, K. P., Ogar, J. M., Phengrasamy, L., Rosen, H. J., et al. (2004). Cognition and anatomy in three variants of primary progressive aphasia. *Annals of Neurology, 55,* 335–346.

Gorno-Tempini, M. L., Hillis, A. E., Weintraub, S., Kertesz, A., Mendez, M., Cappa, S. F., et al. (2011). Classification of primary progressive aphasia and its variants. *Neurology, 76,* 1006–1014.

Greene, J. D., Patterson, K., Xuereb, J., & Hodges, J. R. (1996). Alzheimer disease and nonfluent progressive aphasia. *Archives of Neurology, 53,* 1072–1078.

Greener, J., Enderby, P., & Whurr, R. (2001). Pharmacological treatment for aphasia following stroke. *Cochrane Database of Systematic Reviews,* (4), CD000424.

Hadar, U., Ticehurst, S., & Wade, J. P. (1991). Crossed anomic aphasia: Mild naming deficits following right brain damage in a dextral patient. *Cortex, 27,* 459–468.

Hamilton, R. H., Chrysikou, E. G., & Coslett, B. (2011). Mechanisms of aphasia recovery after stroke and the role of noninvasive brain stimulation. *Brain and Language, 118,* 40–50.

Hanlon, R., Lux, W. E., & Dromerick, A. W. (1999). Global aphasia without hemiparesis: Language profiles and lesion distribution. *Journal of Neurology, Neurosurgery, and Psychiatry, 66,* 365–369.

Hecaen, H., & Albert, M. (1978). Human neuropsychology. New York: John Wiley and Sons.

Heilman, K. M., Rothi, L., Campanella, D., & Wolfson, S. (1979). Wernicke's and global aphasia without alexia. *Archives of Neurology, 36,* 129–133.

Heilman, K. M., Tucker, D. M., & Valenstein, E. (1976). A case of mixed transcortical aphasia with intact naming. *Brain, 99,* 415–426.

Heiss, W. D., Kessler, J., Thiel, A., Ghaemi, M., & Karbe, H. (1999). Differential capacity of left and right hemispheric areas for compensation of poststroke aphasia. *Annals of Neurology, 45,* 430–438.

Helm-Estabrooks, N., Fitzpatrick, P. M., & Barresi, B. (1982). Visual action therapy for global aphasia. *Journal of Speech and Hearing Disorders, 47,* 385–389.

Henry, M. L., & Gorno-Tempini, M. L. (2010). The logopenic variant of primary progressive aphasia. *Current Opinion in Neurology, 23,* 633–637.

Herderschee, D., Stam, J., & Derix, M. M. A. (1987). Aphemia as a first symptom of multiple sclerosis. *Journal of Neurology, Neurosurgery, and Psychiatry, 50,* 499–500.

Hillis, A. E. (2007). Pharmacological, surgical, and neurovascular interventions to augment acute aphasia recovery. *American Journal of Physical Medicine and Rehabilitation, 86,* 426–434.

Hillis, A. E., Barker, P. B., Wityk, R. J., Aldrich, E. M., Restrepo, L., Breese, E. L., et al. (2004). Variability in subcortical aphasia is due to variable sites of cortical hypoperfusion. *Brain and Language, 89,* 524–530.

Hodges, J. R., Patterson, K., Oxbury, S., & Funnell, E. (1992). Semantic dementia: Progressive fluent aphasia with temporal lobe atrophy. *Brain, 115,* 1783–1806.

Holland, A. L., Fromm, D. S., DeRuyter, F., & Stein, M. (1996). Treatment efficacy: Aphasia. *Journal of Speech and Hearing Research, 39,* S27–S36.

Iizuka, O., Suzuki, K., Endo, K., Fujii, T., & Mori, E. (2007). Pure word deafness and pure anarthria in a patient with frontotemporal dementia. *European Journal of Neurology, 14,* 473–475.

Inskip, P. D., Tarone, R. E., Hatch, E. E., Wilcosky, T. C., Selker, R. G., Fine, H. A., et al. (2003). Laterality of brain tumors. *Neuroepidemiology, 22,* 130–138.

Iragui, V. J. (1990). Ataxic hemiparesis associated with transcortical motor aphasia. *European Neurology, 30,* 162–166.

Jackson, J. H. (1868). On the physiology of language. *Medical Times and Gazette, 2,* 275. (Reprinted from *Brain, 38,* 59–64, 1915.)

Kakuda, W., Abo, M., Kaito, N., Watanabe, M., & Senoo, A. (2010). Functional MRI-based therapeutic rTMS strategy for aphasic stroke patients: A case series pilot study. *International Journal of Neuroscience, 120,* 60–66.

Kaminski, H. J., Adams, N., Burnstine, T. H., Civil, R. H., & Ruff, R. L. (1992). Relation of aphemia and agraphia. *European Neurology, 32,* 302–304.

Kaplan, E. F., Goodglass, H., & Weintraub, S. (2001). *The Boston naming test* (2nd ed.). Philadelphia: Lippincott Williams & Wilkins.

Karussis, D., Leker, R. R., & Abramsky, O. (2000). Cognitive dysfunction following thalamic stroke. A study of 16 cases and review of the literature. *Journal of the Neurological Sciences, 172,* 25–29.

Kelly, H., Brady, M. C., & Enderby, P. (2010). Speech and language therapy for aphasia following stroke. *Cochrane Database of Systematic Reviews,* (5), CD000425.

Kennedy, P. G., Adams, J. H., Graham, D. I., & Clements, G. B. (1988). A clinico-pathological study of herpes simplex encephalitis. *Neuropathology and Applied Neurobiology, 14,* 395–415.

Kertesz, A. (1982). *Western aphasia battery.* San Antonio, TX: Psychological Corporation.

Kertesz, A., Appell, J., & Fisman, M. (1986). The dissolution of language in Alzheimer's disease. *Canadian Journal of Neurological Sciences, 13,* 415–418.

Kertesz, A., Jesso, S., Harciarek, M., Blair, M., & McMonagle, P. (2010). What is semantic dementia? A cohort study of diagnostic features and clinical boundaries. *Archives of Neurology, 67,* 483–489.

Kertesz, A., Lau, W. K., & Polk, M. (1993). The structural determinations of recovery in Wernicke's aphasia. *Brain and Language, 44,* 153–164.

Kertesz, A., & McCabe, P. (1977). Recovery patterns and prognosis in aphasia. *Brain, 100,* 1–18.

Kertesz, A., & Munoz, D. G. (2003). Primary progressive aphasia and Pick complex. *Journal of the Neurological Sciences, 206,* 97–107.

Kertesz, A., Sheppard, A., & MacKenzie, R. (1982). Localization in transcortical sensory aphasia. *Archives of Neurology, 39,* 475–478.

Kessler, J., Thiel, A., Karbe, H., & Heiss, W. D. (2000). Piracetam improves activated blood flow and facilitates rehabilitation of poststroke aphasic patients. *Stroke, 31,* 2112–2116.

Khan, O. A., & Ramsay, A. (2006). Herpes encephalitis presenting as mild aphasia: Case report. *BMC Family Practice, 7,* 22.

Kim, E. J., Suh, M. K., Lee, B. H., Park, K. C., Ku, B. D., Chung, C. S., et al. (2009). Transcortical sensory aphasia following a left frontal lobe infarction probably due to anomalously represented language areas. *Journal of Clinical Neuroscience, 16,* 1482–1485.

Kirshner, H. S. (2004). Aphasia. In W. C. Bradley, R. B. Daroff, G. M. Fenichel, & J. Jankovic (Eds.), *Neurology in clinical practice: Principles of diagnosis and management* (4th ed., pp. 141–160). Boston: Butterworth-Heinemann.

Kirshner, H. S., & Webb, W. G. (1982a). Alexia and agraphia in Wernicke's aphasia. *Journal of Neurology, Neurosurgery, and Psychiatry, 45,* 719–724.

Kirshner, H. S., & Webb, W. G. (1982b). Word and letter reading and the mechanism of the third alexia. *Archives of Neurology, 39,* 84–87.

Kirshner, H. S., Webb, W. G., & Duncan, G. W. (1981). Word deafness in Wernicke's aphasia. *Journal of Neurology, Neurosurgery, and Psychiatry, 44,* 197–201.

Knopman, D. S., Selnes, O. A., Niccum, N., Rubens, A. B., Yock, D., & Larson, D. (1983). A longitudinal study of speech fluency in aphasia: CT correlates of recovery and persistent nonfluency. *Neurology, 33,* 1170–1178.

Krishnan, G., Rao, S. N., & Rajasekar, B. (2009). Apraxic agraphia: An insight into the writing disturbances of posterior aphasia. *Annals of Indian Academy of Neurology, 12,* 120–123.

Ku, A., Lachmann, E. A., & Nagler, W. (1996). Selective language aphasia from herpes simplex encephalitis. *Pediatric Neurology, 15,* 169–171.

Kuljic-Obradovic, D. C. (2003). Subcortical aphasia: Three different language disorder syndromes? *European Journal of Neurology, 10,* 445–448.

Kumar, R., Masih, A. K., & Pardo, J. (1996). Global aphasia due to thalamic hemorrhage: A case report and review of the literature. *Archives of Physical Medicine and Rehabilitation, 77,* 1312–1315.

Kure, K., Park, Y. D., Kim, T. S., Lyman, W. D., Lantos, G., Lee, S., et al. (1989). Immunohistochemical localization of an HIV epitope in cerebral aneurismal arteriopathy in pediatric acquired immunodeficiency syndrome (AIDS). *Pediatric Pathology, 9,* 655–667.

Lacour, A., De Seze, J., Revenco, E., Lebrun, C., Masmoudi, K., Vidry, E., et al. (2004). Acute aphasia in multiple sclerosis: A multicenter study of 22 patients. *Neurology, 62,* 974–977.

Lebrun, Y. (1987). Anosognosia in aphasics. *Cortex, 23,* 251–263.

Lecours, A. R., & Lhermitte, F. (1976). The pure form of the phonetic disintegration syndrome (pure anarthria): Anatomo-clinical report of an historical case. *Brain and Language, 3,* 88–113.

Legatt, A. D., & Brust, J. C. (1992). Global aphasia without hemiparesis. *New England Journal of Medicine, 327,* 1244.

Legatt, A. D., Rubin, M. J., Kaplan, L. R., Healton, E. B., & Brust, J. C. (1987). Global aphasia without hemiparesis: Multiple etiologies. *Neurology, 37,* 201–205.

Lendrem, W., & Lincoln, N. B. (1985). Spontaneous recovery of language in patients with aphasia between 4 and 34 weeks after stroke. *Journal of Neurology, Neurosurgery, and Psychiatry, 48*, 743–748.

Lendrem, W., McGuirk, E., & Lincoln, N. B. (1988). Factors affecting language recovery in aphasic stroke patients receiving speech therapy. *Journal of Neurology, Neurosurgery, and Psychiatry, 51*, 1103–1110.

Levin, H. S., Grossman, R. G., & Kelly, P. J. (1976). Aphasic disorder in patients with closed head injury. *Journal of Neurology, Neurosurgery, and Psychiatry, 39*, 1062–1070.

Li, E. C., & Williams, S. E. (1991). An investigation of naming errors following semantic and phonemic cueing. *Neuropsychologia, 29*, 1083–1093.

Liu, G. T., Moore, M. R., & Goldman, H. (1991). Transcortical motor aphasia due to a subdural hematoma. *American Journal of Emergency Medicine, 9*, 620–622.

Maeshima, S., Kuwata, T., Masuo, O., Yamaga, H., Okita, R., Ozaki, F., et al. (1999). Transcortical sensory aphasia due to a left frontal subcortical haemorrhage. *Brain Injury, 13*, 927–933.

Maeshima, S., Osawa, A., Nakayama, Y., & Miki, J. (2004). Transcortical sensory aphasia following infarction in the left frontal lobe. *European Neurology, 52*, 125–128.

Maeshima, S., Toshiro, H., Sekiguchi, E., Okita, R., Yamaga, H., Ozaki, F., et al. (2002). Transcortical mixed aphasia due to cerebral infarction in the left inferior frontal lobe and temporo-parietal lobe. *Neuroradiology, 44*, 133–137.

Maeshima, S., Uematsu, Y., Terada, T., Nakai, K., Itakura, T., & Komai, N. (1996). Transcortical mixed aphasia with left frontoparietal lesions. *Neuroradiology, 38*, S78–S79.

Marshall, R. C., Wertz, R. T., Weiss, D. G., Aten, J. L., Brookshire, R. H., Garcia-Bunuel, L., et al. (1989). Home treatment for aphasic patients by trained nonprofessionals. *Journal of Speech and Hearing Disorders, 54*, 462–470.

Masdeu, J. C., Schoene, W. C., & Funkenstein, H. (1978). Aphasia following infarction of the left supplementary motor area: A clinicopathologic study. *Neurology, 28*, 1220–1223.

Mazzocchi, F., & Vignolo, L. A. (1979). Localisation of lesions in aphasia: Clinical-CT scan correlations in stroke patients. *Cortex, 15*, 627–653.

McFarling, D., Rothi, L. J., & Heilman, K. M. (1982). Transcortical aphasia from ischaemic infarcts of the thalamus: A repot of two cases. *Journal of Neurology, Neurosurgery, and Psychiatry, 45*, 107–112.

Mega, M. S., & Alexander, M. P. (1994). Subcortical aphasia: The core profile of capsulostriatal infarction. *Neurology, 44*, 1824–1829.

Meinzer, M., Harnish, S., Conway, T., & Crosson, B. (2011). Recent developments in functional and structural imaging of aphasia recovery after stroke. *Aphasiology, 25*, 271–290.

Mendez, M. F. (2004). Aphemia-like syndrome from a right supplementary motor area lesion. *Clinical Neurology and Neurosurgery, 106*, 337–339.

Mendez, M. F., & Benson, D. F. (1985). Atypical conduction aphasia: A disconnection syndrome. *Archives of Neurology, 42*, 886–891.

Mesulam, M. M. (1982). Slowly progressive aphasia without generalized dementia. *Annals of Neurology, 11*, 592–598.

Mesulam, M. M. (2001). Primary progressive aphasia. *Annals of Neurology, 49*, 425–432.

Mohr, J. P., Pessin, M. S., Finkelstein, S., Funkestein, H. H., Duncan, G. W., & Davis, K. R. (1978). Broca aphasia: Pathologic and clinical. *Neurology, 28*, 311–324.

Moss, A., & Nicholas, M. (2006). Language rehabilitation in chronic aphasia and time postonset: A review of single-subject data. *Stroke, 37*, 3043–3051.

Moster, M. L., Johnston, D. E., & Reinmuth, O. M. (1983). Chronic subdural hematoma with transient neurological deficits: A review of 15 cases. *Annals of Neurology, 14*, 539–542.

Mouridsen, S. E. (1995). The Landau-Kleffner syndrome: A review. *European Child and Adolescent Psychiatry, 4*, 223–228.

Murdoch, B. E., Chenery, H. J., Wilks, V., & Boyle, R. S. (1987). Language disorders in dementia of the Alzheimer type. *Brain and Language, 31*, 122–137.

Nadeau, S. E., & Crosson, B. (1997). Subcortical aphasia. *Brain and Language, 58*, 355–402.

Naeser, M. A. (1994). Neuroimaging and recovery of auditory comprehension and spontaneous speech in aphasia with some implications for treatment in severe aphasia. In A. Kertesz (Ed.), *Localization and neuroimaging in neuropsychology* (pp. 245–295). San Diego, CA: Academic Press.

Naeser, M. A., Alexander, M. P., Helm-Estabrooks, N., Levine, H. L., Laughlin, S. A., & Geschwind, N. (1982). Aphasia with predominantly subcortical lesion sites: Description of three capsular/putaminal aphasia syndromes. *Archives of Neurology, 39*, 2–14.

Naeser, M. A., & Hayward, R. W. (1978). Lesion location in aphasia with cranial computed tomography and the Boston Diagnostic Aphasia Exam. *Neurology, 28*, 545–551.

Naeser, M. A., Helm-Estabrooks, N., Haas, G., Auerbach, S., & Srinivasan, M. (1987). Relationship between lesion extent in "Wernicke's area" on computed tomographic scan and predicting recovery of comprehension in Wernicke's aphasia. *Archives of Neurology, 44*, 73–82.

Naeser, M. A., Martin, P. I., Nicholas, M., Baker, E. H., Seekins, H., Helm-Estabrooks, N., et al. (2005). Improved naming after TMS treatments in a chronic, global aphasia patient—Case report. *Neurocase, 11*, 182–193.

Naeser, M. A., Martin, P. I., Treglia, E., Ho, M., Kaplan, E., Bashir, S., et al. (2010). Research with rTMS in the treatment of aphasia. *Restorative Neurology and Neuro-science, 28,* 511–529.

Naeser, M. A., Palumbo, C. L., Helm-Estabrooks, N., Stiassny-Eder, D., & Albert, M. L. (1989). Severe non-fluency in aphasia: Role of the medial subcallosal fasciculus and other white matter pathways in recovery of spontaneous speech. *Brain, 112,* 1–38.

Nakamura, M., Roser, F., Bundschuh, O., Vorkapic, P., & Samii, M. (2003). Intraventricular meningiomas: A review of 16 cases with reference to the literature. *Surgical Neurology, 59,* 491–503.

Nathan, P. W. (1947). Facial apraxia and apraxic dysarthria. *Brain, 70,* 449–478.

Neary, D., Snowden, J. S., Gustafson, L., Passant, U., Stuss, D., Black, S., et al. (1998). Frontotemporal lobar degeneration: A consensus on clinical diagnostic criteria. *Neurology, 51,* 1546–1554.

Norton, A., Zipse, L., Marchina, S., & Schlaug, G. (2009). Melodic intonation therapy: Shared insights on how it is done and why it might help. *Annals of the New York Academy of Science, 1169,* 431–436.

Oelschlaeger, C., Dziewas, R., Reichelt, D., Minnerup, J., Niederstadt, T., Ringelstein, E. B., et al. (2010). Severe leukoencephalopathy with fulminant cerebral edema reflecting immune reconstitution inflammatory syndrome during HIV infection: A case report. *Journal of Medical Case Reports, 4,* 214.

Ojha, P. K., Nandavar, S., Pearson, D. M., & Demchuk, A. M. (2011). Aphemia as a presenting symptom in acute stroke. *Neurology India, 59,* 432–434.

Otsuki, M., Soma, Y., Sato, M., Homma, A., & Tsuji, S. (1998). Slowly progressive pure word deafness. *European Neurology, 39,* 135–140.

Ottomeyer, C., Reuter, B., Jager, T., Rossmanith, C., Hennerici, M. G., & Szabo, K. (2009). Aphemia: An isolated disorder of speech associated with an ischemic lesion of the left precentral gyrus. *Journal of Neurology, 256,* 1166–1168.

Pachalska, M., Macqueen, B. D., Jastrzebowska, G., & Pufal, A. (2004). Disturbances of speech and language in patients aroused from long-term coma subsequent to traumatic brain injury. *Ortopedia, Traumatologia, Rehabilitacja, 30,* 472–482.

Pai, M. C. (1999). Supplementary motor area aphasia: A case report. *Clinical Neurology and Neurosurgery, 101,* 29–32.

Palumbo, C. L., Alexander, M. P., & Naeser, M. A. (1992). CT scan lesion sites associated with conduction aphasia. In S. Kohn (Ed.), *Conduction aphasia* (pp. 51–75). Hillsdale, NJ: Erlbaum.

Parkinson, B. R., Raymer, A., Chang, Y. L., Fitzgerald, D. B., & Crosson, B. (2009). Lesion characteristics related to treatment improvement in object and action naming for patients with chronic aphasia. *Brain and Language, 110,* 61–70.

Plowman, E., Hentz, B., & Ellis, C. (in press). Post-stroke aphasia prognosis: A review of patient-related and stroke-related factors. *Journal of Evaluation in Clinical Practice.*

Poncet, M., Habib, M., & Robillard, A. (1987). Deep left parietal lobe syndrome: Conduction aphasia and other neurobehavioral disorders due to a small subcortical lesion. *Journal of Neurology, Neurosurgery, and Psychiatry, 50,* 709–713.

Porch, B. E. (1983). *Porch index of communicative ability.* Palo Alto, CA: Consulting Psychologist Press.

Poser, C. M. (1987). Aphemia as a first symptom of multiple sclerosis. *Journal of Neurology, Neurosurgery, and Psychiatry, 50,* 1388.

Price, C. J., & Crinion, J. (2005). The latest on functional imaging studies of aphasic stroke. *Current Opinion in Neurology, 18,* 429–434.

Profitlich, T., Hoppe, C., Reuber, M., Helmstaedter, C., & Bauer, J. (2008). Ictal neuropsychological findings in focal nonconvulsive status epilepticus. *Epilepsy and Behavior, 12,* 269–275.

Rahimi, A. R., & Poorkay, M. (2000). Subdural hematomas and isolated transient aphasia. *Journal of the American Medical Directors Association, 1,* 129–131.

Raymer, A. M., Bandy, D., Adair, J. C., Schwartz, R. L., Williamson, D. J., Gonzalez Rothi, L. J., et al. (2001). Effects of bromocriptine in a patient with crossed nonfluent aphasia: A case report. *Archives of Physical Medicine and Rehabilitation, 82,* 139–144.

Reeves, R. R., & Panguluri, R. L. (2011). Neuropsychiatric complications of traumatic brain injury. *Journal of Psychosocial Nursing and Mental Health Service, 49,* 42–50.

Rheims, S., Nighoghossian, N., Hermier, M., Formaglio, M., Cakmak, S., Derex, L., et al. (2006). Aphemia related to a premotor cortex infarction. *European Neurology, 55,* 225–226.

Roberts, M., Sandercock, P., & Ghadiali, E. (1987). Pure word deafness and unilateral right temporo-parietal lesions: A case report. *Journal of Neurology, Neurosurgery, and Psychiatry, 50,* 1708–1709.

Robey, R. R. (1994). The efficacy of treatment for aphasic persons: A meta-analysis. *Brain and Language, 47,* 582–608.

Robey, R. R. (1998). A meta-analysis of clinical outcomes in the treatment of aphasia. *Journal of Speech, Language, and Hearing Research, 41,* 172–187.

Robinson, R. G., Kubos, K. L., Starr, L. B., Rao, K., & Price, T. R. (1984). Mood disorders in stroke patients: Importance of location of lesion. *Brain, 107,* 81–93.

Rolak, L. A., Rutecki, P., Ashizawa, T., & Harati, Y. (1992). Clinical features of Todd's post-epileptic paralysis. *Journal of Neurology, Neurosurgery, and Psychiatry, 55,* 63–64.

Rosche, J., Schley, A., Schwesinger, A., Grossmann, A., Mach, H., Benecke, R., et al. (2011). Recurrent aphasic status epilepticus after prolonged generalized tonic-clonic

A

seizures versus a special feature of Todd's paralysis. *Epilepsy and Behavior, 20,* 132–137.

Ruff, R. L., & Arbit, E. (1981). Aphemia resulting from a left frontal hematoma. *Neurology, 31,* 353–356.

Sabe, L., Salvarezza, F., Garcia Cuerva, A., Leiguarda, R., & Starkstein, S. (1995). A randomized, double-blind, placebocontrolled study of bromocriptine in nonfluent aphasia. *Neurology, 45,* 2272–2274.

Safaz, I., Alaca, R., Yasar, F., Tok, F., & Yilmaz, B. (2008). Medical complications, physical function and communication skills in patients with traumatic brain injury: A single center 5-year experience. *Brain Injury, 22,* 733–739.

Sahaya, K., Dhand, U. K., Goyal, M. K., Soni, C. R., & Sahota, P. K. (2010). Recurrent epileptic Wernicke aphasia. *Journal of the Neurological Sciences, 291,* 98–99.

Sakurai, Y., Murayama, S., Fukusako, Y., Bando, M., Iwata, M., & Inoue, K. (1998). Progressive aphemia in a patient with Pick's disease: A neuropsychological and anatomic study. *Journal of the Neurological Sciences, 159,* 156–161.

Sarno, M. T., & Levita, E. (1979). Recovery in treated aphasia in the first year post-stroke. *Stroke, 10,* 663–670.

Schiff, H. B., Alexander, M. P., Naeser, M. A., & Galaburda, A. M. (1983). Aphemia: Clinical-anatomic correlations. *Archives of Neurology, 40,* 720–727.

Schlaug, G., Marchina, S., & Norton, A. (2008). From singing to speaking: Why singing may lead to recovery of expressive language function in patients with Broca's aphasia. *Music Perception, 25,* 315–323.

Schramm, J., & Aliashkevich, A. F. (2008). Surgery for temporal mediobasal tumors: Experience based on a series of 235 patients. *Neurosurgery, 62,* 1272–1282.

Schuell, H. (1965). *The Minnesota test for differential diagnosis of aphasia.* Minneapolis: University of Minnesota Press.

Seliger, G. M., Lefever, F., Lukas, R., Chen, J., Schwartz, S., Codeghini, L., et al. (1991). Word deafness in head injury: Implications for coma assessment and rehabilitation. *Brain Injury, 5,* 53–56.

Selnes, O. A., Knopman, D. S., Niccum, N., Rubens, A. B., & Larson, D. (1983). Computed tomographic scan correlates of auditory comprehension deficits in aphasia: A prospective recovery study. *Annals of Neurology, 13,* 558–566.

Servan, J., Verstichel, P., Catala, M., Yakovleff, A., & Rancurel, G. (1995). Aphasia and infarction of the posterior cerebral artery territory. *Journal of Neurology, 242,* 87–92.

Sethi, N. K., Burke, L., Torgovnick, J., & Arsura, E. (2007). Transcortical sensory aphasia as a result of left frontal cortical-subcortical infarction: A case report. *European Neurology, 57,* 52–53.

Shallice, T., & Warrington, E. K. (1977). Auditory-verbal short-term memory impairment and conduction aphasia. *Brain and Language, 4,* 479–491.

Shivashankar, N., Shashikala, H. R., Nagaraja, D., Jayakumar, P. N., & Ratnavalli, E. (2001). Pure word deafness in two patients with subcortical lesions. *Clinical Neurology and Neurosurgery, 103,* 201–205.

Short, R. A., Broderick, D. F., Patton, A., Arvanitakis, Z., & Graff-Radford, N. R. (2005). Different patterns of magnetic resonance imaging atrophy for frontotemporal lobar degeneration syndromes. *Archives of Neurology, 62,* 1106–1110.

Signoret, J. L., Castaigne, P., Lhermitte, F., Abelanet, R., & Lavorel, P. (1984). Rediscovery of Leborgne's brain: Anatomical description with CT scan. *Brain and Language, 22,* 303–319.

Silveri, M. C., & Colosimo, C. (1995). Hypothesis on the nature of comprehension deficit in a patient with transcortical mixed aphasia with preserved naming. *Brain and Language, 49,* 1–26.

Singer, E. J., Stoner, G. L., Singer, P., Tomiyasu, U., Licht, E., Fahy-Chandon, B., et al. (1994). AIDS presenting as progressive multifocal leukoencephalopathy with clinical response to zidovudine. *Acta Neurologica Scandinavica, 90,* 443–447.

Slevc, L. R., Martin, R. C., Hamilton, A. C., & Joanisse, M. F. (2011). Speech perception, rapid temporal processing, and the left hemisphere: A case study of unilateral pure word deafness. *Neuropsychologia, 49,* 216–230.

Smith Doody, R., Hrachovy, R. A., & Feher, E. P. (1992). Recurrent fluent aphasia associated with a seizure focus. *Brain and Language, 42,* 419–430.

Sonobe, N., Yashima, Y., Takahashi, Y., Katayose, K., & Kumashiro, H. (1991). Three cases of anomic aphasia after lesions in and/or around the basal ganglia. *Fukushima Journal of Medical Science, 37,* 29–40.

Sparks, R., Helm, N., & Albert, M. (1974). Aphasia rehabilitation resulting from melodic intonation therapy. *Cortex, 10,* 303–316.

Staff, N. P., Lucchinetti, C. F., & Keegan, B. M. (2009). Multiple sclerosis with predominant, severe cognitive impairment. *Archives of Neurology, 66,* 1139–1143.

Steele, R. D., Weinrich, M., Wertz, R. T., Kleczewska, M. K., & Carlson, G. S. (1989). Computer-based visual communication in aphasia. *Neuropsychologia, 27,* 409–426.

Steinlein, O. K. (2009). Epilepsy-aphasia syndromes. *Expert Review of Neurotherapeutics, 9,* 825–833.

Strauss, E., Sherman, E. M. S., & Spreen, O. (2006). *A compendium of neuropsychological tests: Administration, norms, and commentary.* New York: Oxford University Press.

Swanberg, M. M., Nasreddine, Z. S., Mendez, M. F., & Cummings, J. L. (2007). Speech and language. In G. G. Goetz (Ed.), *Textbook of clinical neurology* (3rd ed., pp. 88–92). Philadelphia: Saunders Elsevier.

A

Szaflarski, J. P., Vannest, J., Wu, S. W., DiFrancesco, M. W., Banks, C., & Gilbert, D. L. (2011). Excitatory repetitive transcranial magnetic stimulation induces improvements in chronic post-stroke aphasia. *Medical Science Monitor, 17*, CR132–CR139.

Szirmai, I., Farsang, M., & Csuri, M. (2003). Cortical auditory disorder caused by bilateral strategic cerebral bleedings. Analysis of two cases. *Brain and Language, 85*, 159–165.

Takahashi, N., Kawamura, M., Shinotou, H., Hirayama, K., Kaga, K., & Shindo, M. (1992). Pure word deafness due to left hemisphere damage. *Cortex, 28*, 295–303.

Takeda, M., Tachibana, H., Shibuya, N., Nakajima, Y., Okuda, B., Sugita, M., et al. (1999). Pure anomic aphasia caused by a subcortical hemorrhage in the left temporo-parieto-occipital lobe. *Internal Medicine, 38*, 293–295.

Tanaka, Y., Yamadori, A., & Mori, E. (1987). Pure word deafness following bilateral lesions: A psychophysical analysis. *Brain, 110*, 381–403.

Thiel, A., Habedank, B., Herholz, K., Kessler, J., Winhuisen, L., Haupt, W. F., et al. (2006). From the left to the right: How the brain compensates progressive loss of language function. *Brain and Language, 98*, 57–65.

Tijssen, C. C., Tavy, D. L., Hekster, R. E., Bots, G. T., & Endtz, L. J. (1984). Aphasia with a left frontal interhemispheric hematoma. *Neurology, 34*, 1261–1264.

Toledo, M., Munuera, J., Sueiras, M., Rovira, R., Alvarez-Sabin, J., & Rovira, A. (2008). MRI findings in aphasic status epilepticus. *Epilepsia, 49*, 1465–1469.

Tranel, D., Biller, J., Damasio, H., Adams, H. P., Jr., & Cornell, S. H. (1987). Global aphasia without hemiparesis. *Archives of Neurology, 44*, 304–308.

Tyler, L. K., Marslen-Wilson, W. D., Randall, B., Wright, P., Devereux, B. J., Zhuang, J., et al. (2011). Left inferior frontal cortex and syntax: Function, structure and behaviour in patients with left hemisphere damage. *Brain, 134*, 415–431.

Udgirkar, V. S., Tullu, M. S., Bavdekar, S. B., Shaharao, V. B., Kamat, J. R., & Hira, P. R. (2003). Neurological manifestations of HIV infection. *Indian Pediatrics, 40*, 230–234.

Vignolo, L. A., Boccardi, E., & Caverni, L. (1986). Unexpected CT-scan finding in global aphasia. *Cortex, 22*, 55–69.

Vukovic, M., Vuksanovic, J., & Vukovic, I. (2008). Comparison of the recovery patterns of language and cognitive functions in patients with post-traumatic language processing deficits and in patients with aphasia following a stroke. *Journal of Communication Disorders, 41*, 531–552.

Weiduschat, N., Thiel, A., Rubi-Fessen, I., Hartmann, A., Kessler, J., Merl, P., et al. (2011). Effects of repetitive transcranial magnetic stimulation in aphasic stroke: A randomized controlled pilot study. *Stroke, 42*, 409–415.

Weinrich, M. (1991). Computerized visual communication as an alternative communication system and therapeutic tool. *Journal of Neurolinguistics, 6*, 159–176.

Wells, C. R., Labar, D. R., & Solomon, G. E. (1992). Aphasia as the sole manifestation of simple partial status epilepticus. *Epilepsia, 33*, 84–87.

Wernicke, C. (1908). The symptom of complex aphasia. In E. D. Church (Ed.), *Modern clinical medicine: Diseases of the nervous system* (pp. 265–324). New York: Appleton-Century-Crofts.

Wertz, R. T., Collins, M. J., Weiss, D., Kurtzke, J. F., Friden, T., Brookshire, R. H., et al. (1981). Veterans administration cooperative study on aphasia: A comparison of individual and group treatment. *Journal of Speech and Hearing Research, 24*, 580–594.

Wilkinson, G. S., & Robertson, G. J. (2006). *Wide Range Achievement Test 4 professional manual.* Lutz, FL: Psychological Assessment Resources.

Wirkowski, E., Echausse, N., Overby, C., Ortiz, O., & Radler, L. (2006). I can hear you yet cannot comprehend: A case of pure word deafness. *Journal of Emergency Medicine, 30*, 53–55.

You, D. S., Kim, D. Y., Chun, M. H., Jung, S. E., & Park, S. J. (2011). Cathodal transcranial direct current stimulation of the right Wernicke's area improves comprehension in subacute stroke patients. *Brain and Language, 119*, 1–5.

Zakzanis, K. K., & Boulos, M. I. (2001). Posterior cortical atrophy. *Neurologist, 7*, 341–349.

Ziegler, W., Kilian, B., & Deger, K. (1997). The role of the left mesial frontal cortex in fluent speech: Evidence from a case of left supplementary motor area hemorrhage. *Neuropsychologia, 35*, 1197–1208.

APRAXIA

DESCRIPTION

"Apraxia," the Greek term for inactivity, was initially used in 1891 by Heyman Steinthal. It is a higher order movement disorder characterized by inability to perform purposeful actions and the incorrect use of objects (Binkofski & Reetz, 2008). In 1920, Hugo Liepmann further established apraxia as a distinct disorder, which led to a classification of subtypes as well as the development of theory with regard to normal and abnormal praxis. Apraxia is further defined negatively by ruling out the presence of other deficits such as akinesia, abnormal tone or posture, weakness, uncooperativeness, intellectual deterioration, deafferentation, poor comprehension,

A

or other movement disorders (Petreska, Adriani, Blanke, & Billard, 2007). To simplify, apraxia describes an inability to execute a voluntary motor movement despite being able to demonstrate normal muscle function. The desire and the capacity to move are present, but the person simply cannot execute the act. It is not related to a lack of understanding or to any kind of physical paralysis but is caused by a problem in the cortex of the brain.

In general, apraxia is believed to be caused by a lesion in the neural pathways of the brain that contain the learned patterns of movement. It is often a symptom of neurological, metabolic, or other disorders. Disorders that are associated with apraxia injure or destroy areas of the cerebral cortex and thalamus including trauma, tumors, and stroke (hemorrhage or infarction). Various degenerative diseases may also result in apraxia. Specifically, ideomotor, conceptual, and ideational apraxias are commonly seen in Alzheimer disease and limb-kinetic and ideomotor apraxia are often seen in corticobasal degeneration (Heilman & Rothi, 2003). As described in the following sections, apraxia is noted in disorders that affect the brain diffusely, particularly those that impair frontal lobe function. It is most commonly derived from a lesion in post-Rolandic neural pathways that retain memories of learned movement patterns resulting in an inability to conceptualize and perform the desired action. Apraxic errors are also noted in parietal lobe lesions. Most parietal lobe apraxias are related to loss of the area's capacity to recognize spatially executed tasks, even well-learned ones, such as dressing. As an example, corticobasal ganglionic degeneration affects elderly patients in particular and impairs parietal lobe functions. In these cases, spatial awareness of the arm is sometimes lost, and the arm may become incapable of performing previously learned motor tasks.

PRIMARY TYPES OF APRAXIA

Ideomotor Apraxia

DESCRIPTION

Ideomotor apraxia is the inability to carry out or mimic limb or head movements performed or suggested by others. It was originally called motor apraxia and later ideokinetic apraxia. It is characterized by an inability to perform skilled movements secondary to spatial organizational, time, and sequencing errors in the context of spared manual dexterity and comprehension (Heilman & Rothi, 2003).

NEUROPATHOLOGY/PATHOPHYSIOLOGY

Many theories exist regarding the pathophysiology of ideomotor apraxia. Kimura (1979) in discussing Liepmann's theory reported certain areas in the left hemisphere are thought to contain "movement formulas" responsible for skilled purposeful movements as well as a "time-space-form picture of the movement" (as cited in Heilman & Rothi, 2003, p. 220). In order to perform a learned skilled act, body parts must be placed in specific spatial positions in certain order and at a certain time. When a lesion occurs in the corpus callosum, a disconnect occurs not only between the hemisphere dominant for language and the hemisphere responsible for left hand control but also between the areas containing these movement formulas and right hemisphere motor areas. However, it should be noted that apraxia does not always occur with callosal lesions and depends largely on the motor dominance and language patterns of each particular patient.

Other hypotheses include damage to the left primary motor association cortex, arcuate fasciculus, dominant parietal lobe, supramarginal or angular gyrus, cortex anterior to the supramarginal or angular gyrus, supplementary motor area in the frontal lobe, and basal ganglia and thalamus. However, little support for these hypotheses is available at the present (Heilman & Rothi, 2003).

NEUROPSYCHOLOGICAL/CLINICAL
PRESENTATION

Ideomotor apraxia will likely not be noticed in typical living activities. Difficulties are more often associated with imitation of a movement followed by a visual or verbal cue. However, in vivo, when presented with different objects/tools, the patient with ideomotor apraxia will be able to use these without difficulty. Behaviors characteristic of ideomotor apraxia include perseveration, substitution, surplus movements, "verbal overflow," omission, conduite d'approche, and "body part as object errors." With perseveration, the patient with ideomotor apraxia will perform movements either completely or partially that were performed previously in the examination. With substitution, the patient will replace the intended action with some other movement. Surplus movements are characterized by the addition of some other action to the intended task. For example, when asked to wrinkle the nose, the patient may also purse the lips. In cases of verbal overflow, the patient will try to explain the use of an object rather than performing it. Errors of omission are characterized by only partial completion of a movement such as running fingers through hair rather than demonstrating combing or brushing. Conduite d'approche is described as the patient's continuous attempts at completing a movement (with multiple approximation errors) until it is done correctly. Finally, a "body part as object" error is seen when a patient uses a body part despite the presence of the object, such as a fist instead of a hammer, to complete a movement (Binkofski & Reetz, 2008).

Ideational Apraxia

DESCRIPTION

Ideational apraxia is described by impairment in the basic conceptual organization and planning of tasks. It involves complex actions or sequences in which the patient may be able to perform the individual components of a task but fails to perform the movements in sequence. Patients with ideational apraxia are able to complete the movements required to perform the intended action but exhibit inappropriate use of the presented objects or perform the acts out of sequence. This is most often seen in patients with dementing disorders or in confusional states (Gross & Grossman, 2008; Heilman & Rothi, 2003; Petreska et al., 2007). Ideational apraxia is often confused with conceptual apraxia in which a patient may be unable to discriminate gestures, match objects with actions, or understand the mechanical advantage of tools.

NEUROPATHOLOGY/PATHOPHYSIOLOGY

Ideational apraxia is most commonly observed in dementing disorders, specifically vascular dementia and early Alzheimer's Disease. Functional imaging and lesion analyses show the frontal lobes play a crucial role in this disorder. However, little evidence is available to support most frequently associated forms of dementia or determine the presence of ideational apraxia in the case of an isolated lesion (Heilman & Rothi, 2003).

NEUROPSYCHOLOGICAL/CLINICAL PRESENTATION

Patients with ideational apraxia are unable to complete tasks in a series or tasks in which a plan is necessary to completion. Heilman and Rothi (2003) provide an example where a patient, rather than cleaning the pipe, putting tobacco in, lighting it, and smoking it, would instead first put tobacco in, then clean it (Heilman & Rothi, 2003). In essence, the sequence of the activity is faulty. Patients with ideational apraxia exhibit improved performance when using actual objects.

Limb-Kinetic Apraxia

DESCRIPTION

Limb-kinetic apraxia is the inability to make precise or exact movements with a finger, an arm or a leg. It is further described as a stiffness or slowness of movements (Petreska et al., 2007). In contrast to ideomotor apraxia, limb-kinetic apraxia occurs unilaterally and is the least frequently diagnosed apraxia. An example is the inability to use a tool despite the fact that the person affected understands what is to be done and has done so in the past.

NEUROPATHOLOGY/PATHOPHYSIOLOGY

Although the specific neuroanatomical correlates are unclear in limb-kinetic apraxia, it is often a unilateral deficit. According to Liepmann's early work and cited more recently (e.g., Heilman & Rothi, 2003), sensory motor cortex lesions are likely to cause the disorder. However, further studies in monkeys determined that corticospinal tract and pyramidal lesions may also be responsible for deficits observed in limb-kinetic apraxia (Heilman & Rothi, 2003).

NEUROPSYCHOLOGICAL/CLINICAL PRESENTATION

Limb-kinetic apraxia is more evident in the evaluation of independent distal movements than in proximal movements. It is most easily seen when asking a patient to perform a finger tapping task or pinching movements. For example, a patient may not be able to pick up a coin from a surface that is flat using a pincer grasp. Instead, the patient will slide the coin to the end of the flat surface and grasp it using the fingers and palm. The patient will additionally be unable to rotate a coin through the fingers effectively (Heilman & Rothi, 2003).

ADDITIONAL TYPES OF APRAXIA

Several additional types of apraxias have been identified; however, the literature regarding these is relatively vague. A brief description will be given of each below.

Orofacial Apraxia (Buccofacial Apraxia)

Orofacial apraxia (sometimes called buccofacial or facial-oral apraxia) is considered by some a subcategory of ideomotor apraxia characterized by impairments in skilled facial, tongue, mouth, larynx, or pharynx movements. Impairments can be seen on such tasks as blowing a kiss, whistling, winking,

A

coughing, and so forth on command. This form includes verbal or speech developmental apraxia, which is perhaps the most common form of the disorder. In general, orofacial apraxia is commonly seen along with limb apraxia. Performance improves significantly upon using or seeing an actual object (i.e., seeing a match with the command to blow out a match) but not with imitation. Primary associated neurological involvement includes lesions of the inferior frontal cortex, insula, or basal ganglia, or subcortical deep frontal lesions (Gross & Grossman, 2008; Heilman & Rothi, 2003).

Conceptual Apraxia

Conceptual apraxia is characterized by an inability to perform actions associated with a specific tool, object, or utensil. These errors are in the context of content (i.e., hammering motion with a screwdriver) rather than an inability to identify the object. Impairments may also exist in the ability to identify a tool associated with a certain object (i.e., a hammer goes with a nail) or the ability to choose an alternative tool in the absence of the correct one (i.e., using a handsaw that is flexible to hammer a nail in the absence of a hammer rather than a wrench or pliers). It is most often associated with a lesion of the posterior left hemisphere, likely in the caudal parietal lobe or temporoparietal junction (Gross & Grossman, 2008).

Constructional Apraxia

Constructional apraxia is characterized by an inability to copy images, draw objects, or build blocks spontaneously. It is reflective of bilateral impairments including portions of the brain responsible for perceptual processing, constructive planning, and coordination of spatial relations (Gross & Grossman, 2008).

Speech Apraxia

Speech apraxia is characterized by a disturbance of the articulatory movements required to produce words and sounds. When speaking, patients often seem as if conscious control of mouth movements is required along with conscious control of respiration and the speech apparatus. This occurs in the absence of dysarthria or aphasia. Normal speed and strength exist in mouth movements, but coordination required for fluency is impaired. Speech apraxia most often results from a lesion in the left frontal cortex, within or near the gyrus precentralis, but may also involve subcortical structures or intrasylvian structures (Binkofski & Reetz, 2008).

Conduction Apraxia

This type of apraxia is described as the ability to pantomime following verbal command but not imitation. Although the pathophysiology of this type of apraxia is relatively unknown, it is likely that impairment exists in the association between the input praxicon and output praxicon, leaving the ability to understand the gesture intact (Binkofski & Reetz, 2008; Heilman & Rothi, 2003).

Tactile Apraxia

Tactile apraxia is characterized by the discoordination and inadequacy of finger movements used in exploration of objects, such that finger movements are inappropriate relative to the shape and size of the object being explored, and is often accompanied by astereognosia. Tactile apraxia exists in the absence of sensory deficits, deficits in expressive and intransitive movements, and paresis. It most often involves an impaired interaction between premotor and parietal areas of the brain and likely is a result of a lesion occurring in the anterior intraparietal sulcus and/or the cotralateral superior parietal lobulus (Binkofski & Reetz, 2008).

DIAGNOSIS

Because patients with apraxia are often not aware of their deficits, apraxic errors may be excused by patients (or clinicians) by attributing them to clumsy use of the nondominant hand in right hemisphere lesions with hemiparesis or to intellectual decline in the cases of dementing disorders. As such, the diagnosis of apraxia must be made on examination and not based on patient or family history. Both hands should be examined and the following tests can be used to determine the presence of an apraxic disorder:

- Gesture to command using transitive (i.e., flip a coin, blow out a match) and intransitive movements (i.e., salute, stick out your tongue)
- Gesture to imitation, gesture with tool presentation, gesture with presentation of object with which a tool works (i.e., a nail that is partially driven)
- Actual use of tool, imitation of examiner tool use, discrimination between incorrect and correct tool use by examiner (i.e., "Is this the correct way to use scissors?")
- Gesture comprehension (i.e., "Am I using a saw or a hammer?")
- Serial acts (i.e., "Fold a letter, put it in the envelope, seal it, and place a stamp on it," or "Show me how you would make a sandwich")

- Tool-action associations (i.e., which tool from an array goes with the action displayed by the examiner)
- Object-tool association (i.e., which tool from an array goes with the displayed object)
- Conceptual knowledge (i.e., what is an alternative tool that would accomplish the same task).

In addition to the evaluation of the patient's performance, the examiner should also determine the level of recognition/disturbance experienced by the patient when he or she commits an error. Many apraxic patients also present with aphasia or some other language disorder that makes it difficult to determine the presence of a true apraxia. Because of this, it is important to evaluate apraxia using a variety of different testing methods, such as using commands as well as asking questions the patient can answer using yes/no or pointing. The overall performance on the mentioned tasks allows the clinician to determine the presence of an apraxia, in general. However, further differentiation is made based on the characteristics mentioned in the individual descriptions of the various types of apraxias mentioned above (Heilman & Rothi, 2003).

TREATMENT

It is possible for spontaneous recovery to occur over a 6-month period following a stroke or other acquired neurologic lesion. However, patients with an apraxia resulting from posterior lesions seem to have a poorer prognosis than those with anterior lesions. It is possible that recovery may occur in damaged areas of the brain responsible for apraxia or remediation may occur as uninjured portions of the brain take over for injured portions of the brain. However, specific areas of the brain responsible for functional recovery have not been identified. In addition, because anosagnosia often exists in apraxic patients and apraxic errors are not often seen in functional daily activities, patients do not often seek treatment for apraxia. In addition, there is little information regarding the efficacy or methods of treatment available at the present (Heilman & Rothi, 2003).

Katherine Meredith
Mark T. Barisa

Binkofski, F., & Reetz, K. (2008). Apraxia. In S. F. Cappa, J. Abutalebi, J. Demonet, P. Fletcher, & P. Garrard (Eds.), *Cognitive neurology: A clinical textbook* (pp. 67–88). New York: Oxford.

Gross, R., & Grossman, M. (2008). Update on Apraxia. *Current neurology and neuroscience reports, 8,* 490–496.

Heilman, K., & Rothi, L. (1993). Apraxia. In K. Heilman & E. Valenstein (Eds.), *Clinical neuropsychology* (5th ed., pp. 215–235). New York: Oxford.

Heilman, K. & Rothi, L.J. (2003). Apraxia. In K. Heilman & E. Valenstein (Eds.), *Clinical neuropsychology* (4th ed., pp. 215–235). Boston: Oxford.

Kimura, D. (1979). Neuromotor mechanisms in the evolution of human communication. In H. D. Steklis & M. J. Raleigh (Eds.), *Neurobiology of social communication in primates: An evolutionary perspective* (pp. 183–198). New York: Academic Press.

Liepman, H. (1920). Apraxia. *Ergebn. Ges. Med.,* 1, 516–543.

Petreska, B., Adriani, M., Blanke, O., & Billard, A. (2007). Apraxia: A review. In C. von Hofsten & K. Rosander (Eds.), *Progress in brain research* (Vol. 164, pp. 61–83). Amsterdam: Elsevier.

ARACHNOID CYSTS

DESCRIPTION

Arachnoid cysts are benign cysts found in the arachnoid layer. Primary, congenital arachnoid cysts are developmental anomalies and are distinguished from secondary arachnoid cysts that might arise from multiple etiologies such as infection or trauma (Choi & Kim, 1998). Arachnoid cysts are found along the craniospinal axis but most commonly (approximately two-thirds of the time) are found in the temporal fossa (Erman et al., 2004). Approximately 1% of the population manifest arachnoid cysts (Vernooij et al., 2007).

NEUROPATHOLOGY/PATHOPHYSIOLOGY

Primary arachnoid cysts result from aberrations of cerebrospinal fluid (CSF) flow during early stages of embryonic development (Choi & Kim, 1998). Although arachnoid cyst development is not fully understood, it is likely an extremely slow process as evidenced by the progressive onset of symptoms in adult and elderly cases, as brain plasticity initially accommodates the growing presence of a cyst (Yamasaki et al., 2003). Minor trauma, so slight that the patient may not recall the incident, might trigger cyst enlargement, which produces signs and symptoms (Watanabe, Kameyama, Takeda, & Tanaka, 1994). Arachnoid cysts can compress nearby cortical gyri, CSF compartments, or cause a midline shift (Wester, 2008). Some researchers have found that arachnoid cysts may decrease metabolism and perfusion in surrounding cortical regions (De Volder, Michel, Thauvoy, Willems, & Ferriere, 1994; Horiguchi & Takeshita, 2000; Martinez-Lage et al., 2006; Sgouros & Chapman, 2001; Tsurushima et al., 2000). Metabolism and perfusion to these surrounding cortical regions have been shown to return to normal levels following surgical decompression, and this correlates with the cognitive improvement seen in postsurgical patients (De Volder et. al., 1994; Martinez-Lage et al., 2006; Sgouros & Chapman, 2001; Tsurushima et al., 2000).

Though some arachnoid cyst patients are symptomatic, others, though presenting with startling radiological findings, are not (Wester, 2008). Wester notes that one explanation for the mismatch between clinical symptoms and radiological findings is that the cyst creates its own intracranial space. During normal child development, the skull is molded after the content inside has grown. This content, in healthy persons, is mostly brain. Alternatively, in the arachnoid cyst patient, the cyst will create surplus space as the skull grows, and this may allow the cyst to exist without resulting symptoms, as there is space for both the cyst and normal brain tissue. This cystic growth, however, may result in an increase of intracystic and intracranial pressure over time (Kumagai et al., 1986; Rao, Anderson, Feldstein, & Brockmeyer, 2005; Wester & Moen, 2000).

NEUROPSYCHOLOGICAL/CLINICAL PRESENTATION

Cases typically present to clinicians with the effects of hydrocephalus. Children may present with delayed motor and intellectual development (Fitzpatrick & Barlow, 2001), and adults often present with instability when walking (Erdincler, Kaynar, Bozkus, & Ciplak, 1999), headaches, dizziness, and vomiting (Fitzpatrick & Barlow, 2001). Cysts appear on CT scans as low-density, uncalcified masses; on MRI scans, the arachnoid cyst content has signal characteristics like that of cerebrospinal fluid (Erdincler et al., 1999).

Arachnoid cysts have been linked to cognitive dysfunction (Bahk, Pae, Chae, Jun, & Kim, 2002; Blackshaw & Bowen, 1987; Deonna, Davidoff, Maeder-Ingvar, Zesiger, & Marcoz, 1997; Hodges, 1991; Kuhnley, White, & Granoff, 1981; Stracciari, Ciucci, & Bissi, 1987), and several have found preoperative cognitive dysfunction will often normalize following surgical decompression (Gundersen, Helland, Rader, Hugdahl, & Wester, 2007; Raeder, Helland, Hugdahl, & Wester, 2005; Soukup, Patterson, Trier, & Chen, 1998; Wester & Hugdahl, 1995, 2003). Such findings indicate that the cyst does not destroy brain tissue, but as noted by Raeder et al., (2005) creates a reversible

suppression of function. In a literature review by Wester (2008), it is noted that various psychiatric symptoms occur among cyst patients, including attention deficit hyperactivity disorder (Millichap, 1997; von Gontard & Muller, 1991), delirium (Cohen, 1989), depression (Escalona, Coffey, & Maus-Feldman, 1991), delusions of hallucination and persecution (Bahk et al., 2002; da Silva et al., 2007; Gulsun, Sabanci, & Ozdemir, 2007; Kohn, Lilly, Sokol, & Malloy, 1989; Wong, Ko, & Wai, 1993), organic dementia syndrome (Clavel, Taborga, & Onzain, 1985; Cohen, 1989; Golaz & Bouras, 1993; Kotil, Balci, & Bilge, 2007), and insomnia and irritability (Ure et al., 1999). Of the six studies giving accounts of postoperative psychiatric functioning, five found normalization of symptoms (Clavel et al., 1985; Krzyzowski, Koziarski, Wejroch, Delimat, & Podgorski, 1998; Kuhnley et al., 1981; Vakis, Koutentakis, Karabetsos, & Kalostos, 2006; Zeegers et al., 2006).

Among patients with temporal arachnoid cysts, Helland and Wester (2007) found a significant correlation between intracystic pressure and preoperative level of patient complaints, even when intracystic pressure remained within the limits of normal intracranial pressure. Wester (2008) notes that symptoms are likely a result of the cyst's pressure on surrounding areas of brain tissue, leptomeninges, and/or cranial nerves, as such pressure can interfere with functions in the surrounding tissues, including the higher brain functions of cognition and emotion. Significant thinning of the cerebral cortex has been observed in areas adjacent to arachnoid cyst (Hund-Georgiadis, Yves Von Cramon, Kruggel, & Preul, 2002), and functional imaging has demonstrated subsequent reorganization of cortical function (Alkadhi, Crelier, Imhof, & Kollias, 2003; Caruso & Colonnese, 2006; Stowe et al., 2000).

Wester's (2008) review noted that among symptomatic patients with arachnoid cysts, some show blatant cognitive or behavioral problems (Deonna et al., 1997; De Volder et al., 1994; Hodges, 1991; Ramtahal, 2006), whereas others' cognitive problems were revealed only following neuropsychological testing (Horiguchi & Takeshita, 2000; Lebowitz, Schefft, Marc Testa, Patton, & Yeh, 2006; Tsurushima et al., 2000). Several types of dyscognition were noted including agraphia (Hodges, 1991), organic dementia syndrome (Clavel et al., 1985; Cohen, 1989; Golaz & Bouras, 1993), mental retardation (Deonna et al., 1997; Martinez-Lage, Poza, Sola, & Puche, 1992; Sztriha & Gururaj, 2005), learning problems and delayed language development in children (da Silva et al., 2007; Deonna et al., 1997; Horiguchi & Takeshita, 2000; Sztriha & Gururaj, 2005), memory deficits (Horiguchi & Takeshita, 2000; Soukup et al., 1989; Tsurushima et al., 2000), and deficits in verbal learning, visual perception, conceptual shifting, psychomotor speed, and constructional skills (Horiguchi & Takeshita, 2000; Soukup et al., 1998; Tsurushima et al., 2000). Few of these cases received surgical decompression; all five such studies using neuropsychological testing described postsurgical normalization of cognition (De Volder et al., 1994; Horiguchi & Takeshita, 2000; Oka, Kumon, Kohno, Saitoh, & Sakaki, 1996; Soukup et al., 1998; Tsurushima et al., 2000).

In addition, Wester and Hugdahl (1995) examined pre- and postoperative verbal memory and verbal perception among 13 adult patients presenting with a left temporal arachnoid cyst. Preoperatively, patients showed impaired total recall versus healthy controls. Further, right ear recall was significantly impaired. Patients also showed impaired abilities on a forced attention, dichotic listening task. Postsurgery, all patients showed improvement in both memory and perception, and memory improvement has been documented as soon as 4 hr postsurgery. In line with these findings (Raeder et al., 2005) compared 54 patients with 32 healthy controls on four pre- and postoperative cognitive tests for both complex verbal and visuospatial tasks (Benton Visual Retention Test, Trails Test A and B, Stroop Test, and Street Gestalt Test). Preoperatively, patients' performances were significantly lower than controls on all four tests. Three to 6 months postsurgery, patients significantly improved on three of the four tests, whereas control scores did not change.

DIAGNOSIS

Differential diagnosis includes ruling out cystic lesions such as cystic astrocytomas, cystic hemangioblastomas, hydatid cysts, abscesses, and epidermoid or dermoid tumors. Typically the appearance of low-density, uncalcified, extra-axial mass with typical borders that do not enhance upon administration of contrast medium allow for differential diagnosis from infectious and neoplastic disorders (Erdincler et al., 1999). Arachnoid cysts displace nearby structures whereas epidermoid tumors engulf arteries and cranial nerves and are slightly hyperintense in proton density-weighted MRI scans (Quint, 1992).

TREATMENT

Arachnoid cyst treatment has been the subject of much debate (Erman et al., 2004; Parsch, Krauss, Hofmann, Meixensberger, & Roosen, 1997; Sommer & Smit, 1997). Even in the presence of significant neuroimaging findings in patients with arachnoid cysts, some contest that operation is unnecessary given the relative paucity of clinical symptoms (Wester, 2008). Choi and Kim (1998) note endoscopic fenestration as the treatment of choice, as this gives the advantage of avoiding craniotomy or complications from cystoperitoneal shunting, as patients can remain shunt dependent (Aoki, Sakai, & Umezawa, 1990; Rappaport, 1993). As noted, patients typically show improvement following surgical cyst decompression.

Audrey L. Baumeister
William Drew Gouvier

Alkadhi, H., Crelier, G. R., Imhof, H. G., & Kollias, S. S. (2003). Somatomotor functional MRI in a large congenital arachnoid cyst. *Neuroradiology, 45,* 153–156.

Aoki, N., Sakai, T., & Umezawa, Y. (1990). Slit ventricle syndrome after cyst-peritoneal shunting for treatment of intracranial arachnoid cyst. *Child's Nervous System, 6,* 41–43.

Bahk, W. M., Pae, C. U., Chae, J. H., Jun, T. Y., & Kim, K. S. (2002). A case of brief psychosis associated with an arachnoid cyst. *Psychiatry Clinical Neurosciences, 56,* 203–205.

Blackshaw, S., & Bown, R. C. (1987). A case of atypical psychosis associated with alexithymia and a left frontotemporal lesion: Possible correlations. *Canadian Journal of Psychiatry, 32,* 688–692.

Caruso, R., & Colonnese, C. (2006). Somatomotor functional MRI in a hypertensive arachnoid cyst. *Acta Neurochirurgica, 148,* 801–803.

Choi, J., & Kim, D. (1998). Pathogenesis of arachnoid cyst: Congenital or traumatic? *Pediatric Neurosurgery, 29,* 260–266.

Clavel, M., Taborga, F. G., & Onzain, I. (1985). Arachnoid cysts as a cause of dementia in the elderly. *Acta Neurochirurgica, 78,* 28–32.

Cohen, A. J. (1989). Localized neuropsychiatric symptoms of an intracranial cyst. *Journal of Neuropsychiatry and Clinical Neurosciences, 1,* 445–446.

da Silva, J. A., Alves, A., Talina, M., Carreiro, S., Guimaraes, J., & Xavier, M. (2007). Arachnoid cyst in a patient with psychosis: Case report. *Annals of General Psychiatry, 6,* 16.

De Volder, A. G., Michel, C., Thauvoy, C., Willems, G., & Ferriere, G. (1994). Brain glucose utilisation in acquired childhood aphasia associated with a sylvian arachnoid cyst: Recovery after shunting as demonstrated by PET. *Journal of Neurology, Neurosurgery, & Psychiatry, 57,* 296–300.

Deonna, T., Davidoff, V., Maeder-Ingvar, M., Zesiger, P., & Marcoz, J. P. (1997). The spectrum of acquired cognitive disturbances in children with partial epilepsy and continuous spike-waves during sleep. A 4-year follow-up case study with prolonged reversible learning arrest and dysfluency. *European Journal of Paediatric Neurology, 1,* 19–29.

A

Erdincler, P., Kaynar, M. Y., Bozkus, H., & Ciplak, N. (1999). Posterior fossa arachnoid cysts. *British Journal of Neurosurgery, 13*(1), 10–17.

Erman, T., Gocer, A. I., Tuna, M., Ergin, M., Zorludemir, S., & Cetinalp, E. (2004). Intracranial arachnoid cysts – clinical features and management of 35 cases and review of the literature. *Neurosurgery Quarterly, 14,* 84–89.

Escalona, P. R., Coffey, C. E., & Maus-Feldman, J. (1991). Electroconvulsive therapy in a depressed patient with an intracranial arachnoid cyst: A brain magnetic resonance imaging study. *Convulsive Therapy, 7,* 133–138.

Fitzpatrick, M. O., & Barlow, P. (2001). Endoscopic treatment of prepontine arachnoid cysts. *British Journal of Neurosurgery, 15*(3), 234–238.

Golaz, J., & Bouras, C. (1993). Frontal arachnoid cyst. A case of bilateral frontal arachnoid cyst without clinical signs. *Clincial Neuropathology, 12,* 73–78.

Gulsun, M., Sabanci, U., & Ozdemir, B. (2007). Neurological signs in a case with arachnoid cyst, localized in the left temporal region, and psychotic disorder: A case report. *Turkiye Klinikleri Tip Bilimleri Dergisi, 27,* 615–617.

Gundersen, H., Helland, C. A., Rader, M. B., Hugdahl, K., & Wester, K. (2007). Visual attention in patients with intracranial arachnoid cysts. *Journal of Neurology, 254,* 60–66.

Helland, C. A., & Wester, K. (2007). Intracystic pressure in patients with temporal arachnoid cysts. A prospective study of pre-operative complaints and post-operative outcome. *Journal of Neurology, Neurosurgery, and Psychiatry, 78,* 620–623.

Hodges J. R. (1991). Pure apraxic agraphia with recovery after drainage of a left frontal cyst. *Cortex, 27,* 469–473.

Horiguchi, T., & Takeshita K. (2000). Cognitive function and language of a child with an arachnoid cyst in the left frontal fossa. *World Journal of Biological Psychiatry, 1,* 159–163.

Hund-Georgiadis M., Yves Von Cramon, D., Kruggel, F., & Preul, C. (2002). Do quiescent arachnoid cysts alter CNS functional organization?: A fMRI and morphometric study. *Neurology, 59,* 1935–1939.

Kohn, R., Lilly, R. B., Sokol, M. S., & Malloy, P. F. (1989). Psychiatric presentations of intracranial cysts. *The Journal of Neuropsychiatry and Clinical Neurosciences, 1,* 60–66.

Kotil, K., Balci, N., & Bilge, T. (2007). Intracranial symptomatic giant arachnoid cyst of the interhemispheric fissure presenting with frontal lobe syndrome. *Turkish Neurosurgery, 17,* 147–151.

Krzyzowski, J., Koziarski, A., Wejroch, A., Delimat, L., & Podgorski, J. K. (1998). A case of schizophrenia-like psychosis in a patient with arachnoid cyst. *Polish Journal of Neurology and Neurosurgery, 32,* 433–440.

Kuhnley, E. J., White, D. H., & Granoff, A. L. (1981). Psychiatric presentation of an arachnoid cyst. *Journal of Clinical Psychiatry, 42,* 167–168.

Kumagai, M., Sakai, N., Yamada, H., Shinoda, J., Nakashima, T., Iwama, T., et al. (1986). Postnatal development and enlargement of primary middle cranial fossa arachnoid cyst recognized on repeat CT scans. *Child's Nervous System, 2,* 211–215.

Lebowitz, B. K., Schefft, B. K., Marc Testa, S., Patton, J. A., & Yeh, H. S. (2006). Neurocognitive sequelae of a giant arachnoid cyst: Case study. *Neurocase, 12,* 339–345.

Martinez-Lage, J. F., Poza, M. Sola, J., & Puche, A. (1992). Congenital arachnoid cyst of the lateral ventricles in children. *Child's Nervous System, 8,* 203–206.

Martinez-Lage, J. F., Valenti, J. A., Piqueras, C., Ruiz-Espejo, A. M., Roman, F., & Nuno de la Rosa, J. A. (2006). Functional assessment of intracranial arachnoid cysts with TC99 m-HMPAO SPECT: A preliminary report. *Child's Nervous System, 22,* 1091–1097.

Millichap, J. G. (1997). Temporal lobe arachnoid cyst-attention deficit disorder syndrome: Role of the electroencephalogram in diagnosis. *Neurology, 48,* 1435–1439.

Oka, Y., Kumon, Y., Kohno, K, Saitoh, M., & Sakaki, S. (1996). Treatment of suprasellar arachnoid cyst-two case report. *Neurologia Medico-Chirurfica, 36,* 721–724.

Parsch, C. S., Krauss, J., Hofmann, E., Meixensberger, J., & Roosen, K. (1997). Arachnoid cysts associated with subdural hematomas and hygromas: Analysis of 16 cases, long-term follow-up and review of the literature. *Neurosurgery, 40,* 483–490.

Quint, D. J. (1992). Retroclival arachnoid cysts. *American Journal of Neuroradiology, 13,* 1503–1504.

Raeder, M. B., Helland, C. A., Hugdahl, K., & Wester, K. (2005). Arachnoid cysts cause cognitive deficits that improve after surgery. *Neurology, 64,* 160–162.

Ramtahal, J. (2006). Arachnoid cyst mimicking normal pressure hydrocephalus. A case report and review of the literature. *Journal of Neurosurgical Sciences, 50,* 79–81.

Rao, G., Anderson, R. C., Feldstein, N. A., & Brockmeyer, D. L. (2005). Expansion of arachnoid cysts in children: Report of two cases and review of the literature. *Journal of Neurosurgery, 102,* 314–317.

Rappaport, Z. H. (1993). Suprasellar arachnoid cysts: Options in operative management. *Acta Neurochirurgica, 122,* 71–75.

Sgouros, S., & Chapman, S. (2001). Congenital middle fossa arachnoid cysts may cause global brain ischaemia: A study with 99Tc-hexamethylpropyleneamineoxime single photon emission computerized tomography scans. *Pediatric Neurosurgery, 35,* 188–194.

Sommer, I. E., & Smit, L. M. (1997). Congenital supratentorial arachnoidal and giant cysts in children: A clinical study with arguments for a conservative approach. *Child's Nervous System, 13,* 8–12.

Soukup, V. M., Patterson, J., Trier, T. T., & Chen, J. W. (1998). Cognitive improvement despite minimal arachnoid cyst decompression. *Brain and Development, 20,* 589–593.

Stowe, L. A., Go, K. G., Pruim, J. Den Dunnen, W., Meiners, L. C., & Paans, A. M. (2000). Language localization in cases of left temporal lobe arachnoid cyst: Evidence against interhemispheric reorganization. *Brain and Language, 75,* 347–358.

Stracciari, A., Ciucci, G., & Bissi, G. (1987). Transient global amnesia associated with a large arachnoid cyst of the middle cranial fossa of the non dominant hemisphere. *Italian Journal of Neurological Sciences, 8,* 609–611.

Sztriha, L., & Gururaj, A. (2005). Hippocampal dysgenesis associated with temporal lobe hypoplasia and arachnoid cyst of the middle cranial fossa. *Journal of Child Neurology, 20,* 926–930.

Tsurushima, H., Harakuni, T., Saito, A., Tominaga, D., Hyodo, A., & Yoshii, Y (2000). Symptomatic arachnoid cyst of the left frontal convexity presenting with memory disturbance-case report. *Neurologia Medico-Chirurfica, 40,* 339–341.

Ure, J., Giudice, F., Videla, H., Ollari, J., Diez, M., Delembert, W., et al. (1999). Partial agenesis of the temporal lobe Behavioral correlations. *International Journal of Neuroradiology, 5,* 225–231.

Vakis, A. F., Koutentakis, D. I., Karabetsos, D. A., & Kalostos, G. N. (2006). Psychosis-like syndrome associated with intermittent intracranial hypertension caused by a large arachnoid cyst of the left temporal lobe. *British Journal of Neurosurgery, 20,* 156–159.

Vernooij, M. W., Ikram, M. A., Tanghe, H. L., Vincent, A. J., Hofman, A., Krestin, G. P., et al. (2007). Incidental findings on brain MRI in the general population. *New England Journal of Medicine, 357,* 1821–1828.

Von Gontard, A., & Muller, U. (1991). Psychiatric and neuropsychological symptoms in children with arachnoid cysts-a case report. *Zeitschrift fur Kinder und Jugendpsychiatrie und Psychotherapie, 19,* 30–37.

Watanabe, M., Kameyama, S., Takeda, N., & Tanaka, R. (1994). Two cases of symptomatic interhemispheric arachnoid cyst in the elderly. *Surgical Neurology, 42,* 346–351.

Wester, K. (2008). Intracranial arachnoid cysts-do they impair mental functions? *Journal of Neurology, 255,* 1113–1120.

Wester, K., & Hugdahl, K. (1995). Arachnoid cysts of the left temporal fossa: Impaired preoperative cognition and postoperative improvement. *Journal of Neurology, Neurosurgery, and Pyschiatry, 59,* 293–298.

Wester, K., & Hugdahl, K. (2003). Verbal laterality and handedness in patients with intracranial arachnoid cyst. *Journal of Neurology, 250,* 36–41.

Wester, K., & Moen, G. (2000). Documented growth of a temporal arachnoid cyst. *Journal of Neurology, Neurosurgery, and Psychiatry, 69,* 699–700.

Wong, C. W., Ko, S. F., & Wai, Y. Y. (1993). Arachnoid cyst of the lateral ventricle manifesting positional psychosis. *Neurosurgery, 32,* 841–843.

Yamasaki, F., Kodama, Y., Hotta, T., Taniguchi, E., Educhi, K., Yoshioka, H., et al. (2003). Interhemispheric arachnoid cyst in the elderly: Case report and review of the literature. *Surgical Neurology, 59*(1), 68–74.

Zeegers, M., Van Der Grond, J., Durston, S., Nievelstein, R. J., Witkamp, T., Van Daalen, E., et al. (2006). Radiological findings in autistic and developmentally delayed children. *Brain and Development, 28,* 495–499.

ARACHNOIDITIS

DESCRIPTION

Arachnoiditis is a disease caused by inflammation and scarring of the arachnoid membrane surrounding the spinal cord. The inflammation can stem from infection, trauma, tumors, and/or genetics (Wright & Denney, 2003), though the most common causes of arachnoiditis are failed back surgeries, intraspinal hemorrhage, spinal steroid administration, and oil-based myelograms (Fast & Goldsher, 2007). Arachnoiditis often presents as chronic lower back and/or leg pain (Martin & Yuan, 1996).

The arachnoid is the deepest, most delicate membrane of the three membranes that cover and protect the spinal cord (Wright & Denney, 2003). It does not easily heal on its own because it lacks innervation and vascularization. Furthermore, the constant flow of cerebrospinal fluid washes away the phagocytes and enzymes that prevent scar tissue from forming (Wright & Denney, 2003). Damage occurs when an inflammatory response causes nerve roots to adhere to themselves or to the thecal sac or meninges, causing fibrosis (Martin & Yuan, 1996). These adhesions put pressure on the arachnoid, which causes scarring (Wright & Denney, 2003), and this buildup of scar tissue can restrict the blood supply, resulting in neural atrophy (Fast & Goldsher, 2007). It can also interfere with the flow of cerebrospinal fluid in the spine, which can lead to interstitial edema and/or syringomyelia (Fast & Goldsher, 2007). Symptoms of depression and anxiety may also develop as a result of the patient's response to symptoms of chronic pain (Aldrete, 2000).

NEUROPATHOLOGY/PATHOPHYSIOLOGY

There are three methods of classification for arachnoiditis, based on its appearance. The first was developed by Jorgensen, Hansen, Steenskov, and Ovesen (1975) and describes two groups: Type I, described as the

A

"sleeveless" appearance, in which the nerve roots adhere to the meninges; and Type II, in which building scar tissue produces blockage and results in narrowing, shortening, and occlusion in the thecal sac (Wright & Denney, 2003). The second method of classification was developed by Delamarter and describes three groups ranked according to severity (Wright & Denney, 2003). Group I is considered mild and appears as a group of nerve roots adhered centrally in the thecal sac (Wright & Denney, 2003). Group II is considered moderate, and appears as nerve roots and the empty sac adheres to the meninges (Wright & Denney, 2003). Group III is considered severe, and appears as a soft-tissue mass filling the subarachnoid space (Wright & Denney, 2003). The third method of classification divides myelographic images into four groups based on their specific appearance (Wright & Denney, 2003); however, because myelographies can further exacerbate the spinal lesion, these classifications are no longer widely used (Aldrete, 2000). Instead, MR and CT scans are used to get an idea of the progression of the disease (Martin & Yuan, 1996).

NEUROPSYCHOLOGICAL/CLINICAL PRESENTATION

Physical symptoms of arachnoiditis include burning pain in the lower back and legs, numbness, spasms of the back and legs, tingling sensations that proceed from the lower back down the legs, persistent pain, unexplained skin rashes or itching, loss of sensation below the afflicted area, and/or burning sensations in the ankles and feet (Wright & Denney, 2003). Symptoms of arachnoiditis can also include changes in reflex, tension, weakness, and sensory deficits (Martin & Yuan, 1996). Neurological symptoms may include weakness in the lower extremities, hypaesthesia, abnormal gait, and/or loss of control of the sphincter (Fast & Goldsher, 2007).

The most common complaint of arachnoiditis patients is chronic back pain (Fast & Goldsher, 2007). Pain is almost always described as burning or aching and worsens with movement (Aldrete, 2000). The pain may shift but most often is bilateral (Aldrete, 2000). Pain in the extremities can be indicative of adhesions higher up in the spinal cord (Aldrete, 2000).

DIAGNOSIS

Diagnosis of arachnoiditis can be difficult since its symptoms mimic those of many other spinal disorders, and the original cause of the disorder may overlap with symptoms of arachnoiditis (Aldrete, 2000). Clinical diagnosis of arachnoiditis involves reviewing the patient's records, identifying key symptoms (such as chronic pain, numbness, gait abnormalities, etc.), and confirming the hypothesis with radiological imaging (Aldrete, 2000). In the past, myelography has been used for diagnosing, but it has recently been shown that the oil-based dyes used in myelography can contribute to inflammation, thereby promoting a trend toward using less invasive tests (Martin & Yuan, 1996). MRI or CT scans with contrast are now typically utilized as they provide a means by which adhesions can be located (Wright & Denney, 2003). MRIs seem to be the most sensitive and specific scan for arachnoiditis and provide the most conclusive evidence (Fast & Goldsher, 2007). Physical examination often reveals changes in reflex, sensory deficits, tension, and/or weakness (Martin & Yuan, 1996).

Differential diagnoses can include spinal cord tumors, arachnoiditis ossificans, cauda equina syndrome, syringomyelia, and failed back syndrome (Wright & Denney, 2003). These conditions must be ruled out when diagnosing arachnoiditis, which can be problematic, as many of them can arise as complications in later stages of the disease (Wright & Denney, 2003).

TREATMENT

There is no cure for arachnoiditis (Fast & Goldsher, 2007), and treatment usually demands a multimodal approach focused on symptom relief. A combination of pharmacological, psychological, and/or surgical treatments are often prescribed (Aldrete, 2000). Corticosteroids may be prescribed if the initial inflammation was the result of a bacterial infection (Aldrete, 2000). However, these can be very detrimental if administered incorrectly (Aldrete, 2000). Anti-inflammatory drugs such as NSAIDs are often prescribed to help manage the pain, as are certain opioids (Aldrete, 2000). Antidepressant drugs may also be prescribed to treat depressive symptoms (such as withdrawal, apathy, sadness) that can result from chronic symptoms (Aldrete, 2000). Furthermore, pharmacological therapies such as tricyclics and MAOIs have been shown to reduce insomnia, restore the sleep cycle, and possibly create a muscle relaxing effect, in addition to decreasing depressive symptoms (Aldrete, 2000).

Surgical interventions can be extremely risky, and in general, are not recommended (Fast & Goldsher, 2007) considering most cases of arachnoiditis originally result from surgeries. However, limited myelotomies can be effective in restricting the lesions and minimizing some of the damage (Aldrete, 2000). Neurolysis can relieve pain and temporarily restore neurologic function, but there is a risk of damaging healthy nerve fibers and worsening the condition (Aldrete, 2000).

Electrical stimulation at a low level has been shown to relieve pain and induce calmness (Aldrete, 2000). Electrodes can be implanted under local anesthesia and activated to see if the electrical stimulation covers the entire afflicted area and then adjusted if necessary (Martin & Yuan, 1996). Electrical stimulation treatment usually lasts from 2 to 3 days, and if it is ineffective the electrodes can be easily removed (Martin & Yuan, 1996).

Many patients with arachnoiditis benefit from the addition of a psychological approach that will assist the patient in learning pain management and relaxation techniques, as it is probable that pain symptoms will never completely subside (Aldrete, 2000; Wright & Denney, 2003). Physical therapy is also essential in helping patients with arachnoiditis retain function, restore motion, and remain active (Aldrete, 2000). Behavioral modification may be necessary to achieve functional goals (Aldrete, 2000). Some patients with severe, late-stage arachnoiditis may benefit from cognitive or behavioral interventions in conjunction with psychotherapy to help relieve symptoms of depression and/or anxiety (Aldrete, 2000).

Courtney Lund
Raymond S. Dean

Aldrete, A. (2000). *Arachnoiditis: The silent epidemic.* Birmingham, AL: Future Med.

Fast, A., & Goldsher, D. (2007). *Navigating the adult spine: Bridging clinical practice & neuroradiology.* New York: Demos Medical Publishing.

Jorgensen, J., Hansen, P. H., Steenskov, V., & Ovesen, N. (1975). A clinical and radiological study of chronic lower spinal arachnoiditis. *Neuroradiology, 9,* 139–144.

Martin, R. J., & Yuan, H. A. (1996). Neurological care of spinal epidural, subdural, and intramedullary abscesses and arachnoiditis. *The Orthopedic Clinics of North America, 27,* 125–136.

Wright, M. H., & Denney, L. C. (2003). A comprehensive review of spinal arachnoiditis. *Orthopaedic Nursing, 22,* 215–221.

ARTERIOVENOUS MALFORMATIONS

DESCRIPTION

Arteriovenous malformations (AVMs) are vascular malformations comprising a complex tangle of abnormal arteries and veins that are linked by one or more fistulas (Arteriovenous Malformation Study Group [AMSG], 1999). They are one of several different forms of vascular malformations that also include capillary telangiectasia, cavernous angiomas, dural ateriovenous fistulae, and venous angiomas. The course of AVMs may be variable, remaining static, growing, or even regressing (Abdulrauf, Malik, & Awad, 1999). The location may also vary, but AVMs are often located in the border areas between vascular regions and as a result may have common circulation from the anterior, middle, and posterior cerebral arteries (Stapf et al., 2001). The location may be cortical, subcortical, or with large AVMs may extend from the cortex to subcortical structures (AMSG, 1999). Research has identified two types of vascular lesions associated with arteriovenous shunting. The first includes pial AVMs that are located in the cerebrum and are thought to be congenital. Dural AVMs, in contrast, are located in the meningeal coverings of the brain and are thought to develop later in life (Lantz & Meyers, 2008). AVMs may also be classified as hemorrhagic and nonhemorrhagic (Stapf et al., 2001), and many patients also have aneurysms (Redekop, TerBrugge, Montanera, & Willinsky, 1998).

NEUROPATHOLOGY/PATHOPHYSIOLOGY

Congenital in nature, intracranial AVMs represent the most common vascular malformations that cause symptomatic intracranial bleeding. As reported, AVMs comprise clustered arteries and veins that may be of different size and location, without intervening capillaries (Chung & Caplan, 2007). Approximately half result in hemorrhage, most commonly intracranial hemorrhage (ICH), although subarachnoid hemorrhage (SAH) and intraventricular hemorrhage occur as well. ICH secondary to AVMs commonly appears wedge shaped, presenting from the cortex down to the ventricles, potentially extending into the intraventricular and/or subarachnoid spaces; SAH is usually due to cortically based AVMs (Brown, Wiebers, Torner, & O'Fallon, 1996; Maeda et al., 1997).

NEUROPSYCHOLOGICAL/CLINICAL PRESENTATION

Many patients with AVMs experience ICH (Choi & Mohr, 2005), and this constitutes perhaps the most frequent symptom of AVMs (Brown et al., 1990). Patients with AVMs that are fed by more than one artery may be at increased risk for hemorrhage (Langer et al., 1998). Seizures may also be the initial symptom in many patients with nonhemorrhagic AVMs, with most being partial or partial complex (Hofmeister et al., 2000; Osipov et al., 1997). In addition, AVMs may be associated with headache (Hofmeister et al., 2000) and are predominantly nonpulsating and ipsilateral to the AVM, with pain experienced in the vicinity of the AVM (Ghossoub et al., 2001). Focal neurological deficits in the absence of hemorrhage have also been reported in many patients (AMSG, 1999), which may include movement disorders such as tremor and dystonia (Krauss, Kiriyanthan, & Borremans, 1999).

Many researchers suggest that few patients with AVMs experience neuropsychological deficits in the absence of hemorrhage (Lazar, 2001). However, some have reported reversible dementia caused by a tentorial dural AVM (Ito, Sonokawa, Mishina, & Sato, 1995). Visuospatial neglect and neglect of the left hemibody have also been reported (Buklina, 2002). Wenz et al. (1998) reported that patients with AVMs exhibited lower scores on tests of attention, memory, and general IQ. Other researchers have also reported lower scores on tests of attention, memory, and IQ (Steinvorth et al., 2002) as well as impairments in verbal or visuospatial processing depending upon whether the left or right hemisphere was involved (Mahalick, Ruff, & U, 1991). Mahalick and colleagues reported differences between AVM patients and normal controls on a range of neuropsychological tests, including those assessing attention and concentration, motor speed, memory, and fluency (Mahalick, Ruff, Heary, & U, 1993). Finally, Whigham and O'Toole (2007) reported that children with AVMs exhibited problems on tests of executive functioning regardless of the location of the AVM.

There have been a number of investigations examining the effects of treatment on neurological and neuropsychological functioning. Mahalick et al. (1993) reported improvements in neuropsychological functioning following surgical treatment, including measures of learning and memory. Baker, McCarter, and Porter (2004) reported the case of an individual with a right temporal AVM and who experienced improved cognitive functioning following excision of the AVM. Jaillard, Peres, and Hommel (1999) reported two cases of dural AVMs associated with subacute dementia whose functioning improved following treatment. Radiosurgery has also been associated with improved intelligence, memory, and attention following treatment (Steinvorth et al., 2002). Further, reduction in seizures and headaches have been reported following complete removal of AVMs (Zimmerman, Lewis, & Tew, 2000). Not all investigators have found improved neuropsychological

functioning, with some finding no significant changes following treatment (Blonder, Hodes, Ranseen, & Schmitt, 1999; Riva et al., 1997).

DIAGNOSIS

Imaging is essential in the diagnosis of AVMs, particularly cerebral angiography. Angiography provides details regarding the arterial supply and venous drainage of the AVM, as well as the vessels supplying the normal surrounding brain (Lantz & Meyers, 2008). Also, angiography provides important information on morphological characterization and treatment planning (Stapf et al., 2001). CT is another important imaging procedure as CT scans may be used to assess changes in the brain due to the AVM, such as hemorrhage and hydrocephalus (Riina & Gobin, 2001). In addition, MRI provides information regarding the size, location, and topographic features of AVMs (Ogilvy et al., 2001). Functional MRI may be used to assess functional brain reorganization associated with AVMs (Lazar et al., 2000), which may be helpful for the purpose of treatment planning (Cannestra et al., 2004).

TREATMENT

Treatment for AVMs include endovascular embolization, radiosurgery (e.g., gamma knife), and craniotomy for surgical resection. Embolization may be warranted in cases where the AVM is surgically inaccessible, deep in the brain, or characterized by dural feeding (Lantz & Meyers, 2008). Removal of the AVM through craniotomy may be warranted when the risk of neurosurgery is less than the risk of hemorrhage (Lunsford et al., 1991; Spetzler & Martin, 1986) and may also reduce the risk of rehemorrhage (Heros et al., 1990). Radiosurgery may include a gamma knife, proton beam, or linear accelerator and involves directing focused beams at the fistula with the intention of causing vascular injury and thrombosis (AMSG, 1999). However, radiosurgery may be more effective with smaller AVMs and complete removal is not always possible (Lantz & Meyers, 2008).

Paul S. Foster
Valeria Drago

Abdulrauf, S. I., Malik, G. M., & Awad, I. A. (1999). Spontaneous angiographic obliteration of cerebral arteriovenous malformations. *Neurosurgery, 44,* 280–287.

Arteriovenous Malformation Study Group. (1999). Arteriovenous malformations of the brain in adults. *New England Journal of Medicine, 340,* 1812–1818.

Baker, R. P., McCarter, R. J., & Porter, D. G. (2004). Improvement in cognitive function after right temporal arteriovenous malformation excision. *British Journal of Neurosurgery, 18*, 541–544.

Blonder, L. X., Hodes, J. E., Ranseen, J. D., & Schmitt, F. A. (1999). Short-term neuropsychological outcome following Gamma Knife radiosurgery for arteriovenous malformations: A preliminary report. *Applied Neuropsychology, 6*, 181–186.

Brown, R. D., Jr., Wiebers, D. O., & Forbes, G. S. (1990). Unruptured intracranial aneurysms and arteriovenous malformations: Frequency of intracranial hemorrhage and relationship of lesions. *Journal of Neurosurgery, 73*, 859–863.

Brown, R. D., Jr., Wiebers, D. O., Torner, J. C., & O'Fallon, W. M. (1996). Frequency of intracranial hemorrhage as a presenting symptom and subtype analysis: A population-based study of intracranial vascular malformations in Olmstead Country, Minnesota. *Journal of Neurosurgery, 85*, 29–32.

Buklina, S. B. (2002). The unilateral spatial neglect phenomenon in patients with arteriovenous malformations of deep brain structures. *Neuroscience and Behavioral Physiology, 32*, 555–560.

Cannestra, A. F., Pouratian, N., Forage, J., Bookheimer, S. Y., Martin, N. A., & Toga, A. W. (2004). Functional magnetic resonance imaging and optical imaging for dominant-hemisphere perisylvian arteriovenous malformations. *Neurosurgery, 55*, 804–812.

Choi, J. H., & Mohr, J. P. (2005). Brain arteriovenous malformations in adults. *Lancet Neurology, 4*, 299–308.

Chung, C. S., & Caplan, L. R. (2007). Stroke and other neurovascular disorders. In C. G. Goetz (Ed.), *Textook of Clinical Neurology* (3rd ed., pp. 1019–1052). Philadelphia: Saunders Elsevier.

Ghossoub, M., Nataf, F., Merienne, L., Devaux, B., Turak, B, & Roux, F. X. (2001). Characteristics of headache associated with cerebral arteriovenous malformations. *Neurochirurgie, 47*, 177–183.

Heros, R. C., Korosue, K., & Diebold, P. M. (1990). Surgical excision of cerebral arteriovenous malformations: Late results. *Neurosurgery, 26*, 570–577.

Hofmeister, C., Stapf, C., Hartmann, A., Sciacca, R. R., Mansmann, U., terBrugge, K., . . . Meisel, J. (2000). Demographic, morphological, and clinical characteristics of 1289 patients with brain arteriovenous malformation. *Stroke, 31*, 1307–1310.

Ito, M., Sonokawa, T., Mishina, H., & Sato, K. (1995). Reversible dural arteriovenous malformation-induced venous ischemia as a cause of dementia: Treatment by surgical occlusion of draining dural sinus: Case report. *Neurosurgery, 37*, 1187–1191.

Jaillard, A. S., Peres, B., & Hommel, M. (1999). Neuropsychological features of dementia due to dural arteriovenous malformation. *Cerebrovascular Diseases, 9*, 91–97.

Krauss, J. K., Kiriyanthan, G. D., & Borremans, J. J. (1999). Cerebral arteriovenous malformations and movement disorders. *Clinical Neurology and Neurosurgery, 101*, 92–99.

Langer, D. J., Lasner, T. M., Hurst, R. W., Flamm, E. S., Zager, E. L., & King, J. T., Jr. (1998). Hypertension, small size, and deep venous drainage are associated with risk of hemorrhagic presentation of cerebral arteriovenous malformations. *Neurosurgery, 42*, 481–486.

Lantz, E. R., & Meyers, P. M. (2008). Neuropsychological effects of brain arteriovenous malformations. *Neuropsychology Review, 18*, 167–177.

Lazar, R. M. (2001). Neuropsychological function and brain arteriovenous malformations: Redefining eloquence as a risk for treatment. *Neurosurgical Focus, 15*, e4.

Lazar, R. M., Marshall, R. S., Pile-Spellman, J., Duong, H. C., Mohr, J. P., Young, W. L., . . . DeLaPaz, R. L. (2000). Interhemispheric transfer of language in patients with left frontal cerebral arteriovenous malformation. *Neuropsychologia, 38*, 1325–1332.

Lunsford, L. D., Kondziolka, D., Flickinger, J. C., Bissonette, D. J., Jungreis, C. A., Maitz, A. H., . . . Coffey, R. J. (1991). Stereotactic radiosurgery for arteriovenous malformations of the brain. *Journal of Neurosurgery, 75*, 512–524.

Maeda, K., Kurita, H., Nakamura, T., Usui, M., Tsutsumi, K., Morimoto, T., et al. (1997). Occurrence of severe vasospasm following intraventricular hemorrhage from an arteriovenous malformation: Report of two cases. *Journal of Neurosurgery, 87*, 436–439.

Mahalick, D. M., Ruff, R. M., Heary, R. F., & U, H. S. (1993). Preoperative versus postoperative neuropsychological sequelae of arteriovenous malformations. *Neurosurgery, 33*, 563–570.

Mahalick, D. M., Ruff, R. M., & U, H. S. (1991). Neuropsychological sequelae of arteriovenous malformations. *Neurosurgery, 29*, 351–357.

Ogilvy, C. S., Stieg, P. E., Awad, I., Brown, R. D., Jr., Kondziolka, D., Rosenwasser, R., . . . Special Writing Group of the Stroke Council, American Stroke Association. (2001). AHA scientific statement: Recommendations for the management of intracranial arteriovenous malformations: A statement for healthcare professionals from a special writing group of the Stroke Counsel, American Stroke Association. *Stroke, 32*, 1458–1471.

Osipov, A., Koennecke, H. C., Hartmann, A., Young, W. L., Pile-Spellman, J., Hacein-Bey, L., . . . Mast, H. (1997). Seizures in cerebral arteriovenous malformations: Type, clinical course, and medical management. *Interventional Neuroradiology, 30*, 37–41.

Redekop, G., TerBrugge, K., Montanera, W. & Willinsky, R. (1998). Arterial aneurysms associated with cerebral

A

arteriovenous malformations: Classification, incidence, and risk of hemorrhage. *Journal of Neurosurgery, 89,* 539–546.

Riina, H. A., & Gobin, Y. P. (2001). Grading and surgical planning for intracranial arteriovenous malformations. *Neurosurgical Focus, 15,* e3.

Riva, D., Pantaleoni, C., Devoti, M., Lindquist, C., Steiner, L., Giorgi, C. (1997). Radiosurgery for cerebral AVMs in children and adolescents: The neurobehavioral outcome. *Journal of Neurosurgery, 86,* 207–210.

Sapf, C., Mohr, J. P., Pile-Spellman, J., Solomon, R. A., Sacco, R. L., & Connolly, E. S., Jr. (2001). Epidemiology and natural history of arteriovenous malformations. *Neurosurgical Focus, 11,* 1–5.

Spetzler, R. F., & Martin, N. A. (1986). A proposed grading system for arteriovenous malformations. *Journal of Neurosurgery, 65,* 476–483.

Steinvorth, S., Wenz, F., Wildermuth, S., Essig, M., Fuss, M., Lohr, F., . . . Hacke, W. (2002). Cognitive function in patients with cerebral arteriovenous malformations after radiosurgery: Prospective long-term follow-up. *International Journal of Radiation Oncology, Biology, Physics, 54,* 1430–1437.

Wenz, F., Steinvorth, S., Wildermuth, S., Lohr, F., Fuss, M., Debus, J., . . . Wannenmacher M. (1998). Assessment of neuropsychological changes in patients with arteriovenous malformation (AVM) after radiosurgery. *International Journal of Radiation Oncology, Biology, Physics, 42,* 995–999.

Whigham, K. B., & O'Toole, K. (2007). Understanding the neuropsychologic outcome of pediatric AVM within a neurodevelopmental framework. *Cognitive and Behavioral Neurology, 20,* 244–257.

Zimmerman, G., Lewis, A. I., & Tew, J. M., Jr. (2000). Pure sylvian fissure arteriovenous malformations. *Journal of Neurosurgery, 92,* 39–44.

ASPERGER'S SYNDROME

DESCRIPTION

Asperger's syndrome represents an autistic spectrum disorder that is primarily characterized by deficits in social reciprocity, diminished nonverbal communication skills, restricted or circumscribed interests, and repetitive and/or stereotyped behaviors. In comparison, autism is also associated with verbal language delays, whereas Asperger's syndrome is not.

Asperger's syndrome was first described by Hans Asperger, a Viennese pediatrician, in 1944, who published a clinical description of a group of children who shared an unusual combination of developmental weakness and strengths. These children had severe social and communication abnormalities, restricted interests, motor delays, and clumsiness. Asperger initially named this syndrome autistic psychopathy (Miller & Ozonoff, 2000). However, although he noted the aforementioned deficits, this group of children acquired language at normal or earlier age and had normal intelligence and some specific strong abilities such as visuospatial skills and verbal abstraction abilities. In 1943, the child psychiatrist Leo Kanner published a description of a group of children with similar characteristics but with no mention of motor deficits as a core symptom of the syndrome.

NEUROPATHOLOGY/PATHOPHYSIOLOGY

The neuropathological basis of Asperger's syndrome remains unclear. Studies have assumed that Asperger's syndrome is part of the autism spectrum disorders, and the causes and mechanisms to explain the symptoms would be essentially the same and the differences would be attributable to the severity (Wicker et al., 2008). Overall, it is accepted that Asperger's syndrome is a polygenetic disorder, and several neurological findings of children with autism spectrum disorder have been described including deficits in intrahemispheric neural connectivity, reductions in the size of the corpus callosum, reductions in the inhibitory cortical activity, abnormal development of gray and white matter, increased activation in Wernicke's area, diminished activation in Broca's area during cognitive processing, decreased connectivity between the inferior frontal gyrus and the limbic system, and a significant deficit in the connectivity between the primary sensory cortex and the association cortex (Minshew & Williams, 2007). In summary, more recent findings support the hypothesis of Asperger's syndrome as a large-scale neural systems disorder in which deficits in cortical connectivity and abnormal balance between excitatory and inhibitory mechanisms might play the main role. For instance, one of the mechanisms that explain the social interaction impairment found in autism spectrum disorders is the deficit in emotional processing of face expressions. This weakness can be explained by the lack of neural connectivity (Wicker et al., 2008). Wicker et al. (2008) in a recent publication found that adults with autism spectrum disorder, when observing angry and happy faces, have an abnormally low activation of the areas involved in the processing of high-order emotional information: dorsomedial prefrontal cortex (DMPFC) and right ventrolateral prefrontal cortex. However, normal activity was found in the areas that are usually activated during perceptual analysis of facial features and expressions such as superior temporal sulcus and fusiform gyrus. This lack of synchrony in the activation of these areas and the deficit of signals from the amygdala to the DMPFC might explain the failure in relating the emotional features of faces with the initiation of socially appropriate behaviors.

NEUROPSYCHOLOGICAL/CLINICAL PRESENTATION

Early language development delays are not expected in children with Asperger's syndrome (Miller and Ozonoff, 2000). In fact, earlier development of language, even before children walk appears to be common. However, later during preschool years some abnormalities may appear such as echolalia, pronoun reversal, repetitive speech, low speech initiative, and limited play. During adulthood, language can be stilted, gauche, or pedantic. Individuals may demonstrate an odd use of words while also demonstrating idiosyncratic gestural accompaniments (Perlman, 2000). The Boston Naming Test, the Rapid Automatized Naming Test, and the Verbal Fluency Test have been used to assess language (Saalasti et al., 2008).

Motor impairment is present even in children with no mental retardation measured by the Movement Assessment Battery for Children (Green et al., 2002), and performance is also poor in tests of apraxia, one-leg balance with eyes closed, tandem gait, and repetitive finger thumb apposition. However, no differences on tests of finger tapping, grooved pegboard, trail making, or visual integration have been found (Weimer, Schatz, Lincoln, Bellantyne, & Trauner, 2001).

Overall, cognitive abilities appear to be normal with higher scores in verbal scales of the Wechsler Intelligence Scale for Children in comparison with nonverbal/performance scales (Miller & Ozonoff, 2000). Consequently, wide variability in cognitive profiles of children with Asperger's syndrome is not uncommon and, in turn, cognitive giftedness is rare (Chiang & Lin, 2007; Edgin & Pennington, 2005). Some memory problems can be observed during free recall tasks, but the deficit disappears when cues are provided (Bowler, Gardiner, & Berthollier, 2005). Creativity and imagination are impoverished when using a test of imaginative fluency (Craig & Baron-Cohen, 1999). Executive functioning is the area more affected in this syndrome as evidenced for defective performance in tasks of response selection/inhibition, flexibility, planning, working memory, abstract problem solving, visual memory, and multitasking (Christ, Holt, White, & Green, 2007; Edgin & Pennington, 2005; Happé, Booth, Charlton, & Hughes, 2006; Hill & Bird, 2006).

The social challenges that individuals with Asperger's syndrome have seem to be related with their inability to attribute mental states to themselves and others in order to explain and anticipate behaviors. This cognitive skill has been called "theory of mind" (Duverger, Da Fonseca, Bailly, & Deruelle, 2007). The social interaction impairment involves deficits in empathy, poor eye contact, isolation, physical contact defensiveness, and generally inappropriate social behavior. These features as well as other clinical characteristics are successfully assessed by different instruments such as the Autism Diagnostic Interview-Revised, the Autism Diagnostic Observation Schedule (Miller & Ozonoff, 2000), and the Autism Spectrum Screening Questionnaire (Saalasti et al., 2008).

DIAGNOSIS

Diagnosis of Asperger's syndrome is largely dependent upon clinical interview and developmental history. In addition, neuropsychological and psychological assessment, both with performance-based measures and self-report or observer rating, may offer further insight into the diagnostic picture. Today, modern systems of diagnosis such as the *Diagnostic and Statistical Manual of Mental Disorders* (*DSM-IV*, American Psychiatric Association [APA], 2000) and the International Classification of Diseases (ICD) (Isaac, Janca, & Sartorius, 1994) place Asperger's syndrome in the category of Pervasive Developmental Disorders. Both diagnostic systems define this syndrome with similar features that were earlier noticed by Leo Kanner and Hans Asperger, including impairment in social interaction and restricted and stereotyped patterns of behavior, interests, and activities. However, the *DSM-IV* requires the criteria of absence of clinical delay in language, cognitive development, and self-help skills to make the diagnosis. The diagnosis of autistic disorder has to be assigned when these cognitive delays and deficits of adaptive skills are present.

Besides the differences in the diagnostic criteria that exist between Asperger's syndrome and autism, both the *DSM-IV* and *ICD-9* point out that there is an overlap among symptoms and features. As such, children with autism who demonstrate high performance in social and cognitive skills can be easily misdiagnosed with Asperger's syndrome. Miller and Ozonoff (2000) explored the external validity of Asperger's disorder by comparing a group of children previously diagnosed with high-functioning autism with another group of children with Asperger's syndrome. In their research, they used clinical measures of autism, intelligence, motor skills, visuoperceptual skills, executive functioning, and cognitive flexibility. The results

A

showed that both groups were not different in most of the measures and the variable that explained the differences between groups was intellectual ability. Overall, the group of children with diagnosis of Asperger's syndrome performed better than children with autism only in intellectual ability. Coinciding with the idea that the difference between these two disorders accounts for severity of symptoms, one approach that is being adopted is to treat autism and Asperger's disorders as being part of a continuum or a spectrum of symptoms that varies in severity. Consequently, children with low language, cognitive, intellectual, and adaptive skills would be located on one side of the spectrum. In the other more adaptive extreme of the spectrum, children with Asperger's syndrome and high-functioning autism would be placed. This approach has been challenged by several publications that found important variability in cognitive and adaptive profiles of both groups (i.e., high-functioning autism and Asperger's syndrome) yet only few essential differences (Chiang & Lin, 2007). These differences between Asperger's syndrome and high-functioning autism remain controversial, and it is suggested that high-functioning autism and Asperger's syndrome would be the same disorder. Moreover, the differences that have been found, appear to be minor or only based on clinical symptoms profiles from a clinical perspective (Paul, Orlovski, Marcinko, & Volkmar, 2008; Schultz et al., 2000). Williams, Goldstein, Kojkowski, and Minshew (2008) when studying IQ profiles of high-functioning autistic children with nonverbal learning disabilities suggested that clinical scales such as the Autism Diagnostic Observation Schedule are more reliable and accurate than IQ profiles in diagnosing autism. Similarly, Spek, Scholte, and Van Berckelaer-Onnes (2008) found that differences between verbal IQ and performance IQ cannot help differentiate adults with Asperger's syndrome from high-functioning autism even though the Asperger's syndrome group performed slightly better in verbal IQ than the autistic subjects. The same difference is found when comparing Asperger's disorder with pervasive developmental disorder not otherwise specified (Koyama & Kurita, 2008).

TREATMENTS

Most of the treatments have been focused on social skills development, even in the school setting (Williams, Keoning, & Scahill, 2007). However, psychotherapy in adults with this disorder is also possible as reviewed by Ramsay, Brodkin, Cohen, Listerud, and Rostain (2005). This review describes how social skills groups and cognitive behavior-based interventions can be useful not only in treating frequent comorbid conditions such as depression and anxiety but also negative beliefs and social aversions that are common in these individuals. Pharmacotherapy is also useful in treating comorbid obsessive-compulsive, mood, sleep, and anxiety problems. The families of the children with this disorder should be assessed for therapeutic and psychosocial interventions as evidenced by the high percentage of mothers who are at higher risk of physical and mental illnesses because of the high stress that they face in their role as caregivers (Allik, Larsson, & Smedje, 2006).

Javier Gontier
Antonio E. Puente

Allik, H., Larsson, J., & Smedje, H. (2006). Health-related quality of life in parents of school-age children with Asperger syndrome or high-functioning autism. *Health and Quality of Life Outcomes.* Retrieved January 12, 2008, from http://www.hqlo.com/content/4/1/1

American Psychiatric Association. (2000). *Diagnostic and statistical manual of mental disorders* (4th ed., text revision). Washington, DC: Author.

Bowler, D. M., Gardiner, J. M., & Berthollier, N. (2004). Source memory in adolescents and adults with Asperger's syndrome. *Journal of Autism and Developmental Disorders, 34* (5), 533–542.

Chiang, H., & Lin, Y. (2007). Mathematical ability of students with Asperger syndrome and high-functioning autism: A review of literature. *Autism, 11* (6), 547–556.

Christ, S. E., Holt, D. D., White, D. A., & Green, L. (2007). Inhibitory control in children with autism spectrum disorder. *Journal of Autism and Developmental Disorders, 37* (6), 1155–1165.

Craig, J., & Baron-Cohen, S. (1999). Creativity and imagination in autism and Asperger syndrome. *Journal of Autism and Developmental Disorders, 29* (4), 319–326.

Duverger, H., Da Fonseca, D., Bailly, D., & Deruelle, C. (2007). Theory of mind in Asperger syndrome. *Encephale, 33* (4, Pt. 1), 592–597.

Edgin, J. O., & Pennington, B. F. (2005). Spatial cognition in autism spectrum disorders: Superior, impaired, or just intact? *Journal of Autism and Developmental Disorders, 35* (6), 729–745.

Green, D., Baird, G., Barnett, A. L., Henderson, L., Huber, J., & Henderson, S. E. (2002). The severity and nature of motor impairment in Asperger's syndrome: A comparison with specific developmental disorder of motor function. *Journal of Child Psychology and Psychiatry and Allied Disciplines, 43* (5), 655–668.

Happé, F., Booth, R., Charlton, R., & Hughes, C. (2006). Executive function deficits in autism spectrum disorders and attention-deficit/hyperactivity disorder: Examining profiles across domains and ages. *Brain and Cognition, 61* (1), 25–39.

Hill, E. L., & Bird, C. M. (2006). Executive processes in Asperger syndrome: Patterns of performance in multiple case series. *Neuropsychologia, 44* (14), 2822–2844.

Isaac, M., Janca, A., Sartorius, N. (1994). ICD-10 symptom glossary for mental disorders. Geneva, Division of Mental Health, World Health Organization.

Koyama, T., & Kurita, H. (2008). Cognitive profile difference between normally intelligent children with Asperger's disorder and those with pervasive developmental disorder not otherwise specified. *Psychiatry and Clinical Neurosciences, 62* (6), 691–696.

Miller, J. N., & Ozonoff, S. (2000). The external validity of Asperger disorder: Lack of evidence from the domain of neuropsychology. *Journal of Abnormal Psychology, 109* (2), 227–238.

Minshew, N. J., & Williams, D. L. (2007). The new neurobiology of autism. *Archives of Neurology*. Retrieved January 12, 2009, from http://www.pubmedcentral.nih.gov/articlerender.fcgi?artid = 2597785

Paul, R., Orlovski, S. M., Marcinko, H. C., & Volkmar, F. (2008). Conversational behaviors in youth with high-functioning ASD and Asperger syndrome. *Journal of Autism and Developmental Disorders, 39* (1), 115–125.

Perlman, L. (2000). Adults with Asperger disorder misdiagnosed as schizophrenic. *Professional Psychology: Research and Practice, 31* (2), 221–225.

Ramsay, J. R., Brodkin, E. S., Cohen, M. R., Listerud, J., & Rostain, A. L. (2005). "Better strangers": Using the relationship in psychotherapy for adult patients with Asperger syndrome. *Psychotherapy: Theory, Research, Practice, Training, 42* (4), 483–493.

Saalasti, S., Lepisto, T., Toppila, E., Kujala, T., Laakso, M., Nieminen-von Wendt, T., et al. (2008). Language abilities of children with Asperger syndrome. *Journal of Autism and Developmental Disorders, 38,* 1574–1580.

Schultz, R. T., Gauthier, I., Klin, A., Fulbright, R. K., Anderson, A. W., Volkmar, F., et al. (2000). Abnormal ventral temporal cortical activity during face discrimination among individuals with autism and Asperger syndrome. *Archives of General Psychiatry, 57* (4), 331–340.

Spek, A. A., Scholte, E. M., & van Berckelaer-Onnes, I. A. (2008). Brief report: The use of WAIS-III in adults with HFA and Asperger syndrome. *Journal of Autism and Developmental Disorders, 38* (4), 782–787.

Weimer, A. K., Schatz, A. M., Lincoln, A., Ballantyne, A. O. & Trauner, D. A. (2001). "Motor" impairment in Asperger syndrome: Evidence for a deficit in proprioception. *Journal of Developmental Behavioral Pediatrics, 22* (2), 92–101.

Wicker, B., Fonlupt, P., Hubert, B., Tardif, C., Gepner, B., & Deruelle, C. (2008). Abnormal cerebral effective connectivity during explicit emotional processing in adults with autism spectrum disorder. *Social Cognitive and Affective Neuroscience, 3* (2), 135–143.

Williams, D. L., Goldstein, G., Kojkowski, N., & Minshew, N. J. (2008). Do individuals with high-functioning autism have the IQ profile associated with nonverbal learning disability? *Research in Autism Spectrum Disorders, 2* (2), 353–361.

Williams, W. S., Keonig, K., & Scahill, L. (2007). Social skills development in children with autism spectrum disorders: A review of the intervention research. *Journal of Autism and Developmental Disorders, 37* (10), 1858–1868.

ATAXIA TELANGIECTASIA

DESCRIPTION

Ataxia telangiectasia (AT), also known as Louis-Bar's syndrome, is a rare, childhood neurological disorder characterized by acute sensitivity to ionizing radiation, immunodeficiency, inability to coordinate voluntary muscle movements (ataxia), poor balance, inability to intentionally shift one's gaze to objects in the visual field (oculomotor ataxia), slurred speech, and telangiectasias (dilated small blood vessels) that are typically present in the corners of the eyes, on the bridge of the nose, or the surface of the ears (Webster, 1998). Estimates of the prevalence of the disorder suggests that it occurs in 1 out of 40,000 live births in the United States, affecting males and females equally (Chun & Gatti, 2004). The earliest symptoms of the disorder include limb and truncal ataxia (swaying of the head and trunk while standing or sitting), which are often apparent before the age of 3. The degree of limb and truncal ataxia gradually progresses over time with most children confined to a wheelchair by age 10 (Di Donato, Gellera, & Mariotti, 2001; Perlman, Becker-Catania, & Gatti, 2003; Webster, 1998). By age 5, speech becomes slurred and slowed (Perlman et al., 2003), and the child displays involuntary movements, such as spontaneous writhing and jerking movements of the limbs and intentional tremors (Di Donato et al., 2001). As the motor symptoms of the disorder progress, children with AT eventually lose the ability to use written forms of communication due to significantly decreased motor control and coordination resulting in illegible handwriting (Crawford, 1998).

Children with AT are at an increased risk (38%) for developing cancer, particularly acute lymphocytic leukemia or lymphoma (Perlman et al., 2003; Di Donato et al., 2001). Due to underdevelopment of the thymus with subsequently weakened immune systems, these children are susceptible to recurrent sinopulmonary infections (Di Donato et al., 2001; Webster, 1998). Other features of AT include mild diabetes mellitus, premature graying of the hair, difficulty swallowing, and delayed physical and sexual development. Individuals with AT do not usually survive beyond their teens or early 20s, but some individuals with AT live well into their 50s (Broccoletti et al., 2008; Webster, 1998). The most common causes of death are malignancy, nonspecific pulmonary failure, and infection (Perlman et al., 2001).

NEUROPATHOLOGY/PATHOPHYSIOLOGY

The gene responsible for AT is known as ataxia-telangiectasia mutated (ATM) and is responsible for making a serine-threonine kinase that activates other proteins, which control cell cycle, DNA repair, and cell death (Perlman et al., 2003; Onodera, 2006). The absence of this protein is what leaves DNA susceptible to damages from ionizing radiation, one of the key features of AT. In addition, the ATM protein has been shown to play a role in blocking cell division of Purkinje's cells (Yang & Herrup, 2005), which are a class of neurons located in the cerebellum that are inhibitory in nature due to their GABAergic function. Consequently, the motor symptoms associated with AT are a result of the loss of Purkinje and granular cells in the cerebellum (Ball & Xiao, 2005; Broccoletti et al., 2008; Perlman et al., 2003; Mostofsky, Kunze, Cutting, Lederman, & Denckla, 2000).

Tavani et al. (2003) compared MRI scans from 19 patients with AT of varying ages and found that cerebellar atrophy begins in the most lateral portions and subsequently progresses to the inferior and posterior areas of the cerebellar cortex. In the later stages of the progression of the disorder, atrophy is observed in the cerebrum, brainstem, spinal cord, peripheral nerves, and muscles. This degeneration causes accelerated aging in 90% of individuals with AT, which leads to such characteristics as gray hair and wrinkled or discolored skin in adolescence (Webster, 1998).

NEUROPSYCHOLOGICAL/CLINICAL PRESENTATION

Individuals with AT have normal or above normal intelligence (Di Donato et al., 2001; Perlman et al., 2003), but some researchers have found that performance on intelligence tests drops after approximately age 9 (Mostofsky et al., 2000). Given the development of motor impairment in children with AT, it is likely that at least a portion of this decline is secondary to fine motor control and coordination deficits,

which can attenuate scores on performance-based measures of intelligence. However, increasing motor impairment alone is not responsible for the drop in reported intellectual ability as some affected individuals may experience retarded intellectual growth during the early stages of the disorder (Webster, 1998). Due to the motor and speech deficits experienced by individuals with AT, traditional measures of intellectual ability are often ill-suited to appropriately measure intellectual functions as the disorder progresses (Webster, 1998).

From a functional standpoint, initial concerns often involve difficulties with fine and gross motor functioning and speech articulation problems, which render physical and occupational therapies the most appropriate initial intervention strategies for this population (Webster, 1998). Furthermore, patients with AT often present with deficits in diction, handwriting, reading, and mobility and often require long-term help with personal hygiene and bathing (Perlman et al., 2003). As children with AT enter school, special education services are typically required and recurrent infections can often lead to the need for homebound education (Webster, 1998).

In addition to motor and speech deficits, Mostofsky et al. (2000) found that individuals with AT demonstrate deficits in judgment of explicit time intervals. The cerebellum also plays a critical role in learning secondary to classical conditioning. Furthermore, Mostofsky, Green, Meginley, Christensen, and Woodruff-Pak (1999) conducted a study demonstrating the presence of deficits in nondeclarative learning in individuals with AT. Finally, more recent research regarding the role of the cerebellum in general cognition and executive functions have found that deficits that were previously believed to be "frontal" in nature can many times be due to lesions or disorders of the cerebellum. This has given rise to the recognition of what is referred to as the cerebellar cognitive affective syndrome (CCAS). Although there are no formally agreed upon diagnostic criteria for CCAS, most researchers typically include aspects of impairment in executive functions, visuospatial ability, emotional regulation, social skills, and linguistic ability (Schmahmann, 2004; Schmahmann, Weilburg, & Sherman, 2007). Consequently, neuropsychological evaluation of individuals with AT should include assessment measures capable of reliably measuring these different skill sets over time.

DIAGNOSIS

The most prominent features of the disease are the truncal and limb ataxia, oculomotor ataxia, and the telangiectasia (Lewis, Lederman, & Crawford, 1999). In addition to these features, AT can be diagnosed through genetic testing to assess for the presence of mutations on the ATM gene. Further clinical findings that can be used in the diagnosis of AT include: cerebellar atrophy on MRI, laboratory evidence of immune deficiency, elevated levels of serum alpha-fetoprotein (AFP), and lymphocyte radiosensitivity (Di Donato et al., 2001). Malignancy is sometimes present before any other signs of AT, and, for this reason, some recommend that a diagnosis of AT be considered in all young children presenting with cancer (Perlman et al., 2003). Three routine tests that are often used for the diagnosis of AT in young children are: serum AFP, karyotyping, and immune status of B-cell and T-cell compartments (T-cell levels are usually low, γ/δ T-cell levels are elevated, and B-cells are normal or slightly elevated) (Perlman et al., 2003).

AT initially resembles Friedreich's ataxia and is often misdiagnosed as such until the emergence of the telangiectasia (Webster, 1998). Another feature of AT that is found in other progressive neuropathies are varus and equinus foot demormities. AT can be differentiated from other disorders because these foot deformities are often exaggerated with walking in AT, and it is not associated with an inflexible high arch, forefoot atrophy, or hammer toe (Crawford, 1998). AT can be differentiated from ataxia oculomotor apraxia by having an increase in chromosome breaks and marked radiation sensitivity (Gascon, Abdo, Sigut, Hemidan, & Hannan, 1995). AT-like disorder can be diagnosed when there are neurological signs of AT and radiosensitivity, but the ATM protein is present and there are no mutations of the ATM gene (Taylor & Byrd, 2005).

TREATMENT

Unfortunately, there is currently no cure for AT and no way to slow its progression (Broccoletti et al., 2008). Therefore, treatment mainly consists of medical management and neurorehabilitation (Perlman et al., 2003). Occupational and physical therapy is used to maintain flexibility, whereas speech therapy is used to help with articulation problems and general communication deficits (Webster, 1998). As the motor and speech problems worsen, the child may need to learn alternative ways of communicating, such as sign language or use of a communication board (Webster, 1998). There are some preliminary findings that treatment with corticosteroids leads to the amelioration of some of the neurological signs of AT, especially speech disturbance, stance, and performance on finger chase tests (Broccoletti et al., 2008).

Gamma-globulin injections and high-dose vitamin regimens are sometimes given to strengthen the immune system. Respiratory infections can be treated with antibiotic medications and valium or antilirium can be used for the treatment of speech problems, such as slurring and muscle disorders (Webster, 1998). Severe contractures can be corrected with surgery to improve the quality of life and increase mobility (Perlman et al., 2003).

Teachers may need to be educated about the typical physical, behavioral, and emotional symptoms associated with AT to assist with general social adjustment and acceptance (Webster, 1998). Patients with AT may also require individual psychotherapy to address emotional problems associated with the social and physical limitations of the disorder (Perlman et al., 2003). Families of children with AT should be offered psychoeducation, genetic counseling, individual and family counseling, referral to support and advocacy groups, and online resources (Perlman et al., 2003).

Sophia Zavrou
Jon C. Thompson

Ball, L. G., & Xiao, W. (2005). Molecular basis of ataxia telangiectasia and related diseases. *Acta Pharmacologica Sinica, 26*(8), 897–907.

Broccoletti, T., Del Giudice, E., Amorosi, S., Russo, I., Di Bonito, M., Imperati, F., et al. (2008). Steroid-induced improvement of neurological signs in ataxia-telangiectasia patients. *European Journal of Neurology, 15,* 223–228.

Chun, H. H., & Gatti, R. A. (2004). Ataxia-telangiectasia, an evolving phenotype. *DNA Repair (Amst), 3,* 1187–1196.

Crawford, T. O. (1998). Ataxia telangiectasia. *Seminars in Pediatric Neurology, 5*(4), 287–294.

Di Donato, S., Gellera, C., & Mariotti, C. (2001). The complex clinical and genetic classification of inherited ataxias. II. Autosomal recessive ataxias. *Neurological Sciences, 22*(3), 219–228.

Gascon, G. G., Abdo, N., Sigut, D., Hemidan, A., & Hannan, M. A. (1995). Ataxia-oculomotor apraxia syndrome. *Journal of Child Neurology, 10*(2), 118–122.

Lewis, R. F., Lederman, H. M., & Crawford, T. O. (1999). Ocular motor abnormalities in ataxia telangiectasia. *Annals of Neurology, 46*(3), 287–295.

Mostofsky, S. H., Green, J. T., Meginley, M., Christensen, J. R., & Woodruff-Pak, D. S. (1999). Conditioning in identical twins with ataxia-telangiectasia. *Neurocase, 5,* 425–433.

Mostofsky, S. H., Kunze, J. C., Cutting, L. E., Lederman, H. M., & Denckla, M. B. (2000). Judgment of duration in individuals with ataxia-telangiectasia. *Developmental Neuropsychology, 17*(1), 63–74.

Onodera, O. (2006). Spinocerebellar ataxia with ocular motor apraxia and DNA repair. *Neuropathology, 26,* 361–367.

Perlman, S., Becker-Catania, S., & Gatti, R. A. (2003). Ataxia-telangiectasia: Diagnosis and treatment. *Seminars in Pediatric Neurology, 10*(3), 173–182.

Schmahmann, J. D. (2004). Disorders of the cerebellum: Ataxia, dysmetria of thought, and the cerebellar cognitive affective syndrome. *Journal of Neuropsychiatry & Clinical Neurosciences, 16,* 367–378.

Schmahmann, J. D., Weilburg, J. B., & Sherman, J. C. (2007). The neuropsychiatry of the cerebellum – insights from the clinic. *The Cerebellum, 6,* 254–267.

Tavani, F., Zimmerman, R. A., Berry, G. T., Sullivan, K., Gatti, R., & Bingham, P. (2003). Ataxia-telangiectasia: The pattern of cerebellar atrophy on MRI. *Neuroradiology, 45,* 315–319.

Taylor, A. M., & Byrd, P. J. (2005). Molecular pathology of ataxia telangiectasia. *Journal of Clinical Pathology, 58*(10), 1009–1015.

Yang, Y., & Herrup, K. (2005). Loss of neuronal cell cycle control in ataxia-telangiectasia: A unified disease mechanism. *The Journal of Neuroscience, 25*(10), 2522–2529.

Webster, R. E. (1998). Louis-Bar syndrome (Ataxia Telangiectasia). In L. Phelps (Ed.), *Health-related disorders in children and adolescents: A guidebook for understanding and educating* (pp. 400–404). Washington, DC: American Psychological Association.

ATTENTION DEFICIT HYPERACTIVITY DISORDER

DESCRIPTION

Attention deficit hyperactivity disorder (ADHD) is a developmental disorder that emerges in childhood that sometimes continues through adulthood. ADHD is the most common diagnosed child psychological disorder (Cherkasova & Hechtman, 2009), with an estimated occurrence in 2% to 7% (Hervey, Epstein, & Curry, 2004) of the childhood population, with boys being overrepresented 3:1 (Barkley, 1997). According to the Centers for Disease Control and Prevention (CDC), 4.5 million children were diagnosed with ADHD as of 2006. The frequency of diagnosis has increased 3% per year from 1997 to 2006, again with boys being diagnosed more frequently than girls. However, some individuals are not diagnosed until adulthood. The prevalence of these disorders is not as well understood nor documented.

The *Diagnostic and Statistical Manual for Mental Disorders* (*DSM-IV-TR;* American Psychiatric Association [APA], 2000) notes that the frequent descriptive patterns in individuals with ADHD are inattentiveness, impulsivity, and/or hyperactivity. A person with a deficit in attention may become easily distracted, dissociate from reality, make careless mistakes and/or have difficulty listening, sustaining attention, and organizing tasks. Individuals with impulsivity are characterized by interrupting, acting without regard for consequences, being impatient, and/or having difficulty waiting. People with ADHD demonstrate hyperactivity by fidgeting, talking excessively, demonstrating difficulty while doing quiet tasks and/or activities, and having trouble staying still. Based on predominant symptoms, the *DSM-IV-TR* (APA, 1994) divided ADHD into three subtypes: predominantly inattentive type, predominantly hyperactive-impulsive type, and the combined type.

The prevalence of these disorders has increased exponentially. In 1981, almost no articles were written on ADHD according to Lopez-Munoz, Alamo, Quintero Gutierrez, and Garcia (2008). By 2005, over 850 articles were being published each year. The top five journals where publications on ADHD were found were psychiatric ones. Interestingly, none of the top 20 journals were neuropsychological, though over 40% were from U.S. journals.

NEUROPATHOLOGY/PATHOPHYSIOLOGY

The cognitive deficits associated with ADHD can be attributed to dysfunction in the frontostriatal circuitry, along with regions outside of this area including the cerebellum and the temporoparietal lobes (Cherkasova & Hechtman, 2009; Schmahmann, 2010; Vaidya & Stollstorff, 2008). These areas interconnect to mediate aspects of attention (Arnsten, 2009). The cognitive deficits extend beyond executive functioning to include spatial, temporal, and lower-level "nonexecutive" functions. In addition to differences in selective regions, there are global brain differences in ADHD (Vaidya & Stollstorff, 2008). The pathophysiology of ADHD has also been shown to involve dysfunction of the catecholaminergic neurotransmitters, dopamine (DA) and norepinephrine (NE), especially in the prefrontal cortex (PFC) (Arnsten, 2009; Vaidya & Stollstorff, 2008).

The frontostriatal circuitry, including the dorsolateral prefrontal cortex, ventrolateral prefrontal cortex, dorsal anterior cingulate cortex, as well as the caudate nucleus and putamen, is the region of brain circuitry that has attracted the most attention from neuroimaging researchers in ADHD (Cherkasova & Hechtman, 2009). This circuitry regulates attention based on relevance (i.e., top-down attention) and mediates task-relevant response selection both with and without affective value (Arnsten, 2009; Vaidya & Stollstorff, 2008). Much research has shown evidence suggesting structural abnormalities in the frontal lobes and striatal structures of people with ADHD (Arnsten, 2009; Cherkasova & Hechtman, 2009; Vaidya & Stollstorff, 2008). Such studies have reported prefrontal volume and cortical thickness reductions as well in the caudate nucleus and pallidum, significant regional gray matter reduction, and hypoactivation of the network as a whole (Cherkasova & Hechtman, 2009; Vaidya & Stollstorff, 2008). The right hemisphere of the PFC is especially important for "top-down" attentional processes and for impulse control. Imaging studies have shown reduced size and functional activity of the right PFC in patients with ADHD (Arnsten, 2009). Research involving the use of stimulant medications resulted in heightened activity in these areas after usage (Cherkasova & Hechtman, 2009).

Recent evidence has implicated that the cerebellum has many cognitive and affective functions and demonstrates cerebellar-cortical connections with regions involved in higher order cognitive operations including those of the cerebellum with the PFC (Cherkasova & Hechtman, 2009). The cerebellum is involved in several executive and nonexecutive functions affected in ADHD. Studies have documented structural and functional abnormalities of the cerebellum, including reduced volumes and cortical thinning, as well as decreased activity during certain cognitive tasks (Cherkasova & Hechtman, 2009; Vaidya & Stollstorff, 2008). Cerebellar input into prefrontal regions that are involved in ADHD related functions are also suggested to be weakened or impaired (Cherkasova & Hechtman, 2009).

Parietal regions are relevant to attentional functioning, and executive functions are thought to be subserved by a network of regions including parietal structures. ADHD-related dysfunction may be found in many of the parietal lobe's functional units (Cherkasova & Hechtman, 2009). Neuroimaging studies have shown structural and functional abnormalities in the parietal lobes of people with ADHD (Arnsten, 2009; Cherkasova & Hechtman, 2009; Vaidya & Stollstorff, 2008). Overall parietal volume reductions have been noted, as well as reductions in gray matter, white matter, and cortical thickness (Cherkasova & Hechtman, 2009). Cherkasova and Hechtman (2009) and Vaidya and Stollstorff (2008) report reduced activity in many parietal regions, especially in the right hemisphere. This altered parietal activity in ADHD has also been seen in the context of numerous cognitive functions. Conversely, there is some evidence of compensatory recruitment of parietal structures in ADHD in the face of frontal-anterior cingulated deficits (Cherkasova & Hechtman, 2009).

The temporal lobe may be of interest in ADHD research because of its role in the auditory processing of linguistic information, as linguistic skill impairments have been reported in ADHD (Cherkasova & Hechtman, 2009). Several structural imaging studies have documented decreases in temporal lobe total volume as well as decreases in gray matter volume, and cortical thickness (Cherkasova & Hechtman, 2009; Vaidya & Stollstorff, 2008). These structural abnormalities are thought to be attributed to the potential delayed maturation of temporal lobes in children with ADHD (Cherkasova & Hechtman, 2009). Although there is some evidence of temporal lobe abnormalities in ADHD, the evidence is not as strong as that of cerebellar or parietal dysfunction (Vaidya & Stollstorff, 2008).

The catecholamines DA and NE have recently been recognized as playing a role in the pathophysiology of ADHD. In 2009, Arnsten stated that "DA and NE are so critical to PFC function that depleting them is as detrimental as removing the cortex itself. Small changes in these catecholamines can have marked effects on PFC function" (p. 36). The dopaminergic and norepinephrinergic systems modulate and determine the balance between sensory/reactive and control processes (Vaidya & Stollstorff, 2008). Neuroreceptor imaging has noted weaker transmission of DA in the striatum, PFC, and limbic structures, which likely reflects global reductions in DA release throughout the brain (Arnsten, 2009; Vaidya & Stollstorff, 2009). Weaker production of NE has also been seen in the PFC of people with ADHD (Arnsten, 2009).

NEUROPSYCHOLOGICAL/CLINICAL PRESENTATION

Deficits in executive functions such as working memory, planning, and inhibitory control have been reported to be neuropsychological factors that contribute to ADHD symptoms (Wahlstedt, 2009). In 1997, Barkley stated that executive functions shift control from one to another context by internal representations regarding possible outcomes. Among many factors, executive function involves the acts of planning, decision making, implementing strategies, and working memory (Wahlstedt, 2009). More specifically, inhibitory control has been reported to be a fundamental aspect of the later emergence of other domains in executive function (Wiersema, van der Meere, Antrop, & Roeyers, 2006). Other neuropsychological factors such as temporal information processing and reinforcement sensitivity have been associated with individuals with ADHD (Luman et al., 2009). Interestingly, other possible neuropsychological deficits may also be playing a role as well (Wahlstedt, 2009).

Research studies have shown that several neuropsychological deficits have been widely reported in adults with ADHD. In a meta-analysis conducted by Hervey et al. (2004), neuropsychological deficits in attention, response inhibition, memory, processing speed, motor speed, and overall intelligence were widely noted among an adult sample with ADHD, with attention and response inhibition being the most notably affected domains. Although individuals generally report these deficits, neuropsychological tests such as Conners' Continuous Performance Test, Wechsler Adult Intelligence Scale, Test of Auditory Discrimination (TOAD), and Rey-Osterrieth are commonly used to address these deficits. It was noted that adults with ADHD performed worse in the following domains of function: behavioral inhibition, attention, and memory. Overall, some of the general findings in the meta-analysis showed that adults with ADHD performed poorly compared with the adults in the control group when there was a verbal presentation of stimuli rather than a visual presentation and when the test required higher cognitive demands or increased complexity (Hervey et al., 2004).

Other studies have aimed to look at the neuropsychological factors associated in children with ADHD. Barkley (1997) explains that the behavioral deficits associated with ADHD (i.e., poor sustained attention, impulsiveness, and hyperactivity) arise relatively early, typically before the age of seven, and are fairly persistent over development. In a study conducted by Wahlstedt (2009), neuropsychological factors such as delay aversion, inhibitory control, and reaction time were investigated to see if they played significant roles in ADHD. Results showed that (1) inhibitory control and reaction time variability were mainly associated with symptoms of inattention and that (2) significant interaction effects of delay aversion and reaction time were associated with inattention and hyperactivity/impulsivity symptoms. In a study that looked at children with ADHD, children with ADHD+ODD (Oppositional Defiant Disorder), and children without ADHD, Luman et al. (2009) found that inhibition problems were only seen among those children diagnosed with ADHD. It was also noted that children with ADHD only showed neurocognitive deficits in (1) temporal information: children were more likely to show time underestimations and deficits (2) reinforcement sensitivity: children were more likely to profit less from penalty (Luman et al., 2009).

Overall, there seems to be numerous studies indicating that neuropsychological deficits such as response inhibition, delay aversion, temporal information, reinforcement sensitivity, as well as neuropsychological deficits seem to be significant in individuals with ADHD.

DIAGNOSIS

The *Diagnostic and Statistical Manual for Mental Disorders (DSM-IV-TR;* APA, 2000) provides the widely accepted criteria for diagnosis of ADHD. Patients must present with six or more of the following symptoms of inattention, which have been present for at least 6 months to a point that is disruptive and inappropriate for the developmental level:

Often does not give close attention to details or makes careless mistakes in schoolwork, work, or other activities; often has trouble keeping attention on tasks or play activities; often does not seem to listen when spoken to directly; often does not follow instructions and fails to finish schoolwork, chores, or duties in the workplace (not due to oppositional behavior or failure to understand instructions); often has trouble organizing activities; often avoids, dislikes, or does not want to do things that take a lot of mental effort for a long period of time (such as schoolwork or homework); often loses things needed for tasks and activities; is often easily distracted; is often forgetful in daily activities

If the patient does not present with symptoms of inattention, the individual must present six or more of the following symptoms of hyperactivity-impulsivity that have been present for at least 6 months to an extent that is disruptive and inappropriate for developmental level:

Often fidgets with hands or feet or squirms in seat; often gets up from seat when remaining in seat is expected; often runs about or climbs when and where it is not appropriate (adolescents or adults may feel very restless); often has trouble playing or enjoying leisure activities quietly; is often "on the go" or often acts as if "driven by a motor"; often talks excessively; often blurts out answers before questions have been finished; often has trouble waiting one's turn; often interrupts or intrudes on others (e.g., butts into conversations or games)

The symptoms presented that cause impairment must be seen before the age of 7, and must be displayed in two or more settings (i.e., home, school, work, etc.);

however, it is not uncommon for impairments to present with different severity across settings. For example, the more sedentary and continuous a situation the more likely symptoms will be noticeable. There must be clear evidence of impairment in social, school, and work functioning. These symptoms must not happen during a psychotic episode, and they must not be better accounted for by another mental disorder.

The World Health Organization (WHO) has determined ADHD diagnosis occurs when an individual presents several of the following symptoms and if these symptoms have been prominently seen for several months:

Being fidgety, restless, and hyperactive most of the time; having poor concentration in activities, leaving tasks unfinished, and frequently shifting from one activity to another; impulsive behavior such as often interrupting others or doing dangerous things; being distracted from activities by minor events and happenings; easy excitability, overtalkativeness, and aggressive behavior

The diagnosis of ADHD is dependent upon documenting a childhood history of the disorder, along with a document of the patient's early adult history and current functioning (Resnick, 2000; Weiss, Hechtman, & Weiss, 1999). ADHD is associated with executive dysfunction; therefore, the task of describing one's childhood presents a challenge that may be more revealing of deficits in these areas than any other aspect of the assessment (Holmes et al., 2010; Weiss et al., 1999). Triolo (1999) states that it is important to have the patient undergo a routine medical exam in order to rule out any medical problems that may mimic the symptoms of ADHD. The medical assessment should also include the patient's documented medical history (Newill, Goyette, & Fogarty, 1984). Comorbidity of ADHD with other psychiatric disorders is as high as 77% (Biederman et al., 1993), and many of these other disorders are associated with attention deficits in their own right. It is essential to do a complete screen for other psychiatric disorders (Weiss et al., 1999).

Cognitive measures of executive function may be used to help identify those with ADHD (Holmes et al., 2010). By using psychological testing, information such as the patient's intellectual potential, academic achievement, and possible comorbid learning disabilities, will be provided. The components of such testing will vary according to what areas the psychologist feels may be impaired (Weiss et al., 1999). It is possible to enhance clinical diagnosis of ADHD by employing neuropsychological/cognitive tests of executive functioning, brief tests of response

inhibition, and working memory. Such neuropsychological testing can provide high levels of discrimination between individuals with and without ADHD (Holmes et al., 2010).

TREATMENT

Although medication is the main approach to treating patients with ADHD, education, psychotherapy, and environmental modification are also used as treatments. Educating patients with ADHD about their condition should include the latest information available regarding each patient's diagnosis, treatment, prognosis, and outcome (Resnick, 2000; Wender, 1995).

The drug treatment of ADHD is of both practical and theoretical importance. The use of medications must always be carefully considered (Resnick, 2000; Wender, 1995). Stimulant medications are the best-researched and most effective drugs available to specifically target symptoms related to ADHD. Interestingly, methylphenidate was prescribed three times more frequently than any other medication for the treatment of ADHD (Lopez Munoz et al., 2008). Medication for ADHD normalizes the under-arousal of the frontal lobe and permits some increased inhibition of the problem behavior (Resnick, 2000). However, Weiss et al. (1999) explain that if these drugs are ineffective or give rise to more serious somatic or psychiatric side effects, second-line drugs should be considered. Generally speaking, in adults as in children, stimulants are the first line of pharmacological treatment. Although 70% to 80% of school-aged children will respond positively to stimulant medication, the percentage drops somewhat to between 50% and 78% in adults (Wilens, Biederman, & Spencer, 1998). Antidepressants are effective and may be the pharmacological treatment of choice when there is a comorbid finding of depression or anhedonia, when stimulants are ineffective, or when there are unpleasant side effects from stimulants (Resnick, 2000). In Wender's experience (1995), drug treatment frequently produces a near complete remission of symptoms. Wender's drug-responsive ADHD patients often claim that they function better than they ever have in their lives.

Psychotherapy helps patients deal with personal, family, interpersonal, and work problems that tend to develop because of ADHD-related behaviors (Resnick, 2000). A significant part of the impairment from ADHD comes from its secondary impact on self-esteem, self-comfort, quality of life, hopefulness, and family burden. Psychotherapy is the treatment of choice to address these secondary effects of

A

psychosocial disability (Weiss et al., 1999). Often, the amount of psychotherapy needed will be brief but intermittent. Common types of psychotherapy generally used include individual, focused psychoeducational, marital, and group therapies (Resnick, 2000). For some patients improvement in actual functioning is accentuated when pharmacotherapy of core symptoms is combined with psychotherapy. Given that adults with ADHD experience considerable psychosocial impairment and given that these patterns are embedded in lifetime histories of dysfunction, addressing a form of psychological therapy as a therapeutic option is crucial (Weiss et al., 1999).

Research by Resnick (2000) suggests that an important component of the treatment plan for adults with ADHD will necessarily focus on a review of needed environmental changes and adjustments that can reduce the expression of symptoms and their impact on the individual. In order to do this, the patient must understand what constitutes an optimal environment and lifestyle for individuals with ADHD. Practitioners often help identify behavioral problem areas, and restrict their current environment and lifestyle to minimize and control ADHD symptoms.

Margie Hernandez
Hannah Lindsey
Antonio E. Puente

American Psychological Association. (1994). *Diagnostic and statistical manual of mental disorders* (4th ed.). Washington, DC: Author.

American Psychiatric Association. (2000). *Diagnostic and statistical manual of mental disorders* (4th ed., text rev). Washington, DC: Author.

Arnsten, A. F. T. (2009). Toward a new understanding of attention-deficit hyperactivity disorder pathophysiology: An important role for prefrontal cortex dysfunction. *CNS Drugs, 23*, 33–41.

Barkley, R. A. (1997). Behavioral inhibition, sustained attention, and executive functions: Constructing a unifying theory of ADHD. *Psychological Bulletin, 121*(1), 65–94.

Biederman, J., Faraone, S. V., Spencer, T., Wilens, T., Norman, D., & Lapey, K. A., et al. (1993). Patterns of psychiatric comorbidity, cognition, and psychosocial functioning in adults with attention deficit hyperactivity disorder. *American Journal of Psychiatry, 150*(12), 1792–1798.

Cherkasova, M. V., & Hechtman, L. (2009). Neuroimaging in attention-deficit hyperactivity disorder: Beyond the fronto-striatal circuitry. *The Canadian Journal of Psychiatry, 54*(10), 651–662.

Hervey, A., Epstein, J., & Curry, J. (2004). Neuropsychology of adults with attention-deficit/hyperactivity disorder: A meta-analytic review. *Neuropsychology, 18*(3), 485–503.

Holmes, J., Gathercole, S., Place, M., Alloway, T., Elliott, J., & Hilton, K. (2010). The diagnostic utility of executive function assessments in the identification of ADHD in children. *Child and Adolescent Mental Health, 15*(1), 37–43.

Lopez-Munoz, F., Alamo, C., Quintero-Gutierriez, F. J., & Garcia, P. (2008). A bibliometric study of international scientific productivity in attention-deficit hyperactivity disorder covering the period 1980–2005. *European Journal of Child and Adolescent Psychiatry, 17*(6), 381–391.

Luman, M., van Noesel, S., Papanikolau, A., Van Oostenbruggen-Scheffer, J., Veugelers, D., Sergeant, J., et al. (2009). Inhibition, reinforcement sensitivity and temporal information processing in ADHD and ADHD+ODD: Evidence of a separate entity? *Journal of Abnormal Child Psychology, 37*(8), 1123–1135.

Newill, B. H., Goyette, C. H., & Fogarty, T. W. (1984). Diagnosis and assessment of the adult with specific learning disabilities. *Journal of Rehabilitation, 8*, 188–189.

Resnick, R. J. (2000). *The hidden disorder: A clinician's guide to attention deficit hyperactivity disorder in adults*. Washington, DC: American Psychological Association.

Schmahmann, J. D. (2010). The role of the cerebellum in cognition and emotion: Personal reflections since 1982 on the dysmetria of thought hypothesis, and its historical evolution from theory to therapy. *Neuropsychology Review, 20*(3), 236–260.

Triolo, S. (1999). *Attention deficit hyperactivity disorder in adulthood: A practitioner's handbook* (pp. 73–76). Philadelphia, PA: Brunner/Mazel.

Vaidya, C. J., & Stollstorff, M. (2008). Cognitive neuroscience of attention deficit hyperactivity disorder: Current status and working hypotheses. *Developmental Disabilities Research Reviews, 14*, 261–267.

Wahlstedt, C. (2009). Neuropsychological deficits in relation to symptoms of ADHD: Independent contributions and interactions. *Child Neuropsychology, 15*(3), 262–279.

Weiss, M., Hechtman, L. T., & Weiss, G. (1999). *ADHD in adulthood*. Baltimore and London: The Johns Hopkins University Press.

Wender, P. H. (1995). *Attention-deficit hyperactivity disorder in adults* (pp. 122–142). New York: Oxford UP.

Wiersema, R., van der Meere, J., Antrop, I., & Roeyers, H. (2006). State regulation in adult ADHD: An event-related potential study. *Journal of Clinical and Experimental Neuropsychology, 28*(7), 1113–1126.

Wilens, T. E., Biederman, J., & Spencer, T. J. (1998). Pharmacotherapy of attention deficit hyperactivity disorder in adults. *Disease Management, 9*, 347–356.

AUTISM

DESCRIPTION

Autism is a complex neurodevelopmental disorder that affects aspects of learning, communication, and socialization. It presents as deficits in social interaction and communication and restricted stereotyped and repetitive behaviors, interests, and activities (American Psychiatric Association [APA], 2000). Reported prevalence rates range from 2 to 20 cases per 10,000 individuals with males being 4–5 times more likely to present with the disorder (APA, 2000).

First described by Kanner in 1943, initially many felt autism was psychogenic and perhaps a result of cold mothering. Kanner states that many of the parents were emotionally cold, perhaps because they were along the autism spectrum themselves (including Asperger's syndrome and pervasive developmental disorder not otherwise specified). Consequently, autism does have a strong genetic component. However, any social coldness per se on the part of the parents clearly did not cause the autism of the children. It is obvious today that autism is a neurological disorder, with no direct relation to the effects of postnatal parenting. The core feature of autism in particular and autistic spectrum disorders in general is a deficit in the ability to take the perspective of another and to appreciate that this other's perspective could differ from their own. Baron-Cohen (1995) provided us with a substantial insight into the mind of a person with autism with the theory of mind concept. Most of us have a theory of mind in that we can guess what others are thinking and how that might differ from what we are thinking. Those with autism can be thought of as mindblind in that they cannot imagine what others might be thinking, or even that those others are thinking. One extension of this is that we can make guesses as to why someone entered a room, but to those with autism, the person simply entered it, with no rhyme or reason. More to the point, we make guesses or conclusions about the mentations of someone who assumes a given body posture or facial expression. Those with autism cannot do this, and this is the basis for the often-seen poor eye contact among those with autism. To them it would be like looking at the headlights of a car to determine why the car just did what it did, or what information it is trying to convey to us.

NEUROPATHOLOGY/PATHOPHYSIOLOGY

Minshew, Sweeney, Bauman, and Webb (2005) have reviewed the gross neuropathological findings related to autism. They report anomalies in the cerebellum, inferior olive, hippocampus, amygdala, mammillary bodies, anterior cingulate gyrus, and medial nucleus of the septum. Additional research has suggested these alterations appear to precede onset of behavioral symptoms (Courchesne, Redcay, & Kennedy, 2004). Megalencephaly and increased neuronal density have been reported in many cases (Bailey et al., 1998; Schumann & Amaral, 2006), potentially related to brain overgrowth as this can be seen as early as 2–3 years of age (Courchesne, Carper, & Akshoomoff, 2003; Courchesne, 2004).

Microscopic reviews have demonstrated loss of Purkinje cells within the cerebellum (Kern, 2003), cortical dysgenesis (Bailey et al., 1998), disrupted neuronal migration (Levitt, Eagleson, & Powell, 2004), minicolumnar organization and laminae of the neocortex with laminae (Casanova, Buxhoeveden, Switala, & Roy, 2002; Mukaetova-Ladinska, Arnold, Jaros, Perry, & Perry, 2004), and astroglial activation (Vargas, Nascimbene, Krishnan, Zimmerman, & Pardo, 2005).

On occasion, anomalies in other areas have been associated with autism. The anomalous areas are known to be involved with learning, memory, behavior, and emotion. To date none of these anatomical findings have really helped to understand the disorder per se. Many other aspects of neurophysiology have also been investigated, but there is some recent work which shows potential for illuminating the impairment in the ability to relate to others. Work with monkeys (Fogassi et al., 2005) showed that certain neurons, mirror neurons, respond similarly to the intentions of the monkey itself and to the perceived intention of an observed monkey. Mirror neurons have been found in normal developing individuals, but not in those with autism spectrum disorders (Oberman, Hubbard, McCleery, Altschuloer, Ramachandran, & Pineda, 2005). In control subjects, the electrical response is the same whether they move their own hands or they observe others moving their hands. The electrical response to self-performed hand movements was not found when observing hand movements in others for those with autism spectrum disorders. One can easily understand how these mirror neurons provide a basis for empathy, taking the perspective of others, pragmatics, and theory of mind, all of which are aspects missing among those with autism. To go further, such results provide a basis for the contention that those with this spectrum of disorders have a severe impairment in reading, or appreciating the existence of the minds of others. Joseph (1999) suggested links between structural abnormalities in the medial temporal lobe and focal areas of the limbic system (e.g., amygdala) and the deficits exhibited in socialization and communication.

A

NEUROPSYCHOLOGICAL/CLINICAL
PRESENTATION

As expected of a neurodevelopmental disorder, there is a high concordance with other neurological disorders. For example, the *Diagnostic and Statistical Manual of Mental Disorders*, Fourth Edition of the APA (2000) states that about 75% of those with autism also have mental retardation, and Minshew et al. (2005) estimate that about a third have epilepsy. In line with this, although many do show specific neuropsychological disorders (e.g., executive dysfunction), there does not appear to be any classic neuropsychological deficits that are universally seen among those with autism (Soper, Canavan, & Wolfson, 2007). Consequently, areas indicted are seen as most vulnerable to dysfunction in correspondence with autism but are not always seen.

Prefrontal cortical dysfunction, and consequently, executive dysfunction have long been linked with autism (Hughes, Russell, & Robbins, 1994; Pennington & Ozonoff, 1996). However, this may be age dependent as studies in early childhood have failed to show consistent deficits within the executive domain (e.g., Dawson et al., 2002). This has been linked to individuals' tendency for cognitive rigidity and concrete thinking (e.g., pronominal reversal; the picture is not on the wall, but next to it; you mean Snow White and the seven little miners?) that may be further related to their rigidity in behavioral actions and preference for environmental structuring. This is not as noticeable among those of higher intellectual abilities, but abstract reasoning is difficult for even these people. They are also unable to generate a perspective other than their own (e.g., telling the story of Snow White from Grumpy's perspective, pointing out something of interest to someone else but not of interest to themselves).

In conjunction with this domain, deficits in attention modulation also show strong association with the disorder. Dawson (1996) noted that though sustained attention may be often spared in autism, selective attention and set shifting are often impaired. This pattern may coincide with above suggestions of cognitive rigidity. This also may commonly present as deficits in joint attention within these individuals (Dawson et al., 2002). Of interest, as stimuli takes on a more socially oriented basis, these deficits increase (Dawson, Meltzoff, Osterling, Rinaldi, & Brown, 1998).

Language is potentially the most commonly discussed domain of neurocognitive functioning discussed in autism as it is often used diagnostically to differentiate autism and Asperger's syndrome. Specifically, the presentations are in many ways differentiated based on early language development. Autism is associated with language deficits often presenting on testing as discrepancies between verbal IQ (VIQ) and performance IQ (PIQ) favoring the latter over the prior. Joseph, Tager-Flusberg, & Lord (2002) confirmed this but indicated that as individuals age the extent of the discrepancy dissipates to some extent. Anatomically, autism is commonly seen as causing more left-hemispheric interference than Asperger's. Consistent with this, research has shown that autism is linked with reduced lateral preference compared with normal controls (Escalante-Mead, Minshew, & Sweeny, 2003). It is also worth noting that this VIQ/PIQ discrepancy remains even in high functioning autism (Lincoln, Courchesne, Allen, Hanson, & Ene, 1998). Performance-based skills such as block design are often relative strengths for individuals with autism.

Memory deficits have been noted in autism, but they remain fairly specific. Dawson (1996) found that though rote memorization and cued recall remain relatively spared in individuals with autism, deficits remain in working memory and free delayed recall. Additional deficits were also noted in learning strategies, potentially owning to the pattern of preserved cued recall versus impeded free recall.

Finally, developmental delays in motor skills are commonly seen in conjunction with autism. Children with autism present with a general degree of deficits in motor coordination and smoothness, both at a gross and fine motor level (Jasmin et al., 2009; Molloy, Dietrich, & Bhattacharya, 2003; Provost, Lopez, & Heimerl, 2007). In fact, these features may be some of the earliest identifiable discrepancies between children with autism and their peers with motor anomalies noticed as early as the first year of life (Teitelbaum et al., 2004).

These features go beyond the clinical presentation that is the hallmark of autism which, again, includes deficits in social interaction and communication and restricted stereotyped and repetitive behaviors, interests, and activities (APA, 2000).

DIAGNOSIS

Although there are some who would quibble over minor points, the industry standard for the diagnosis of autism comes from the *DSM-IV-TR* (APA, 2000). In order to give a diagnosis of autism, the individual must show deficit in social interaction, communication, and restricted and stereotyped patterns of behaviors, interests, and activities. It is generally accepted that all within the autism spectrum of disorders manifest the deficits in social interaction (APA, 2000). Briefly, those diagnosed with Asperger's syndrome do not show the developmental communication deficits, and, generally, those diagnosed with Pervasive Developmental Disorder not otherwise specified do not show the language and behavioral deficits to an extent that they interfere with overall functioning, though they still do have the social interaction deficits. In addition, there are many who may meet the diagnostic criteria for one of these autism spectrum disorders but who are able to function within normal bounds in society and hence do not carry the diagnosis. Because of their limitations at times they come to the attention of the courts and are then given the diagnosis (Soper & Pelz-Sherman, in press).

Beyond the above-mentioned diagnostic criteria, neuropsychological evaluation aids in the identification of neurocognitive deficits that may be associated with the presentation. In addition, the literature has identified a number of diseases or disorders in which autism is a potential symptom. As a result, there can be utility in utilizing neuroimaging, metabolic analysis, and/or genetic testing on a case by case basis as concerns arise of autism being a secondary feature.

TREATMENT

To date there is no accepted or recognized cure for autism. Rather, interventions are symptom based. For example, Lovaas (1987) outlined a program that has demonstrated relative efficacy in improving behavior, especially prosocial behavior. Although claims of total recovery may be an exaggeration, many at a wide range of levels of functioning have been helped by such programs. In addition, concurrent conditions (e.g., ADHD) should be treated symptomatically. Individual education plans in school can be devised to assist in learning and the development of acceptable behavior (Sherman, 2007).

Henry V. Soper
Monica O. Murray

American Psychiatric Association. (1980). *Diagnostic and statistical manual of mental disorders* (3rd ed.). Washington, DC: Author.

Bailey, A., Luthert, P., Dean, A., Harding, B., Janota, I., Montgomery, M., et al. (1998). A clinicopathological study of autism. *Brain, 121,* 889–905.

Baron-Cohen, S. (1995). *Mindblindness: An essay on autism and theory of mind.* Cambridge, MA: MIT Press.

Baron-Cohen, S. (1999). *Mindblindness: An essay on autism and theory of mind.* Cambridge, MA: MIT Press.

Casanova, M. F., Buxhoeveden, D. P., Switala, A. E., & Roy, E. (2002). Minicolumnar pathology in autism. *Neurology, 58,* 428–432.

Courchesne, E. (2004). Brain development in autism. Early overgrowth followed by premature arrest of growth. *Mental Retardation and Developmental Disabilities Research Reviews, 10,* 106–111.

Courchesne, E., Carper, R., & Akshoomoff, N. (2003). Evidence of brain overgrowth in the first year of life in autism. *Journal of the American Medical Association, 290,* 337–344.

Courchesne, E., Redcay, E., & Kennedy, D. P. (2004). The autistic brain: Birth through adulthood. *Current Opinion in Neurology, 17,* 489–496.

Dawson, G. (1996). Brief report: Neuropsychology of autism: A report on the state of the science. *Journal of Autism and Development Disorders, 26*(2), 179–184.

Dawson, G., Meltzoff, A., Osterling, J., Rinaldi, J., & Brown, E. (1998). Children with autism fail to orient to naturally occurring social stimuli. *Journal of Autism and Developmental Disorders, 28,* 479–485.

Dawson, G., Munson, J., Estes, A., Osterling, J., McPartland, J., Toth, K., et al. (2002). Neurocognitive function and joint attention ability in young children with autism spectrum disorder versus developmental delay. *Child Development, 73,* 345–358.

Escalante-Mead, P. R., Minshew, N. J., & Sweeny, J. A. (2003). Abnormal brain lateralization in high-functioning autism. *Journal of Autism and Development Disorders, 33*(5), 539–543.

Fogassi, L., Ferrari, P. F., Gesierich, B., Rozzi, S., Chersi, F., & Rizzolatti, G. (2005). Parietal lobe: Action organization to intention understanding. *Science, 308,* 662–667.

Hughes, C., Russell, J., & Robbins, T. W. (1994). Evidence for executive dysfunction in autism. *Neuropsychologia, 32,* 477–492.

Jasmin, E., Couture, M., McKinley, P., Reid, G., Fombonne, E., & Gisel, E. (2009). Sensori-motor and daily living skills of preschool children with autism spectrum disorders. *Journal of Autism and Development Disorders, 39*(2), 231–241. (Epub 2008 July 16).

Joseph, R. M. (1999). Neuropsychological frameworks for understanding autism. *International Review of Psychiatry, 11,* 309–325.

Joseph, R. M., Tager-Flusberg, H., & Lord, C. (2002). Cognitive profiles and social communicative functioning in children with autism spectrum disorder. *The Journal of Child Psychology and Psychiatry, 43*(6), 807–821.

Kanner, L. (1943). Autistic disturbances of affective contact. *Nervous Child, 2,* 217–250.

Kern, J. K. (2003). Purkinje cell vulnerability and autism: A possible aetiological connection. *Brain and Development, 25,* 377–382.

Levitt, P., Eagleson, K. L., & Powell, E. M. (2004). Regulation of neocortical interneuron development and the implications for neurodevelopmental disorders. *Trends in Neuroscience, 27,* 400–406.

Lincoln, A., Courchesne, E., Allen, M., Hanson, E., & Ene, M. (1998). Neurobiology of Asperger syndrome: Seven cases studies and quantitative magnetic resonance imaging findings. In E. Schopler, G. Mesibov, & L. J. Kunce (Eds.), *Asperger syndrome or high functioning autism?* (pp. 145–163). New York: Plenum.

Lovaas, O. I. (1987). Behavioral treatment and normal educational and intellectual functioning in young autistic children. *Journal of Consulting and Clinical Psychology., 55,* 3–9.

Minshew, N. J., Sweeney, J. A., Bauman, M. L., & Webb, S. J. (2005). Neurologic aspects of autism. In F. R. Volkmar, R. Paul, A. A. Klin, & D. Cohen (Eds.), *Handbook of autism and pervasive developmental disorders: Vol 1. Diagnosis, development, neurobiology, and behavior* (3rd ed., pp. 473–514). Hoboken, NJ: Wiley.

Molloy, C. A., Dietrich, K. N., & Bhattacharya, A. (2003). Postural stability in children with autism spectrum disorder. *Journal of Autism and Development Disorders, 33*(6), 643–652.

Mukaetova-Ladinska, E. B., Arnold, H., Jaros, E., Perry, R., & Perry, E. (2004). Depletion of MAP2 expression and laminar cytoarchitectonic changes in dorsolateral prefrontal cortex in adult autistic individuals. *Neuropathology and Applied Neurobiology, 30,* 615–623.

Oberman, L. M., Hubbard, E., M., McCleery, J. P., Altschuler, E. L., Ramachandran, V. S., & Pineda, J. A. (2005). EEG evidence for mirror neuron dysfunction in autism spectrum disorders. *Cognitive Brain Research, 24,* 190–198.

Pennington, B. F., & Ozonoff, S. (1996). Executive functions and developmental psychopathology. *Journal of Child Psychology and Psychiatry and Allied Disciplines, 37,* 51–87.

Provost, B., Lopez, B. R., & Heimerl, S. (2007). A comparison of motor delays in young children: Autism spectrum disorder, developmental delay, and developmental concerns. *Journal of Autism and Development Disorders, 37*(2), 321–328.

Schumann, C. M., & Amaral, D. G. (2006). Stereological analysis of amygdala neuron number in autism. The *Journal of Neuroscience, 26,* 7674–7679.

Sherman, D. A. (2007). *Autism: Asserting your child's right to a special education.*

Soper, H. V., Canavan, F., & Wolfson, S. S. (2007). Neuropsychology of autism spectrum disorders. In A. M. Horton & D. Wedding (Eds.), *Neuropsychology handbook* (3rd ed., pp. 681–703). Philadelphia: Elsevier.

Soper, H. V., & Pelz-Sherman, P. J. (2010). Special difficulties of autism spectrum disorders in the forensic arena. In A. M. Horton & L. Hartlage (Eds.), *Handbook of forensic neuropsychology* (2nd ed.). New York: Springer.

Teitelbaum, O., Benton, T., Shah, P. K., Prince, A., Kelly, J. L., & Teitelbaum, P. (2004). Eshkol-Wachman movement notation in diagnosis: The early detection of Asperger's syndrome. *Proceeding of the National Academy of Sciences USA, 101,* 11909–11914.

Vargas, D. L., Nascimbene, C., Krishnan, C., Zimmerman, A. W., & Pardo, C. A. (2005). Neuroglial activation and neuroinflammation in the brain of patients with autism. *Annals of Neurology, 57,* 67–81.

Batten's Disease

DESCRIPTION

Batten's disease is part of a group of disorders called neuronal ceroid lipofuscinoses (NCLs). These are the most common neurodegenerative disorders in children. This disease is an inherited disorder that turns fatal usually by the late teen or 20s. Symptoms are first noticeable between the ages of 5–10 and present as visual and mental impairment, seizures, and motor skills difficulties. It occurs in 2 to 4 of every 100,000 births in the United States, approximately. NCLs seem to be more common in northern Europe, Finland, Sweden, and Canada. They are also more prevalent in families that carry the mutation (Chamberlin & Narins, 2005; National Institute of Neurological Disorders [NINDS], 2003; National Organization for Rare Disorders [NORD], 2008). Batten's disease was first diagnosed by a British pediatrician, Frederick Batten's in 1903, and it was named after him; it is also known as Sjörgen-Batten's disease, juvenile NCL, Vogt-Spielmeyer disease (NINDS, 2003; NORD, 2008).

NEUROPATHOLOGY/PATHOPHYSIOLOGY

Batten's disease is transmitted as a recessive gene, and the disorder only develops if the child inherits both defective genes from his/her parents. Symptoms are related to an accumulation of lipofuscins or lipopigments in different parts of the body including but not limited to eyes, brain, skin, and muscles. These substances form different shapes within the cells; in Batten's disease, a fingerprint profile prevails. The gene affected in this disorder has been identified as *CLN3* (Chamberlin & Narins, 2005, pp. 145–147). The most prominent mutation is a 1-kb deletion in the gene; this mutation is found in most of the defective chromosomes, approximately in 85% of them (Mole, Williams, & Goebel, 2005).

This disorder is characterized by a significant loss of neurons, predominantly in the cerebral and cerebellar cortices and a massive build up of lipopigments. The mutations can be homozygous, the most common one, where the patient has the 1-kb mutation alone, or it can have a heterozygous presentation and this includes different possible mutations in NCLs. The homozygous cases typically begin with visual loss and results in a diagnosis of retinitis pigmentosa or cone dystrophy due to pigmentary retinopathy. The severity and location where the mutations take place impact the clinical features of the disorder; a classical Batten's disease symptomatology is caused by acute damage to the *CLN3* structures or its critical parts; conversely, damage to less critical parts result in a delay of symptom progression, mentally and physically (Mole et al., 2005).

NEUROPSYCHOLOGICAL/CLINICAL PRESENTATION

The initial symptoms of Batten's disease are usually progressive vision difficulties; later, speech is affected presenting as stuttering and/or echolalia. A distinctive characteristic of the disorder is the loss of already attained milestones. Initially, the children attend schools for the blind, but their academics suffer as the disease progresses. There is a decline in motor and cognitive skills resulting in frustration, depression, and aggression. As patients reach their teen years there is more profound emotional, cognitive, and motor deterioration with symptoms such as aggressiveness, psychosis, mood disturbance, anxiety, reduced mobility, and parkinsonian features develop along with dementia. Eventually, they lose their ability to take care of their basic needs or activities of daily living and become bedridden. Not all cases present the same, and some may appear with more subtle symptoms, including clumsiness, imbalance, and behavioral or personality changes (Adams et al. 2006; Mole, Mitchison, & Munroe, 1999; NINDS, 2003; NORD, 2008).

The standardized assessment data for Batten's disease is limited. However, some studies have been done in order to identify and track the progression as well as attempt to treat the psychiatric symptoms of Batten's disease. In a study carried out by Backman, Santavuori, Aberg, and Aronen (2005), it was reported that IQ scores of patients decline to low average or borderline; symptoms prevalent in most patients are anxiety, aggression, hallucinations, depression, and psychotic symptoms; the cause of these symptoms is unclear, it can be due to the progression of the disease or as a way to cope with the mental and physical deterioration.

It was also found that more people who were taking psychotropic drugs, most common being the antidepressant citalopram and the antipsychotic risperidone, had more social, thought, and attention problems. In addition, females had more depression or anxiety and attention problems than males. Overall, females and patients on psychotropic drugs seemed to have more psychiatric symptoms.

However, these symptoms cannot be placed in a single category; they vary by case, hence the challenge in treating patients with this disorder. In this particular study, the available standardized measures used to assess the symptoms of Batten's disease were Children's Depression Inventory (CDI), Teacher Report Form (TRF), and Child Behavior Checklist (CBCL) (Backman et al., 2005).

In a longitudinal study, the Unified Batten's Disease Rating Scale (UBDRS) was developed in order to quantify the physical, behavioral, and functional characteristics of Batten's disease. This scale includes the CBCL, the Children's Yale-Brown obsessive-compulsive scale, and the Scale of Independent Behavior-Revised (SIB-R). As in the previous study, the most common problems were social, thought, attention, and behavior; however, no sex differences were found. Although obsessions and compulsions were part of the symptomatology, criteria for obsessive-compulsive disorder was not met in any of the cases. In these patients, the obsessions and compulsions were not disturbing, and their behaviors were not goal directed. Further studies are needed to distinguish certain Batten's disease symptoms from those present in other conditions such as autism, developmental delay, and other psychiatric and neurological diseases (Adams et al., 2006).

In a study designed to follow the course of juvenile neuronal ceroid-lipofuscinosis (JNCL) for 5 years after diagnosis, a special psychometric battery was created using an adaptation of Luria's neuropsychological test for children, the Developmental Neuropsychological Assessment (NEPSY) modified for the visually impaired, and the Wechsler Intelligence Scale for Children-Revised (WISC-R [verbal]). Areas assessed were general attention, verbal skills, motor functions, speech, acoustic rhythms, reading and writing, arithmetic, mnestic processes, stereognosis, spatial orientation, and quality of performances. It was found that different abilities deteriorate at different rates; however, all patients had a drop in IQ. During the first years, the WISC-R was the subtest of the battery showing the most abnormal findings, but as the disease advanced the other subtest provided more relevant information on cognitive deficits. Short-term memory and digit span were impaired at an early stage, spatial orientation was affected in all of them, and motor function declined around 10 years of age (Lamminranta et al., 2001).

Progress has been made in using standardized measures to assess children with JNCL; however, tools to assess these patients are very limited due to the fact that there are scarce measures to assess children with visual impairments (Adams et al., 2006).

DIAGNOSIS

There are three types of NCLs; they differ in three main characteristics: age of onset, order in which clinical features appear, and profiles of the buildup inside the cell. For example, infantile NCL is characterized by an onset at 6 months with motor difficulties and mental retardation, late infantile NCL has an onset of 2 years of age and the symptoms are seizures, and Batten's disease has an onset of about 6 years of age and initially presents with visual loss (Mole et al., 1999).

The use of fluorescent light microscopy and electron microscopy allows for NCLs to be distinguished from gangliosidoses and permits for a more accurate distinction among NCLs. And even though the dementia in the late stages of Batten's disease is severe, there is a structural difference when compared with infantile and late-infantile disorders; in Batten's disease, the accumulation of lipopigments in cerebro-cortical neurons is significant and obvious, but the loss of neurons in this area is less and not as advanced as in the other two forms of NCLs. Another differential diagnosis is mental retardation (it may be difficult to differentiate in the early stage of the disease); however, this changes when the mental deterioration becomes apparent in the form of dementia (Mole et al., 2005; Tolnay & Probst, 2001, pp. 212–217).

Recent advancements have shown that the accumulation of lipopigments is initiated before birth; therefore, it is possible to reach a prenatal diagnosis in families that have children already diagnosed with NCL disorders (Mole et al., 1999).

Tests to diagnose Batten's disease are (1) blood/urine tests (elevated levels of dolichol are found in the urine of many NCL patients); (2) skin/tissue sampling (under an electron microscope NCL deposits can be identified); (3) electroencephalography; (4) electrical studies of the eyes (which aids in detecting eye problems in NCL patients); (5) brain scans (CT and MRI); (6) DNA analysis.

TREATMENT

At the present time, there is no treatment to stop or reverse the progression of Batten's disease. Anticonvulsant drugs are used to reduce or control seizures, and other symptoms are treated as they present. Physical and occupational therapy seem to delay the loss of physical function. Also, there are reports that claim that a modified diet with vitamins C and E and low vitamin A slows down the progress of the disorder. Support groups help patients and their families to share their experiences. Support and encouragement are used to help patients and their relatives cope with the detrimental course of the disease (NINDS, 2003).

An important suggestion based on the result of the longitudinal study carried out by Lamminranta et al., (2001) is to teach children Braille before the age of 10, even if their vision is not greatly impaired at the time. Furthermore, gross and fine motor skills should be practiced at a young age; due to the decline in cognitive and motor abilities, learning new tasks becomes very difficult or impossible.

Efforts in research are being made to have a better understanding of the role of normal functioning as well as mutated proteins in NCLs. There are different teams working on various aspects of the disease; one team is working on identifying the content of the lipopigments; others are working on animal models e.g., the usefulness of bone marrow transplant on a sheep model and on mice models — to reach a more clear understanding of the genetics of the disorder (NINDS, 2003).

Luz M. Restrepo
Charles Golden

Adams, H., de Blieck, E. A., Mink, J. W., Marshall, F. J., Kwon, J., Dure, L., et al. (2006). Standardized assessment of behavior and adaptive living skills in juvenile neuronal ceroid lipofuscinosis. *Developmental Medicine and Child Neurology, 48,* 259–264.

Backman, M. L., Santavuori, P. R., Aberg, L. E., & Aronen, E. T. (2005). Psychiatric symptoms of children and adolescents with juvenile neuronal ceroid lipofuscinosis. *Journal of Intellectual Disability Research, 49,* 25–32.

Chamberlin, S. L., & Narins, B. (2005). *The Gale encyclopedia of neurological disorders* (Vol. 1). Detroit, MI: Gale.

Lamminranta, S., Aberg, L. E., Autti, T., Moren, R., Laine, T., Kaukoranta, J., et al. (2001). Neuropsychological test battery in the follow-up of patients with juvenile neu-

ronal ceroid lipofuscinosis. *Journal of Intellectual Disability Research, 45,* 8–17.

Mole, S. E., Mitchison, H. M., & Munroe, P. B. (1999). Molecular basis of the neuronal ceroid lipofuscinoses: Mutations in cln1, cln2, cln3, and cln5. *Human Mutation, 14,* 199–215.

Mole, S. E., Williams, R. E., & Goebel, H. H., (2005). Correlations between genotype, ultrastructural morphology and clinical phenotype in the neuronal ceroid lipofuscinoses. *Neurogenetics, 6,* 107–126.

National Institute of Neurological Disorders and Stroke. (2003, April). *Batten disease fact sheet.* Retrieved December 20, 2008, from www.ninds.nih.gov/disorders/batten/detail_batten.htm

National Organization for Rare Disorders. (2008, November 26). *Batten disease.* Retrieved December 20, 2008, from www.rarediseases.org/search/rdbdetail_abstract.html?disname = Batten Disease

Tolnay, M., & Probst, A. (Eds.). (2001). *Neuropathology and genetics of dementia* (pp. 212–217). New York: Kluwer Academic/Plenum Publishers.

BEHÇET'S DISEASE

DESCRIPTION

Behçet's disease (BD) is a recurrent, multisystem inflammatory disease that can affect the eyes, skin and mucous membranes, joints, vascular system, lungs, heart, gastrointestinal tract, and nervous system (Akman-Demir, Serdaroglu, Tasci, & Neuro-Behçet Study Group, 1999; Al-Araji, Sharquie, & Al-Rawi, 2003; Tunc et al., 2006). The disease was first described in 1937 by a Turkish dermatologist named Hulusi Behçet (Al-Araji et al., 2003; Tunc et al., 2006). BD is more prevalent in an area extending from the Mediterranean basin to Japan (Al-Araji et al., 2003; Gul, 2005). The prevalence of BD does not differ by gender, but symptomology is often more severe in males (Gul, 2005; Ozdimir, Ozsoylar, Candansayar, Cosar, & Onder, 2004).

When there is neurological involvement in the manifestation of BD, it is sometimes referred to as neuro-BD (Akman-Demir et al., 1999; Al-Araji et al., 2003; Tunc et al., 2006). Neuro-BD has been examined by multiple studies that have resulted in two variants of the disease being identified. The first type is consistently found across the research and presents with parenchymal central nervous system (CNS) involvement. The second type is inconsistent in the research but never has parenchymal CNS involvement

(Akman-Demir et al., 1999; Al-Araji et al., 2003; Tunc et al., 2006).

NEUROPATHOLOGY/PATHOPHYSIOLOGY

The etiology of BD remains unknown. Although viral, environmental, and autoimmune etiologies have all been alluded to, it has been further specified that these factors are merely relevant in genetically susceptible individuals (Gul, 2005; Kalayclyan & Zouboulis, 2007). Familial cases identified have shown an association between the disease and HLA-B5 and HLA-B1 antigens (Moore & Calabrese, 1994; O'Duffy, 1990) but only in the Middle East and Mediterranean region. This antigen is reportedly present in approximately 84% of BD patients in Turkey; however, it is not found in British or North American patients (Akman-Demir et al., 1999; Ozdimir et al., 2004). Originally theorized as a hypocoagulate state, research has now demonstrated that elevation of procoagulation factors actually represents a secondary feature of BD (Bartt & Topel, 2007).

Pathologically, BD presents as chronic and recurrent vasculitis, primarily affecting small vessels (Ropper & Brown, 2005). The brainstem and diencephalic regions are the most commonly affected on a neurological level (Al-Fahad & Al-Araji, 1999; Kidd, Steuer, Denman, & Rudge, 1999). Spinal cord lesions can also been seen at an intramedullary level, although this is more rare (Kidd et al., 1999). Cerebrospinal fluid (CSF) analysis will commonly show pleocytosis, elevated protein, and normal glucose but is not clinically consistent as negative findings have still been recorded in the literature even in the presence of abnormal MRI (Wechsler et al., 1993).

NEUROPSYCHOLOGICAL/CLINICAL PRESENTATION

There are many symptoms associated with BD, particularly genital and oral ulcers as well as uveitis (swelling and irritation of the middle layer of the eye). Vasculitis, or inflammation of the blood vessels, is considered a major feature of the disease (Gul, 2005; Tunc et al., 2006). In addition, ocular symptoms occur in 90% of patients (Miller & Jubelt, 1989). Other features commonly seen in patients with BD include thrombophlebitis (blood clot in a vein deep in the body), oligoarthritis (a type of arthritis), gastrointestinal ulcerations, and neurological involvement (Akman-Demir et al., 1999). Erythema nodosum and polyarteritis are also prevalent (Ropper & Brown, 2005) as are migraines and tension-type headaches (Al-Araji et al., 2003).

The neurological features associated with BD may vary but most commonly include recurrent meningoencephalitis, cranial nerve palsies with abducens involvement being the most common, cerebellar ataxia, and corticospinal tract signs (Ropper & Brown, 2005). Consequently, brainstem involvement due to the aforementioned meningoencephalitis is the most commonly reported location of parenchymal disease (Al-Fahad & Al-Araji, 1999; Kidd et al., 1999). Thrombosis may be seen at higher rates due to the aforementioned vasculitis.

DIAGNOSIS

There are no definite diagnostic tests for BD. As a result, the diagnosis is based on the recognition of the clinical features of the disease in combination with ruling out competing diagnostic considerations (Al-Araji et al., 2003). According to the International Study Group for BD, the diagnostic criteria for BD is the presence of recurrent oral ulcers accompanied by any two of the following: genital ulcerations, skin lesions, eye involvement (i.e., anterior and posterior uveitis), or a skin pathergy reaction such as skin hypersensitivity to a nonspecific physical insult (Akman-Demir et al., 1999; Al-Araji et al., 2003).

When neuro-BD is suspected, cranial MRI and magnetic resonance venography are useful for categorizing neurological involvement. Some patients have an asymptomatic presentation, meaning that they do not complain of neurological involvement but have neurological signs. Therefore, a neurological examination should be considered when diagnosing BD (Akman-Demir et al., 1999; Al-Araji et al., 2003). Findings have shown subclinical neurological involvement in patients with BD (Tunc et al., 2006). The main differential diagnosis for neuro-BD is multiple sclerosis. Differential diagnosis may also include other diseases of the CNS including systemic lupus erythematosus, polyarteritis nodosa, bacterial endocarditis, meningitis, encephalitis, and even stroke (Akman-Demir et al., 1999; Al-Araji et al., 2003). Given the potential competing diagnoses, clinical workup may include CSF analysis, metabolic panels, and neuroimaging (Wechsler et al., 1993).

TREATMENT

In the past, treatment for BD has included various antibiotics, chemotherapy, and corticosteroids. Immunosuppressive therapy was considered when the neurologic components of the disease were life-threatening (Miller & Jubelt, 1989). Although corticosteroids are still commonly used to address the noted inflammation, they have demonstrated little to no effectiveness in preventing blindness or the morbidity or mortality associated with neuro-BD (Wechsler et al., 1993). The combination of prednisone and alkylating agents can help ward off and treat vessel occlusion. Anticoagulation can also be used in emergent situations but is contraindicated in individuals with pulmonary vasculitis (Bartt & Topel, 2007).

Amy E. Zimmerman
Chad A. Noggle

Akman-Demir, G., Serdaroglu, P., Tasci, B., & the Neuro-Behçet Study Group (1999). Clinical patterns of neurological involvement in Behçet's disease: Evaluation of 200 patients. *Brain, 122,* 2171–2181.

Al-Araji, A., Sharquie, K., & Al-Rawi, Z. (2003). Prevalence and patterns of neurological involvement in Behçet's disease: A prospective study from Iraq. *Journal of Neurology, Neurosurgery, and Psychiatry, 74,* 608–613.

Al-Fahad, S. A., & Al-Araji, A. H. (1999). Neuro-Behçet's disease in Iraq: A study of 40 patients. *Journal of Neurological Science, 170,* 105–111.

Bartt, R. E., & Topel, J. L. (2007). Autoimmune and inflammatory disorders. In C. G. Goetz (Ed.), *Textbook of clinical neurology* (3rd ed., pp. 1155–1184). Philadelphia: Saunders Elsevier.

Gul, A. (2005). Behçet's disease as an autoinflammatory disorder. *Current Drug Targets — Inflammation & Allergy, 4,* 81–83.

Kalayciyan, A., & Zouboulis, C. C. (2007). An update on Behçet's disease. *Journal of the European Academy of Dermatology and Venereology, 21,* 1–10.

Kidd, D., Steuer, A., Denman, A. M., & Rudge, P. (1999). Neurological complications in Behçet's syndrome. *Brain, 122,* 2183–2194.

Miller, J. R., & Jubelt, B. (1989). Bacterial infections. In Lewis P. Rowland (Ed.), *Merritt's textbook of neurology* (8th ed., pp. 63–88). Philadelphia: Lea & Febiger.

Moore, P. M., & Calabrese, L. H. (1994). Neurological manifestations of systemic vasculitides. *Seminal Neurology, 14,* 300–306.

O'Duffy, J. D. (1990). Vasculitis in Behçet's disease. *Rheumatic Disease Clinics of North America, 16,* 423–431.

Ozdimir, D., Ozsoylar, G., Candansayar, S., Cosar, B., & Onder, M. (2004). Psychiatric findings related to neurological complications in Behçet's disease: A short review and a case presentation. *International Journal of Psychiatry in Clinical Practice, 8,* 185–190.

Ropper, A. H., & Brown, R. H. (2005). *Adams and Victor's principles of neurology* (8th ed., pp. 660–746). New York: McGraw-Hill.

Tunc, T., Ortapamuk, H., Naldoken, S., Ergun, U., Ciliz, D., Atasoy, H. T., et al. (2006). Subclinical neurological involvement in Behçet's disease. *Neurology India, 54,* 4, 408–411.

Wechsler, B., Dell'Isola, B., Vidailhet, M., Dormont, D., Piette, J. C., Blétry, O., et al. (1993). MRI in 31 patients with Behçet's disease and neurological involvement: Prospective study with clinical correlation. *Journal of Neurology, Neurosurgery, and Psychiatry, 56,* 793–798.

BELL'S PALSY

DESCRIPTION

Bell's palsy represents an acute lower motor neuron condition involving peripheral and transient paralysis of the facial nerve (cranial nerve VII), unilaterally. Bell's palsy was named after the Scottish surgeon and anatomist, Charles Bell, during the 19th century (Carmichael, 1926). The etiology of Bell's palsy remains unclear, though viral infections, most commonly herpes simplex virus Type 1 (HSV-1), are often considered as a potential cause. As such, Bell's palsy is believed to occur due to edema and ischemia involving compression of the facial nerve passing through the fallopian canal, the bony passage in the temporal bone through which the cranial nerve passes (Peitersen, 2002). Although some patients' symptoms completely remit, a small percentage of patients experience ongoing sequelae (Minnerop et al., 2008). In addition to facial paralysis, sense of taste, hyperacusis (abnormally acute hearing due to neural irritation), tear, and saliva production might also be problematic in these patients.

The incidence of Bell's palsy is thought to be 20–30: 100,000 annually (Minnerop et al., 2008; Rowlands, Hooper, Hughes, & Burney, 2002), occurring equally between genders and sides of the face. Age distribution of Bell's palsy suggests that individuals between the ages of 15 and 45 are more likely to be affected and that the occurrence for those under 15 and over 60 is quite low. Bell's palsy is most common during the second, third, and fourth decades of life (Peitersen, 2002).

NEUROPATHOLOGY/PATHOPHYSIOLOGY

Occasional familial incidence of Bell's palsy has been reported within the literature, though the precise genetic link remains uncertain and the evidence for familial link remains debatable (Rowlands et al., 2002). Although this has been noted, in general, Bell's palsy is viewed as idiopathic in nature as no

B

underlying cause is identified following clinical workup in 60% to 75% of cases (Bauer & Coker, 1996). However, the literature has demonstrated that herpes simplex infection is the most commonly reported cause. In addition, pregnant women as well as patients with diabetes mellitus and/or multiple sclerosis have been found to demonstrate heightened risk of the presentation (Brackman & Fetterman, 2007).

Bell's palsy occurs as a result of infringement on the seventh cranial nerve, either due to edema or ischemia at the point of the meatal foramen, at the beginning of the labyrinthine segment (Brackman & Fetterman, 2007).

NEUROPSYCHOLOGICAL/CLINICAL PRESENTATION

No neuropsychological findings have been reported within the literature as the presentation is typically sudden in onset and transient with full recovery commonly being noted. In fact, 85% of patients will spontaneously improve within 3 weeks of onset, even without treatment; the remaining generally improve within 3–6 months (Adour, Byl, Hilsinger, Kahn, & Sheldon, 1978; Peitersen, 2002). Clinically, Bell's palsy, as suggested, is primarily characterized by peripheral cranial nerve VIII dysfunction leading to a sudden onset of facial weakness with most severe paralysis being seen several days later. This can be seen in conjunction with numbness or pain of the ear, tongue, and/or face, reduced ipsilateral tear and/or saliva production, impeded acoustic reflex, and irritation of the chorda tympani nerve (May & Klein, 1991).

The facial palsy involved with Bell's palsy may present as complete or partial paralysis. Those with partial paralysis have a greater chance of complete recovery (94%), though a majority of all patients regain full recovery. Peitersen (2002), in his study of more than 1,700 patients, suggested that 71% experienced full recovery during the first 3 weeks. Furthermore, age appears to be a risk factor for incomplete recovery of facial function, as the likelihood of full recovery declines with age; above 45 years of age, the chances for full recovery diminish significantly. Rate of remission of symptoms is another parameter influencing recovery with patients showing signs of remission early on tending to have better outcomes (Peitersen, 2002). Another factor that appears to influence recovery involves auricular pain; those complaining of auricular pain have a poor prognosis for complete recovery than those without (Peitersen, 2002). A number of patients may experience recurrence of facial palsy on the same or opposite side of the face. Finally, increased incidence of Bell's palsy and poorer outcomes have been associated with patients having hypertension and diabetes mellitus, though this link remains controversial.

DIAGNOSIS

Bell's palsy is idiopathic and diagnosis is based on exclusionary information. Diagnosis of Bell's palsy is difficult due to the sudden onset and often spontaneous and complete recovery of symptoms reported in a majority of patients. Bell's palsy is the most common cause of peripheral facial palsy, though certainly other causes should be considered (e.g., focal tumor, stroke, Lyme disease) with monosymptomatic presentation required for diagnosis. Thorough examination including cranial nerve and neurological evaluations along with continued follow-up are essential. The presence of antibodies within the cerebrospinal spinal fluid and serum examination (e.g., Epstein-Barr virus, HSV-1, mumps, measles, etc.) is another method (Minnerop et al., 2008). Because a link between hypertension and diabetes mellitus is not yet fully understood, glucose tolerance and monitoring of blood pressure should be established in patients identified as having Bell's palsy.

TREATMENT

Corticosteriods as well as anti-viral and anti-inflammatory agents are among the preferred treatments for facial nerve paralysis to reduce swelling and further degeneration of the facial nerve and in rare cases surgical intervention for decompression (Engström, Jonsson, Grindlund, & Stålberg, 1998), though the efficacy of the aforementioned treatments remains controversial. Surgical intervention is only reserved for those who do not have good functional recovery and involves decompression of the entire infratemporal facial nerve by taking both a middle cranial fossa and a transmastoid approach (Friedman, 2000; Gantz, Runbinstein, Gidley, & Woodworth, 1999).

Facial exercises are often recommended for patients with Bell's palsy, though the efficacy of these treatments has not been clear (Peitersen, 2002). If the patient experiences difficulty closing the affected eye, efforts to protect the eye from irritants and maintain moisture within the affected eye are important. Early intervention is preferred and associated with better outcomes. Finally, anxiety has been commonly reported in Bell's palsy (Peitersen, 2002), and treatment of this may be warranted in some cases.

Michelle R. Pagoria
Chad A. Noggle

Adour, K. K., Byl, F. M., Hilsinger, R. L. Jr., Kahn, Z. M., & Sheldon, M. I., (1978). The true nature of Bell's palsy: Analysis of 1000 consecutive patients. *Laryngoscope, 88,* 787–801.

Bauer, C. A., & Coker, N. J. (1996). Update on facial nerve disorders. *Otolaryngological Clinics of North America, 29,* 3, 445–454.

Brackmann, D. E., & Fetterman, B. L. (2007). Cranial nerve VII: Facial nerve. In C. G. Goetz (Ed.) *Textbook of clinical neurology* (3rd ed., pp. 185–198). Philadelphia, PA: Saunders Elsevier.

Carmichael, L. (1926). Sir Charles Bell: A contribution to the history of physiological psychology. *Psychological Review, 33,* 188–217.

Engström, M., Jonsson, L., Grindlund, M., & Stålberg, E. (1998). House-Brackmann and Yanagihara grading scores in relation to electroneurographic results in the time course of Bell's palsy. *Acta Otolaryngologica, 118,* 783–789.

Friedman, R. A. (2000). The surgical management of Bell's palsy: A review. *American Journal of Olotaryngology, 21,* 1, 139–144.

Gantz, B. J., Rubinstein, J. T., Gidley, P., & Woodworth, G. G. (1999). Surgical management of Bell's palsy. *Laryngoscope, 109,* 1177–1188.

May, M., & Klein, S. R. (1991). Differential diagnosis of facial nerve palsy. *Otolaryngological Clinics of North America,* 24, 3, 613–645.

Minnerop, M., Herbst, M., Fimmers, R., Matz, B. M., Klockgether, T., & Wüllner, U. (2008). Bell's palsy: Combined treatment of famciclovir and prednisone is superior to prednisone alone. *Journal of Neurology, 255,* 1176–1730.

Peitersen, E. (2002). Bell's palsy: The spontaneous course of 2,500 peripheral facial nerve palsies of different etiologies. *Acta Otolaryngologica, 549,* 4–30.

Rowlands, S., Hooper, R., Hughes, R., & Burney, P. (2002). The epidemiology and treatment of Bell's palsy in the UK. *European Journal of Neurology, 9,* 63–67.

BENIGN ROLANDIC EPILEPSY

DESCRIPTION

Benign Rolandic epilepsy (BRE) is considered the most common idiopathic partial epilepsy in childhood (Northcott et al., 2005). As a benign focal seizure disorder, it is characterized by brief (up to 1–2 min), simple, partial hemifacial motor seizures that are often accompanied by somatosensory symptoms (Ferrie, Nordli, & Panayiotopoulos, 2008; Perkins et al., 2008). Behavioral semiology suggests onset in the lower portions of the pre-and postcentral gyrus (Blume, 2001). Hemifacial motor symptoms include clonic contractions of the lower lip and ipsilateral tonic deviation of the mouth (Ferrie et al., 2008). Somatosensory symptoms include numbness and paresthesia (Ferrie et al., 2008). Oropharyngolaryngeal symptoms can result in gurgling and grunting noises ("mouth death rattle"). Speech arrest and hypersalivation can also occur. Seizures tend to evolve into generalized tonic-clonic seizures, particularly with seizures occurring during sleep (Ferrie et al., 2008). Consciousness is retained in the majority of seizures; however, impaired consciousness occurs with secondary generalization.

Seizures are typically infrequent (most will have fewer than 10 seizures) and often occur during sleep, particularly during non-REM (rapid eye movement) sleep, or shortly after awakening (Ferrie et al., 2008; Perkins et al., 2008). Mean age at onset is 8–9 years, and boys are more often affected (3:2) (Ferrie et al., 2008). Onset prior to 3 years of age has been identified as a predictor of more frequent seizure occurrence (Kramer, Zelnik, Lerman-Sagie, & Shahar, 2002). The term "benign" refers to the ultimate remission of seizures commonly occurring within 1–3 years from onset and before age 16 years (Ferrie et al., 2008). A 3% risk of epilepsy in adulthood has been reported (Ferrie et al., 2008).

Estimates for the incidence of BRE range from 5% to 15% of childhood epilepsy syndromes (Perkins et al., 2008). Several studies emphasize a genetic basis, suggesting an association of BRE with chromosome 15q14. Family history is estimated to range from 21% to 32% (Loiseau, 2001); however, modes of inheritance are complicated. Although an EEG trait is thought to follow an autosomal dominant mode of inheritance (Loiseau, 2001), not all children with this EEG trait exhibit clinical seizures. Noninherited factors may play a major role (Vadlamude et al., 2006) based on research failing to show concordant twin pairs of BRE. Notably, about 10% have exhibited either birth or neurological complications, including CNS infections, head trauma, or other minor pathologic events (Louiseau, 2001).

Because seizures are typically infrequent and nocturnal, there is no clear consensus regarding treatment of BRE with antiepileptic drugs (AEDs). However, antiepileptic medications are generally initiated when seizures are frequent, occur during the daytime, are unpleasant, or are secondarily generalized (Ferrie et al., 2008; Perkins et al., 2008). AEDs may significantly decrease secondary generalized seizures, whereas focal seizures may not be impacted (Ferrie et al., 2008). The decision to treat with AEDs has no clear impact on spontaneous remission.

B

NEUROPATHOLOGY/PATHOPHYSIOLOGY

BRE is associated with a characteristic EEG pattern involving sleep-activated, high-amplitude centrotemporal/Rolandic spikes. This discharge pattern is typically followed by slow waves, that are unilateral, bilateral, synchronous, or asynchronous (Ferrie et al., 2008). It is important to highlight that spikes are rarely located in temporal electrodes (Ferrie et al., 2008). Epileptogenic involvement of both the precentral and the postcentral gyri accounts for the simultaneous expression of motor and sensory phenomena (Blume, 2001). Epileptiform activity can spread from side to side (Treiman & Treiman, 2001). Background activity and sleep architecture are normal. There are very few ictal EEG recordings of Rolandic seizures. Before the onset of ictal discharge, centrotemporal spikes become sparse (Ferrie et al., 2008).

Dipole potentials are common and attributed to the horizontal orientation along the sylvian or Rolandic fissures (Noachtar & Wyllie, 2001). Horizontal frontal dipole is typical (Perkins et al., 2008). Magnetoencephalography may show a higher resolution of dipole localization compared with conventional electroencephalography (Perkins et al., 2008).

Most seizures occur in non-REM sleep either shortly after sleep initiation or shortly before waking. Secondary generalizing seizures occur later in the sleep cycle. Imaging studies do not identify significant structural abnormalities on CT or MRI (Gaillard et al., 2009; McAbee & Wark, 2000).

NEUROPSYCHOLOGICAL/CLINICAL PRESENTATION

Although BRE has long been associated with an excellent prognosis, largely based on seizure outcome, recent literature has suggested that some patients may have cognitive difficulties (Northcott et al., 2005). Although one study has suggested some children experience a significant decline in language and other areas of cognitive functioning, which can improve with AEDs (Berroya et al., 2004), the preponderance of research suggests that transient cognitive impairment can occur with centrotemporal spike activity (Ferrie et al., 2008).

Studies of children with BRE tend to demonstrate intelligence within normal limits (Northcott et al., 2005; Perkins et al., 2008; Piccinelli et al., 2008). However, some studies have shown significantly lower IQ scores in children with BRE when compared with control groups matched for age, gender, and SES (Northcott et al., 2005). Domain-specific difficulties including memory (Northcott et al., 2005), language

processing (Northcott et al., 2005; Perkins et al., 2008), learning disability (Piccinelli et al., 2008), fine motor (Perkins et al., 2008), visual-motor integration (Perkins et al., 2008), and sustained attention (Piccinelli et al., 2008) have been documented. One study reported mild neurocognitive difficulty in at least one domain in approximately 78% and in more than one domain in almost 56% of their sample of children with BRE (Perkins et al., 2008). Impairment has been inconsistent across studies, however, likely due to a combination of methodological factors (e.g., heterogeneity in samples, absence of control groups, differences in measures, variability in how deficits are defined).

In their relatively large sample of 42 children with BRE, Northcott et al. (2005) reported mean IQ scores that were in fact significantly higher than normative means. This study identified, however, specific memory and phonological awareness impairment (based on scores falling below two standard deviations) among a notable proportion of their sample. Specifically, on the Wide Range Assessment of Memory and Learning (WRAML), mean index scores were significantly lower than normative data, with 10% obtaining impaired verbal memory index scores and 5% obtaining impaired visual memory index scores. Thirty-three percent obtained impaired range scores on the Rey Figure Delay, an additional memory of visual memory. The mean phonological awareness scores in Northcott et al.'s (2005) study were significantly lower than normative data on the Queensland University Inventory of Literacy, despite average language scores on the Clinical Evaluation of Language Fundamentals — Third Edition. Moreover, phonological scores were positively correlated with reading and spelling scores on the Wechsler Individual Achievement Test.

Other studies have documented moderate rates of language processing difficulties and academic underachievement. Perkins et al. (2008) identified impaired language involving receptive, expressive, or fluency skills among four out of nine children in their case series. Dyslexia and dysgraphia were identified in 9 out of 20 children with BRE in a study by Piccinelli et al. (2008), which was significantly higher than the corresponding rate in their control group. Among their group of children with BRE, Piccinelli et al. (2008) reported that 5 of 16 exhibited dyscalculia and 11 of 20 exhibited sustained attention deficits (characterized by slowness and easy fatigue); however, these rates were not significantly higher than the corresponding rates in their control group.

It is important to highlight that cognitive impairment in BRE has not been consistently associated with seizure frequency (Northcott et al., 2005; Piccinelli et al., 2008) or location of seizure focus (Northcott et al.,

2005). There is some evidence to suggest that there is an increased risk of learning disabilities in children who have seizure onset prior to age 8 or in children who have persistent epileptiform discharges during sleep (over more than a year) (Piccinelli et al., 2008). Although neuropsychological functioning may improve with normalization of EEG over time or improved seizure control (Northcott et al., 2005; Piccinelli et al., 2008), further research is warranted with longitudinal samples to verify this relation.

DIAGNOSIS

Diagnosis of BRE relies upon identification of a characteristic EEG pattern involving the centro-temporal region that corresponds with clinical seizures that manifest as brief, simple partial seizures involving hemifacial sensorimotor symptoms. With the exception of the EEG, other clinical assessments are typically normal, including the neurological examination (Ferrie et al., 2008). Many practitioners would not consider neuroimaging necessary if the clinical picture is typical, taking into account age, the absence of any comorbidities, seizure semiology, and EEG features.

It is noteworthy that centrotemporal spikes occur in 2% to 3% of normal children and are also common in children with neurologic deficits who do *not* have epileptic seizures (Ferrie et al., 2008). In fact, one study (van der Meij, Wienecke, Van Huffelen, Schenk-Rootlieb, & Willemse, 1993) revealed that the morphology of the centrotemporal spikes did not distinguish among five different clinical groups (of different epileptogenicity and presence of an organic cerebral lesion). Therefore, the presence of the characteristic EEG pattern has been described as possibly incidental when considering the likelihood that many children with this pattern do not have clinical seizures (Noachtar & Wyllie, 2001). Differential diagnoses include fragile X syndrome; however, these disorders are differentiated by neurological examinations that are normal for children with BRE and EEG findings that normalize earlier in fragile X (Tatum, Genton, Bureau, Dravet, & Roger, 2001).

TREATMENT

When antiepileptic drug (AED) treatment is initiated for children whose seizures are unusually frequent or unpleasant, it is expected that seizures will be easily controlled in most cases. Oxcarbazepine and carbamazepine are considered treatments of choice (Lee, 2010). There is currently no information, however, about whether treatment with AEDS can help prevent or minimize neurocognitive difficulties associated with BRE.

Neuropsychological evaluation is not only helpful for assessing the impact of epilepsy and its treatment on neurobehavioral functioning, but also for developing an appropriate intervention plan (Blackburn, Zelko, & Shurtleff, 2007). Such an intervention plan can help minimize the impact of identified neurobehavioral difficulties on daily functioning and, subsequently, the need for further services. Depending on the neuropsychological profile of a child with epilepsy, intervention may include a combination of remediation, accommodation, psychotherapy or pharmacological treatment approaches.

Among available research, the examination of the effectiveness of specific intervention or rehabilitation approaches for the cognitive or educational impact of BRE is scarce. In clinical practice, it is common to recommend intervention programs based on findings from available literature for children exhibiting the cognitive deficit alone (without epilepsy). For example, much research has been published about the efficacy of different remedial programs for reading disabilities including the phonological processing deficits that can underlie them (for a review, see Wills, 2007). However, Blackburn et al. (2007) caution that there are no studies assessing the effectiveness of reading remediation techniques in learning-disabled children who also have epilepsy. As such, one cannot assume that documented improvements or, in contrast, lack of response seen in healthy children to any given intervention program would generalize to children with epilepsy.

Nicole Cruz
Jeffrey B. Titus

Berroya, A.G., McIntyre, J., Webster, R., Lah, S., Sabaz, M., Lawson, J., et al. (2004). Speech and language deterioration in benign retrorolandic epilepsy. *Journal of Child Neurology, 19*(1), 53–58.

Blackburn, L., Zelko, F., & Shurtleff, H. (2007). Seizure disorders. In S. Hunter & J. Donders (Eds.), *Pediatric neuropsychological intervention* (pp. 133–150). Cambridge, UK: Cambridge University Press.

Blume, W. (2001). Focal motor seizures and epilepsia partialis continua. In E. Wyllie (Ed.), *The treatment of epilepsy: Principles and practice* (3rd ed., pp. 329–344). Philadelphia: Lippincott Williams & Wilkins.

Ferrie, C. D., Nordli, D. R., & Panayiotopoulos, C. P. (2008). Benign focal epilepsies of childhood. In J. Pellock, B. Bourgeois, W. E. Dodson, D. Nordli, & R. Sankar (Eds.), *Pediatric epilepsy: Diagnosis and therapy* (3rd ed., pp. 335–350). New York: Demos Medical Publishing.

B

Gaillard, W. D., Chiron, C., Cross, J. H., Harvey, A. S., Kuzniecky, R., Hertz-Pannier, L., et al. (2009). Guidelines for imaging infants and children with recent-onset epilepsy. *Epilepsia, 50*(9), 2147–2153.

Kramer, U., Zelnik, N., Lerman-Sagie, T., & Shahar, E. (2002). Benign childhood epilepsy with centrotemporal spikes: Clinical characteristics and identification of patients at risk for multiple seizures. *Journal of Child Neurology, 17*(1), 17–19.

Lee, G. (2010). *Neuropsychology of epilepsy and epilepsy surgery (Oxford workshop series American Academy of Clinical Neuropsychology).* New York: Oxford University Press.

Loiseau, P. (2001). Idiopathic and benign partial epilepsies. In E. Wyllie (Ed.), *The treatment of epilepsy: Principles and practice* (3rd ed., pp. 475–484). Philadelphia: Lippincott Williams & Wilkins.

McAbee, G. N., & Wark, J. E. (2000). A practical approach to uncomplicated seizures in children. *American Family Physician, 62*(5), 1109–1116.

Noachtar, S., & Wyllie, E. (2001). Electroencephalographic atlas of epileptiform abnormalities. In E. Wyllie (Ed.), *The treatment of epilepsy: Principles and practice* (3rd ed., pp. 225–286). Philadelphia: Lippincott Williams & Wilkins.

Northcott, E., Connolly, A. M., Berroya, A., Sabaz, M., McIntyre, J., Christie, J., et al. (2005). The neuropsychological and language profile of children with benign rolandic epilepsy. *Epilepsia, 46*(6), 924–930.

Perkins, F. F., Breier, J., McManis, M., Castillo, E., Wheless, J., McGregor, A., et al., (2008). Benign Rolandic epilepsy — perhaps not so benign: Use of magnetic source imaging as predictor of outcome. *Journal of Child Neurology, 23*(4), 389–393.

Piccinelli, P., Borgatt, R., Aldini, A., Bindelli, D., Ferri, M., Perna S., et al. (2008). Academic performance in children with rolandic epilepsy. *Developmental Medicine & Child Neurology, 50,* 353–356.

Tatum, W., Genton, P, Bureau, M., Dravet, C., & Roger, J. (2001). Less common epilepsy syndromes. In E. Wyllie (Ed.), *The treatment of epilepsy: Principles and practice* (3rd ed., pp. 551–576). Philadelphia: Lippincott Williams & Wilkins.

Treiman, L. J., & Treiman, D. M. (2001). Genetic aspects of epilepsy. In E. Wyllie (Ed.), *The treatment of epilepsy: Principles and practice* (3rd ed., pp. 115–130). Philadelphia: Lippincott Williams & Wilkins.

Vadlamudi, L., Kjeldsen, M., Corey, L., Solaas, M., Friis., Pellock, J., et al. (2006). Analyzing the etiology of BRE: A multicenter twin collaboration. *Epilepsia, 47*(3), 550–555.

van der Meij, W., Wieneke, G. H., Van Huffelen, A. C., Schenk-Rootlieb, A. J., & Willemse, J. (1993). Identical morphology of the rolandic spike-and-wave complex in different clinical entities. *Epilepsia, 34*(3), 540–550.

Wills, K. (2007). Remediating specific learning disabilities. In S. Hunter & J. Donders (Eds.), *Pediatric Neuropsychological Intervention* (pp. 224–252). Cambridge, UK: Cambridge University Press.

BERNHARDT–ROTH SYNDROME

DESCRIPTION

Bernhardt–Roth syndrome, also named lateral femoral cutaneous nerve entrapment or meralgia paresthetica, which translated from Greek means "thigh pain involving anomalous perception," is a sensory entrapment neuropathy (Pearce, 2006). The condition was initially identified by Hagar in 1885 with subsequent publications delineating the specifics of the condition by Bernhardt and Roth in two independent publications in 1895 (Lee, 1936). As the name of the syndrome suggests, this disorder is the result of compression of a single nerve that results in numbness, burning, and/or tingling in the lateral and anterior portion of the thigh. Prevalence is approximately 3–4 per 10,000 and typically occurs in those who are middle aged and overweight (Pearce, 2006). Males are three times more likely to develop this condition than females. Recent attention to this syndrome has been catalyzed by the introduction of tight clothing styles (Ivins, 2000). However, this diagnosis continues to be ambiguous to many practitioners and may be misdiagnosed (Ivins, 2000).

NEUROPATHOLOGY/PATHOPHYSIOLOGY

Bernhardt–Roth syndrome is a chronic disorder caused by entrapment or compression of the lateral femoral cutaneous nerve, which is a peripheral sensory nerve that passes between the ilium (upper anterior pelvis) and the inguinal ligament attached to the anterior superior iliac spine (upper point of pelvis) that supplies the anterolateral regions of the thigh (Ivins, 2000).The compression/entrapment occurs at the regional point where the nerve passes between the two prongs of attachment of the inguinal ligament (Ropper & Brown, 2005). The lateral femoral cutaneous nerve contains vasomotor, pilomotor, and sudomotor transmitters originating from a variety (five documented variations) of lumbar nerves (L1, L2, and/or L3) depending on the individual (Ivins, 2000). However, more commonly than not the nerve originates from the second and third lumbar roots (Ropper & Brown, 2005). Tingling, numbness, and burning are often experienced as painful and in a focal and unilateral manner; however, bilateral sensory symptoms may exist secondary to etiology.

Although nerve entrapment or compression from tight clothing or obesity is paramount, other less common causes include damage from diabetes, neuropathy, or trauma (Ivins, 2000). Regarding the latter, injuries from seatbelts following motor vehicle accidents tend to be most common, but surgery has resulted in an increase in prevalence (Macnichol & Thompson, 1990).

NEUROPSYCHOLOGICAL/CLINICAL PRESENTATION

The clinical presentation of Bernhardt–Roth syndrome typically includes a unilateral area of sensitive and sometimes painful tingling (dysesthesia) as well as numbness (paresthesia) ranging from slight hyperesthesia to total anesthesia in the anterior lateral aspect of the thigh. Symptoms can present bilaterally but do so in only 20% of cases. Although a reduction of perception is commonly seen in the detection of touch and discrimination of pinpricks, increased sensitivity has also been noted in cases (Ivins, 2000). Although these symptoms are most commonly mild in their presentation, occasionally a persistent and distressing (moderate to severe) burning sensation or pain may be experienced (Ropper & Brown, 2005). Hair loss in this region may also occur (Ivins, 2000). Individuals who suffer from this condition typically report worsening of symptoms in certain positions, specifically walking or standing, or when wearing tight clothing (Ivins, 2000). These symptoms may also be associated with weight gain, diabetes mellitus, or pregnancy (Grossman, Ducey, Nadler, & Levy, 2001).

Neuropsychological presentation of this condition will typically include the sensory symptoms described above, often with a unilateral arrangement, within the context of other generally intact cognitive and other sensorimotor functions. Symptoms may be mild and spontaneously resolve or may be chronic and severe. Patients typically may have difficulty describing symptoms, which may result in the cluster of symptoms being treated as psychiatric or incorrectly treating back, hip, or groin pathology (Ivins, 2000). Bernhardt–Roth syndrome is ruled out if sensory symptoms are associated with radiating pain and weakness in the back (Ivins, 2000).

DIAGNOSIS

Diagnosis of Bernhardt–Roth syndrome is completed through interview and sensory evaluation. Interview will elucidate possible trauma, medical conditions, or other factors described above that could result in nerve entrapment or submission. Sensory examination could utilize light touch to the affected area to determine level of sensitivity. Also, in unilateral involvement differences in sensation between legs may be conducted.

Typically, a pelvic and abdominal exam will be utilized to rule out other possible causes for the sensory symptoms (Grossman et al., 2001). Other studies include electromyography (EMG), X-rays, CT, or MRI in order to respectively determine nerve conduction, rule out bone abnormalities entrapping or compressing the nerve, or rule out soft tissue etiologies (i.e., tumor) (Grossman et al., 2001). Nerve conduction studies may be inconclusive due to transmission dysfunction (Ivins, 2000).

TREATMENT

Treatment of Bernhardt–Roth syndrome varies based on etiology. Behavioral modification with pain relief is often used simultaneously. In regard to the former, rest, modification of tight fitting clothing, weight loss programs, and exercise typically alleviate symptoms. For those with symptoms secondary to pregnancy, delivery of the child typically improves symptoms. In regard to pain management, heat, ice, or electrical stimulation may be utilized for temporary relief. Medication for neuralgic pain (such as amitriptyline, carbamazepine, or gabapentin) is often used but provides little benefit for those suffering from Bernhardt–Roth syndrome (Grossman et al., 2001).

For those with persisting symptoms, cortisone injections may reduce inflammation and the resulting pressure on the nerve (Grossman et al., 2001). Nerve blocks at the inguinal ligament with local anesthetic and corticosteroids may provide short-term relief (Grossman et al., 2001). If symptoms remain, surgery may be considered to resect tissue that may compress or entrap the nerve or resecting a section of the nerve itself. This treatment often results in permanent numbness in the area (Grossman et al., 2001). As such, performing a short-term block is preferable initially as it provides an opportunity for patients to determine whether the pros outweigh the cons: specifically, whether avoiding the pain is worth permanent numbness.

Javan Horwitz
Natalie Horwitz
Chad A. Noggle

Grossman, M., Ducey, S., Nadler, S., & Levy, A. (2001). Meralgia paresthetica: Diagnosis and treatment. *Journal of the American Academy of Orthopaedic Surgeons, 9:5,* 336–344.

Ivins, G. (2000). Meralgia paresthetica, the elusive diagnosis: Clinical experience with 14 adult patients. *Annals of Surgery*, 232(2), 281–286.

Lee, F. (1936). Meralgia paresthetica. *International Clinics*, 1, 210.

Macnichol, M., & Thompson, W. (1990). Idiopathic meralgia paresthetica. *Clinical Orthopaedics*, 254, 270–274.

Pearce, J. (2006). Meralgia paraesthetica: Bernhardt-Roth syndrome. *The Journal of Neurology, Neurosurgery, and Psychiatry*, 77(1), 84.

Ropper, A. H., & Brown, R. H. (2005). *Adams and victor's principles of neurology* (8th ed.). New York: McGraw-Hill.

BINSWANGER'S DISEASE

DESCRIPTION

Binswanger's disease is considered a type of vascular dementia associated with subcortical white matter disease. It has been somewhat controversial since first being identified more than a century ago. In 1894, Otto Binswanger described a type of dementia marked by slowly progressing decline of intellect, associated with sporadic stroke-like events and/or seizure episodes. He termed the disorder *encephalitis subcorticalis chronica progressiva* (Ortiz & Knight, 1994). In 1902, Alois Alzheimer furthered the understanding of the disorder by describing arteriosclerotic subcortical white matter changes, and he renamed it *Binswanger's disease*. There has since been controversy and debate over (1) the appropriateness of the name of the disease, (2) whether Binswanger's disease should even be considered a unique subtype of vascular dementia, and (3) whether there needs to be further differentiating between dementias associated with white matter disease (Caplan, 1995; Hurley, Tomimoto, Akiguchi, Fisher, & Taber, 2000).

NEUROPATHOLOGY/PATHOPHYSIOLOGY

Binswanger's disease is a disorder of the cerebral white matter; however, the etiology is not fully understood (Caplan, 1995; Ortiz & Knight, 1994). It is thought that lesions are caused by repeated hypoxic-ischemic events that occur in the arterioles that supply blood flow to the deep white matter (Caplan, 1995). The external surface of the brain is typically normal in appearance, whereas white matter may be firm, rubbery, puckered, granular, wrinkled, and discolored in severe cases (Caplan, 1995; Ortiz & Knight, 1994). Often white matter lesions are located in the periventricular and deep cerebral tissues (Hurley et al., 2000). Within the lesions, the nerve fibers are often observed to be reduced in density, and axonal damage is apparent (Hurley et al., 2000). There is often a widespread loss of myelin, particularly in the periventricular regions (Caplan, 1995). The corpus callosum may appear thinner compared with normal controls. Lacunar infarcts are also common in the basal ganglia, thalamus, pons, internal capsule, and occasionally in the cerebellum (Caplan, 1995; Ortiz & Knight, 1994). In addition, the disease is often characterized by diffuse atrophy and enlarged ventricles (Caplan, 1995; Shyu et al., 1996). Evidence of vascular disease is apparent in those with Binswanger's disease, including thickening of the walls of the arterioles and small vessel disease (lipohyalinosis) (Hurley et al., 2000; Ortiz & Knight, 1994).

Although imaging techniques can provide clear visuals of white matter lesions and infarcts, they do not enable one to judge more specifically the nature of the pathology or the clinical impact of the damage. Positron emission tomography scans have indicated that individuals with Binswanger's disease have reduced cerebral blood flow and metabolic rate compared with controls, as well as compared with persons who have white matter disease without dementia (Hurley et al., 2000).

NEUROPSYCHOLOGICAL/CLINICAL PRESENTATION

The average age of onset for Binswanger's disease is in the 50s or 60s (Caplan, 1995; Hurley et al., 2000). The disease equally affects both genders (Caplan, 1995). It has been reported that on autopsy, the characteristic pattern of lesions of Binswanger's disease is apparent in 4% of the general population and 35% of those with previously diagnosed dementias (Hurley et al., 2000). Typically, there is a stepwise decline of functioning over a 5–10 year span, with motor, cognitive, and behavioral deficits becoming apparent and worsening with time (Caplan, 1995).

The clinical presentation overlaps with other types of dementias, including Alzheimer's disease, normal pressure hydrocephalus, and multi-infarct dementia (Ortiz & Knight, 1994). Common symptoms associated with Binswanger's disease are cognitive deficits, behavioral changes, and neurological abnormalities, such as motor, sensory, visual, and/or atypical reflexes (Caplan, 1995). Presentation often includes executive dysfunction, psychotic thinking, slow processing speed, mild memory difficulties, apathy, mood disturbances, and gait deficits (Hurley et al., 2000). Extent of subcortical white matter degeneration, cerebral hypoperfusion, and cerebral atrophy have been observed to be associated with the extent of cognitive and motor deficits in Binswanger's disease (Shyu et al., 1996). However, a correlation between pathological markers (e.g., number of lesions, cerebral blood flow) and extent of cognitive impairment has not been firmly established (Hurley et al., 2000).

Deficits in cognitive functioning are variable but often include dysfunction of the frontal systems. Problems with memory, language, and visuospatial functioning are apparent to a much lesser degree than in other dementias (e.g., Alzheimer's disease, Pick's disease) (Caplan, 1995). In addition, individuals often have limited insight into their deficits and have poor judgment. Common motor symptoms are parkinsonian in nature, including slowed walking, unsteadiness, taking small steps, flexion posture, rigidity, and pseudobulbar palsy (Caplan, 1995; Ortiz & Knight, 1994). Behaviorally and emotionally, individuals with Binswanger's disease often appear depressed, as they become disinterested in previously enjoyed activities and interests, have decreased spontaneity in action and conversation, and are generally apathetic (Caplan, 1995; Ortiz & Knight, 1994).

DIAGNOSIS

Making a diagnosis of Binswanger's disease is based on the individual's health history; risk factors; cognitive, behavioral, and motor symptoms; and neuroimaging information. The criteria for diagnosis include evidence of a subcortical dementia based on neurocognitive testing, bilateral abnormalities (e.g., lesions, infarcts) on imaging (CT or MRI), and two or more of the following: (a) vascular risk factors or vascular disease (e.g., hypertension); (b) focal cerebrovascular disease (e.g., evidence of stroke); and/or (c) subcortical cerebral deficits (e.g., gait abnormalities) (Thakur, Verma, Mokta, Aggarwal, & Sharma, 2007).

TREATMENT

Because Binswanger's disease is a chronic, progressive dementia, treatment is limited to maintaining cognitive functioning as long as possible and addressing any psychological or behavioral problems. There is no known treatment to reverse or cure the disease (Thakur et al., 2007). It is therefore important to treat the individual symptoms, which may include focusing on the behavioral and motor manifestations. Some promise has come from medication trials that have been observed to maintain or even improve some aspects of cognitive function for a brief period

of time (up to a year), but no definitive treatment has been identified (Hurley et al., 2000). It can be helpful to promote cardiovascular health (e.g., blood pressure) generally, including treating some of the associated vascular risk factors (Thakur et al., 2007).

Shane S. Bush
Kathryn M. Lombardi Mirra

Caplan, L. R. (1995). Binswanger's disease—Revisited. *Neurology, 45*, 626–633.

Hurley, R. A., Tomimoto, H., Akiguchi, I., Fisher, R. E., & Taber, K. H. (2000). Binswanger's disease: An ongoing controversy. *Journal of Neuropsychiatry and Clinical Neuroscience, 12*, 301–304.

Ortiz, J., & Knight, P. V. (1994). Review: Binswanger's disease, leukoaraiosis, and dementia. *Age and Ageing, 23*, 75–81.

Shyu, W. C., Lin, J. C., Shen, C. C., Hsu, Y. D., Lee, C. C., Shiah, I. S., et al. (1996). Vascular dementia of Binswanger's type: Clinical, neuroradiological, and tc-hmpao spect study. *European Journal of Nuclear Medicine, 23*, 1338–1344.

Thakur, S., Verma, B., Mokta, J., Aggarwal, P., & Sharma, A. (2007). Binswanger's disease. *Journal of The Association of Physicians of India, 55*, 285.

BLEPHAROSPASM

DESCRIPTION

Blepharospasm (BEB) is a neurological disorder that affects 36 per 1,000,000 individuals (Troung, Comella, Fernandez, & Ondo, 2008). The disorder is classified as a focal cranial dystonia and occurs more commonly in the elderly and women (Troung et al., 2008). The disease occurs sporadically, but there can also be a familial pattern of movement disorders associated with the development of BEB (Walsh et al., 2007). The key feature of this focal dystonia is that the orbicularis oculi muscles contract involuntarily (Reimer, Gilg, Karow, Esser, & Franke, 2005). Characteristic symptoms include Charcot's sign, sensitivity of light, ocular pain, and orbicularis oculi spasms. Symptoms are exacerbated by emotional stress and fatigue (Gorlin, Cohen, & Hennekam, 2001). The etiology of BEB is unknown.

NEUROPATHOLOGY/PATHOPHYSIOLOGY

Although the pathophysiology of this focal dystonia is unknown, structural changes occurring in BEB have been suggested. Imaging has shown activation in the anterior visual cortex, anterior cingulated cortex, primary motor cortex, central region of the thalamus, and superior cerebellum. This is suggestive of a hyperactive cortical circuit. Activation in these areas is greater during voluntary blinking than for spontaneous blinking (Baker, Andersen, Morecraft, & Smith, 2003). Past research has found increased bilateral activation in the ventral lateral nucleus of the thalamus. Increased bilateral activation has also been discovered in the lateral globus pallidus, caudate nucleus, and putamen, suggesting a basal-ganglia involvement in BEB (Obermann et al., 2008). Basal-ganglia involvement is further supported by the evident increase in gray matter in the putamen in this disease. Patients with BEB show a decrease of gray matter in the left inferior parietal lobe, which is thought to reflect a secondary cause of the disease (Etgen, Mühlau, Gaser, & Sander, 2006).

NEUROPSYCHOLOGICAL/CLINICAL PRESENTATION

Clinical features of BEB include depression, obsessive-compulsive behavior, stress, anxiety, and sensitivity to light (Difasio & Livrea, 2004; Judd, Digre, Warner, Schulman, & Katz, 2007; Reimer et al., 2005). Patients tend to find the depression and anxiety more difficult to live with than the actual disease (Ochudlo, Bryniarski, & Opala, 2007). Due to the debilitating symptoms, BEB has been highly correlated to general anxiety disorder (Hall et al., 2005). BEB may interfere with the patient's independence, making it difficult to walk alone. The disorder may interrupt daily activities such as driving, reading, and recreational activities (Reimer et al., 2005). BEB can create occupational difficulties (Walsh et al., 2007). In severe cases, the person is not able to work at all. Contractions appear to become more intense when the person relaxes but can partially disappear when the person concentrates. However, the symptoms can fluctuate at times (Difasio & Livrea, 2004). Behavioral observations include facial grimacing, yawning, humming, neck extensions, forced jaw opening, or touching of the eye area. These may all be attempts by the person to keep the eyes open (Lishman, 1998). Consideration of limited vision is important at neuropsychological testing, and if the BEB has progressed enough, visual tests may be impossible to administer effectively. Apraxia of the eyelid opening (AEO) is often concurring with the disease.

DIAGNOSIS

The onset of BEB is usually insidious. Early symptoms of the disorder include increased blink rate to stimuli, unpleasant sensations, and eyelid fluttering (Troung et al., 2008). The symptoms could start unilaterally but tend to become bilateral. The orbicularis oculi spasms start subtle and sparse, but increasingly become more intense and occur more often (De Groot, De Wilde, Smet, & Tassignon, 2000). Dystonic movements of the jaw, face, and cervical muscles may accompany the chronic involuntary spasms that evolve as the disorder progresses (Difasio & Livrea, 2004). The orbicularis oculi muscle is constructed by three distinct parts: the orbital, the preseptal, and the pretarsal areas. As the orbital and preseptal areas contract, the action results in Chariot's sign, a main clinical feature of BEB. Characteristic of Chariot's sign is the lowering of the brow below the superior orbital rim (Difasio & Livrea, 2004). Due to sensitivity to light, patients can develop photophobia. They become fearful of light since it triggers the symptoms, making them worse (Judd et al., 2007).

The clinician should assess the patient carefully, focusing on the physical and neurological history of the patient. Imaging and laboratory work are not useful unless the patient is younger than 50 years of age because an identifiable cause is rarely present. If the patient is below 50 years of age, Wilson's disease and structural causes need to be excluded from the etiology (Difasio & Livrea, 2004). Common differential diagnoses are AEO, Tourette's syndrome, bilateral hemifacial spasm, facial myokymia, facial synkinesia, and dry eye. AEO is a movement disorder with similar symptoms that can occur concurrently with BEB, making it difficult to separate the two disorders. Patients with BEB, experiencing eyelid closures due to dysfunction in the pretarsal orbicularis oculi, are able to reopen their eyes after they voluntarily closed their eyes in between spasms, but patients with AEO are not able to perform such action (Difasio & Livrea, 2004). Tics in Tourette's syndrome can be mistaken for BEB, but Tourette's syndrome has a childhood onset whereas BEB symptoms show up in the 50s (McCann, Ugurbas, & Goldberg, 2002). Bilateral hemifacial spasm is easily confused with BEB.

Both diseases can occur in the elderly and become worse with stress. However, the spasms in bilateral hemifacial spasm can be distinguished from BEB since the bilateral hemifacial spasms do not occur at the same time (Difasio & Livrea, 2004). Another difference is that light sensitivity and ocular surface irritation does not commonly occur in hemifacial spasm (McCann et al., 2002). Dry eye is often mistaken for BEB due to the excessive blinking and closure of the eyelids in dry eye. Dry eye can be diagnosed if the symptoms improve with warm compresses, eye ointment, and artificial tears (Difasio & Livrea, 2004). The involuntary contractions of the orbicularis oculi muscles occurring in BEB arise from the central nervous system. This particular origin of eyelid closure dysfunction is unique to BEB and can distinguish the disease from facial myokymia or facial synkinesia (Difasio & Livrea, 2004). An additional difference is that the latter two present symptoms unilaterally (McCann et al., 2002).

TREATMENT

BEB symptoms can improve without treatment; symptoms disappear after 5 years in 11% of patients with BEB (Walsh et al., 2007). However, most patients need some type of treatment to improve their condition. There are several types of treatments to improve the condition, but none will cure the disease. The most efficient treatment is botulinum toxin type A (BoNT-A) (Troung et al., 2008). BoNT-A prevents the release of acetylcholine causing a transient muscle paralysis (Fante & Frueh, 2001). The treatment lasts for 3 months and past research has shown a 90% success rate (McCann et al., 2002). BoNT-A has also shown to have an indirect positive effect on depressive symptoms (Ochudlo et al., 2007). Side effects from the treatment include dry eye, ptosis, mild facial weakness, and diplopia. However, these side effects are transient (Reimer et al., 2005).

Pharmacological treatment is most commonly used in BEB when the person does not respond to BoNT-A, which occurs in 4–15% of treatment cases (Grivet et al., 2005). Pharmacological interventions are not very efficient and are therefore not the first choice of treatment. Trihexyphenidyl and clonazepam may relieve symptoms but have side effects such as sedation, confusion, memory difficulty, and hallucinations (Difasio & Livrea, 2004). If BoNT-A treatment is not successful, myectomy surgery is another option for treatment of BEB (McCann et al., 2002). Therapy can help the person make adjustments to living with the disease and its psychosocial burdens. Because of visual and psychological impairments, patients with BEB sometimes withdraw from social interaction and become isolated (Ochudlo et al., 2007). The clinician can offer solutions to symptom and stress relief, such as the use of tinted sunglasses to address light sensitivity (McCann et al., 2002).

Lena M. F. Prinzi
Charles Golden

Baker, R. S., Andersen, A. H., Morecraft, R. J., & Smith, C. D. (2003). A functional magnetic resonance imaging study in patients with benign essential blepharospasm. *Journal of Neuro-Ophthalmology, 23,* 11–15.

Defasio, G., & Livrea, P. (2004). Primary blepharospasm. *Drugs, 64,* 237–244.

De Groot, V., De Wilde, F., Smet, L., & Tassingnon, M. J. (2000). Frontalis suspension combined with blepharoplasty as an effective treatment for blepharospasm associated with apraxia of eyelid opening. *Ophthalmic Plastic and Reconstructive Surgery, 16,* 34–38.

Etgen, T., Mühlau, M., Gaser, C., & Sander, D. (2006). Bilateral grey-matter increase in the putamen in primary belpharospasm. *Journal of Neurology, Neurosurgery, and Psychiatry, 77,* 1017–1020.

Fante, R. G., & Frueh, B. R. (2001). Differential section of the seventh nerve as a tertiary procedure for the treatment of benign essential blepharospasm. *Ophthalmic Plastic and Reconstructive Surgery, 17,* 276–280.

Gorlin, R. J., Cohen, M. M., & Hennekam, R. C. M. (2001). *Syndromes of the head and neck* (4th ed.). New York: Oxford University Press.

Grivet, D., Robert, P. Y., Thuret, G., De Feligonde, O. P., Gain, P., Maugery, J., et al. (2005). Assessment of blepharospasm surgery using an improved disability scale: Study of 138 patients. *Ophthalmic Plastic and Reconstructive Surgery, 21,* 230–234.

Hall, T. A., McGwin, G., Searcy, K., Xie, A., Hupp, S. L., Owsley, C., et al. (2005). Benign essential blepharospasm: Risk factors with reference to hemifacial spasm. *Journal of Neuro-Ophthalmology, 25,* 280–285.

Judd, R. A., Digre, K. B., Warner, K. E. A., Schulman, S. F., & Katz, B. J. (2007). Shedding light on blepharospasm: A patient-researcher partnership approach to assessment of photophobia and impact on activities of daily living. *Neuro-Ophthalmology, 31,* 49–54.

Lishman, W. A. (1998). *Organic psychiatry: The psychological consequences of cerebral disorder.* Malden, MA: Blackwell Publishing.

McCann, J. D., Ugurbas, S. H., & Goldberg, R. A. (2002). Benign essential blepharospasm. *International Ophthalmology Clinics, 42,* 113–121.

Obermann, M., Yaldizli, O., de Greiff, A., Konczak, J., Lachenmayer, M. L., Tumczak, F., et al. (2008). Increased basal-ganglia activation performing a non-dystonia-related task in focal dystonia. *European Journal of Neurology, 15,* 831–838.

Ochudlo, S., Bryniarski, P., & Opala, G. (2007). Botulinum toxin improves the quality of life and reduces the intensification of depressive symptoms in patients with blepharospasm. *Parkinsonism and Related Disorders, 13,* 505–508.

Reimer, J., Gilg, K., Karow, A., Esser, J., & Franke, G. H. (2005). Health-related quality of life in blepharospasm or hemifacial spasm. *Acta Neurologica Scandinavica, 111,* 64–70.

Troung, D., Comella, C., Fernandez, H. H., & Ondo, W. G. (2008). Efficacy and safety of purified botulinum toxin type A (Dysport®) for the treatment of benign essential blepharospasm: A randomized, placebo-controlled, phase II trial. *Parkinsonism and Related Disorders, 14,* 407–414.

Walsh, F. B., Miller, N. R., Newman, N. J., Hoyt, W. F., Biousse, V., & Kerrison, J. B. (2007). *Walsh and Hoyt's clinical neuro-ophthalmology: The essentials.* Philadelphia: Lippincott Williams & Wilkins.

BLOCH–SULZBERGER SYNDROME

DESCRIPTION

Bloch–Sulzberger syndrome, also known as incontinentia pigmenti (IP), is a rare, dominant, X-linked genetic disorder seen almost entirely in females. Although affected males usually die in utero, Bloch–Sulzberger syndrome has been diagnosed in males with Klinefelter's syndrome (Ormerod, White, McKay, & Johnston, 1987). IP is a multisystemic disorder with dermatological, ocular, dental, and central nervous system (CNS) symptoms. Clinical presentation can vary greatly among patients, ranging from mild symptomatology to severe, life-threatening manifestations. Diagnosis is usually made in infancy, as dermatologic symptoms are frequently present at birth or soon after.

NEUROPATHOLOGY/PATHOPHYSIOLOGY

The NEMO (NF-kappa-B essential modulator) gene has been identified as the mutated gene in individuals with Bloch–Sulzberger syndrome. This gene is responsible for producing the proteins that regulate inflammation and provide protection against apoptosis. A cell with a mutated copy of the NEMO gene will not properly produce this protein, leading to the death of the cell. Some neurological symptoms commonly seen in IP are thought to be due to hypersensitivity to inflammation, which leads to cell death (Loh, Jadresic & Whitelaw, 2008). Similarly, the hypersensitivity to inflammation and subsequent apoptosis is thought to cause the dermatologic lesions frequently seen in the disorder (Smahi et al., 2000).

Common MRI findings in individuals with Bloch–Sulzberger syndrome include callosal and cerebellar hypoplasia, periventricular white matter damage, and neuronal heterotopias (Vicente-Villa et al., 2001). These are thought to occur prenatally and to cause some of the CNS and neuropsychological symptoms seen in IP (Mangano & Barbagallo, 1993).

NEUROPSYCHOLOGICAL/CLINICAL PRESENTATION

Mental retardation and delayed psychomotor development are the most common neuropsychological symptoms seen in IP, although compared with the frequency of other symptoms they are rare occurrences (Phan, Wargon, & Turner, 2005). The incidence of neuropsychological dysfunction in Bloch–Sulzberger syndrome is a function of the onset of CNS symptoms. Earlier onset and increased frequency of seizures has been associated with poorer outcomes (Hadj-Rabia et al., 2003; Landy & Donnai, 1993). In addition, CNS symptomatology, particularly seizure activity, has been positively associated with greater dermatological involvement (Happle, 2003). Thus, the severity of the cutaneous lesions may be associated with cognitive dysfunction.

DIAGNOSIS

Dermatological symptoms are the key feature in most IP cases; however, a diagnosis can be made in their absence. Cutaneous features have been grouped into four stages, although some stages may present simultaneously or not at all (Landy & Donnai, 1993). Stage 1 consists primarily of pus-filled lesions that can occur anywhere on the body except the face. Papular lesions, frequently seen on the limbs, characterize Stage 2. The hyperpigmentation seen in Stage 3 is characteristic of Bloch–Sulzberger syndrome and appears most often on the trunk. In Stage 4 of IP, the lesions have healed and hyperpigmentation has faded leaving pale, hairless patches of skin (Landy & Donnai, 1993; Vicente-Villa et al., 2001).

Ocular symptoms in Bloch–Sulzberger syndrome have been reported in anywhere from 25% to 77% of cases. The most commonly reported of the ocular symptoms are vascular abnormalities of the retina. These frequently lead to micro-aneurysms, hemorrhages, and retinal detachment. Nystagmus, cataracts, and optic atrophy have also been reported in IP patients (Jandeck, Kellner, & Foerster, 2004).

Dental abnormalities are seen in 60% of IP cases. Peg-like and conical shaped teeth are most commonly reported dental symptoms. Missing teeth and late or incomplete eruption of teeth is also frequently seen. In addition, poorly mineralized teeth leading to tooth decay is seen as patients age (Minic, Novotny, Trpinac, & Obradovic, 2006).

Although neurological symptoms do not occur as frequently as many of the other symptoms, they are the most serious (Jandeck et al., 2004). Seizures occur most frequently and are a poor prognostic sign. Spastic paralysis and, rarely, microcephaly are seen with IP.

Differential diagnosis of IP is complicated due to the variety of presentations. Differential diagnoses include a large number of disorders that manifest with dermatological, ocular, dental, and CNS symptoms. An examination of symptoms as well as genetic testing can be used to rule out other disorders.

TREATMENT

Currently, there is no known cure for Bloch–Sulzberger syndrome. Selection of treatments should be done on a case-by-case basis and consist mainly of symptom management. Many of the dermatological abnormalities will disappear on their own by adulthood or will appear as pale areas compared with surrounding skin (Stage 4). Earlier stages of dermatological symptoms should be covered with sterile dressings to prevent infection (Berlin, Paller, & Chan, 2002). Ocular symptoms are often treated with corrective lenses or medication. For more severe vascular abnormalities, laser coagulation or surgery may be required (Jandeck et al., 2004). Dental symptoms are rarely life threatening and can be treated by dental specialists (Minic et al., 2004). CNS sequelae including seizures, muscle spasms, and hemiparesis, should be managed by a neurologist using standard treatment protocols.

Daniel L. Frisch
Charles Golden

Berlin, A. L., Paller, A. S., & Chan, L. S. (2002). Incontinentia pigmenti: A review and update on the molecular basis of pathophysiology. *Journal of the American Academy of Dermatology, 47*(2), 169–187.

Hadj-Rabia, S., Froidevaux, D., Bodak, N., Hamel-Teillac, D., Smahi, A., Touil, Y., et al. (2003). Clinical study of 40 cases of incontinentia pigmenti. *Archives of Dermatology, 139*(9), 1163–1170.

Happle, R. (2003). A fresh look at incontinentia pigmenti. *Archives of Dermatology, 139*(9), 1206–1208.

Jandeck, C., Kellner, U., & Foerster, M. H. (2004). Successful treatment of severe retinal vascular abnormalities in incontinentia pigmenti. *Retina, 24*(4), 631–633.

Landy, S. J., & Donnai, D. (1993). Incontinentia pigmenti (Bloch-Sulzberger Syndrome). *Journal of Medical Genetics, 30*(1), 53–59.

Loh, N., Jadresic, L. P., & Whitelaw, A. (2008). A genetic cause for neonatal encephalopathy: Incontinentia pigmenti with NEMO mutation. *Acta Paediatrica, 97*(3), 379–381.

Mangano, S., & Barbagallo, A. (1993). Incontinentia pigmenti: Clinical and neuroradiologic features. *Brain Development, 15*, 362–366.

Minic, S., Novotny, G. E. K., Trpinac, D., & Obradovic, M. (2006). Clinical features of incontinentia pigmenti with emphasis on oral and dental abnormalities. *Clinical Oral Investigations, 10*(4), 343–347.

Ormerod, A. D., White, M. I., McKay, E., & Johnston, A. W. (1987). Incontinentia pigmenti in a boy with Klinefelter's syndrome. *Journal of Medical Genetics, 24*(7), 439–441.

Phan, T. A., Wargon, O., & Turner, A. M. (2005). Incontinentia pigmenti case series: Clinical spectrum of incontinentia pigmenti in 53 female patients and their relatives. *Clinical and Experimental Dermatology, 30*(5), 474–480.

Smahi, A., Courtois, G., Vabres, P., Yamaoka, S., Heuertz, S., Munnich, A., et al. (2000). Genomic rearrangement in NEMO impairs NF-kappaB activation and is a cause of incontinentia pigmenti. *Nature, 405*(6785), 466–472.

Vicente-Villa, A., Lamas, J. V., Pascual, A. M., Cuesta, D. L., Marfa, M. P., & González-Enseñat, M. A. (2001). Incontinentia pigmenti: A report of ten cases. *European Journal of Pediatrics, 160*(1), 64–65.

BRAIN TUMORS

DESCRIPTION

A tumor is a mass of new tissue that persists and grows independently of its surrounding structures and has no physiological use. They vary in pathological origin as discussed in the following. The rate of the tumor's growth varies greatly depending upon the type of cell from which it grows. They are distinguished as being either primary or secondary, benign or malignant. Furthermore, malignancy is divided into low grade and high grade. A primary tumor is defined as a tumor that arises from substances within the brain itself. A secondary or metastatic tumor is carried through the blood to the nervous system from a primary tumor elsewhere (e.g., lungs or breasts). Brain metastasis actually represents the most common intracranial tumor.

For both primary and secondary tumors, the brain is the second most common site of tumors with the uterus being the first. Brain tumors are most common in early to middle adulthood. The overall incidence is nearly equal for males and females.

Functionally, variability is seen in neuropsychological presentation and outcome. Although there is a tendency to conceptualize malignant tumors as most devastating from this perspective as well as from a mortality standpoint, benign tumors may be as serious as malignant tumors because the site of the tumor may be inaccessible to the surgeon without risk to life. As noted by Anderson and Ryken (2008), clinical presentation is consistent with a patterning consistent with expanding mass lesioning. As the authors note, progressive neurologic deficit (68%), motor deficits or weakness (45%), headache (54%), and seizures (36%) are all common features across tumor types. In addition to the sequelae associated the tumor itself, there may be deficits arising from treatment, including surgical approach and chemotherapeutic and/or radiation therapy in cases of malignancy.

NEUROPATHOLOGY/PATHOPHYSIOLOGY

As suggested, an initial means of classification is whether the tumor is primary or secondary, which coincides with its pathological origin. In addition, the area or tissue of invasion suggests underlying physiology. The combination of these factors results in various tumor classes including those discussed below. Tumor locality can be divided into (1) the skull, (2) the meninges, (3) the cranial nerves, (4) the supporting tissue, (5) the pituitary or pineal body, and (6) congenital origin. The various tumors are discussed individually for clarity's sake.

A tumor may develop as a distinct entity in the brain (encapsulated tumor) and put pressure on the rest of the brain. These are known as cystic tumors because they produce a fluid-filled cavity in the brain, usually lined with the tumor cells. The additional space occupied by these tumors compresses the brain, resulting in dysfunction. A second type of tumor is the infiltrating tumor. These tumors are not clearly marked off from the surrounding tissue. They may destroy normal cells and occupy their place or they may surround existing cells and interfere with normal functioning.

The gliomas are likely the most discussed tumors as they constitute the greatest portion of primary tumors. They arise from glial cells and are classified as low grade or high grade. They are further divided into specific tumor types. These include astrocytomas, glioblastomas, oligodendrogliomas, medulloblastomas, and ependymomas.

Beyond the gliomas, a multitude of other tumors are important to mention. These include meningiomas, schwannomas, pituitary adenomas, primary central nervous system (CNS) lymphoma, and metastatic tumors. Table 1 outlines the pathological features associated with these tumors.

Emerging literature has suggested the potential role of genetics in the manifestation of primary CNS tumors, particularly malignant gliomas. Janus and Yung (2007) reported that, to date, the most common alterations along these lines include deletions in chromosome 17p, 9p, 10q, and multiple copies of chromosome 7 across all types; 1p, 9p, 10p, 10q, 11p, 13q, and 17p in relation to astrocytomas; 19q in oligodendrocytes; and 22q in meningiomas.

NEUROPSYCHOLOGICAL/CLINICAL PRESENTATION

There is no unitary profile for intracranial brain tumors. Consequently, neuropsychological features vary. Anderson and Ryken (2008) said it best in noting that such tumors involve the potential for "virtually any neurological or neuropsychological sign." However, as shown in Table 2, there are certain characteristics most commonly seen based on the locality of the tumor. Although these features largely adhere to regional activation/localization theory, this is not always the case (Anderson, Damasio, & Tranel, 1990). Sometimes tumors do not produce the symptoms one would expect given its locality (e.g., a left frontal tumor may have only subtle effects on language based on the subtleties in its regional infiltrate). Often, sensory and motor features can be the first clinical symptoms seen and may serve as the most effective means of localization from pure functional assessment (not that this is needed per se given imaging techniques).

Symptoms result from regional infiltration of the tumor, mass effect, and increased intracranial pressure caused by the growth of the tumor and blockage of the flow of cerebrospinal fluid (CSF) through the ventricles. In some cases, the tumor presses upon or destroys parts of the brain, which produces effects that become gradually worse as the tumor grows. Consequently, common symptoms of intracranial tumors include headaches, especially after lying flat, increased by coughing or stooping; vomiting, which usually occurs at the peak of the headache; diplopia: blurred vision when moving the head; slowing of the pulse; increased drowsiness that progresses to coma; dilation of the pupils, which fail to react to light; and papilledema. Convulsive seizures, focal or generalized, occur with cerebral hemisphere tumors and may precede other symptoms by months or years. They are most common with meningiomas and the slow growing astrocytomas (see Table 2).

Table 1
PATHOLOGICAL FEATURES OF BRAIN TUMORS

Neuropathology/Pathophysiology	*Additional Description*
Astrocytomas	
Infiltrate and invade vital neural systems.	Usually develop slowly.
Characterized by increased cell number and nuclear pleomorphism without necrosis.	Account for about 40% of gliomas.
Mitotic figures should not be present.	Most common in adults over 30 years of age.
Uniformity of cells closely resembling mature resting or reactive, nonanaplastic astrocytes.	At times all the tumorous infiltrates can be removed, which can coincide with prognosis.
Anaplastic astrocytoma	
Increased cellular and nuclear pleomorphism.	
Increased cell density.	
Increased mitoses.	
Vascular endothelial proliferation.	
Pilocytic astrocytoma	
Most commonly found in the cerebellum, brainstem, thalamus, and optic nerve.	
Gelatinous appearance, often well circumscribed and can be fully removed if in an acceptable surgical plane.	
Histologically marked by fibrillary astrocytes and stellate cells and often Rosenthal fibers and microcystic changes.	
Glioblastomas	
Present with all of the same features of astrocytomas and anaplastic astrocytomas.	Rapidly growing gliomas.
Grow far more rapidly.	They are highly malignant.
Demonstrate foci of coagulative necrosis.	Represent about 30% of gliomas.
Infiltrate and migrate along white matter pathways.	Most common in men over 35 years of age.
	Sometimes considered a malignant form of astrocytomas.
	Prognosis is poor, life expectancy is short, usually less than 1 year after surgery.
Oligodendrogliomas	
Arise from oligodendrocytes and thus develop in the white matter of the cerebrum.	Generally slow growing hemispheric tumors.
Most commonly present in frontotemporal regions simply due to the prominence of white matter and thus oligodendrocytes in these areas.	The grade may vary from 1 to 4 with Grade 4 being rare. Survival may extend to 15 years. Oligodendrogliomas represent about 5% of gliomas.
Demonstrate significant overlap with astrocytomas making differentiation difficult at times. When differentiation cannot be made, it is termed a ligoastrocytoma.	
Tumor cell infiltration in the cortex is seen in most cases.	
Many tumors show an artifactual halo around the nucleus.	
Vascular channels are common.	
Medulloblastomas	
The cerebellum is the most common site of origin.	Highly malignant tumor.
Appears on macroscopic examination as friable tumor with central necrosis.	Most commonly found in children and is the most common form of brain tumor in children.
Proposed as arising from the germinal neuroepithelium during embryogenesis permitting differentiation between tumor cells with neuronal, glial, or ependymal characteristics.	Approximately 80% of all cases occur during the first 15 years of life and mainly during the first decade.
Small blue cell tumors with little cytoplasm and pseudorosettes.	Boys are affected more than girls.
	They account for about 10% of gliomas. Survival beyond 5 years of age ranges between 18% and 38%.

(cont.)

B

Table 1
PATHOLOGICAL FEATURES OF BRAIN TUMORS (*cont.*)

Neuropathology/Pathophysiology	*Additional Description*
Ependymomas Associated with and arise in the cerebral ventricles from ependymal cells, particularly from the fourth ventricle. Marked by pseduorosettes, often located in the perivascular region. Blepharoplasts are present. *Anaplastic ependymomas* Have increasing features of nuclear atypia, necrosis, and mitotic figures. *Myxopapillary ependymomas* Usually confined to the filum terminale and have a distinctive fibrillary pattern with mucin secretion.	Represent about 10% of gliomas. Slow growing and tend to block the fourth ventricle, thus preventing the flow of CSF resulting in hydrocephalus. Such tumors are usually benign. Ependymomas constitute about 10% of all intracranial tumors in children with a peak incidence during the first decade. The 5-year survival rate in children with postoperative treatment is about 40% to 50%.
Meningiomas These are extrinsic tumors that grow from the arachnoid matter. They irritate the surface and compress the brain. Have a firm off-white appearance and are well demarcated from surrounding tissue as they are extra-axial in positioning. Demonstrate a whorled pattern with calcifications. Brain invasion and mitotic activity can be seen in aggressive tumors. Classified as fibroblastic, syncytial, transitional, and angioblastic.	They are the most benign of all brain tumors. Meningiomas can occur between the hemispheres. When surgically removed they generally will not recur.
Schwannomas Sex hormone influence has been suggested due to predominance in females. Most commonly involve cranial nerves VIII, V, VII.	Tend to be slow growing. Benign Intervention is not always needed beyond sequential monitoring of the tumor if individuals are not overly troubled by symptoms. Often found incidentally.
Pituitary adenomas These are neuroepithelial tumors of the pituitary region. Appear acophilic, basophilic, or chromophobic on staining. Vary in whether they secrete hormones.	A variety of problems arise with respect to growth characteristics of these tumors, including obesity, hairiness of the face, and amenorrhoea. If they develop before puberty, the child may demonstrate gigantism. They can also cause acromegaly after puberty. These tumors are treatable and can be removed. Develop in a stepwise fashion.
Primary CNS lymphomas Mass lesion presenting in the periventricular white matter. Diffuse histological activity, even in tissues appearing normal macroscopically. Mechanisms of transformation largely unknown given there are no lymphatics in the CNS. Considered a non-Hodgkin's lymphoma, of B cell origin, which is perplexing as these cells are not usually present in the CNS. Aggregate near blood vessels. Stain positive for appropriate immunohistological B cell or T cell markers.	Commonly associated with immunocompromise or immunosuppression.

(*cont.*)

Table 1
PATHOLOGICAL FEATURES OF BRAIN TUMORS (*cont.*)

Neuropathology/Pathophysiology	Additional Description
Metastases	
Can present throughout the CNS.	The most common intracranial tumor.
Associated with cancerous presentations of different organ sites with breast and lung cancers being the most common preceding cancer presentations.	
Also can occur in relation to skin, colorectal, and renal cancers.	

Data compiled from *Textbook of Clinical Neurology* (3rd ed., pp.1053–1080), by T. J. Janus and W. F. A. Yung, 2007, Philadelphia: Saunders Elsevier and *Textbook of Clinical Neuropsychology* (pp. 578–587), by S. W. Anderson and T. C. Ryken, 2008, New York: Taylor & Francis.

Table 2
TUMOR CHARACTERISTICS BASED ON LOCATION

Tumor Location	Symptoms
Cerebral hemispheres Frontal lobes	Hemiplegia, focal or generalized seizures, and mental changes. Expressive aphasia may be present with tumors present in the dominate hemisphere. Precipitate urination may be associated with a tumor on the medial surface. Inattention, loss of motivation, and ataxic gait may be exhibited as the tumor spreads to both lobes.
Parietal lobes	Astereognosis and sensory impairment contralaterally. Seizures may be either generalized or focal. Anosognosia, apraxia, and denial of illness may be present. Speech disturbances may be associated with a tumor in the dominant hemisphere.
Temporal lobes	Usually show few indications except for seizures. Tumors involving the dominate hemisphere may produce mixed expressive and receptive aphasia or more pure receptive aphasia. Memory deficits can occur.
Occipital lobes	Result in contralateral quadrant defect in the visual field. Convulsion may have an aura of flashing lights.
Subcortical	Commonly contralateral hemiparesis is present. Tumors that invade the thalamus produce contralateral cutaneous sensory impairment. With basal ganglia involvement, there is sometimes athetosis, bizarre tremors, or dystonic posturing.
Pituitary and suprasellar region	Headache and visual field defects, usually bitemporal hemianopia, are common. Other endocrinopathies resulting from tumors of this region were mentioned under pituitary adenomas above.
Pineal area	Precocious puberty may result, more commonly in boys. Hydrocephalus and papilledema result from compression of the aqueduct of Sylvius. Paralysis of upward gaze, ptosis, and loss of pupillary light and accommodation reflexes result from compression of the pretectum. There may be unilateral or bilateral paralysis of the 5th, 6th, 7th, and 10th cranial nerves and of lateral gaze. Hemiplegia, hemianesthesia, ataxia, nystagmus, or intention tremor may be present.
Cranial fossas	Symptoms of increased intracranial pressure appear early. Posterior fossa tumor has primary signs of ataxia and intention tremor. Anterior fossa can have more cognitive issues similar to executive dysfunction and poor attention. Hemiparesis, language deficits, and personality changes may present.
Cerebellopontine fossa	Produce tinnitus, unilateral hearing impairment, and vertigo. There will be loss of corneal reflex, facial palsy, anathesia, and signs of cerebellar dysfunction.

B

In many instances, cognitive features are seen later as unrecognized tumors continue to grow and become more infiltrating and potentially causing mass effect. Yet, interestingly, subtle changes in cognition can be predictive of recurrence and/or tumor growth prior to it even being recognized on imaging (Armstrong, Goldstein, Shera, Ledakis, & Tallent, 2003; Meyers & Hess, 2003).

Cognitive issues have likely been historically underreported as neurologists and neurosurgeons who primarily serve these patients do not regularly seek neuropsychological consultation, relying on traditional mental status checks such as the mini-mental state examination. Emerging literature has demonstrated the relative insensitivity of such measures and practices to identifying cognitive deficits in tumors due to low ceiling effects (Pahlson, Elk, Ahlstronm, & Smits, 2003). Newer data suggest that nonspecific neurocognitive deficits present in upward of 90% of patients (Tucha, Smely, Preier, & Lange, 2000) with nondominant hemisphere lesions constituting the majority of cases that do *not* present with cognitive deficits (Hahn et al., 2003).

Beyond deficits associated with the tumors themselves, negative neuropsychological outcomes have also been linked with treatment modalities. In general, those clinical features apparently related to the hemispheric origin of the tumor often remain even following resection but are sometimes to a lesser extent. Where improvement is seen is in the reduction of mass effect and those residuals related to it (Duffau, 2006). This is in comparison with focal deficits that present immediately following surgery and recover gradually over the course of 3–6 months (Duffau et al., 2003).

Surgery contributes to focal deficits that are not necessarily new features, but likely a continuation of deficits owing to the location of the tumor, whereas radiation and chemotherapy coincide with more diffuse and potentially new deficits. Radiation of the brain has been associated with demyelination and small vessel damage that coincide with a diffuse subcortical pattern of cognitive dysfunction. The most common features include slowed reaction time, diminished processing speed, retrieval-based memory deficits, diminished working memory capacity, slowed or impeded problem-solving skills, diminished reading comprehension, reduced initial learning capacity, and varied executive deficits. Of interest, although some of these features present early in relation to the demyelinating effects, some deficits do not come to light until months after treatment and are related to a diffuse encephalopathy (Armstrong et al., 2002). When it comes to chemotherapy, a similar diffuse pattern may be seen. This has included changes in working memory, executive

functions, processing speed, and memory (Ahles & Saykin, 2002; Anderson-Hanley, Sherman, Riggs, Agocha, & Compas, 2003; Ferguson & Ahles, 2003; Tannock, Ahles, Ganz, & Van Dam, 2004). Although such deficits are most commonly noted acutely during chemotherapy (Ahles & Saykin, 2002; Ferguson & Ahles, 2003), some may persist at lesser levels following treatment discontinuation. Research in this area has, however, been plagued by flaws in methodology in addition to difficulties in controlling for confounds. There needs to be recognition that the idea of "chemobrain" is not necessarily restricted to direct effect. Indirect effects due to fatigue, metabolic changes, and so forth must also be considered.

DIAGNOSIS

Diagnostic procedures should be multifaceted and comprehensive to aid in the proper understanding of not only the tumor type but its impact. Workup should include complete neurologic examination, testing of visual acuity and visual fields, audiometric tests, a CT scan or MRI, and neuropsychological testing. Biopsy may be performed through a burr hole placement, but sometimes surgical removal is simply done at the outset based on the locality of the tumor and its symptom. Pathological review is then undertaken following surgical removal. Then, the pathology determines what if any additional treatment options should be considered. X-rays of the chest and/or positron emission tomography/CT of the body should be sought in cases of metastases. A CSF examination is only necessary if preliminary tests do not provide clear results. If papilledema is present, the use of a lumbar puncture is contraindicated because the pressure change could cause a herniation syndrome. Neuropsychological testing is best completed pre- and posttreatment and potentially on an annual basis as it can prove sensitive to identifying recurrence even prior to it being recognized on imaging. Furthermore, it may suggest broader issues prior to surgery than may be purely indicated based on imaging due to capabilities in detecting tumor spread that is not yet massed to the point the imaging recognizes it.

TREATMENT

Treatment involves factors related to location and type of tumor. Infiltrating tumors may require surgical removal as soon as possible after diagnosis. In most cases, the infiltrate cannot be completely removed. Radiation and chemotherapy follow the surgery in cases of malignancy. In cases in which surgery is ruled out, due to the location of thalamic or brainstem tumors, radiation therapy and chemotherapy are the primary treatment. A postoperative period of anticonvulsant therapy is usually included.

Encapsulated tumors are generally benign and nonresponsive to radiation therapy. They are generally surgically removed. Pituitary tumors may be treated by surgery and radiation therapy or radiation therapy alone. Tumors that obstruct the flow of CSF may be treated with the placement of a shunt prior to surgical or radiation therapy.

Neuropsychological assessment can elucidate what areas present with dysfunction and thus require neuropsychological rehabilitation. Cognitive rehabilitation may be undertaken. In the case of children, this may also need to incorporate components of special education services. Physical and occupational therapy may be warranted based on the functional outcomes.

The prognosis for recovery from a brain tumor depends on the grade, type, rate of growth, the patient's age, the presence of other diseases, the responsiveness of the tumor to radiation or chemotherapy, and so forth. Primary tumors generally have a poor prognosis for complete recovery, with glioblastomas having the least favorable survival rates, whereas hemangiomas and meningiomas have the best survival rates. With the exception of hemangiomas and meningiomas, patients with the other primary tumors show a rapid decline in functioning during the first 2 years after diagnosis; thereafter decline is more gradual. Decline is more rapid in glioblastomas with median survival below a year.

In the case of inoperable tumors, the therapy involves treatment of symptoms such as headache and seizures. Increased intracranial pressure can be treated temporarily with dexamethasone. At the terminal stage, skilled nursing care is required. In the case of benign tumors, intervention may involve supportive therapy or more specialized therapy, marital or family, in cases where recovery of function is feasible. In the case of malignant tumors, support therapy for the family should be considered. In the latter stages of the disease, hospice care may prove beneficial.

Chad A. Noggle
Raymond S. Dean

Ahles, T. A., & Saykin, A. J. (2002). Breast cancer chemotherapy-related cognitive dysfunction. *Clinical Breast Cancer, 3*(3), 84–90.

Anderson, S. W., Damasio, H., & Tranel, D. (1990). Neuropsychological profiles associated with lesions caused by tumor or stroke. *Archives of Neurology, 47*, 397–405.

Anderson, S. W., & Ryken, T. C. (2008). Intracranial tumors. In J. E. Morgan & J. H. Ricker (Eds.), *Textbook of clinical neuropsychology* (pp. 578–587). New York: Taylor & Francis.

Anderson-Hanley, C., Sherman, M. L., Riggs, R., Agocha, V. B., & Compas, B. E. (2003). Neuropsychological effects of treatments for adults with cancer: A meta-analysis and review of the literature. *Journal of the International Neuropsychological Society, 9*(7), 967–982.

Armstrong, C. L., Goldstein, B., Shera, D., Ledakis, G. E., & Tallent, E. M. (2003). The predictive value of longitudinal neuropsychologic assessment in the early detection of brain tumor recurrence. *Cancer, 97*, 649–656.

Armstrong, C. L., Hunter, J. V., Ledakis, G. E., Cohen, B., Tallent, E. M., Goldstein, B. H., et al. (2002). Late cognitive and radiographic changes related to radiotherapy: Initial prospective findings. *Neurology, 59*, 40–48.

Duffau, H. (2006). New concepts in surgery of WHO grade II glioma: Functional brain mapping, connectionism and plasticity review. *Journal of Neurooncology, 79*, 77–115.

Duffau, H., Capelle, L., Denvil, D., Sichez, N., Gatignol, P., Lopes, M., et al. (2003). Functional recovery after surgical resection of low-grade glioma in eloquent brain: Hypothesis of brain compensation. *Journal of Neurology, Neurosurgery, and Psychiatry, 74*(7), 901–907.

Ferguson, R. J., & Ahles, T. A. (2003). Low-neuropsychologic performance among adult cancer survivors treated with chemotherapy. *Current Neurology and Neuroscience Reports, 3*, 215–222.

Hahn, C. A., Dunn, R. H., Logue, P. E., King, J. H., Edwards, C. L., & Halperin, E. C. (2003). Prospective study of neuropsychologic testing and quality of life assessment of adults with primary malignant brain tumors. *International Journal of Radiation Oncology, Biology, Physics, 55*, 992–999.

Janus, T. J., & Yung, W. F. A. (2007). Primary neurological tumors. In C. G. Goetz (Ed.), *Textbook of clinical neurology* (3rd ed., pp. 1053–1080). Philadelphia: Saunders Elsevier.

Meyers, C. A., & Hess, K. R. (2003). Multifaceted end points in brain tumor clinical trials. Cognitive deterioration precedes MRI progression. *Neuro-oncology, 5*, 89–95.

Pahlson, A., Elk, L., Ahlstronm, G., & Smits, (2003). Pitfalls in the assessment of disability individuals with low-grade gliomas. *Journal of Neuro-oncology, 65*, 149–158.

Tannock, I. F., Ahles, T. A., Ganz, P. A., & Van Dam, F. S., (2004). Cognitive impairment associated with chemotherapy for cancer: Report of a workshop. *Journal of Clinical Oncology, 22*(11), 2233–2239.

Tucha, O, Smely, C., Preier, M., & Lange, K. W. (2000). Cognitive deficits before treatment among patients with brain tumors. *Neurosurgery, 47*, 324–333.

BROWN-SÉQUARD SYNDROME

DESCRIPTION

Brown-Séquard syndrome is a rare clinical presentation arising from unilateral spinal cord or medullary lesioning. The pathological basis of Brown-Séquard syndrome causes ipsilateral motor and proprioceptive loss. Simultaneously, contralateral pain and temperature loss occurs. The face is spared.

The syndrome was first described in 1849 by Charles Edouard Brown-Séquard and revisited in the case report he submitted in 1869 (Tattersall & Turner, 2000). In his report, Brown-Séquard discussed a patient with a lesion in one of the lateral halves of the spinal cord that caused paralysis of muscular sense and movement on the same side of the lesion while creating an anesthesia to touch, tickling, pain, and temperature sensation on the opposite side. Based on his description, the syndrome now bears his name.

NEUROPATHOLOGY/PATHOPHYSIOLOGY

Brown-Séquard syndrome manifests secondary to a lesion affecting one half of the spinal cord, which interrupts transmission of the descending corticospinal tract, ascending fibers in the posterior columns, and the crossed spinothalamic tract. Case reports have demonstrated both traumatic and nontraumatic etiologies as a potential cause of the syndrome. In regard to trauma (e.g., stab wounds, gunshot wounds, motor vehicle accidents [MVAs], disc herniation, etc.), the particular mechanism in all cases must be through laceration or compression of one half of the spinal cord.

Historically, extramedullary lesions such as tumors have been the most common basis for Brown-Séquard syndrome. Abcesses and intrinsic lesions such as vasculitis in this area have also been associated with the presentation. When the syndrome arises from an extramedullary lesion, segmental lower motor neuron and sensory sign may also be observed (Hammerstad, 2007).

The locality of the lesion is directly linked to the localization of the symptoms. Loss of pain and temperature sensation begins one or two segments below the lesion. When segmental lower motor neuron and sensory signs are seen, they present at the level of the lesion. As noted, these latter features are more commonly seen in association with an extramedullary lesion. Tactile sensation remains generally intact as fibers are distributed in multiple tracks including the posterior columns, as well as the anterior and

lateral spinothalamic tracts on both sides of the cord (Ropper & Brown, 2005).

The perplexing clinical symptoms are directly related to the differential manner in which the corresponding tracts ascend or descend. Ipsilateral paralysis of voluntary motor movements and proprioception is seen because the corresponding corticospinal tract descends from the cortex and crosses over at the point of the medulla (i.e., the pyramidal decussation) and enters the spinal cord via the dorsal root ganglion. Thus, a lesion below the pyramids will not permit the impulse to travel further down the spine activating the muscles on that side nor will their proprioceptive feedback be able to ascend beyond the lesion, which would eventually cross over to the contralateral side. In comparison, pain and temperature fibers enter the spinal cord from peripheral regions, and almost immediately cross over (2–3 segments above entry) to the contralateral spinothalamic tract that would then normally ascend up to the thalamus, but would in these cases not go beyond the lesion.

NEUROPSYCHOLOGICAL/CLINICAL PRESENTATION

The characteristic pattern seen in Brown-Séquard syndrome involves both sensory and motor features of a mixed ipsilateral-contralateral pattern. Spastic weakness and loss of proprioception below the lesion on the ipsilateral side is seen whereas loss of pain and temperature sensation is observed on the contralateral side of the lesion. As suggested, segmental lower motor neuron and sensory sign may be seen if the presentation arises from extramedullary lesioning.

Mentation is not affected as the dysfunction arises outside the cortex. Although there is not adequate literature on the psychological impact of Brown-Séquard syndrome, one might presume from the general literature on spinal cord injuries that there may be an increased risk of psychiatric features in the form of depression and anxiety related to their adjustment. As patients recover from the underlying presentation or injury, improvement may be seen that can offset this to some extent.

DIAGNOSIS

Diagnosis of Brown-Séquard syndrome itself is symptom based requiring the aforementioned constellation of features of contralateral loss of pain and temperature sensation in combination with ipsilateral loss of proprioception and spastic weakness. Imaging involving either MRI or CT demonstrating hemi-dissection of the spinal cord or extramedullary lesioning is required. Again, if the latter serves as the underlying pathological origin, segmental lower motor neuron and sensory signs are likely to be seen. Although the clinical features define the syndrome, importance is placed on identifying the underlying cause, which suggests the importance of imaging. MRI best visualizes the spine and any potential injury and/or edema.

TREATMENT

Treatment varies depending on the underlying etiology. When arising from a penetrating trauma such as a gunshot or stab wound, antibiotics and tetanus boosters as well as other medicinal interventions may be employed to prevent meningitis. Wound debridement may be utilized in stab wounds whereas surgical intervention is commonly employed in gunshot wounds or in stab wounds if symptoms worsen, which may suggest epidural hematoma. Physical and occupational therapy may then be utilized over the long term for rehabilitation. Surgical intervention is also utilized when the syndrome arises from herniations. Radiotherapy may at times be used for extramedullary

tumors or abcesses, although surgical intervention may at times be attempted. In general, Brown-Séquard syndrome is associated with a favorable pattern of recovery for patients (Little & Halar, 1985; Roth, Park, Pang, Yarkony, & Lee, 1991).

Chad A. Noggle
Michelle Pagoria

Hammerstad, J. P. (2007). Strength and reflexes. In C. G. Goetz (Ed.), *Textbook of clinical neurology* (3rd ed., pp. 243–288). Philadelphia: Saunders Elsevier.

Little, J. W., & Halar, E. (1985). Temporal course of motor recovery after Brown-Séquard spinal cord injuries. *Paraplegia, 23*, 39–46.

Ropper, A. H., & Brown, R. J. (2005). *Adams and Victor's principles of neurology* (8th ed., pp. 129–143). New York: McGraw-Hill.

Roth, E. J., Park, T., Pang, T., Yarkony, G. M., & Lee, M. Y. (1991). Traumatic cervical Brown-Séquard and Brown-Séquard-plus syndromes: The spectrum of presentations and outcomes. *Paraplegia, 29*, 582–589.

Tattersall, R., & Turner, B. (2000). Brown-Séquard and his syndrome. *Lancet, 356*, 61–63.

CANAVAN'S DISEASE

DESCRIPTION

Canavan's disease is an autosomal-recessive illness, presenting in infancy and is characterized by a spongy degeneration of the white matter throughout the nervous system. Canavan's disease is among the most common cerebral degenerative diseases in infancy (Rowland, 2005; Shoji, 2007). Although it has been documented in several ethnic groupings, it is most commonly seen in Ashkenazi Jews with 1 in 40 individuals presenting as carriers.

Progressive in nature, initial symptoms are seen in the form of a loss of previously acquired skills, hypotonia or hypertonia, feeding difficulties, and mental retardation. As the disease progresses, greater impairments along these lines may eventually be seen including, but not limited to, paralysis, blindness, severe mental retardation, and hearing loss. Eventually death occurs, usually before age four, although some children may survive into their teens and twenties.

NEUROPATHOLOGY/PATHOPHYSIOLOGY

Canavan's disease originates from a defect in the ASPA gene on chromosome 17p13 (Tahmaz et al., 2001) indirectly causing demyelination within the brain. This is due to the fact that the ASPA gene regulates production of aspartoacylase, which is an enzyme essential to breaking down N-acetylaspartate (NAA) into aspartic and acetic acid. This defect in activity and excessive levels of N-actylaspartic acid in the urine, plasma, and cerebrospinal fluid (CSF) is considered the hallmark of Canavan's disease. (Hagenfeldt et al., 1987; Matalon et al., 1988). Aspartoacylase deficiencies are detectable in skin fibroblast cultures (Matalon et al., 1988).

The elevated levels of NAA prove toxic to the system, particularly the white matter, causing demyelination throughout subcortical regions as can be seen through MRI (Pastores, 2008; Shoji, 2007; United Leukodystrophy Foundation [ULF], 2007). This decay most commonly occurs early in infancy although cases of adolescent onset have been noted. However,

diagnosis has been made as early as the prenatal period as assay of amniotic fluid can sometimes demonstrate the noted anomalies in NAA levels. (Bennett et al., 1993)

From a neuropathological standpoint, the subcortical white matter is most affected with numerous vacuoles often being noted on microscopic investigation creating the spongy presentation. Similar findings may be noted in other areas including the deeper cortex, deep white matter, and superficial cortex although to a lesser degree. This vacuolation develops secondary to swelling of astrocytes and splitting of thin myelin lamellae due to fluid accumulation (Gascon et al., 1990). This creates an increase in brain volume and weight. Given astrocytes present throughout the cortex, so too can the vacuoles associated with Canavan's disease (Adachi et al., 1973). Over time, the preferential degeneration of the white matter is of such a degree that there is poor differentiation between it and the cortex (Lake, 1997). There is a general sparing of oligodendroglia and axonal fibers centrally in addition to peripheral nerves.

NEUROPSYCHOLOGICAL/CLINICAL PRESENTATION

Degenerative in nature, upon onset of symptoms, the clinical picture over time deteriorates with more symptoms developing or becoming worse. Physically, infants often present with megalencephaly in the absence of hydrocephalus over the course of the first 2 years of life (Maertens & Dyken, 2007). This often corresponds with poor head control. In later onset forms, such as during adolescence, megalencephaly is not seen. Of interest, the brain itself is commonly normal in size. Feeding and/or swallowing difficulties are also common physical deficits (ULF, 2007).

Infants and toddlers commonly present with normal development for some period of time aside from potentially poorer head control due to megalencephaly. Following symptom onset, previously acquired motor skills are lost and hypotonia commonly develops. Choreoathetotic or dystonic movements may occur. As further degeneration is seen, spasticity develops. In later stages of the disease process, decorticate and decerebrate posturing,

C

dysautonomia (e.g., vomiting, hyperthermia, hypotension), blindness (usually preceded by optic atrophy and nystagmus), and deafness may occur prior to death (Zelnik et al., 1993; Feigelman et al., 1991). Seizures, focal and/or myoclonic, develop in more than 50% of patients over the course of the disease (Rowland, 2005; Lake, 1997). Cognitively, mental retardation develops early in the course of the disease with impairments increasing with progression. Death usually occurs prior to 5 years of age.

The neonatal form is more limited from a presentation standpoint as death usually occurs within a few weeks from birth. Following birth, infants are observed as overly lethargic, hypotonic, and demonstrating minimal spontaneous or reflexive movements.

The juvenile form manifests after 5 years of age. Initial symptoms appear posterior in origin. Cerebellar dysfunction resulting in ataxia is one of the initial symptoms. Tremor, dysarthria, seizures, spasticity and gradual loss of vision are also commonly seen (Maertens & Dyken, 2007). Dementia develops as mentation deteriorates further.

DIAGNOSIS

Diagnosis is initially suggested based on the clinical features that arise characterized by a developmental pattern of a plateau and regression. Confirmation is then made through a combination of laboratory analysis and neuroimaging workup. On MRI, Canavan's disease will present with diffuse, high signal intensity on T2-weighted images, whereas on CT, attenuation of cerebral and cerebellar white matter in an enlarged head with normal-sized ventricles is noted (Ropper & Brown, 2005). This is due to the characteristic pattern of fluid accumulation in the astrocytes, as discussed above. When seen in combination with elevated urinary levels of NAA, diagnosis is seen as definitive.

TREATMENT

There is no cure for Canavan's disease nor standard means of treatment. Prognosis is poor with death usually occurring prior to age four in the infant form, although some survive into adolescence or even early adulthood (Shoji, 2007). The neonatal form is associated with death commonly within a month of birth, although they may survive past their first birthday in rare cases. Children with the juvenile form commonly survive into adolescence before succumbing to the progressive nature of the disease.

Following symptom onset and prior to death, treatment is symptom based and supportive. Anticonvuslants may be used to address seizures if they develop. A feeding tube may be required depending on the severity of feeding and swallowing difficulties if they are present. Counseling for parents and family members can prove essential and should be encouraged to address their coping. This should include thorough education so they may be better informed of what to expect as their child's disease progresses.

J. Aaron Albritton
Chad A. Noggle

Adachi, M., Schneck, L., Cara, J., Volk, B.W. (1973). Spongy degeneration of the central nervous system: A review. Human Pathology, 4, 331–347.

Feigelman, T., Shih, V.E., & Buyse, M.L. (1991). Prolonged survival in Canavan disease. Dysmorphic Clinical Genetics, 5, 107–110.

Gascon, G.G., Ozand, P.T., Mahdi, A., et al., (1990). Infantile CNS spongy degeneration-14 cases: Clinical update. Neurology, 40, 1876–1882.

Hagenfeldt, L., Bollgren, I., Venizelos, N. (1987). N-acetylaspartic aciduria due to aspartoacylase deficiency-a new etiology of childhood leukodystrophy. Journal of Inherited Metabolic Disorders, 10, 134–141.

Lake, B. (1997). Lyosomal and peroxisomal disorders. In D. Graham & P. Lantos (Eds.). Greenfield's Neuropathology (6th Ed.). Oxford University Press: New York (pp. 657–753).

Maertens, P & Dyken, R.P. (2007). Storage diseases: Neuronal Ceroid-Lipofuscinoses, Lipidoses, Glycogenoses, and Leukodystrphies. In C.G. Goets (Ed.) Textbook of Clinical Neurology. Saunders Elsevier: Philadelphia (pp. 613–640)

Matalon, R., Michals, K., Sebesta, D., et al., (1988). Aspartoacylase deficiency in N-acetylaspartic aciduria in patients with Canavan disease. American Journal of Medical Genetics, 29, 463–471.

Pastores, Gregory M. (2008). Chapter 66: Inborn Errors of Metabolism of the Nervous System. In: Bradley, Walter G., et al. Neurology in Clinical Practice, 5th Ed. Butterworth-Heinemann

Ropper, A.H. & Brown, R.H. (2005). Adams and Victor's Principles of Neurology (8th Edition). McGraw-Hill: New York (pp.797–849)

Rowland, Lewis P. (Ed.). (2005). Merritt's Neurology: 11th Ed. Philadelphia, PA: Lippincott Williams & Wilkins.

Shoji Tsuji, (2007). Leukodystrophies. In: Sid Gilman, MD, FRCP, Editor(s), Neurobiology of Disease (Pages 43–49). Burlington: Academic Press.

Tahmaz, F.E., Sam, S., Hognason, G.E., Quan, F. (2001). A partial deletion of aspartoacylase gene is the cause of Canavan disease in a family from Mexico. Journal of Medical Genetics, 38, E9.

United Leukodystrophy Foundation (2007, Aug 2). Types of Leukodystrophy: Canavan Disease. Retrieved May 3, 2009, Web site: http://www.ulf.org/types/Canavan.html

Zelnik, N., Luder, A.S., Elpeleg, O.N., et al. (1993). Protracted clinical course for patient with Canavan Disease. Developmental Medicine and Child Neurology, 35, 355–358.

FURTHER READING

Canavan, M. M. (1931). Schilder's encephalitis periaxialis diffusa. Report of a case in a child aged sixteen and one-half months. Archives of Neurology and Psychiatry, 25, 299–308.

Canavan Research Foundation. Our story: The search for a cure. Retrieved May 14, 2009.

Janson, C., Mcphee, S., Bilaniuk, L., Haselgrove, J., Testaiuti, M., Freese, A., et al. (2002, July). Clinical protocol. Gene therapy of Canavan disease: AAV-2 vector for neurosurgical delivery of aspartoacylase gene (ASPA) to the human brain. Human Gene Therapy, 13(11), 1391–412. doi:10.1089/104303402760128612. PMID 12162821.

Mathew, R., Arun, P., Madhavarao, C. N., Moffett, J. R., & Namboodiri, M. A. (2005). Progress toward acetate supplementation therapy for Canavan disease: Glyceryl triacetate administration increases acetate, but not N-acetylaspartate, levels in brain. The Journal of Pharmacology and Experimental Therapeutics, 315(1), 297–303. doi:10.1124/jpet.105.087536. PMID 16002461. http://jpet.aspetjournals.org/cgi/reprint/315/1/297.pdf

Namboodiri, A. M., Peethambaran, A., Mathew, R., Sambhu, P. A., Hershfield, J., Moffett, J. R., et al. (2006, June). Canavan disease and the role of N-acetylaspartate in myelin synthesis. Molecular and Cellular Endocrinology, 252(1–2), 216–223. doi:10.1016/j.mce.2006.03.016. PMID 16647192. Online Mendelian Inheritance in Man. 271900

CAPGRAS'S SYNDROME

DESCRIPTION

Capgras's syndrome (CS) is characterized by a delusional misidentification wherein an individual believes that a person, most often a loved one, has been replaced by an identical looking imposter. The individual with CS recognizes the close relation and strong resemblance, but denies his or her identity and often uses subtle misperceived differences in behavior, personality, or physical appearance to differentiate the "imposter" from the actual person. The presentation may be transient or persistent and may include more than one subject of misidentification (Mendez, 1992; Todd, Dewhurst, & Wallis, 1981). Despite the similarities, CS is not the same syndrome as prosopagnosia where the patient loses the inability to identify patients. Patients with CS can perceive faces, and recognize that they look an identified individual, but they do not make the emotional or identity connection with the resemblance (Ellis & Young, 1990). In other words, the person object looks like the patient's spouse, but the patient does not believe the person actually is the spouse.

CS was first described by Joseph Capgras and Jean Reboul-Lachaux, who described a patient who was convinced that her family and neighbors had all been replaced by look-alikes (Capgras & Reboul-Lachaux, 1923). It was assumed to be a rare phenomenon, initially reported to be associated only with psychiatric disturbance. It is estimated to occur in about 4% of psychotic patients, most commonly observed in patients with the paranoid subtype of schizophrenia (Christodoulou, 1991; Frazer & Roberts, 1994). More recent literature has found the syndrome to be more common than initially thought with CS identified in a variety of neurologic conditions including epilepsy, cerebrovascular disease, traumatic brain injury, pituitary tumors, and other diagnoses (Collins, Hawthorne, Gribbin, & Jacobson, 1990; Frazer & Roberts, 1994). Even more recently, a strong relationship has been noted in patients with neurodegenerative conditions such as Alzheimer's disease, Parkinson's disease, and Lewy body dementia. In a review article by Bourget and Whitehurst (2004), they cite indications that CS may be present in 20–30% of patients with Alzheimer's disease. Josephs more recent study of 2007 provides even stronger support for CS in neurodegenerative conditions, particularly Lewy body dementia. When CS occurs in the context of neurodegeneration, there is likely an older age at onset in comparison to other neurologic/psychiatric manifestations. CS occurring in the context of dementia where visual hallucinations are also present was suggestive of Lewy body disease (Joseph, 2007).

NEUROPATHOLOGY/PATHOPHYSIOLOGY

Ellis and Young (1990) describe a disconnect between the areas in the brain that are responsible for facial recognition and those involved in emotions and memory. In patients with neurologic damage, this disconnect is believed to occur by damage to the ventromedial frontal cortex, which causes impairment of automatic arousal responses, and damage to the right frontal lobe, which causes an inability to evaluate beliefs and impairs reasoning. Ellis and Young posit that to rationalize the strange feeling produced by the inability to recognize a face, the patient develops a delusion that the loved one is an imposter. This is consistent with Joseph's review of the literature (2007) indicating that CS may be more the result of a disconnection of other lobes from the frontal lobes. Specifically, bilateral frontal lobe disturbance with additional involvement of the right hemisphere temporal and/or parietal lobes was noted across several cases. Results of neuroradiological studies for patients with known underlying neurologic disturbance in the absence of psychiatric history provide further support for this organic-based etiology. Bourget and Whitehurst (2004) and Ellis (1994) cite numerous studies showing right hemisphere along with bilateral frontal lobe dysfunction in most of the study patients. Regarding the right hemisphere disturbance, temporal and parietal disturbance, individually or in combination, were noted. Global atrophy has also been found but typically in combination with specific abnormalities in the bilateral frontal lobes and right hemisphere. Despite the variability noted in diagnostic populations, most research points to involvement of the bilateral frontal lobes along with some aspect of the right hemisphere in cases of CS (Ellis, 1994). However, there is no single lesion location that has been identified to be specific to CS.

Similarly, in CS cases involving psychiatric disturbance, there is no single neurologic anatomic area associated with the misidentification syndrome, but some posit that neurologic disturbance underlies the development of the syndrome in psychiatric patients. As noted by Bourget and Whitehurst (2004), the syndrome has been linked to dopaminergic overactivity and serotonin abnormality in some psychiatric cases. In addition, neuropsychological and neuroradiologic studies again point to frontal and right hemispheric disturbance in these cases.

NEUROPSYCHOLOGICAL/CLINICAL PRESENTATION

As described previously, CS is characterized by a delusional misidentification wherein an individual believes that a person, most often a loved one, has been replaced by an identical looking imposter. In essence, it is a sign or symptom of underlying neurologic disturbance, but is not specific to any single diagnostic group. Neuropsychological test results highlight the frontal/executive deficits expected with frontal lobe disturbance along with right hemispheric disturbance in terms of visual spatial processing, reasoning, and memory (Alexander, Stuss, & Benson, 1977). Interestingly, neuropsychological

studies have consistently differentiated the phenomena of CS from prosopagnosia (Bauer, 1984).

DIAGNOSIS

It is important to note that CS is a sign or symptom of underlying neurologic disturbance but is not specific to any single diagnostic group. Identification of CS is based on observation and patient and collateral reporting of the misidentification phenomena. Follow-up interview and observation are valuable to distinguish transient from more chronic forms of the syndrome and to guide treatment as needed. Observation of the symptoms of CS should prompt a systematic search for cerebral lesions, electric disorders on electroencephalography, and organic disorders (infectious, toxic, metabolic), even in a defined psychiatric case, to guide treatment.

TREATMENT

The main treatment of CS is pharmacotherapy with antipsychotics and cognitive behavioral therapy (CBT) to help with fixed delusions (Denes, 2007). Psychotherapeutic interventions require significant persistence along with reality testing methods to challenge the delusions. Success is limited without additional psychopharmacological treatments.

Mark T. Barisa

Alexander, M. P., Stuss, D. T., & Benson, D. F. (1979). Capgras syndrome: A reduplicative phenomenon. *Neurology, 29,* 334–339.

Bauer, R. M. (1984). Autonomic recognition of names and faces in prosopagnosia: A neuropsychological application of the guilty knowledge test. *Neuropsychologia, 22,* 457–469.

Bourget, D., & Whitehurst, L. (2004). Capgras syndrome: A review of the neurophysiological correlates and presenting features in cases involving physical violence. *Canadian Journal of Psychiatry, 49,* 719–725.

Capgras, J., & Reboul-Lachaux, J. (1923). Illusions des sosies dans un délire systematize chronique. *Bulletin de la Société Clinique de Médicine Mentale, 23,* 6–16.

Christodoulou, G. N. (1991). The delusional misidentification syndromes. *British Journal of Psychiatry, 159,* 65–69.

Collins, M. N., Hawthorne, M. E., Gribbin, N., & Jacobson, R. (1990). Capgras' syndrome with organic disorders. *Postgraduate Medicine Journal, 66,* 1064–1067.

Denes, G. (2007). Capgras delusion. *Neurological Science, 28,* 163–164.

Ellis, H. D. (1994). The role of the right hemisphere in the Capgras delusion. *Psychopathology, 27,* 177–185.

Ellis, H., & Young, A. W. (1990). Accounting for delusional misidentifications. *British Journal of Psychiatry, 157*, 239–248.

Frazer, S. J., & Roberts, J. M. (1994). Three cases of Capgras' syndrome. *British Journal of Psychiatry, 164*, 557–559.

Josephs, K. A. (2007). Capgras syndrome and its relationship to neurodegenerative disease. *Archives of Neurology, 64*(12), 1762–1766.

Mendez, M. F. (1992). Delusional misidentification of persons in dementia. *British Journal of Psychiatry, 160*, 414–416.

Todd, J., Dewhurst, K., & Wallis, G. (1981). The syndrome of Capgras. *British Journal of Psychiatry, 39*, 319–327.

CAUSALGIA

DESCRIPTION

Causalgia, also known as complex regional pain syndrome Type 2, is a chronic, progressive, peripheral neuralgia. It differs from complex regional pain syndrome Type 1, or reflex sympathetic dystrophy, in that causalgia presents with damage to the nerve. Causalgia is frequently caused by an illness, traumatic injury, or as a side effect of surgery. Patients with causalgia often report burning sensations in their extremities and are extremely sensitive to even the lightest touch or draft of air (Ropper & Brown, 2005). Prognosis for causalgia is good if treatment is begun before the neuralgia can spread. However, if left untreated, permanent nerve, muscle, and bone damage may occur.

NEUROPATHOLOGY/PATHOPHYSIOLOGY

The pathophysiology of causalgia is not known, although the cause of the disorder is thought to be related to an electrical short circuit in the peripheral nerves. Recent research on the effects of neurotransmitters has led to the belief that the disorder is chemically based, rather than electrically. One prevailing theory that implicates peripheral nerves holds that abnormal sensitivity to adrenergic neurotransmitters develops in the injured nerve endings responsible for the perception of pain. Pain signals in the nerve are then constantly triggered by neurotransmitters secreted at the site or circulating around the nerve. Proponents of a central nervous system pathophysiology propose that continuous afferent activity from the extremities sensitizes the central nervous system (Ropper & Brown, 2005).

Functional magnetic resonance imaging findings of patients with causalgia reveal diffuse activation in contralateral primary somatosensory and motor cortices, parietal association cortices, bilateral secondary somatosensory cortex, insular cortex, frontal cortices, and anterior and posterior parts of the cingulate cortex (Peyron et al., 2004). This indicates that causalgia involves pain, motor, and cognitive processing areas of the brain (Maihofner, Handwerker, & Birklein, 2006).

NEUROPSYCHOLOGICAL/CLINICAL PRESENTATION

Causalgia does not in and of itself have any neuropsychological symptoms. However, chronic pain has been shown to cause cognitive deficits (Apkarian et al., 2004). Working memory and attention are adversely affected by chronic pain. These deficits are not alleviated by administration of short-term localized analgesics (Dick & Rashiq, 2007). In addition, processing and executive function are two of the other most commonly affected neuropsychological domains (Martelli, Zasler, Bender, & Nicholson, 2004).

DIAGNOSIS

There is no test to directly diagnose causalgia; rather, diagnosis is typically based on symptomatology. Due to the differentiation between causalgia from reflex sympathetic dystrophy, causalgia is usually suspected after a traumatic injury. In addition, neuropathy is often seen not only in the damaged nerve, but also throughout the affected region. Increased sensitivity to both painful and nonpainful stimuli in the periphery is a hallmark sign of the disorder. The fingers, toes, palms of the hands, and soles of the feet are most commonly affected. Edema and sweating are also seen at the site of the nerve damage. Abnormal skin blood flow in the region causes irregular skin temperature as well as shiny and smooth or scaly and discolored skin (Bruehl et al., 1999).

A combination of technique is used to confirm the diagnosis of causalgia. Temperature changes due to abnormal blood flow can be seen through thermographic images of the affected areas. Results of quantitative sweat tests have also shown to be related to the clinical presentation of causalgia (Sandroni et al., 1998). The severe pain experienced often leads to disuse of the affected limb. Through lack of use, muscles atrophy and bones become less dense. Although not a direct symptom of causalgia, X-rays, bone scans, and electromyography are frequently used to detect changes in the density of the bone and in the electrical signals within the muscles.

Diagnosis of causalgia is also often based on ruling out other conditions. Vascular abnormalities, inflammatory diseases, neuropathies, diseases of the spine, and tumors should all be ruled out. Specific disorders within these categories should be examined depending where the pain is located (Burton, Bruehl, & Harden, 2005).

TREATMENT

Treatment of causalgia involves combining a number of different treatment modalities. Pharmacologically, local anesthetics are often used to treat the acute symptoms of causalgia (Devers & Galer, 2000). Antidepressants, anti-inflammatories, alpha- and beta-blockers, and drugs designed specifically for the treatment of neuropathic pain are used to treat the chronic symptoms (Ropper & Brown, 2005). Recently, ketamine has been used experimentally to treat causalgia. Results are promising although future research and approval from the FDA is required before it can be used clinically (Correll, Maleki, Gracely, Muir, & Harbut, 2004).

Surgical techniques can be helpful for pain modulation. Spinal cord stimulators can be implanted to help reduce pain. They directly stimulate the spinal cord and long-term follow-up has shown them to be effective (Kemler, De Vet, Barendse, Van Den Wildenberg, & Van Kleef, 2004). Drug pumps are also occasionally implanted. They allow medication to be directly released into the cerebrospinal fluid so that more of the medication reaches the affected area through administration of a lower dose.

Nerve pain often causes the patient to stop using the affected limb, which leads to the progression of the neuropathy. As a result, physical therapy is an integral part of the treatment process to slow, or even reverse, the spread of causalgia. Research has demonstrated that high intensity and long duration physical therapy yields the best outcomes (Lee et al., 2002).

In addition to the medical treatments, psychotherapy plays a role in recovery from causalgia. The majority of the research has been conducted with cognitive behavioral therapy, and results have been promising (Lee et al., 2002). Relaxation techniques, hypnosis, and neurofeedback are also frequently parts of the treatment regimen for causalgia (Gainer, 1992).

Daniel L. Frisch
Charles Golden

Apkarian, A. V., Sosa, Y., Krauss, B. R., Thomas, P. S., Fredrickson, B. E., Levy, R. E., et al. (2004). Chronic pain patients are impaired on an emotional decision-making task. *Pain, 108*(1–2), 129–136.

Bruehl, S., Harden, R. N., Galer, B. S., Saltz, S., Bertram, M., Backonja, M., et al. (1999). External validation of IASP diagnostic criteria for Complex Regional Pain Syndrome and proposed research diagnostic criteria. *Pain, 81*(1–2), 147–154.

Burton, A. W., Bruehl, S., & Harden, R. N. (2005). Current diagnosis and therapy of complex regional pain syndrome: Refining diagnostic criteria and therapeutic options. *Expert Review of Neurotherapies, 5*(5), 643–651.

Correll, G. E., Maleki, J., Gracely, E. J., Muir, J. J., & Harbut, R. E. (2004). Subanesthetic ketamine infusion therapy: A retrospective analysis of a novel therapeutic approach to complex regional pain syndrome. *Pain Medicine, 5*(3), 263–275.

Devers, A., & Galer, B. S. (2000). Topical lidocaine patch relieves a variety of neuropathic pain conditions: An 0open-label study. *Clinical Journal of Pain, 16*(3), 205–208.

Dick, B. D., & Rashiq, S. (2007). Disruption of attention and working memory traces in individuals with chronic pain. *Anesthesia and Analgesia, 104*(5), 1223–1229.

Gainer, M. J. (1992). Hypnotherapy for reflex sympathetic dystrophy. *American Journal of Clinical Hypnosis, 34*(4), 227–232.

Kemler, M. A., De Vet, H. C., Barendse, G. A., Van Den Wildenberg, F. A., & Van Kleef, M. (2004). The effect of spinal cord stimulation in patients with chronic reflex sympathetic dystrophy: Two years' follow-up of the randomized controlled trial. *Annals of Neurology, 55*(1), 13–18.

Lee, B. H., Scharff, L., Sethna, N. F., McCarthy, C. F., Scott-Sutherland, J., Shea, A. M., et al. (2002). Physical therapy and cognitive-behavioral treatment for complex regional pain syndromes. *Journal of Pediatrics, 141*(1), 135–140.

Maihofner, C., Handwerker, H. O., & Birklein, F. (2006). Functional imaging of allodynia in complex regional pain syndrome. *Neurology, 66*(5), 711–771.

Martelli, M. F., Zasler, N. D., Bender, M. C., & Nicholson, K. (2004). Psychological, neuropsychological, and medical considerations in assessment and management of pain. *Journal of Head Trauma Rehabilitation, 19*(1), 10–28.

Peyron, R., Schneider, F., Faillenot, I., Convers, P., Barral, F. G., Garcia-Larrea, L., et al. (2004). An fMRI study of cortical representation of mechanical allodynia in patients with neuropathic pain. *Neurology, 63*(10), 1838–1846.

Ropper, A. H., & Brown, R. H. (2005). *Adams and Victor's principles of neurology* (8th ed.). New York: McGraw-Hill.

Sandroni, P., Low, P. A., Ferrer, T., Opfer-Gehrking, T. L., Willner, C. L., & Wilson, P. R. (1998). Complex regional pain syndrome I (CRPS I): Prospective study and laboratory evaluation. *Clinical Journal of Pain, 14*(4), 282–289.

C

CENTRAL CORD SYNDROME

DESCRIPTION

Central cord syndrome (CCS) is an incomplete cervical spinal cord injury characterized by a disproportionately greater amount of motor impairment in the upper extremities versus the lower extremities. Symptoms typically include loss of fine motor control and movements in the arms and hands but relatively less impairment of leg movements. A variable amount of sensory loss below the site injury and bladder dysfunction is also commonly associated with CCS. The overall functional impairment is dependent upon the severity of the injury (Schneider, Cherry, & Pantek, 1954). CCS is one of the most common types of traumatic spinal cord injuries, accounting for approximately 9% of these injuries (McKinley, Santos, Meade, & Brooke, 2007). Although CCS can occur in persons of any age due to various etiologies, injury mechanisms, and predisposing factors, CCS may develop in older persons over the age of 50 due to cervical spondylosis, a chronic degenerative condition marked by the gradual weakening and deterioration of the vertebrae and discs, causing the compression of the spinal cord (McCormack & Weinstein, 1996; Schneider et al., 1954).

NEUROPATHOLOGY/PATHOPHYSIOLOGY

CCS tends to result from trauma in persons of all ages, whereas in older individuals with longstanding cervical spondylosis it is typically caused by hyperextension injuries (McCormack & Weinstein, 1996). The mechanism of injury involves the pinching of the spinal cord amid the ligamentum lavum, intervertebral disc, and posterior vertebral body osteophytes (bone spurs) resulting in compression of adjacent white matter tracts. This compression of the spinal cord leads to edema and hemorrhage, or ischemia into the centre of the spinal cord. The site of most injuries is located in the mid-to-lower cervical spinal cord. The syndrome also may be associated with a fracture-dislocation or compression fracture injury, especially among those with a congenitally narrowed spinal canal. Specific motor impairments in CCS result from the pattern of the corticospinal and spinothalamic tract lamination (Quencer et al., 1992).

NEUROPSYCHOLOGICAL/CLINICAL PRESENTATION

Due to the anatomical lamination of the corticospinal tract with the upper limb fibers medially, and the lower limb fibers laterally, the arms are affected more so than the legs. Symptoms include loss of upper extremity pain, temperature sensation, and strength. Damage to the gray matter produced by the pinching effect of osteophytes anteriorly and buckled ligamentum flavum posteriorly, produces severe flaccid lower motor neuron paralysis of fingers, hands, and arms. The more peripheral positioning of lower extremity axons within the spinal cord tracts accounts for the injury pattern. Damage to the central portion of the corticospinal and spinothalamic long tracts in the white matter produces upper motor neuron spastic paralysis of the trunk and lower extremity, causing bladder and/or bowel dysfunction, and variable loss of sensation of the lower extremities (Maroon, Abla, Wilberger, Bailes, & Sternau, 1991; Schneider et al., 1954). Some patients may develop dysphagia secondary to anterior cervical spine fusion or cervical orthoses (Alpert, 2007). Although no specific cognitive impairments are associated with CCS, secondary impairments can occur as a result of co-occurring traumatic brain injury.

DIAGNOSIS

A complete neurological examination, a thorough history, and brain and cervical spine imaging will facilitate the diagnosis of CCS and will help to rule out other syndromes or types of injuries (e.g., Bell's cruciate paralysis, bilateral brachial plexus injury, cervical root avulsion [Alpert, 2007]). MRI can provide direct evidence of spinal cord impingement from bone, disc, or hematoma (Dai, 2001) and CT can identify spinal canal compromise and facilitates indirect approximation of the degree of spinal cord impingement. X-rays can identify the structure of the vertebrae and the outline of the joints and can delineate fractures and dislocations, as well as the degree and extent of spondylitic changes. Flexion/extension views in CT scans and X-rays can assist in evaluation of ligamentous stability (Song, Mizuno, Inoue, & Nakagawa, 2006).

TREATMENT

There is no cure for CCS or even a standard course of treatment. However, rehabilitative therapy, medication and pain management, rest, and in some circumstances surgery are typical interventions to improve the quality of life in patients with CCS (Roth, Lawler, & Yarkony, 1990). Physical therapy focuses on the preservation of range of motion, enhancement of mobility skills, and strengthening of any preserved lower extremity and trunk functions for improved balance and stabilization. Occupational therapy addresses the upper extremity weakness and the restoration of basic activities of daily living. Surface electromyelogram (EMG) biofeedback can help patients to isolate specific weak muscles in the upper extremities. For patients presenting with dysphagia, speech therapy can address swallowing problems to prevent aspiration as well as improving speech (Alpert, 2007; Tow & Kong, 1998). Surgery can be beneficial in individuals with persistent compression of the spinal cord and ongoing neurological deterioration (Chen et al., 1997).

Darla J. Lawson

Alpert, M. (2007). Central cord syndrome. *EMedicine.* Retrieved March 12, 2009, from http://www.emedicine.medscape.com/article/321907-media

Chen, T. Y., Lee, S. T., Lui, T. N., Wong, C. W., Yeh, Y. S., Tzaan, W. C., et al. (1997). Efficacy of surgical treatment in traumatic central cord syndrome. *Surgical Neurology, 48*(5), 435–440.

Dai, L. (2001). Magnetic resonance imaging of acute central cord syndrome: Correlation with prognosis. *Chinese Medical Sciences Journal, 16*(2), 107–110.

Maroon, J. C., Abla, A. A., Wilberger, J. I., Bailes, J. E., & Sternau, L. (1991). Central cord syndrome. *Clinical Neurosurgery, 37*, 612–621.

McCormack, B. M., & Weinstein, P. R. (1996). Cervical spondylosis: An update. *Western Journal of Medicine, 165*(1–2), 43–51.

McKinley, W., Santos, K., Meade, M., & Brooke, K. (2007). Incidence and outcomes of spinal cord injury clinical syndromes. *Journal of Spinal Cord Medicine, 30*(3), 215–224.

Quencer, R. M., Bunge, R. P., Egnor, M., Green, B. A., Puckett, W., Naidich, T. P., et al. (1992). Acute traumatic central cord syndrome: MRI-pathological correlations. *Neuroradiology, 34*(2), 85–94.

Roth, E. J., Lawler, M. H., & Yarkony, G. M. (1990). Traumatic central cord syndrome: Clinical features and functional outcomes. *Archives of Physical Medicine and Rehabilitation, 71*(1), 18–23.

Schneider, R. C., Cherry, G., & Pantek, H. (1954). The syndrome of acute central cervical spinal cord injury; with special reference to the mechanisms involved in hyperextension injuries of cervical spine. *Journal of Neurosurgery, 11*(6), 546–577.

Song, J., Mizuno, J., Inoue, T., & Nakagawa, H. (2006). Clinical evaluation of traumatic central cord syndrome: Emphasis on clinical significance of prevertebral hyperintensity, cord compression, and intramedullary high-signal intensity on magnetic resonance imaging. *Surgical Neurology, 65*(2), 117–123.

Tow, A. M., & Kong, K. H. (1998). Central cord syndrome: Functional outcome after rehabilitation. *Spinal Cord, 36*(3), 156–160.

CENTRAL PONTINE MYELINOLYSIS AND EXTRAPONTINE MYELINOLYSIS

DESCRIPTION

Central pontine myelinolysis (CPM) is a neurological disorder that most commonly arises from rapid correction of hyponatremia (Estol, Faris, Martinez, Ahdab-Barmada, 1989; Ghidoni, Di Bella, Masini, Paone, & Matturri, 1994). This rapid correction causes a homeostatic shift that eventually results in myelinolysis. Although a variety of areas have shown susceptibility to this process, the pons has demonstrated particular susceptibility. The term central pontine myelinolysis arises from the anatomical finding of internal (i.e., central) demyelination of the pons with a relatively preserved rim of white matter. When more expansive demyelination occurs in addition to this central region, often involving the basal ganglia, as well as other regions, the presentation is termed *extrapontine myelinolysis* (EPM).

Approximately 24–72 hours after the abrupt correction of hyponatremia, individuals manifest initial symptoms that commonly involve dysphagia and dysarthria in addition to potential weakening of voluntary motor strength. Over the course of the following days to weeks, motor deficits may increase to widespread weakness and rigidity preventing ambulation. Sensation may also be diminished. Locked-in syndrome and death are possible in severe cases.

Adams, Victor, and Mancall (1959) are attributed with the identification of the presentation following their summary of four cases observed between 1950 and 1959. The presentations name arose from the distinctive pathological picture of pontine-only demyelination while other areas were spared. The understanding of the mechanism by which this occurs was determined later, although some aspects of the process remains unknown.

The presentations have not been linked with any genetic marker, making individuals more susceptible to the presentation. No sex differences exist and both adults and children may develop the presentation (McKee, Winkelman, & Banker, 1988). However, other studies have identified possible risk factors for CPM and EPM including malnutrition often resulting from chronic alcoholism or an eating disorder, orthotopic liver transplant, dialysis, and hepatic encephalopathy (Amann, Schafer, Sterr, Arnold, & Grunze, 2001; Lawson & Niedermeyer, 2002; Lee et al., 2009; Ozgur-Ilhan, Demirbas, Yalcin, Yucesan, & Dogan, 2005). Although the majority of individuals improve over the course of several months, some are left with persisting deficits.

NEUROPATHOLOGY/PATHOPHYSIOLOGY

Rapid correction of hyponatremia serves as the primary mechanism by which CPM or EPM develop, although others suggest a possible role of hypoxia (Lee, Cheung, Lau, Mak, & Li, 2003). At the point of correction for hyponatremia, high doses of sodium serve to draw water out of brain cells and cause associated movement of small molecules. This initiates a demyelinating process to which the pons is particularly susceptible. Consequently, those at risk receive a rapid increase of serum sodium levels. In particular, chronic alcoholics, burn victims, anorexics or bulimics, and those undergoing dialysis are at higher risk. In addition, use of diuretics can increase risk when used in excess.

On autopsy, lesions vary in size with the largest occupying almost the entire pons. The center of the pons is characterized by a rim of intact myelin that surrounds a grayish center and demonstrates fine granularity. On microscopic examination, demyelination is seen throughout the lesion whereas axons and nerve cells of the pontine nuclei remain spared. Phagocytes and glial cells remain reactive in the demyelinated area whereas oligodendrocytes are depleted (Ropper & Brown, 2005). In addition, lesions to the corticospinal tract, corticobulbar tract, and the pontocerebellar tracts have been proposed as potential areas of associated damage secondary to CPM and EPM as well (Lee et al., 2003).

As suggested, in the case of CPM, the lesions remain confined within the central pons; however, extension to and involvement of other structures can be observed resulting in an associated EPM. When this occurs, it most commonly involves the medial lemniscus and/or other tegmental structures as well as basal ganglion areas, although it may also involve the midbrain in severe cases (Ropper & Brown, 2005). Wright et al. (1979) when discussing cases of EPM reported potential widespread lesioning of the diencephalon structures, internal capsule, corpus callosum, striatum, amygdala, cerebellum, and white and gray matter of the cortex.

Advances in neuroimaging have made visualization of CPM and EPM more readily possible. The characteristic pattern of CPM consists of a bat-wing lesion of the pons that may be observed as early as 2–3 days following symptom onset. This is seen as brightness on T2-weighted imaging. EPM is marked by the general finding of CPM in combination with more extensive foci of demyelination that develops rapidly in response to hyponatremic correction and is not better explained by other "acute" demyelinating processes such as multiple sclerosis.

NEUROPSYCHOLOGICAL/CLINICAL PRESENTATION

Clinical presentation is largely based on motor deficits in CPM although sensory symptoms may be observed in more moderate to severe cases. Residual systems are generally consistent with the anatomical origin or impairment. Over the first few days, patients gradually develop bilateral paralysis of upper and lower extremities in conjunction with dysarthria and dysphagia. These symptoms may become so severe that individuals often appear to be presenting with a locked-in syndrome in which voluntary movement and speech is severely compromised. However, throughout all degrees of severity, voluntary eye movements remain generally intact.

Although cognitive and emotional impairments are not often thought of as potential sequelae of CPM and EPM given the anatomical location, the few studies examining cognitive deficits secondary to CPM and EPM have indeed demonstrated evidence of significant deficit (Lee et al., 2003; Price & Mesulam, 1987; Soek, Lee, Kang, & Park, 2007). Lee et al. (2003) identified global cognition and impaired higher cortical functions. Frontal striatal dysfunction has been reported in EPM , presumably due to involvement of the basal ganglia (Seok, Lee, Kang, & Park, 2007). Specifically, Seok et al. (2007) reported evidence of significant deficits related to attention, confrontational naming, aspects of both verbal and visual memory, visuospatial ability and, in general, executive functions in a case report of a 69-year-old man with EPM in the absence of CPM. Lee et al. reported evidence of global executive function impairment, including poor mental flexibility, significant perseveration, and poor visual fluency in a patient with CPM. Deficits related to aspects of visuospatial ability, simple directed verbal attention, and general processing speed were also reported whereas verbal list learning appeared to be relatively spared in their patient (Lee et al., 2003).

Theories abound in terms of explaining this with the authors themselves suggesting the potential role of corticopontine networks, including upstream transmission to the dorsolateral prefrontal area and dopaminergic and cholinergic pathways, which have all been established in the literature (Schmahmann & Pandya, 1997; Torack & Morris, 1988; Williams, Murphy, Reynolds, Welch, & King, 1996). Given the presence of relatively extensive neurological lesions

C

seen in patients with EPM in comparison with CPM, these patients typically demonstrate greater cognitive and emotional impairment relative to patients with CPM alone.

DIAGNOSIS

Diagnosis involves a combination of clinical examination, neurological workup, and a history. As patients present with the aforementioned motor deficits, bilaterally expressed, CT and/or MRI are indicated. This is necessary to evaluate for the possibility of symptoms arising from an acute cerebrovascular event with particular attention given to the areas supplying posterior circulation. Upon ruling out cerebrovascular accident (CVA), simultaneous evaluation of the pons on MRI in conjunction with record review to determine the patient's sodium level at initial presentation as well as the intervention provided is recommended. Aforementioned clinical symptoms arising following rapid correction of hyponatremia in the absence of a cerebrovascular event is enough to suggest probable CPM. MRI may then be used to confirm the diagnosis, but it may not be achieved until 2–3 days following symptom onset. In the case of EPM, more widespread foci are observed in addition to pontine involvement. However, it is largely distinguished from presentations such as multiple sclerosis from a historical standpoint (i.e., the patient did not present with the symptoms or findings, rather they developed following the aforementioned intervention).

TREATMENT

The most appropriate intervention for both CPM and EPM has been good prevention. When individuals present with hyponatremia, specific guidelines should be followed to gradually and effectively raise serum sodium levels. This correction should be by no more than 10 mEq/L in the initial 24 hours and no more than 21mEq/L in the following 48 hours (Karp & Laureno, 1993). In those instances where CPM or EPM develop, treatment is primarily supportive as no treatment after the fact has proven to be consistently effective. Physical and occupational therapy is often recommended as is speech therapy. Recovery is variable and often protracted. Although some individuals may experience near complete spontaneous remission of symptoms, the majority present with chronic dysfunction of varying levels of severity. In the most severe cases, patients may exhibit permanent locked-in syndrome, coma, or death.

Chad A. Noggle
Jon C. Thompson

Adams, R. D., Victor, M., & Mancall, E. L. (1959). Central pontine myelinolysis. *Archives of Neurology and Psychiatry, 81,* 154.

Amann, B., Schafer, M., Sterr, A. Arnold, S., & Grunze, H. (2001). Central pontine myelinolysis in a patient with anorexia nervosa. *International Journal of Eating Disorders, 30*(4), 462–466.

Estol, C. J., Faris, A. A., Martinez, A. J., Ahdab-Barmada, M. (1989). Central pontine myelinolysis after liver transplantation. *Neurology, 39,* 493–498.

Ghidoni, P., Di Bella, C., Masini, T., Paone, G., & Matturri, L. (1994). Central pontine and extrapontine myelinolysis after orthotopic liver transplantation. *Transplantation Proceedings, 26,* 3602–3603.

Karp, B. I., & Laureno, R. (1993). Pontine and extrapontine myelinolysis: A neurologic disorder following rapid correction of hyponatremia. *Medicine, 72,* 359.

Lawson, A., & Niedermeyer, E. (2002). Central pontine myelinolysis: Clinical and EEG considerations. *American Journal of Electroneurodiagnostic Technology, 42*(3), 151–158.

Lee, E. M., Kang, J. K., Yun, S., Kim, K., Kim, S. J., Hwang, K., & Lee, S. (2009). Risk factors for central pontine and extrapontine myelinolysis following orthotopic liver transplantation. *European Neurology, 62,* 362–368.

Lee, T. M., Cheung, C. C., Lau, E. Y., Mak, A., & Li, L. S. (2003). Cognitive and emotional dysfunction after central pontine myelinolysis. *Behavioral Neurology, 14,* 103–107.

McKee, A. C., Winkelman, M. D., & Banker, B. Q. (1988). Central pontine myelinolysis in severely burned patients: Relationship to serum hyperosmolality. *Neurology, 38,* 1211.

Ozgur-Ilhan, I., Demirbas, H., Yalcin, G. A., Yucesan, C., & Dogan, Y. B. (2005). Alcoholic case of central pontine myelinolysis with mainly cerebellar signs. *European Addiction Research, 11,* 155–156.

Price, B. H., & Mesulam, M. M. (1987). Behavioral manifestations of central pontine myelinolysis. *Archives of Neurology, 44,* 671–673.

Ropper, A. H., & Brown, R. J. (2005). *Adams and Victor's principles of neurology* (8th ed., pp. 959–982). New York: McGraw-Hill.

Schmahmann, J. D., & Pandya, D. N. (1997). Anatomic organization of the basilar pontine projections from prefrontal cortices in rhesus monkey. *Journal of Neuroscience, 17,* 438–458.

Seok, J. I., Lee, D. K., Kang, M. G., & Park, J. H. (2007). Neuropsychological findings of extrapontine myelinolysis without central pontine myelinolysis. *Behavioural Neurology, 18,* 131–134.

Torack, R., & Morris, J. (1988). The association of ventral tegmental area histopathology with adult dementia. *Archives of Neurology, 45,* 497–501.

Williams, J. B., Murphy, D. M., Reynolds, K. E., Welch, S. J., & King, M. S. (1996). Demonstration of a bilateral projection from the rostral nucleus of the solitary tract to the medial parabrachial nucleus in the rat. *Brain Research 737*, 231–237.

Wright, D.G., Laureano, R., & Victor, M. (1979). Pontine ad extrapotine myelinolysis. *Brain*, 10, 361

CEREBELLAR HYPOPLASIA

DESCRIPTION

The diagnosis of cerebellar hypoplasia, made as early as 1940, was based primarily on clinical and postmortem findings (deSouza, Chaudhuri, Bingham, & Cox, 1993). Norman (1940) reported the clinical and pathological findings in two patients with primary atrophy of the granular layer of the cerebellum; the remarkable feature was the small size of the cerebellum. Cerebellar hypoplasia has been further studied and is now considered a neurological developmental disorder distinguished by the underdevelopment or incomplete development of the cerebellum. Evidence has shown that cerebellar hypoplasia may occur sporadically or may have a genetic link. The cerebellum is integral in controlling many functions, therefore cerebellar hypoplasia may cause developmental delay, hypotonia, ataxia, seizures, mental retardation, and involuntary eye movements (nystagmus). Cerebellar hypoplasia may also be related to headaches, vertigo, imbalance, and hearing impairment later in life.

NEUROPATHOLOGY/PATHOPHYSIOLOGY

The proposed mechanism for cerebellar hypoplasia is in utero vascular compromise with hypoplastic posterior circulation structures due to associated craniovertebral junction anomalies (Tabarki, Al-Malki, & Al-Ghamdi, 2007). According to Stagno et al. (1982), cerebellar hypoplasia is known to occur in congenital cytomegalovirus infection due to maternal infection in the first trimester. Diffuse cerebellar hypoplasia occurs in a wide variety of neurological and systemic disorders, in most of which it is only one of many characteristic features. It may be associated with an uncommon neurological syndrome with autosomal recessive inheritance or may be sporadic (deSouza et al., 1993).

Cerebellar hypoplasia may be found with other structural brain abnormalities such as absence of the corpus callosum or communicating hydrocephalus. The brainstem, especially the pons, may be atrophic in association with cerebellar hypoplasia (deSouza et al., 1993). According to deSouza et al. (1993), clinical features help differentiate cerebellar hypoplasia associated with such diverse disorders as spinal muscular atrophy, Tay-Sachs' disease, Menke's disease, and Leber's congenital amaurosis.

NEUROPSYCHOLOGICAL/CLINICAL PRESENTATION

The cerebellum has traditionally been conceptualized as being involved predominantly in motor control (Gilman, 1992). The existence of acquired cerebellar lesions in various disease states has established that the cerebellum plays an integral role in posture maintenance and in the execution of smoothly controlled movements (Shevell & Majnemer, 1996). Functional involvement of the cerebellum beyond traditional concepts of motor control and coordination has been provided by demonstration in both imaging and pathologic studies of selective hypoplasia and hyperplasia of regional cerebellar structures in patients with autism (Courchesne, Townsend, & Saitoh, 1994). Shevell and Majnemer (1996) postulate that the cerebellum may play a role in normal cognitive, social, and language development, though this has yet to be clearly defined. According to a study by Shevell and Majnemer (1996), the developmental delay in regard to cerebellar hypoplasia in their patient population was not limited merely to motor findings but extended in variable degree to speech/language, social, cognitive, and attentional domains. Therefore, the cerebellum is now believed to have a much larger role in overall functioning than was once thought.

Cerebellar hypoplasia is considered a fairly rare condition; however, this disorder has been shown to occur concomitantly with severe visual loss, ataxia, mental retardation, Joubert syndrome, Dandy-Walker syndrome, Walker-Warburg syndrome, and Williams syndrome. According to Parmeggiani, Posar, and Scaduto (2008), cerebellar congenital abnormalities represent a risk factor for epileptic seizure occurrence and/or cognitive and behavior disorders; mental retardation and autism are more frequent in cases with cerebellar hypoplasia as well.

As indicated by the National Institutes of Neurological Disorders and Stroke (NINDS) (2007), cerebellar hypoplasia is a feature of a number of congenital malformation syndromes present at birth, such as Williams syndrome, and some of the neurodegenerative disorders that begin in early childhood, such as ataxia telangiectasia. In an infant or young child, symptoms of a disorder that features cerebellar hypoplasia might include floppy muscle tone, developmental or speech delay, problems with walking and balance, seizures, mental retardation, and involuntary side-to-side movements of the eyes. In an older child, symptoms might include headache, dizzy spells, clumsiness, and hearing impairment.

DIAGNOSIS

Technological advances have significantly enhanced the clinician's ability to ascertain an underlying etiology of the disorder. Most frequently, a cerebral malformation will be documented: one which often is not suspected on clinical grounds alone (Majenemer & Shevell, 1995). Technological advances also offer the hope of greater diagnostic precision, permitting the identification of particular subtypes of developmental delay unified by clinical, genetic, imaging, and natural history factors (Shevell & Majnemer, 1996).

MRI clearly documents the size of the cerebellum and any associated abnormalities, providing accurate diagnosis in individual patients and allowing for genetic counseling. This then gives a better appreciation of the prognosis for the patient (deSouza et al., 1993), though the prognosis for each patient will vary based on the underlying etiology of symptoms. Some of the disorders that are associated with cerebellar hypoplasia are progressive, which means the condition will worsen over time, and will most likely have a poor prognosis. Other disorders that feature cerebellar hypoplasia are not progressive, such as those that are the result of abnormal brain formation during fetal development, and might have a better outcome (NINDS, 2007).

TREATMENT

There is currently no universally recommended course of treatment for patients suffering from cerebellar hypoplasia. Current treatment procedures include treating the underlying symptoms caused by cerebellar hypoplasia. The NINDS conducts research related to cerebellar hypoplasia and its associated disorders in its laboratories at the National Institutes of Health and also supports additional research through grants to major medical institutions across the country. Much of this research focuses on finding better ways to prevent, treat, and ultimately cure disorders that feature cerebellar hypoplasia (NINDS, 2007).

Justin Boseck
Raymond S. Dean

Courchesne, E., Townsend, J., & Saitoh, O. (1994). The brain in infantile autism: Posterior fossa structures are abnormal. *Neurology, 44*, 214–223.

deSouza, N., Chaudhuri, R., Bingham, J., & Cox, T. (1993). MRI in cerebellar hypoplasia. *Neuroradiology, 36*, 148–151.

Gilman, S. (1992). Cerebellum and motor dysfunction. In A. Asbury, G. M. McKhann, & W. I. McDonald (Eds.), *Diseases of the nervous system: Clinical neurobiology*. Philadelphia: W.B. Saunders.

Majnemer, A., & Shevell, M. I. (1995). Diagnostic yield of the neurological assessment of the globally delayed child. *Journal of Pediatrics, 127*, 193–199.

National Institute of Neurological Disorders and Stroke. (2007, December). *NINDS cerebellar hypoplasia information sheet*. Retrieved April 4, 2009, from NINDS via: http://www.ninds.nih.gov/disorders/cerebellar_hypoplasia/cerebellar_hypoplasia.htm

Norman, R. M. (1940). Primary degeneration of the granular cell layer of the cerebellum: An unusual form of familial cerebellar atrophy occurring in early life. *Brain, 63*, 365–379.

Parmeggiani, A., Posar, A., & Scaduto, M. C. (2008). Cerebellar hypoplasia, continuous spike-waves during sleep, and neuropsychological and behavioral disorders. *Journal of Child Neurology, 23*(12), 1472–1476.

Shevell, M. I., & Majnemer, A. (1996). Clinical features of developmental disability associated with cerebellar hypoplasia. *Pediatric Neurology, 15*(3), 224–229.

Stagno, S., Pass, R. F., Dworsky, M. E., Henderson, R. E., Moore, E. G., Walton, P. D., et al. (1982). Congenital CMV infection, the relative importance of primary and recurrent maternal infection. *New England Journal of Medicine, 306*, 945–949.

Tabarki, B., Al-Malki, S., & Al-Ghamdi, H. (2007). Severe cerebellar hypoplasia associated with osteogenesis imperfect Type III. *Journal of Pediatrics, 151*, 325.

CEREBRAL ANOXIA/HYPOXIA

DESCRIPTION

Although often used interchangeably, cerebral *anoxia* is defined as the complete lack of oxygen supply to tissue or in the arterial blood, whereas *hypoxia* is decreased oxygen supply to tissue. *Hypoxemia* occurs when oxygen saturation is reduced in the arterial blood. Although the most common cause of cerebral anoxia is cardiac arrest, other etiologies include obstructive sleep apnea (OSA), chronic obstructive pulmonary disease, carbon monoxide (CO) poisoning, attempted hanging, suffocation, exposure to high altitudes, near drowning, acute respiratory distress syndrome, asthma, and cardiac disease or surgery.

NEUROPATHOLOGY/PATHOPHYSIOLOGY

More so than any other organ, the brain requires an abundant and continuous supply of oxygen. Although it comprises less than 2.5% of total body weight, it utilizes 20% of the body's total oxygen consumption at rest (Greenfield, 1997). Oxygen is primarily transported to the brain via hemoglobin. Therefore, either reduced blood flow to the brain or reduced oxygen content in the blood can produce an anoxic or hypoxic state. When blood circulation is normal, the percentage of oxygen saturation of the hemoglobin molecule is the most essential component for adequate oxygen supply to the brain.

There are two main mechanisms of anoxic/hypoxic brain injury: (1) a circulatory deficiency that reduces the amount of arterial oxygen to the brain, resulting in an *ischemic hypoxia* and (2) oxygen deficiency in the red blood cells, resulting in an *anemic hypoxia*. Given that perfusion failure, or an *ischemia*, is one common cause of anoxia/hypoxia, the terms "anoxia," "hypoxia," and "ischemia" are often used interchangeably (Caine & Watson, 2000). When oxygen supply to the brain is disrupted, regulatory mechanisms are activated that work to maintain cerebral blood flow. With sustained oxygen deprivation, however, these regulatory mechanisms become exhausted and the potential for brain damage occurs. At the neuronal level, damage occurs secondary to the release of excitatory neurotransmitters that cause an influx of sodium, resulting in cellular swelling and injury. More irreversible damage, including cell death, is attributed to massive calcium overloading (White, Wiegenstein, & Winegar, 1984) that can occur by way of ionic pump failure due to energy failure or excessive release of excitatory neurotransmitters (e.g., glutamate) resulting in excitotoxicity (Hopkins & Bigler, 2008).

There has been much discussion on the selective vulnerability of different areas of the brain to cerebral anoxia. Although hippocampal damage has been long regarded as the prototypical injury from anoxia, a review of 43 cases of cerebral anoxia by Caine and Watson (2000) found that the hippocampus was the sole affected structure in only 8 of the 43 cases (18%), whereas 31 cases had lesions in either the pallidum, striatum, or both. In other reports, the hippocampus, basal ganglia, thalamus, neocortex, cerebellum, primary visual cortex, and "watershed zones" have been identified as being the most vulnerable areas

(e.g., Hopkins & Bigler, 2008). Generally, it is accepted that the neuropathological outcomes of anoxia are highly variable and depend, in part, upon the specific etiology. For instance, anoxia secondary to high-altitude exposure or CO poisoning can affect brain regions that are more resistant to other types of anoxia, such as that secondary to cardiac arrest or sudden asphyxia (Lampert, 1961).

In their review of neuroradiological studies, Caine and Watson (2000) found that edema or atrophy of the cerebrum was the most common finding, occurring in 40 of the 90 cases reviewed. Changes were also noted in the cerebral and cerebellar cortices, caudate, lentiform nuclei, and thalamus. Interestingly, only two cases showed isolated hippocampal abnormalities.

NEUROPSYCHOLOGICAL/CLINICAL PRESENTATION

Given that cerebral anoxia/hypoxia can come by way of several different mechanisms of injury, the pathological outcomes and pattern of neuropsychological deficits can also be highly varied. Both generalized and focal impairment can be observed. With milder cases, symptoms may include difficulties with attention, new learning, motor coordination, cyanosis, and increased heart rate. Continued oxygen deprivation results in loss of consciousness, coma, seizures, and brain death.

Despite recent evidence that the hippocampus may not be the most selectively vulnerable brain structure, memory problems remain the most common sequelae following anoxic/hypoxic injuries. In a review of 67 cases, Caine and Watson (2000) found that an amnesic syndrome was the most frequently cited disturbance, reported in 36 of the 67 cases (54%). Anterograde memory loss was recorded in all 67 cases. In addition to memory, other common domains of neurocognitive impairment include executive functions (Devine, Kirkley, Palumbo, & White, 2002; Parkinson et al., 2002), language (see Caine & Watson, 2000 for a review), visuospatial abilities (e.g., Parkinson et al., 2002), and estimated baseline intellect (e.g., Bigler & Alfano, 1988; Dunham & Johnstone, 1999).

Personality changes and behavioral difficulties are also frequently observed sequelae. Among the 67 individual cases reviewed by Caine and Watson (2000), 31 (46.2%) had changes in personality and behavior, with emotional lability and impulsivity being the most commonly endorsed changes. Other reported symptoms include irritability, disinhibition, loss of judgment, apathy, flattened affect, and loss of initiative. Of note, the onset of personality and emotional changes can be delayed, as has been found in a

C

number of CO poisoning cases (Dunham & Johnstone, 1999).

Motor disturbances are common as well, particularly for those cases involving cerebellar damage. Sequelae include ataxia, balance and postural instability, gait disturbance, and difficulties initiating purposeful movements.

DIAGNOSIS

The etiology of anoxia/hypoxia is generally easily determined by the circumstances surrounding the injury (e.g., cardiac arrest, drowning, high-altitude exposure, etc.). Diagnosis can be more challenging with mechanisms such as CO poisoning, as the circumstances of injury may be unclear and patients commonly present with nonspecific symptoms. Given the nature of cerebral anoxia, patients are often unconscious or comatose upon discovery and require cardiopulmonary resuscitation. The exact nature and extent of cerebral damage, however, can be made via neuroimaging, EEG, and neuropsychological testing. Electrocardiograms are beneficial as well. Neuroimaging findings, however, may be normal in the initial acute stages. Caine and Watson (2000) reviewed 11 CT and MRI studies of cerebral anoxia involving a total of 90 patient cases and found that imaging was typically normal in the early acute postanoxic period. Following a prolonged anoxic episode, however, abnormalities were found to be evident as early as 24–48 hr. Gale et al. (1999) also found quantitative MRI and single photon emission computed tomography to be sensitive in identifying neuropathological changes following CO poisoning. Diagnosis of CO poisoning, in particular, is used by measuring carboxyhemoglobin levels in the venous blood using a CO oximeter, with elevated levels indicating CO poisoning.

TREATMENT

Treatment is generally dependent upon the underlying cause of the anoxia/hypoxia but is similar among the various etiologies in that the primary goal is to restore oxygen supply to the brain. Mechanical ventilation may be used with patients who are experiencing hypoxia secondary to breathing difficulties. In cases of hypoxia secondary to OSA, treatment generally involves the use of a continuous positive airway pressure machine. Oxygen supplementation is used for cases involving hypoxia secondary to high-altitude exposure. With CO poisoning, treatment typically includes 100% mask oxygen and/or hyperbaric oxygen therapy. In regard to pharmacological

interventions, a recent case study found that administration of zolpidem twice daily was effective in improving the level of alertness, speech, and gait of a patient following anoxic brain injury (Cohen & Duong, 2008). There is also emerging evidence that induced hypothermia may have neuroprotective effects and help decrease neurological deficits following cardiac arrest (Zeitzer, 2005).

Anita H. Sim
Sarah M. Viamonte

Bigler, E. D., & Alfano, M. (1988). Anoxic encephalopathy: Neuroradiological and neuropsychological findings. *Archives of Clinical Neuropsychology, 3,* 383–396.

Caine, D., & Watson, J. D. G. (2000). Neuropsychological and neuropathological sequelae of cerebral anoxia: A critical review. *Journal of the International Neuropsychological Society, 6,* 86–99.

Cohen, S. I., & Duong, T. T. (2008). Increased arousal in a patient with anoxic brain injury after administration of zolpidem. *American Journal of Physical Medicine & Rehabilitation, 87,* 229–231.

Devine, S. A., Kirkley, S. M., Palumbo, C. L., & White, R. F. (2002). MRI and neuropsychological correlates of carbon monoxide exposure: A case report. *Environmental Health Perspectives, 110,* 1051–1055.

Dunham, M. D., & Johnstone, B. (1999). Variability of neuropsychological deficits associated with carbon monoxide poisoning: Four case reports. *Brain Injury, 13,* 917–925.

Gale, S. D., Hopkins, R. O., Weaver, L. K., Bigler, E. D., Booth, E. J., & Blatter, D. D. (1999). MRI, quantitative MRI, SPECT, and neuropsychological findings following carbon monoxide poisoning. *Brain Injury, 13,* 229–243.

Greenfield, S. A. (1997). *The human brain: A guided tour.* New York: Basic Books.

Hopkins, R. O., & Bigler, E.D. (2008). Hypoxic and anoxic conditions of the CNS. In J. E. Morgan & J. H. Ricker (Eds.), *Textbook of clinical neuropsychology* (pp. 521535). New York: Taylor & Francis.

Lampert, P. (1961). Selective vulnerability of brain to anoxia. *Canadian Medical Association Journal, 84,* 1172–1176.

Parkinson, R. B., Hopkins, R. O., Cleavinger, H. B., Weaver, L. K., Victoroff, J., Foley, J. F., et al. (2002). White matter hyperintensities and neuropsychological outcome following carbon monoxide poisoning. *Neurology, 58,* 1525–1532.

White, B. C., Wiegenstein, J. G., & Winegar, C. D. (1984). Brain ischemic anoxia. *Journal of the American Medical Association, 251,* 1586–1590.

Zeitzer, M. B. (2005). Inducing hypothermia to decrease neurological deficit: Literature review. *Journal of Advanced Nursing, 52,* 189–199.

CEREBRAL ARTERIOSCLEROSIS

DESCRIPTION

Cerebral arteriosclerosis is a disease of the blood vessels that supply the brain and is a type of organic brain damage. Cerebral arteriosclerosis involves the hardening and thickening of the walls of the arteries in the brain. This thickening can be seen under a microscope (Shepherd, Lader, Wing, Wing, & Russell, 1983). The disease begins to develop between the ages of 60 and 70 with the individual suffering from heart attack or stroke within 3–4 years (Aiken, 1994). Research suggests that the condition of an individual's heart and blood vessels has a significant impact on the intactness of brain function (Hersen, Turner, & Beidel, 2007). Cerebrovascular diseases affect older adults by altering brain structure and are ultimately responsible for producing cognitive decline (Kuczynski et al., 2008). Cerebrovascular disease affects around 3 million Americans and kills approximately 150,000 in the United States per year (Aiken, 1994).

NEUROPATHOLOGY/PATHOPHYSIOLOGY

In cerebral arteriosclerosis, the walls of the arteries in the brain become thickened and the width of vessels is reduced due to fatty deposits or plaque. The plaque clogs the arteries and blocks the circulation of blood (Aiken, 1994). Without the circulation of blood due to plaque buildup, the brain is unable to get enough oxygen (Hersen et al., 2007) and other needed nutrients and vitamins, which increases the chances of artery blockage and rupture (Aiken, 1994).

If a blockage occurs in the brain, it can lead to cerebral thrombosis, or a stroke (Shepherd et al., 1983). The most common symptom experienced after a stroke is hemiplegia, or paralysis of one side of the body. A person may experience a mild stroke called a transient ischemic attack (TIA). Over time these small TIAs can lead to cognitive impairment and may result in vascular dementia (Hersen et al., 2007).

The changes in the arteries due to the hardening of the walls and the buildup of plaque can cause the development of infarction in brain tissue, brain necrosis in some areas, liquefaction, and finally cavity formation (Shepherd et al., 1983). In cerebral arteriosclerosis, cardiac arrhythmias, electrocardiographic (ECG) abnormalities, and elevated pulse have been shown to be indicators that cerebral infarcts will be exposed upon postmortem examination. (Shepherd

et al., 1983). Despite these changes to the brain, imaging of the brain shows a lack of changes in white matter. (Sahlas, Bilbao, Swartz, & Black, 2002)

NEUROPSYCHOLOGICAL/CLINICAL PRESENTATION

A number of symptoms can be present in patients with cerebral arteriosclerosis. Patients are usually between 60 and 70 years of age and tend to manifest organic brain syndrome symptoms of confusion, disorientation, incoherence, restlessness, and sometimes hallucinations. Individuals may also complain of having headaches, dizziness, and fatigue. Often any maladaptive personality characteristics and behaviors that were present before the onset of the disorder may become accentuated after the disease begins to progress. As the disorder will often eventually lead to occlusions of the arteries in the brain, patients may develop any cognitive symptom commonly seen with stroke. The most prominent of these arise from middle cerebral artery disorders that can lead to paralysis, aphasia, ataxia, and visuospatial disorders.

Dementia may also be present with cerebral arteriosclerosis. A history of stroke has been shown to be a distinguishing feature of dementia associated with cerebral arteriosclerosis (Shepherd et al., 1983). By promoting arteriosclerosis, hypertension might be the cause of a stroke and therefore is a contributing factor to the early expression of subclinical Alzheimer's disease. Hypertension predisposes an individual to cognitive decline and the development of dementia. It may impair cognitive functions and is related to the occurrence of not only Alzheimer's disease but also vascular dementia. (Kuczynski et al., 2008).

In early cases, patients may be asymptomatic. The neuropsychological and neurological symptoms do not arise until the blood flow to a given area of the brain has been significantly compromised. Due to the redundancy of the vascular system and its ability to adapt to slow changes in blood flow, a slow onset of arteriosclerosis will allow the brain to compensate until the impairment becomes more pervasive.

DIAGNOSIS

MRI or CT can be helpful in identifying cerebral arteriosclerosis and differentiating it from Alzheimer's disease (Collins, 2002). Electroencephalogram changes are not typically seen in individuals with cerebral arteriosclerosis (Niedermeyer & Lopes da Silva,

C

2004). Arteriosclerosis, the hardening and thickening of the arteries, can be seen using a microscope, and cardiac arrhythmias, ECG abnormalities, and elevated pulse are signs that softened areas of the brain caused by blood supply deprivation will be seen postmortem in cerebral arteriosclerosis (Shepherd et al., 1983).

Techniques like functional magnetic resonance imaging (fMRI), positron emission tomography (PET), angiography, and single-photon emission computed tomography (SPECT) can measure blood flow to the brain and indicate problems not seen on structural techniques like MRI or CT. These techniques may be more sensitive to earlier stages of arteriosclerosis. fMRI is similar to MRI but uses the magnetic images to detect the tiny metabolic changes that take place in an active part of the brain. Angiography is a procedure in which an X-ray visible dye is injected into blood vessels to allow them to be imaged on an X-ray, allowing the cerebral vessels to be more clearly visualized.

PET traces an injected radiotracer where it gives off energy in the form of gamma rays. This energy is detected by a gamma camera that monitors the emissions of the radiotracer that is used to determine blood flow in specific areas of the brain. The SPECT scan works in a similar manner. Each of these techniques can identify impairment in blood flow that is characteristic of arteriosclerosis.

Early forms of other dementing disorders such as Alzheimer's disease can mimic the early forms of arteriosclerosis and later forms of this disorder can lead to full dementia. In many cases, these disorders can be difficult to separate without neuroradiological evaluations that show clear differences in most cases.

TREATMENT

Taking action to prevent cerebral arteriosclerosis can prevent vascular cognitive impairment (Erkinjuntti & Gauthier, 2002). Statins are used to lower cholesterol and as a secondary prevention of cardiovascular disease. Older individuals who smoke are at an increased risk; therefore, quitting smoking would be an important part of treatment (Kuczynski et al., 2008). Weight is a significant risk factor, so weight reduction and exercise are often helpful. Changes in diet are often essential. Following a "heart healthy" diet will often slow the development of arteriosclerosis in the brain. Although there are genetic tendencies for the development of arteriosclerosis and related vascular disorders, a combination of medication, diet, and exercise make this one of the more controllable and preventable disorders, especially if a healthy lifestyle begins before the disorder has significantly progressed.

However, even in later stage the progression of the disorder can be slowed or even stopped.

Jessi Robbins
Charles Golden

Aiken, L. (1994). *Aging: An introduction to gerontology*. Thousand Oaks, CA: Sage Publications.

Collins, R. D. (2002). *Algorithmic diagnosis of symptoms and signs: A cost-effective approach*. Philadelphia, PA: Lippincott Williams & Wilkins.

Erkinjuntti, T., & Gauthier, S. (2002). *Vascular cognitive impairment*. London: Martin Dunitz, Ltd.

Hersen, M., Turner, S. M., & Beidel, D. C. (2007). *Adult psychopathology and diagnosis*. Hoboken, NJ: John Wiley and Sons.

Kuczynski, B., Reed, B., Mungas, D., Weiner, M., Chui, H., & Jagust, W. (2008). Cognitive and anatomic contributions of metabolic decline in Alzheimer disease and cerebrovascular disease. *Vascular Health and Risk Management, 4*, 363–381.

Niedermeyer, E., & Lopes da Silva, F. H. (2004). *Electroencephalography*. Philadelphia, PA: Lippincott Williams & Wilkins.

Sahlas, D., Bilbao, J. M., Swartz, R., & Black, S. (2002). Clasmatodendrosis correlating with periventricular hyperintensity in mixed dementia. *Annals of Neurology, 52*, 378–381.

Shepherd, M., Lader, M. H., Wing, J. K., Wing, L., & Russell, G. (1983). *Handbook of psychiatry*. New York: Cambridge University Press.

CEREBRAL AUTOSOMAL DOMINANT ARTERIOPATHY WITH SUBCORTICAL INFARCTS AND LEUKOENCEPHALOPATHY

DESCRIPTION

Cerebral autosomal dominant arteriopathy with subcortical infarcts and leukoencephalopathy (CADASIL) is an inherited small vessel disease of the brain. It is a common but underdiagnosed cause of inherited stroke in young patients lacking other established cardiovascular risk factors (Andreadou, Papadimas, & Sfagos, 2008). The most common clinical manifestations of CADASIL include recurrent subcortical ischemic stroke, TIAs, cognitive decline, migraine with aura, and mood disorders (Dichgans, 2009; Liem et al., 2007). Dementia is often diagnosed at the end stage of the disorder and is associated with motor dysfunction, pseudobulbar palsy, and incontinence. The mean age of onset is 40.3 ± 13.8 years with the mean age of death at 64.5 ± 10.6 years.

NEUROPATHOLOGY/PATHOPHYSIOLOGY

CADASIL is a nonarteriosclerotic, nonamyloid arteriopathy that primarily affects small cerebral arteries and arterioles. CADASIL develops due to a hereditary mutation of the *NOTCH3* gene on chromosome 19 (Buffon et al., 2006). The *NOTCH3* gene is responsible for encoding a transmembrane receptor that is predominantly expressed in arterial smooth muscle cells (Andreadou et al., 2008). In general, NOTCH signaling is essential for vascular development. Hereditary mutations in *NOTCH3*, most often missense point mutations, lead to an odd number of cysteine residues within the *NOTCH3* extracellular domain. Although the mechanism by which mutations in *NOTCH3* become pathogenic is unknown, the odd number of cysteine residues suggests abnormalities in protein folding and disulphide bridging (Federico, Bianchi, & Dotti, 2005), potentially disrupting ligand binding and consequently, receptor activation and signal transduction. As *NOTCH3* functions during vascular development and homestasis, disruption of this molecular pathway results in the progressive degeneration of arteriole smooth muscle within the skin and cerebrum, which is replaced with fibrotic deposits. Ultimately, these vessels grow narrower, and blood flow to the brain is diminished (Rein Gustavsen, Reinholt, & Schlosser, 2006).

Brain changes of patients with CADASIL typically include three separate lesion types including white matter hyperintensities (WMH), lacunar lesions, and cerebral microhemorrhages (Federico et al., 2005; Jouvent et al., 2007). However, MRIs of symptomatic as well as asymptomatic adult mutation carriers often reveal WMH without evidence of definitive infarctions (Liem et al., 2007). Lesions associated with CADASIL are characteristically present in the anterior temporal lobes, periventricular caps, and frontal lobes.

NEUROPSYCHOLOGICAL/CLINICAL PRESENTATION

Individuals with CADASIL typically demonstrate cognitive deficits by the age of 35, and in more than 80% of cases there is a progressive decline in cognitive functions before 60 years of age (Liem et al., 2007). Because cortical causes of dementia such as Alzheimer's disease do not play a significant role at this age, it is likely that the cognitive decline seen in these individuals is caused by subcortical cerebral damage that is specific to CADASIL. It has been found that lacunar infarct lesion load, rather than WMH or microbleeds, is the most important MRI finding associated with the severity of cognitive

dysfunction in individuals with CADASIL. The number of infarcts is significantly associated with neuropsychological test results of global cognitive functioning, including language, praxis, memory, and executive functions. Furthermore, individuals who have had multiple strokes demonstrate declines in perceptual speed, visuospatial skills, and working memory (Rein Gustavsen et al., 2006). Episodic and semantic memory, however, appear to be fairly well preserved. The severity of cognitive deficits in individuals carrying the *NOTCH3* mutation appears to vary, from no cognitive decline in individuals under 35 years of age to progressive cognitive difficulties such as dementia. Changes in executive function and working memory have also been found among mutation carriers in the prestroke phase, which is an early and common feature in vascular dementia. In addition, it is possible that white matter infarcts, also seen in vascular dementia, may cause cortical cholinergic denervation; this finding may be important for the potential therapeutic use of acetylcholine esterase (AChE) inhibitors.

Apathy is commonly present in patients with CADASIL with evidence to suggest that the presence and degree of apathy demonstrated is related to the volume of subcortical lesions present and the overall clinical severity of subsequent cognitive and motor disability (Reyes et al., 2009). Moreover, a vast majority of individuals demonstrating significant apathy also demonstrate evidence of other neuropsychiatric disturbances including irritability, depression, agitation, and aggressive behaviors (Reyes et al., 2009).

DIAGNOSIS

A diagnosis of CADASIL can be obtained through the use of brain MRI, gene testing, skin biopsy, and neuropsychological testing. Some individuals with CADASIL have been initially diagnosed with multiple sclerosis; however, MRI results showing no spinal cord involvement and the absence of oligoclonal bands in CSF provide a means of differentiation (Andreadou et al., 2008). In addition, MRI of individuals with CADASIL will show symmetrical and extensive WMH on T-2 weighted images and well-defined hypointense lesions on T-1 images (Jouvent et al., 2007). MRI can also distinguish CADASIL from ischemic leukoaraiosis, as white matter changes in the anterior temporal lobe and hyperintensities in the external capsule are highly specific for CADASIL. Lesions may also be present in the frontal lobe region as well as the brainstem (Rein Gustavsen et al., 2006).

A diagnosis of CADASIL may also be obtained through mutational screening, which may identify

C

presymptomatic or early symptom cases (Peters et al., 2005). The absence of vascular risk factors and a family history consistent with autosomal dominant inheritance also increases the possibility of CADASIL (Andreadou, 2008). Skin biopsy, examined by electron microscopy, can also detect the degeneration and loss of smooth muscle cells as well as deposits of GOM in the external basal lamina in the extracellular matrix of arterioles and small arteries (Reid Gustavsen et al., 2006). Due to the younger age of individuals diagnosed with CADASIL, a concurrent disorder that could impact cognition would be unusual; therefore, understanding the cognitive profile that is typical of CADASIL and vascular dementia is important for diagnosis.

TREATMENT

There is currently no evidence-based treatment available for CADASIL. Most interventions focus on treating associated symptoms of the disorder, including migraine and mood disorders. There has been some link to cholinergic deficits in patients with CADASIL (Keverne et al., 2007), which suggests that AChE inhibitors such as donepezil may be an effective treatment to address the cognitive deficits associated with CADASIL. Consequently, donepezil is often given as an off-label use for multi-infarct dementia. Unfortunately, donepezil has not been shown to be effective in treatment of patients with CADASIL (Dichgans et al., 2008).

Alyssa M. Maulucci
Jon C. Thompson

Andreadou, E., Papadimas, G., & Sfagos, C. (2008). A novel heterozygous mutation in the *NOTCH3* gene causing CADASIL. *Swiss Medical Weekly, 138,* 614–617.

Buffon, F., Porcher, R., Hernandez, K., Kurtz, A., Pointeau, S., Vahedi, K., et al. (2006). Cognitive profile in CADA-SIL. *Journal of Neurology, Neurosurgery, and Psychiatry, 77,* 175–180.

Dichgans, M. (2009). Cognition in CADASIL. *Stroke, 40*(1), 45–47.

Dichgans, M., Markus, H. S., Salloway, S., Verkkoniemi, A., Moline, M., Wang, Q., et al. (2008). Donepezil in patients with subcortical vascular cognitive impairment: A randomized double-blind trial in CADASIL. *Lancet Neurology, 7*(4), 310–318.

Federico, A., Bianchi, S., & Dotti, M. T. (2005). The spectrum of mutations for CADASIL diagnosis. *Neurological Sciences, 26,* 117–124.

Jouvent, E., Viswanathan, A., Mangin, J., O'Sullivan, M., Guichard, J., Gschwendtner, A., et al. (2007). Brain

Atrophy is related to lacunar lesions and tissue microstructural changes in CADASIL. *Stroke, 38,* 1786–1790.

Keverne, J. S., Low, W. C. R., Ziabreva, I., Court, J. A., Oakley, A. E., & Kalaria, R. N. (2007). Cholinergic neuronal deficits in CADASIL. *Stroke, 38,* 188–191.

Liem, M. K., van der Grond, J., Haan, J., van der Boom, R., Ferrari, M. D., Knapp, Y. M., et al. (2007). Lacunar infarcts are the main correlate with cognitive dysfunction in CADASIL. *Stroke, 38,* 923–928.

Peters, N., Opherk, C., Danek, A., Ballard, C., Herzog, J., & Dichgans, M. (2005). The pattern of cognitive performance in CADASIL: A monogenic condition leading to subcortical ischemic vascular dementia. *American Journal of Psychiatry, 162,* 2078–2085.

Rein Gustavsen, W., Reinholt, F. P., & Schlosser, A. (2006). Skin biopsy findings and results of neuropsychological testing in the first confirmed cases of CADASIL in Norway. *European Journal of Neurology, 13,* 359–362.

Reyes, S., Viswanathan, A., Godin, O., Dufouil, C., Benisty, S., Hernandez, K., et al. (2009). Apathy: A major symptom in CADASIL. *Neurology, 72,* 905–910.

CEREBRAL CAVERNOUS MALFORMATIONS

DESCRIPTION

Cerebral cavernous malformations (CCMs) are small blood vessels in the brain that become distended and weakened. The walls of the vessels are thin and lack elastin, making them prone to stretching. They also have a tendency to leak (Rothbart et al., 1996). There are two types of CCMs — sporadic and familial. Interestingly, CCMs occur mostly in Hispanic families where an ancestor had the disorder; however, anyone can develop CCMs regardless of ethnicity (Gunel et al., 1996). It occurs in 0.4% to 0.5% of the population (Rigamonti et al., 1988).

NEUROPATHOLOGY/PATHOPHYSIOLOGY

CCMs appear most often in the brain, but they can also emerge in the spinal cord, retina, and on the skin (Eerola et al., 2000). It is generally hypothesized that they are caused by "errors occurring during blood vessel formation or maintenance" (Baev, Issam, & Awad, 1988, p. 3). The defining features of CCMs are vascular malformations consisting of dilated capillaries (caverns) with decreased blood flow. The vascular caverns become filled with blood and the surrounding blood vessels, weak and lacking elastin and smooth muscle, become enlarged (Moriarity, Clatterbuck, & Rigamonti, 1999).

CCMs also can occur sporadically in individuals with no family history of the disorder, but the specific cause or causes are still not understood. Clatterbuck, Eberhart, Rain, and Rigamonti (2001) suggest that all CCMs could be the result of defects within KRIT1 (Krev interaction-trapped 1 protein) and other protein-encoding genes. However, acquired CCMs are most often preceded by trauma to the brain or spinal cord (Moriarity et al., 1999; Sahoo et al., 1999), indicating that the etiology is a combination of genetic and environmental factors.

In familial CCMs, the disorder manifests by genes mutating throughout the body, rather than just one cell mutating, as is seen in sporadic CCMs. The familial condition is autosomal dominant in that a gene from only one parent is needed to pass the disorder to the children.

The prevailing theory on the organic basis of familial CCMs proposes genetic mutations in the KRIT1, CCM2, and PDCD10 genes. The KRIT1 protein is necessary for life. It seems to assist in designing the structure of the endothelial cells in the blood vessels of the brain. CCM2 assists in controlling the production of the protein malcavernin, which in turn seems to determine where the endothelial cells (KRIT1) become active in the body. It is estimated that 20% of familial CCMs involve CCM2 mutation (Liquori et al., 2003). The third gene, CCM3, creates PDCD10, or programmed cell death 10 proteins (Bergametti et al., 2005), but it is still unclear what role this protein plays in the development of CCM.

NEUROPSYCHOLOGICAL/CLINICAL PRESENTATION

The sporadic form of CCMs most often presents with a single lesion, and there is no family history of neurological problems. Familial CCMs presents with multiple lesions and there is a long family history of neurological problems. It is estimated that 25% of individuals with CCMs do not experience symptoms (Johnson, 2006). In those that do, the most common are seizures, occurring in approximately 40% to 70% of cases. The next most common symptoms include focal neurological deficits, occurring in approximately 35% to 50% of cases; nonspecific headaches, occurring in approximately 10% to 32% of cases; and cerebral hemorrhaging, occurring in roughly 32% of cases (Denier et al., 2004; Siegel, 1998). Other common neurological dysfunctions can occur, such as paralysis, muscle weakness, and hearing and vision abnormalities (Selman, Tarr, & Ratcheson, 2000).

DIAGNOSIS

The preferred diagnostic tool for detecting CCMs is an MRI. The CCMs present with a mixed signal inside the lesion (Awad & Jabbour, 2006). The lesions also appear as vascular sinusoids lined with endothelial cells embedded in a thick fibrous substance. The lesions are characterized by the absence of, or abnormalities in, the blood/brain barrier (Tu, Stoodley, Morgan, & Storer, 2005).

Once the lesions are detected, a biopsy will help to further clarify the diagnosis. In some cases, it is also clinically useful to perform genetic testing to provide additional confirmation of the diagnosis, assist with prenatal diagnosis, and obtain a prognosis (Johnson, 2006).

From a differential diagnosis standpoint, cerebral arteriovenous malformations, moyamoya disease, blue rubber bleb nevus disorder, and von Hippel–Lindau's disease all present with characteristics similar to CCM and must be ruled out clinically. Briefly, moyamoya disease is characterized by constricted blood vessels, most notably in the circle of Willis and surrounding arteries (Gosalakkal, 2002). Blue rubber bleb nevus syndrome is characterized by a bluish or reddish-purple swelling that commonly occurs under the skin or on the surface of internal organs (Park, Park, & Chung, 2006). von Hippel–Lindau's disease is characterized by malformations known as hemangioblastomas or angiomas, which can occur anywhere in the body. The primary symptoms are headache, vomiting, ataxia, and severe high blood pressure (Molino, Sepe, Anastasio, & De Santo, 2006).

TREATMENT

The treatment of CCMs focuses on the symptoms resulting from their location. Therapy decisions must be based on comparing the risks associated with the malformation itself and the risks associated with its surgical removal. Factors such as age, gender, lesion location, presence of seizures, and the possibility of hemorrhaging should always be taken into account (Folkersma & Mooij, 2001). The treatment options for CCM are not abundant. If seizures occur, they are best treated with antiepileptic medication. On the other hand, if the seizures are intractable or there is frequent hemorrhaging resulting in focal deficits, surgery is recommended to remove the lesions associated with these symptoms (Folkersma & Mooij, 2001; Heros, & Heros, 2000).

Teri J. McHale
Henry V. Soper

Awad, I., & Jabbour, P. (2006). *Cerebral cavernous malformations and epilepsy. Neurological focus*. Retrieved from http://www.medscape.com/viewarticle/547601.

Baev, N., Issam, A., & Awad, M. (1998). Endothelial cell culture from human cerebral cavernous malformations. *Stroke, 29*, 2426–2434.

Bergametti, F., Denier, C., Labauge, P., Arnoult, M., Boetto, S., Clanet, M., et al. (2005). Mutations within the programmed cell death 10 gene cause cerebral cavernous malformations. *American Journal of Human Genetics, 76(1)*, 42–51.

Clatterbuck, R., Eberhart, C., Crain, B., & Rigamonti, D. (2001). Ultrastructural and immunocytochemical evidence that an incompetent blood-brain barrier is related to the pathophysiology of cavernous malformations. *Journal of Neurosurgery and Psychiatry, 71*, 188–192.

Denier, C., Labauge, P., Brunereau, L., Cavé-Riant, F., Marchelli, F., Arnoult, M., et al. (2004). Clinical features of cerebral cavernous malformations patients with KRIT1 mutations. *Annals of Neurology, 55*, 213–220.

Eerola, I., Plate, K., Spiegel, R., Boon, L., Mulliken, J., & Vikkula, M. (2000). KRIT 1 is mutated in hyperkeratotic cutaneous capillary-venous malformation associated with cerebral capillary malformation. *Human Molecular Genetics, 9*, 1351–1355.

Folkersma, H., & Mooij, J. (2001). Follow-up of 13 patients with surgical treatment of cerebral cavernous malformations: Effect on epilepsy and patient disability. *Clinical Neurology and Neurosurgery, 103*, 67–71.

Gosalakkal, J. (2002). Moyamoya disease: A review. *Neurology India, 50(1)*, 6–10.

Gunel, M., Awad, I., Finberg, K., Steinberg, G., Craig, H., Cepeda, O., et al. (1996). Genetic heterogeneity of inherited cerebral cavernous malformation. *Neurosurgery, 38*, 1265–1271.

Heros, R., & Heros, D. (2000). *Principles of neurosurgery*. In W. Bradley, R. Daroff, G. Fenichel, & C. Marsden (Eds.), *Neurology in clinical practice* (Vol. 1, pp. 931–958), Boston: Butterworth Heinemann.

Johnson, E. (2006). Cerebral cavernous malformation, familial. *Gene Reviews*. Retrieved from http://www.ncbi.nlm.nih.gov/bookshelf/br.fcgi?book=gene&part=ccm

Liquori, C., Berg, M., Siegel, A., Huang, E., Zawistowski, J., Stoffer, T., et al. (2003). Mutations in a gene encoding a novel protein containing aphosphotyrosine-binding domain cause type 2 cerebral cavernous malformations. *American Journal of Human Genetics, 73(6)*, 1459–1464.

Molino, D., Sepe, J., Anastasio, P., & De Santo, N. (2006). The history of von Hippel-Lindau disease. *Journal of Nephrology, 19(10)*, S119–S123.

Moriarity, J. L., Clatterbuck, R. E., & Rigamonti, D. (1999). The natural history of cavernous malformations. *Neurosurgery Clinics of North America, 10*, 411–417.

Park, C., Park, J., & Chung, K. (2006). Blue rubber bleb nevus syndrome with central nervous system involvement. *Journal of Dermatology, 33(9)*, 649–651.

Rigamonti, D., Hadley, M., Drayer, B., Johnson, P., Hoenig-Rigamonti, K., Knight, J., et al. (1988). Cerebral cavernous malformation. Incidence and familial occurrence. *New England Journal of Medicine, 319*, 343–347.

Rothbart, D., Awad, I., Lee, J., Kim, J., Harbaugh, R., & Criscuolo, G. (1996). Expression of angiogenic factors and structural proteins in central nervous system vascularmalformations. *Neurosurgery, 38*, 915–924.

Sahoo, T., Johnson, E. W., Thomas, J. W., Kuehl, P. M., Jones, T. L., Dokken, C., et al. (1999). Mutations in the gene encoding KRIT1, a Drev-1/rap1a binding protein, cause cerebral cavernous malformations (CCM1). *Human Molecular Genetics, 8(12)*, 2325–2333.

Selman, W., Tarr, R., & Ratcheson, R. (2000). Arteriovenous malformation. In W. Bradley, R. Daroff, G. Fenichel, & C. Marsden (Eds.), *Neurology in clinical practice* (Vol. 1). Boston: Butterworth Heinemann.

Siegel, A. (1998). Familial cavernous angioma: An unknown, known disease. *Acta Neurologica Scandinavica, 98*, 369–371.

Tu, J., Stoodley, M., Morgan, M., & Storer, K. (2005). Ultrastructural characteristics of hemorrhagic, nonhemorrhagic, and recurrent cavernous malformations. *Journal of Neurosurgery, 103*, 903–909.

CEREBRAL PALSY

DESCRIPTION

Cerebral palsy (CP) refers to a group of nonprogressive motor impairment syndromes that involve compromise of movement, posture, and muscle control caused by static lesions or anomalies of the brain arising in the early stages of its development. In other words, CP is an "umbrella term" that encompasses a number of neurodevelopmental conditions rather than a specific disorder (Bax & Brown, 2004). The manifestations of CP are variable and can range from subclinical abnormalities to severe impairments (Blondis, 2004). With a prevalence of 2–2.5 out of every 1,000 live births, CP is a leading cause of physical disability in childhood (Ashwal et al., 2004). Many children with CP also experience nonmotor problems of clinical significance (Bax, Tydeman, & Flodmark, 2006). Approximately 90% of cases stem from damage that occurs in the prenatal or perinatal period (Blondis, 2004). Prenatal risk factors include maternal infection during pregnancy (which in one multicenter study was found in nearly 40% of cases; Bax, Tydeman, & Flodmark, 2006) and multiple birth gestation. Perinatal risk factors include premature birth (although just over half of children with CP are born at term) and low birth weight. Contrary to popular belief, a history of anoxic damage to the brain during difficult labor or delivery is present in only a minority of cases. Postnatal risk factors include infection or head trauma (Bax et al., 2006; Winter, 2007).

NEUROPATHOLOGY/PATHOPHYSIOLOGY

CP can affect either or both of the two semi-independent motor systems of the brain: (a) The pyramidal system, comprised of precentral motor cortex and spinal motor neurons and the corticospinal tract that connects the two, is responsible for initiating and carrying signals for voluntary muscle contractions that enable skilled movements, and (b) the extrapyramidal system, which includes the cerebellum, basal ganglia, and brainstem areas, and "fine tunes" the movements of the pyramidal system by making adjustments to posture and coordination (Tupper & Sondell, 2004; Winter, 2007). The most widely accepted classification system for CP specifies two main types of the syndrome based on which motor system is damaged.

1. Damage to the pyramidal system results in spastic CP, which represents the majority (70% to 85%) of cases. Spastic CP is characterized by abnormally high muscle tone. Within that, subtypes of spastic CP that reflect the distribution of the affected limbs are delineated: hemiplegic CP involves the arm and leg on one side of the body, diplegic CP involves the lower extremities although the upper extremities often are affected to a lesser degree, and quadriplegic CP involves all four extremities (Tupper, 2007; Warschausky, 2006; Winter, 2007)

2. Damage to the extrapyramidal system is associated with two main subtypes of CP. Dyskinetic CP accounts for 10% to 20% of cases and is characterized by athetoid (slow, writhing, involuntary movements that can affect any part of the body, including the extremities, mouth and tongue) or dystonic (twisting and repetitive movements or abnormal postures caused by sustained muscle contractions) features. Ataxic CP accounts for 5% to 10% of cases and is characterized by weakness, incoordination, and intention tremor that affect balance and coordination and result in unsteadiness, a wide-based gait, and difficulty with rapid or fine movements (Blondis, 2004). In actuality, mixed forms of CP are common, tone abnormalities can vary within and across days (Tupper, 2007), and classifications of CP based on topography do not provide much-needed information about functional abilities. Including a

formal measure of mobility can therefore facilitate efforts to identify clinical needs, determine appropriate treatments, and track progress. One such widely used system is the Gross Motor Functional Classification Scale—Expanded and Revised, which rates overall mobility on a 5-level ordinal scale (Palisano, Rosenbaum, Bartlett, & Livingston, 2008).

In addition to specifying phenotypical features of the syndrome, CP can be classified based upon etiology. Toward that end, neuroimaging is of value since strong correlations exist between brain pathology and motor symptomatology in children with CP (Bax et al., 2006). For example, the most common MRI finding ("white matter damage of prematurity" involving periventricular leukomalacia or intraventricular hemorrhage) corresponds to the most common (spastic) type of CP (Bax et al., 2006). Basal ganglia lesions, cortical/subcortical lesions, malformations, and focal infarcts are present in the minority of cases, and some children with CP have normal imaging studies (Bax et al., 2006).

Given that CP is a disorder of the brain, the higher incidence of mental retardation, learning disabilities, ophthalmologic defects such as strabismus, amblyopia, nystagmus, and refractive errors, articulation and speech disorders, and hearing impairment in this population is not surprising (Russman & Ashwal, 2004). A much higher incidence of epilepsy (28% to 45%) also occurs in children with CP and represents a major risk factor for lower cognitive status (Fennell & Dikel, 2001). Secondary medical problems that can result from the sensory-motor impairments of CP include poor nutrition, oral dysphagia, dental problems, growth delays, orthopedic musculoskeletal deformities and contractures, pathological fractures, osteoporosis, respiratory illness, gastroesophageal reflux disease, constipation, urinary tract problems, pain, sleep disturbance, and fatigue. Importantly, although CP results from a static brain insult and is nonprogressive, symptoms often change over time. For example, a gradual and premature deterioration of functional skills due to the chronic stress that CP places on the motor system can occur in adulthood (Edwards, 2004).

NEUROPSYCHOLOGICAL/CLINICAL PRESENTATION

Children with CP demonstrate a full spectrum of cognitive abilities, from severe impairment to giftedness. Reflecting the neuroanatomical interconnectedness of the cognitive and motor systems, the degree of cognitive impairment is positively correlated with the degree of motor disability (i.e., mental retardation occurs more frequently in children with quadriplegia than diplegia or hemiplegia; Russman & Ashwal, 2004). However, standardized cognitive assessment can be complicated, if not precluded, by the auditory, communication, visual, and motor impairments that exist in children with CP since most available tests rely upon verbal and visual-motor responses. As a result, clinicians often must resort to using measures that may result in an underestimation of true abilities or, conversely, must forgo formal testing at the risk of leaving important needs unidentified (Fennell & Dikel, 2001; Warschausky, 2006). The most robust finding across studies that have addressed those confounds is significant visual-perceptual and visuospatial impairments beyond what can be accounted for by visual acuity alone. Those impairments typically occur in the context of relatively better-developed language-based processes (Fennell & Dikel, 2001; Jacobson, Ek, Fernell, Flodmark, & Broberger, 1996; Pueyo, Junqué, Vendrell, Narberhaus, & Segarra, 2009; Stiers, Vanneste, Coene, De Rammalaere, & Vandenbussche, 2002). Recent efforts to examine specific neuropsychological domains in children with CP have yielded preliminary evidence of particular problems with executive aspects of learning and memory (White & Christ, 2005) and abstract reasoning (Pueyo et al., 2009). Higher rates (25% to 30%) of specific learning disabilities in children with CP, compared with typically developing children, also have been found (Winter, 2007), including in studies that demonstrated normal measured intelligence and adequate visual acuity (Jacobson et al., 1996).

Children with CP experience a spectrum of physical disabilities that can limit their ability to initiate and participate in communication, interact with others, explore the environment, and take part in leisure activities, all of which are important for social development and psychological well-being (Larkin & Summers, 2004; Murphy & Such-Neibar, 2003). Indeed, children with CP are at increased risk for social-emotional and adjustment problems, including feelings of loneliness, social difficulties, low self-esteem, and depression. Behavior problems also are more likely (Warschausky, 2006). In addition, motor disability can result in difficulty performing daily living activities (Larkin & Summers, 2004), which in turn restricts opportunities for independence and increases demands on caregivers and stress in the family system.

DIAGNOSIS

The American Academy of Neurology has published an algorithm for diagnosing CP (Ashwal et al., 2004).

A standard neurological examination represents an important first step in the workup and helps discriminate between normal and abnormal development, determine the distribution of limb involvement, and direct additional workup (Roy, Bottos, Pryde, & Dewey, 2004). However, the assessment should be expanded to include formal observation of dynamic motor movements and postural control, which is not part of a traditional neurological examination but is essential for eliciting many of the abnormalities associated with CP (Winter, 2007). Serial developmental assessments often are necessary to confirm a diagnosis since outward signs of an underlying brain insult may not be apparent during the newborn period (Murphy & Such-Neibar, 2003; Russman & Ashwal, 2004). Abnormal muscle tone, persistent infantile reflex patterns, and delays in motor development often are the first outward signs of the disorder making it difficult to establish the presence of CP during early infancy. Serial examinations also are useful for providing prognostic information by tracking the age at which pivotal milestones are achieved (e.g., sitting independently by 2 years of age is predictive of future ambulation; Murphy & Such-Neibar, 2003) and for identifying children who "outgrow" their motor deficits due to ongoing brain development (Winter, 2007). Although neuroimaging is a routine part of the diagnostic workup, EEG studies are not recommended unless there are features suggestive of epilepsy (Russman & Ashwal, 2004). In all cases, screening for ophthalmologic, hearing, oral-motor, speech-language and cognitive problems is essential (Russman & Ashwal, 2004).

TREATMENT

CP is not curable but management and treatment can help minimize impairment, prevent secondary disabilities, maximize independence within the limits of motor and associated disabilities, and improve quality of life for patients and their families (Winter, 2007). Beyond general agreement that early institution of intervention using an interdisciplinary and family-centered approach should be provided, there is no proven best practice model (Murphy & Such-Neibar, 2003; Polatajko, Rodger, Dhillon, & Hirji, 2004; Tupper, 2007). Thus, an individually tailored and comprehensive treatment plan is recommended.

Several evidence-based surgical interventions with unique applications to individuals with CP have improved treatment efficacy in recent years. Selective dorsal rhizotomy is a neurosurgical procedure that reduces lower extremity spasticity and improves functional mobility in select children when followed by a physical therapy program (McLaughlin et al., 2002; Murphy & Such-Neibar, 2003). The procedure may also result in improved cognitive efficiency (Craft et al., 1995). Deep Brain Stimulation, typically to the globus pallidus, has been used to treat dystonia with some success (Lundy, Lumsden, & Fairhurst, 2009). Pharmacological interventions include use of muscle relaxants (most commonly, baclofen and Botox) to reduce spasticity and improve neuromuscular coordination by modulating the lower motor neuron system (Edwards, 2004). Hyperbaric oxygen therapy and many complementary and alternative medical approaches remain controversial because their validity has not been supported by available research (Babcock et al., 2009; Edwards, 2004). Several potential treatments for CP involving neuroprotective interventions and stem-cell-based therapies are in the very early stages of research and development but hold promise (Babcock et al., 2009).

Physical, occupational, and speech/language therapies to optimize gross and fine motor functioning, mobility, daily living skills, swallowing, and communication are the cornerstones of intervention for children with CP and usually are most effective when started at a young age (Tupper, 2007). Constraint-induced movement therapy in individuals with hemiplegia has been shown to increase use of the involved upper extremity by restraint of the preferred or dominant upper extremity (Murphy & Such-Neibar, 2003; Tupper, 2007). Specialized equipment, adaptive devices, and mechanical aids can be used to help increase or maintain independent functioning and include orthotic devices and augmentative communication systems (Polatajko et al., 2004). Recreational therapies such as therapeutic horsemanship and adaptive sports not only improve gross motor functioning and endurance, but also can help increase social participation, self-esteem, and physical and emotional well-being (Polatajko et al., 2004). In addition, therapists play a key role in removing barriers to participation by recommending changes in the physical environment at home, school, and the community. Physical and occupational therapies that do not have strong research evidence to support claims of their efficacy and are considered controversial include neurodevelopmental treatment, patterning, conductive education, and sensory integration therapy (Murphy & Such-Neibar, 2003; Polatajko et al., 2004).

School-based services and supports are of paramount importance for children with CP. In that context, applying "universal design" concepts to the classroom environment and curriculum can be instrumental in providing true access to educational opportunities. Presenting information in varied formats, providing different ways to reach goals and demonstrate understanding, and incorporating assistive technology are several such strategies (Ferguson, 2006). Although social skills training for children with physical disabilities can be helpful, preliminary research suggests that intervention is most effective when integrated into the school setting (Miyahara & Cratty, 2004). Psychological interventions play a critical role in addressing social-emotional, behavioral, and parenting issues and should be tailored based on presenting problems and needs. On a broader level, outreach and advocacy to improve services, systems and policies that affect individuals with disabilities, and provide education to correct public misperceptions about CP that shape negative attitudes can result in a meaningful increase in acceptance and integration of individuals with CP into their communities (Feldman-Winter, Krueger, Neyhart, & McAbee, 2002; Mihaylov, Jarvis, Colver, & Beresford, 2004).

Tara V. Spevack

Ashwal, S., Russman, B. S., Blasco, P. A., Miller, G., Sandler, A., Shevell, M., et al. (2004). Practice parameter: Diagnostic assessment of the child with cerebral palsy: Report of the Quality Standards Subcommittee of the American Academy of Neurology and the Practice Committee of the Child Neurology Society. *Neurology, 62*, 851–863.

Babcock, M. A., Kostova, F. V., Ferriero, D. M., Johston, M. V., Brunstrom, J. E., Hagberg, H., et al. (2009). Injury to the preterm brain and cerebral palsy: Clinical aspects, molecular mechanisms, unanswered questions, and future research directions. *Journal of Child Neurology, 24*(9), 1064–1084.

Bax, M., & Brown, J. K. (2004). The spectrum of disorders known as cerebral palsy. In D. Scrutton, D. Damiano, & M. Mayson (Eds.), *Management of the motor disorders of children with cerebral palsy* (2nd ed., pp. 9–21). London: Mac Keith Press.

Bax, M., Tydeman, C., & Flodmark, O. (2006). Clinical and MRI correlates of cerebral palsy: The European cerebral palsy study. *Journal of the American Medical Association, 296*(13), 1602–1608.

Blondis, T. A. (2004). Neurodevelopmental motor disorders: Cerebral palsy and neuromuscular diseases. In R. A. Bornstein (Series Ed.), D. Dewey, & D. E. Tupper (Eds.), *Developmental motor disorders: A neuropsychological perspective* (pp. 113–136). New York: Guilford Press.

Craft, S., Park, T. S., White, D. A., Schatz, J., Noetzel, M., & Arnold, S. (1995). Changes in cognitive performance in children with spastic diplegic cerebral palsy following selective dorsal rhizotomy. *Pediatric Neurosurgery, 23*, 68–75.

C

Edwards, S. (2004). Cerebral palsy in adult life. In D. Scrutton, D. Damiano, & M. Mayson (Eds.), *Management of the motor disorders of children with cerebral palsy* (2nd ed., pp. 170–182). London: Mac Keith Press.

Feldman-Winter, L., Krueger, C. J., Neyhart, J. M., & McAbee, G. N. (2002). Public perceptions of cerebral palsy. *The Journal of the American Osteopathic Association*, *102*(9), 471–475.

Fennell, E. B., & Dikel, T. N. (2001). Cognitive and neuropsychological functioning in children with cerebral palsy. *Journal of Child Neurology*, *16*(1), 58–63.

Ferguson, P. M. (2006, July). *Strategies for inclusive approaches to the education of students with physical disabilities: What to notice—what to ask.* Presented at the Third Annual Cerebral Palsy Conference, St. Louis, MO.

Jacobson, L., Ek, U., Fernell, E., Flodmark, O., & Broberger, U. (1996). Visual impairment in preterm children with periventricular leukomalacia—visual, cognitive, and neuropaediatric characteristics related to cerebral imaging. *Developmental Medicine and Child Neurology*, *38*, 724–735.

Larkin, D., & Summers, J. (2004). Implications of movement difficulties for social interaction, physical activity, play, and sports. In R. A. Bornstein (Series Ed.), D. Dewey, & D. E. Tupper (Eds.), *Developmental motor disorders: A neuropsychological perspective* (pp. 443–460). New York: Guilford Press.

Lundy, C., Lumsden, D., & Fairhurst, C. (2009). Treating complex movement disorders in children with cerebral palsy. *The Ulster Medical Journal*, *78*(3), 157–163.

McLaughlin, J., Bjornson, K., Temkin, N., Steinbok, P., Wright, V., Reiner, A., et al. (2002). Selective dorsal rhizotomy: Meta-analysis of three randomized controlled trials. *Developmental Medicine and Child Neurology*, *44*, 17–25.

Mihaylov, S. I., Jarvis, S. N., Colver, A. F., & Beresford, B. (2004). Identification and description of environmental factors that influence participation of children with cerebral palsy. *Developmental Medicine and Child Neurology*, *46*, 299–304.

Miyahara, M., & Cratty, B. J. (2004). Psychosocial functions in children and adolescents with movement disorders. In R. A. Bornstein (Series Ed.), D. Dewey, & D. E. Tupper (Eds.), *Developmental motor disorders: A neuropsychological perspective* (pp. 427–442). New York: Guilford Press.

Murphy, N., & Such-Neibar, T. (2003). Cerebral palsy diagnosis and management: The state of the art. *Current problems in pediatric and adolescent health care*, *33*(5), 146–169.

Palisano, R. J., Rosenbaum, P., Bartlett, D., & Livingston, M. H. (2008). Content validity of the expanded and revised Gross Motor Function Classification System. *Developmental medicine and child neurology*, *50*, 744–750.

Polatajko, J. J., Rodger, S., Dhillon, A., & Hirji, F. (2004). Approaches to the management of children with motor problems. In R. A. Bornstein (Series Ed.), D. Dewey, & D. E. Tupper (Eds.), *Developmental motor disorders: A neuropsychological perspective* (pp. 461–486). New York: Guilford Press.

Pueyo, R., Junqué, C., Vendrell, P., Narberhaus, A., & Segarra, D. (2009). Neuropsychologic impairment in bilateral cerebral palsy. *Pediatric Neurology*, *40*(1), 19–26.

Roy, E. A., Bottos, S., Pryde, K., & Dewey, D. (2004). Approaches to understanding the neurobehavioral mechanisms associated with motor impairments in children. In R. A. Bornstein (Series Ed.), D. Dewey, & D. E. Tupper (Eds.), *Developmental motor disorders: A neuropsychological perspective* (pp. 44–65). New York: The Guilford Press.

Russman, B. S., & Ashwal, S. (2004). Evaluation of the child with cerebral palsy. *Seminars in Pediatric Neurology*, *11*(1), 47–57.

Stiers, P., Vanneste, G., Coene, S., De Rammalaere, M., & Vandenbussche, E. (2002). Visual-perceptual impairment in a random sample of children with cerebral palsy. *Developmental Medicine and Child Neurology*, *44*, 370–382.

Tupper, D. E. (2007). Management of children with disorders of motor control. In S. J. Hunter & J. Donders (Eds.), *Pediatric neuropsychological intervention* (pp. 338–365). Cambridge, UK: Cambridge University Press.

Tupper, D. E., & Sondell, S. K. (2004). Motor disorders and neuropsychological development: A historical appreciation. In R. A. Bornstein (Series Ed.), D. Dewey, & D. E. Tupper (Eds.), *Developmental motor disorders: A neuropsychological perspective* (pp. 3–25). New York: Guilford Press.

Warschausky, S. (2006). Physical impairments and disability. In J. E. Farmer, J. Donders, & S. Warschausky (Eds.), *Treating neurodevelopmental disabilities: Clinical research and practice* (pp. 81–97). New York: Guilford Press.

White, D. A., & Christ, S. E. (2005). Executive control of learning and memory in children with bilateral spastic cerebral palsy. *Journal of the International Neuropsychological Society*, *11*, 920–924.

Winter, S. (2007). Cerebral palsy. In M. C. Roberts & L. Peterson (Series Eds.) & J. W. Jacobson, J. A. Mulick, & J. Rojahn (Eds.), *Handbook of intellectual and developmental disabilities* (pp. 61–80). New York: Springer.

CEREBRO-OCULO-FACIO-SKELETAL SYNDROME

DESCRIPTION

Cerebro-oculo-facio-skeletal (COFS) syndrome or Pena–Shokeir II is an uncommon neurodegenerative disorder first presented by Pena and Shokeir in 1974

(Longman, Sewry, & Mutoni, 2004; Sakai, Kikuchi, Takashima, Matsuda, & Watanabe, 1997). They concluded that the disorder was of autosomal recessive inheritance and could be mainly observed among families in Manitoba that were socially isolated. This isolation resulted in marriages within the same bloodline and therefore the propagation of COFS in their offspring (Graham et al., 2001).

The disorder is characterized by rapid degeneration of the spinal cord and brain as well as such physical and mental abnormalities as microcephaly (an abnormally small head), cataracts, nystagmus (quick and involuntary movements of the eyes), prominent nasal bridge and ears, failure to thrive (inadequate physical growth and weight gain in infancy), severe retardation, problems with kidneys and feeding, and hypotonia (low muscle tone), among other symptoms (Longman et al., 2004; Sakai et al., 1997).

NEUROPATHOLOGY/PATHOPHYSIOLOGY

COFS syndrome is characterized by neuropathological symptoms including significant reductions of the myelin sheath and white matter in the brain and spinal cord and discoloration of gray matter (Lee et al., 2001). Severe deterioration of the layers of the cerebellum was noted in children who were older (Graham et al., 2001).

Some researchers believe that a fetus's inability to move in the womb may cause some of these problems. For this reason, this disorder may also be known as fetal akinesia-hypokinesia deformation sequence (FADS) (Torii, Morikawa, Tanaka, & Takahashi, 2002). This idea was proposed after many autopsies (conducted on those who had succumbed to COFS) showed a decrease in motor neurons in the spine (Torii et al., 2002). It is uncertain, however, whether the diminution in movement had a neurological or myogenic (muscular) origin (Torii et al., 2002).

NEUROPSYCHOLOGICAL/CLINICAL PRESENTATION

Physically, a person with this disorder will exhibit a smaller than normal head (microcephaly), deep-set eyes, failure to thrive because of feeding problems, "rocker bottom" feet, and other abnormalities of the body (Graham et al., 2001). MRIs and brain CT scans show atrophy of the brain, myelin sheaths, and optic nerve, as well as a reduction in white matter, discoloration of gray matter, and calcifications within the cranium (Lee et al., 2007). The severe muscle weakness caused by this disorder leads to a significant reduction

in movement (Lee et al., 2007). A patient will most likely spend most of his or her life in a hospital because extensive ailments leave the patient considerably handicapped.

DIAGNOSIS

Clinically, COFS will present as a rare birth defect, affecting both males and females. This means that patients will most likely be very young and therefore quite vulnerable because of the excessive number of systems affected. In fact, infants with this disorder will most likely die within the first 5 years of their life (Lee et al., 2007).

Degeneration of the brain is believed to begin while the fetus is in the womb. Many infants may be born seemingly normal, but after a few weeks or months will exhibit physical symptoms such as failure to thrive and hypotonia. Because of the extensive damage done to the brain, patients become severely mentally handicapped. Problems with feeding and infections of the respiratory tract (which lead to difficulties in breathing) are just some of the factors in potential early death (Graham et al., 2001).

A significant overlap between the characteristics of other autosomal recessive disorders (such as Cockayne syndrome) may make diagnosing COFS quite a task. There are many prenatal disorders whose symptoms include degeneration of the brain and eyes. However, special attention should be given to the differences in symptoms in order to make an accurate diagnosis of COFS syndrome. Eye defects in COFS are considered more severe than those in Cockayne syndrome (optic atrophy in COFS v. pigmentary retinopathy in Cockayne syndrome) (Graham et al., 2001).

A prenatal diagnosis can be done, which plays an important role for patients with this disorder. In a prenatal ultrasound, a fetus with COFS will exhibit a combination of micrognathia (an undersized jaw), contractures on many joints, and "rocker bottom" feet (Lee et al., 2007).

TREATMENT

Children born with this disorder have a poor prognosis. They will inevitably continue to deteriorate until they are affected in most aspects of their health, leading to their incapacitation and eventual death. For this reason, treatment is usually "symptomatic and supportive" and made so that the person is as comfortable as possible. Most patients undergo a gastrostomy, a procedure in which the stomach is surgically opened for the purposes of installing a feeding tube (Lee et al., 2008).

Genetic counseling may be pursued by parents who believe they are at risk of transmitting an inherited (genetic) disorder to their offspring. By finding the probabilities of transmission and therefore having the ability to plan accordingly, parents may feel that they have some control of their situation (Graham et al., 2001).

Josie Bolanos
Charles Golden

Graham, J. M., Anyane-Yeboa, K., Raams, A., Appeldoorn, E., Kleijer, W. J., Garritsen, V. J., et al. (2001). Cerebro-oculo-facio-skeletal syndrome with a nucleotide excision – repair defect and a mutated *XPD* gene, with prenatal diagnosis in a triplet pregnancy. *American Journal of Human Genetics, 69*, 296–297.

Lee, S. H., Hong, S. J., Lee, J. H., Oh, S. Y., Kim, S. H., Kim, S. H., et al. (2007). Cerebro-oculo-facio-skeletal syndrome: A case report. *Korean Journal of Pediatrics, 51*(4), 436–437.

Longman, C., Sewry, C. A., & Muntoni, F. (2004). Muscle involvement in the cerebro-oculo-facio-skeletal syndrome. *Pediatric Neurology, 30*(2), 125. Retrieved from Elsevier.

Sakai, T., Kikuchi, F., Takashima, S., Matsuda, H., & Watanabe, N. (1997). Neuropathological findings in the cerebro-oculo-facio-skeletal (Pena-Shokeir) syndrome. *Brain Development, 19*, 58. Retrieved from Elsevier.

Torii, I., Morikawa, S., Tanaka, J., & Takahashi, J. (2002). An autopsy case of Pena-Shokeir syndrome: Severe retardation of skeletal muscle development compared with neuronal abnormalities. *Pediatric Pathology and Molecular Medicine, 21*, 468. Retrieved from Taylor and Francis Health Sciences.

CEREBROVASCULAR ACCIDENTS

DESCRIPTION

The World Health Organization (WHO) defines a cerebrovascular accident (CVA) as "rapidly developing clinical signs of focal (or global) disturbance of cerebral function, with symptoms lasting 24 hr or longer, or leading to death, with no apparent cause other than that of vascular origin" (Birkett, 1998). By applying this definition, ischemic stroke (infarction), hemorrhagic stroke, and subarachnoid hemorrhage are included, whereas transient ischemic attack (TIA) is excluded. Another definition is that of Adams, Victor, and Ropper (1999) that stipulates that a CVA is any encephalic anomaly that occurs as a result of a pathological blood vessel process. Consequently, the term pathologic process is inclusive, consisting of thrombotic or embolic (light) occlusion, vessel rupture, and injury or permeability disorders on the vascular wall, with an increase on the viscosity and other changes on blood quality.

The classification system proposed by the National Institute of Neurological Disorders and Stroke (NINDS) (1990) divides CVAs based on whether their clinical presentation is asymptomatic or symptomatic. Asymptomatic CVAs do not cause any neurological or retinal symptoms but damage to the neuronal network. On the other hand, symptomatic CVA causes neurological or retinal symptoms, such as TIA, ischemic stroke and hemorrhage, vascular dementia (VD), and hypertensive encephalopathy.

According to this classification, ischemic strokes are divided into focal and global. A general cut on the blood flow that affects the entire brain is called global ischemic stroke, whereas blood supply problems that only affect a brain area cause focal ischemia. In turn, focal ischemia is divided into two big groups: TIA and ischemic stroke or cerebral infarction, with the main difference being their length. According to its classical definition, TIA has a length of less than 24 hr and the recovery of the neurological deficit is totally reversible. Nevertheless, it has been redefined as a brief episode of neurological dysfunction caused by cerebral or retinal ischemia, with clinical symptoms that typically last for less than an hour, and without evidence of an acute infarction (Easton, Albers, Caplan, Saver, & Sherman, TIA Working Group, 2004). TIA is caused by a disruption of the blood flow to the brain, and its symptoms appear suddenly, last between 2 and 15 min, and depend on the affected area. Cerebral infarction refers to the set of clinical manifestations that appear as a consequence of the quantitative or qualitative disturbance of the blood supply to an encephalic area, producing necrosis of the brain tissue that results in a neurological deficit lasting more than 24 hr.

NEUROPATHOLOGY/PATHOPHYSIOLOGY

There are several forms of classifying ischemic stroke (Martí-Vilalta & Martí-Fábregas, 2004). One classification option attends to pathologic characteristics that can be thrombotic (when a thrombus in an artery obstructs the blood flow), embolic (when an embolus [whose origin can be arterial or cardiac] comes off), or hemodynamic (produced by an important decrease of arterial pressure that diminishes cerebral blood flow). Another classification is based on the affected vascular area (arterial, venous, or border areas origin). Ischemic stroke can also be classified by attending to the involved artery size: large-vessel infarction (large arteries) or small vessel infarction (less than 15 mm, called lacunar infarction). According to their etiology, infarctions can be artherothrombotic (large artery arterioscleroses), cardioembolic, lacunar (small vessel occlusive disease), infarctions of unusual cause, and infarctions of undetermined origin (Díez-Tejedor, Del Brutto, Álvarez-Sabín, Muñoz, & Abiusi, 2001).

Hemorrhagic strokes are characterized by the presence of blood in the brain due to the rupture of a blood vessel or other causes. As with ischemic diseases, symptoms will depend on their location and the magnitude of the blood extravasation. They can be divided into two groups: intracerebral hemorrhage (blood leaks into the brain) and subarachnoid hemorrhage (blood leaks into the subarachnoid space). There are other hemorrhages that occur less frequently, such as epidural or extradural hemorrhage (blood is found in the space found between the bones and the dura mater, most frequently caused by a traumatic injury) and subdural hemorrhage (blood is found between the arachnoid and dura mater layers) (Martí Vilalta, Matías-Guiu Guía, Arboix Damún, & Vázquez Cruz, 1989). Intracerebral or intracranial hemorrhages can be divided into parenchymal and ventricular hemorrhages. The fundamental difference between these two hemorrhages is their location. Parenchymal hemorrhage is a blood extravasation into the cerebral parenchyma, and they can be either primary or secondary (Díez-Tejedor et al., 2001). In primary parenchymal hemorrhages a degenerative process (such as arteriosclerosis or myeloid angiopathy) causes the vessel rupture. Secondary parenchymal hemorrhage is due to other causes, such as congenital abnormalities (vascular malformation), intratumoral hemorrhages or modified vessels because of inflammatory processes (vasculitis or mycotic aneurysms). Ventricular hemorrhage consists of blood accumulation in the ventricles. This can be, in turn, primary (blood is located only in the ventricles) or secondary (blood comes from another place, such as the parenchyma or subarachnoid space). Primary ventricular hemorrhage has a very low frequency.

A subarachnoid hemorrhage, however, is located in the subarachnoid space, and it can be primary and secondary. Primary subarachnoid hemorrhage consists of a vessel rupture located in the subarachnoid space, producing the invasion of space with blood under high pressure. Secondary subarachnoid hemorrhage is produced when blood comes from the ventricles or the parenchyma. Hemorrhages found in the subarachnoid space rapidly enter the ventricular system through cerebrospinal fluid flow. The most common symptoms are severe headaches that start suddenly, decreased consciousness, vomiting, and stiff neck (Díez-Tejedor et al., 2001). Different factors affect those symptoms, such as extent of bleeding, arterial pressure during bleeding, affected brain area, patient's premorbid status, blood expansion to ventricles, subdural space or parenchyma, bleeding etiology, and complications (Cardentey-Pereda & Pérez-Falero, 2002). Subarachnoid hemorrhage can be classified as traumatic and nontraumatic (spontaneous) depending on the event that causes the bleeding (Nathal & Yasui, 1998). Causes of the traumatic subarachnoid hemorrhage can be traumatic brain injury, electrical injuries, or surgical manipulations. In the nontraumatic group, (spontaneous) causes are cerebral aneurysms, vascular malformations and, less frequently, a consequence of a vasculitis, hematological alterations, neoplasia, arterial or venal hemorrhagic infarction, and infections. The most common is subarachnoid hemorrhage due to an aneurysm rupture, comprising the 77.2% of all subarachnoid hemorrhages (Cardentey-Pereda & Pérez-Falero, 2002), although there are also subarachnoid hemorrhages, whose causes cannot be determined, called subarachnoid hemorrhages from an unknown origin.

NEUROPSYCHOLOGICAL/CLINICAL PRESENTATION

There are two concepts that cover cognitive deficits caused by CVA: VD and vascular cognitive deficit. In 1993, the Association International pour la Recherche et l'Enseignement en Neurosciences (NINDS-AIREN) (Roman et al., 2004) published diagnostic criteria for VD based on Alzheimer's type dementia. This definition is one of the most employed because of its high specificity, although there are others that are more global, such as ICD-10 and *DSM-IV* criteria. VD does not have a specific clinical framework because it is a very heterogeneous syndrome in its etiology and physiopathogenesis. According to Roman (2003), its characteristics are personality preservation, emotional liability and incontinency, night confusional states, depression, and heterogeneous cognitive deficit. VD can be cortical (with neurological and neuropsychological focal signs such as aphasia, apraxia, and agnosia) and subcortical (with memory loss, depression, moderate cognitive deficits, apathy, motor disorders, and frontal and pseudobulbar signs). VD is the

C

second most common dementia, after Alzheimer (Roman, 2002).

According to the NINDS-AIREN VD classification (Erkinjuntti, Roman, Gauthier, Feldman, & Rockwood, 2004), there are different types of dementia. Multi-infarct or poststroke dementia consists of several cortical infarctions, resulting in a cortical cognitive deficits such as aphasia, apraxia, or agnosia. Dementia due to a unique infarct in a strategic area is characterized by a small infarct located in specific brain areas such as the thalamus, basal forebrain, or caudate, and their clinical manifestations can vary depending on the injury location (cortical vs. subcortical): memory and executive function deficits, conscious fluctuations, and behavioral changes (apathy, lack of spontaneity, and perseveration). Subcortical ischemic VD includes mainly small vessel dementia and hypoperfusion dementia, resulting in focal and diffuse lesions on the white matter that usually appears on the prefrontal-subcortical circuit, leading to executive function deficits (Price, Jefferson, Merino, Heilman, & Libon, 2005; Yuspeh, Vanderplog, Crowel, & Mullan, 2002), attention and concentration disorders, initiative loss, and lack of motivation (Delgado, 1992). Mixed dementia is a combination of Alzheimer disease (AD) and lesions produced by a CVA. There are also other types of dementia, such as hemorrhagic, small vessel dementia (multiple lacunar infarction, Binswanger's disease, cerebral autosomal dominant arteriopathy with subcortical infarcts and leukoencephalopathy, cerebral amiloyd angiopathy), hypoperfusion dementia, and dementia caused by other vascular mechanisms.

Bowler and Hachinsky (2002) expressed their arguments against the term VD and set up the use of a more accurate term: vascular cognitive impairment (VCI). Their first argument refers to the fact that VD is based on AD diagnostic criteria, and therefore requires a loss of memory and a progressive and irreversible cognitive deficit as criteria. The second argument implies that two or more affected cognitive functions should exist, besides the memory deficit, to diagnose the disorder, which complicates the identification of cases with mild deficits. These authors defend the term VCI because it includes cognitive deficits of vascular origin, being unnecessary to match dementia criteria, but establishing a continuum where the VCI constitutes a previous stage of VD characterized by a pattern of cognitive deficit with affected frontal-subcortical areas that result in an executive dysfunction. There are no specific criteria to define the VCI (Bowler, 2007). Black (2007) affirms that the concept VCI is dynamic and covers VD, VCI-no dementia (VCIND), and mixed dementia (AD and CVA).

Stephan, Matthews, Khaw, Dufouil, and Brayne (2009) define VCI as a cognitive deficit due to vascular causes that covers the initial stages of cognitive deficit to VD. These authors, for their part, describe a term for those patients who do not match dementia criteria called VCIND, a preclinical stage related to a high risk of developing dementia. Therefore, this term includes a big group of patients to treat therapeutically and preventively. Risk factors that increase the probability of suffering cognitive deficit or dementia are arterial hypertension, cholesterol, diabetes, or cardiac disease (Erkinjuntti, 2007), as well as obesity and smoking (Reitz, Luchsinger, & Mayeux, 2008).

Several factors influence cognitive alteration, such as the patient's age, the interval between CVA and rehabilitation, type of CVA (hemorrhagic, ischemic), injury size, and location (Zillmer & Spiers, 2001). In general, there are neuropsychological differences attending to the affected brain hemisphere. If the left hemisphere is affected, problems usually include language expression and comprehension, apraxia, and alexia. On the other hand, if the right hemisphere is damaged, visuoperceptive problems are common (calculating the distance between objects and between oneself and other people and/or objects) as well as emotional liability (manifesting emotions from indifference to euphoria), anosognosia, and difficulties driving a car, walking up stairs, and so forth (Zillmer & Spiers, 2001). There are also differences between the anterior and posterior brain regions. If lesions are located in the anterior brain, some common symptoms are sensorial and motor deficits on the legs, disinhibition, and executive function problems. Posterior lesions cause a loss of vision and sensory problems on the opposite side of the body (Zillmer & Spiers, 2001).

According to Weinstein and Swenson (1998), neuropsychological alterations depend exclusively on the implicated cerebral artery. Medial cerebral artery supplies the area of language, and therefore could result in Broca aphasia (if the lesion is located on the inferior frontal gyrus of the dominant hemisphere) or Wernicke's aphasia (if the lesion is located on the superior temporal gyrus of the dominant hemisphere). The medial cerebral artery is also implicated in visual perception, resulting in visual integration problems, neglect and visual agnosia (parieto-occipital lobe of the nondominant hemisphere); constructive apraxia and dressing apraxia (parietal lobe of the nondominant hemisphere); Gerstmann's syndrome that includes agraphia, acalculia, alexia, finger agnosia, and left-right confusion) (angular gyrus of the dominant hemisphere). Medial, posterior, anterior choroidal, and posterior communicating cerebral arteries are related to short and long-term memory problems (hippocampus, medial temporal lobe, frontal lobe, cerebral base, and medial thalamus). Working memory is related to the anterior cerebral artery (dorsolateral frontal lobe). Executive functions depend on the medial cerebral artery for maintenance and planning of behaviors, problem solving, self-evaluation, and ability to modify behaviour (dorsolateral frontal lobe); on the anterior cerebral artery for inhibition and emotional regulation (orbitofrontal cortex); and on the anterior choroid and medial arteries for akinesia, bradikinesia, and diskinesia (basal ganglia, putamen, globus pallidus, caudate, and amygdala).

Junqué and Barroso (2001) make a distinction between neuropsychological problems due to ischemia and those due to hemorrhage. Ischemic CVA significantly destroys gray matter, whereas a cerebral hemorrhage causes an affectation that is basically subcortical, such as gray nucleus and white matter, resulting in a disconnection deficit because of an interruption of the cortico cortical and cortico subcortical circuits. Given that the gray substance remains intact and therefore neural bodies, new circuits can be established that totally or partially restore the function. From a survival point of view, hemorrhages have a worse prognosis than infarctions, but related to the recovery of focal neuropsychological deficits hemorrhages have a better prognosis (Junqué & Barroso, 2001). In addition to the aforementioned destruction of tissue, hemorrhages produce neuropsychological symptoms due to the effect of the blood extravasation compressing surrounding tissue. This compression can even affect the contralateral hemisphere, producing contralateral hemisphere symptoms. As soon as the clot disintegrates, these symptoms disappear (Junqué & Barroso, 2001).

Neuropsychological consequences of subarachnoid hemorrhage deserve special mention. The most frequent symptoms are memory problems (especially verbal, both short and long term), attention, concentration, mental flexibility, language, information processing, and cognitive speed.

DIAGNOSIS

Diagnosis is twofold. First, in the acute stages, neuroimaging is the gold-standard diagnostic tool. Upon initial presentation, CT is utilized for a more rapid viewing of the brain so as to provide the quickest suggestion for neurosurgical intervention, if needed, in those instances of hemorrhage. If not contraindicated, MRI is commonly utilized as a follow-up to offer better resolution of the images to more accurately identify the area(s) of involvement. Magnetic resonance angiography may be employed to offer better evaluation of vascular integrity. In addition, carotid ultrasound is sometimes employed if the presentation is suggestive of an embolic or thrombus origin to consider the potential precipitating variable.

In the later stages, once CVA has been confirmed, diagnosis of residuals is essential. Given deficits may arise across a number of domains, often such diagnostic workup is multidisciplinary. Physical therapy/occupational therapy (OT) evaluations are crucial to identifying potential residuals that impede motor functioning in day-to-day activities. Speech therapy evaluations are commonly employed to not only evaluate language and speech but to also evaluate for dysphagia. In many institutions, stroke protocols are in place that automatically initiate these evaluations.

Beyond these domains, assessment to determine neuropsychological status is necessary. Due to the variability of neuropsychological deficits due to CVAs, assessment should cover all possible neuropsychological disorders (memory, attention, language, visuospatial functions, dementia, and depression) (Prigatano & Pliskin, 2003). Of the people who suffer a stroke 64% present cognitive damage (Hachinski et al., 2006). Although there is no unanimous protocol to assess cognitive deficits after a CVA, a recent article published by the NINDS and the Canadian Stroke Network (CNS) (Hachinski et al., 2006) recommends gathering together the demographic data and medical records of the patient and his/her family. Selective tests should cover all the cognitive functions, especially executive functions that are usually affected in these patients. Both institutions proposed protocols to assess patients who suffered a CVA. These protocols vary in length (one lasts 60 min, another 30 min, and the last 5 min). The 60-min protocol assesses frontal functions through semantic fluency (animals), phonetic fluency (Controlled Oral Word Association Test), Digits (WAIS-III), Hopkins Verbal Learning Test, and Trail Making Test; visuospatial abilities are assessed with the Rey Complex Figure Test; language with the Boston Naming Test; memory with the California Verbal Learning Test; and neuropsychiatric/depressive symptoms through the Center for Epidemiologic Studies-Depression Scale and Neuropsychiatric Inventory. Lastly, the Informant Questionnaire for Cognitive Decline in the Elderly assesses premorbid status. To complete the protocol, the Mini-Mental State Examination can be administered.

TREATMENT

The main objectives on the VCI and VD treatment are the improvement of cognitive, neuropsychiatric,

C

behavioral, and functional symptoms, as well as the slowing down of the symptoms' progression. Some cholinesterase inhibitors, such as donepezil and galantamine, yielded improvements on cognitive and behavioral levels, and on daily life activities (Erkinjuntti et al., 2004). For example, Malouf and Birks (2004) concluded that donepezil improves cognitive function, general clinical status and daily life activities in patients with VCI after a 6-month period of treatment. Regarding nonpharmacological treatment, two different possibilities exist: OT and neuropsychological rehabilitation (NR). OT facilitates the execution of activities, improving the necessary abilities, or developing compensatory strategies to overcome lost abilities. NR is concerned with the amelioration of cognitive, emotional, psychosocial, and behavioral deficits caused by an insult to the brain (Wilson, 2008). Some studies proved the efficacy of NR in patients with CVA in cognitive functions such as memory (Blanchet, Belleville, Noreau, Fougeyrollas, & Crepeau, 2007), working memory (Westerberg et al., 2007), and attention (Maeshima & Osawa, 2007).

Sandra Santiago Ramajo
Raquel Vilar López
Antonio E. Puente

Adams, R. D., Victor, M., & Ropper, A. H. (1999). *Principios de neurología*. Mexico: McGraw-Hill Interamericana Editores, S. A.

Birkett, D. P. (1998). *Psiquiatría clínica y accidente vascular cerebral*. Barcelona: Masson S. A.

Black, S. E. (2007). Therapeutic issues in vascular dementia: Studies, designs and approaches. *The Canadian Journal of Neurological Sciences, 34*(1), 125–130.

Blanchet, S., Belleville, S., Noreau, L., Fougeyrollas, P., & Crépeau, F. (2007). Impact of cognitive rehabilitation on episodic memory and life habits in persons with stroke. *Brain and Cognition, 63*(2), 200–201.

Bowler, J. V. (2007). Modern concept of vascular cognitive impairment. *British Medical Bulletin, 83*, 291–305.

Bowler, J. V., & Hachinski, V. C. (2002). The concept of vascular cognitive impairment. In T. Erkinjuntti & S. Gauthier (Eds.), *Vascular cognitive impairment*. London: Dunitz.

Cardentey-Pereda, A. L., & Pérez-Falero, R. A. (2002). Hemorragia subaracnoidea. *Revista de Neurología, 35*(8), 954–966.

Delgado, D. (1992). Enfermedad vascular subcortical en pacientes con demencia. In S. Lopez-Pousa, J. M. Manubens, & W. A. Rocca (Eds.), *Epidemiología de la demencia*

vascular. Controversias en su diagnóstico (pp. 77–90). Barcelona: Prous Science.

Díez-Tejedor, E., Del Brutto, O., Álvarez-Sabín, J., Muñoz, M., & Abiusi, G., (2001). Clasificación de las enfermedades cerebrovasculares. Sociedad Iberoamericana de Enfermedades Cerebrovasculares. *Revista de Neurología, 33*(5), 455–464.

Easton, J. D., Albers, G. W., Caplan, L. R., Saver, J. L., & Sherman, D. G, TIA Working Group. (2004). Discussion: Reconsideration of TIA terminology and definitions. *Neurology, 62*(8), 29–34.

Erkinjuntti, T. (2007). Vascular cognitive deterioration and stroke. *Cerebrovascular Diseases, 24*(1), 189–194.

Erkinjuntti, T., Román, G., Gauthier, S., Feldman, H., & Rockwood, K. (2004). Emerging therapies for vascular dementia and vascular cognitive impairment. *Stroke, 35*(4), 1010–1017.

Hachinski, V., Iadecola, C., Peterson, R. C., Breteler, M., Nyenhuis, D. L., Black, S. E., et al. (2006). National Institute of Neurological Disorder and Stroke Canadian Stroke Network vascular cognitive impairment harmonization standards. *Stroke, 37*(9), 2220–2241.

Junqué, C., & Barroso, J. (2001). *Neuropsicología*. Madrid: Editorial Síntesis, S. A.

Maeshima, S., & Osawa, A. (2007). Stroke rehabilitation in a patient with cerebellar cognitive affective syndrome. *Brain Injury, 21*(8), 877–883.

Malouf, R., & Birks, J. L., J. (2004). Donepezil for vascular cognitive impairment. *Cochrane Database System Review, 1*, CD004395.

Martí Vilalta, J. L., Matías-Guiu Guía, J., Arboix Damún, A., & Vázquez Cruz, J. (1989). Enfermedades Vasculares. In N. Acarín Tusell, J. Álvarez Sabin, & J. Pérez Serra (Eds.), *Glosario de Neurología* (pp. 145–160). Sociedad Española de Neurología. Editorial MCR, SA.

Martí-Vilalta, J. L., & Martí-Fabregas, J. (2004). Nomenclatura de las enfermedades vasculares cerebrales. In J. R. Martí-Fabregas (Ed.), *Enfermedades vasculares cerebrales* (pp. 453–458). España: Prous Science.

National Institute of Neurological Disorder and Stroke. (1990). Special report from the National Institute of Neurological Disorders and Stroke. Classification of cerebrovascular disease III. *Stroke, 21*(4), 637–741.

Nathal, E., & Yasui, N. (1998). Hemorragia subaracnoidea. In F. Barrinagarrementería & C. Cantú (Eds.), *Enfermedad vascular cerebral* (pp. 327–346). Mexico: McGraw-Hill Interamericana Editores, S. A.

Price, C. C., Jefferson, A. L., Merino, J. G., Heilman, K. M., & Libon, D. J. (2005). Subcortical vascular dementia. Integrating neuropsychological and neuroradiological data. *Neurology, 65*(3), 376–382.

Prigatano, G., & Pliskin, N. H. (2003). *Clinical neuropsychology and cost outcome research: A beginning*. New York: Psychology Press.

Reitz, C., Luchsinger, J. A., & Mayeux, R. (2008). Vascular disease and cognitive impairment. *Expert Review of Neurotherapeutics, 8*(8), 1171–1174.

Roman, G. C. (2002). Vascular dementia revisited. Diagnosis, pathogenesis, treatment, and prevention. *The Medical Clinics of North America, 86*(3), 477–499.

Roman, G. C. (2003). Demencia vascular: Conceptos actuales, diagnósticos & tratamiento. In J. C. Arango Lasprilla, S. Fernandez Guinea, & A. Ardila (Eds.), *Las demencias. aspectos clínicos, neuropsicológicos and tratamiento* (pp. 209–235). España: Díaz Santos.

Roman, G. C., Sachdev, P., Royall, D. R., Bullock, R. A., Orgogozo, J. M., Lopez-Pousa, S., et al. (2004). Vascular cognitive disorder: A new diagnostic category updating vascular cognitive impairment and vascular dementia. *Journal of Neurological Science, 226*(1–2), 81–87.

Stephan, B. C., Matthews, F. E., Khaw, K. T., Dufouil, C., & Brayne, C. (2009). Beyond mild cognitive impairment: Vascular cognitive impairment, no dementia (VCIND). *Alzheimer's Research & Therapy, 1*(1), 4. [Epub ahead of print].

Weinstein, A., & Swenson, R. A. (1998). Cerebrovascular disease. In P. J. Snyder & P. D. Nussbaum (Eds.), *Clinical neuropsychology*. Washington: American Psychological Association.

Westerberg, H., Jacobaeus, H., Hirvikoski, T., Clevberger, P., Ostensson, M. L., Bartfai, A., et al. (2007). Computerized working memory training after stroke—a pilot study. *Brain Injury, 21*(1), 21–29.

Wilson, B. A. (2008). Neuropsychological rehabilitation. *Annual Review of Clinical Psychology, 4*, 141–162.

Yuspeh, R. L., Vanderplog, R. D., Crowel, T. A., & Mullan, M. (2002). Differences in executive functioning between Alzheimer's disease and subcortical ischemic vascular dementia. *Journal of Clinical and Experimental Neuropsychology, 24*(6), 745–754.

Zillmer, E. A., & Spiers, M. V. (2001). *Principles of neuropsychology*. Belmont, CA: Wadsworths: Thomson Learning.

Charçot–Marie–Tooth Disease

DESCRIPTION

Charçot–Marie–Tooth (CMT) disease is a genetically heterogeneous disorder involving gradually progressive muscular atrophy and sensory neuropathy. A typical feature of CMT is known as "foot drop" resulting from weakness in the lower leg and foot. As a result of muscular degeneration and loss of sensation in limbs, lessened manual dexterity, weakness, gait problems, and loss of balance occur as the disease

progresses. Other common features of CMT disease include loss of sensation in hands and feet, and muscle cramps and pain (Arnold, McEntagart, & Younger, 2005) that worsen at variable rates over time.

Primarily affecting distal body parts, the disease causes muscle atrophy that may result in debilitating deformities of extremities. Physical manifestations of the disease include high-arched feet or flat feet, claw-hand deformities, and, in more severe cases, scoliosis or kyphosis and vocal cord paralysis may exist (Arnold et al., 2005; Scriver, Beaudet, Sly, & Valle, 2001). It is the most common hereditary peripheral neuropathy and usually presents in adolescence or early adulthood with mild initial symptoms such as clumsiness and numbness. CMT is not life threatening, although age of onset, rate of progression, and severity of the disease are variable and unpredictable even among family members, making prognosis difficult.

NEUROPATHOLOGY/PATHOPHYSIOLOGY

Pathological mechanisms of CMT disease involve inherited mutated autosomal dominant genes most commonly but may also involve mutated autosomal recessive or X-linked dominant genes (Arnold et al., 2005). There are four subtypes of CMT that have been distinguished based upon the disease pathophysiology: CMT1, CMT2, CMT3, and CMT4. CMT1 is characterized by demyelination and motor nerve conduction velocities below 35 m/s (Stojkovic et al., 2003). Unlike CMT2, nerve biopsies of patients with CMT1 reveal an "onion bulb" formation (Arnold et al., 2005). CMT1A is the most common CMT1 subcategory and has been linked to a duplication on the peripheral myelin protein *PMP22* gene, whereas CMT1B is associated with mutations in the myelin protein zero (*MPZ*) gene and motor nerve conduction velocities of below 25 m/s (Stojkovic et al., 2003).

CMT2 involves axonal dysfunction and motor nerve conduction velocities that fall within normal limits. The mutated genes discovered in CMT2 are responsible for the integrity of the axon, and axonal degeneration occurs when these genes malfunction. Degeneration of the axons in CMT2 is associated with mutations in the mitochondrial fusion protein mitofusin 2 (MFN2) (Baloh, Schmidt, Pestronk, & Milbrandt, 2007). Axonal mitochondrial transport is disrupted in CMT2 and a lack of energy due to an insufficient supply of mitochondria in peripheral axons exists, leading to neuronal dysfunction in distal regions of the body (Baloh et al., 2007).

CMT3, also known as Dejerine–Sottas's disease, begins in infancy and involves severe sensory

C

abnormalities and muscle degeneration. Mutations in the *PO* gene or the *PMP22* gene are believed to be responsible for CMT3 pathology. CMT4 encompasses an array of demyelinating subcategories, each of which cause motor and sensory abnormalities involving leg weakness that progresses to paralysis by adolescence.

CMTX, the X-linked form of CMT, is linked to a mutation in the gene encoding connexin 32, a gap junction protein having multiple roles in the Schwann cell and present in various tissues throughout the body (Abrams et al., 2003). The pathology of CMTX includes axonal loss, partially failed regeneration, and myelin abnormalities (Abrams et al., 2003; Hahn, Ainsworth, Bolton, Bilbao, & Vallat, 2001). Mutations in the connexin 32 gene may explain the variable pattern of muscular abnormalities across patients..

NEUROPSYCHOLOGICAL/CLINICAL PRESENTATION

Involvement of cranial nerves is rare and cognitive changes are usually not related to the disease itself, although they may occur secondary to psychological distress. For example, fatigue is common in CMT and associated with slowed mental processing. Psychological aspects of CMT are usually related to decreased mobility. As the disease progresses, the patient becomes increasingly dependent on others to assist them with simple tasks that they no longer are able to accomplish independently given muscle and sensory dysfunction (i.e., buttoning a shirt, walking on uneven surfaces).

The CMT patient may react to increasingly demanding daily activities with altered perceptions of self-efficacy and feelings of inferiority, guilt, and fear. A significant deterioration in quality of life is found in patients with CMT, particularly in older, unemployed women (Padua et al., 2006) who typically report most of the symptoms. Feelings of shame and embarrassment may result from the need to ask others for assistance with simple physical tasks, frequent tripping, unusually shaped feet or hands, and/or awkward gait. Body image, self-esteem, and self-worth are also greatly impacted by the altered physical appearance that accompanies muscle atrophy and the use of orthopedic devices (Arnold et al., 2005).

CMT patients may display anger toward their disability and frustration that they are no longer able to perform simple tasks as efficiently as they once did. CMT patients have a sense of emotional loss that accompanies physical degeneration that may lead to hopelessness and depression. Anxiety is a common psychological feature of the disease based upon the

patient's perceived dependence, worry regarding disease progression, and concern about the potential for genetic transmission to offspring. Given the progressive nature of the disease, patients are often uncertain of the future and apprehensive toward goal-making for fear of failure due to physical limitations imposed by CMT disease.

Patients with CMT disease also experience prejudices related to the stigma of having a disability. They may be viewed as less attractive, incompetent, or clumsy. Patients may attempt to hide their disability for fear of job jeopardy or social rejection. Slowed job performance, social isolation, and medical expenses contribute to emotional distress in CMT patients. Adequate resources, social support, and personal beliefs are influential in determining patients' levels of adjustment to their disability (Arnold et al., 2005; Marshak, Seligman, & Prezant, 1999). CMT patients often choose to cope with their illness by modifying their environment to the level of their disability (i.e., replacing staircases with ramps, buying shoes with Velcro rather than laces) in order to maintain a relative amount of independence.

DIAGNOSIS

Sensory and motor neuropathy is a common feature of various diseases with multiple causes. CMT disease may mimic acquired neuropathies such as alcoholism and vitamin B12 deficiency, other genetic neuropathies (i.e., amyloid neuropathy), or occur in association with chronic illnesses (i.e., diabetic neuropathy) (Arnold et al., 2005). It is important to distinguish CMT from other neuropathies by its defining clinical features. For the diagnosis of CMT disease, patients undergo a physical examination, electromyography and nerve conduction velocity testing, nerve biopsy, and a comprehensive family and medical history is gathered (Bird, 2004; De Jonghe et al., 1999). MRI and CT are frequently used to diagnose CMT disease by identifying nerve root enlargement within the lumbosacral portion of the spine (Aho, Wallace, Pitt, & Sivakumar, 2004).

TREATMENT

Patients with CMT disease should receive social support to assist them in dealing with strong emotions such as depression and anxiety, which commonly accompany the diagnosis of disabling diseases such as CMT. Cognitive restructuring regarding their perception of the level and extent of their disability may improve self-efficacy and the ability to cope effectively. Psychiatric medications such as antidepressants may be necessary in addition to therapy to improve the patient's psychological well-being. Access to resources such as specialty devices and medications to assist with physical discomfort will improve their ability to function motorically, foster independence, and aid in job security. Orthopedic braces and other devices for hands, legs, and feet provide alternate ways of functioning in order to increase independence and efficiency during everyday activities. These devices can be molded to the individual needs of the patient and modified as the disease progresses. Some patients may elect to have reconstructive surgery to correct deformities caused by muscular degeneration and may require rehabilitation and occupational therapy to regain usage of the affected limb.

Patients with CMT disease will benefit from a variety of medical professions including geneticists, neurologists, social workers, psychiatrists, neurological rehabilitation specialists, occupational therapists, orthopedists, and support groups to assist them in adjusting physically and emotionally to their level of disability (Arnold et al., 2005). Patients themselves may contribute to the treatment of CMT and receive free medical resources while increasing their sense of self-worth by becoming research participants in the search for a cure for CMT. Genetic information and testing is available for patients who wish to be informed of the likelihood of passing on CMT to offspring. Education regarding the disease and the transmission of CMT to offspring will help reduce the patient's anxiety and assist them in making informed decisions regarding treatment and future planning.

Stephanie Lei Santiso
Charles Golden

Abrams, C. K., Freidin, M., Bukauskas, F., Dobrenis, K., Bargiello, T. A., Verselis, V. K., et al. (2003). Pathogenesis of X-linked Charcot-Marie-Tooth disease: Differential effects of two mutations in connexin 32. *Journal of Neuroscience, 23*(33), 10548–10558.

Aho, T. R., Wallace, R. C., Pitt, A. M., & Sivakumar, K. (2004). Charcot-Marie-Tooth disease: Extensive cranial nerve involvement on CT and MR Imaging. *American Journal of Neuroradiology, 25*, 494–497.

Arnold, A., McEntagart, M., & Younger, D. S. (2005). Psychosocial issues that face patients with Charcot-Marie-Tooth disease: The role of genetic counseling. *Journal of Genetic Counseling, 14*(4).

Baloh, R. H., Schmidt, R. E., Pestronk, A., & Milbrandt, J. (2007). Altered axonal mitochondrial transport in the pathogenesis of Charcot-Marie-Tooth disease from mitofusin 2 mutations. *Journal of Neuroscience, 27*(2), 422–430.

Bird, T. D. (2004). *Charcot-Marie-Tooth hereditary neuropathy overview.* In GeneReviews at GeneTests-GeneClinics: Medical genetics information resource [database online]. Copyright, University of Washington, Seattle. 1997–2001. Available from http://www.geneclinics.org or http://www.genetests.org

De Jonghe, P., Nelis, E., Timmerman, V., Lofgren, A., Martin, J. J., & Van Broeckhoven, C. (1999). Molecular diagnostic testing in Charcot-Marie-Tooth disease and related disorders. Approaches and results. *Annals of the New York Academy of Sciences, 883*, 389–396.

Hahn, A. F., Ainsworth, P. J., Bolton, C. F., Bilbao, J. M., & Vallat, J. M. (2001). Pathological findings in the x-linked form of Charcot-Marie-Tooth disease: A morphometric and ultrastructural analysis. *Acta Neuropathologica (Berlin), 101*, 129–139.

Marshak, L. E., Seligman, M., & Prezant, F. (1999). Chapter 1: Families coping with disability. Foundational and conceptual issues. In S. McDaniel, J. Hepworth, & W. F. Doherty (Eds.), *Disability and the family life cycle* (pp. 1–37). Portland, OR: Book News.

Padua, L., Aprile, I., Cavallaro, T., Commodari, I., La Torre, G., Pareyson, D., et al. (2006). Variables influencing quality of life and disability in Charcot Marie Tooth (CMT) patients: Italian multicentre study. *Journal of the Neurological Sciences, 27*, 417–423.

Scriver, C. R., Beaudet, A. L., Sly, W. S., & Valle, D. (2001). Charcot-Marie-Tooth peripheral neuropathies and related disorders. In C. R. Scriver, A. L. Beaudet, W. S. Sly, & D. Valle (Eds.), *Metabolic and molecular bases of inherited disease* (8th ed., Vol. 4, pp. 63–38). New York: McGraw-Hill.

Stojkovic, T., de Seze, J., Dubourg, O., Arne-Bes, M. C., Tardieu, S., Hache, J. C., et al., (2003). Autonomic and respiratory dysfunction in Charcot-Marie-Tooth disease due to Thr124Met mutation in the myelin protein zero gene. *Clinical Neurophysiology, 114*, 1609–1614.

CHIARI MALFORMATIONS

DESCRIPTION

Chiari malformations, sometimes referred to as Arnold-Chiari malformations, are a type of structural defect where the cerebellar tonsils protrude through the bony space at the bottom of the skull, the foramen magnum. This compression can cause blockage of the cerebral spinal fluid (CSF), which leads to hydrocephalus

C

(Gilbert, Jones, Rorke, Chernoff, & James, 1986). Symptoms associated with hydrocephalus are therefore common, including urinary incontinence, mental status change, gait disturbance, numbness, headache, and muscle weakness. Chiari malformations are broken down into four subtypes in order of severity, I through IV, with IV being the most severe.

Chiari malformations were first described by Hans Chiari in the 1880s and later more clearly defined by Dr. Julius Arnold. Dr. Chiari specifically described abnormalities of the hindbrain, addressing forms I through III (Koehler, 1991). The fourth type, a general disruption in brain development, was later added by his predecessors (Bejjani, 2001). Types III and IV are reportedly rarer whereas type I is the most common. Type I is seen in adults and becomes evident as the brain develops whereas type II, sometimes referred to as Arnold-Chiari malformation, is congenital and is the most common childhood form of the malformation (Funk & Siegel, 1988). Overall, Chiari malformations are more common in women, have a prevalence of around 1 in 1000, and average age of diagnosis is around 27.

NEUROPATHOLOGY/PATHOPHYSIOLOGY

As previously mentioned, Chiari malformations are characterized by improper development of the brain or skull leading to potential herniation of the cerebellum. Classically, Chiari malformations are defined as tonsillar herniations greater than 3–5 mm; the herniation is large enough to move beyond the foramen magnum (Aboulezz, Sartor, Geyer, & Gado, 1985; Caldarelli & Di Rocco, 2004). Given the nature of the brain abnormalities, comorbid conditions are common. Specifically, comorbid conditions may include hydrocephalus, syringomyelia, spina bifida, Ehlers–Danlos syndrome, and Marfan's syndrome (Wit et al., 2008).

NEUROPSYCHOLOGICAL/CLINICAL PRESENTATION

Overall, symptoms manifest as either medullary (pyramidal signs, spasticity, disrupted gait), cerebellar (poor balance, poor coordination, dysmetria), brainstem (sleep disturbance [e.g., apnea], dysphagia, dizziness, basic bodily functions, ocular problems), or those related to hydrocephalus (urinary incontinence, mental status change, gait disturbance, headache, etc.) (Taricco & Melo, 2008). Despite general similarities in presentation, there is some variation in symptoms based on the type of Chiari malformation.

Chiari type I involves herniation of the cerebellar tonsils and the inferior portions of the cerebellum,

crowding of the structures within the posterior cranial fossa with impaction against the foramen magnum, and is often associated with abnormalities of the craniovertebral junction (Caldarelli & Di Rocco, 2004). Type I is often asymptomatic and is typically discovered by accident during examination for other reasons (Henriques-Filho & Prates, 2008). If passages of CSF are blocked, symptoms of hydrocephalus may occur (e.g., headache, gait changes, etc.). Specifically, symptoms of type I Chiari malformations typically include headache (sometimes mistaken for migraines), neck pain and pressure behind the head, gait disturbance, poor fine motor coordination, numbness, dizziness, difficulty swallowing, diplopia, and dysarthria. Tinnitus, chest pain, urinary incontinence, scoliosis are less common, but can occur (Quigley, Iskander, Quigley, Nicosia, & Haughton, 2004).

Chiari types II through IV involve a greater level of hindbrain disturbance than type I and are therefore associated with greater symptom severity. Type II, often discovered during ultrasounds or at birth, is a result of the spinal canal and spinal cord not closing during birth (myelomeningocele) and thus protruding through the back leading to poor development of the cerebellum and medulla. The medulla, fourth ventricle (which is elongated), and pons are displaced into the cervical spinal canal resulting in hydrocephalus (and related symptoms) at least 70% of the time (Cai & Oakes, 1997). Type II is often seen in combination with spina bifida, specifically myelomeningocele-a, and paralysis below the defect is common (Wit et al., 2008).

Types III and IV are also generally discovered during ultrasound. By definition, Chiari type III involves dislocations and herniation of large portions of the cerebellum and brainstem with the fourth ventricle opening into the cervical canal (Taricco & Melo, 2008). Spina bifida in the first few cervical vertebrae has also been commonly described. Type III leads to severe neurological impairment and is often seen with encephalocele, an extremely rare cranial malformation involving failure of the bones of the skull to fully close and fuse allowing the brain, CSF, and meninges to protrude through the hole in a sac-like fashion (Furtado, Anantharam, Reddy, & Hegde, 2009). Encephalocele has high mortality rates, depending on location of the "sac," and should the child survive, development of mental skills is almost always compromised.

Type IV Chiari malformations are extremely severe and result from failure of the brain to develop. Specifically, they are characterized by underdevelopment of the cerebellum without displacement of the brainstem (Taricco & Melo, 2008). Prominent and pervasive neurological signs, especially those related to cerebellar function, are seen.

DIAGNOSIS

Chiari malformations are typically diagnosed via neuroimaging in combination with clinical presentation. Neuroimaging is most often conducted via T1 MRI, which is effective in revealing herniation associated with the Chiari malformation and as well as defects due to potentially related conditions, such as syringomyelia (Caldarelli & Di Rocco, 2004). Downward herniation of the cerebellar tonsils is evident on scans, with displacement below the foramen magnum. In addition, MRI cerebral spinal fluid flow studies are helpful in determining the impact of herniation on CSF flow (Taricco & Melo, 2008). CT, although used less often, can be helpful in examining the details of unusual bone formations, especially around the foramen magnum and the upper cervical spinal cord.

TREATMENT

Treatment of Chiari malformations depends on type and symptom severity. Medication and surgery are often utilized, although sometimes the herniation is not severe enough to warrant any type of intervention.

Posterior fossa decompression is often utilized for treating types I and II; this procedure involves removal of the second and sometimes third cervical vertebrae along with a portion of the occipital bone in order to release pressure and allow CSF to drain. Shunt placement is also sometimes used for a similar purpose. Approximately 80% of patients improve following these procedures (Guo et al., 2007; Lam, Irwin, Poskitt, & Steinbok, 2009). Also, when the brainstem compression is more ventral, transoral clivus-odontoid resection is performed.

Treatment for types III and IV vary depending on the nature of the cerebral/spinal abnormalities (Furtado et al., 2009). Overall, surgery is designed to recreate the cisterna magnum, reestablish CSF flow, and decompress brain structures.

Jeremy Hertza
Andrew S. Davis

Aboulezz, A., Sartor, K., Geyer, C., & Gado, M. (1985). Position of cerebellar tonsils in the normal population and in patients with Chiari malformation: A quantitative approach with MR imaging. *Journal of Computer Assisted Tomography, 9.*

Bejjani, G. (2001). Definition of the adult Chiari malformation: A brief historical overview. *Neurosurgical Focus, 11*(1).

Cai, C., & Oakes, W. (1997). Hindbrain herniation syndromes: The Chiari malformations (I and II). *Pediatric Neurology, 4.*

Caldarelli, M., & Di Rocco, C. (2004). Diagnosis of Chiari I malformation and related syringomyelia: Radiological and neuropsychological studies. *Child Nervous System, 20.*

Funk, K., & Siegel, M. (1988). Sonography of congenital midline brain malformations. *RadioGraphics, 8*(1).

Furtado, S., Anantharam, B., Reddy, K., & Hegde, A. (2009). Repair of Chiari III malformation using cranioplasty and an occipital rotation flap: Technical note and review of literature. *Surgical Neurology, 13.*

Gilbert, J., Jones, K., Rorke, L., Chernoff, G., & James, H. (1986). Central nervous system anomalies associated with meningomyelocele, hydrocephalus, and the Arnold-Chiari malformation: Reappraisal of theories regarding the pathogenesis of posterior neural tube close defects. *Neurosurgery, 18.*

Guo, F., Wang, M., Long, J., Wang, H., Sun, H., Yang, B., et al. (2007). Surgical management of Chiari malformation: Analysis of 128 cases. *Pediatric Neurosurgery, 43*(5).

Henriques-Filho, P., & Prates, R. (2008) Sleep apnea and REM sleep behavioral disorder in patients with Chiari malformations. *Arquivos de Neuropsiquiatria, 66.*

Koehler, P. (1991). Chiari's description of cerebellar ectopy (1891) with a summary of Cleland's and Arnold's contributions and some early observations on neural tube defects. *Journal of Neurosurgery, 75.*

Lam, F., Irwin, B., Poskitt, K., & Steinbok, P. (2009). Cervical spine instability following cervical laminectomies for Chiari II malformation: A retrospective study. *Child Nervous System, 25*(1).

Quigley, M., Iskander, B., Quigley, M., Nicosia, M., & Haughton, V. (2004). Cerebrospinal fluid flow in foramen magnum: Temporal and spatial patterns at MR imaging in volunteers and in patients with Chiari I malformation. *Radiology, 232.*

Taricco, M., & Melo, L. (2008). Retrospective study of patients with Chiari malformation submitted to surgical treatment. *Arquivos de Neuropsiquiatria, 2.*

Wit, O., Dunnen, W., Sollie, K., Munoz, R., Meiners, L., Brouwer, O., et al. (2008). Pathogenesis of cerebral malformations in human fetuses with meningomyelocele. *Cerebrospinal Fluid Research, 5*(4).

CHILDHOOD ABSENCE EPILEPSY

DESCRIPTION

Absence epilepsy (also termed "petit mal epilepsy") is a form of idiopathic generalized epilepsy in which seizures involve sudden cessation in activity as well as impaired consciousness and responsiveness (Lee, 2010). Automatisms such as lip smacking are common. Lack of recall of the seizure event is typical, and patients often resume previous activity with little or no postictal effects (Lee, 2010; Pearl & Holmes, 2008). Seizures are typically brief (about 2–10 seconds), thus making them difficult to detect, and they occur multiple times per day (as often as 10–100 times per day) (Hughes, 2009; Siren et al., 2007). Absence seizures can be either typical or atypical, with the latter being differentiated by less abrupt onset and termination (Hughes, 2009). Typical absences are characteristic of other idiopathic generalized epilepsies including juvenile absence epilepsy and, less often, juvenile myoclonic epilepsy (Berkovic & Benbadis, 2001); however, this article will focus on childhood absence epilepsy given its much more prominent attention in the epilepsy literature. Atypical absences are associated with more severe syndromes that can involve mental retardation and multiple other seizure types, particularly Lennox–Gastaut's syndrome (Berkovic & Benbadis, 2001). Generalized tonic–clonic seizures can also occur, though much more frequently in juvenile absence epilepsy than childhood absence epilepsy (Siren et al., 2007).

Seizure onset usually occurs between ages 4 and 10, and onset is uncommon after age 14 (Annegers, 2001; Siren et al., 2007). An average incidence rate of 10% of pediatric epilepsy cases has been reported across multiple studies (Hughes, 2009). Girls are more often affected (Hughes, 2009; Pearl & Holmes, 2008). Although etiological processes are likely multifactorial, inherited factors are thought to play a larger role than acquired factors (Berkovic & Benbadis, 2001; Pearl & Holmes, 2008). Moreover, the generalized spike-and-wave EEG pattern associated with absence seizures is thought to be an inherited trait (Pearl & Holmes, 2008). Most patients experience remission of seizures by mid-adolescence, though persistence into adulthood may occur, even de novo in adulthood (Berkovic & Benbadis, 2001; Lee, 2010).

Absence epilepsy has long been considered a benign form of epilepsy due to remission in adolescence and good functional outcomes. Children with absence epilepsy tend to exhibit normal development and normal intelligence (Siren et al., 2007). Unfavorable prognostic indicators include appearance of generalized tonic–clonic seizures in the active stage of absences, myoclonic jerks, eyelid myoclonia, EEG features atypical of childhood absence epilepsy, and limited response to treatment (Grosso et al., 2005).

NEUROPATHOLOGY/PATHOPHYSIOLOGY

Typical absence epilepsy is associated with a characteristic EEG pattern involving a sudden onset of 3-Hz generalized, symmetrical spike-or multiple spike-and-slow-wave complexes that are superimposed on a normal background, with voltage that is often strongest in the frontocentral regions (Pearl & Holmes, 2008). Abrupt onset of the 3-Hz spike-wave discharges impairs the child's responsiveness and cessation of the spike-wave discharge results in immediate return to baseline behaviors (Browne, Penry, Porter, & Dreifuss, 1974). Clinical symptoms are generally perceived when discharges last longer than 3 seconds (Pearl & Holmes, 2008). Compared with typical absences, atypical absences are characterized by discharges that are more irregular morphologically, lower in amplitude, and occur with broader and blunter spikes (Berkovic & Benbadis, 2001). The interictal background is abnormal in atypical absences—characterized by a diffusely slow background and focal or multifocal spikes (Berkovic & Benbadis, 2001; Pearl & Holmes, 2008).

Although typical absences are not associated with structural anomalies of the brain, microdysgenesis can occur (Berkovic & Benbadis, 2001). Absence seizures are not associated with global cortical involvement but rather involve select cortical networks, including the frontal and thalamocortical circuits (Hughes, 2009; Pearl & Holmes, 2008). Numerous functional MRI studies emphasize ictal activation in the thalamus and decreased activity in the precuneus, frontal, and parietal regions of the cortex, as well as subcortical structures, especially in the caudate (Hamandi et al., 2006; Laufs, Lengler, Hamandi, Kleinschmidt, & Krakow, 2006; Li et al., 2009; Moeller et al., 2008). This pattern of decreased activity is associated with the arrest of activity and loss of awareness in absence seizures (Hughes, 2009).

Possible mechanisms underlying absence seizures include dysfunction of the GABAergic systems (Hughes, 2009). Absence seizures have been associated with the T-calcium channel gene *CACNA1H*, *CACNG3*, chloride gene *CLCN2*, genes on chromosomes 3p and 18P, and the *EGR1* and *RCN2* genes (Hughes, 2009).

NEUROPSYCHOLOGICAL/CLINICAL PRESENTATION

Absence epilepsy has typically been associated with normal intelligence and the absence of significant functional impairment. Complaints of academic difficulties are rare and any cognitive difficulties that occur are typically subtle (Siren et al., 2007). When comparing 69 school-age children with absence epilepsy with controls, Caplan et al. (2008) identified lower, though still average range, intellectual functioning on the *Wechsler Intelligence Scale for Children-Revised*, Third Edition, with similar rates of verbal and nonverbal abilities among the two groups.

Although intelligence is typically intact, children with absence epilepsy may present with domain-specific weaknesses in areas such as attention, language, verbal memory, verbal fluency, and fine motor coordination (Bhise, Burack, & Mandelbaum, 2009; Henkin et al., 2005). Children with idiopathic generalized epilepsy, regardless of subtype, have shown a vulnerability to attention problems (Henkin et al., 2005; Levav et al., 2002; Parisi, Moavero, Verrotti, & Curatolo, 2010). Caplan et al., in their 2008 study, found children with absence epilepsy exhibited lower, though still average range language processing on the Test of Language Development. Notably, however, significantly more children with absence epilepsy demonstrated below average IQ (27% vs. 6%) and Spoken Language Quotient scores (43% vs. 15%) than the control group. Bhise et al., in their 2009 study of children with new-onset idiopathic epilepsy, found that children with absence epilepsy performed worse on the story memory subtest of the Wide Range Assessment of Memory and Learning than children classified with other types of epilepsy. Likewise, within their Israeli sample of children with idiopathic generalized epilepsy, Henkin et al. (2005) reported poorer performance among the children with absence epilepsy compared with controls on the California Verbal Learning Test, word fluency test, and the finger tapping test. In contrast, performance differences between children with generalized tonic–clonic seizures and controls tended to be non-significant. Future research with larger, longitudinal samples is required to clarify the presence of domain-specific neurocognitive impairment among children with absence epilepsy.

Children with absence epilepsy have been shown to exhibit elevated rates of emotional and behavioral comorbidities. Attention deficit hyperactivity disorder (ADHD) is the most commonly reported psychiatric diagnosis among children with absence epilepsy (Parisi et al., 2010). Caplan et al. (2008) reported that 61% of their sample had some kind of psychiatric diagnosis. Of these children, 30% were diagnosed with ADHD (52% of them with the inattentive subtype) and 29% were diagnosed with a mood disorder. Among this latter group, 75% had an anxiety disorder, 20% had depression, and 5% exhibited both anxiety

and depression. After controlling for IQ and demographic variables, children with absence epilepsy were rated significantly higher on indices measuring attention problems, somatic problems, social problems, and thought problems on the Child Behavior Checklist.

The mechanisms underlying cognitive and social-emotional dysfunction among children with absence epilepsy are unclear. However, attentional deficits may reflect abnormalities in the frontal and thalamo-cortical circuits (Holmes, Brown, & Tucker, 2004). Caplan et al. (2008) mention several studies in which the frontal lobe, thalamus, and 5HT are implicated in both absence seizures and anxiety disorders.

Seizure variables are associated with cognitive or social-emotional outcomes in a few studies. Longer duration of the generalized 3-Hz spike wave complexes have been correlated with poorer performance on the visual memory task (Siren et al., 2007). Likewise, children with absence epilepsy or anxiety may have more frequent or longer duration of seizures (Caplan et al., 2008).

DIAGNOSIS

Reports of staring spells by caregivers often precipitate an evaluation for absence epilepsy. Typical absence seizures are effectively activated (clinically and electrographically) through hyperventilation (Pearl & Holmes, 2008). Hyperventilation is less effective at inducing atypical absences (Berkovic & Benbadis, 2001). Diagnosis requires the presence of a characteristic EEG pattern involving spike and slow-wave discharges. EEG findings can help discriminate between typical or atypical absences, as described above. Imaging studies show a structurally normal brain. Patients do not typically present with focal abnormalities upon examination.

Brief complex partial seizures can mimic absence seizures. It is particularly difficult to distinguish between complex partial seizures of temporal lobe origin and absence seizures (Berkovic & Benbadis, 2001). The latter, however, are distinguished by briefer duration, more frequent occurrence, absence of an aura, limited/no postictal confusion, and generalized discharges on interictal EEG instead of temporal spikes (Berkovic & Benbadis, 2001). Complex partial seizures of frontal origin can also mimic absence seizures and are differentiated by clinical, EEG, and radiological features of a frontal focus. More rarely, absences can be seen in specific diffuse cerebral disorders such as metabolic encephalopathies or benzodiazepine withdrawal, though seizure occurrence is more isolated with these disorders (Berkovic & Benbadis, 2001).

Finally, distinguishing between variations in attention, daydreaming, and absence seizures can be challenging, even for the most seasoned clinicians (Berkovic & Benbadis, 2001). This is best done by completing a detailed history and obtaining an EEG. Although assessing the degree of responsiveness during the episodes is clinically useful, this may be more difficult when absence seizures are very brief. A neuropsychological evaluation may be helpful in this regard as the extended one-to-one observations and interactions provide opportunities to observe for episodes and assess responsiveness. It is also important for the clinician to remember that attention problems have a high rate of comorbidity with absence epilepsy, so it is not uncommon for patients to display a combination of absence seizures and episodes of inattention.

TREATMENT

Valproic acid, lamotrigine, and ethosuximide are often considered first-line treatment options for absence epilepsy (Hughes, 2009; Wheless, Clarke, & Carpenter, 2005). Carbamazepine can worsen seizures (Berkovic & Benbadis, 2001). More recent research has suggested that transcranial magnetic stimulation may hold some promise for decreasing the duration of slow-wave activity (Hughes, 2009). There is limited information regarding whether treatment with antiepileptic drugs (AEDs) can help prevent or minimize neurocognitive difficulties associated with absence epilepsy. Following introduction of AEDs (ethosuximide and sodium valproate), with subsequent attainment of seizure freedom, children with absence epilepsy observed by Siren et al. (2007) exhibited improved sustained attention, fine motor coordination, and rote visual memory. Intellectual ability remained stable. Atypical absence seizures may be more difficult to control initially (Hughes, 2009), which may contribute to poorer outcomes.

Neuropsychological evaluation is not only helpful for assessing the impact of epilepsy and its treatment on neurobehavioral functioning but also for developing an appropriate intervention plan (Blackburn, Zelko, & Shurtleff, 2007). Such an intervention plan can help minimize the impact of identified neurobehavioral difficulties on daily functioning and, subsequently, the need for further services. Depending on the neuropsychological profile of a child with epilepsy, intervention may include a combination of remediation, accommodation, psychotherapy, or pharmacological treatment approaches.

Among the available research, there is minimal information about the effectiveness of specific interventions or rehabilitation approaches for individuals with absence epilepsy. In clinical practice, it is common to recommend intervention programs based on findings from available literature for children without epilepsy, but the effectiveness of such programs have not been extensively examined in the epilepsy population. For example, much research has been published about the efficacy of different remedial programs for reading disorders, specifically targeting the underlying deficits in phonological processing that tend to accompany the disorders (for a review, see Wills, 2007). However, Blackburn et al. (2007) caution that there are no studies assessing the effectiveness of reading remediation techniques in children with epilepsy.

Nicole Cruz
Jeffrey B. Titus

Annegers, J. F. (2001). Absence seizures. In E. Wyllie (Ed.), *The treatment of epilepsy: Principles and practice* (3rd ed., pp. 357–368). Philadelphia: Lippincott Williams & Wilkins.

Berkovic, S. F., & Benbadis, S. (2001). Absence seizures. In E. Wyllie (Ed.), *The treatment of epilepsy: Principles and practice* (3rd ed., pp. 357–368). Philadelphia: Lippincott Williams & Wilkins.

Bhise, V. V., Burack, G. D., & Mandelbaum, D. E. (2009). Baseline cognition, behavior, and motor skills in children with new-onset, idiopathic epilepsy. *Developmental Medicine and Child Neurology, 52,* 22–26.

Blackburn, L., Zelko, F., & Shurtleff, H. (2007). Seizure disorders. In S. Hunter & J. Donders (Eds.), *Pediatric neuropsychological intervention* (pp. 133–150). Cambridge, UK: Cambridge University Press.

Browne, T. R., Penry, J. K., Porter, R. J., & Dreifuss, F. E. (1974). Responsiveness before, during and after spike-wave paroxysms. *Neurology, 24,* 659–665.

Caplan, R., Siddarth, P., Stahl, L., Lanphier, E., Vona, P., Furbani, S. (2008). Childhood absence epilepsy: Behavioral, cognitive and linguistic comorbidities. *Epilepsia, 49,* 11, 1838–1846.

Grosso, S., Galimberti, D., Vezzosi, P., Farnetani, M., Di Bartolo, R. M., Bazzoti, S., et al. (2005). Childhood absence epilepsy: Evolution and prognostic factors. *Epilepsia, 46,* 11, 1796–1801.

Hamandi, K., Salek-Haddadi, A., Laufs, H., Liston, A., Friston, K., Fish, D. R., et al. (2006). EEG/fMRI of idiopathic and secondary generalized epilepsies. *Neuroimage, 31,* 1700–1710.

Henkin, Y., Sadeh, M., Kivity, S., Shabtal, E., Kishon-Rabin, L., & Gadoth, N. (2005). Cognitive function in idiopathic generalized epilepsy of childhood. *Developmental Medicine & Child Neurology, 47,* 126–132.

Holmes, M. D., Brown, M., & Tucker, D. M. (2004). Are "generalized" seizures truly generalized? Evidence of localized mesial frontal and frontopolar discharges in absence. *Epilepsia, 45,* 1568–1579.

Hughes, J. R. (2009). Absence seizures: A review of recent reports with new concepts. *Epilepsy & Behavior, 15,* 404–412.

Laufs, H., Lengler, U., Hamandi, K., Kleinschmidt, A., & Krakow, K. (2006). Linking generalized spike-and-wave discharges and resting state brain activity by using EEG/fMRI in a patient with absence seizures. *Epilepsia, 47,* 444–448.

Lee, G. (2010). Neuropsychology of epilepsy and epilepsy surgery. Oxford University Press.

Levav, M., Mirsky, A. F., Herault, J., Xiong, L., Amir, N., & Andermann, E. (2002). Familial association of neuropsychological traits in patients with generalized and partial seizures disorders. *Journal of Clinical and Experimental Neuropsychology, 24,* 311–326.

Li, Q., Luo, C., Yang, T., Yao, Z., He, L., Liu, L., et al. (2009). EEG-fMRI study on the interictal and ictal generalized spike-wave discharges in patients with childhood absence epilepsy. *Epilepsy Research, 87,* 2–3, 160–168.

Moeller, F., Siebner, H. R., Wolff, S., Muhle, H., Granert, O., Jansen, O., et al. (2008). EEG-fMRI in drug-naïve children with newly diagnosed absence epilepsy. *Epilepsia 49,* 1510–1519.

Parisi, P., Moavero, R., Verrotti, A., & Curatolo, P. (2010). Attention deficit hyperactivity disorder in children with epilepsy. *Brain and Development, 32,* 10–16.

Pearl, P. L., & Holmes, G. L. (2008). Childhood absence epilepsies. In J. Pellock, B. Bourgeois, W. E. Dodson, D. Nordli, & R. Sankar (Eds.), *Pediatric epilepsy: Diagnosis and therapy* (3rd ed., pp. 323–334). New York: Demos Medical Publishing.

Siren, A., Kylliainen, A., Tenhunen, M., Hirvonen, K., Riita, T., & Koivikko, M. (2007). Beneficial effects of antiepileptic medication on absence seizures and cognitive functioning in children. *Epilepsy and Behavior, 11,* 85–91.

Wheless, J. W., Clarke, D. F., & Carpenter, D. (2005). Treatment of pediatric epilepsy: Expert opinion. *Journal of Child Neurology, 20,* S1–S56.

Wills, K. (2007). Remediating specific learning disabilities. In S. Hunter & J. Donders (Eds.), *Pediatric neuropsychological intervention* (pp. 224–252). Cambridge, UK: Cambridge University Press.

CHILDHOOD ANXIETY DISORDERS

DESCRIPTION

General anxiety can be defined as a feeling of uneasiness or distress of the mind, caused from a specific life event, or an overarching feeling of constant nervousness. Minimal levels of anxiety are normal and likely occur in both children and adults at some point in their lifetime. Some form of anxiety disorder is the most common of all mental health disorders among children (Morrison & Anderson, 2001). Childhood anxiety disorders are a topic in pediatric research which has sometimes been overlooked due to the perception of a transient component to the impairment. Nevertheless, those disorders that comprise the general term, childhood anxiety, can include Attention Deficit Hyperactivity Disorder (ADHD), Separation Anxiety Disorder (SAD), Generalized Anxiety Disorder (GAD), Social Phobia, Posttraumatic Stress Disorders (PTSDs), Agoraphobia, Panic Disorder, and Obsessive-Compulsive Disorder (OCD) (American Psychiatric Association [APA], 2000).

During infancy and toddlerhood, anxiety is a part of human development, arising in situations involving strangers, heights, and separation, and largely disappearing during the preschool years (Eley et al., 2003; King, Hamilton, & Ollendick, 1988; Muris, Meesters, Merckelbach, Sermon, & Zwakhalen, 1998). Continuous feelings of anxiety may affect the daily functioning of a patient, which may warrant a diagnosis of an anxiety-related disorder. However, there can be ambiguity in distinguishing "normal" worries and fears (Eley et al., 2003), leading to difficulties in diagnosing disorders, particularly in children.

Childhood anxiety can manifest in a variety of ways and can be diagnosed differently based on the presentation. It can be challenging because it is difficult to differentiate short-term developmental phasic anxiety, such as stranger or separation anxiety, from symptoms that warrant a diagnosis of an anxiety disorder (Langley, Bergman, & Piacentini, 2002). Prevalence has been reported between 8% and 21% (Anderson, Williams, McGee, & Silva, 1987; Eley et al., 2003); however, controversy on the exact prevalence of childhood anxiety disorders exists, particularly because most children show varying symptoms of anxiety normally (Gregory & Eley, 2007). For example, they are fearful and nervous when they have to take a standardized test but do not display any anxious symptoms when they are not taking an exam.

Determining the exact origin of childhood anxiety has proven to be a daunting task within the literature. There have been links to biological markers (Gregory & Eley, 2007), neuropathological implications (Pine, 1999), and environmental factors (Grant, Bagnell, Chambers, & Stewart, 2009; Messer & Beidel, 1994). Particularly, due to the nature of development, it is likely there are a number of factors that contribute to the overall emotional behavior of a child. Laucht

C

et al. (2000) noted it is more likely that the cumulative effects of multiple factors or the developing general emotional difficulties contribute to the development of clinical anxiety rather than any one single precursor in isolation.

As research is continuing to narrow the true etiology of childhood anxiety, research has already illuminated a number of risk factors in its development. Identifying risk factors or predispositions for anxiety can assist in understanding the triggers that in turn increase a child's level of anxiety. Current studies have focused on a child's temperaments, including the mental, physical, and emotional traits of a patient (Grant et al., 2009). Different temperamental characteristics predispose children to react in a specific way to a given situation (Rothbart, Ahadis, & Evans, 2000).

Grant et al. (2009) defined two negative temperaments: behavioral inhibition and fussy-difficult temperaments. Behaviorally inhibited children are unable to adapt to new people or situations and are emotionally restrained from new people or new situations, whereas fussy-difficult children are irritable, easily upset, difficult to soothe, and illustrate "negative affect" (Grant et al., 2009). Grant et al. (2009) used the National Longitudinal Survey of Children and Youth to track the development of the Canadian population living in the 10 provinces. The authors used the telephone or an in person computer-assisted interview; however, the child-reported anxiety information from subjects aged 10–11 were provided with a written questionnaire. Using 768,600 participants, their research indicated both behavioral inhibition and fussy-difficult temperaments as predictors of anxiety later in childhood. Thus, it seems underlying temperaments may be a good predictor in detecting childhood anxiety and the development of anxious symptoms later in life.

Perez-Edgar and Fox (2005) reported similar findings with regard to temperament and the development of anxiety. A rising number of studies have found a consistent link between temperament and negative affect in early childhood with the development of anxiety in mid to late adolescence (Kagan & Snidman, 1999; Perez-Edgar & Fox, 2005; Schwartz, Snidman, & Kagan, 1999). Parents and their parenting style can also influence the presence of negative temperament and its impact on anxiety in children (Perez-Edgar & Fox, 2005). For instance, parents who are overprotective and have controlling behavior, as well as who lack warmth, tend to be linked with the surfacing of anxiety in children (Goldin, 1969; Parker, 1990; Perez-Edgar & Fox, 2005). Parents who have an intrusive parenting style may interfere with the

development of a child's self-regulation, which may increase a child's vulnerability (Calkins, Hungerford, & Dedmon, 2004; Perez-Edgar & Fox, 2005).

Intraindividual characteristics of children may be influenced by the family environment in which they are raised, which in turn can affect the level of anxiety in a child. Specifically, an assessment of the parent–child relationship can provide insight and perhaps help determine children at risk for anxiety (Messer & Beidel, 1994). Some examples include parent–child relationships that are marked with hostility and/or dependency (Messer & Beidel, 1994). Understanding a parent–child relationship may be beneficial in predicting antecedents of the various subtypes of anxiety behaviors in children. For example, children with parents who have panic disorders reported less structure and independence and reported more conflict and control (Messer & Beidel, 1994; Sylvester, Reichler, & Hyde, 1987). Environmental control and independence are also critical in understanding the etiology of anxiety disorders, as it has been found that higher traits of anxiety were correlated with lower self-competence (Messer & Beidel, 1994). This may suggest that family dynamics play a critical role in the influence on how anxiety affects the internal workings of a child.

Diagnosing anxiety disorders in children can be very challenging for a number of reasons. Primarily, it is difficult to differentiate between developmentally appropriate fears and true anxiety (Weems & Costa, 2005). In addition, without appropriate knowledge of these developmental stages, clinicians may misinterpret appropriate fears to be pathological. Another difficulty in diagnosis is related to the comorbidity of childhood anxiety disorders with other common emotional difficulties. This has lead to discussions about whether there is a single underlying shared risk of anxiety or several features that are specific to a different disorder (Eley et al., 2003). For instance, patients who are diagnosed with anxiety often also experience several symptoms of depression, including a diminished ability to think or concentrate, recurrent thoughts of death, insomnia or hypersomnia, or feelings of sadness/emptiness (APA, 2000). Another commonly misinterpreted manifestation of anxiety is symptoms associated with ADHD. Symptoms of ADHD can include avoiding things that take a lot of mental effort; losing items needed for tasks and activities (i.e., toys, pencils, or books); not listening when being spoken directly to; or not giving close attention to details or making careless mistakes in schoolwork and activities (APA, 2000). Though the underlying symptoms of ADHD may be rooted in anxiety, treatment for anxiety and ADHD are quite different, warranting careful consideration prior to a definitive diagnosis.

Over the past decade there has been an increase in assessment procedures to simplify our understanding of anxious children (Labellarte, Ginsburg, Walkup, & Riddle, 1999; Langley et al., 2002; Ollendick & King, 1998; Pine, 1997). This historical neglect of childhood anxiety may have been due to the perceived difficulties in the assessment of these disorders (Greenhill, Pine, March, Birmaher, & Riddle, 1998; Langley et al., 2002). In many instances, the presence of comorbid symptoms makes it challenging to provide a diagnosis. Using various assessment methods allow clinicians to understand information about the specific symptoms of a disorder (Langley et al., 2002). Specifically, using a structured or semistructured diagnostic interview (respondent-based interviews) offers a reliable and objective diagnostic profile (Langley et al., 2002). Some assessment tools (Muris & Broeren, 2009) to measure anxiety disorder symptoms from the child and parent perspective include the Spence Child Anxiety Scale (Spence, 1998) and the screen for child anxiety related emotional disorders (SCARED) (Birmaher et al., 1999). Social Phobia (subtype of anxiety disorders) can be measured using the Social Anxiety Scale for Children Revised (LaGreca & Stone, 1993) and the Social Phobia and Anxiety Inventory for Children (Beidel, Turner, & Morris, 1995; Muris & Broeren, 2009).

The DSM-IV-based interviews appear to be the most acceptable and reliable psychometric tool for diagnosing anxiety (Langley et al., 2002). For instance, an effective DSM-IV-based interview, the Anxiety Disorders Interview Schedule for DSM-IV (ADIS-IV), is a semistructured interview developed to evaluate anxiety disorders from ages 6–17 (Langley et al., 2002). It relies on the DSM-IV criteria for anxiety disorders and uses an interviewer–observer format. The ADIS-IV offers developmentally appropriate language, along with visual prompts to supplement the child's verbal abilities (Langley et al., 2002). It takes approximately 1–1.5 hr per interview and offers excellent test–retest reliability, specifically illustrating sensitivity to treatment effects for children and adolescents with anxiety disorders (Langley et al., 2002; Silverman, Saavedra, & Pina, 2001). Another beneficial DSM-IV-based interview is the K-schedule for affective disorders and schizophrenia for school-aged children — present and lifetime version (K-SADS-PL). It is a semistructured diagnostic interview used to create clinical diagnosis in research settings (Langley et al., 2002). This interview takes approximately 1 hr to complete and is used on children 6–18 years of age. It has illustrated positive test–retest reliability; however, the scores of anxiety disorders show a lower reliability versus

externalizing disorder (Kaufman et al., 1997; Langley et al., 2002). In comparison with the ADIS-IV, the K-SADS-PL does not provide specific details of symptoms as opposed to ADIS-IV (Langley et al., 2002). Another effective psychometric tool for the diagnosis of anxiety is the DISC-IV (National Institute of Mental Health Diagnostic Interview Schedule for Children — fourth version) (Langley et al., 2002). It is a respondent-based diagnostic measure incorporating both the DSM-IV and the ICD-10 (World Health Organization) diagnoses (Langley et al., 2002). It is a structured interview, which can last from 70–120 min, and is best used by beginner clinicians because it does not require clinical judgment (versus K-SADS-PL) (Langley et al., 2002).

Children with anxiety disorders often exhibit various sleeping problems that can include bedtime resistance, sleep anxiety, and nightmares (Gregory & Eley, 2005). About 10% of children show signs of anxiety disorders by age 16 (Costello, Mustillo, Erkanli, Keeler, & Angold, 2003), with 25% of adolescents exhibiting a sleep problem (Gregory & Eley, 2005; Stores & Wiggs, 1998). Gregory and Eley (2005) conducted a study to determine any associations between anxiety, sleep problems, and cognition (e.g., anxiety sensitivity and attributional styles). Seventy-nine children aged 8–11 participated in this study, with 48% of subjects males and 70% of the children Caucasian (Gregory & Eley, 2005). A 13-item sleep self-report (Owens, Maxim, Noblie, McGuinn, & Msall, 2000) was utilized to measure sleep problems in children (Gregory & Eley, 2005). For instance, did the participant have difficulties in going to bed or falling asleep, or daytime sleepiness, or waking up during the night (Gregory & Eley, 2005). Anxiety was measured by using the SCARED (Birmaher et al., 1997, 1999), which consists of a 41-item questionnaire, rated on a 3-point Likert scale (Gregory & Eley, 2005). The results indicate associations between sleep problems and anxiety, features of anxiety sensitivity, and attributional style (Gregory & Eley, 2005). The study also illustrated anxiety to be strongly correlated with specific types of sleep problems (e.g., sleep anxiety), whereas sleep problems display a stronger relationship with certain types of anxiety (e.g., school phobias) (Gregory & Eley, 2005). A child with inadequate sleep may exhibit increased amounts of stress and anxiety since his or her body is physically and mentally unable to get rest (Gregory & Eley, 2005; Gregory, Eley, O'Connor, & Plomin, 2004a).

NEUROPATHOLOGY/PATHOPHYSIOLOGY

Although there is a substantial amount of research on childhood anxiety disorders, there is a relatively small amount of research studying the neuropathology of childhood anxiety. Modern research has emphasized a genetic component as an antecedent of anxiety (Gregory & Eley, 2007). Behavioral-genetic research has shown that there is a genetic transmission of childhood anxiety disorders (Muris & Broeren, 2009). Eley and Gregory's (2004) study depict up to 50% of anxiety problems being hereditary. In an earlier study, Eley and colleagues examined phenotype and genetic structure of mother-reported anxiety-related behaviors in 4,564 4-year-old twin pairs (Eley et al., 2003). The study found that it is possible to distinguish anxiety-related behaviors in children as young as 4 years old. In relation to twins, the behavior of one twin has the direct effect on decreasing the same behavior in the co-twin (Eley et al., 2003). For instance, if one child is shy it may cause the other child to be more sociable (Eley et al., 2003). Eley et al. (2003) are currently conducting follow-up assessments of their sample to determine specificity of development over the years of middle childhood.

Biologically, serotonin is a neurotransmitter that assists in relaying messages from one area of the brain to another (Brouchez, 2009). It can influence psychological and other body functions (such as the cardiovascular system, muscles, and various elements of the endocrine system) (Bouchez, 2009). Males tend to have more serotonin than females (which might explain why women have a higher rate of anxiety and depression than men) (Bouchez, 2009). Raised levels of serotonin are called 5-HT. When 5-HT is further from the outside of the nerve cell (extracellular of the neuron), it benefits the patient in reducing anxiety disorders (particularly with OCDs) (Blier & Mansari, 2007).

The availability of 5-HT is controlled by several elements. The 5-HT reuptake transporter carries 5-HT outside the neurone into the cell body and a presynaptic terminal to regulate 5-HT levels in the synaptic cleft (Blier & Mansari, 2007). The 5-HT1A autoreceptor binds 5-HTand makes an "inhibitory effect" on the neurons (Blier & Mansari, 2007). The 5-HT1B autoreceptor regulates 5-HT levels in the synaptic cleft (Blier & Mansari, 2007). The last serotonin system, postsynaptic 5-HT receptors, includes the 5-HT1A and 5-HT1B subtypes located on the cell body of the neurone (Blier & Mansari, 2007). When there is an irregular/unbalanced level of serotonin, medication is provided to patients to regulate serotonin levels.

Frontal brain activation can determine the level of anxiousness in a child as well. The left frontal brain region is associated with positive emotions and readiness to approach the environment, versus the right frontal brain region that corresponds to negative emotions and withdrawal reactions (Baving, Laucht, & Schmidt, 2002). Children with anxiety have higher brain activity on the right side of their brain, and tend to be shy and fearful—often experiencing stronger emotions in response to negative events (Davidson, Jackson, & Kalin, 2000).

Gender differences can also determine the level of anxiety in children while in school. Boys are more likely to exhibit disruptive behavior disorders, whereas girls exhibit more emotional disorders (Baving et al., 2002). Gender differences in the frontal brain activation can determine differences in basic affective styles (Baving et al., 2002). For example, increased levels of left-sided orbitofrontal glucose metabolism have been found in women compared with men (Baving et al., 2002). In relation to childhood anxiety, Baving et al. (2002) measured anxious symptoms with 8- and 11-year-old children. Their results indicated no gender differences when comparing anxious children with healthy children with aggressive symptoms (Baving et al., 2002). Gender differences may not be a predictor for anxious children, but it may prove significant when comparing adults. Left frontal activation in highly defensive women are associated with reduced negative effect, versus right frontal activation in highly defensive men (Baving et al., 2002; Kline, Allen, & Schwartz, 1998).

NEUROPSYCHOLOGICAL/CLINICAL PRESENTATION

There are several physical signs that accompany anxiety. These can include sweating, vomiting, dizziness, weakness in the legs, palpitations, difficulty breathing, and dryness of the mouth (Lader, 1975). Children with anxiety can also exhibit a fear of losing control, dying, and panic attacks (Fong & Silien, 1999). Panic attacks, episodes of intense fear, are generally uncued and unexpected, whereas anxious symptoms related to panic disorders are typically cued or situationally bound (Fong & Silien, 1999). Depressive symptoms are also common manifestations of childhood anxiety. Children with depression illustrate behaviors such as crying, social withdrawal, dependency, psychomotor retardation, and suicidal acts (Essau & Petermann, 1999). Somatic signs with depression can consist of fatigue, sleep disturbance, weight loss/gain, and gastrointestinal upset (Essau & Petermann, 1999).

Research has established various cognitive biases believed to play a role in the development of childhood anxiety disorders (Muris & Broeren, 2009). Specifically, studies have shown anxious children display hyperattention toward potentially threatening materials, and frequently interpret ambiguous situations in a threatening way (Muris & Broeren, 2009). However, the various symptoms of children with anxiety vary based on the child's age group (Geller et al., 2001; Kendall & Pimentel, 2003; Muris & Broeren, 2009). For instance, childhood GAD typically has an onset around the age of 9, whereas children with a specific phobia such as dental phobia, typically begin displaying symptoms at around age 12 (Morrison & Anderson, 2001). Anxiety is also most common among children with PTSD and OCDs; thus, when a child presents with a history of these diagnoses, it would be expected that anxiety would accompany his or her presentation of symptoms (Muris & Broeren, 2009).

Weems, Silverman, Rapee, and Pina (2003) investigated the role of control in childhood anxiety disorders. To study this topic, the authors used Barlow's model of control and anxiety, which suggests that the lack of control over external threats and/or the control over internal threats are central to experience anxiety (Barlow, 1998, 2002; Weems et al., 2003). For example, the belief anxiety experiences are uncontrollable is part of the obstacle for patients with anxiety disorders (Weems et al., 2003). Weems et al. (2003) collected data from 117 participants, from ages 9–17. The majority of the participants were Hispanic/Latino (57%) and Caucasian (34%), with 51% of the sample female (Weems et al., 2003). To assess "control" over anxiety, a set of 14 questions were used to determine external threats (such as fear-producing situations) and another set of 16 questions to measure a patient's control over negative internal reactions (such as trembling or shaking) (Rapee, Craske, Brown, & Barlow, 1996; Weems et al., 2003). To measure self-reported anxiety levels, the 37-item revised children's manifest anxiety scale was given to participants (Reynolds & Richmond, 1978; Weems et al., 2003). Results indicated that participants who were clinically referred for anxiety problems illustrated lower perceived control over their internal reactions to anxiety (Weems et al., 2003). The results are also consistent with Barlow's model of anxiety disorders (Barlow, 1988), indicating that the perceived lack of control over external threats and control over internal threats are important to the experience/awareness of anxiety in youths (Rapee et al., 1996; Weems et al., 2003). Adolescents and children may not characterize internal and external threats as adults — requiring further research to identify youths understanding of control beliefs (Weems et al., 2003).

DIAGNOSIS

It is important to have multi-informant methods when assessing childhood anxiety. Family influence such as parenting style may affect the emotional development of a child including expectations and coping approaches of parents (Langley et al., 2002). For example, parents of anxious children are more controlling, confrontational, and do not encourage independence as opposed to parents of nonanxious children (Barrett, Rapee, Dadds, & Ryan, 1996; Langley et al., 2002; Whaley, Pinto, & Sigman, 1999). Assessing a child's environment can be beneficial to determine triggers that increase their level of anxiety. Specifically, assessing a child's family can establish reinforcements for anxious behaviors (Langley et al., 2002).

There are various types of anxiety disorders. Under the DSM (APA, 2000), anxiety can consist of agoraphobia, OCDs, GADs, as well as anxiety disorder due to a general medical condition. These are all commonly diagnosed in adults, whereas SAD is more commonly diagnosed in children. Children with SAD often experience significant emotional distress when a child is separated from their home or a significant other (usually a separation from a parent). Children may become severely homesick when leaving home and may express a fear of being lost, which results in the child refusing to be away from the house alone (APA, 2000). Children could also develop nightmares based on these fears (i.e., their family being killed or murdered) (APA, 2000).

As mentioned, children diagnosed with anxiety disorder can often exhibit signs of depression, OCDs, or PTSD. A child exhibiting depressive symptoms may feel emotional dejection and withdrawal, which can lead to anxiety disorders (i.e., complaints of somatic systems or elevated levels of blood pressure) (Rapee, Schniering, & Hudson, 2009). In many instances anxiety disorders are comorbid with other disorders such as depression. There are about 40% to 60% of anxious children having more than one anxiety disorder (Benjamin, Costello, & Warren, 1990; Kashani & Orvaschek, 1990; Last, Hersen, Kazdin, Francis, & Grubb, 1987; Rapee et al., 2009). There may be a high comorbidity with anxiety and other disorders due to poor diagnosis and an overlap of common risk factors (Rapee et al., 2009). For example, boys with anxiety disorders are significantly at a lower risk of displaying substance abuse disorders (Costello et al., 2003; Rapee et al., 2009).

Though less commonly diagnosed in children, agoraphobia and OCD can create significant intrapersonal and interpersonal difficulties. According to the APA (2000), agoraphobia is diagnosed when the patient experiences intense anxiety that is the result of being in situations where escape might be difficult or embarrassing; and/or if the patient experiences a

C

panic attack, help may not be immediately available. In children, agoraphobia may be diagnosed if the child avoids a situation or place that triggers these anxious feelings and emotions, requiring companionship when in the situation; and/or enduring the situation with significant distress (Morrison & Anderson, 2001). Patients with OCD exhibit obsessions, compulsions, or both (Morrison & Anderson, 2001). For a child to meet the criteria for an obsession, all of these symptoms must be present: recurring, persisting thoughts, impulses, or images intrude into the awareness and cause distress/anxiety; insight that these ideas are products of the patient's mind; the ideas are not just excessive worries about ordinary problems; and the patient tries to ignore or suppress these ideas (Morrison & Anderson, 2001). For compulsions, patients display the need to repeat physical or mental behaviors; the goal of these behaviors are to reduce distress or prevent from doing something that is dreaded; the behaviors are a response to an obsession with strict rules; and either of the behaviors are not realistically related to the events they are supposed to (Morrison & Anderson, 2001). Patients usually recognize obsession or compulsive behaviors, but unfortunately, this is untrue for children (Morrison & Anderson, 2001). Children are not developmentally mature enough to be able to recognize the abnormality in their ritualistic behaviors.

PTSD is the one disorder that is experienced similarly throughout the lifespan, where children and adolescents exhibit similar symptoms as adults (Morrison & Anderson, 2001). PTSD occurs when the patient has witnessed or experienced a traumatic event that has both these components: The actual event was either life-threatening or could result in serious physical injury to the patient or others; and the patient responded with intense fear or helplessness (Morrison & Anderson, 2001). The symptoms last longer than 1 month, as opposed to acute stress disorder (ASD), which requires exactly the same criteria, except symptoms only last from 2 days to 4 weeks with ASD (Morrison & Anderson, 2001).

Children with GAD worry about several situations or events, including those at home, at school, or in the community. For instance, they may feel anxious in situations where their behavior or performance is being assessed, like in school when doing a presentation or taking a test (Morrison & Anderson, 2001). Symptoms of GAD include having more than half the day where the patient experiences excessive anxiety and worry about several events (in at least 6 months) and trouble controlling one's feelings (Morrison & Anderson, 2001). There are also three (at least one is required for the diagnosis of

children) or more of the following symptoms associated with this anxiety and worry: feelings of being restless, easily tired, trouble concentrating, irritability, increased muscle tension, and/or trouble sleeping (initial insomnia or restless sleep) (Morrison & Anderson, 2001).

As a general rule, it is important to remember that anxiety occurs at various levels for patients. It can be a normal and valuable emotion that goes through a series of changes in a person's lifetime. The *DSM-IV* offers several subtypes of anxiety that protect clinicians from the impulse to overdiagnose mental disorders (Morrison & Anderson, 2001). This is particularly beneficial when working with children since they can have difficulty expressing (both physically and verbally) their feelings and emotions. When a child does not qualify for any distinct *DSM-IV* anxiety disorder they are usually diagnosed as Anxiety Disorders Not Otherwise Specified (Morrison & Anderson, 2001).

TREATMENT

The most common therapy for children with anxiety is cognitive-behavioral therapy (CBT) and pharmacotherapy (Muris & Broeren, 2009). CBT focuses on coping styles and aims to assist children in identifying their anxiety, in hopes of facing situations that make them anxious (Rapee et al., 2009). Various techniques include verbal instructions, activities, role plays, and modeling to provide children with the skills needed to reduce their level of anxiety (Rapee et al., 2009). The effectiveness of CBT is influenced by the child's age and gender, type of disorder and severity, and the parent's role in therapy. A majority of CBT programs include the involvement of a child's parent (i.e., providing positive reinforcement to their child) (Rapee et al., 2009).

The majority of CBT programs involve the child's parents, either as active participants or as indirect recipients of information (Rapee et al., 2009). For instance, some programs inform parents of the various behavior management strategies that encourage positive reinforcement for a child (Rapee et al., 2009). To reduce any interference of the parents' own anxiety onto their child, several CBT programs offer a component to target parental anxiety (Cobham, Dadds, & Spence, 1998; Rapee et al., 2009). This is beneficial for both the parent and the child, since it allows clarification for both the parent and the child's emotions and feelings. At times, a parent may be encouraging or influencing a child's behavior and anxiety, particularly if the child frequently mimics the parents' behavior. Parents' encouragement and assistance enables the child to be independent, which reduces controlling or overprotective parenting (Rapee, 2000; Rapee et al., 2009). Several research studies have indicated that parents' anxiety can constrict a child's outcome, particularly with younger children (Berman, Weems, Silverman, & Kurtines, 2000; Rapee et al., 2009). A family history of anxiety can also influence the success of treatment (Rapee et al., 2009). Pharmacotherapy is used typically as a secondary option when children do not respond adequately to CBT (Muris & Broeren, 2009).

Khanna and Kendall (2009) explored the role of parent training in the treatment of childhood anxiety using CBT. Several studies have indicated parent training to predict improved outcomes (Crawford & Manassis, 2001; Khanna & Kendall, 2009; Wood, Piacentini, Southam-Gerow, Chu, & Sigman, 2006); however, some studies report little or no benefit of these strategies in CBT (Khanna & Kendall, 2009; Nauta, Scholing, Emmelkamp, & Minderaa, 2003; Spence, Donovan, & Brechman-Toussaint, 2000). Khanna and Kendall's study found no significant improvement on parental training in the treatment of childhood anxiety. External factors may have an influential impact on a parents training in CBT. For example, having a single parent assist with treatment versus both parents encouraging their child, a parents' history with anxiety, or having other family members with anxiety.

Parents who are skeptical of CBT treatments and rather work with their child independently may decide to use a less costly treatment such as bibliotherapy. This form of therapy requires little or no clinician contact, and parents implement treatment with the aid of written materials. According to Rapee, Abbott, and Lyncham (2006) parent bibliotherapy was effective for children on a wait list but was not as effective as a standard group treatment. Having a therapist provide input (via telephone or email) to parents using bibliotherapy has shown improved outcomes (Lyneham & Rapee, 2006; Rapee et al., 2009).

Various medications are recommended and given to children with anxiety disorders. Sometimes the medications can be too strong and carry severe side effects when given to children, as not all medications are produced by manufacturers for use with children. Physicians and psychiatrists often closely monitor a child's behavior when taking these medications for the first time to minimize prolonged negative side effects. Fluoxetine has been shown to be effective in the acute treatment of children and adolescents with GAD, SAD, and social phobia (Birmaher et al., 2003). The most common antidepressant medication given to children is Prozac (with serotonin–norepinephrine reuptake inhibitors of fluoxetine) (Schoenstadt, 2009). It is the only medication approved by the FDA for treating depression in children 8 years or older (Schoenstadt, 2009). Some other common medications are Zoloft (sertraline), Paxil (paroxetine), Celexa (citalopram), Lexapro (escitalopram), and Luvox (fluvoxamine) (Schoenstadt, 2009).

Several studies aim to provide children with early interventions to prevent the development of anxiety. Research has indicated a great reduction in the symptoms of anxiety with children who are engaged in active interventions; however, the symptoms of depression have not shown significant improvement (Rapee et al., 2009). For example, Mifsud and Rapee (2005) researched children from a low socioeconomic background who were not given previous treatment for their symptoms. Children from the active intervention (according to teachers and self-reports) displayed greater reduction of anxiety symptoms versus children in the monitoring-only intervention group (Mifsud & Rappee, 2005; Rapee et al., 2009). Unfortunately replications of interventions with positive results have been challenging. Many of the interventions do not produce the same outcome, requiring further research to improve the results of early interventions (Rapee et al., 2009).

Melissa Singh
Beth Trammell
Chad A. Noggle

American Psychiatric Association. (2000). *Diagnostic and statistical manual of mental disorders* (4th ed.). Washington, DC: Author.

Anderson, J. C., Williams, S., Mcgee, R., & Silva, A. (1987). DSM-III disorders in preadolescent children. *Archives of General Psychiatry, 44*, 69–80.

Barlow, D. H. (1988). *Anxiety and its disorders: The nature and treatment of anxiety and panic.* New York: Guilford Press.

Barlow, D. H. (2002). *Anxiety and its disorders: The nature and treatment of anxiety and panic* (2nd ed.). New York: Guildford Press.

Barrett, P., Rapee, R., Dadds, M., & Ryan, S. (1996). Family enhancement of cognitive styles in anxious and aggressive children. *Journal of Abnormal Child Psychology, 24*, 187–203.

Baving, L., Laucht, M., & Schmidt, M. H. (2002). Frontal brain activation in anxious school children. *Journal of Child Psychology and Psychiatry, 43*(2), 265–274.

Beidel, D. C., Turner, S. M., & Morris, T. L. (1995). A new inventory to assess childhood social anxiety and phobia: The social phobia and anxiety inventory for children. *Psychological Assessment, 7*, 73–79.

Benjamin, R. S., Costello, E. J., & Warren, M. (1990). Anxiety disorders in a pediatric sample. *Journal of Anxiety Disorders, 4*, 293–316.

C

Berman, S., Weems, C. F., Silverman, W. K., & Kurtines, W. M. (2000). Predictors of outcome in exposure-based cognitive behavioral treatments for phobic and anxiety disorders in children. *Journal of Consulting and Clinical Psychology, 64*, 333–342.

Birmaher, B., Axelson, D. A., Monk, K., Kalas, C., Clark, D. B., Ehmann, M., et al. (2003). Fluoxetine for the treatment of childhood anxiety disorders. *Journal of the American Academy of Child & Adolescent Psychiatry, 42*(4), 415–423.

Birmaher, B., Brent, D., Chiappetta, L., Bridge, J., Monga, S., & Baugher, M. (1999). Psychometric properties of the screen for child anxiety related emotional disorders (SCARED): A replication study. *Journal of the American Academy of Child and Adolescent Psychiatry, 38*, 1230–1236.

Birmaher, B., Khetarpal, S., Brent, D., Cully, M., Balach, L., Kaufman, J., et al. (1997). The screen for child anxiety related emotional disorders (SCARED): Scale construction and psychometric characteristics. *Journal of the American Academy of Child and Adolescent Psychiatry, 36*, 545–553.

Blier, P., & Mansari, M. E. (2007). The importance of serotonin and noradrenaline in anxiety. *International Journal of Psychiatry in Clinical Practice, 11*, 16–23.

Brouchez, C. (2009). *Serotonin: 9 questions and answers-WebMD*. Retrieved November 3, 2009, from http://www.webmd.com/depression/recognizing-depression-symptoms/serotonin

Calkins, S. D., Hungerford, A., & Dedmon, S. E. (2004). Mothers' interactions with temperamentally frustrated infants. *Infant Mental Health Journal, 25*, 219–240.

Cobham, V. E., Dadds, M. R., & Spence, S. H. (1998). The role of parental anxiety in the treatment of childhood anxiety. *Journal of Consulting and Clinical Psychology, 66*, 893–905.

Costello, E. J., Mustillo, S., Erkanli, A., Keeler, G., & Angold, A. (2003). Prevalence and development of psychiatric disorders in childhood and adolescence. *Archives of General Psychiatry, 60*, 837–844.

Crawford, A. M., & Manassis, K. (2001). Familial predictors of treatment outcome in childhood anxiety disorders. *Journal of the American Academy of Child and Adolescent Anxiety, 40*, 1182–1189.

Davidson, R. J., Jackson, D. C., & Kalin, N. H. (2000). Emotions, plasticity, context, and regulation: Perspective from affective neuroscience. *Psychological Bulletin, 126*, 890–909.

Eley, T. C., Bolton, D., O'Connor, T. G., Perrin, S., Smith, P., & Plomin, R. (2003). A twin study of anxiety-related behaviours in pre-school children. *Journal of Child Psychology and Psychiatry, 44*(7), 945–960.

Eley, T. C., & Gregory, A. M. (2004). Behavioral genetics. In T. L. Morris & J. S. March (Eds.), *Anxiety disorders in children and adolescents* (pp. 71–97). New York: Guildford.

Essau, C. A., & Petermann, F. (Eds.). (1999). *Depressive disorders in children and adolescents*. North Bergen, NJ: Jason Aronson.

Fong, M. L., & Silien, K. A. (1999). Assessment and diagnosis of DSM-IV anxiety disorders. *Journal of Counseling & Development, 77*, 209–217.

Geller, D. A., Biederman, J., Faraone, S., Agranat, A., Cradock, K., Hagermoser, L., et al. (2001). Developmental aspects of obsessive-compulsive disorder: Findings in children, adolescents, and adults. *The Journal of Nervous and Mental Disease, 189*, 471–477.

Goldin, P. C. (1969). A review of children's reports of parent behaviors. *Psychological Bulletin, 77*, 222–236.

Grant, V. V., Bagnell, A. L., Chambers, C. T., & Stewart, S. H. (2009). Early temperament prospectively predicts anxiety in later childhood. *The Canadian Journal of Psychiatry, 54*(5), 320–329.

Greenhill, L., Pine, D., March, J., Birmaher, B., & Riddle, M. (1998). Assessment issues in treatment research of pediatric anxiety disorders: What is working, what is not working, what is missing, and what needs improvement. *Psychopharmacology Bulletin, 34*, 155–164.

Gregory, A. M., & Eley, T. C. (2005). Sleep problems, anxiety, and cognitive style in school-aged children. *Infant and Child Development, 14*, 435–444.

Gregory, A. M., & Eley, T. C. (2007). Genetic influence on anxiety in children: What we've learned and where we're heading. *Clinical Child and Family Psychology, 10*(3), 199–212.

Gregory, A. M., Eley, T. C., O'Connor, T. G., & Plomin, R. (2004a). Etiologies of associations between childhood sleep and behavioral problems in a large twin sample. *Journal of the American Academy of Child and Adolescent Psychiatry, 43*, 744–751.

Kagan, J., & Snidman, N. (1999). Early childhood predictors of adult anxiety disorders. *Biological Psychiatry, 46*, 1536–1541.

Kashani, J. H., & Orvaschel, H. (1990). A community study of anxiety in children and adolescents. *American Journal of Psychiatry, 147*, 313–318.

Kaufman, J., Birmaher, B., Brent, D., Rao, U., Flynn, C., Moreci, P., et al. (1997). Schedule for affective disorders and schizophrenia for school-aged children present and lifetime version (KSADS-PL): Initial reliability and validity data. *Journal of the American Academy of Child & Adolescent Psychiatry, 36*, 980–989.

Kendall, P. C., & Pimentel, S. S. (2003). On the physiological symptom constellation in youths with generalized anxiety disorder. *Journal of Anxiety Disorders, 17*, 211–221.

Khanna, M. S., & Kendall, P. C. (2009). Exploring the role of parent training in the treatment of childhood anxiety. *Journal of Consulting and Clinical Psychology, 77*(5), 981–986.

King, N. J., Hamilton, D. I., & Ollendick, T. H. (1988). *Children's phobias: A behavioural perspective.* New York: John Wiley.

Kline, J. P., Allen, J. J. B., & Schwartz, G. E. (1998). Is left frontal brain activation in defensiveness gender specific? *Journal of Abnormal Psychology, 107,* 149–153.

Labellarte, M. J., Ginsburg, G. S., Walkup, J. T., & Riddle, M. A. (1999). The treatment of anxiety disorders in children and adolescents. *Biological Psychiatry, 46,* 1567–1578.

Lader, M. (1975). *The psychophysiology of mental illness.* London: Routledge and Kegan Paul.

LaGreca, A. M., & Stone, W. L. (1993). Social anxiety scale for children-revised: Factor structure and concurrent validity. *Journal of Clinical Child Psychology, 22,* 17–27.

Langley, A. K., Bergman, R. L., & Piacentini, J. C. (2002). Assessment of childhood anxiety. *International Review of Psychiatry, 14,* 102–113.

Last, C. G., Hersen, M., Kazdin, A. E., Francis, G., & Grubb, H. J. (1987). Psychiatric illness in the mothers of anxious children. *American Journal of Psychiatry, 144,* 1580–1583.

Laucht, M., Esser, G., Baving, L., Gerhold, M., Hoesch, I., Ihle, E., et al. (2000). Behavioral sequelae of perinatal insults and early family adversity at 8 years of age. *Journal of the American Academy of Child & Adolescent Psychiatry, 39,* 1229–1237.

Lyneham, H. J., & Rapee, R. M. (2006). Evaluation of therapist supported parent-implemented CBT for anxiety disorders in rural children. *Behaviour Research and Therapy, 44*(9), 1287–1300.

Messer, S. C., & Beidel, D. C. (1994). Psychosocial correlates of childhood anxiety disorders. *Journal of the American Academy of Child and Adolescent Psychiatry, 33*(7), 975–983.

Mifsud, C., & Rapee, R. M. (2005). Early intervention for childhood anxiety in a school setting: Outcomes for an economically disadvantaged population. *Journal of the American Academy of Child & Adolescent Psychiatry, 44*(10), 996–1004.

Morrison, J., & Anderson, T. H. (2001). *Interviewing children and adolescents: Skills and strategies for effective DSM-IV diagnosis.* New York: The Guildford Press.

Muris, P., & Broeren, S. (2009). Twenty-five years of research on childhood anxiety disorders: Publication trends between 1982 and 2006 and a selective review of the literature. *Journal of Child and Family Studies, 18,* 388–395.

Muris, P., Meesters, C., Merckelbach, H., Sermon, A., & Zwakhalen, S. (1998). Worry in normal children. *Journal of American Academy of Child and Adolescent Psychiatry, 37,* 703–710.

Nauta, M. H., Scholing, A., Emmelkamp, P. M. G., & Minderaa, R. B. (2003). Cognitive-behavioral therapy for children with anxiety disorders in a clinical setting: No additional effect of a cognitive parent training. *Journal of the American Academy of Child and Adolescent Psychiatry, 42,* 1270–1278.

Ollendick, T. H., & King, N. J. (1998). Empirically supported treatments for children with phobic and anxiety disorders: Current status. *Journal of Clinical Child Psychology, 27*(2), 156–167.

Owens, J. A., Maxim, R., Noblie, C., McGuinn, M., & Msall, M. (2000). Parental and self-report of sleep in children with attention-deficit/hyperactivity disorder. *Archives of Pediatrics and Adolescent Medicine, 154,* 549–555.

Parker, G. A. (1990). A decade of research. *Social Psychiatry and Psychiatric Epidemiology, 25*(6), 281–282.

Perez-Edgar, K., & Fox, N. A. (2005). Temperament and anxiety disorders. *Journal of Child and Adolescent Psychiatric Clinics of North America, 14,* 681–706.

Pine, D. S. (1997). Childhood anxiety disorders. *Current Opinion in Pediatrics, 9,* 329–338.

Rapee, R. M. (2000). Group treatment of children with anxiety disorders: Outcomes and predictors of treatment response. *Australian Journal of Psychology, 52*(3), 125–130.

Rapee, R. M., Abbott, M., & Lyneham, H. (2006). Bibliotherapy for children with anxiety disorders using written materials for parents: A randomized controlled trial. *Journal of Consulting and Clinical Psychology, 74,* 436–444.

Rapee, R. M., Craske, M. G., Brown, T. A., & Barlow, D. H. (1996). Measurement of perceived control over anxiety related events. *Behavior Therapy, 27,* 279–293.

Rapee, R. M., Schniering, C. A., & Hudson, J. L. (2009). Anxiety disorders during childhood and adolescence: Origins and treatment. *Annual Review of Clinical Psychology, 5,* 311–341.

Reynolds, C. R., & Richmond, B. O. (1978). What I think and feel: A revised measure of children's manifest anxiety. *Journal of Abnormal Child Psychology, 6,* 271–280.

Rothbart, M. K., Ahadis, S. A., & Evans, D. E. (2000). Temperament and personality: Origins and outcomes. *Journal of Personality and Social Psychology, 78,* 122–135.

Schoenstadt, R. (2009). *Antidepressants in children page – eMedTV.* Retrieved November 3, 2009, from http://depression.emedtv.com/childhood-depression/antidepressants-in-children.html

Schwartz, C. E., Snidman, N. S., & Kagan, J. (1999). Adolescent social anxiety as an outcome of inhibited temperament in childhood. *Journal of American Academy of Child & Adolescent Psychiatry, 53,* 1008–1015.

Silverman, W. K., Saavedra, L. M., & Pina, A. A. (2001). Test-retest reliability of anxiety symptoms and diagnoses with anxiety disorders interview schedule for DSM-IV: Child and parent versions. *Journal of the American Academy of Child & Adolescent Psychiatry, 20,* 162–168.

Spence, S. H. (1998). A measure of anxiety symptoms among children. *Behaviour Research and Therapy, 36*(5), 545–566.

Spence, S. H., Donovan, C., & Brechman-Toussaint, M. (2000). The treatment of childhood social phobia: The effectiveness of a social skills training-based, cognitive-behavioural intervention, with and without parental involvement. *Journal of Child Psychology and Psychiatry, 41*, 713–726.

Stores, G., & Wiggs, L. (1998). Clinical services for sleep disorders. *Archives of Disease in Childhood, 79*, 495–497.

Sylvester, C. E., Hyde, T. S., & Reichler, R. J. (1987). The Diagnostic Interview for Children and Personality Inventory for Children in studies of children at risk for anxiety disorders or depression. *Journal of the American Academy of Child and Adolescent Psychiatry, 26*, 668–675.

Weems, C. F., & Costa, N. M. (2005). Developmental differences in the expression of childhood anxiety symptoms and fears. *Journal of the American Academy of Child and Adolescent Psychiatry, 44*, 656–663.

Weems, C. F., Silverman, W. K., Rapee, R. M., & Pina, A. A. (2003). The role of control in childhood anxiety disorders. *Cognitive Therapy and Research, 27*(5), 557–568.

Whaley, S. E., Pinto, A., & Sigman, M. (1999). Characterizing interaction between anxious mothers and their children. *Journal of Clinical Child Psychology, 67*, 826–836.

Wood, J. J., Piacentini, J. C., Southam-Gerow, M., Chu, B., & Sigman, M. (2006). Family cognitive behavioral therapy for child anxiety disorders. *Journal of the American Academy of Child and Adolescent Psychiatry, 45*, 314–321.

CHILDHOOD MOOD DISORDERS

DESCRIPTION

Childhood mood disorders encompass several psychological disorders that disrupt one's affect and mood. Specifically, such disorders include Major Depressive Disorder (MDD), Bipolar Disorder, and other specified affect disorders, such as Cyclothymic Disorder and Dysthymic Disorder. Although mood disorders are listed in the adult disorders section of the *Diagnostic and Statistical Manual of Mental Disorders* (*DSM-IV-TR*; American Psychiatric Association [APA], 2000), the aforementioned mood disorders may also occur in children, but symptoms and duration may differ from that of adults (Essau, Petermann, & Reynolds, 1999).

Depressed affect refers to periods of sadness, unhappiness, or dysphoric mood that occur in approximately one-third of children and adolescents, often peaking during the middle adolescent years (Brooks-Gunn, Auth, Petersen, & Compas, 2001). However, it is only when the depressive symptoms are persistent and severe that they are considered pathological. Oftentimes, older children and adolescents are more likely to report experiencing a depressed mood. Interestingly, depression has been found to have a higher prevalence in girls during adolescence, yet childhood depression appears to be more common in boys (Angold & Castello, 2001). Although many individuals report experiencing periods of negative affect, to be labeled as a disorder, the disturbance in mood must be characterized by a change that is persistent, severe, and pathological.

MDD is characterized by the primary symptoms of (1) dysphoria, or feeling bad, and/or apathetic mood, (2) a loss or decrease in the strength of stimuli, and (3) anhedonia, which is described as the chronic inability to experience pleasure. Though depression typically appears through affective and behavioral reports and observations, neurobiological associates may also be indicative of MDD. In children, symptoms of MDD appear to be associated with dysregulation in growth hormone, peripheral hormone secretion (specifically cortisol and prolactin hormones), and hypothalamic–pituitary regulation of hormones (Birhamer & Ryan, 1999; Brooks-Gunn et al., 2001).

When an individual demonstrates depressive symptoms but does not meet the *DSM-IV-TR* (2000) criteria for MDD, his/her symptoms may be indicative of dysthymic disorder. This is diagnosed when the depressed mood occurs for more days than not in a period of 2 years (in adults). Although Dysthymic Disorder is chronic, it often appears in a less severe form than Depressive Disorder. Children diagnosed with Dysthymic Disorder demonstrate chronic depressive and/or irritable symptoms for at least 1 year (compared with 2 years in adults) without a period of more than 2 symptom-free months (Essau, Petermann et al., 1999).

Bipolar Disorder, which can be differentiated from MDD as a unipolar disorder, has historically been referred to as manic-depressive psychosis, and consists of two major types. Bipolar I Disorder is characterized by the existence of at least one manic or one mixed episode (Essau, Petermann et al., 1999). Essau, Petermann et al. (1999) describe a manic episode as a substantial period of persistently high or irritable mood and the presence of three of seven characteristics listed in the *DSM-IV-TR* (APA, 2000) for at least 1 week. In contrast, a mixed episode occurs when the criteria for manic or major depressive episodes appear nearly every day, for a period of at least 1 week. Bipolar II Disorder, on the other hand, occurs when at least one major depressive episode is accompanied by one or more hypomanic episodes, which refer to periods of elevated, expansive, or irritable mood that occurs persistently for at least 4 days during a given week (Essau, Petermann et al., 1999). Like adults, children with Bipolar Disorder meet the same diagnostic criteria described in the *DSM-IV-TR* in experiencing mixed, manic, and major depressive episodes. Interestingly, childhood Bipolar Disorder has been suggested to be highly comorbid with Attention Deficit Hyperactivity Disorder (ADHD) (Angold & Costello, 2001).

Cyclothymic Disorder, an additional mood disorder listed in the *DSM-IV-TR* (APA, 2000), is characterized by numerous periods of hypomanic and depressive symptoms in a span of at least 2 years (in adults) that do not meet the criteria for a manic episode or major depressive episode. Cyclothymic Disorder is considered a bipolar mood disorder that involves chronic and fluctuating mood disturbances. Children and adolescents who are identified as having cyclothymic disorder must meet the hypomanic and depressive symptoms for at least 1 year (compared with 2 years in adults). Such symptoms are likely to cause significant impairments in both social and occupational functioning (Essau, Petermann et al., 1999). Specific to children, impairments in functioning may be evident in levels of energy, school performance (specific cognitive problems with processing speed, attention, and memory), sleep disturbances, and problems maintaining friendships (Davis, 2006).

Further mood disorders listed in the *DSM-IV-TR* (APA, 2000) include mood and bipolar disorders not otherwise specified, in which an individual's symptoms fail to meet the criteria for classifying mood disorders, and mood disorders related to a general medical condition or self-induced drug use. Mood disorder related to a general medical condition occurs when a persistent disturbance in mood is directly related to the physiological effects of a general medical condition. The disturbance in mood is not related to another mental disorder but causes impairments in functional ability. In substance-induced mood disorder, prominent and persistent mood disorders are the direct result of the physiological effects of a substance. The symptoms associated with substance-induced mood disorder occur during or within 1 month of substance intoxication or withdrawal (Essau, Petermann et al., 1999). Although mood disorders related to substance abuse during childhood are rare, such disorders may particularly be prevalent during adolescence, a time in which drug and alcohol use serve as powerful predictive factors of depression and suicidal behavior (Kienhorst et al., 1990; de Wilde, Kienhorst, & Diekstra, 2001). In Mood Disorders Related to a General Medical Condition, children demonstrate a depressed, expansive, or irritable mood as a result of a previously determined medical condition (Essau, Petermann et al., 1999).

NEUROPATHOLOGY / PATHOPHYSIOLOGY

In general, differences in neuroanatomy and brain function are suggestive of mood disorders in children, though depressive disorders have historically been attributed to environmental, emotional, or intrapsychic issues (Davis, 2006). Reviewed and relevant studies examining depression and brain structure and functioning have indicated organic differences, specifically in the amygdala and hippocampus of depressed children. Rosso et al. (2005) confirmed decreased volumes in the left and right amygdala in children with mood disorders. Further, decreased volumes in the hippocampus of children with depression may cause additional resistance to treatment (Vythilingam et al., 2002). Additional neuropsychological studies through the use of positron emission tomography, single photon emission computed tomography, and functional magnetic resonance imaging have further indicated differences in glucose metabolism and regional cerebral blood flow in children with mood disorders (Davis, 2006). For example, differences in right- and left-hemisphere activity (i.e., right-hemisphere dominance) in children with depression may explain a tendency to demonstrate increased attention and sensitivity to negative stimuli (Surguladaze et al., 2005).

Major Depressive Disorder. Besides the behavioral demonstrations and reports that are suggestive of mood disorders, studies on physiological processes associated with MDD suggest neurological underpinnings and predictive factors of such mood disorders. Brooks-Gunn et al. (2001) suggest implications of biological dysregulation in children and adolescents with clinical depression, specifically in changes that occur in the hypothalamic–pituitary axes and neurotransmitter regulation associated with this structure during puberty.

Much of the research associated with the physiological implications of depression has focused on studying the limbic system, which has involved an emphasis on the hypothalamic–pituitary axes (Graber, 2009). As children transition to adolescence through puberty, specific changes occur in the hypothalamic–pituitary–gonadal (HPG), hypothalamic–pituitary–thyroidal (HPT), and the hypothalamic–pituitary–adrenal (HPA) axes. Although all children experience such neurological changes, children with depression have demonstrated varying degrees of regulation during periods of depression, as well as during periods of recovery (Brooks-Gunn et al., 2001).

In adult patients, studies have consistently found dysregulation in the HPA axis, which is evident through hypersecretion and dysfunctional responses of the hormone cortisol, which is released by the adrenal gland. However, a lack of support has been found in the same studies of depressed children and adolescents (Brooks-Gunn et al., 2001). Although adults with depression demonstrate a hypersecretion of cortisol, this finding has been inconsistent in studies of children and adolescents (Birhamer, & Ryan, 1999). Studies of children and adolescents have, however, indicated that hyposecretion and control of cortisol may instead be related to depression based on the time of day in which cortisol and other hormones are secreted. For example, evening hyposecretion of cortisol and morning hyposecretion of dehydroepiandrosterone (DHEA) appear to be associated with depression in childhood and adolescence. Further, hyposecretion of cortisol and DHEA during late evening and midnight seem to be associated with depression.

In examining difference in the HPT axis, research suggests that thyroid-stimulating hormone may be lower in both child and adult depressed patients. The final area of the hypothalamic–pituitary axes that has been examined in relation to depression is the HPG axis. Though little research focuses on the role of the HPG axis in depression, pubertal studies have consistently found HPG hormones (specifically estradiol or testosterone) to be predictive of depression in girls (Angold & Castello 2001).

Studies of neurotransmitter systems have also suggested important findings related to depression in children and adolescents. Such studies have primarily examined the serotonergic, cholinergic, and noradrenergic systems in relation to depression, focusing on both the presynaptic and postsynaptic events, and the role of pharmacological agents in controlling depressive symptoms. Brooks-Gunn et al. (2001) explain that depression has generally been associated with an activated locus ceruleus–noradrenaline system, which is a norepinephrine system. In addition, the cholinergic system seems to be hyper-responsive in depressed patients, whereas the aminobutyric acid, GABA, and serotonin exhibit low levels in such patients.

Dysthymic Disorder. Though little research regarding neurological implications associated with dysthymic disorder exists, it is likely that many of the aforementioned neuroanatomical differences that contribute to depressive symptoms (e.g., differences in amygdala and hippocampus volume) are also present in children with dysthymic disorder. Like MDD, imbalances in neurotransmitter function, specifically serotonergic and noradrenergic, in the central nervous system have been suggestive of Dysthymic Disorder in children (Flory, Vance, Birelson, & Luk, 2002). Further, similar to the research on children with MDD, activation differences in the hypothalamic–pituitary–adrenal–gonadal axes may be indicative of dysthymic disorder in children (Rogeness, Javors, & Pliszka, 1992). Still, suggested findings regarding brain dysfunction and Dysthymic Disorder should be interpreted with caution due to the lack of consistent research using child participants.

Bipolar Disorder. Controversy exists regarding the recent increased prevalence of Bipolar Disorder during childhood. Because children with Bipolar Disorder demonstrate behavior that includes irritability, mood instability, irregular temper, and hyperactivity, some clinicians may associate such symptoms with a more common diagnosis of ADHD (Smith, 2007). Due to the comorbidities that are frequently present, the diagnosis of juvenile Bipolar Disorder may be clouded, and clinicians may be faced with difficulties in determining diagnoses and treatment (Smith, 2007). Still, studies of neurological anatomy and functioning consistently suggest organic differences that exist between children with Bipolar Disorder and typically functioning children.

In addition to the affective behaviors demonstrated in individuals diagnosed with Bipolar Disorder, several neurochemical and anatomical differences have been suggested in studies of Bipolar Disorder in children. Geller and DelBello (2003) first suggested differences in neurotransmitter regulation that appear in children with Bipolar Disorder, specifically in hypofunction on the NMDA (N-methyl-D-aspartate) receptor. Next, neuroimaging studies indicated neuroanatomical discrepancies in children and adolescencents with Bipolar Disorder compared with healthy child participants (Geller & DelBello, 2003). Though minimal neuroimaging studies exist on children with Bipolar Disorder compared with those of adults with Bipolar Disorder, functional and structural brain differences seem to appear in the amygdala, prefrontal cortex, thalamus, striatum, and cerebellar vermis.

Hypofunction of the NMDA receptor has been consistently found in studies of adults with bipolar disorder (Farber & Newcomer,). Because the NMDA neurotransmitter system is understood to be related to memory, cognitive function, and sensory information processing, NMDA receptor blockage is associated with psychiatric symptoms. Underexcitation, or hypofunction of NMDA, which is called NRHypo, has significant effects on CNS functioning and is further related to psychiatric impairments. NRHypo is a hypothesized neurological underpinning of adult Bipolar Disorder but cannot be generalized to the developing brain of a child due to the low prevalence of psychotic disorders during childhood and an onset during adolescence. Still, the relationship of NRHypo and psychotic symptoms may suggest a deeper understanding of cognitive and behavioral symptoms in children, which are predictive of future psychiatric disorders.

Besides understanding the role of NMDA receptors in bipolar patients, the use of neuroimaging has been used to further examine structural and functional brain differences in cases of pediatric Bipolar Disorder. Advances in brain imaging techniques have allowed for an increase in noninvasive brain studies, but most findings still exist among studies of adults with by Bipolar Disorder, rather than children. Though not all findings in adult clients can be applied to children with Bipolar Disorder, some significant findings regarding functional and structural neurology do exist. Botteron et al. (1995) conducted a study comparing children and adolescents with Bipolar Disorder with healthy participants, using MRI to examine neuroanatomical differences. Though the study was limited by a small sample size, the results demonstrated reduced structural asymmetry of the cerebral hemispheres and ventricular abnormalities (deep white matter hyperintensities) in bipolar children (DelBello & Kowatch, 2003). Additional MRI studies of pediatric Bipolar Disorder have indicated significantly reduced intracranial volumes, enlarged frontal and temporal fluid and lateral ventricular volumes, and decreased brain circumferences and thalamic volumes compared with control participants (Dasari et al., 1999).

NEUROPSYCHOLOGICAL/CLINICAL
PRESENTATION

Though the aforementioned neuropsychological implications associated with mood disorders may be useful in understanding such disorders, they often present themselves in ways that are directly observed by oneself or others.

Major Depressive Disorder. Although the *DSM-IV-TR* (2000) lists features of MDD as it applies to adults, children manifest depression in a way that is analogous to adults, though some differences do exist in developmental appropriateness and age-specific features (Stark, 1990). Children with MDD display five of

the following symptoms nearly every day for a period of at least 2 weeks and present a change in the level of previous functioning: Depressed mood (or irritable mood in children and adolescents); markedly diminished interest or pleasure in all or almost all activities; significant weight loss or weight gain, or decrease or increase in appetite (in children, consider failure to make expected weight gains); insomnia or hypersomnia; psychomotor agitation or retardation; fatigue or loss of energy; feelings of worthlessness or excessive or inappropriate guilt; indecisiveness or diminished ability to think or concentrate; and recurrent thoughts of death or suicide (with or without a specific suicidal plan), or a suicide attempt (APA, 2000; Essau, Petermann et al., 1990).

Besides the qualifying symptoms of MDD as listed in the *DSM-IV-TR* (APA, 2000), depressive episodes may be classified according to the severity. Depending on the number of symptoms, the symptom severity, and the degree of functional distress or disability, major depressive episodes may be classified as mild, moderate, or severe (Essau, Petermann et al., 1999). The *DSM-IV-TR* (APA, 2000) describes mild episodes as a period in which five to six depressive symptoms are observed, causing a minor impairment in occupational, social, or interpersonal functioning. Moderate episodes occur when the severity of one's symptoms and functional ability lies between mild and severe classification. During severe episodes, more symptoms than needed to meet the diagnostic criteria are present, which significantly interferes with occupational, social, or interpersonal functioning (APA, 2000).

Dysthymia. When an individual displays depressive symptoms but does not meet the criteria for MDD or other mood disorder, their symptoms may describe dysthymic disorder. Classified as a mood disorder in the *DSM-IV-TR* (APA, 2000), dysthymia occurs when an individual experiences a depressed mood for most of the day, for more days than not, during a period of at least 2 years (though children need only meet the criteria during a shorter duration of at least 1 year). The disorder requires two of the following six symptoms: poor appetite or overeating; insomnia or hypersomnia; low energy or fatigue; low self-esteem; poor concentration or difficulty making decisions; and feelings of hopelessness (Kolvin and Sadowski, 2001).

Bipolar Disorder. In identifying Bipolar I Disorder, an individual must demonstrate at least one manic or mixed episode, often having at least one major depressive episode, as well (Essau, Petermann et al., 1999). In addition to the presence of such episodes, bipolar individuals must also exhibit at least three of the seven symptoms identified in the *DSM-IV-TR* (APA, 2000), including grandiosity, decreased need for sleep, increased talkativeness, flight of ideas, distractibility, increased goal-directed activity and excessive involvement in pleasurable activities that have a high risk for dangerous or painful consequences. In Bipolar II Disorder, an individual demonstrates one or more major depressive episodes, at least one hypomanic episode, and at least three of the following symptoms: inflated self-esteem, decreased need for sleep, pressure of speech, flight of ideas, distractibility, increased involvement in goal-directed activities, and excessive involvement in pleasurable activities with high potential for painful consequences.

Beyond the behavioral and mood-based features that constitute the primary clinical features of the mood disorders, neurocognitive and motor deficits are also noted. Cognitively, deficits are commonly noted in areas of attention and concentration, executive functioning, abstract thinking and problem solving, mental flexibility, memory consolidation, organization and retrieval, control and shift of attention, and working memory and processing speed. In addition, motoric retardation has been commonly linked with depressive features. Although these cognitive and motoric symptoms are reported, it is emphasized that their appearance is more varied in children than in adults.

DIAGNOSIS

Diagnosis of mood disorders often involves the integration of knowledge gained from the client, observations made by a practitioner, and information gathered from individuals interacting and working directly with the child, such as teachers and parents. Specific to childhood psychopathology, many practitioners utilize a multimethod/multi-informant approach in order to develop a thorough understanding of the client's symptoms and needs. Parents and teachers are likely to provide useful information regarding the client's daily functioning.

A primary disturbance in mood and the aforementioned symptoms presented in each disorder serve as the primary means of diagnosing a mood disorder. The number, severity, and duration of depressive symptoms allow clinicians to then differentiate between various types of mood disorders (Stark, 1990).

In assessing mood disorders, advances have been made in the development of assessments, interviews, and questionnaires specific to children and adolescents. Essau, Hakim-Larson, et al. (1999) suggests the battery of assessment to include home and school performance, multiple domains of depressive symptoms (including affect, cognitions, and behavior), and

overall adjustment. In addition, the authors suggest that the battery of measurement used for diagnosing mood disorders should be appropriate to the developmental level of the child/client. Such assessment measures are suggested to include parent reports, teacher reports, cognitive assessment, physical assessment, self-assessment, and a structured diagnostic interview (Essau, Hakim-Larson, et al., 1999). In order to gain a comprehensive understanding of a child's maladaptive behavior and symptoms, a *Diagnostic Interview Schedules for Children* (DISC) may be used by a clinician. The DISC is used for children aged 9–17 and may be applied to the diagnosis of mood disorders or many other psychiatric disorders that occur during childhood, such as attachment disorders, eating disorders, anxiety, schizophrenia, or substance abuse (Essau, Hakim-Larson et al., 1999). During the DISC, the examiner presents a "stem" question that asks about the presence of maladaptive behavior, and the child (and/or parent) will then respond by answering "Yes," "No," or "Maybe" (Essau, Hakim-Larson et al., 1999). At the conclusion of the interview, the clinician will examine the symptoms reported by the client in order to determine whether a mood disorder is present.

In other cases, ratings by clinicians are used to assess mood disorders in children. Such as the *Children's Depression Rating Scale-Revised* (CSDRS-R; Poznanski et al., 1985). Clinician ratings involve a less-specific interview than the DISC and more general questions.

Clinicians may also assess a child through a self-report questionnaire that examines reports of self-worth, depressive thoughts, and underlying somatic symptoms. Self-report questionnaires that have been found to be reliable and valid in measuring mood disorders in children include the *Reynolds Child Depression Scale* (Reynolds, 1989; Reynolds and Graces, 1989), *The Depression Self-Rating Scale* (Birleson, 1981; Birleson et al., 1981), and *the Children's Depressive Inventory* (CDI; Kovas, 1992). Because not all children are fully capable of completing a self-report questionnaire, clinicians may include ratings completed by teachers and parents, who generally play a role referring a child for a psychological evaluation (Essau, Hakim-Larson, et al., 1999). Such ratings include the *Child Behavior Checklists* (CBCL, Achenbach, 1991, as cited in Essau, Hakim-Larson et al., 1999) or the *Behavior Assessment System for Children* (BASC), which includes both teacher and parent rating scales.

TREATMENT

The use of psychotherapy is a widely utilized and researched approach to treating children with mood disorders. Because some parents may resist the use of psychopharmacological treatment for their children, and because some children may not physically respond to psychotropic medication, therapy may be a useful tool in treating mood disorders during childhood. Though a variety of psychological treatments exist, psychotherapy is generally used to identify and adjust maladaptive behavior and characteristics in order to enhance one's cognitive, behavioral, and emotional management skills that contribute to the ability to cope with present and future life stressors (Nobile, Cataldo, Marino, & Molteni, 2003). Commonly used psychological treatments for childhood mood disorders include group, family, and individual therapy.

During group therapy, clients are able to listen to their peers and gain educational and problem-solving insights, in addition to general support from knowing they are not alone in experiencing difficulties with mood. Family therapy is used to promote healthy and positive relations between the parents and the child. Family therapy focuses on decreasing parental criticism and child isolation, encouraging a sense of family cohesion and support, and providing parents with information and support (Weis, Valeri, McCarthy, & Moore, 1999). Most commonly, the use of individual therapy is applied to the treatment of a child dealing with a mood disorder.

Individual therapy encompasses a variety of frameworks and techniques that can be used to treat a client. In treating children with mood disorders, one commonly used individual treatment includes cognitive behavioral therapy, which often involves a time-limited intervention that seeks to replace negative and depressive thoughts and behaviors for adaptive coping skills (Nobile et al., 2003). Interpersonal therapy may also be used to treat mood disorders. Here, the therapist encourages the client to identify links between negative moods with current problem areas (Nobile et al., 2003). Specific to children with mood disorders, the use of play therapy may be implemented, which involves unstructured and nondirective play in which a child is free to express difficult feelings which they are unable to articulate verbally (Weisz et al., 1999).

In addition to suggested psychotherapy, mood disorders in children are often treated using psychopharmacological agents. Many of the same medications used in adults with mood disorders are used to treat children. However, much caution is used in considering the dosage and side effects of the drug. In MDD, selective serotonin reuptake inhibitors (SSRIs), which are antidepressant drugs, and monoamine oxidase inhibition (MAOI) drugs are used to chemically balance neurotransmitters (Schultz & Remschmidt,

2001). In addition, though tricyclic antidepressants (TCAs) are commonly used in adult patients, children with mood disorders have demonstrated inconsistent responses to this treatment (Ryan et al., 1986, as cited in Schulz & Remschmidt, 2001).

Though the aforementioned medications (SSRIs, MAOIs, & TCAs) may be useful in treating depressive symptoms, such medications tend to be less effective in treating children with bipolar disorders. Like adults, children with bipolar disorder have consistently responded best to the use of lithium for psychopharmacological treatment (Ryan, 2003). Further, anticonvulsants, such as valproate, divalproex, and carbamazepine are also currently being used to treat children with bipolar disorder, though such medications possess significant potential side effects (Ryan, 2003).

Sarah Connolly
Chad A. Noggle

American Psychiatric Association. (1994). *Diagnostic and statistical manual of mental disorders* (4th ed., text revision). Washington, DC: Author.

Angold, A., & Castello, E. J. (2001). The epidemiology of depression in children and adolescents. In I. M. Goodyer (Ed.), *The depressed child and adolescent* (2nd ed., pp. 143–178). Cambridge, UK: Cambridge University Press.

Birhamer, B., & Ryan, N. D. (1999). Neurobiological factors. In C. A. Essau & F. Petermann (Eds.), *Depressive disorders in children and adolescents* (pp. 287–318). New Jersey: Jason Aronson.

Botteron, K. N., Vannier, M. W., Geller, B., Todd, R. D., & Lee, B. C. (1995). Preliminary study of magnetic resonance imaging characteristics in 8- to 16-year-olds with mania. *Journal of American Academy of Child Adolescent Psychiatry, 34*, 742–749.

Brooks-Gunn, J. B., Auth, J. J., Petersen, A. C., & Compas, B. E. (2001). Physiological processes and the development of childhood and adolescent depression. In I. M. Goodyer (Ed.), *The depressed child and adolescent* (2nd ed., pp. 79–118). Cambridge, UK: Cambridge University Press.

Dasari, M., Friedman, L., Jesberger, J., Stuve, T. A., Findling, R. L., Swales, T, P., et al. (1999). A magnetic resonance imaging study of thalamic area in adolescent patients with either schizophrenia or bipolar disorder as compared to healthy controls. *Psychiatry research, 91*(3), 155–162.

Davis, A. S. (2006). The neuropsychological basis of childhood psychopathology. *Psychology in the Schools, 43*(4), 503–512.

Delbello, M. P., & Kowatch, R. A. (2003). Neuroimaging in pediatric bipolar disorder. In B. Geller & M. P. DelBello (Eds.), *Bipolar disorder in childhood and early adolescence* (pp. 158–192). New York: Guilford Press.

C

de Wilde, E. J., Kienhorst, I. C. W. M., & Diekstra, R. F. W. (2001). Suicidal behaviour in adolescents. In I. M. Goodyer (Ed.), *The depressed child and adolescent* (2nd ed., pp. 143–178). Cambridge, UK: Cambridge University Press.

Essau, C. A., Hakim-Larson, J., Crocker, A., & Petermann, F. (1999). Assessment of depressive disorders in children and adolescents. In C. A. Essau & F. Petermann (Eds.), *Depressive disorders in children and adolescents* (pp. 27–67). New Jersey: Jason Aronson.

Essau, C. A., Petermann, F., & Reynolds, W. M. (1999). Classification of depressive disorders. In C. A. Essau & F. Petermann (Eds.), *Depressive disorders in children and adolescents* (pp. 3–25). New Jersey: Jason Aronson.

Flory, V., Vance, A. L. A., Birelson, P., & Luk, E. S. (2002). Early onset dysthymic disorder in children and adolescents: Clinical implications and future directions. *Child and Adolescent Mental Health, 7*(2), 79–84.

Geller, B., & DelBello, M. P. (Eds.). (2003). *Bipolar disorder in childhood and early adolescence*. New York: Guilford.

Graber, J. A. (2009). Pubertal and neuroendocrine development and risk for depression. In N. B. Allen & L. B. Sheeber (Eds.), *Adolescent emotional development and the emergence of depressive disorders* (pp. 74–91). Cambridge, UK: Cambridge University Press.

Kolvin, I., & Sadowski, H. (2001). Childhood depression: Clinical phenomenology and classification. In I. M. Goodyer (Eds.), *The depressed child and adolescent* (2nd ed., pp. 119–142). Cambridge, UK: Cambridge University Press.

Nobile, M., Cataldo, G. M., Marino, C., & Molteni, M. (2003). Diagnosis and treatment of dysthymia in children and adolescents. *CNS Drugs, 17*(13), 927–946.

Poznanski, E. O., & Mokros, H. B. (1996). *Children's depression rating scale, revised (CDRS-R)*. Los Angeles, CA: Western Psychological Services. Retrieved from http://openlibrary.org/search?publisher_facet = Western%20Psychological%20Services

Rogeness, G. A., Javors, M. A., & Pliszka, S. R. (1992). Neurochemistry and child and adolescent psychiatry. *Journal of the American Academy of Child and Adolescent Psychiatry, 31*, 765–781.

Rosso, I. M., Cintron, C. M., Steingard, R. J., Renshaw, P. F., Young, A. D., & Yurgelun-Todd, D. A. (2005). Amygdala and hippocampus volumes in pediatric major depression. *Biological Psychiatry, 57*, 21–26.

Ryan, N. D. (2003). The pharmacological treatment of child and adolescent bipolar disorder. In B. Geller & M. P. DelBello (Eds.), *Bipolar disorder in childhood and early adolescence* (pp. 247–271). New York: Guilford Press.

Schulz, E., & Remschmidt, H. (2001). Psychopharmacology of depressive states in childhood and adolescence. In I. M. Goodyer (Eds.), *The depressed child and adolescent* (2nd ed., pp. 292–324). Cambridge, UK: Cambridge University Press.

Smith, D. H. (2007). Controversies in childhood bipolar disorders. *The Canadian Journal of Psychiatry, 52*(7), 407–408.

Stark, K. D. (1990). *Childhood depression*. New York: Guilford Press.

Surguladze, S., Brammer, M. J., Keedwell, P., Giampietro, V., Young, A. W., Travis, M. J., et al. (2005). A differential pattern of neural response toward sad versus happy facial expressions in major depressive disorder. *Biological Psychiatry, 57*, 201–209.

Vythilingam, M., Heim, C., Newport, J., Miller, A. H., Anderson, B. A., Bronen, R., et al. (2002). Childhood trauma associated with smaller hippocampal volume in women with major depression. *American Journal of Psychiatry, 159*, 2072–2080.

Weis, J. R., Valeri, S. M., McCarthy, C. A., & Moore, P. S. (1999). Interventions for depression: Features, effects, and future directions. In C. A. Essau & F. Petermann (Eds.), *Depressive disorders in children and adolescents* (pp. 383–431). New Jersey: Jason Aronson.

CHOLESTERYL ESTER STORAGE DISEASE

DESCRIPTION

Cholesteryl ester storage disease (CESD), a type of lysosomal storage disease, is a rare condition involving the inappropriate breakdown and storage of fats and cholesterol causing harmful amounts of lipids to accumulate in cells and tissues throughout the body (the blood, lymph, and lymphoid tissues). The liver is most severely affected. Disease onset typically takes place during childhood or adolescence, though milder forms of CESD are not identified until adulthood (Assman & Seedorf, 2001).

NEUROPATHOLOGY/PATHOPHYSIOLOGY

CESD is inherited as an autosomal recessive trait. CESD results from an accumulation or storage of cholesteryl esters and triglycerides in the blood, lymph cells, and lymphoid tissues throughout the body. Cholesteryl esters and triglycerides remain in the blood and tissues and are unable to be transported to the liver for excretion. CESD is due to a deficiency in lysosomal acid lipase, the enzyme that breaks down both cholesteryl esters and triglycerides. Although both cholesteryl esters and triglycerides build up in the body, cholesteryl esters accumulate more than triglycerides (Aslanidis et al., 1996; Cox, 2005). The complete absence of lysosomal acid lipase activity causes

Wolman's disease, which is normally fatal within the first 6 months of life, whereas mutations resulting in CESD retain some enzyme activity of lysosomal acid lipase. Researchers have identified mutations in the lysosomal acid lipase gene contributing to CESD. The underlying gene is located on chromosome 10q23.2-q23.3 (Assman & Seedorf, 2001; Muntoni et al., 2007).

NEUROPSYCHOLOGICAL/CLINICAL PRESENTATION

The symptoms of CESD are highly variable. Some individuals present with liver dysfunction in early childhood, whereas others present with only minimal symptoms and are not diagnosed until adulthood. The expected lifespan of patients with CESD can vary and depend on the severity of associated complications (Assman & Seedorf, 2001). Hepatomegaly (enlarged liver) is one of the major symptoms of CESD. In addition, cirrhosis and chronic liver failure often occur before adulthood (Lageron & Polonovski, 1988). Elevated low density lipoprotein (LDL) and reduced high density lipoproteins (HDL) may also be present in CESD (Assman & Seedorf, 2001). Atherosclerosis (an accumulation of fatty deposits on the artery walls) is often seen early in life, increasing the chance of having a heart attack or stroke (Longhi et al., 1988). As CESD advances, patients may present with jaundice and calcium deposits in the adrenal glands. Although neuropsychological impairments are associated with some forms of lysosomal storage diseases (e.g., progressive encephalopathy and dementia in Tay-Sachs disease and metachromatic leukodystrophy), CESD does not necessarily present with any specific neurocognitive impairments since accumulation is typically seen in the liver, spleen, lymph nodes, and other tissues, rather than accumulating in the central nervous system (Assman & Seedorf, 2001; Cox, 2005). However, due to the increased risk of a stroke, secondary neurocognitive impairments and vascular dementia are highly likely.

DIAGNOSIS

Diagnosis is based on specific clinical features and evidence of acid lipase deficiency. Performing an enzyme assay, which identifies a deficiency of the enzyme acid lipase in liver cells, cultured white blood cells, or tissue specimens, facilitates a diagnosis of CESD. If there is evidence of significant family history for CESD, a prenatal diagnosis can be conducted to ascertain whether there is an absence of acid lipase activity in the fetus (Assman & Seedorf, 2001; Boldrini, Devito, Biselli, Filocamo, & Bosman, 2007).

TREATMENT

There is no cure for CESD. However, treating secondary hypercholesterolemia, hypertriglyceridemia, and HDL deficiency can be effective in reducing the symptoms of CESD. Cholesterol-reducing drugs, low cholesterol diet, and blood thinners to prevent clots are often the first line of treatment (Assman & Seedorf, 2001; Dalgc et al., 2006). Angioplasty with stenting can reduce angina or other symptoms of coronary artery disease, whereas an endarterectomy may be used to remove plaque buildup from atherosclerosis (Longhi et al., 1988). A transplant is the treatment of choice for patients presenting with advanced cirrhosis (Ferry, Whisennand, Finegold, Alpert, & Glombicki, 1991).

Darla J. Lawson

Aslanidis, C., Ries, S., Fehringer, P., Büchler, C., Klima, H., & Schmitz, G. (1996). Genetic and biochemical evidence that CESD and Wolman disease are distinguished by residual lysosomal acid lipase activity. *Genomics, 33*, 85–93.

Assman, G., & Seedorf, U. (2001). Acid lipase deficiency: Wolman disease and cholesteryl ester storage disease. In C. R. Scriver, A. L. Beaudet, W. S. Sly, D. Vale, B. Childs, K. W. Kinzler, et al. (Eds.), *The metabolic and molecular bases of inherited disease* (8th ed., pp. 8551–8572). New York: McGraw-Hill.

Boldrini, R., Devito, R., Biselli, R., Filocamo, M., & Bosman, C. (2007). Wolman disease and cholesteryl ester storage disease diagnosed by histological and ultrastructural examination of intestinal and liver biopsy. *Pathology: Research and Practice, 200*(3), 231–240.

Cox, T. M. (2005). Biomarkers in lysosomal storage diseases: A review. *Acta Paediatrica, 94*(447), 39–42.

Dalgc, B., Sar, S., Gunduz, M., Ezgu, F., Tumer, L., Hasanoglu, A., et al. (2006). Cholesteryl ester storage disease in a young child presenting as isolated hepatomegaly treated with simvastatin. *The Turkish Journal of Pediatrics, 48*(2), 148–151.

Ferry, G. D., Whisennand, H. H., Finegold, M. J., Alpert, E., & Glombicki, A. (1991). Liver transplantation for cholesteryl ester storage disease. *Journal of Pediatric Gastroenterology and Nutrition, 12*, 376–378.

Lageron, A., & Polonovski, J. (1988). Histochemical abnormalities in liver and jejunal biopsies from a case of cholesterol ester storage disease. *Journal of Inherited Metabolic Disease, 11*, 139–142.

Longhi, R., Vergani, C., Valsasina, R., Riva, E., Galluzzo, C., Agostoni, C., et al. (1988). Cholesteryl ester storage disease: Risk factors for atherosclerosis in a 15-year-old boy. *Journal of Inherited Metabolic Disease, 11*, 143–145.

Muntoni, S., Wiebusch, H., Jansen-Rust, M., Rust, S., Seedorf, U., Schulte, H., et al. (2007). Prevalence of cholesteryl ester storage disease. *Arteriosclerosis, Thrombosis, and Vascular Biology, 27*, 1866–1868.

CHRONIC INFLAMMATORY DEMYELINATING POLYNEUROPATHY

DESCRIPTION

Chronic inflammatory demyelinating polyneuropathy (CIDP) is a neurological disorder where certain autoantibodies infiltrate the peripheral myelin leading to progressive weakness and impaired sensory function in the legs and arms. Diagnosis is made in patients that present with a chronically progressive or relapsing symmetric sensorimotor disorder with cytoalbuminologic dissociation as well as interstitial and perivascular endoneurial infiltration by lymphocytes and macrophages (Lewis, 2009; Rajabally, Jacob, & Abbott, 2006).

Rare in occurrence, epidemiological research suggests a prevalence of only 2–7 per 100,000 (McLeod et al., 1999; Mygland & Monstad, 2001). Although cases have been documented across the life span, even in childhood, the disease most commonly presents in young adults and in men slightly more than females.

NEUROPATHOLOGY/PATHOPHYSIOLOGY

CIDP occurs secondary to an immunologic antibody-mediated reaction with interstitial and perivascular infiltration of the endoneurium and epineurium of peripheral nerve fibers with inflammatory T cells and macrophages (Prineas & McLeod, 1976). Furthermore, human leukocyte antigens Dw3, DRw3, A1, and B8 are found in higher rates in individuals with CIDP when compared with the healthy population. The collective result of these features is a segmental demyelination of the peripheral nerves and spinal roots with a variable degree of inflammatory infiltration (Lewis, 2009). Additional pathological changes have been noted to involve the plexuses, proximal nerve trunks, and, occasionally, cranial nerves and sympathetic trunks as well as some autonomic nerves (Dyck, Prineas, & Pollard, 1993). Intrafascicular edema and hypertrophic changes are often seen (Graham & Lantos, 1997).

Although CIDP predominately impacts peripheral nerves, CNS involvement has also been reported in 5% to 50% of cases consisting of white matter lesions of diffuse orientation (Hawke, Hallinan, & McLeod, 1990; Ormerod, Waddy, Kermode, Murry, & Thomas, 1990; Uncini et al., 1991). For example, Fee and Fleming (2003) reported the case of a 45-year-old left-handed woman with CIDP that on MRI-FLAIR sequencing was found to have four or more lesions including a prominent lesion in the left superior frontal gyrus involving the gray–white matter junction and three smaller lesions involving the white matter in the left frontal, left parietal, and right frontal lobes respectively. As such, though CNS involvement is possible, no specific pattern is noted.

Pathologically, research has suggested that CIDP has been found to be accompanied by several systematic diseases such as systemic lupus erythematosus (SLE), HIV infection, diabetes mellitus, and monoclonal gammopathy. Furthermore, Hashimoto's thyroiditis, thyroxicosis, hepatitis, urticaria, eczema, Sjogren's syndrome, and melanoma have also been linked with CIDP (Haq, Pendlebury, Fries, & Tandan, 2003; Parry, 1993). It suggests that CIDP has a heterogeneous pathogenesis or is a clinical syndrome that can result from several photogenic mechanisms (Nakajima et al., 2005).

NEUROPSYCHOLOGICAL/CLINICAL PRESENTATION

CIPD initially presents as proximal-to-distal limb weakness in combination with sensory symptoms including tingling sensation or numbness. However, additional symptoms may also develop including facial weakness, areflexia described as loss of deep tendon reflexes, fatigue and abnormal sensations, as well as dysphasia, speech impairment, muscle atrophy, coordination difficulties, bladder dysfunction, and difficulties breathing. Muscle weakness may affect mobility such as walking or turning, whereas sensory impairments may exhibit a negative influence on balance and aspects of coordination. Although motor deficits are the most commonly seen feature (Dyck et al., 1975; McCombe, McManis, Frith, Pollard, & McLeod, 1987), primary sensory variants can occur (Oh, Joy, & Kuruoglu, 1992). Sensory features most commonly manifest as paresthesia, numbness, decreased tactile sensitivity, and even sensory ataxia in more severe instances. Infrequent muscle cramping and fasciculations as well as general pain and irritation may occur. Diplopia, dysarthria, and dysphagia may develop in the face of cranial nerve infiltration, whereas incontinence and erectile dysfunction may occur related to autonomic dysfunction (Dyck et al., 1993; Prineas & McLeod, 1976).

C

Oftentimes the onset of the disease is mostly subtle yet alarming, followed by a chronic progressive (over 60% of patients) or relapsing (33% of patients) course of illness. It is believed that 16% of patients present with an acute or subacute onset of the disease, with steady or fluctuating disease course. In fact, the presentation is closely linked with Guillain-Barré syndrome and is considered the chronic form of that presentation. In other words, Guillain–Barré syndrome is a prodromal state of CIDP, with the patients who develop it being classified as having CIDP as they continue to present with symptoms chronically. Consequently, complete remissions are seldom probable in CIDP in comparison to Guillain–Barré syndrome. On rare occasions, the disease is associated with quadriplegia, respiratory failure, and death.

Neurocognitive effects are not commonly seen as primary manifestations. Some deficits may present secondary to slowed graphomotor performance or due to general fatigue. However, in those rare cases where CNS involvement is noted, no specific profile emerges as the pathology varies.

DIAGNOSIS

CIDP is considered when patients present with a symmetric proximal and distal motor-predominant disorder. Diagnostic workup should include neurological examination to detect sensory impairment and weakness as well as nerve biopsy to detect the cause of the inflammation and to rule out other nerve diseases. Additional tests include spinal tap to detect levels of CSF total protein and EMG and nerve conduction tests to detect loss of myelin sheath and erosion of nerve cell (Lewis, 2009). Koski et al. (2009) suggested diagnostic criteria for CIDP to include the presence of a chronic nongenetic polyneuropathy, progressive for the duration of at least 8 weeks, without a serum paraprotein, and either recordable compound muscle action potentials in more than 75% of motor nerves or abnormal F wave latency in more than 50% of nerves, or a symmetrical onset of motor symptoms in all four limbs, and proximal weakness in one limb or more.

Electrophysiology findings suggest that in order to differentiate between the following neuropathies: myelin-associated glycoprotein (MAG), sulphated glucuronyl paragloboside (SGPG) and CIDP, CIDP had at least two nerves with TLI 0.25 and no conduction block (CB). CIDP was reported to have poorer response for therapy. Anti-MAG/SGPG neuropathy was reported to have a length-dependent process with a likely centripetal evolution. Moreover, the presence of disproportionate slowing of conduction in distal segments of motor nerves suggests MAG/SGPG (Capasso et al., 2002).

TREATMENT

The course of CIDP varies widely among individuals. Some may have a bout of CIDP followed by spontaneous recovery, whereas others may have many bouts with partial recovery in between relapses. The disease is a treatable cause of acquired neuropathy, and initiation of early treatment to prevent loss of nerve axons is recommended. However, some individuals are left with some residual numbness or weakness.

Treatment begins with proper identification. Rajabally et al. (2006) noted the importance of awareness of benign forms of CIDP and its diverse presentation, as it can be functionally disabling and may progress to severe symptomatology. Once identified, treatment for CIDP includes corticosteroids, such as prednisone, which may be prescribed alone or in combination with immunosuppressant drugs (Dyck et al., 1982; Hadden & Hughes, 2003). Corticosteroids are useful not only in reducing inflammation but also in general symptom relief. Plasmapheresis (plasma exchange) and intravenous immunoglobulin (IVIg) therapy are effective as a means of removing the problematic autoantibodies. IVIg may be used even as a first-line therapy (Mehndiratta & Hughes, 2002). Physical therapy is recommended to improve function and mobility, increase muscle strength, and reduce the shrinkage of tendons, muscles, and distortions of the joints (Muley & Parry, 2009; Kuntzer, 2006).

Shira Louria
Chad A. Noggle

Capasso, M., Torrieri, F., Di Muzio, A., De Angelis, M. V., Lugaresi, A., & Uncini, A. (2002). Can electrophysiology differentiate polyneuropathy with anti-MAG/SGPG antibodies from chronic inflammatory demyelinating polyneuropathy? *Clinical Neurophysiology, 113,* 346–353.

Dyck, P. J., Lais, A. C., Ohta M., Bastron, J. A., Okazaki, H., & Groover, R. V., (1975). Chronic inflammatory polyradiculoneuropathy. *Mayo Clinic Proceedings, 50,* 621–637.

Dyck, P. J., O'Brien, P. C., Oviatt, K. F., Dinapoli, R. P., Daube J. R., Bartleson J. D., Mokri B., Swift, T., Low, P. A., & Windebank, A. J. (1982). Prednisone improves chronic inflammatory demyelinating polyradiculoneuropathy more than no treatment. *Annals of Neurology, 11,* 136–141.

Dyck, P. J., Prineas, J., & Pollard, J. (1993). Chronic inflammatory demyelinating polyradiculoneuropathy. In P. J.

C

Dyck & P. K. Thomas (Eds.), *Peripheral neuropathy* (pp. 1498–1517). Philadelphia: Saunders.

Fee, D. B., & Fleming, J. O. (2003). Resolution of chronic inflammatory demyelinating polyneuropathy-associated central nervous system lesions after treatment with intravenous immunoglobulin. *Journal of the Peripheral Nervous System, 8*, 155–158.

Hadden, R. D., & Hughes, R. A. (2003). Management of inflammatory neuropathies. *Journal of Neurology Neurosurgery and Psychiatry, 74*, 9–14.

Haq, R. U., Pendlebury, W. W., Fries, T. J., & Tandan, R. (2003). Chronic inflammatory demyelinating polyradiculoneuropathy in diabetic patients. *Muscle Nerve, 27*, 465–470.

Hawke, S., Hallinan, J., & McLeod, J. (1990). Cranial magnetic resonance imaging in chronic demyelinating polyneuropathy. *Journal of Neurology, Neurosurgery and Psychiatry, 53*, 794–796.

Koski, C. L., Baumgarten, M., Magder, L. S., Barohn, R. J., Goldstein, J., Graves, M., et al. (2009). Derivation and validation of diagnostic criteria for chronic inflammatory demyelinating polyneuropathy. *Journal of the Neurological Sciences, 277*(1/2), 1–8.

Kuntzer, T. (2006). Treatment options for chronic inflammatory demyelinating polyradiculoneuropathy. *Review Neurology, 162*(4), 539–543.

Lewis, R. A. (2009). *Chronic inflammatory demyelinating polyradiculoneuropathy*. The emedicine Web. Retrieved March 19, 2009, from http://emedicine.medscape.com/article

McCombe, P. A., McManis, P. E., Frith, J. A., Pollard, J. D., & McLeod, J. G. (1987). Chronic inflammatory demyelinating polyradiculoneuropathy associated with pregnancy. *Annals of Neurology, 21*, 102–104.

McLeod, J. G., Pollard, J. D., Macaskill, P., Mohamed, A., Spring, P., & Khurana, V. (1999). Prevalence of chronic inflammatory demyelinating polyneuropathy in New South Wales, Australia. *Annals of Neurology, 46*, 910–913.

Mehndiratta, M. M., & Hughes, R. A. C. (2002). Corticosteroids for chronic inflammatory demyelinating polyradiculoneuropathy. *Cochrane Database of Systematic Reviews*, (1). Art No. CD002062. doi:10.1002/14651868. CD002062

Muley, S. A., & Parry, G. J. (2009). Inflammatory demyelinating neuropathies. *Current Treatment Options in Neurology, 11*(3), 221–227.

Mygland, A., & Monstad, P. (2001). Chronic polyneuropathies in Vest-Agder, Norway. *European Journal of Neurology, 8*, 157–165.

Nakajima, H., Shinoda, K., Doi, Y., Tagami, M., Furutama, D., Sugino, M., et al. (2005). Clinical manifestation of chronic inflammatory demyelinating polyneuropathy with anti-cardiolipin antibodies. *Acta Neurologica Scandinavia, 111*, 258–263.

Oh, S. J., Joy, S. L., & Kuruoglu, R. (1992). Chronic sensory demyelinating neuropathy: Chronic inflammatory demyelinating polyneuropathy presenting as a pure sensory neuropathy. *Journal of Neurology, Neurosurgery and Psychiatry, 55*, 677–680.

Ormerod, I., Waddy, H., Kermode, A., Murry, N., & Thomas, P. (1990). Involvement of the central nervous system in chronic inflammatory demyelinating polyneuropathy: A clinical, electrophysiological and magnetic resonance imaging study. *Journal of Neurology, Neurosurgery and Psychiatry, 53*, 789–793.

Parry, G. J. (1993). *Guillain-Barré syndrome*. New York: Thieme Medical Publishers.

Prineas, J. W., & McLeod, J. G. (1976). Chronic relapsing polyneuritis. *Journal of Neurological Science, 27*, 427–458.

Rajabally, Y. A., Jacob, S., & Abbott, R. J. (2006). Clinical heterogeneity in mild chronic demyelinating polyneuropathy. *European Journal of Neuropathy, 13*, 958–962.

Uncini, A., Gallucci, M., Lugaresi, A., Porrini, A., Onofrj, M., & Gambi, D. (1991). CNS involvement in chronic inflammatory demyelinating polyneuropathy: An electrophysiological and MRI study. *Electromyography and Clinical Neurophysiology, 31*, 365–371.

CHRONIC PAIN SYNDROME

DESCRIPTION

Chronic pain syndrome is a disorder that is characterized by a combination of chronic pain as well as reduced daily functioning and depressive symptoms. Though injury may be the initial cause of the syndrome, pain can also occur in the absence of tissue damage (Clifford, 1993). Depression and anxiety stem from long-term pain perception and functioning decreases over time (Weitz, Witt, & Greenfield, 2000).

When categorizing or diagnosing the disorder, chronic pain must be distinguished from acute pain (Clifford, 1993). Acute pain is precise and localized and likely the result of tissue damage, whereas chronic pain is pain that persists beyond the reasonable time it takes for damaged tissues to heal (Clifford, 1993). It is also important to distinguish chronic organic pain from chronic inorganic pain (Clifford, 1993). Chronic organic pain generally follows tissue damage or dysfunction, whereas chronic inorganic pain occurs in the absence of tissue damage (Clifford, 1993). Furthermore, chronic organic pain can be established using diagnostic tests or clinical findings, whereas chronic inorganic pain lies outside the realm of diagnostic tests (Clifford, 1993). Generally speaking, in chronic pain syndrome, pain tends to be inorganic (Clifford, 1993). Over time, such pain becomes diffuse and difficult to treat and feelings of depression and anger can both stem from, and exacerbate, the perception of pain (Clifford, 1993). Certain personality disorders, such as narcissistic personality disorder and borderline personality disorder, are sometimes associated with chronic pain syndrome (Pawl, 1998).

NEUROPATHOLOGY/PATHOPHYSIOLOGY

Chronic pain syndrome is a difficult disorder to identify and understand because it has no clear pathophysiological basis (Mostoufi, 2008). Its etiology is presumed based on the initial injury, but as chronic pain symptoms exist beyond the scope of tissue damage, a clear etiology is difficult to determine (Clifford, 1993). There is no diagnostic test available to screen for it (Mostoufi, 2008), though diagnostic tests are often given in order to rule out other undiagnosed causes of pain (Mostoufi, 2008). A diagnosis of chronic pain syndrome is made by excluding all other possible diagnoses (Clifford, 1993).

NEUROPSYCHOLOGICAL/CLINICAL PRESENTATION

Typical complaints of chronic pain patients are of back pain, specifically of the spinal axial muscle groups, and/or pain or tenderness where muscles attach to bones elsewhere in the body (Pawl, 1998). Since pain is a subjective experience that varies from patient to patient, the true severity of pain is difficult to verify, though it is generally either localized to a specific body part or generalized throughout the entire body (Mostoufi, 2008). Behavioral observations such as abnormal gait, poor posture, facial grimacing, and stiff movements can be helpful in diagnosing (Mostoufi, 2008). Emotional responses of fear or avoidance are also commonly observed, which can lead to deconditioning. Depressive symptoms such as withdrawal, decreased functioning, insomnia, decreased libido, and suicidal ideations are also common presentations (Weitz et al., 2000). Insomnia is a particular problem with chronic pain patients and relates to both the physical pain and anxiety about the pain (Mostoufi, 2008). Anxiety can increase the experienced intensity of pain as well as create physical tension (Weitz et al., 2000).

Often, patients who have chronic pain syndrome have a high rate of somaticization (manifest physical symptoms secondary to psychological distress),

making comprehensive evaluation an imperative part of diagnosis (Pawl, 1998). Individuals who do somaticize tend to believe that there is some organic cause for their pain and deny any psychological disturbance (Pawl, 1998).

DIAGNOSIS

Chronic pain syndrome is a diagnosis of exclusion and several disorders must be ruled out in order to diagnose it accurately. First, a physical examination must be given in order to determine the extent of the patient's functioning. Such examinations are geared toward discovering problems that are treatable (Mostoufi, 2008). A musculoskeletal and neurological examination is necessary, and depending upon the complaint, other areas may be examined (e.g., gastrointestinal complaints) to rule out physiological courses (Mostoufi, 2008). Diagnostic testing for chronic pain syndrome may include laboratory work, MRI or CAT scans, and/or electrodiagnostics (Mostoufi, 2008). Such tests often come back negative or inconclusive. The Minnesota Multiphasic Personality Inventory (MMPI) (or some other personality inventory) is sometimes given to gain an understanding of the patient's emotional state (Mostoufi, 2008). Inconclusive results from the physical battery coupled with results indicative of depression and/or anxiety from the emotional battery lead to a diagnosis of chronic pain syndrome. Differential diagnoses include somatoform disorders, somatization disorder, conversion disorder, hypochondriasis, and malingering (Mostoufi, 2008).

TREATMENT

There are two methods of treatment for chronic pain syndrome. The first is a pharmacological approach, which focuses mainly on symptom alleviation. Prescribed pain relief medication generally falls into three categories that are ranked according to potency (Weitz et al., 2000). The first category includes analgesics such as NSAIDs. The second category includes low-potency opioids, and the third category includes high-potency opioids (Weitz et al., 2000). Antidepressants may also be prescribed, particularly if the chronic pain individual is withdrawn, low functioning, has disrupted sleep patterns, or exhibits anhedonia (Weitz et al., 2000). Anxiolytics are sometimes prescribed if the individual expresses symptoms of daytime anxiety (Weitz et al., 2000).

It has been found, however, that treatment plans for chronic pain should focus more on rehabilitation and return of function rather than symptom alleviation (Clifford, 1993). Pharmacological approaches treat only the symptoms of chronic pain, which are unlikely to subside completely in chronic pain syndrome, and potential side effects deter the patient from adhering to a pharmacological regimen (Clifford, 1993). Exercise is especially helpful and has been shown to decrease reported pain levels, as activity level increases (Clifford, 1993). If perceptions of pain exist beyond the scope of medical management, then a functional restoration program must be installed. The goal of such a program is not relief of pain but increased functionality (Clifford, 1993). Functional restoration programs are based on exercise regimens that increase in small, controlled steps, slowly maximizing function and minimizing further tissue damage (Clifford, 1993). The program must also include emotional and psychological support, as it is likely pain will subside slowly, if ever (Clifford, 1993). Continually, the program should integrate vocational aspects in order to increase the individual's functions in the workplace (Clifford, 1993). Rehabilitation therapies such as functional restoration are most effective when undergone for 2–3 hr per day, 3 days a week, for 6–12 weeks (Mostoufi, 2008). Engaging in weekly therapy with a mental health counselor may also be beneficial (Mostoufi, 2008). With a multidisciplinary approach to rehabilitation, it is still recommended that a pain specialist oversee the entire rehabilitation process based on the specialist's expertise in this area (Mostoufi, 2008).

There are many methods of treating the psychological aspects of chronic pain syndrome. The goals of mental health treatment for chronic pain patients are to provide them with techniques to manage pain and decrease pain behaviors (Mostoufi, 2008). One important technique is relaxation training, as it helps ease anxiety and provides reprieve from discomfort (Weitz et al., 2000). Other therapeutic techniques include electromyelographic biofeedback, clinical hypnosis, and developing coping mechanisms (Mostoufi, 2008). Cognitive-behavioral therapy and interpersonal therapy have also been shown to be effective in treating individuals with chronic pain syndrome, particularly when it includes educating the individual and his or her family to help encourage an active role in treating the syndrome (Weitz et al., 2000).

Courtney Lund
Raymond S. Dean

Clifford, J. C. (1993). Successful management of chronic pain syndrome. *Canadian Family Physician, 39,* 549–559.

Mostoufi, S. A. (2008). Chronic pain syndrome. In W. R. Frontera, J. K. Silver, & T. J. Rizzo (Eds.), *Essentials of physical medicine and rehabilitation: Musculoskeletal disorders, pain, and rehabilitation* (2nd ed., pp. 505–509). Philadelphia: Saunders, an imprint of Elsevier.

Pawl, R. P. (1998). Chronic pain syndrome. *Surgical Neurology, 50,* 200–201.

Weitz, S. E., Witt, P. H., & Greenfield, D. P. (2000). Treatment of chronic pain syndrome. *New Jersey Medicine, 97,* 63–67.

CHURG–STRAUSS SYNDROME

DESCRIPTION

Churg–Strauss syndrome (CSS) is a rare form of systemic autoimmune vasculitis, also known as allergic angiitis and allergic granulomatosis. It is characterized by angiitis—inflammation of blood vessels throughout the body. CSS often occurs in middle-aged patients with a history of asthma or allergy (Churg, 2001; Churg & Strauss, 1951).

NEUROPATHOLOGY/PATHOPHYSIOLOGY

Vasculitis is caused by the inflammation of blood vessels. In CSS, small- to medium-sized blood vessels (i.e., arteries, arterioles, venules) become inflamed from an invasion of eosinophils, white blood cells. Granulomatosis form when eosinophils cluster together and release harmful granules that cause inflammatory lesions in the lungs, skin, kidneys, heart, gastrointestinal tract, and nerves. These inflammatory lesions can impair blood flow to various organ systems. Asthma and eosinophilic inflammation are key features of CSS (Guillevin, Pagnoux, & Mouthon, 2004). The cause of CSS is unknown, but it is speculated to be due to a variety of factors including genetics, environment, and infection. There is evidence to support causal factors related to autoimmunity due to the presence of hypergammaglobulinemia (increased levels of immunoglobulin in the blood). CSS often develops after steroid withdrawal in asthma patients who are treated with leukotriene receptor antagonists and who are steroid dependent (Churg, 2001; Lanham, Elkon, Pusey, & Hughes, 1984; Wechsler, Pauwels, & Drazen, 1999).

NEUROPSYCHOLOGICAL/CLINICAL PRESENTATION

Clinical presentation of CSS is progressive, consisting of three distinct stages. First is the allergic stage characterized by asthma, allergic rhinitis, and sinusitis. Patients often experience allergic inflammation of the nose, sinuses, skin, and lungs. Patients with childhood-onset asthma and allergies may present with a sudden worsening of symptoms, whereas other patients are often diagnosed with late-onset asthma. Second is the hypereosinophilic stage characterized by an excess of eosinophils in the blood and in certain organs causing inflammation of the lungs, skin, kidneys, heart, gastrointestinal tract, and nerves. Patients often develop chronic eosinophilic pneumonia and/or eosinophilic gastroenteritis. Symptoms include shortness of breath, coughing, weight loss, fever, abdominal pain, bloating, vomiting, diarrhea, ulcers, nausea, and night sweats. Esophageal inflammation may contribute to dysphagia or difficulty swallowing. Third is the systemic vasculitis stage characterized by inflammation and damage of blood vessels throughout the body. General symptoms include fever, weight loss, adenopathy (swollen lymph nodes), skin rashes, sores, joint pain, abdominal pain, vomiting, diarrhea, and chest pain. If the nerves are involved, patients exhibit mononeuritis multiplex—a form of peripheral neuropathy involving severe pain, numbness, tingling, and muscle wasting of the hands and feet (Boyer, Vargas, Slattery, Rivera-Sanchez, & Colin, 2006; Churg, 2001; Lanham et al., 1984). Not all patients diagnosed with CSS experience all three phases or experience them sequentially. Intervention can assist or even prevent CSS from progressing to advanced stages (Solans et al., 2001).

DIAGNOSIS

The symptoms of CSS vary widely from patient to patient and are similar to other syndromes, thus its diagnosis can be difficult. Nonetheless, a diagnosis is based on specific clinical features and a thorough history. CSS is often considered with late-onset asthma or worsening asthma, pain or numbness in the extremities, symptoms of cardiac involvement, sinus difficulty, persistent cough, skin rash, or lasting stomach problems. The American College of Rheumatology has proposed six criteria for diagnosing CSS. The six criteria include asthma, eosinophilia, mononeuropathy or polyneuropathy, pulmonary infiltrates, history of acute or chronic sinus pain, and extravascular eosinophils. CSS is generally considered if a person presents with four of the six criteria, though a diagnosis can be made if a patient only presents with two or three of the criteria (Masi et al., 1990). There are no specific tests to confirm CSS; however, a variety of tests can be used to facilitate a diagnosis of CSS. Blood tests can detect certain autoantibodies—an increase of eosinophils in the blood. Imaging tests such as X-rays, CT, and MRI can detect abnormalities in the lungs, sinuses, and other tissues and organs. Biopsy of affected tissue is often used to determine the presence of vasculitis (Noth, Strek, & Leff, 2003).

TREATMENT

There is no cure for CSS, and if left untreated, it is almost always fatal. However, effective drug therapy can treat the presenting symptoms of CSS, and patients often achieve medically maintained remission. Because there is no cure, relapses are common (Guillevin et al., 1996). Management of CSS symptoms involves suppressing the immune system and addressing inflammation of the affected blood vessels. The first line of treatment typically involves corticosteroids. Those who do not respond to steroids or those with more severe complications often require other immunosuppressive drugs such as cytotoxic drugs to reduce the body's immune response (Churg, Brallas, Cronin, & Churg, 1995; Guillevin et al., 2004). Severe complications of the gastrointestinal tract, worsening of asthma, or cardiopulmonary failure are the primary causes of mortality (Guillevin et al., 1996; Solans et al., 2001).

Darla J. Lawson

Boyer, D., Vargas, S. O., Slattery, D., Rivera-Sanchez, Y. M., & Colin, A. A. (2006). Churg-Strauss syndrome in children: A clinical and pathologic review. *Pediatrics, 118*(3), 914–920.

Churg, A. (2001). Recent advances in the diagnosis of Churg-Strauss syndrome. *Modern Pathology, 14*(12), 1284–1293.

Churg, A., Brallas, M., Cronin, S. R., & Churg, J. (1995). Formes frustes of Churg-Strauss syndrome. *American College of Chest Physicians, 108*(2), 320–323.

Churg, J., & Strauss, L. (1951). Allergic granulomatosis, allergic angiitis, and periarteritis nodosa. *American Journal of Pathology, 27*(2), 277–301.

Guillevin, L., Lhote, F., Gayraud, M., Cohen, P., Jarrousse, B., Lortholary, O., et al. (1996). Prognostic factors in polyarteritis nodosa and Churg-Strauss syndrome. A prospective study in 342 patients. *Medicine, 75*(1), 17–28.

Guillevin, L., Pagnoux, C., & Mouthon, L. (2004). Churg-Strauss syndrome. *Seminars in Respiratory and Critical Care Medicine, 25*(5), 535–545.

Lanham, J. G., Elkon, K. B., Pusey, C. D., & Hughes, G. R. (1984). Systemic vasculitis with asthma and eosinophilia: A clinical approach to the Churg-Strauss syndrome. *Medicine, 63*(2), 65–81.

Masi, A. T., Hunder, G. G., Lie, J. T., Michel, B. A., Bloch, D. A., Arend, W. P., et al. (1990). The American College of Rheumatology 1990 criteria for the classification of

Churg-Strauss syndrome (allergic granulomatosis and angiitis). *Arthritis and Rheumatism, 33*(8), 1094–1100.

Noth, I., Strek, M., & Leff, A. (2003). Churg-Strauss syndrome. *The Lancet, 361,* 587–594.

Solans, R., Bosch, J. A., Pérez-Bocanegra, C., Selva, A., Huguet, P., Alijotas, J., et al. (2001). Churg–Strauss syndrome: Outcome and long-term follow-up of 32 patients. *Rheumatology,* 40, 763–771.

Wechsler, M. E., Pauwels, R., & Drazen, J. M. (1999). Leukotriene modifiers and Churg-Strauss syndrome. *Drug Safety, 21*(4), 241–251.

CLUSTER HEADACHES

DESCRIPTION

A cluster headache (CH) is a severe pain syndrome characterized by unilateral headaches localized around the eye orbit and temporal areas and often accompanied by ipsilateral autonomic symptoms. The attacks are relatively brief in duration (15–180 min) and may occur up to eight times per day (Headache Classification Committee of the International Headache Society, 2004; Leone et al., 2009). A side shift is mentioned in about 15% of cases (Manzoni, 1983). The autonomic symptoms may include ptosis, miosis, lacrimation, conjunctival injection rhinorrhea, and nasal congestion during the attack (May, 2005), with increased sweating and blood flow on the side experiencing pain (Drummond, 1994).

CH differs from migraine headache in that patients with CH are often restless, preferring to rock back and forth or pace. They may also exert pressure and rub the affected eye and temple (May, 2005). The attacks are characterized by a circadian rhythmicity, typically experienced at consistent hours during the day or night (Leone et al., 2009).

CHs have been described for over 300 years. The 20th century saw several different descriptions of unilateral headaches with a variety of proposed names (Bussone, 2008). Currently, two different forms of CH are generally recognized. The episodic form is characterized by daily headaches that occur in bouts lasting from 6–12 weeks (i.e., a cluster period). Remissions may last up to 12 months. This is the most common form of the disorder, affecting 80% to 90% of the patients with CH. The chronic form is characterized by headaches that occur with no periods of notable remission, often on a daily basis for years. Chronic CH is diagnosed after the patient has experienced headaches for a year without remission or a remission that has lasted fewer than 30 days in duration. Also, the chronic form may either arise in isolation or evolve from the episodic form (Leone, 2004; Leone et al., 2009; May, 2005).

NEUROPATHOLOGY/PATHOPHYSIOLOGY

Although CH have been well defined as a clinical syndrome, the pathophysiological basis is not as well understood (Goadsby, 2002). Pathophysiological explanations for CH should address three major features, including the trigeminal distribution of the pain, the ipsilateral cranial autonomic features, and the episodic or circadian pattern of headaches (May, 2005).

The vascular theory was based on an inflammation of the walls of the cavernous sinus (Hardebo, 1991, 1994). Evidence for a vascular basis was thought to be provided by the efficacy of ergot derivatives in treating short-lasting headaches, given the potent vasoconstrictive action of these derivatives (Boes et al., 2002; Ekbom, 1975; Matthew, 1992). However, researchers are now aware that the vascular changes observed in the cavernous sinus of CH patients are of a peripheral origin and represent a aspecific aspect of the pathophysiology of CH (Bussone, 2008). Hence, the vascular theory has been replaced by a central pathogenic theory that recognizes the importance of neurovascular events and a central impulse generator. This model posits that the unilateral pain is mediated by activation of the first division of the trigeminal nerve, and the autonomic features result from activation of the cranial parasympathetic outflow from the seventh cranial nerve (Goadsby & Edvinsson, 1994). Further, research has also implicated the locus coeruleus and dorsal raphe nucleus in the pathogenesis of CH (Basbaum et al., 1983; Hodge et al., 1981).

Recently, the hypothalamus has been identified as playing a central role in CH. Anomalies in the hypothalamus have been demonstrated in patients with CH (May et al., 1999; May et al., 2000; Spenger et al., 2004). Morelli et al. (2009) reported significant activation of the hypothalamus ipsilateral to the side of pain. Activation of the hypothalamic gray matter during spontaneous headache has been reported by other investigators as well (Sprenger et al., 2004). May et al. (2000) triggered CH attacks in patients with nitroglycerin and found activation within the posterior inferior hypothalamic gray matter. A number of other regions of the brain were also activated in the May et al. (2000) study, including the contralateral ventroposterior thalamus, anterior cingulated, ipsilateral basal ganglia, right anterior frontal lobe, and bilateral insular cortices. Sprenger et al.

(2007) compared CH patients with normal controls using PET and found hypometabolism at the perigenual anterior cingulated cortex as well as the prefrontal and orbitofrontal cortex, during both "in bout" and "out of bout" episodes of CH. Research using voxel-based morphometry also has shown structural differences in gray matter in the inferior posterior hypothalamus in patients with CH as compared with normal controls (May, 1999).

NEUROPSYCHOLOGICAL/CLINICAL PRESENTATION

Given the previously noted research findings that CHs are associated with activation in the prefrontal and orbitofrontal lobes, it seems reasonable to conclude that this disorder may affect neuropsychological functioning. However, a rather surprising paucity of research has been conducted to examine how CH might affect memory, cognitive, and mood functioning. Some research has suggested that, as compared with normal controls, patients with CH are more prone to anxiety (Levi et al., 1992). Jorge et al. (1999) reported that nearly one-quarter of episodic CH patients met the DSM-IV criteria for an anxiety disorder, with additional patients meeting criteria for panic disorder (10%) and generalized anxiety disorder (14%). In addition, Jorge et al. (1999) reported a significant difference between episodic CH patients and patients with tension headache on their scores on the Hamilton Anxiety Rating Scale.

The investigation by Jorge et al. (1999) also examined neuropsychological functioning in CH patients by administering a number of tests of memory, visuospatial, and executive functioning. The results indicated that, as compared with patients with tension headache, patients with episodic CH evidenced significantly lower scores on the Auditory Verbal Learning Test. No differences were noted on the other tests of neuropsychological functioning. Meyer et al. (2000) reported significant declines on the Cognitive Capacity Screening Examination and Mini Mental Status Examination during headache intervals. Evers (2005) also reported a reversible decline in memory in CH patients during an attack and that based on long-term observations there did not appear to be progressive cognitive decline in patients with CH. Others have reported no significant differences between CH patients and normal controls in neuropsychological functioning (Sinforiani et al., 1987). Given the relative paucity of research examining neuropsychological functioning in patients with episodic or chronic CH, there is clearly a need for further research in this area. A comparison between the episodic and chronic forms of CH in terms of neuropsychological functioning may be beneficial. Also, examination of neuropsychological functioning may be useful in helping to determine suitability for the more invasive deep brain stimulation treatment. Further research will need to be conducted to determine the veracity of this proposition.

DIAGNOSIS

The diagnosis of CH is based on aforementioned clinical criteria/features and exclusion of secondary causes. A CT or MRI of the head should be strongly considered for the initial diagnosis, particularly if the neurological examination is abnormal (May, 2005). Neuroimaging is imperative to rule out potential secondary causes of CH. Mass lesions have been described in patients with CH (Hannerz, 1989; Purdy & Kirby, 2004), as have intracranial aneurysms (Valenca et al., 2007).

TREATMENT

The demonstrated role of the hypothalamus has led to the use of deep brain stimulation, targeting the hypothalamus as a treatment for CH (Grover et al., 2009; Sillay et al., 2010). A number of investigations have used deep brain stimulation of the posterior hypothalamic gray matter to treat intractable chronic CH (Bussone et al., 2007; Leone et al., 2001; Leone et al., 2004; Schoenen et al., 2005). However, a recent investigation by Pinsker et al. (2008) failed to find lasting effects of deep brain stimulation. Recently, occipital nerve stimulation has emerged as an effective treatment for CH patients as well (Grover et al., 2009; Leone et al., 2009; Sillay et al., 2009).

Pharmacological interventions represent a first-line treatment for CH patients and may be divided into those for treating an acute attack or for prophylactic treatment (McGeeney, 2005). Inhalation of pure oxygen is known to be effective in treating an acute CH attack (Fogan, 1985; Kudrow, 1981), with about 60% of patients responding to this treatment in the span of 20–30 minutes (Ekbom, 1995; Gallagher et al., 1996). Another effective acute treatment consists of subcutaneous injection of sumatriptan (Ekbom et al., 1993; Stovner & Sjaastad, 1995). Oral ergotamine has a demonstrated history of effectively treating CH when administered early in an attack (Ekbom, 1947). The nasal application of lidocaine is effective in the acute treatment of CH for many patients (Markley, 2003; Mills & Scoggin 1997; Robbins, 1995). Finally, a number of pharmacological agents have demonstrated effectiveness in preventive or prophylactic treatment. Specifically, verapamil is an established treatment of choice in preventing CH attacks (Bussone et al., 1990; Leone et al., 2000; Matharu et al., 2003; May, 2003). Other medicines for prophylactic treatment have included lithium (Ekbom, 1981; Reilly, 1998) and methysergide (Campbell, 1993; Dodick & Capobianco, 2001).

Paul S. Foster
Valeria Drago

Basbaum, A. I., Moss, M. S., & Glazer, E. J. (1983). Opiate and stimulation produced analgesia: The contribution of monoamines. *Advances in Pain Research and Therapy, 5,* 323–339.

Boes, C. J., Capobianco, D. J., Matharu, M. S., & Goadsby, P. J. (2002). Wilfred Harris' early description of cluster headache. *Cephalalgia, 22,* 320–326.

Bussone, G. (2008). Cluster headache: From treatment to pathophysiology. *Neurological Sciences, 29,* S1–S6.

Bussone, G., Franzini, A., Proietti Cecchini, A., Mea, E., Curone, M., Tullo, V., et al. (2007). Deep brain stimulation in craniofacial pain: Seven years' experience. *Neurological Sciences, 28*(Suppl. 2), S146–S149.

Bussone, G., Leone, M., Peccarisi, C., Micieli, G., Granella, F., Magri, M., et al. (1990). Double blind comparison of lithium and verapamil in cluster headache prophylaxis. *Headache, 30,* 411–417.

Campbell, J. K. (1993). Diagnosis and treatment of cluster headache. *Journal of Pain and Symptom Management, 8,* 155–164.

Dodick, D. W., & Capobianco, D. J. (2001). Treatment and management of cluster headache. *Current Pain and Headache Reports, 5,* 83–91.

Drummond, P. D. (1994). Sweating and vascular responses in the face: Normal regulation and dysfunction in migraine, cluster headache, and harlequin syndrome. *Clinical Autonomic Research, 4,* 273–285.

Ekbom, K. A. (1947). Ergotamine tartrate orally in Horton's 'Histaminic cephalgia' (also called Harris's 'ciliary neuralgia'). *Acta Psychiatrica Scandinavica, 46*(Suppl.), 106–113.

Ekbom, K. (1975). Some observations on pain in cluster headache. *Headache, 14,* 219–225.

Ekbom, K. (1981). Lithium for cluster headache: Review of the literature and preliminary results of long-term treatment. *Headache, 21,* 132–139.

Ekbom, K. (1995). Treatment of cluster headache: Clinical trials, design and results. *Cephalalgia, 15*(Suppl.), 33–36.

Ekbom, K., Monstad, I., Prusinski, A., Cole, J. A., Pilgrim, A. J., & Noronha, D. (1993). Subcutaneous sumatriptan in the acute treatment of cluster headache: A done comparison study. The Sumatriptan Cluster Headache Study Group. *Acta Neurological Scandinavica, 88,* 63–69.

Evers, S. (2005). Cognitive processing in cluster headache. *Current Pain and Headache Reports, 9,* 109–112.

Fogan, L. (1985). Treatment of cluster headache. A double-blind comparison of oxygen v air inhalation. *Archives of Neurology, 42,* 362–363.

Gallagher, R. M., Mueller, L., & Ciervo, C. A. (1996). Analgesic use in cluster headache. *Headache, 36,* 105–107.

Goadsby, P. J. (2002). Pathophysiology of cluster headache: A trigeminal autonomic cephalgia. *Lancet Neurology, 1,* 251–257.

Goadsby, P. J., & Edvinsson, L. (1994). Human in vivo evidence for trigeminovascular activation in cluster headache. Neuropeptide changes and effects of acute attacks therapies. *Brain, 117,* 427–434.

Grover, P. J., Pereira, E. A., Green, A. L., Brittain, J. S., Owen, S. L., Schweder, P., et al. (2009). Deep brain stimulation for cluster headache. *Journal of Clinical Neuroscience, 16,* 861–866.

Hannerz, J. (1989). A case of parasellar meningioma mimicking cluster headache. *Cephalalgia, 9,* 265–269.

Hardebo, J. E. (1991). On pain mechanisms in cluster headache. *Headache, 31,* 91–106.

Hardebo, J. E. (1994). How cluster headache is explained as an intracavernous inflammatory process lesioning sympathetic fibers. *Headache, 34,* 125–131.

Headache Classification Subcommittee of the International Headache Society. (2004). The International Classification of Headache Disorders, 2nd edition. *Cephalagia, 24*(Suppl. 1), 9–160.

Hodge, C. J., Jr., Apkarian, A. V., Stevens, R., Vogelsang, G., & Wisnicki, H. J. (1981). Locus coeruleus modulation of dorsal horn unit responses to cutaneous stimulation. *Brain Research, 204,* 415–420.

Jorge, R. E., Leston, J. E., Arndt, S., & Robinson, R. G. (1999). Cluster headaches: Association with anxiety disorders and memory deficits. *Neurology, 53,* 543–547.

Kudrow, L. (1981). Response of cluster headache attacks to oxygen inhalation. *Headache, 21,* 1–4.

Leone, M. (2004). Chronic cluster headache: New and emerging treatment options. *Current Pain and Headache Reports, 8,* 347–352.

Leone, M., D'Amico, D., Frediani, F., Moschiano, F., Grazzi, L., Attanasio, A., et al. (2000). Verapamil in the prophylaxis of episodic cluster headache: A double-blind study versus placebo. *Neurology, 54,* 1382–1385.

Leone, M., Franzini, A., Broggi, G, May, A., & Bussone, G. (2004). Long-term follow-up of bilateral hypothalamic stimulation for intractable cluster headache. *Brain, 127,* 2259–2264.

Leone, M., Franzini, A., & Bussone, G. (2001). Stereotactic stimulation of posterior hypothalamic gray matter in a patient with intractable cluster headache. *New England Journal of Medicine, 345,* 1428–1429.

Leone, M., Franzini, A., Cecchini, A. P., Mea, E., Broggi, G., & Bussone, G. (2009). Cluster headache: Pharmacological treatment and neurostimulation. *Nature Clinical Practice. Neurology, 5*, 153–162.

Levi, R., Edman, G. V., Ekbom, K., & Waldenlind, E. (1992). Episodic cluster headache. I: Personality and some neuropsychological characteristics in male patients. *Headache, 32*, 119–125.

Manzoni, G. C., Terzano, M. G., Bono, G., Micieli, G, Martucci, N., & Nappi, G. (1983). Cluster headache — clinical findings in 180 patients. *Cephalalgia, 3*, 21–30.

Markley, H. G. (2003). Topical agents in the treatment of cluster headache. *Current Pain and Headache Reports, 7*, 139–143.

Matharu, M. S., Boes, C. J., & Goadsby, P. J. (2003). Management of trigeminal autonomic cephalgias and hemicranias continua. *Drugs, 63*, 1637–1677.

Mathew, N. T. (1992). Cluster headache. *Neurology, 42*(Suppl 2), 22–31.

May, A. (2003). Headaches with (ipsilateral) autonomic symptoms. *Journal of Neurology, 250*, 1273–1278.

May, A. (2005). Cluster headache: Pathogenesis, diagnosis, and management. *Lancet, 366*, 843–855.

May, A., Ashburner, J., Buchel, C., McGonigle, D. J., Friston, K. J., Frackowiak, R. S., et al. (1999). Correlation between structural and functional changes in brain in an idiopathic headache syndrome. *Nature Medicine, 5*, 836–838.

May, A., Bahra, A., Buchel, C., Frackowiak, R. S., & Goadsby, P. J. (2000). PET and MRA findings in cluster headache and MRA in experimental pain. *Neurology, 55*, 1328–1335.

McGeeney, B. E. (2005). Cluster headache pharmacotherapy. *American Journal of Therapeutics, 12*, 351–358.

Meyer, J. S., Thornby, J., Crawford, K., & Rauch, G. M. (2000). Reversible cognitive decline accompanies migraine and cluster headache. *Headache, 40*, 638–646.

Mills, T. M., & Scoggin, J. A. (1997). Intranasal lidocaine for migraine and cluster headaches. *Annals of Pharmacotherapy, 31*, 914–915.

Morelli, N., Pesaresi, I., Cafforio, G., Maluccio, M. R., Gori, S., Di Salle, F., et al. (2009). Functional magnetic resonance imaging in episodic cluster headache. *Journal of Headache and Pain, 10*, 11–14.

Pinsker, M. O., Bartsch, T., Falk, D., Volkmann, J., Herzog, J., Steigerwald, F., et al. (2008). Failure of deep brain stimulation of the posterior inferior hypothalamus in chronic cluster headache — report of two cases and review of the literature. *Zentralblatt fur Neurochirurgie, 69*, 76–79.

Purdy, R. A., & Kirby, S. (2004). Headaches and brain tumors. *Neurologic Clinics, 22*, 39–53.

Reilly, D. (1998). Lithium vs placebo in cluster headache. *Cephalalgia, 18*, 1.

Robbins, L. (1995). Intranasal lidocaine for cluster headache. *Headache, 35*, 83–84.

Schoenen, J., Di Clemente, L., Vandenheede, M., Fumal, A., De Pasqua, V., Mouchamps, M., et al. (2005). Hypothalamic stimulation in chronic cluster headache: A pilot study of efficacy and mode of action. *Brain, 128*, 940–947.

Sillay, K. A., Sani, S., & Starr, P. A. (2010). Deep brain stimulation for medically intractable cluster headache. *Neurobiology of Disease, 38*, 361–368.

Sinforiani, E., Farina, S., Mancuso, A., Manzoni, G. C., Bono, G., & Mazzucchi, A. (1987). Analysis of higher nervous functions in migraine and cluster headache. *Functional Neurology, 2*, 69–77.

Sprenger, T., Boecker, H., Tolle, T. R., Bussone, G., May, A., & Leone, M. (2004). Specific hypothalamic activation during a spontaneous cluster headache attack. *Neurology, 62*, 516–517.

Sprenger, T., Ruether, K. V., Boecker, H., Valet, M., Berthele, A., Pfaffenrath, V., et al. (2007). Altered metabolism in frontal brain circuits in cluster headache. *Cephalalgia, 27*, 1033–1042.

Stovner, L. J., & Sjaastad, O. (1995). Treatment of cluster headache and its variants. *Current Opinion in Neurology, 8*, 243–247.

Valenca, M. M., Andrade-Valenca, L. P., Martins, C., de Fatima Vasco Aragao, M., Batista, L. L., Peres, M. F., et al. (2007). Cluster headache and intracranial aneurysm. *Journal of Headache and Pain, 8*, 277–282.

COFFIN–LOWRY SYNDROME

DESCRIPTION

Coffin–Lowry is an X-linked recessive disorder caused by a variety of mutations on the *RPS6KA3* (ribosomal protein S6 kinase, 90 kDa, polypeptide 3) (*RSK2*) gene (Abidi et al., 1999; Field et al., 2006). Delaunoy, Dubos, Marques, and Hanauer (2006) reported at least 128 known mutations on the *RSK2* gene resulting in phenotypic expression of Coffin–Lowry. The RSK2 protein kinase gene is associated with regulation of growth factor (David et al., 2005). Coffin–Lowry is characterized by mental retardation, progressive skeletal abnormalities, hypotonia (low muscle tone), and physical irregularities. This disorder was first described independently by Coffin, Siris, and Wegienka (1966) and Lowry, Miller, and Fraser (1971). Occurrence rate is likely to be 1 in every 50,000–100,000 males (Jacquot, Zeniou, Touraine, & Hanauer, 2002).

NEUROPATHOLOGY/PATHOPHYSIOLOGY

Males typically have more severe symptomatology than females as a result of their only X-chromosome being affected, whereas female carriers have one affected X-chromosome and one unaffected X-chromosome.

C

The phenotypic expression of the syndrome ranges from mild to severe (Field et al., 2006). Some aspects of the phenotypic presentation of Coffin–Lowry are a result of deficiencies in proteins in the chromatin-remodeling pathway (Ausió, Levin, de Amorim, Bakker, & Maclead, 2003). Chromatin is the material in a cell nucleus consisting of protein, RNA, and DNA, which comprises eukaryotic chromosomes.

NEUROPSYCHOLOGICAL/CLINICAL PRESENTATION

Skeletal abnormalities include tapering fingers, kyphosis (curvature of the upper spine), and scoliosis (lateral spine curvature). Less frequent skeletal abnormalities include pectus carinatum (prominent breastbone) or pectus excavatum (inverted breastbone), narrow pelvis, and abnormally short bones in the lower extremities (Touraine, Zeniou, & Hanauer, 2002). These skeletal abnormalities may progress in severity through the course of the patient's life. Skeletal abnormalities seen in Coffin–Lowry are a result of a defect in the functionality of osteoblasts (bone-forming cells) due to deficiencies in RSK2, which plays a role in proper osteoblast activity (David et al., 2005).

Physical characteristics seen in males with Coffin–Lowry may include a prominent forehead, palpebral fissures (down-slanting eyelid folds), hypertelorism (abnormally wide-set eyes), nares (protruding nostrils), a thick nose, and thick lips (Touraine et al., 2002). Female carriers typically exhibit fewer physical irregularities. The most common symptoms in carrier females include obesity, finger tapering, and milder facial coarsening than is seen in affected males (Touraine et al., 2002).

Cognitive abilities are more significantly impaired in affected males than carrier females, and both affected males and carrier females are more significantly impaired than nonaffected males and females (Simensen, Abidi, Collins, Schwartz, & Stevenson, 2002). Carrier females may present with normal or near-normal intelligence (Jacquot et al., 1998). Affected males frequently have an IQ in the range of 15–60 and retarded language acquisition (Poirier et al., 2007). In a study of mice deficient in RSK2, Poirier et al. (2007) found impairments in spatial working memory, spatial memory acquisition, and long-term spatial memory.

There is a wide variety of movement disorder and drop attacks in individuals with Coffin–Lowry, including epilepsy, cataplexy (sudden temporary paralysis), hyperekplexia (startle reaction with increase of muscle tone), and increased startle response. An affected individual may also exhibit a combination of these movement disorders, with onset at about 5 years of age (Stephenson et al., 2005). Cardiac implications

may also arise, including congestive heart failure and mitral regurgitation, the leaking of blood from the mitral valve from the left ventricle into the left atrium of the heart (Massin, Radermecker, Verloes, Jacquot, & Grenade, 1999). Development of the corpus callosum may also be defective (Kondoh, Matsumoto, Ochi, Sukegawa, & Tsuji, 1998).

DIAGNOSIS

Coffin–Lowry is primarily diagnosed through clinical examination. In young children, it may present similarly to Fragile X syndrome, Sotos syndrome, Williams syndrome, lysosomal storage disease, and α-thalassaemia (Jacquot et al., 2002). A differential diagnosis may also include Opitz–Kaveggia syndrome (Martinez-Garay et al., 2003). A definitive diagnosis can be made by genetic screening for known mutations.

Kaphzan, Doron, and Rosenblum (2007) proposed that the mutations in the RSK2 protein kinase gene known to cause Coffin–Lowry do so either by diminishing the capacity of RSK2 to bind with other proteins, specifically extracellular regulated kinase (ERK), or by affecting RSK2's induction properties. Kaphzan et al. (2007) also noted that it is not clear whether this is the sole explanation for phenotypic expression of Coffin–Lowry.

TREATMENT

There is no cure and no standard method of treatment for individuals with Coffin–Lowry syndrome. Treatment is supportive and may include physical rehabilitation for movement difficulties and a supportive and enriching educational environment geared toward special education. Benzodiazepines may be useful in decreasing frequency of drop attacks when applicable (Jacquot et al., 2002). The parents of a patient may be referred for genetic counseling or supportive therapy.

Maryellen C. Dougherty
Charles Golden

Abidi, F., Jacquot, S., Lassiter, C., Trivier, E., Hanauer, A., & Schwartz, C. E. (1999). Novel mutations in Rsk-2, the gene for Coffin-Lowry syndrome (CLS). *European Journal of Human Genetics, 7,* 20–26.

Ausió, J., Levin, D. B., de Amorim, G. V., Bakker, S., & Macleod, P. M. (2003). Syndromes of disordered chromatin remodeling. *Clinical Genetics, 64,* 83–95.

Coffin, G. S., Siris, E., & Wegienka, L. C. (1966). Mental retardation with osteocartilaginous anomalies. *American Journal of Diseases of Children, 112,* 205–213.

David, J., Mehic, D., Bakiri, L., Schilling, A. F., Mandic, V., & Priemel, M. (2005). Essential role of RSK2 in c-Fos-dependent osteosarcoma development. *The Journal of Clinical Investigation, 115,* 664–672.

Delaunoy, J. P., Dubos, A., Marques, P. P., & Hanauer, A. (2006). Identification of novel mutations in the RSK2 gene (RPS6KA3) in patients with Coffin-Lowry syndrome. *Clinical Genetics, 70,* 161–166.

Field, M., Tarpey, P., Boyle, J., Edkins, S., Goodship, J., Luo, Y., et al. (2006). Mutations in the RSK2 (RPS6KA3) gene cause Coffin-Lowry syndrome and nonsyndromic X-linked mental retardation. *Clinical Genetics, 70,* 509–515.

Jacquot, S., Merienne, K., Pannetier, S., Blumenfeld, S., Schinzel, A., & Hanauer, A. (1998). Germline mosaicism in Coffin-Lowry syndrome. *European Journal of Human Genetics, 6,* 578–582.

Jacquot, S., Zeniou, M., Touraine, R., & Hanauer, A. (2002). X-linked Coffin-Lowry syndrome (CLS, MIM 303600, RPS6KA3 gene, protein product known under various names: pp90^{rsk2}, RSK2, ISPK, MAPKAP1). *European Journal of Human Genetics, 10,* 2–5.

Kaphzan, H., Doron, G., & Rosenblum, K. (2007). Co-application of NMDA and dopamine-induced rapid translation of RSK2 in the mature hippocampus. *Journal of Neurochemistry, 103,* 388–399.

Kondoh, T., Matsumoto, T., Ochi, M., Sukegawa, K., & Tsuji, Y. (1998). New radiological finding by magnetic resonance imaging examination of the brain in Coffin-Lowry syndrome. *Journal of Human Genetics, 43,* 59–61.

Lowry, B., Miller, J. R., & Fraser, F. C. (1971). A new dominant gene mental retardation syndrome: Association with small stature, tapering fingers, characteristic facies, and possible hydrocephalus. *American Journal of Diseases of Children, 121,* 496–500.

Martinez-Garay, I., Ballesta, M. J., Ottra, S., Orellana, C., Palomeque, A., Moltó, M. D., et al. (2003). Intronic L1 insertion and F268S, novel mutations in RPS6KA3 (RSK2) causing Coffin-Lowry syndrome. *Clinical Genetics, 64,* 491–496.

Massin, M. M., Radermecker, M. A., Verloes, A., Jacquot, S., & Grenade, T. (1999). Cardiac involvement in Coffin-Lowry syndrome. *Acta Paediatrica, 88,* 468–470.

Poirier, R., Jacquot, S., Vaillend, C., Soutthiphong, A. A., Libbey, M., Davis, S., . . . Wolfer, D. P. (2007): Deletion of the Coffin-Lowry syndrome gene Rsk2 in mice is associated with impaired spatial learning and reduced control of exploratory behavior. *Behavioral Genetetics, 37,* 31-50.

Simensen, R. J., Abidi, F., Collins, J. S., Schwartz, C. E., & Stevenson, R. E. (2002). Cognitive function in Coffin-Lowry syndrome. *Clinical Genetics, 61,* 299–304.

Stephenson, J. B., Hoffman, M. C., Russell, A. J., Falconer, J., Beach, R. C., Tolmie, J. L., et al. (2005). The movement disorders of Coffin-Lowry syndrome. *Brain and Development, 27,* 108–113.

Touraine, R., Zeniou, M., & Hanauer, A. (2002). A syndromic form of X-linked mental retardation: The Coffin-Lowry syndrome. *European Journal of Pediatrics, 161,* 179–187.

COLPOCEPHALY

DESCRIPTION

Colpocephaly is a disorder of abnormal neurological development corresponding with enlargement of the occipital horns of the lateral ventricles and microcephaly. One of the cephalic disorders, the neurological disruption associated with colpocephaly is of such a degree that mental retardation is commonly noted. Motor and sensory anomalies, particularly visual disturbance are also common as are seizures. Most commonly diagnosed after birth, there is no known cure. Rather, treatment is symptom based with anticonvulsant medication commonly employed to address seizures. A variety of behavioral and academic interventions as well as physical, occupational, and/or speech therapies may be utilized to address deficits.

NEUROPATHOLOGY/PATHOPHYSIOLOGY

Colpocephaly is characterized by a significant dilation of the posterior (i.e., occipital) horns of the lateral ventricles, thickening of the overlying rim of cortical gray matter, and thinning of the white matter (Ropper & Brown, 2005). This has been proposed to result from a disturbance of intrauterine development occurring sometime over the course of the late first trimester through the second. Although the pathological basis is presumed to be multifactorial, the presentation has been linked with mosaicism for trisomy 8 (Herskowitz, Rosman, & Wheller, 1985). Optic nerve hypoplasia is quite common and serves as the basis for visual abnormalities commonly noted.

As noted by Norman and Armstrong (1998), early in the development of the fetus, the cerebral mantle is thin and the lateral ventricles are relatively large. Although both grow, the mantle grows proportionately more resulting in the adult-like appearance of a thick cerebral mantle and smaller ventricles, comparatively. Colpocephaly has been used generally to describe the appearance of a thinner mantle and large ventricles, not explained by hydrocephalus. However, as suggested, the most accurate definition of colpocephaly is the enlarged posterior horns of the lateral ventricle.

C

NEUROPSYCHOLOGICAL/CLINICAL PRESENTATION

Aside from the structural anomalies noted in the cerebrum (i.e., dilation of the occipital horns of the lateral ventricles and microcephaly), clinically, colpocephaly is associated with an array of sequelae including mental retardation, spasticity, optic nerve hypoplasia, and seizures (Ropper & Brown, 2005). The severity of these features and overall prognosis is dependent upon the degree of structural compromise. No unitary profile exists.

DIAGNOSIS

Neuroradiological examination remains the most efficient means of diagnosis. Although structural abnormalities may be seen on prenatal ultrasound, findings may be nondefinitive. The presentation is distinguishable from hydrocephalus as there should not be an appearance of compression on the cortical surface.

TREATMENT

Prognosis for individuals with colpocephaly is dependent upon the degree of neurological disruption. There is no unitary profile nor method of care. Treatment is directed at addressing symptoms that present. Given the high prevalence of seizures, anticonvulsant agents are often employed. Various interventions may be used to address orthopedic and ambulatory issues related to spasticity as well as visual defects related to optic nerve hypoplasia. There are no specific guidelines or established recommendations for this population in regard to these interventions; thus, standard practices should be considered as starting points to address those symptoms that present. Special education services will likely be warranted in all cases.

Chad A. Noggle
Javan Horwitz

Herskowitz, J., Rosman, P., & Wheller, C. B. (1985). Colpocephaly: Clinical, radiologic, and pathogenetic aspects. *Neurology, 35,* 1594.

Norman, M. G., & Armstrong, D. D. (1998). Disturbances of brain development. In C. E. Coffey & R. A. Brumback (Eds.), *Textbook of pediatric neuropsychiatry* (pp. 43–64). Washington, DC: American Psychiatric Press.

Ropper, A. H., & Brown, R. H. (2005). *Adams and Victor's principles of neurology* (8th ed., pp. 850–894). New York: McGraw-Hill.

COMA AND PERSISTING VEGETATIVE STATE

DESCRIPTION

Coma (from the Greek word *koma* — deep sleep or trance) is defined as a state of unresponsiveness in which the individual lies with eyes closed and cannot be aroused to respond appropriately to stimuli even with vigorous stimulation (Posner, Saper, Schiff, & Plum, 2007). The end result of coma can be recovery, vegetative state, or death. A persisting vegetative state is a state of mind when there is total loss of awareness in the setting of intact sleep–wake cycles, which has persisted long enough to make improvement improbable statistically.

NEUROPATHOLOGY/PATHOPHYSIOLOGY

Coma requires significant disruption of the reticular activating system, which stretches from brainstem to thalamus or bilateral cerebral hemispheres (Posner et al., 2007). Coma can be due to such etiologies as trauma, raised intracranial pressure, generalized seizure, hypoxic injury, or toxic/metabolic perturbations. Persisting vegetative state, on the other hand, requires sparing of the reticular activating system, which is essential for the sleep–wake cycle, and thus instead involves profound disruption of the bilateral cerebral hemispheres. Persisting vegetative state shares similar underlying etiologies with coma and in fact is one of the major possible outcomes of coma.

For prognostic purposes, coma and vegetative states are often differentiated between traumatic and nontraumatic coma. In general, trauma can have a much lengthier recovery period, and although the prognosis in nontraumatic coma is typically known by the end of a month, that of traumatic coma can be as long as a year.

NEUROPSYCHOLOGICAL/CLINICAL PRESENTATION

Before we mention the diagnosis of coma and vegetative state we will discuss awareness and wakefulness. Wakefulness is the normal condition of the mind when it is not in sleep. With eyes open, responding appropriately with motor and sensory skills, it is usually associated with awareness but need not be. Awareness is the bodily perception of the surroundings with usually intact memory, thoughts, intentions, and emotions. The brainstem is the center for the former and the cerebral hemispheres are controlling the latter. In vegetative state, usually there is dissociation between these two conditions but some components of awareness can be spared.

Any insult of the CNS, irrespective of the etiology, can have diverse effects ranging from clouding of consciousness to brain death. In between these lies a large spectrum of disorders of consciousness, namely delirium, obtundation, stupor, abulia, akinetic mutism, sleep/memory disorders, locked-in syndrome, minimally conscious state, persistent vegetative state and coma depending upon the type, extent, and site of injury.

Since the introduction of the term apallic syndrome (or Kretschmer's syndrome) describing vegetative state by German psychiatrist Ernst Kretschme in 1940, and formal coining of the term persistent vegetative state by Jennet and Plum in 1972, there has been extensive debate and research in this field.

Vegetative state is a state of mind when there is loss of self-awareness, loss of communication capabilities, and no purposeful motor activities with or without response to painful stimuli, startle auditory and visual response, intact sleep–wake cycles, no intentional motor activities, withdrawing or posturing for painful stimulus, reduced cerebral metabolism, and suppressed electoencephalogram (EEG) (Jennet, 2002). The major difference between coma and vegetative state is the preserved sleep–wake cycle, some auditory and visual response, and intact respiratory function (Bryan Young, Ropper, & Bolton, 1998; Report of a working party of the Royal College of Physicians, 2003; The Multi-Society Task Force on PVS, 1994).

When vegetative state persists for more than 4 weeks, it is called persistent vegetative state, and when it is irreversible, it is called permanent vegetative state (Bryan Young et al., 1998; Report of a Working Party of the Royal College of Physicians, 2003; The Multi-Society Task Force on PVS, 1994). Hypoxia, medications (including those with sedative effect), metabolic derangements, and reversible structural brain insults should be ruled out before a patient is labeled as vegetative state (Report of a Working Party of the Royal College of Physicians, 2003).

DIAGNOSIS

Diagnosis is solely made by the clinical presentation as outlined previously. Traumatic causes may include hemorrhage, contusion, and diffuse axonal injury from shearing. Nontraumatic causes include hypoxia, seizure, intracranial hypertension, metabolic disturbances, toxins/medication effect, neoplasia, and CNS infection.

TREATMENT

The primary treatment in coma is to correct, where possible, the underlying cause and to provide superior supportive care to allow the optimal chance of recovery. There is no treatment other than supportive care for persisting vegetative state. Coma and vegetative state remain among the biggest challenges in intensive care management in terms of outcome, resources, and dealing with the family and the ethical issues involved. Per the statistics from the Nationwide Inpatient Sample for 1993 Hospital Inpatient Stays, total discharges, mean length of stay, and mean total charges were 10,524/5.01/7,214, respectively for nontraumatic coma and for traumatic coma it was 22,055/6.50/12,847, which was quiet significant when compared with other diagnosis (HCUP-3 Nationwide Inpatient, 1993).

Hospital mortality in cases of coma, stupor, and brain damage is 16.3 as per the 1997 census in U.S. hospitals (Department of Health). Also, from time to time there appear sporadic clinical cases in the media wherein a patient awakes from long-term coma, and this is often used to make a case for being optimistic and aggressive in our approach toward these patients. Even though there is extensive research in these fields, there is still no clear-cut standardized guidelines that have been accepted throughout the world satisfying all the clinicians and families in the care of these unfortunate patients.

Glen R. Finney
Abhay Kumar
Vishnumurthy S. Hedna

Bryan Young, G., Ropper, A. H., & Bolton, C. F. (1998). *COMA and impaired consciousness.* New York: McGraw Hill.

Department of Health, http://ftp.ahrq.gov/data/hcup/factbk1/fctbk4.htm

F:\Statistics from the HCUP-3 Nationwide Inpatient Sample for 1993 Diagnosis-Related Groups.htm

Jennet, B. (2002). *Vegetative state.* Cambridge: Cambridge University Press.

Posner, J. B., Saper, C. B., Schiff, N. D., Plum, F. (2007). *Plum and Posner's diagnosis of stupor and coma* (4th ed.). Oxford University Press.

Report of a working party of the Royal College of Physicians. (2003). The vegetative state, guidance on diagnosis and management. *Clinical Medicine, 3,* 249–254.

The Multi-Society Task Force on PVS. (1994). *The New England Journal of Medicine, 330,* 1499–1508.

C

Conduct Disorder and Oppositional Defiant Disorder

DESCRIPTION

Conduct disorder (CD) and oppositional defiant disorder (ODD), along with attention deficit hyperactivity disorder (ADHD), are considered "disruptive behavior disorders" (American Psychiatric Association [APA], 2000, p. 85) that are "usually first diagnosed in childhood or adolescence" (p. 39). They characterize a range of behaviors that many clinicians believe to lie on a continuum in terms of severity and/or development or evolution, and cause "clinically significant impairment in social, academic, or occupational functioning" (APA, 2000, p. 99 and 102).

The *Diagnostic and Statistical Manual of Mental Disorders*, Fourth Edition, with Text Revision (*DSM-IV-TR*; APA, 2000) describes the essential feature of ODD as a recurring pattern, persisting for at least 6 months, of negative, defiant, disobedient, and hostile behavior toward authority. Problematic behaviors in ODD occur more often than expected for the child's developmental level and can include temper outbursts, arguing with adults, defiance toward authority, annoying and/or being easily annoyed, blaming and/or resentfulness, and spitefulness and/or vindictiveness. Onset is typically prepubertal, often by age 8, and often precedes development of CD, although most children diagnosed with ODD do not develop CD. Operationalized developmental criteria and rating of severity are proposed for *DSM-5* (http://www.dsm5.org/ProposedRevisions).

According to the *DSM-IV-TR* (APA, 2000), the essential feature of CD is described as a repetitive, persistent pattern of behavior lasting at least 12 months where the basic rights of others or age-appropriate societal norms or rules are violated. This wording is similar to the *DSM-IV-TR* essential feature of antisocial personality disorder (APD), and, in fact, meeting diagnostic criteria for CD prior to age 15 is a prerequisite for a diagnosis of APD (APA, 2000). However, less than half of children diagnosed with severe CD go on to meet diagnostic criteria for APD (Webster-Stratton & Dahl, 1995). Problematic behaviors in CD are categorized as (1) aggression toward people and animals, (2) destruction of property (nonphysically aggressive), (3) deceitfulness or theft, and (4) serious violations of rules (APA, 2000, pp. 98–99). Age of onset prior to 10 (childhood-onset type), evidenced by at least one symptom in retro-

spect, suggests a more severe and chronic course than does onset after 10 (adolescent-onset type). CD can also be classified as mild (i.e., few symptoms), moderate, or severe (i.e., many symptoms). Other than potentially adding a Callous and Unemotional specifier, no major revisions are currently proposed for CD in *DSM-5* (as of May 2010; see http://www.dsm5.org/ProposedRevisions). The diagnosis of CD can be applied beyond age 18 only if *DSM-IV-TR* criteria for APD are not met.

In instances in which *DSM-IV-TR* criteria are met for both CD and ODD, CD is diagnosed alone. However, there is an increasing expert opinion that ODD and CD are sufficiently unique and predictive to constitute distinct diagnostic entities that should be diagnosed simultaneously if comorbid (Rowe, Maughan, Costello, & Angold, 2005; see also Nock, Kazdin, Hiripi, & Kessler, 2007), and that not doing so may obscure research into the long-range consequences of ODD. In factor analytic studies, for example, symptoms of ODD and CD consistently load separately (see Loeber, Burke, & Pardini, 2009, for a brief summary). In addition, when CD and ODD are comorbid and the diagnosis of CD precludes a diagnosis of ODD, prevalence rates in boys reach a high of between 4% and 5% at age 7 and decline to less than 1% by age 15, but when CD and ODD are comorbid and a diagnosis of CD does not preclude a diagnosis of ODD, the prevalence of ODD in boys at age 7 is between 5% and 6% and at age 15 is between 4% and 5% (Maughan, Rowe, Messer, Goodman, & Meltzer, 2004). For girls, the prevalence of ODD peaks at close to 2% at age 8 and again at age 12, and then declines to less than 1% at age 15. However, when diagnosing ODD in addition to CD in girls, prevalence rates hover around 2% from age 7 to 15 (Maughan et al., 2004). These prevalence rates suggest that the presumed substantial decline in ODD as a function of age is an artifact of diagnostic criteria and bolsters the argument that ODD and CD should be diagnosed comorbidly. Nock et al. (2007) reported lifetime prevalence rates for ODD in boys/men at 11.2% and in girls/women at 9.2%.

Prevalence rates for *DSM-IV-TR* CD increase with age, steadily for boys (from about 2% at age 10 to between 5% and 6% at age 15), with a milder slope for girls until about age 12 (from <1% at age 12 to between 3% and 4% at age 15; Maughan et al., 2004). Other prevalence estimates for ODD range from 2.6% to 15.6% in the community, and from 28% to 65% in clinical samples (Boylan, Vaillancourt, Boyle, & Szatmari, 2007), whereas other prevalence rates for CD range from 1.8% to 16% for boys, and

0.8% to 9.2% for girls (Loeber, Burke, Lahey, Winters, & Zera, 2000). Base rates for CD among delinquent populations range from about 50% to 60% (Otto et al., 1992 as recounted in Grisso, 1998). Base rates for ODD and CD vary, and will continue to vary, because they are sample-, definition-, and measurement-dependent, factors that plague epidemiological research in general (cf. Wynkoop, Capps, & Priest, 1995).

NEUROPATHOLOGY/PATHOPHYSIOLOGY

The early age of onset of ODD suggests the possibility of biological constitutional factors (Burke, Loeber, & Birmaher, 2004), and genetic linkage studies suggest that early onset of CD is associated with parental sociopathy (Lahey et al., 1998). However, the totality of the underlying contributions to constitution and temperament are not yet well understood when taking into account various biological and environmental influences (Burke et al., 2004).

Twin studies have demonstrated genetic linkage across gender for ODD and CD (Eaves et al., 2000). Same-sex sibling pair and adoption studies demonstrate biological trends for negativity and adolescent antisocial behavior and aggression and CD, respectively (Cadoret, Yates, Troughton, Woodworth, & Stewart, 1995; Pike, McGuire, Hetherington, Reiss, & Plomin, 1996). Maternal alcohol use (Fast, Conry, & Loock, 1999; Olsen et al., 1997; Streissguth, Barr, Bookstein, Sampson, & Olsen, 1999) and smoking (Brennan, Grekin, & Mednick, 1999; Rantakallio, Laara, Isohanni, & Moilanen, 1992) have also been linked with CD and/or with violent behavior in children, with up to a four-fold increase (Weissman, Warner, Wickramaratne, & Kandel, 1999) even when controlling for social and medical confounds (see Burke et al., 2004; Wynkoop, 2008, for more thorough discussions).

The development of disruptive behaviors observed in ODD and CD has been the subject of some debate and investigation, with developmental (e.g., ODD evolving into CD) and various path models being proposed (see Burke et al., 2004, for a review). Of the range of CD symptoms that may be biologically related, aggression and violence have gained the most attention in recent years. In general, studies have also linked gestation/birth complications, early malnutrition (in utero or early infancy), early maternal rejection, sympathetic under-arousal (e.g., slow resting heart rate has one of the strongest correlations), neurotransmitters, and functional imaging results to aggressive and violent behavior in children and adults (see Raine, 2002; Raine, Brennan, & Mednick, 1994; Raine, Venables, & Mednick, 1997; also, see Juvenile Delinquency by Wynkoop in this text for more detail). Abnormal frontal EEG findings in children diagnosed with ODD are believed to reflect the negativism often associated with the disorder (Baving, Laucht, & Schmidt, 2000). Early onset of CD has been associated with reduced right temporal lobe and right temporal gray matter volumes on MRI, more striking than slightly reduced prefrontal volumes, when compared with age, sex, and handedness-matched controls (Kruesi, Casanova, Mannheim, & Johnson-Bilder, 2004).

Common comorbidities with ODD include disorders of mood (45.8%), anxiety (62.3%), disorders of impulse control (68.2%), and substance use (47.2%; Nock et al., 2007). Common comorbidities with CD include ADHD (50%–75%) and internalizing anxiety and/or depression (almost 50%), and 90% of young drug-abusing offenders are also diagnosed with CD (Children's Mental Health Ontario [CMHO], 2001). Other comorbidities with CD include depression (for which children with CD are at higher risk of self-harm including suicide; CMHO, 2001), developmental disorders, lower IQ scores, academic delay, head injuries, psychomotor seizures, soft neurological signs and/or nonspecific EEG findings, history of febrile seizures, and vague and/or transient psychotic symptoms (Bock & Goode, 1996; Carey, DiLalla, & Plomin, 1994; Plomin, 1994). Barklay, Fischer, Edelbrock, and Smallish (1990) found that 80% of young children diagnosed with ADHD maintained their hyperactivity into adolescence and that 60% had developed ODD or CD. A note of caution is in order with regard to assuming that symptoms of restlessness and distractibility in ODD or CD are related to comorbid ADHD, as high bone lead levels at ages 6–8 are known to predict distractibility, restlessness, and cognitive problems by ages 12–13 (Fergusson, Horwood, & Lynskey, 1993). In other words, the etiology of comorbid symptoms should not be taken at face value in ODD or CD.

NEUROPSYCHOLOGICAL/CLINICAL PRESENTATION

Both ODD and CD present clinically as behavioral disorders. There is no neurocognitive profile for ODD or CD per se, nor should one be reasonably expected given the heterogeneity of causes and contributing factors. The clinical presentation involves the behavioral problems described in the *DSM-IV-TR* along with the Neuropathology/Pathophysiology section above and in the chapter on Juvenile Delinquency by Wynkoop in this text.

Unfortunately, the majority of neurocognitive studies that we reviewed for this chapter, although initially encouraging, were fraught with fatal flaws (e.g., attributing superior performance on executive functioning measures to control groups with substantially higher mean IQ scores, not controlling for ADHD or recent substance abuse among ODD/CD participants while comparing their test performances with normal control groups, not controlling for test taking motivation or effort). For example, although a meta-analysis of the relationship between executive functioning and antisocial behavior in teens and adults revealed a 0.62 effect size (Morgan & Lilienfeld, 2000), when controlling for attention deficit in 13 year olds (the youngest age group represented, and the only study in the meta-analysis that controlled for attention deficit) the individual effect sizes were much more modest (0.23–0.25 on Trails B time, impulsive responses on Wechsler Intelligence Scale for Children-III Mazes, and Wisconsin Card Sorting Test perseverative errors; Moffitt & Henry, 1989). Unfortunately, neither substance abuse/dependence (controlled in only 25% of the individual studies) nor ADHD (controlled in only one study) could be controlled in the meta-analysis, as they were not controlled in the majority of the individual studies.

There is at least a complex relationship between ODD/CD and intelligence, if a relationship exists at all when controlling for fatal research confounds (e.g., ADHD, effort; cf. Hogan, 1999; see the Juvenile Delinquency article by Wynkoop in this text for additional discussion regarding IQ and cognition in relation to delinquency in general). However, one rather consistent neurocognitive finding is that deficit(s) in reading, independent of race and income, often accompany CD from a very early age (Maguin, Loeber, & LeMahiew, 1993; Sanson, Prior, & Smart, 1996). In addition, ODD contributed to poor impulse control as measured on a Go/No-go procedure over and above the controlled effects of ADHD in a European sample (Van der Meere, Marzocchi, & Meo, 2005).

Behavioral impulsivity is associated with early onset of CD and antisocial behavior (Tremblay, Pihl, Vitaro, & Dobkin, 1994; White et al., 1994, respectively), whereas lack of social skills and social withdrawal place boys at increased risk for antisocial behaviors (Dodge, Pettit, Bates, & Valente, 1995). There may also be a tendency on the part of aggressive boys to impute malevolence toward others when not called for (Dodge, 1993). Early physical maturation has been associated with ODD/CD in girls (possibly as a risk factor) but not necessarily in boys (see Burke et al., 2004). Although these factors may be associated with and observed clinically in relation to CD, they are not easily quantified. There are also patterns typical of various psychological disorders associated with antisocial and other behavioral disorders that can be assessed via personality assessment (e.g., Minnesota Multiphasic Personality Inventory-Adolescent, Personality Inventory for Children, Second Edition, Personality Assessment Inventory-Adolescent, Adolescent Personality Scale).

DIAGNOSIS

Diagnostic formulation per the DSM-IV-TR (APA, 2000) is made based on history. Comorbidities (e.g., depression, anxiety, posttraumatic stress disorder, ADHD, substance abuse; see CMHO, 2001; Maughan et al., 2004; Nock et al., 2007) and other forms of psychopathology that can mimic or contribute to symptoms of ODD and CD should be ruled out in the process of firming the diagnostic impression (e.g., ADHD, bipolar disorder, phobias, child abuse).

Other syndromes in which disruptive behavior is the primary focus (and that should be considered as alternative diagnoses to ODD and CD) include child or adolescent antisocial behavior, adjustment disorder with disturbance of conduct or with mixed disturbance of emotions and conduct, parent—child and/or sibling relational problem, phase of life problem, and disruptive behavior disorder, and impulse control disorders not otherwise specified (cf. APA, 2000). Problems often associated with ODD or CD include academic problems, physical or sexual abuse of child (with the child patient as victim and/or perpetrator), neglect of child (typically with the child patient as victim), and in some instances physical abuse of adult (by the child; cf. APA, 2000). A thorough history along with personality/behavioral and neurocognitive assessment can be helpful in clarifying the differential diagnosis as well as determining the presence of comorbid disorders.

Some diagnostic caveats are in order (cf. Wynkoop, 2008). First, CD should not be diagnosed if the behavior is "simply a reaction to the immediate social context" (APA, 2000, p. 96). Second, clinicians should avoid the temptation to end the diagnostic process once they observe symptoms of CD (Grisso, 1998). Third, although CD is a prerequisite to APD in adulthood, most children who meet diagnostic criteria for CD do not continue to offend in adulthood and/or meet APD diagnostic criteria (Lahey, Pelham, Loney, Lee, & Willcutt, 2005), and most children diagnosed with ODD do not progress to CD (Loeber et al., 2000, 2009; Nock et al., 2007), thus limiting the predictive utility of these diagnoses.

TREATMENT

Intervention should be symptom focused rather than syndrome focused (akin to working with personality disorders). Consequently, the treatment plan should be based on the results of a comprehensive evaluation including the child's corroborated history (e.g., family, gestation and development, abuse, educational, social, response to previous developmentally appropriate interventions), personality assessment, intelligence, academic achievement, and neurocognitive strengths and weaknesses (e.g., sustained attention, learning and recall, language functions, spatial functions and constructional praxis, executive functions, sensory perception, balance and motor functions). Clinicians should also consider the settings, social aspects, and environmental reinforcers of the disruptive behaviors as well as comorbid disorders. For example, if the child lacks social skills and/or empathy, then training in these areas is indicated. Management of peer contact is useful if peers exert undue negative influence. If the parents lack parenting skills, then training is indicated (demonstrably among the most effective interventions for ODD/CD; Brestan & Eyberg, 1998). Family and multimodal interventions hold more promise than individual therapy, and rational behavior training along with social skills and anger management training is often programed in many youth detention facilities.

Psychopharmacology is often advocated for management of aggression (likely due to the effect of violence on the risk benefit ratio for the patient). However, few medication studies include children, and almost none are randomized (see Burke et al., 2004, for a review). Studies have suggested off-label effectiveness of lithium, haloperidol, molindone, thioridazine, risperidone, and methylphenidate over placebo or other medications to manage aggression in very aggressive youths, most of whom were hospitalized (note: this list should not be used to make medical treatment decisions). School interventions can include individualized education plans or Section 504 plans to accommodate the emotional and academic needs of students. Unfortunately, interment and/or long-term residential intervention remain necessary for a select group of aggressive/violent youth.

Timothy F. Wynkoop
Mary E. Haines
Melissa M. Swanson

American Psychiatric Association. (2000). *Diagnostic and statistical manual of mental disorders, fourth edition, text revision*. Washington, DC: Author.

Barklay, R. A., Fischer, M., Edelbrock, E. S., & Smallish, L. (1990). The adolescent outcome of hyperactive children diagnosed by research criteria, I: An eight year prospective follow-up study. *Journal of the American Academy of Child and Adolescent Psychiatry, 29*, 546–557.

Baving, L., Laucht, M., & Schmidt, M. H. (2000). Oppositional children differ from healthy children in frontal lobe activation. *Journal of Abnormal Child Psychology, 28*, 267–275.

Bock, G., & Goode, J. (1996). *Genetics of criminal and antisocial behavior*. Ciba Foundation Symposium 194, Chichester, West Sussex: Wiley.

Boylan, K., Vaillancourt, T., Boyle, M., & Szatmari, P. (2007). Comorbidity of internalizing disorders in children with oppositional defiant disorder. *European Journal of Child Adolescent Psychiatry, 16*, 484–494.

Brennan, P. A., Grekin, E. R., & Mednick, S. A. (1999). Maternal smoking during pregnancy and adult male criminal outcomes. *Archives of General Psychiatry, 56*, 215–219.

Brestan, E. V., & Eyberg, S. M. (1998). Effective psychosocial treatments of conduct disordered children and adolescents: 29 years, 82 studies, and 5272 kids. *Journal of Clinical Child Psychology, 27*, 180–189.

Burke, J. D., Loeber, R., & Birmaher, B. (2004). Oppositional defiant disorder and conduct disorder: A review of the past 10 years, part II. *Focus: The Journal of Lifelong Learning in Psychiatry, 2*, 558–576.

Cadoret, R. J., Yates, W. R., Troughton, E., Woodworth, G., & Stewart, M. A. (1995). Genetic-environmental interaction in the genesis of aggressivity and conduct disorders. *Archives of General Psychiatry, 52*, 916–924.

Carey, G., DiLalla, D., & Plomin, R. (1994). Personality and psychopathology: Genetic perspectives. *Journal of Abnormal Psychology, 103*, 32–43.

Children's Mental Health Ontario. (2001). *Children and adolescents with Conduct Disorder: Findings from the literature and clinical consultation in Ontario*. Toronto, ON: Author. Retrieved from http://www.kidsmentalhealth.ca/documents/EBP_conduct_disorder_findings.pdf.

Dodge, K. A. (1993). Social-cognitive mechanisms in the development of conduct disorder and depression. *Annual Review of Psychology, 44*, 559–584.

Dodge, K. A., Pettit, G. S., Bates, J. E., & Valente, E. (1995). Social information processing patterns partially mediate the effect of physical abuse on later conduct problems. *Journal of Abnormal Psychology, 104*, 632–643.

Eaves, L., Rutter, M., Silberg, J. L., Shillady, L., Maes, H., & Pickles, A. (2000). Genetic and environmental causes of covariation in interview assessments of disruptive behavior in child and adolescent twins. *Behavioral Genetics, 30*, 321–334.

Fast, D. K., Conry, J., & Loock, C. A. (1999). Fetal alcohol syndrome among youth in the criminal justice system. *Journal of Developmental and Behavioral Pediatrics, 20*, 370–372.

Fergusson, D. M., Horwood, L. J., & Lynskey, M. T. (1993). Early dentine lead levels and subsequent cognitive and behavioural development. *Journal of Child Psychology and Psychiatry, 34*, 215–228.

Grisso, T. (1998). *Forensic evaluation of juveniles*. Sarasota, FL: Professional Resource Press.

Hogan, A. E. (1999). Cognitive functioning in children with oppositional defiant disorder and conduct disorder. In H. C. Quay & A. E. Hogan (Eds.), *Handbook of disruptive behavior disorders* (pp. 317–335). New York: Kluwer/ Plenum.

Kruesi, M. J. P., Casanova, M. F., Mannheim, G., & Johnson-Bilder, A. (2004). Reduced temporal volume in early onset conduct disorder. *Psychiatry Research: Neuroimaging, 132,* 1–11.

Lahey, B. B., Loeber, R., Quay, H. C., Applegate, B. A., Shaffer, D., Waldman, I. D., et al. (1998). Validity of DSM-IV subtypes of conduct disorder based on age of onset. *Journal of the American Academy of Child and Adolescent Psychiatry, 37,* 435–442.

Lahey, B. B., Pelham, W. E., Loney, J., Lee, S. S., & Willcutt, E. (2005). Instability of the DSM-IV subtypes of ADHD from preschool through elementary school. *Archives of General Psychiatry, 62,* 896–902.

Loeber, R., Burke, J., & Pardini, D. A. (2009). Perspectives on oppositional defiant disorder, conduct disorder, and psychopathic features. *Journal of Child Psychology and Psychiatry, 50,* 133–142.

Loeber, R., Burke, J. D., Lahey, B. B., Winters, A., & Zera, M. (2000). Oppositional defiant and conduct disorder: A review of the past 10 years, part 1. *Journal of the American Academy of Child and Adolescent Psychiatry, 39,* 1468–1484.

Maguin, E., Loeber, R., & LeMahiew, P. (1993). Does the relationship between poor reading and delinquency hold for different age and ethnic groups? *Journal of Emotional and Behavioral Disorders, 1,* 88–100.

Maughan, B., Rowe, R., Messer, J., Goodman, R., & Meltzer, H. (2004). Conduct disorder and oppositional defiant disorder in a national sample: Developmental epidemiology. *Journal of Child Psychology and Psychiatry, 45,* 609–621.

Moffitt, T. E., & Henry, B. (1989). Neuropsychological assessment of executive functions self-reported delinquents. *Development and Psychopathology, 1,* 105–118.

Morgan, A. B., & Lilienfeld, S. O. (2000). A meta-analytic review of the relation between antisocial behavior and neuropsychological measures of executive function. *Clinical Psychology Review, 20,* 113–136.

Nock, M. K., Kazdin, A. E., Hiripi, E., & Kessler, R. C. (2007). Lifetime prevalence, correlates, and persistence of oppositional defiant disorder: Results from the National Comorbidity Survey Replication. *Journal of Child Psychology and Psychiatry, 48,* 703–713.

Olsen, H. C., Streissguth, A. P., Sampson, P. D., Barr, H. M., Bookstein, F. L., & Thiede, K. (1997). Association of prenatal alcohol exposure with behavioral and learning problems in early adolescence. *Journal of the American Academy of Child and Adolescent Psychiatry, 36,* 1187–1194.

Pike, A., McGuire, S., Hetherington, E. M., Reiss, D., & Plomin, R. (1996). Family environment and adolescent depressive symptoms and antisocial behavior: A multivariate genetic analysis. *Developmental Psychology, 32,* 590–603.

Plomin, R. (1994). The Emanuel Miller Memorial Lecture 1993. Genetic research and identification of environmental influences. *Journal of Child Psychology and Psychiatry, 35,* 817–834.

Raine, A. (2002). Biosocial studies of antisocial and violent behavior in children and adults: A review. *Journal of Abnormal Child Psychology, 30,* 311–326.

Raine, A., Brennan, P., & Mednick, S. A., (1994). Birth complications combined with early maternal rejection at age 1 year predispose to violent crime at age 18 years. *Archives of General Psychiatry, 51,* 984–988.

Raine, A., Venables, P., & Mednick, S. (1997). Low resting heart rate at age three years predisposes to aggression at age 11 years: Evidence from the Mauritius Child Health Project. *Journal of the Academy of Child and Adolescent Psychiatry, 36,* 1457–1464.

Rantakallio, P., Laara, E., Isohanni, M., & Moilanen, I. (1992). Maternal smoking during pregnancy and delinquency of the offspring. *International Journal of Epidemiology, 21,* 1106–1113.

Rowe, R., Maughan, B., Costello, E. J., & Angold, A. (2005). Defining oppositional defiant disorder. *Journal of Child Psychology and Psychiatry, 46,* 1309–1316.

Sanson, A., Prior, M., & Smart, D. (1996). Reading disabilities with and without behaviour problems at 7–8 years: Prediction from longitudinal data from infancy to 6 years. *Journal of Child Psychology and Psychiatry, 37,* 529–541.

Streissguth, A. P., Barr, H. M., Bookstein, F. L., Sampson, P. D., & Olsen, H. C. (1999). The long term neurocognitive consequences of prenatal alcohol exposure: A 14-year study. *Psychological Science, 10,* 186–190.

Tremblay, R. E., Pihl, R .D., Vitaro, F., & Dobkin, P .L. (1994). Predicting early onset of male antisocial behavior from preschool behavior. *Archives of General Psychiatry, 51,* 732–739.

Van der Meere, J., Marzocchi, G. M., & Meo, T. D. (2005). Response inhibition and attention deficit hyperactivity disorder with and without oppositional defiant disorder screened from a community sample. *Developmental Neuropsychology, 28,* 459–472.

Webster-Stratton, C., & Dahl, R. W. (1995). Conduct disorder. In M. Hersen & R. T. Ammerman (Eds.), *Advanced abnormal child psychology* (pp. 333–352). Hillsdale, NJ: Lawrence Erlbaum Associates.

Weissman, M. M., Warner, V., Wickramaratne, P., & Kandel, D. B. (1999). Maternal smoking during pregnancy and psychopathology in offspring followed to adulthood. *Journal of the American Academy of Adolescent Psychiatry, 38,* 892–899.

White, J. L., Moffitt, T. E., Caspi, A., Bartusch, D. J., Needles, D. J., & Stouthamer-Loeber, M. (1994). Measuring impulsivity and examining its relationship to delinquency. *Journal of Abnormal Psychology, 103,* 192–205.

Wynkoop, T. F. (2008). Neuropsychology in the juvenile justice system. In R. Denney & T. Sullivan (Eds.), *Clinical neuropsychology in the criminal forensic setting* (pp. 295–325). New York: Guilford.

Wynkoop, T. F., Capps, S. C., & Priest, B. J. (1995). Incidence and prevalence of child sexual abuse: A critical review of data collection procedures. *Journal of Child Sexual Abuse, 4,* 49–66.

CONGENITAL AND CHILDHOOD MYASTHENIAS

DESCRIPTION

Myasthenic syndromes all arise from a dysfunction of nerve cells communicating with muscles. The end result is muscle weakness, although there is some variability in the specific muscles affected. Myasthenia gravis (MG) is likely the most common variant, occurring in adults. However, a number of variants present early in life that present either as congenital syndromes (i.e., congenital myasthenia) or related to an autoimmune process (i.e., juvenile myasthenia). Within the pediatric population, both variations are seen in relatively equal frequency (Anlar et al., 1996). Various subtypes exist within these broad groupings involving their own distinct pathology and clinical presentation which are discussed below.

NEUROPATHOLOGY/PATHOPHYSIOLOGY

Although all myasthenic syndromes arise from a lack of communication between nerve cells and muscles, the underlying neuropathology/pathophysiology varies based on the subtype, consequently, corresponding with different clinical presentations. Shen, Fukuda, Ohno, Sine, and Engel (2008) in their review of the literature, synthesized findings suggesting these pathologies include problems with choline acetyltransferase; the collagenic tail subunit of endplate (EP) acetylcholinesterase (AChE); the acetylcholine receptor (AChR); the cytoplasmic protein rapsyn, which concentrates AChR at the crests of the junctional folds; the muscle-specific receptor tyrosine kinase (MuSK), which activates rapsyn; the muscle-intrinsic activator of MuSK known as Dok-7; and the Nav1.4 sodium channel in the troughs of the folds. They also noted that postsynaptic congenital myasthenias (CMs) are caused by mutations in different subunits of AChR that alter its kinetic properties, reduce its expression, or both. When generalized, in the case of CMs, they arise from mutations whereas other myasthenias occurring early in life, similar to MG in adults, arise from an autoimmune process. Across all variants, acetycholine uptake is the primary pathogenesis. These variants are discussed separately for clarity's sake.

Transient Neonatal Myasthenia (TNM)

TNM arises from a placental transmission of transplacental anti-AChR antibodies from the mother, who herself has MG, to the fetus (Tellez-Zenteno, Hernandez-Ronquillo, Salinas, Estanol, & da Silva, 2004). This leads to a short-lived interference in acetylcholine uptake due to receptor blockage. Over the course of a few weeks, spontaneous recovery is often seen as the problematic antibodies are removed naturally from the system. In more severe cases, medicinal intervention or transfusion is required. Permanent damage has not been linked with the presentation. Furthermore, difficulty arises in suggesting "increased risk" of MG in the future, as the infants clearly have a genetic predisposition for this presentation which itself could explain any later development.

Childhood Autoimmune Myasthenia Gravis (AMG)

Similar to the adult form of MG, AMG is caused by autoantibodies that bind to and reduce the number of active AChRs at the postsynaptic membrane through decay, acytosis, and/or blockage, which is considered the prototypical synaptic disorder (Vincent, 2002). Although it demonstrates a genetic basis, as do all of the myasthenic disorders, it is still classified as an acquired disorder, related to the human leukocyte antigen (HLA)-B8 and DR3, which presents in approximately 60% of patients (Toth et al., 2006). The end result of this blockage is reduced uptake of acetylcholine which is why acetylcholinesterase inhibitors are utilized in treatment. The differential between AMG and MG is primarily the time of onset. Debate persists regarding the cutoff between AMG and juvenile myasthenia (JM). Cutoffs may range from 5 to 10 years of age and below. Onset is usually after 12 months of age, and prior to age 10 may be seen as an effective cutoff. In comparison, JM would be the preferred diagnosis when the symptoms onset above this cutoff but prior to 20 years of age at which time it is simply referred to as MG.

The mechanisms behind the degradation of AChRs have been illuminated through clinical research. Sensitized T cells lead to continued stimulation of B cells, which together appear to complement the triggering of anti-AChR antibodies, which bind to, block and attack AChRs at the neuromuscular junction (Richman & Agius, 1994). These activities have been linked with dysfunction of the thymus in adults, either due to hyperplasia or neoplasms (thymomas). However, in general, thymomas are rarer in children thus limiting the utility of surgery. The end result of the process is decreased numbers of active or present AChRs and simplification and reduction/regression of the postsynaptic clefts leading to an overall widening of the synaptic space (Drachman, 1994).

Juvenile Myasthenia Gravis (JM)

As indicated with AMG, JM is essentially traditional MG but with a far earlier onset. Again, variations in these chronological cutoff points can be found, but we describe it as a clinical onset after 10 years of age but prior to 20 years of age. Comparatively, juvenile onset is far rarer than both childhood and adult onsets.

Lambert–Eaton Myasthenic Syndrome (LEMS)

In lieu of reiterating information, the interested reader is recommended to see the entry on Lambert–Eaton Syndrome included in this text for the pathogenesis of this variant and its clinical features. Briefly, this variant rarely presents in childhood or adolescence, but may; thus, it is included here. The pathogenesis is related to degradation of voltage-gated calcium channels secondary to antibody infiltration. It has been most commonly associated with malignancies in adults (e.g., small cell lung cancer), but this has not been commonly seen in pediatrics (Maddison, Lang, Mills, & Newsom-Davis, 2001), which is not surprising given the most common pathogenesis of small cell lung cancer is smoking, which is not a common issue in children aside from second-hand encounter.

Congenital Myasthenias (CMs)

CMs are differentiated from other variants, including MG because the disrupted communication is not caused by antibodies but by genetic defects. They arise from defects in proteins associated with the neuromuscular junction (Middleton, 1996). Parr and Jaya-want (2007) noted that aside from the autosomal dominantly inherited slow-channel syndrome, all CMs are inherited via autosomal recessive mutations. They are subtyped by the nature and point of the

dysfunction. This includes presynaptic defects including defect of acetylcholine resynthesis and/or reduced numbers/amount of presynaptic vesicles and quantal release; combined presynaptic/postsynaptic defects in the form of endplate AChE deficiency; and postsynaptic defects (most common), including kinetic abnormalities with (e.g., slow channel uptake, Epsilon subunit mutations, AChR deficiency combined with short channel opening time) or without (e.g., high-conductance fast channel syndrome or abnormal interactions of acetylcholine and receptors) deficiencies of AChRs (Rose & Griggs, 2007). Although the mechanism causing the disruption may vary, when generalized, the dysfunction remains a dysfunction in the uptake of acetylcholine at the neuromuscular junction.

NEUROPSYCHOLOGICAL/CLINICAL PRESENTATION

As with the underlying neuropathology/pathophysiology, clinical presentations are discussed in relation to the various myasthenic forms. Across all forms, aside from TNM, mentation is traditionally considered spared. However, as fatigue increases, difficulties in sustained attention, concentration, and processing speed and efficiency should be expected. For children, this becomes problematic academically as the sheer act of sitting erect in the classroom, working on assignments in the classroom or at home with prolonged writing or typing, and so forth, can lead to fatigue that can inevitably impede these domains. For adults, similar difficulties may be observed at work.

Transient Neonatal Myasthenia (TNM)

In infants presenting with TNM, the most common clinical manifestations present as poor sucking and feeding, weak crying, and reduced movements. The features are consistent with the concept of weakened muscle activation and increased fatigability. In severe cases, more prominent respiratory distress can be observed requiring ventilation. "Emphasis is placed" on the description of transient as the presentation in most cases resolves after a few weeks spontaneously, whereas severe cases may require medicinal intervention, and, rarely, exchange transfusion.

Childhood Autoimmune Myasthenia Gravis (AMG)

AMG is considered progressive; thus, features discussed may increase in severity over time or even acutely in the presence of systemic compromise as discussed below. Symptom onset is commonly noted after 12 months of age, often first presenting as diplopia and ptosis, with the former being associated with ophthalmoplegia (Afifi & Bell, 1993). Most often, there is increased fatigability of voluntary motor systems, particularly in the extremities as well as bulbar musculature. In the case where symptoms are restricted to ocular muscles, a subdiagnosis of ocular myasthenia may be given (Sommers et al., 1997). However, even in these cases, there is often a tendency for subtle weakness of the rest of the face and possibly even limb involvement and, eventually, the features progress to more prominently involve these other musculature regions/systems. In more severe cases, respiratory weakness can be seen. This can contribute to dysphonia or tendency for respiratory distress that can be misidentified as asthma if other symptoms are ignored or not recognized. Dysphagia and tongue weakness can also manifest as part of the aforementioned bulbar dysfunction.

At times of systemic illness, which itself depletes muscular output and strength, symptoms can become severe. Particular attention should be given to respiratory functioning during systemic illnesses such as the flu as this can cause a myasthenic crisis leading to prominent respiratory distress, potentially requiring hospitalization (Vincent, Palace, & Hilton-Jones, 2001).

Juvenile Myasthenia Gravis (JM)

Clinical symptoms of JM are very much the same as AMG. Generalized weakness of the extremities, particularly following physical exertion, is the hallmark feature of JM. Ocular and bulbar weaknesses commonly manifest and may serve as the initial symptoms (Kupersmith, Latkany, & Homel, 2003). There can also be a tendency for respiratory weakness increasing risks of respiratory distress. Dysphonia can inhibit voice quality, reducing tone and amplitude. Individuals may have difficulties walking long distances with their gait becoming somewhat staggered due to fatigue. Consequently, they can be at risk of falls due to these weaknesses. In more prominent cases, even sitting erect in a classroom can be quite physically draining as individuals must keep their torso and neck muscles engaged to some extent. Furthermore, completing homework can be draining due to lengthy writing or typing. Inevitably, as fatigue increases children are prone to lapses in sustained attention and concentration, which is the primary cognitive finding in this population as well as the others discussed.

Lambert–Eaton Myasthenic Syndrome (LEMS)

As recommended above, the interested reader is recommended to see the entry on Lambert–Eaton syndrome included in this text for discussion on the clinical features associated with this variant. Clinical symptoms primarily include limb weakness, often the legs more so than the arms, in combination with various autonomic symptoms.

Congenital Myasthenias (CMs)

The congenital myasthenias are most commonly first manifested in childhood, although some do not reach observable levels until adulthood. The timeline in which they develop largely determines the clinical symptoms first observed. Infants commonly present with developmental delays in motor functioning. Sitting up, crawling, and walking may all be delayed. Infants may present with a degree of floppiness, poor head and neck control, difficulties feeding due to dysphagia and bulbar weakness, and even respiratory weakness characterized by a weak cry and even pauses in breathing. When symptom onset manifests in early childhood or even toddlers, muscular fatigue on exertion becomes more noticeable. They often cannot play for very long without become noticeably worn-down. Their running and even walking may after short amounts of time begin to appear dyscoordinated or staggered due to this fatigue. Speech can seem slurred or dysarthric with prolonged activation. Ptosis may be observed, and if they can properly describe the features, diplopia may be observed. Similar symptoms are observed in middle to late childhood, adolescence, and even adulthood. The key feature, as with all myasthenic disorders, is that weakness increases with prolonged activity with a return of strength after a period of rest.

DIAGNOSIS

Diagnosis of all variants discussed is relatively similar, although subtle differences exist. Those aspects included for all comprise a combination of clinical history taking including family history, clinical examination (as discussed below), and electrophysiological tests (e.g., EMG). Genetic, pharmacological, and serological tests may also be employed as means of differentiating presentation types.

As with all neurological or psychiatric presentations, clinical history is an essential component. Within this group of disorders, it is particularly useful when considering differences between AMG and JM because of the age of onset criteria. Family history is useful when considering CMs and especially TNM given that it is dependent upon the mother having MG. Beyond this it is essential to determine the severity of the presentation and nature of the symptoms.

C

Clinicians should question the patient on their experience of all potential symptoms to know how widespread the symptoms are and allow for careful determination of whether life-threatening symptoms are possibly involved (i.e., respiratory distress).

Clinical examination can be carried out within a standard office setting although some more extensive evaluation may include tasks such as walking on a treadmill or climbing stairs, which is not as feasible in close quarters. Eye fatigability can be elicited by sustained vertical or horizontal gaze as well as continuous eye tracking. Positional regression or nystagmus may be observed. Gag reflexes may be checked by stimulating the back of the throat. Reading out load a long paragraph may aid in assessing for fatigue-based dysarthria. Various motor exercises such as continuous arm movements (e.g., lifting very light weights) or ambulation (e.g., walking on a treadmill) may add important clinical information, particularly the rate of fatigue.

Beyond clinical evaluation, EMG is one of the more classic measures used in the evaluation of myasthenias. This can assist in gauging rate of fatigue and location of symptoms. Positive findings consist of reduced EMG response with repetitive stimulation. Repetition is the key as initial measurement can often present as normal across most variants except in severe cases. This can be used in both the extremities and face. Single-fiber EMG (SFEMG) may be the most sensitive test for neuromuscular transmission defects as it is almost always abnormal in the clinically affected muscles (Skeie et al., 2006). Positive findings do not suggest definitive myasthenia as other presentations can produce similar results. However, negative findings across the board can be seen as ruling out myasthenia, thus its importance.

Serology tests can be used to evaluate for the presence of AChE receptor antibodies, which are highly suggestive of myasthenia, although positive findings can be found in family members of positive individuals (Gardnerova et al., 1997). This is commonly used in combination with pharmacological tests in which EMG is repeated following administration of AChE-inhibiting agents. Intravenous injections of edrophonium is preferred as it is short acting. Precautions should be observed. For children, neostigmine is preferred as it allows for longer observation time due to it being a bit longer acting then edrophonium thus allowing more time to observe features (Anlar, 2000). Immunocytochemical and molecular genetic investigations on muscle biopsy and DNA samples should be used to distinguish CMs from autoimmune variants (Dooley, Goulden, Gatien, Gibson, & Brown, 1986).

Beyond these methods, imaging is strongly recommended as many symptoms can be mimicked by other entities. MRI of the head, neck, and chest are useful. In regard to the chest, MRI permits evaluation of the thymus. MRI of the head and neck permits ruling out focal lesions. For example, in instances where patients present with purely ocular or bulbar features, brainstem tumors can mimic these features clinically and should thus be considered (Anlar, 2000).

TREATMENT

Treatments largely vary based on the type of myasthenia. In CMs, in which the basis of the presentation is not related to an autoimmune response, treatment primarily focuses on increasing signal strength at the neuromuscular junction by way of pharmacological intervention. The most common agents used include pyridostigmine, fluoxetine, ephedrine, and 3,4-diaminopyridine (Anlar, 2000).

In autoimmune forms, treatment is more expansive as it seeks to also increase signal strength while minimizing the autoimmune response. In regard to the prior, those agents listed above remain those most commonly employed. In terms of regulating the autoimmune features, glucocorticoids or azathioprine is often effective. In addition, corticosteroids may be employed as a boost to treatment. In patients who do not respond to these agents, cyclophosphamide and cyclosporin may be considered but are not often used as first-line treatments as they have a higher propensity for adverse effects.

Plasmapheresis can be used as necessary, often at times of myasthenic crisis, in order to return individuals to therapeutic levels. It is effective by removing the AChR antibodies from the system. Alternatively, intravenous immunoglobulin treatment may also be considered. In cases where the thymus, possibly a thymoma, is seen as the root of the problem, thymectomy may be considered, usually if medicinal interventions have not proven effective. However, this is often reserved for adults but may be used in children in whose case the pros seem to outweigh the cons.

As suggested earlier, ventilation is sometimes required in cases of TNM, but this is short-lived. Feeding tubes may also be required initially. Education of children and parents is essential to avoid potential fatal issues. Respiratory status should be monitored closely during times of systemic illness as things such as fever can elicit myasthenic crises, which can inhibit respiration. In severe cases, hospitalization with ventilation may be required for these individuals as well.

Chad A. Noggle
Javan Horwitz

Afifi, A. K., & Bell, W. E. (1993). Tests for juvenile myasthenia gravis: Comparative diagnostic yield and prediction of outcome. *Journal of Child Neurology, 8,* 403–411.

Anlar B, Özdirim E, Renda Y, (1996). Myasthenia gravis in childhood. Acta Paediatr 85: 838–842

Anlar, B. (2000). Juvenile myasthenia: Diagnosis and treatment. *Pediatric Drugs, 2*(3), 161–169.

Dooley, J. M., Goulden, K. J., Gatien, J. G., Gibson, E. J., & Brown, B. S. (1986). Topical therapy for oropharyngeal symptoms of myasthenia gravis. *Annals of Neurology, 19,* 192–194.

Drachman, D. B. (1994). Myasthenia gravis. *New England Journal of Medicine, 330,* 1797–1810.

Gardnerova, M., Eymard, B., Morel, E., Faltin, M., Zajac, J., Sadovsky, O., et al. (1997). The fetal/adult acetylcholine receptor antibody ratio in mothers with myasthenia gravis as a marker for transfer of the disease to the newborn. *Neurology, 48,* 50–54.

Kupersmith, M. J., Latkany, R., & Homel, P. (2003). Development of generalised disease at 2 years in patients with ocular myasthenia gravis. *Archives of Neurology, 60,* 243–248.

Maddison, P., Lang, B., Mills, K., & Newsom-Davis, J. (2001). Long term outcome in Lambert-Eaton myasthenic syndrome without lung cancer. *Journal of Neurology, Neurosurgery & Psychiatry, 70,* 212–217.

Middleton, L. T. (1996). Congenital myasthenic syndromes. 34th ENMC International Workshop, June10–11, 1995. *Neuromuscular Disorder, 6,* 133–136.

Parr, J. R., & Jayawant, S. (2007). Childhood myasthenia: Clinical subtypes and practical management. *Developmental Medicine & Child Neurology, 49,* 629–635.

Richman, D. P., & Agius, M. A. (1994). Myasthenia gravis: Pathogenesis and treatment. *Seminars in Neurology, 14,* 106–110.

Rose, M., & Griggs, R. C. (2007). Hereditary neurodegenerative neuromuscular disease. In C. G. Goetz (Ed.), *Textbook of clinical neurology* (3rd ed., pp. 813–826). Philadelphia: Saunders Elsevier.

Shen, X. M., Fukuda, T., Ohno, K., Sine, S. M., & Engel, A. (2008). Congenital myasthenia-related AChR subunit mutation interferes with intersubunit communication essential for channel gating. *The Journal of Clinical Investigation, 118*(5), 1867–1876.

Skeie GO, Apostolski S, Evoli A, Gilhus NE, Hart IK, Harms L, Hilton-Jones D, Melms A, Verschuuren J, Horge HW. (2006) Guidelines for the treatment of autoimmune neuromuscular transmission disorders. *Eur J Neurol* 13: 691–699.

Sommer, N., Sigg, B., Melms, A., Weller, M., Schepelmann, K., Herzau, V., et al. (1997). Ocular myasthenia gravis: Response to long-term immunosuppressive treatment. *Journal of Neurology, Neurosurgery, & Psychiatry, 62,* 156–162.

Tellez-Zenteno, J. F., Hernandez-Ronquillo, L., Salinas, V., Estanol, B., da Silva, O. (2004). Myasthenia gravis and pregnancy: Clinical implications and neonatal outcome. *BMC Musculoskeletal Disorders, 5,* 42.

Toth C, McDonald D, Oger J, Brownell K. (2006) Acetylcholine receptor antibodies in myasthenia gravis are associated with greater risk of diabetes and thyroid disease. *Acta Neurol Scand* 114: 124–132.

Vincent, A. (2002). Unravelling the pathogenesis of myasthenia gravis. *Nature Reviews Immunology, 2,* 797–804.

Vincent, A., Palace, J., & Hilton-Jones, D. (2001). Myasthenia gravis. *Lancet, 357,* 2122–2128.

CONGENITAL MYOPATHY

DESCRIPTION

Congenital myopathy describes hundreds of distinct syndromes of neuromuscular disorders occurring at birth or infancy (however, adult versions have been reported) and resulting in muscle weakness. In 1956, congenital myopathy was introduced in a patient who presented with central core disease (CCD) (Laporte et al., 1997). Typical symptoms of congenital myopathy include diminished muscle bulk and tone (hypotonia), which in layman's terms is referred to as "floppy," diminished reflexes (hyporeflexia), and generalized weakness centered in the body (North, 2008). Additional symptoms found in infancy include difficulty breathing, feeding, and delayed achievement of gross motor milestones (i.e., sitting up) (North, 2008). Congenital myopathies result from reduced contractile function rather than progressive dystrophy (muscle death) or inflammation (North, 2008).

Due to the amount of distinct syndromes of congenital myopathy, prevalence rates are uncertain, but are estimated to be approximately 14% of diagnosed cases of hypotonia, with CNS etiology being paramount (Both & Both, 1987). The sexes are equally represented due to the condition being autosomal dominant or recessive. However, there are variations of the congenital myopathies that are translated from the sex chromosomes (X chromosome) (Pierson, Tomczak, Agrawal, Moghadaszadeh, & Beggs, 2004). In these presentations females can be carriers of the disorder, but generally not express the phenotype because the gene is carried on the X chromosome resulting in a higher prevalence of males exhibiting the symptoms of this subtype over females. Congenital myopathies tend to be quite rare with only 180 cases documented over the span of 20 years

(Akiyama & Nonaka, 1996). As noted, there is a plethora of varieties of congenital myopathies. Some subtypes include: congenital fiber-type disproportion or Type 1 fiber predominance (21% of myopathies), nemaline rod myopathy (20%), CCD (16%), centronuclear myopathy (14%), multiminicore myopathy (10%), and other miscellaneous myopathies (comprising the final 19% of myopathies) (Both & Both, 1987). The prognosis of congenital myopathies is as varied as the subtypes and ranges from very poor with rapid death to a grossly normal life span (Sarnat, 1994). In general, cardiovascular or pulmonary complications, which tend to be adversely impacted by malignant hyperthermia and skeletal deformities, often lead to death.

NEUROPATHOLOGY/PATHOPHYSIOLOGY

In regard to the pathophysiology of the disease, there is a change in the genes that encode the actin-myosin structures, which results in diminished contractile abilities and specific morphological features depending on the subtype of congenital myopathy. The muscle weakness is not due to inflammation or degeneration.

Despite the variability of congenital myopathies, seven distinct pathophysiologies have been elucidated. The first subtype, congenital fiber-type disproportion, is described as a rare condition despite accounting for 21% of the congenital myopathies and is characterized by hypotonia, muscle weakness in the face and limbs, and problems with breathing (Sarnat, 1994). The second subtype, nemaline myopathy, is regarded as "the most common" congenital myopathy affecting infants by manifesting as difficulties with breathing and feeding, musculoskeletal complications (i.e., scoliosis), and a chronic yet static muscle weakness (Sarnat, 1994). The third subtype, CCD, affects children with variable severity and decline (Both & Both, 1987). Symptoms tend to be static and typically include mild hypotonia, delayed achievement of gross developmental milestones, and moderate extremity weakness. The fourth subtype, centronuclear myopathy, initiates in infancy or early childhood and is manifested by progressive limb weakness, microcephaly ptosis (droopy eyelids), and abnormal oculomotor movements (Both & Both, 1987). The fifth subtype, multiminicore disease, is comprised of numerous symptom variations, yet most manifest significant limb weakness and scoliosis with less common symptoms involving breathing difficulties and weakness in oculomotor movements (Sarnat, 1994).

Two important subtypes that comprise the other miscellaneous congenital myopathies include myotubular myopathy and hyaline body myopathy. The former subtype, myotubular myopathy, which some researchers consider to be the same as centronuclear myopathy, is a disorder that exclusively affects males and manifests as severe muscle weakness, hypotonia, and osteopenia (weakness of the bones) (Pierson, Tomczak, Agrawal, Moghadaszadeh, & Beggs, 2004). The severity of muscle weakness and hypotonia frequently results in reduced fetal movements that will be experienced by the mother in utero. In addition, the extent of breathing and swallowing difficulties often correspond with early mortality. The latter subtype, hyaline body myopathy, is a condition that is confirmed by muscle biopsy and is thought to have multiple etiologies and a varied phenotype (Both & Both, 1987).

Given the recent improvements in imaging technology, the myopathies have been classified into four categories: myopathies with protein accumulation, myopathies with cores, myopathies with central cores, and myopathies with fiber size variation (North, 2008).

NEUROPSYCHOLOGICAL/CLINICAL PRESENTATION

The clinical presentation of the congenital myopathies is consistent with a genetic etiology, generally static, and typically early onset hypotonia, hyporeflexia, and proximal generalized weakness. Dysmorphia may be evident secondary to muscle weakness. Hypotonia tends to be the primary symptom of the condition, which can be evaluated during the neurobehavioral evaluation. Neurobehavioral evaluation will also reveal diminished reflexes and weakness more proximal than distal.

Given the variety of subtypes of this disorder, many variations in functioning exist. However, in general, cognitive, academic, sensory, and emotional functions may be normal (Bodensteiner, 1994). In addition, there are typically no specific behavioral symptoms associated with the disorder (North, 2008). Regarding emotional functions, it is expected that some individuals may have some difficulties with the adjustment to their medical condition and as a result a mood disorder may develop.

DIAGNOSIS

Muscle weakness may have multiple etiologies such as central and/or peripheral causes. Thus, a neurologist, who performs a comprehensive physical examination and functional analyses to ascertain the cause of muscle weakness, typically identifies a diagnosis of congenital myopathy. If the neurologist alleges that a congenital myopathy is present, tests to definitively diagnose a myopathy include laboratory tests to determine the activity of the enzyme creatine kinase (CK), an electromyogram to assess the electrical conduction of the muscle, a muscle biopsy, and genetic testing (Both & Both, 1987). CK tends to be in the normal ranges, mildly elevated ranges, or moderately elevated ranges—the latter being typical of CCD (Both & Both, 1987). High elevations of CK are atypical and suggest other disorders such as Duchenne–Becker or limb-girdle muscular dystrophy (Both & Both, 1987). Other common differentials include other diseases such as spinal muscular atrophy, congenital myasthenia, hereditary neuropathy, cerebral palsy, congenital muscular dystrophy, metabolic myopathies, and myasthenia gravis (Both & Both, 1987).

Typically, nerve conduction studies are either normal or may demonstrate characteristic potentials consistent with myopathies (Both & Both, 1987). Electrocardiogram may also be used for diagnostic purposes as some myopathies display specific patterns (Both & Both, 1987). Muscle biopsies and pathological studies often confirm differential diagnosis of specific congenital myopathy subtypes (Both & Both, 1987).

TREATMENT

In regard to treatment, there is no cure for congenital myopathy. Treatments tend to be aggressive in nature yet supportive and are comprised of orthopedic involvement to address skeletal abnormalities, surgery or medical treatment to compensate for feeding issues, physical therapy, occupational therapy, and speech therapy (North, 2008). The goal of treatment is to maintain muscle function, including diaphragmatic muscles, which often translates to increased life expectancy and better quality of life. Individuals with congenital myopathies may suffer from hypoxia due to muscle weakness and therefore treatments to address and compensate for these impairments are implemented. Genetic counseling may be beneficial for family planning purposes. Treatment of choice tends to be a multidisciplinary team that can treat the patient in a holistic manner (North, 2008). Ongoing medical assessment for patients with congenital myopathies is warranted to determine the extent and nature of functional abilities.

Javan Horwitz
Natalie Horwitz
Chad A. Noggle

Akiyama, C., & Nonaka, I. (1996). A follow-up study of congenital non-progressive myopathies. *Brain Development, 18*, 404.

Bodensteiner, J. (1994). Congenital myopathies. *Muscle Nerve, 17*, 131.

Both, A., & Both, I. (1987). Congenital myopathies with "diagnostic" pathological features. *Journal of Medicine, 18*(2), 93–107.

Laporte, J., Guiraud-Chaumeil, C., Vincent, M., Mandel, J., Tanner, S., Leichti-Gallati, S., et al. (1997). Mutations in the MTM1 gene implicated in X-linked myotubular myopathy. ENMC International Consortium on Myotubular Myopathy. European Neuro-Muscular Center. *Human Molecular Genetics, 6*(9), 1505–1511.

North, K. (2008). What's new in congenital myopathies? *Neuromuscular Disorders, 18*(6), 433–442.

Pierson, C., Tomczak, K., Agrawal, P., Moghadaszadeh, B., & Beggs, A. (2004). X-linked myotubular and centronuclear myopathies. *Neurology, 62*(9), 1484–1490.

Sarnat, H. (1994). New insights into the pathogenesis of congenital myopathies. *Journal of Child Neurology, 9*(2), 193–201.

CORTICOBASAL DEGENERATION

DESCRIPTION

Corticobasal degeneration (CBD) is a neurodegenerative condition first described by Rebeiz and colleagues (1968) and is classically described as an akinetic-rigid syndrome with asymmetric motor features including rigidity, dystonia, and myoclonus. However, research during the previous decade indicates that CBD encompasses a broader range of motor symptoms and also presents with a fairly consistent cognitive profile, including apraxia, executive dysfunction, and language impairment, with relatively preserved memory function (Graham, Bak, & Hodges, 2003; Murray et al., 2007). Typical age of onset is in the sixth decade, with a median survival time of approximately 7 years from the initial onset of symptoms (Tröster & Fields, 2008).

NEUROPATHOLOGY/PATHOPHYSIOLOGY

CBD is a tauopathy. Tau-positive neurofibrillary tangles are found in the cortex, subcortical nuclei, and brainstem (Cummings, 2003). Among cortical regions, abnormalities—namely ballooned and achromatic neurons—are primarily found in the frontal and superior parietal cortices (Graham et al., 2003; Murray et al., 2007). Autopsy-proven cases of CBD demonstrate moderate-to-severe tau pathology in the gray and white matter of these areas. Severity of tau pathology is less severe and more variable in the inferior parietal lobe and the substantia nigra, and most cases demonstrate mild to no neuronal loss in the temporal lobe (Murray et al., 2007). Spinal cord abnormalities, including neuropil threads predominantly in the cervical gray matter and neuronal inclusions primarily in cervical interneurons, have also been documented in patients with pathologically diagnosed CBD (Iwasaki, Yoshida, Hattori, Hashizume, & Sobue, 2005).

NEUROPSYCHOLOGICAL/CLINICAL PRESENTATION

CBD has historically been viewed primarily as a movement disorder. Most often, patients present with a Parkinsonian syndrome manifested by an asymmetric rigidity. Motor features also typically include dystonia and myoclonus, both of which are usually focal and isolated to one limb. Oculomotor impairment and balance and gait disturbance can be present as well (Belfor et al., 2006; Murray et al., 2007). Not surprisingly, CBD can be misdiagnosed if only the presenting motor symptoms are considered during evaluation (Litvan et al., 2003).

Although the neurocognitive pattern and severity of CBD presentation varies somewhat across patients, reviews by Graham et al. (2003) as well as Belfor et al. (2006) present several generally consistent trends. The most prominent cortical symptom of CBD is an asymmetric ideomotor apraxia, wherein patients are unable to use tools, mime tool use, or imitate mimed tool use. In addition, limb kinetic, ideational, buccofacial, constructional, and truncal apraxias, as well as alien limb phenomena, have been reported as well. However, apraxia is not a universal symptom, as there are some pathologically confirmed cases in which it was not present. Visuospatial impairment, as evidenced by difficulties with judging line orientation and mechanical problem solving, is common (Graham et al., 2003). Other reported visuospatial difficulties include impaired two-dimensional construction abilities, as evidenced by copy of four geometric shapes (Murray et al., 2007).

Impaired executive function, as measured by the Wisconsin Card Sorting Test, Trail Making, and letter and category fluency tests, is well documented (see Graham et al., 2003 for a review). Slowed performances have also been documented on measures of working memory, processing speed, and mental flexibility (Libon et al., 2007). Caregivers most often cite inattention and difficulties with planning as the primary executive deficits, and patients with pathologically defined CBD generally demonstrate executive dysfunction at some point prior to death (Murray et al., 2007). Although somewhat less common, changes in social behavior including disinhibition, increased agitation, aggressiveness, hypersexuality, hyperorality, and inappropriate laughter have also been reported. Interestingly, many patients report awareness of their deficits despite significant impairments in multiple cognitive domains (Murray et al., 2007). O'Keefe et al. (2007), however, completed a more systematic evaluation of patients with CBD (as well as patients with progressive supranuclear palsy [PSP] and frontotemporal dementia [FTD]) and found that all three groups demonstrated impaired metacognitive awareness (i.e., self-appraisal of cognitive ability). In addition, all patient groups demonstrated an impaired ability to detect errors as they emerged (i.e., emergent awareness) and an overestimation of performance ability (i.e., anticipatory awareness). Aphasia is estimated to develop in roughly one-third to one-half of patients with CBD (Graham et al., 2003). The aphasia is most often nonfluent, although sensory, anomic, and mixed aphasia have all been documented as well.

The literature varies regarding the severity of episodic memory impairment, but in general, patients with CBD typically perform more poorly than controls and generally demonstrate a decline in performance as the disease progresses. However, patients with CBD generally perform better than patients with Alzheimer's disease, even when matched by Mini-Mental State Examination scores (Graham et al., 2003). Given the disruption of frontal-subcortical circuits in CBD, patients demonstrate difficulties with encoding and unassisted retrieval abilities but show a benefit with cueing (Graham et al., 2003). Semantic memory has not been extensively studied, but at present it appears that with typical cases of CBD semantic memory function remains relatively intact as measured by tests of information, vocabulary, name–photograph matching, word–picture matching, and a task requiring the patient match conceptually similar pictures (Graham et al., 2003).

Finally, some cognitive abilities have not been systematically researched, but case reports have documented impairments. Language skills, such as naming (e.g., Boston Naming Test), grammatical comprehension (e.g., Token Test), and reading are typically intact in the early stages of CBD but may decline with disease progression (Graham et al., 2003). In addition, others have observed difficulties with spelling skills (distinct from handwriting or oral expression) and acalculia (Murray et al., 2007).

DIAGNOSIS

The diagnosis of CBD generally has low sensitivity but high specificity (Cummings, 2003). Therefore, many patients can go undiagnosed but have features consistent with CBD at autopsy. Differential diagnosis can be challenging given that the neurobehavioral expression of CBD can resemble that of FTD, PSP, and primary progressive aphasia. CBD, FTD, and PSP also share similar radiological features (O'Keefe et al., 2007). As mentioned, CBD can only be definitively determined upon autopsy. Clinically, the most reliable diagnostic features of CBD include limb dystonia, asymmetric Parkinsonism, ideomotor apraxia, executive dysfunction, and balance and gait disturbance (Belfor et al., 2006). Unlike AD, patients generally demonstrate relatively preserved episodic memory. Profound personality changes and changes in social behavior are less common in CBD than in FTD. Although impaired insight has been documented, patients with CBD do not demonstrate the severity of impairment as in FTD (O'Keefe et al., 2007). The hallmark vertical gaze palsy observed in PSP is generally absent, although increased saccade latency can be present (Belfor et al., 2006).

TREATMENT

At present, there are no treatments available to cure or slow the progression of CBD; however, symptom management can provide some benefit to the patient and caregiver. Limited research has been conducted regarding pharmacological treatment outcomes (Belfor et al., 2006). Variable response has been observed with respect to levodopa and other dopaminergic drugs, with some research reporting limited benefit, whereas the majority of reports cite no improvement in motor symptoms. Of note, side effects such as dyskinesias can occur regardless of clinically beneficial response to treatment. Some patients benefit from physiotherapy and occupational therapy, especially given the morbidity and mortality associated with falling. A neurologically informed daily exercise regimen can improve strength and coordination, whereas appropriate mobility assistive devices, as warranted, can provide increased stability (Belfor et al., 2006).

Pharmacological treatment of the cognitive and psychological symptoms of CBD is not well studied. There are no placebo-controlled studies that support the use of cholinesterase inhibitors. The frequent occurrence of depressive symptoms can be treated with serotonin reuptake inhibitors (Belfor et al., 2006).

As CBD progresses, patients can develop dysphasia and thus are at increased risk of aspiration. In these cases, dietary modifications or a feeding tube may become necessary.

The patient with CBD presents unique physical and psychological challenges for caregivers and families. Declines in mobility, cognitive function, and, in particular, language function, can be quite distressing. Caregivers should be encouraged to seek support groups that represent a diversity of neurological conditions. Caregivers should also be encouraged to seek respite care, as necessary.

Anita H. Sim
Sarah M. Viamonte

Belfor, N., Amici, S., Boxer, A. L., Kramer, J. H., Gorno-Tempini, M. L., Rosen, H. J., et al. (2006). Clinical and neuropsychological features of corticobasal degeneration. *Mechanisms of Ageing and Development, 127*, 203–207.

Cummings, J. L. (2003). *The neuropsychiatry of Alzheimer's disease and related dementias.* New York: Taylor & Francis Group

Graham, N. L., Bak, T. H., & Hodges, J. R. (2003). Corticobasal degeneration as a cognitive disorder. *Movement Disorders, 18*, 1224–1232.

Iwasaki, Y., Yoshida, M., Hattori, M., Hashizume, Y., & Sobue, G. (2005). Widespread spinal cord involvement in corticobasal degeneration. *Acta Neuropathologica, 109*, 632–638.

Libon, D. J., Xie, S. X., Moore, P., Farmer, J., Antani, S., McCawley, G., et al. (2007). Patterns of neuropsychological impairment in frontotemporal dementia. *Neurology, 68*, 369–375.

Litvan, I., Bhatia, K. P., Burn, D. J., Goetz, C. G., Lang, A. E., McKeith, I., et al. (2003). Movement Disorders Society Scientific Issues Committee report: SIC Task Force appraisal of clinical diagnostic criteria for Parkinsonian disorders. *Movement Disorders, 18*, 467–486.

Murray, R., Neumann, M., Forman, M. S., Farmer, J., Massimo, L., Rice, A., et al. (2007). Cognitive and motor assessment in autopsy proven corticobasal degeneration. *Neurology, 68*, 1274–1283.

O'Keefe, F. M., Murray, B., Coen, R. F., Dockree, P. M., Bellgrove, M. A., Garavan, H., et al. (2007). Loss of insight in frontotemporal dementia, corticobasal degeneration, and progressive supranuclear palsy. *Brain, 130*, 753–764.

Tröster, A. I., & Fields, J. A. (2008). Parkinson's disease, progressive supranuclear palsy, corticobasal degeneration, and related disorders of the frontostriatal system. In J. E. Morgan & J. H. Ricker (Eds.), *Textbook of clinical neuropsychology*. New York: Taylor & Francis.

C

C

CRANIOSYNOSTOSIS

DESCRIPTION

Craniosynostosis is a condition that can occur both independently, or as part of a syndrome. Craniosynostosis occurs when the cranial sutures fuse prematurely in infancy, causing irregular skull development, potential brain damage, and potential increased intracranial pressure. The prevalence of craniosynostosis is about 1 in 1,800 to 2,200 births (Kabanni & Raguveer, 2004). Cranial sutures are fibrous joints that fuse the cranial bones together and ultimately help protect the central nervous system. These sutures unite the five cranial bones, which are: the paired frontals, the paired parietals, and the interparietal.

Cranial sutures are elastic, allowing for proper brain development and expansion. For this reason, craniosynostosis can detrimentally affect brain growth by not providing the brain proper room to mature and the abrupt closure of fontanelles. Fontanelles are the gaps between the calvarian bones, sometimes known as the "soft spots" on an infant's head. Suture closure reaches maturity at age 12, though continues gradually until the third decade of life.

Craniosynostosis can involve either the premature fusion of one suture (simple craniosynostosis) or the fusion of multiple cranial sutures (compound craniosynostosis). Simple craniosynostosis occurs much more frequently than compound craniosynostosis, anywhere between 85% and 95% of all cases of craniosynostosis (Morris-Kay & Wilkie, 2005). In addition, the involvements of specific cranial (calvarian) sutures are seen in craniosynostosis. Sagittal synostosis occurs in 40–55% of all cases, coronal synostosis is seen 20–25% of the time, and lambdoid synostosis is present in about 5% of all cases (Morris-Kay & Wilkie, 2005). As their names suggest, these various types of craniosynostosis are labeled depending upon which suture is involved.

NEUROPATHOLOGY/PATHOPHYSIOLOGY

Syndromic craniosynostosis occurs as part of a disease or syndrome, rather than an independent event. The two diseases most commonly involving craniosynostosis are Crouzon's disease and Apert syndrome. Crouzon's disease, which is the most frequently occurring syndrome with craniosynostosis, is inherited in an autosomal-dominant pattern. Children can acquire this disease genetically from an affected parent, or from a new genetic mutation, with no family history of the disorder. Among all cases of craniosynostosis, about 5% are directly related to Crouzon's disease. The synostosis in Crouzon's disease presents as very prominent eyes, a beaked nose, and an abnormally large space between the eyes (hypertelorism). Craniosynostosis in this syndrome often involves premature fusion of the coronal suture. This condition known as bradycephaly flattens the head due to early fusion of the coronal suture that connects the frontal calvarian bones to the paired parietal bones.

Apert syndrome, which is caused by a mutation in the gene encoding for *FGFR2* on chromosome 10, also involves craniosynostosis. Specifically, Apert syndrome involves coronal suture synostosis, leading to megalocephaly. Megalocephaly is an abnormally large presentation of the head, without intracranial pressure. Agenesis of the corpus callosum, another serious concern associated with Apert syndrome, is the partial or complete absence of the corpus callosum and can lead to several severe cognitive deficiencies. These deficiencies include poor interhemispheric communication, poor performance on tests of reasoning, and below average concept formation (Morriss-Kay & Wilkie, 2005).

NEUROPSYCHOLOGICAL/CLINICAL PRESENTATION

Past research on neuropsychological differences between control groups and children with craniosynostosis, has delineated that children with craniosynostosis are three to five times more likely to have a learning disorder (Speltz, Kapp-Simon, Cunningham, Marsh, & Dawson, 2004). More specifically, children with craniosynostosis often have a very wide discrepancy between verbal and performance IQ scores (Shipster et al., 2003). These findings indicate deficient visuo spatial processing, poor perceptual organization, and below average working memory scores. One study using a control group and a sagittal synostosis group found that children with craniosynostosis not only obtained discrepant IQ scores but performed significantly lower than the mean, with an average IQ score of 74 (Camfield & Camfield, 1986).

DIAGNOSIS

Nonsyndromic craniosynostosis typically involves one suture, whereas syndromic craniosynostosis most commonly presents as compound craniosynostosis. There are four different types of single suture craniosynostosis: sagittal synostosis, unilateral coronal synostosis, metopic synostosis, and lambdoid synostosis. The physical manifestations of sagittal synostosis include an elongated cranium and a large head circumference. In this condition, the cranial vault is severely impacted, whereas the cranial base remains unaffected. The cranial vault can be thought of as the top portions of the cranium such as the paired frontal and parietal bones, whereas the cranial base makes up the areas beneath the prominent vault bones, as well as occipital area bone.

Unilateral coronal synostosis, which is the premature fusion of the coronal suture, involves several characteristic cranial and craniofacial abnormalities. In children with unilateral coronal synostosis, typically the affected side of the calvaria is significantly depressed, whereas the frontal bone of the unaffected side tends to protrude. The orbital area and frontal region of the calvaria appear flattened (Sakurai, Hirabayashi, Sugawara, & Harii, 1998). Craniofacial anomalies include half of the face appearing higher than the other half with the affected side of the face higher than the unaffected. The affected side may protrude as well, due to abnormal development of the malar bone (Sakurai et al., 1998).

Metopic synostosis remains much more rare than coronal, or sagittal synostosis. Metopic synostosis contorts the calvarial bones in a triangular shape, specifically the paired frontal bones (trigonocephaly). It also causes hypotelorism, defined as abnormally close eyes, due to the malformed frontal bones. In addition, the temporal areas are narrowed, whereas the parietal areas of the calvarium are widened. Past research has indicated that children with metopic synostosis may be particularly vulnerable to mental retardation (Kane, 2004). The metopic suture is the first suture to fuse, beginning in the second year of life (Huang, Mouradian, Cohen, & Gruss, 1998). Due to this rapid fusion, it is important to differentiate malignant metopic synostosis from the much more benign metopic ridging. Similar to metopic synostosis, metopic ridging causes the premature fusion of the paired frontal bones, yet the overall shape of the cranium is normal. Metopic ridging lacks the supraorbital recession, the narrow temporal areas, the widened parietal areas, and the hypotelorism. Metopic ridging usually requires no surgical intervention, due to typical natural correction. In contrast, metopic synostosis may cause increased intracranial pressure due to calvarian deformity and almost always requires extensive surgery (Huang et al., 1998).

Lambdoid synostosis remains the rarest and the most controversial of the four simple types of craniosynostosis. This controversy stems from the similarity between lambdoid synostosis, and deformational plagiocephaly. Past research indicates many cases of surgical intervention in plagiocephaly that were mistakenly assumed to be lambdoid synostosis. The prevalence of lambdoid synostosis is less than 5% of all cases of single-suture craniosynostosis (Kane, 2004).

When assessing for craniosynostosis, it is important to be aware of the commonality between craniosynostosis and deformational plagiocephaly. To differentiate a case of the generally benign plagiocephaly from the malignant craniosynostosis, the clinician must first use CT scan to determine the presence or absence of suture fusion, hydrocephalus, or brain herniation (Kabhanni & Raghuveer, 2004).

TREATMENT

Once craniosynostosis has been confirmed, surgical intervention is necessary. There are currently three major forms of surgery for craniosynostosis. The most common intervention used is a strip craniectomy. The strip craniectomy involves resecting the specific suture that has fused prematurely. One major consequence of this intervention is heavy blood loss, which commonly requires blood transfusion during operation (Kabhanni & Raghuveer, 2004). Recent advancement has provided the endoscopic strip craniectomy, a procedure that emulates the strip craniectomy, without the risk of excessive blood loss. This surgery requires the physician to make a 2–3 cm incision near the fused suture. Once the incision has been made, the endoscope assists in providing visual feedback on the resection process (Cartwright, Jimenz, Barone, & Baker, 2003.) Lastly, cranial vault remodeling is an invasive surgical intervention that involves excising, and restructuring cranial bones, in order to both reduce the potential for neurological problems such as intracranial pressure, as well as cosmetically reshaping the cranium to ensure proper bone development.

Ryan Boddy
Charles Golden

Camfield, M. D., & Camfield, C. S. (1986). Neurologic aspects of craniosynostosis. In M. M. Cohen Jr. (Ed.), *Diagnosis, evaluation, and management.* New York: Raven Press.

Cartwright, C., Jimenez, D., Barone, C., & Baker, L. (2003). Endoscopic strip craniectomy: A minimally invasive treatment for early correction of craniosynostosis. *Journal of Neuroscience Nursing, 35*(3), 130–138.

Huang, M. H., Muoradian, S., Cohen, S. R., & Gruss, J. S. (1998). The differential diagnosis of abnormal head shapes: Separating craniosynostosis from positional de-formities and normal variants. *The Cleft Palate-Craniofacial Jouranl, 35,* 204–211.

Kabbani, H., & Raghuveer, S. (2004). Craniosynostosis. *American Family Physician, 69*(12), 2863–2870.

Kane, A. A. (2004). An overview of craniosynostosis. *Journal of Prosthetics and Orthotics, 16*(4), 50–55.

Morriss-Kay, G. M. &, Wilkie, A. O. (2005). Growth of the normal skull vault and its alteration in craniosynostosis: Insights from human genetics and experimental studies. *Journal of Anatomy, 207*(5), 637–653.

Sakurai, A., Hirabahashi, S., Sugawara, Y., & Harii, K. (1998). Skeletal analysis of craniofacial asymmetries in plagiocephaly (unilateral coronal synostosis). *Scandinavian Journal of Plastic & Reconstructive Surgery & Hand Surgery, 32*(1), 81–89.

Shipster, C., Hearst, D., Somerville, A., Stackhouse, J., Hayward, R., & Wade, A. (2003). Speech, language, and cognitive development in children with isolated sagittal synostosis. *Developmental Medicine and Child Neurology, 45,* 34–43.

Speltz, M. L., Kapp-Simon, K. A., Cunningham, M., Marsh, J., & Dawson, G. (2004). Single-suture craniosynostosis: A review of neurobehavioral research and theory. *Journal of Pediatric Psychology, 29*(8), 651–668.

CREUTZFELDT–JAKOB'S DISEASE

DESCRIPTION

Creutzfeldt–Jakob's disease (CJD) is a rare, neurodegenerative, human transmissible spongiform encephalopathy (TSE) with a rapid, incurable, and fatal course (Knight, 2006). CJD is classified as a prion disease due to the presence of prion protein (*PRNP*) gene. Pathognomonic signs of CJD include myoclonus, ataxia, visual disturbance, progressive dementia, pyramidal and extrapyramidal motor signs (parkinsonism), and akinetic mutism in the final stages. Laboratory findings often reveal characteristic EEG abnormalities and the presence of protein (14-3-3 assay) in the CSF (Iwasaki, Mimuro, Yoshida, Sobue, & Hashizume, 2009; Josephs, Tsuboi, & Dickson, 2004). Other shared features of prion diseases include central nervous system involvement, an incubation period of months to years, rapid disease progression, and fatal prognosis.

Four variants of CJD have been identified and appear to affect both men and women equally. Although sporadic CJD (sCJD) is the most common, compromising approximately 85% of all cases (Krasnianksi et al., 2009), sCJD remains quite rare with a worldwide prevalence of 1–2 cases per million. Onset is typically in the sixth or seventh decade, and disease course is typically between 4 and 6 months, though it may be as rapid as 4 weeks (Knight, 2006; Mendez & Cummings, 2003).

The second most common variant of CJD is familial (fCJD), accounting for approximately 5% to 15% of cases. Familial CJD is an autosomal-dominant disease, caused by gene mutations on the short arm of chromosome 20 with nearly two dozen family specific mutations identified to date. The onset of fCJD is somewhat earlier, though a great deal of variability has been cited within the literature.

Iatrogenic CJD is a third variant and even more rare variant transmitted person to person via exposure to infected human tissues (e.g., improperly cleaned surgical instruments, transplanted tissues etc.).

The fourth variant originating from bovine spongiform encephalitis in cattle in the United Kingdom used for human consumption, variant CJD (vCJD) labeled "mad cow" disease, has perhaps received the most media attention. The age of onset in vCJD is typically younger (mid-20s) with reported adolescent cases and has a disease duration of approximately 14 months. Psychiatric manifestations (e.g., depression, social withdrawal, anxiety) and sensory disturbance may be the presenting symptoms in vCJD followed by more classic symptoms of ataxia, myoclonus, and cognitive impairment (Knight, 2006). Although only 10–15 cases per year have been reported since its emergence in 1996, the full implications of vCJD may have not yet been realized due to the protracted incubation period of prion diseases (McHugh et al., 2007; Mendez & Cummings, 2003).

NEUROPATHOLOGY/PATHOPHYSIOLOGY

Prion protein is a normally occurring protein that is encoded by the *PrP* gene on the short arm of chromosome 20. Prion diseases result from mutations to the *PrP* gene and interact with other macrophages resulting in deposition of amyloid plaques in the brain, a characteristic finding of many prion diseases (Mendez & Cummings, 2003). More specifically, the polymorphism occurs at codon 129 of the *PRNP*, and the *PrPSc* Types 1 and 2 are the basis for a molecular classification of sCJD (Parchi et al., 1996, 1999).

Neuropathological features of CJD include neuronal loss, gliosis, and vacuolation of gray matter (spongiosis) creating a "sponge-like" appearance upon microscopic examination (Aguzzi, 2006; Mendez & Cummings, 2003).

Hyperintensities on T2-weighted images in the basal ganglia are commonly noted, whereas cortical signal increase has also been noted on FLAIR and DWI (Bahn, Kido, Lin, & Pearlman, 1997; Greitz et al., 1992; Meissner et al., 2004; Shiga et al., 2004). When employing methods such as FLAIR and DWI, signal increase in the cortex is actually seen in greater frequency than in the basal ganglia (Kallenberg et al., 2006; Young et al., 2005)

NEUROPSYCHOLOGICAL/CLINICAL PRESENTATION

Clinical presentation may vary between variants of CJD; however, key features include ataxia, myoclonus (present in approximately 80% of sCJD cases and often startle-dependent), pyramidal and extrapyramidal signs, rapidly progressive dementia, and akinetic mutism later on (Iwasaki et al., 2009; Mendez & Cummings, 2003). Parchi et al. (1999) reported that clinical features are to some extent related to the genotype of the disease and such correlation have limited practical utility apart from predicting longer or shorter survival times after onset. Earliest symptoms usually appear gradually over a few weeks but may present more suddenly.

Although neuropsychological data are sparse due to the rapid and progressive course of the disease, cognitive deficits in complex attention, processing speed, executive functioning, memory, and eventually language have been cited (Mendez & Cummings, 2003). Memory loss and either cerebellar or visual oculomotor signs are frequently seen at the outset and as the illness evolves pyramidal and extrapyramidal signs as well as involuntary movements such as myoclonus are seen (Brown, 2007). Mental deterioration progresses in a rapid manner terminating in mutism and global dementia prior to death, which usually occurs within 6–9 months from initial symptom onset. However, a fair number of individuals succumb to the disease after only a few months, whereas a small percentage (i.e., <10%) demonstrate a more extended course of roughly 2 years (Pocchiari et al., 2004).

DIAGNOSIS

Neuropathological confirmation of CJD is made via brain biopsy or postmortem with evidence of gliosis, neuronal loss, and spongiform changes. EEG abnormalities have been identified, including periodic sharp-wave complexes. The presence of 14-3-3 assay or elevated white cell counts in CSF of CJD individuals is another finding, though some researchers have not universally found this analysis to be positive in all cases (Green et al., 2007). MRI findings often reveal high signal intensities within the putamen and head of the caudate, bilaterally in sCJD (Mendez & Cummings, 2003) and high signal intensities in the posterior thalamus ("pulvinar sign") of vCJD (Aguzzi, 2006; Knight, 2006). FLAIR and DWI have proven particularly effective in the imaging of CJD. These techniques have proven beneficial in detecting both cortical and basal ganglion signal increases (7–8). DWI has been found to be the most sensitive technique for detecting alterations in sCJD (10–11). Finally, high concentration of prion protein has been confirmed upon biopsy of the tonsils in vCJD (Aguzzi, 2006). Differential diagnosis varies based on disease stage. At onset infectious, metabolic, and intoxication processes should be ruled out. In addition, cerebrovascular accidents, neoplasms, and normal pressure hydrocephalus should be considered (Brown, 2007). In later stages, cortical dementias and various movement disorders with dementing features may represent the most difficult differentials (e.g., Parkinson's disease with dementia, Lewy body dementia, amyotrophic lateral sclerosis, Pick's disease, Huntington's disease, olivopontocerebellar atrophy, etc.); however, often the rate of progression alone may point toward CJD.

TREATMENT

CJD is a rare, incurable neurodegenerative TSE with a rapid and fatal course. Caution is warranted to avoid transmission. Precautions should be taken when patients are hospitalized in the hand or in disposal of tissues, excretions, and other contaminated material (Brown, 2007).

Pharmacological approaches in certain variants in humans and vaccination procedures in animal models are currently being explored. Although several pharmacological approaches appear useful in symptom reduction, none have been successful in curing the disease. Symptom management is essential. Benzodiazepines and/or anticonvulsant agents may be utilized to suppress myoclonus or seizures (Brown, 2007). Patient and family support, including genetic counseling in fCFJD cases, remain important (Aguzzi, 2006; Mendez & Cummings, 2003).

Michelle R. Pagoria
Chad A. Noggle

Aguzzi, A. (2006). Prion disease of humans and farm animals: Epidemiology, genetics, and pathogenesis. *Journal of Neurochemistry, 97,* 1726–1739.

Bahn, M. M., Kido, D. K., Lin, W., & Pearlman, A. L. (1997). Brain magnetic resonance diffusion abnormalities in Creutzfeldt–Jakob disease. *Archives of Neurology, 54,* 1411–1415.

Brown, P. (2007). Transmissible spongiform encephalopathy. In C. G. Goetz (Ed.), *Textbook of clinical neurology* (3rd ed., pp. 969–979). Philadelphia: Saunders Elsevier.

Green, A., Sanchez-Juan, P., Ladogana, A., Cuadrado-Corrales, N., Sánchez-Valle, R., Mitrová, E., et al. (2007). CSF analysis in patients with sporadic CJD and other transmissible spongiform encephalopathies. *European Journal of Neurology, 14,* 121–124.

Greitz, D., Wirestam, R., Franck, A., Nordell, B., Thomsen, C., & Stahlberg, F. (1992). Pulsatile brain movement and associated hydrodynamics studied by magnetic resonance phase imaging. The Monro-Kellie doctrine revisited. *Neuroradiology, 34,* 370–380.

Iwasaki, Y., Mimuro, M., Yoshida, M., Sobue, G., & Hashizume, Y. (2009). Clinical diagnosis of Creutzfeldt-Jakob disease: Accuracy based on analysis of autopsy-confirmed cases. *Journal of Neurological Sciences, 277,* 119–123.

Josephs, K. A., Tsuboi, Y., & Dickson, D. W. (2004). Creutzfeld-Jakob disease presenting as progressive supranuclear palsy. *European Journal of Neurology, 11,* 343–346.

Kallenberg, K., Schulz-Schaeffer, W., Jastrow, U., Poser, S., Meissner, B., Tschampa, H. J., et al. (2006). Creutzfeldt–Jakob disease: Comparative analysis of MR imaging sequences. *American Journal of Neuroradiology, 27,* 1459–1462.

Knight, R. (2006). Creutzfeldt-Jakob disease: A rare case of dementia in elderly persons. *Aging and Infectious Diseases, 43,* 340–346.

Krasnianski, A., von Ahsen, N., Heinemann, U., Meissner, B., Schulz-Schaeffer, W. J., Kretzschmar, H. A., et al. (2009). Increased frequency of positive family history of dementia in sporadic CJD. *Neurobiology of Aging, 30,* 615–621.

McHugh, J. C., Bradley, B., Hutchinson, M., Brett, F., Heffernan, J., Howley, R., et al. (2007). Variant Creutzfeldt-Jakob disease: First two indigenous cases in Republic of Ireland. Case report and perspective. *European Journal of Neurology, 14,* 467–469.

Meissner, B., Körtner, K., Bartl, M., Jastrow, U., Mollenhauer, B., & Schröter, A., (2004). Sporadic Creutzfeldt–Jakob disease: Magnetic resonance imaging and clinical findings. *Neurology, 63,* 450–456.

Mendez, M. F., & Cummings, J. L. (2003). *Dementia: A clinical approach* (3rd ed.). Philadelphia: Butterworth-Heinemann.

Parchi, P., Castellani, R., Capellari, S., Ghetti, B., Young, K., Chen, S. G., et al. (1996). Molecular basis of phenotypic variability in sporadic Creutzfeldt–Jakob disease. *Annals of Neurology, 39,* 767–778.

Parchi, P., Giese, A., Capellari, S., Brown, P., Schulz-Schaeffer, W., Windl, O., et al. (1999). Classification of sporadic Creutzfeldt-Jakob disease based on molecular and phenotypic analysis of 300 subjects. *Annals of Neurology, 46,* 224–233.

Pocchiari, M., Puopolo, M., Croes, E. A., Budka, H., Gelpi, E., Collins, S., et al., (2004). Predictors of survival in sporadic Creutzfeldt-Jakob disease and other human transmissible spongiform encephalopathies. *Brain, 127,* 2348–2357.

Shiga, Y., Miyazawa, K., Sato, S., Fukushima, R., Shibuya, S., Sato, Y., et al. (2004). Diffusion-weighted MRI abnormalities as an early diagnostic marker for Creutzfeldt–Jakob disease. *Neurology, 63,* 443–449.

Young, G. S., Geschwind, M. D., Fischbein, N. J., Martindale, J. L., Henry, R. G., Liu, S., et al. (2005). Diffusion-weighted and fluid-attenuated inversion recovery imaging in Creutzfeldt–Jakob disease: High sensitivity and specificity for diagnosis. *American Journal of Neuroradiology, 26,* 1551–1562.

CUSHING'S SYNDROME

DESCRIPTION

Cushing's syndrome (CS) is a hormonal disorder caused by prolonged exposure to elevated levels of the stress hormone cortisol in the blood. It is a rare condition, with a prevalence rate of only approximately 1 in 500,000 or 0.0% in the United States. In the majority of cases, the onset is insidious, and it may take years for the full symptomatology to develop (Magiakou, Smyrnaki, & Chrousos, 2006). Recent literature suggests that endogenous hypercortisolism may occur in 0.5% to 1% of patients with hypertension, 3% to 4% with poorly controlled diabetes, 6% to 9% with incidental adrenal masses, and 11% with osteoporosis and vertebral fractures (Newell-Price, Bertagna, Grossman, & Nieman, 2006). CS in children co-occurs with growth retardation (Miyachi, 2000; Newell-Price, Trainer, Besser, & Grossman, 1998).

The hypercortisolism can be due to either endogenous adrenocorticotropic hormone (ACTH)-dependent or exogenous ACTH-independent causes involving treatment with glucocorticoids or adrenocortical tumors that produce cortisol (Newell-Price et al., 1998). Values of 24-hour urinary free cortisol (UFC) excretions higher than 300 µg/day are indicative of CS. False-positive results can be found in individuals with chronic stress, malnutrition, or alcoholism resulting in elevated cortisol levels. In a low-dose dexamethasone overnight suppression screening test (LDDST), serum cortisol levels higher than 5 µg/dL are indicative of CS (Newell-Price et al., 2006).

NEUROPATHOLOGY/PATHOPHYSIOLOGY

CS is caused by various etiologies that can be divided into endogenous corticotropin ACTH-dependent and exogenous ACTH-independent mechanisms. The latter mechanism is often iatrogenic and due to an excessive use of glucocorticoids. The most common form is due to Cushing's disease (CD), which accounts for 60% to 80% of the causes (Newell-Price et al., 2006). It is caused by overproduction of ACTH from a pituitary adenoma, usually a microadenoma (6 mm in diameter). Other causes of ACTH-dependent CS include ACTH-producing nonpituitary tumors and ectopic corticotropin-releasing hormone (CRH)-producing tumors. ACTH-independent CS can be caused by cortisol-producing adrenal benign or malignant tumors, micronodular adrenal hyperplasia, and other adrenal-dependent processes such as McCune–Albright's syndrome and Carney's complex (Newell-Price et al., 1998; Samuels & Loriaux, 1994). Overall, ACTH-dependent causes contribute to 85% of CS cases, whereas 15% to 20% are due to ACTH-independent forms (Ilias et al., 2005). Ectopic corticotropin-caused CS is characterized with rapid onset of symptoms including paraneoplastic wasting syndrome and hypokalemia (Newell-Price et al., 2006).

Prolonged exposure to high levels of glucocorticoids contributes to morphologic brain changes by reducing dendritic length and branching of adult hippocampal pyramidal cells (Woolley, Gould, & McEwen, 1990), which in turn reduce the neuronal capacity of the brain to recover from injuries (DeKorsky, Scheff, & Cotman, 1984). In addition, chronic elevation of cortisol levels may cause cerebral atrophy, ventricular enlargement, and reduced hippocampal volume in patients with CS (Forget, Lacroix, Somma, & Cohen, 2000; Starkman, Gebarski, Berent, & Schteingart, 1992).

NEUROPSYCHOLOGICAL/CLINICAL PRESENTATION

Clinical symptoms of CS include truncal obesity, weight gain, moon facies (rounding of the face), hypertension, hyperlipidemia, insulin resistance, diabetes, muscle weakness, erectile dysfunction in males, menstrual irregularities in women, osteoporosis, and skin conditions involving thinning, bruising, purple striae, facial hair, hyperpigmentation, and acne (Magiakou et al., 2006; Miyachi, 2000). Women are more likely to present with purple striae, muscle atrophy, osteoporosis, and kidney stones than men (Newell-Price et al., 2006). Bone loss maybe more

severe in adrenal-dependent rather than pituitary-dependent CS syndrome (Minetto et al., 2004).

Several psychiatric and psychological disorders are often associated with this condition, regardless of its etiology, including major depressive disorder (MDD), mania, psychosis, irritability, and anxiety disorders. Comorbidity with depression indicates a severe clinical presentation and is prognostically important. Due to a plethora of clinical symptoms, no single symptom is required for a diagnosis (Sonino & Fava, 2001).

Cognitive impairment is seen in several domains, particularly those involving intellectual functioning, attention/concentration, memory, language, and visuospatial abilities. Executive dysfunction commonly involves impaired reasoning, concept formation, and phonemic fluency (Forget et al., 2000). However, perceptual attention and recognition abilities seem to be intact. High levels of cortisol have also been suggested to exacerbate cognitive decline in older adults (Pomara, Greenberg, Branford, & Doraiswamy, 2003). Findings are mixed with regard to recovery of cognitive function following the normalization of cortisol levels (Hook et al., 2007). Patients with CD significantly improve on tests of immediate and delayed recall of verbal memory and auditory attention span (Mauri et al., 1993) 6 months following successful treatment. Patients with a more heterogeneous etiology of CS show improvements on measures of visual organization and phonemic fluency but do not improve on tests of attention, memory, reasoning, language, or visuospatial reasoning (Forget, Lacroix, & Cohen, 2002).

DIAGNOSIS

Cortisol levels normally peak in the morning and fall throughout the day, with the lowest levels occurring overnight. With this cycle in mind, the three most common tests used to screen for CS include the 24-hour UFC test, measurement of midnight plasma cortisol or late-night salivary cortisol, and the low-dose dexamethasone suppression test with a 24-hour UFC and the overnight dexamethasone suppression tests used as screening for presence of hypercortisolism. Diagnosis of CS is required before the differential diagnosis of etiological considerations.

If the corticotropin level is low in the morning, an adrenal tumor is more likely to be diagnosed. Elevated UFC, cortisol serum more than 50 nmol/L on dexamethasone-suppression test, midnight plasma cortisol levels more than 207 nmol/L when awake and more than 50 nmol/L when sleeping, in conjunction with elevated late night salivary cortisol indicate presence of CS (Newell-Price et al., 1998; Newell-Price et al., 2006). The 48-hour low-dose dexamethasone suppression test is used to confirm the overproduction of cortisol (Miyachi, 2000). Concentrations of corticotropin greater than 15 mg/mL indicate presence of ACTH-dependent CS, whereas concentrations of corticotropin lower than 5 pg/mL suggest ACTH-independent CS, and imaging techniques are used to localize the tumors (Newell-Price et al., 2006).

To establish the cause of CS both biochemical tests and imaging techniques are employed. CT scans of the adrenal gland and/or MRI of the pituitary gland are performed to detect adrenal or pituitary adenomas or benign lesions. Scintigraphy of the adrenal gland can also be useful in cases of ACTH-dependent forms and adrenal tumors (see Table 1 for tests used for differential diagnosis of Cushing's syndrome). Genetic testing for mutations of PRKAR1A or evaluation of Carney's complex is performed in the cases of normal adrenal glands on imaging. Physical examinations to detect visual field defects in cases of a pituitary lesion are recommended to examine the cause of typically present bitemporal hemianopia.

TREATMENT

Treatment is employed based on the etiology of CS. The primary goal is to normalize levels of cortisol in the blood. Transphenoidal selective adenomectomy is the most common procedure in the cases of CD with resulting remission rates ranging from 80% to 90% (Newell-Price et al., 2006). However, relapse within 6 months after surgery is common, especially in cases when a pituitary tumor has not been found. Pituitary irradiation or bilateral adrenalectomies are performed in those individuals for whom a second surgery is contraindicated (Newell-Price et al., 2006). Surgical excision is performed for those with ectopic corticotrophin elevations, CRH syndrome, and those with primary adrenal hypersecretion. Drug treatment with corticosteroid inhibitors are used as an adjunctive treatment and are mainly used in either presurgical or postoperative stages of the disease, as well as for those treated with external pituitary irradiation, or those refusing surgical treatment (Newell-Price et al., 2006).

Prolonged exposure to corticosteroids may result in some degree of irreversible pathological damage and subsequently impact psychological functioning. Thus, following the surgical and pharmacological interventions aimed at normalizing cortisol levels, treatment includes psychotherapeutic interventions (e.g., cognitive behavioral therapies that have been empirically shown to be effective in mood disorders) and psychotropic medications, including antidepressants (e.g., selective serotonin reuptake inhibitors and tricyclic agents), and benzodiazepines in small doses for those with severe anxiety symptoms. Corticosteroid inhibitors (e.g., ketoconazole, meyrapone, aminoglutethimide) rather than antidepressant drugs are used to reduce depressive symptoms in patients with co-occurring MDD and CS (Sonino & Fava, 2001).

Anita H. Sim
Maya Yutsis

Table 1
TESTS USED FOR DIFFERENTIAL DIAGNOSIS OF CUSHING'S SYNDROME

Tests	Differential
CRH stimulation	Pituitary adenomas from those with ectopic adrenocorticotropic hormone (ACTH) syndrome or adrenal tumors
High-dose dexamethasone suppression test	Pituitary adenomas from those with ectopic ACTH-producing tumors
Radiologic imaging: CT and MRI	Localization of tumors in adrenal adenomas, carcinomas, or ACTH-independent macronodular adrenal hyperplasia
Somatostatin scintigraphy	Individuals with recurrent disease
Bilateral petrosal sinus sampling	Pituitary vs. non-pituitary causes of Cushing's syndrome in those with normal pituitary gland MRI scans

Adapted from Newell-Price, J., Bertagna, X., Grossman, A. B., & Nieman, L. K. (2006). Cushing's syndrome. *Lancet, 367,* 1605–1617.

DeKorsky, S. T., Scheff, S. W., & Cotman, C. W. (1984). Elevated corticosterone levels. A possible cause of reduced axon sprouting in aged animals. *Neuroendocrinology, 38,* 33–38.

Forget, H., Lacroix, A., & Cohen, H. (2002). Persistent cognitive impairment following surgical treatment of Cushing's syndrome. *Psychoneuroendocrinology, 27,* 367–383.

Forget, H., Lacroix, A., Somma, A., & Cohen, H. (2000). Cognitive decline in patients with Cushing's syndrome. *Journal of the International Neuropsychology Society, 6,* 20–29.

Hook, J. N., Giordani, B., Schteingart, D. E., Cuire, K., Giles, J., Ryan, K., et al. (2007). Patterns of cognitive change over time and relationship to age following successful treatment of Cushing's disease. *Journal of the International Neuropsychology Society, 13,* 21–29.

Ilias, I., Torpy, D. J., Pacak, K., Mullen, N., Wesley, R. A., & Nieman, L. K. (2005). Cushing's syndrome due to ectopic corticotropin secretion: Twenty years' experience at the National Institutes of Health. *Journal of Clinical Endocrinology and Metabolism, 90,* 4955–4962.

Magiakou, M. A., Smyrnaki, P., & Chrousos, G. P. (2006). Hypertension in Cushing's syndrome. *Best Practice & Research Clinical Endocrinology & Metabolism, 20*(3), 467–482.

Mauri, M., Sinforiani, E., Bono, G., Vignati, F., Berselli, M. E., Attansio, R., et al (1993). Memory impairment in Cushing's disease. *Acta Neurologica Scandinavica, 87,* 52–55.

Minetto, M., Reimondo, G., Osella, G., Ventura, M., Angeli, A., & Terzolo, M. (2004). Bone loss is more severe in primary adrenal than in pituitary-dependent Cushing's syndrome. *Osteoporosis International, 15,* 855–861.

Miyachi, Y. (2000). Pathophysiology and diagnosis of Cushing's syndrome. *Biomed and Pharmacotherapy, 54*(1), 113–117.

Newell-Price, J., Bertagna, X., Grossman, A. B., & Nieman, L. K. (2006). Cushing's syndrome. *Lancet, 367,* 1605–1617.

Newell-Price, J., Trainer, P., Besser, M., & Grossman, A. (1998). The diagnosis and differential diagnosis of Cushing's syndrome and pseudo-Cushing's states. *Endocrine Reviews, 19*(5), 647–672.

Pomara, N., Greenberg, W. M., Branford, M. D., & Doraiswamy, P. M. (2003). Therapeutic implications of HPA axis abnormalities in Alzheimer's disease: Review and update. *Psychopharmacology Bulletin, 37,* 120–134.

Samuels, M. H., & Loriaux, D. L. (1994). Cushing's syndrome and the nodular adrenal gland. *Endocrinology and Metabolism Clinics of North America, 23,* 555–569.

Sonino, N., & Fava, G. A. (2001). Psychiatric disorders associated with Cushing's syndrome. *CNS Drugs, 15*(5), 361–373.

Starkman, M. N., Gebarski, S. S., Berent, S., & Schteingart, D. E. (1992). Hippocampal formation volume, memory dysfunction, and cortisol levels in patients with Cushing's syndrome. *Biological Psychiatry, 32,* 756–765.

Woolley, C. A., Gould, E., & McEwen, B. S. (1990). Exposure to excess glucocorticoids alters dendritic morphology of adult hippocampal pyramidal neurons. *Brain Research, 531,* 225–231.

CYTOMEGALOVIRUS

DESCRIPTION

Human cytomegalovirus (CMV) is a variant of the herpes virus. Relatively common, it is estimated that roughly 80% of individuals in the United States by the age of 40 have a latent form of the virus that is held at bay by antibodies (Roos, 2007). The presentation becomes symptomatic at points when there is compromise of the host's immune system, either due to infection or immunosuppressive therapy. Beyond this, congenital forms are also observed in newborns.

Clinical presentation may vary as the virus has the propensity to invade a wide range of cell types (Bissinger, Sinzger, Kaiserling, & Jahn, 2002; Kahl, Siegel-Axel, Stenglein, Jahn, & Sinzger, 2000; Riegler et al., 2000; Sinzger, Grefte, Plachter, Gouw, & Jahn, 1995; Sinzger, Plachter, Grefte, & Jahn, 1996). In most instances, this simply presents as pneumonia, hepatitis, arteriosclerosis, or other forms of systemic infection. However, central nervous system (CNS) involvement is also possible. For adults, this is more commonly noted in populations with severe immune compromise such as those with AIDS. The most common features correspond with encephalitis, ventriculoencephalitis, retinitis, myelitis, and lumbosacral polyradiculopathy. In infants presenting with congenital CMV, features are more widespread and prominent, including seizures, cerebral atrophy, blindness, deafness, microcephaly, spasticity, and intracerebral calcifications (Bale, 1984). This occurs at an estimated rate of 0.4% to 2.4% (Larke et al., 1980; Stagno et al., 1977), with statistics suggesting CNS involvement in these infants ranging anywhere from 10% to 80% (Hanshaw, 1966; Hanshaw et al., 1985; Weller et al., 1957).

NEUROPATHOLOGY/PATHOPHYSIOLOGY

CMV, as with other variants of the herpes virus, is transmitted through bodily secretions (e.g., blood, saliva, semen, cervical secretions) in adults. In infants, transmission occurs either through breast milk or by infants coming in contact with cervical secretions.

When activated during immune compromise in adults, the virus may infiltrate various areas within the CNS. Basal ganglion and cerebellar regions as well as the brainstem (including the cranial nerves) are most prone to invasion as is the gray matter of the cortex and periventricular regions (Haymaker et al., 1954; Mediaris, 1957). Encephalitis associated with CMV presents with diffuse infiltration of these areas by microglial nodules and inclusion-bearing cytomegalic cells (Roos, 2007). In some instances, the spinal cord may also be involved as may be peripheral nerves (McCutchan, 1995). Retinitis, a common feature of CMV is linked with microhemorrhages, most commonly in the peripheral fundus, although they may involve the macula and optic disc in severe cases (Bale, 1984). Infants present with similar neuropathological features. However, in infants, microcephaly and hydrocephalus may present.

Polymicrogyria and cerebellar cortical dysplasia are neurological abnormalities also commonly associated with intrauterine transmission (Marie et al., 1957, Marques Dias et al., 1984).

NEUROPSYCHOLOGICAL/CLINICAL PRESENTATION

Congenital CMV may initially present with microcephaly or hydrocephalus at birth in symptomatic infants whereas others may be completely asymptomatic. Blindness is one of the most common features resulting from atrophy of the optic nerve in combination with the other previously reported ocular lesions. In comparison with CMV in adults, seizures are far more likely to occur in infants. Spasticity may also be seen in relation to basal ganglion involvement. In both adults and infants, paresis of the extremities, involving the legs more than the arms, can be seen. Sensory weakness may also be observed. In children, cerebral palsy may present (Bale, 1984).

When encephalitis manifests, neurocognitive functioning often becomes compromised. In many ways, it presents similar to a diffuse white matter dysfunction. Cognitive efficiency is impacted. Individuals may present with deficits in delayed recall more so than recognition. Sustained attention may demonstrate relative weakness as will processing speed and working memory.

Beyond functional aspects, CMV is related to a variety of systemic features. Multiple organs are vulnerable to the CMV. Adults and infants alike may manifest hepatitis, anemia, thrombocytopenia, and/or splenomegaly. Admittedly, these presentations are more common in infants compared with adults.

DIAGNOSIS

In many instances, individuals with CMV may go undiagnosed as few symptoms may actually present. Confirmation of the diagnosis is established through laboratory analysis of urine, blood, or cerebrospinal fluid (CSF). The particular marker of interest in the diagnosis of CMV is identification of seroconversion or a fourfold elevation increase in CMV antibody titers between the acute and convalescent sera (Roos, 2007). Diagnosis of CMS symptoms varies. MRI remains the gold standard approach for identifying neurological sequelae of the presentation. Subcortical foci predominates with diffuse intercerebral calcification often observed. Attention should also be given to periventricular regions. Furthermore, evaluation of the brainstem and spinal cord is best achieved through MRI. CSF analysis is commonly used to evaluate CMV DNA and lumbosacral polyradiculopathy. The former is essential in patients with a CMV-based neurological syndrome by way of the polymerase chain reaction technique (Holland et al., 1994; Kalayjian et al., 1993).

TREATMENT

In most instances, specific treatment for CMV is unwarranted as most individuals remain asymptomatic. For those who develop clinical features, treatment varies based on the nature of their presentation. Antiviral agents have proven effective in treating CMV. These have included ganciclovir, acyclovir, valganciclovir, and foscarnet. These are most commonly employed in individuals who have a suppressed immune system, such as those with HIV or AIDS. Infected mothers should avoid breast feeding.

When CNS involvement occurs, treatment is therapeutic and symptom based. If seizures manifest in infants, anticonvulsants should be used. The aforementioned antiviral agents are often standard treatment for retinitis as well as the lumbosacral polyradiculopathy. In comparison, encephalitis and ventriculoencephalitis tend to be less receptive to these agents (Berman & Kim, 1994; McCutchan, 1995)

Chad A. Noggle

Bale, J. F., Jr. (1984). Human cytomegalovirus infection and disorders of the nervous system. *Archives of Neurology,* 41, 310–320.

Berman, S. M., & Kim, R. C. (1994). The development of cytomegalovirus encephalitis in AIDS patients receiving ganciclovir. *American Journal of Medicine,* 96, 415–419.

Bissinger, A. L., Sinzger, C., Kaiserling, E., & Jahn, G. (2002). Human cytomegalovirus as a direct pathogen: Correlation of multiorgan involvement and cell distribution with clinical and pathological findings in a case of congenital inclusion disease. *Journal of Medical Virology,* 67(2), 200–206.

Hanshaw, J. B. (1966). Congenital and acquired cytomegalovirus infection. *Pediatric Clinics of North America,* 13, 279–293.

Hanshaw, J. B., Dudgeon, J. A., & Marshall, W. C. (1985). *Viral diseases of the fetus and newborn* (2nd ed.). Philadelphia, PA: W. B. Saunders.

Haymaker, W., Girdany, B. R., Stephens, J., Lillie, R. D., & Fetterman, G. H. (1954). Cerebral involvement with advanced periventricular calcification in generalised cytomegalic inclusion disease in the newborn. *Journal of Neuropathology and Experimental Neurology,* 13, 562–586.

Holland, N. R., Power, C., Matthews, V. P., Glass, J. D., Forman, M., & McArthur, J. C. (1994). Cytomegalovirus encephalitis in acquired immunodeficiency syndrome (AIDS). *Neurology, 44*, 507–514.

Kahl, M., Siegel-Axel, D., Stenglein, S., Jahn, G., & Sinzger, C. (2000). Efficient lytic infection of human arterial endothelial cells by human cytomegalovirus strains. *Journal of Virology, 74*(16), 7628–7635.

Kalayjian, R. C., Cohen, M. L., Bonomo, R. A., & Flanigan, T. P. (1993). Cytomegalovirus ventriculoencephalitis in AIDS: A syndrome with distinct clinical and pathologic features. *Medicine, 72*, 67–77.

Larke, R. P. B., Wheatley, E., Saroj, S., & Chernesky, M. (1980). Congenital cytomegalovirus infection in an urban Canadian community. *Journal of Infectious Diseases, 142*, 647–653.

Marie, J., See, G., Gruner, J., Hebert, S., De Gennes, J. L., & De Fouquet, J. (1957). Manifestations cerebrales de la maladie des inclusions cytomegaliques. *Annales de Pediatrie, 25*, 248–256.

Marques Dias, M. J., Harmant-van Rijckevorsel, G., Landrieu, P., & Lyon, G. (1984). Prenatal cytomegalovirus disease and cerebral microgyria: Evidence for perfusion failure, not disturbance of histogenesis, as the major cause of fetal cytomegalovirus encephalopathy. *Neuropediatrics, 15*, 18–24.

McCutchan, J. A. (1995). Cytomegalovirus infections of the nervous system in patients with AIDS. *Clinical Infectious Diseases, 20*, 747–754.

Mediaris, D. N., Jr. (1957). Cytomegalic inclusion disease. An analysis of the clinical features based on the literature and six additional cases. *Pediatrics, 19*, 466–480.

Riegler, S., Hebart, H., Einsele, H., Brossart, P., Jahn, G., & Sinzger, C. (2000). Monocyte-derived dendritic cells are permissive to the complete replicative cycle of human cytomegalovirus. *Journal of General Virology, 81*(Pt. 2), 393–399.

Roos, K. (2007). Viral infections. In C. G. Goetz (Ed.), *Textbook of clinical neurology* (3rd ed., pp. 920–942). Philadelphia, PA: Saunders Elsevier.

Sinzger, C., Grefte, A., Plachter, B., Gouw, A. S., The, T. H., & Jahn, G. (1995). Fibroblasts, epithelial cells, endothelial cells and smooth muscle cells are major targets of human cytomegalovirus infection in lung and gastrointestinal tissues. *Journal of General Virology, 76*(Pt. 4), 741–750.

Sinzger, C., Plachter, B., Grefte, A., The, T. H., & Jahn, G. (1996). Tissue macrophages are infected by human cytomegalovirus in vivo. *Journal of Infectious Diseases, 173*(1), 240–245.

Stagno, S., Reynolds, D. W., Huang, E. S., Thames, S. D., Smith, R. J., & Alford, C. A., Jr. (1977). Congenital cytomegalovirus infection: Occurrence in an immune population. *New England Journal of Medicine, 296*, 1254–1258.

Weller, T. H., Macauley, J. C., Craig, J. H., & Wirth, P. (1957). Isolation of intranuclear inclusion producing agents from infants with illnesses resembling cytomegalic inclusion disease. *Proceedings of the Society for Experimental Biology New York, 94*, 4–12.

C

Dandy-Walker Malformation/ Syndrome

DESCRIPTION

Dandy-Walker malformation (DWM) is a congenital brain malformation involving abnormal cerebellar development with cyst formation around the base of the skull. Specifically, DWM is a malformation of the paleocerebellum involving complete or partial agenesis of the cerebellar vermis, the cystic dilation of the fourth ventricle, and an enlarged posterior fossa with upward displacement of the tentorium. DWM was first described in 1914 by Dandy and Blackfan and later further detailed by Taggart and Walker in 1942 (Dandy & Blackfan, 1914; Taggart & Walker, 1942). Blenda ascribed the label "Dandy-Walker" in 1954.

There is some disagreement in the literature about the exact diagnostic criteria for DWM. There has also been suggestion of a possible more mild form of the disorder with less severe abnormalities (Barkovich, Kjos, Norman, & Edwards, 1989). Thus, some researchers choose to include similar cystic malformations — not just cysts isolated to posterior cranial fossa, in their definition (Boddaert et al., 2003).

Incidence ranges from 1 in 25,000 to 1 in 35,000 births (Hirsch, Pierre-Kahn, & Renier, 1984). Outcome varies from normal development to mental retardation, central nervous system (CNS) dysfunction, and death (Gerszten & Albright, 1995). Longevity is highly correlated with the severity of the syndrome and the presence of multiple congenital defects.

NEUROPATHOLOGY/PATHOPHYSIOLOGY

DWM is characterized by an enlarged posterior fossa; a large median posterior fossa cyst with dilation of the fourth ventricle; a small, rotated, and raised cerebellar vermis; anteriolaterally displaced tentorium; and normal cerebellar hemispheres with an intact brainstem. Atresia of the foramen of Magendie and the foramen of Luschka may also occur (Cakmak, Zeyrek, Cekin, & Karazeybek, 2008; Richter & Pincus, 2006).

NEUROPSYCHOLOGICAL/CLINICAL PRESENTATION

DWM can present unnoticed or have profound and obvious manifestations. Typically observed in early infancy, motor development is often slow with increased and progressive enlargement of the posterior portion of the skull due to buildup of cerebrospinal fluid. Thus, symptoms of hydrocephalus are common with poor muscle coordination, jerky saccades, unsteadiness, vomiting, possible convulsions, problems with the nerves that control the eyes, neck, and face, breathing difficulties, and changes in mood/ personality (e.g., irritability).

Neurocognitive abnormalities are present in many children with DWM, and mental retardation occurs in roughly half of patients (Hirsch, Pierre-Kahn, Renier, Sainte-Rose, & Hoppe-Hirsch, 1984). According to Boddaert et al. (2003), normal lobulation of the cerebellar vermis in the absence of any supratentorial abnormalities, as evident on MRI, may be a good prognosticator of good intellectual development in DWM. Poor sensory development (hearing or vision), CNS disruption, and seizure activity have been shown to be associated with poorer intellectual prognosis (Bindal, Storrs, & McLone, 1990).

A number of conditions have been suggested to be associated with DWM including, but not limited to, PHACE (an association of symptoms including Posterior fossa malformations, Hemangiomas, Arterial abnormalities, Cardiovascular abnormalities, and Eye anomalies), Klippel-Feil syndrome (congenital fusion of cervical vertebrae), and Down's syndrome (Friden, Resse, & Cohen, 1996). In fact, DWM is often associated with CNS anomalies, extra-CNS abnormalities, and chromosomal irregularities. Agenesis of the corpus callosum and malformation of the heart, face, limbs, fingers, and toes may also occur. Also noted in the literature are interhemispheric cysts, gyral abnormalities, meningoceles, gray matter heterotopias, cardiovascular malformations (e.g., ventricular septal defects), facial malformation (e.g., cleft palate), malformed limbs, and intestinal and urogenital abnormalities (Poetke, Bultmann, & Berlien, 2000).

D

DIAGNOSIS

DWM is diagnosed via MRI with the use of T2-weighted images (Klein, Pierre-Kahn, Boddaert, Parisot, & Brunelle, 2003). Prenatal sonography is also used to detect DWM. Differential diagnosis can be challenging as almost any condition resulting in infracerebellar fluid collection can elevate the cerebellar vermis, open the foramen of magendie, and shift the cerebellar tonsils. Thus, according to Klein and colleagues (2003), careful neuroimaging, a strict diagnostic classification system, and prenatal evaluation are critical toward accurate diagnosis.

TREATMENT

Treatment for DWM consists of symptom management that usually involves placement of a shunt to drain cerebrospinal fluid, reduce pressure, and control swelling. As DWM is a sporadic genetic syndrome, genetic counseling for families intending to have additional children may be helpful. In addition, neuropsychological assessment may prove beneficial in identifying a pattern of strengths and weaknesses that can serve as avenues for intervention.

Jeremy Hertza
Andrew S. Davis

Barkovich, A., Kjos, B., Norman, D., & Edwards, M. (1989). Revised classification of posterior fossa cysts and cystlike malformations based on the results of multiplanar MR imaging. *American Journal of Roentgenology, 153,* 1289–1300.

Bindal, A., Storrs, B., & McLone, D. (1990). Management of the Dandy Walker syndrome. *Pediatric Neurosurgery, 16.*

Blenda, C. (1954). The Dandy-Walker syndrome or the so-called atresia of the foramen of Magendie. *Journal of Neuropathology and Experimental Neurology, 13.*

Boddaert, N., Klein, O., Ferguson, N., Sonigo, P., Parisot, D., Hertz-Pannier, L., et al. (2003). Intellectual prognosis of the Dandy-Walker malformation in children: The importance of vermian lobulation. *Neuroradiology, 45.*

Cakmak, A., Zeyrek, D., Cekin, A., & Karazeybek, H. (2008). Dandy-Walker syndrome together with occipital encephalocele. *Minerva Pediatrics, 60*(4), 465–468.

Dandy, W., & Blackfan, K. (1914). Internal hydrocephalus, and experimental clinical and pathological study. *American Journal of Diseases in Children, 8,* 406–482.

Friden, I., Resse, V., & Cohen, D. (1996). Phace syndrome. *Archives of Dermatology, 132.*

Gerszten, P., & Albright, A. (1995). Relationship between cerebellar appearance and function in children with Dandy-Walker variant. *Pediatric Neurosurgery, 23.*

Hirsch, J. F., Pierre-Kahn, A., & Renier, D. (1984). The Dandy-Walker syndrome and associated abnormalities. *Pediatric Neuroscience, 13.*

Hirsch, J., Pierre-Kahn, A., Renier, D., Sainte-Rose, C., & Hoppe-Hirsch, E. (1984). The Dandy-Walker malformation: A review of 40 cases. *Journal of Neurosurgery, 61.*

Klein, O., Pierre-Kahn, A., Boddaert, N., Parisot, D., & Brunelle, F. (2003). Dandy-Walker malformation: Prenatal diagnosis and prognosis. *Child Nervous System, 19.*

Poetke, M., Bultmann, O., & Berlien, H. (2000). Association of large facial hemangiomas with Dandy-Walker syndrome. Case study concerning three infants. *European Journal of Pediatric Surgery, 10.*

Richter, E. O., & Pincus, D. W. (2006). Development of syringohydromyelia associated with Dandy-Walker malformation: Treatment with cystoperitoneal shunt placement. A case report. *Journal of Neurosurgery, 104*(Suppl. 3), 206–209.

Taggart, J., & Walker, A. (1942). Congential atresia of the foramens of Luschka and Magendie. *Archives of Neurology, 48.*

DAWSON'S DISEASE

DESCRIPTION

Dawson's disease, also called subacute sclerosing panencephalitis, is a rare demyelinating disease of the central nervous system. Specifically, it is a slow-acting viral infection that results in a chronic neurological disease that is caused by a defective measles virus (Jubelt, 2005). It is primarily a disease of childhood and is characterized by cognitive and motor dysfunction. These difficulties may be due to brain inflammation and nerve cell death. Typically, the progression is a downhill course that ultimately results in death within a few years. Since the widespread use of the measles vaccine, this disease has become very rare; however, areas of the world that do not have access to the vaccine have higher rates of incidence (Ropper & Brown, 2005). It has been reported to occur more frequently in Caucasian children from rural areas, specifically those in the southeastern United States, although approximately only five cases are reported every year (Maria & Bale, 2006). It is believed that the disease is caused by wild-type measles rather than the strand of measles that is vaccinated for (Maria & Bale, 2006).

Dawson's disease is much more common in rural areas, with an average age of onset around 10 (Maria & Bale, 2006). In general, boys are more likely affected than girls at a ratio of about 5:3 (Maria & Bale, 2006). Those children who contract the measles virus at a young age, prior to 1 year, are at a greater risk to contract the wild-type measles that causes Dawson's disease (Maria & Bale, 2006). The prognosis for Dawson's disease is poor, and death is likely to occur as early as 6 months after the onset of symptoms; however, individuals have been known to survive up to 5 years after the age of onset (Wolinsky & McArthur, 2000).

NEUROPATHOLOGY/PATHOPHYSIOLOGY

In Dawson's disease, lesions generally appear in the hippocampus, cerebral cortex, cerebellar cortex, thalamus, and brainstem (Roos & Tyler, 2008). In the cerebral cortex, cell loss occurs due to swelling (Roos & Tyler, 2008). There may be inclusions that may be large but occur less frequently, or they may be smaller and occur more frequently (Roos & Tyler, 2008). In chronic cases, demyelinization is more evident (Roos & Tyler, 2008). In the early stages, Dawson's disease primarily affects the occipital areas, spreading to the brainstem and spinal cord (Roos & Tyler, 2008). As the disease progresses, the damage can be seen on a larger scale in multiple areas throughout the brain (Roos & Tyler, 2008).

NEUROPSYCHOLOGICAL/CLINICAL PRESENTATION

Some of the first symptoms include personality change and a slow deterioration of intellect including problems with reading, writing, and processing (Maria & Bale, 2006). Parents may notice a change in behavior and school performance (Maria & Bale, 2006). Seizures, which may develop within the first 2–3 months, are characterized by myoclonic jerks of the head, trunk, and limbs (Maria & Bale, 2006). The seizures do not appear to interfere with consciousness; however, they may cause or contribute to falling episodes (Maria & Bale, 2006). In general the seizures are exacerbated by excitement and do not occur during sleep (Maria & Bale, 2006). In addition to seizures, spontaneous speech and movements decrease though comprehension does not appear to be affected (Maria & Bale, 2006). Other symptoms may include hallucinations, a decrease in ability to perform voluntary movements (i.e., apraxia), difficulty recognizing objects (i.e., agnosia), and dementia (Fallon, 2005). As the illness progresses, the inability to control bodily movements (i.e., extrapyramidal dyskinesia) and body spasms (i.e., spasticity) become more prominent (Fallon, 2005). In addition, swallowing difficulties may develop (i.e., dysphagia). Vision loss will also begin to develop at this stage, specifically cortical blindness (Wolinsky & McArthur, 2000). On rare occasions, optic atrophy has been reported (Wolinsky & McArthur, 2000). In the terminal stages of Dawson's disease, breathing becomes irregular and strenuous (Wolinsky & McArthur, 2000). The individual may become gradually more unresponsive and rigid. Instability, hyperthermia, profuse sweating, and disturbances of blood pressure and pulse have also been noted (Fallon, 2005).

The course of the disease is characterized by a slow deterioration with short periods of remission (Ropper & Brown, 2005). The disease on average has duration of 12 months, generally resulting in death (Ropper & Brown, 2005). Rare cases have been reported of individuals who lived 20 or more years after the onset of symptoms and remission periods lasting up to 25 years (Ropper & Brown, 2005).

DIAGNOSIS

Initial diagnosis may include blood tests, specifically to look for the measles antibody. An electroencephalogram may be used to show an abnormality consisting of periodic bursts of high-voltage waves, followed by a flat pattern in brain activity (Ropper & Brown, 2005). An electrocardiogram, a test that measures the electrical currents through the heart muscle, may be used in order to determine whether normal rhythm is present (Ropper & Brown, 2005). Examination of the cerebrospinal fluid reveals few to no cells, but protein levels are increased (Maria & Bale, 2006). MRI examinations show abnormal signals in the subcortical white matter that reflects the inflammation caused by the disease (Maria & Bale, 2006). Positron emission tomography (PET) has been used to study Dawson's disease, demonstrating inflammation in the basal ganglia that appears to lead to excitation of neuronal activity followed by hypermetabolism (Maria & Bale, 2006). PET and single photon emission computed tomography (SPECT) studies may reveal early subcortical hypermetabolism (Maria & Bale, 2006). Dawson's disease should be differentiated from progressive rubella panencephalitis and other degenerations of white matter (Maria & Bale, 2006).

TREATMENT

Treatment typically is given in order to reduce the discomfort of symptoms; however, there is no cure for the disease at present (Maria & Bale, 2006). Anticonvulsant medications can reduce symptoms such as seizures, and some other medications such as ribavirin, interferon beta, interferon alpha, and inosine pranobex can be used in order to stabilize or delay the progression of Dawson's disease (Maria & Bale, 2006).

Significant efficacy has not been reported for any of these medications. The most common form of treatment is supportive therapy including tube feedings and nursing care when necessary (Maria & Bale, 2006).

Danielle S. Dance
Charles Golden

Fallon, B. A. (2005). Neuropsychiatric aspects of other infectious diseases. In B. J. Sadock & V. A. Sadock (Eds.), *Kaplan & Sadock's comprehensive textbook of psychiatry*. Philadelphia: Lippincott Williams & Wilkins.

Jubelt, B. (2005). Viral infections. In L. P. Rowland (Ed.), *Merritt's neurology*. Philadelphia: Lippincott Williams & Wilkins.

Maria, B. L., & Bale, J. F. (2006). Infections of the nervous system. In J. H. Menkes, H. B. Sarnat, & B. L. Maria (Eds.), *Child neurology*. Philadelphia: Lippincott Williams & Wilkins.

Roos, K. L., & Tyler, K. L. (2008). Meningitis, encephalitis, brain abscess and empyema. In A. S. Fauci, D. L. Kasper, D. L. Longo, E. Braunwald, S. L. Hauser, J. L. Jameson, et al. (Eds.), *Harrison's principles of internal medicine*. McGraw-Hill.

Ropper, A. H., & Brown, R. H. (2005). In *Adams & victors' principles of neurology. McGraw-Hill*.

Wolinsky, J. S., & Mcarthur, J. C. (2000). Slow virus infections in the nervous system, including AIDS. In H. D. Humes et al. (Eds.), *Kelley's textbook of internal medicine*. Philadelphia: Lippincott Williams & Wilkins.

DE MORSIER'S SYNDROME

DESCRIPTION

Also known as septo-optic dysplasia (SOD), septo-optic-pituitary dysplasia, and optic nerve hypoplasia (ONH), de Morsier's syndrome is a rare congenital condition characterized by a heterogeneous cluster of developmental abnormalities involving ONH, hypothalamic-pituitary dysfunction, and agenesis of the septum pellucidum (the membrane separating the anterior horn of the left and right lateral ventricles). Clinical presentation varies significantly. While incidence of de Morsier's syndrome is not currently available, it has been estimated to be no more than $1:10^6$ (Humphreys, 2007).

NEUROPATHOLOGY/PATHOPHYSIOLOGY

Etiology is unknown. In most cases, de Morsier's syndrome occurs as a sporadic birth defect and subsequent pregnancies are not associated with higher risk of developing the disorder. However, on rare occasions, de Morsier's syndrome has been linked to genetic mutation of *HESX1* (Cohen et al., 2003). Familial occurrences are extremely rare but have been reported (Benner, Preslan, Gratz, Joslyn, & Kelman, 1990; Wales & Quarrell, 1996). While de Morsier's syndrome has not been linked to low birth weight, it has been associated with young maternal age and first pregnancy. Maternal alcohol and therapeutic and recreational drug use have also been linked with de Morsier's syndrome, although this association has been disputed (Murray, Patterson, & Donaldson, 2005).

Most cases of de Morsier's syndrome are believed to be caused by an in utero infection or other insult to the forebrain during the very early stage of embryogenesis, between the 4th and 8th week of gestation. During this period, the telencephalic optic vesicles and retinal ganglion cells differentiate. An insult can produce failure of ganglion cell formation with subsequent hypoplasia of optic nerves and chiasm. During this period, the lamina terminalis also thickens and an infection of insult can result in malformation of the anterior commissure. Between the 5th and 6th week of gestation, the development of the pituitary gland occurs; therefore, an infection or insult during this period may result in malformation of the pituitary gland (Humphreys, 2007).

Due to the underdevelopment of the optic nerve, visual impairment is often present, although the severity ranges from mild visual impairment in one eye to complete blindness. Visual impairments may also include amblyopia, nystagmus, hemianopia, and visual field defects in varying degrees of severity (Siatkowski, Sanchez, Andrade, & Alvarez, 1997).

Due to the variety of clinical presentations, Barkovich (2005) postulated three variations of the disorder. The first variation is thought to be associated with malformations of cortical development, particularly schizencephaly and gray matter heterotopia. A second variation is characterized by absence of the septum pellucidum, hypoplasia of the white matter, but normal cortex. This variation is thought to be a mild form of holoprosencephaly as the abnormalities form in the same developmental stage. The third variation is characterized by pituitary abnormalities and hormonal problems. Pituitary abnormalities are not uniform and range from a deficit in one pituitary hormone to panhypopituitarism in which all pituitary hormones are deficit (Barkovich, 2005). The combination of a well-developed posterior pituitary with deficit anterior pituitary or well-developed anterior pituitary with deficit posterior pituitary can occur. Additionally, the expression of hormone deficiency varies depending upon the hormone that is at lower than normal levels. In addition to growth hormone deficiency, common problems include adrenal insufficiency, hypothyroidism, and disturbance in antidiuretic hormone production. Access hormone production has also been reported (Margalith, Jan, McCormick, Tze, & Lapointe, 1984; Polizzi, Pavone, Iannetti, Manfre, & Ruggieri, 2006).

NEUROPSYCHOLOGICAL/CLINICAL PRESENTATION

Seventy-five to eighty percent of cases diagnosed with de Morsier's syndrome demonstrate ONH with approximately 12% of the cases having unilateral ONH and 88% having bilateral ONH. In addition to visual impairments, cognitive problems are often present. Incidence of developmental delay among children with de Morsier's syndrome has been reported to be 39% in children with unilateral ONH and 78% in children with bilateral ONH (Margalith et al., 1984). Cognitive problems range from mild learning disabilities to mental retardation. However, due to the low incidence of the disorder and the wide variety of neuroanatomical and functional deficits that may be present in each patient, a specific cognitive profile associated with de Morsier's syndrome has not been identified. In a clinical sample of patients diagnosed with de Morsier's syndrome, 27% of patients did not present with cognitive or psychiatric impairments (Margalith et al., 1984).

While agenesis of the septum pellucidum at younger than 3 years of age was not associated with higher risk of later delay, both corpus callosum hypoplasia and hypothyroidism were associated with higher risk of delayed language and motor skills at age 5. However, children with ONH, without neuroradiological and endocrinological abnormalities, were also found to demonstrate developmental delays (Garcia-Filion et al., 2008). However, normal cognitive and language development has been reported among children with milder symptom presentation although performance on visual motor tasks and visual attention problems are common problems impacted by visual acuity difficulties (Williams et al., 1993).

In children with severe symptom presentation, including severe bilateral ONH resulting in blindness, high incidence of cognitive and behavioral problems is evident. In younger children, severe tantrums and mood swings are common while sluggish tempo and narrow range of interests subsequently emerge. In addition, empirical research demonstrated 69% of children in a clinical sample had been diagnosed with an autism spectrum disorder and 38% had been diagnosed with mental retardation (Ulla, Fernell, & Jacobson, 2007).

In clinical samples, about two-thirds of patients with bilateral ONH also experience visual impairments and endocrine abnormalities. These abnormalities can lead to precocious puberty or hypogonadism. Neurological symptoms including seizures and hemiparesis are also associated with the cluster of neurological abnormalities (Margalith et al., 1984; Skarf & Hoyt, 1984).

Although research has not been conclusive, it has been suggested that clinical presentation of endocrine dysfunction can be predicted by abnormalities of the septum pellucidum and hypothalamic-pituitary axis evident on neuroimaging. The severity of neuroimaging findings may predict the most common endocrinological symptom, growth hormone deficiency, as well as deficiencies of thyroid-stimulating hormone (TSH) and adrenocorticotropic hormone (ACTH) (Humphries, 2007; Siatkowski et al., 1997).

DIAGNOSIS

A diagnosis of de Morsier's syndrome is usually made if two or more of the hallmark features including ONH, midline brain defects, and/or hypopituitarism are present. Approximately 62% of patients diagnosed with de Morsier's syndrome have hypopituitarism and 60% of patients diagnosed with de Morsier's syndrome have an absent septum pellucidum. Furthermore, roughly 30% of patients diagnosed with de Morsier's syndrome have all three hallmark features (Morishima & Aranoff, 1986).

In general, patients present with varying levels of pituitary hormone deficiencies and visual impairments. These symptoms may or may not be present in conjunction with mental retardation. Usually, the first presenting feature is optic nerve dysplasia, with later onset of endocrine dysfunction; however, because clinical presentation varies significantly, this has been difficult to determine (Humphreys, 2008). Suspicion of de Morsier's syndrome may not occur until direct ophthalmoscopy of optic nerve abnormalities reveals abnormal development in combination with functional impairment. In severe cases, hypopituitarism causes severe jaundice (characterized by conjugated hyperbilirubinemia), hypoglycemia, and mircopenis (in males), and can be diagnosed within days of birth. However, many times endocrine problems do not become apparent until the child is not making age-expected gains in height and weight. MRI of the brain is typically conducted after other symptoms of de Morsier's syndrome become evident (Margalith et al., 1984).

TREATMENT

There is no known cure for de Morsier's syndrome. Furthermore, there is no known treatment to stimulate optic nerve growth or function. As such, strategies to compensate for visual impairments are learned. Parents are often advised to see an endocrinologist to test hormonal levels and to monitor their child's height and weight even if hormone levels are reported to be adequate due to the delayed onset of this symptom. Pituitary deficiencies are often effectively treated with hormone replacement therapy.

Jessica Garcia
Charles Golden

Barkovich, A. J. (2005). Congenital malformations of the brain and skull. In A. J. Barkovich (Ed.), *Pediatric neuroimaging* (4th ed., pp. 291–439). Philadelphia: Lippincott, Williams, & Wilkins.

Benner, J. D., Preslan, M. W., Gratz, E., Joslyn J. S., & Kelman, S. (1990). *American Journal of Ophthalmology, 109,* 632–637.

Cohen, R. N., Cohen, L. E., Botero, D., Yu, C., Sagar, A., Jurkiewicz, M., & Radovick, S. (2003). Enhanced repression of HESX1 as a cause of hypopituitarism and septo-optic dysplasia. *Journal of Clinical Endocrinology & Metabolism, 88,* 4832–4839.

Garcia-Filion, P., Epport, K., Nelson, M., Azen, C., Geffner, M. E., Fink, C., et al. (2008). Neuroradiographic, endocrinologic, and ophthalmic correlates of adverse developmental outcomes in children with optic nerve hypoplasia: A prospective study. *Pediatrics, 121,* 653–659.

Humphreys, P. (2007). Septo-optic-pituitary dysplasia. In H. B. Sarnat & Paolo Curtolo (Eds.), *Malformations of the nervous system: Vol. 87. Handbook of clinical neurology.* Amsterdam: Elsevier.

Margalith, D., Jan, J. E., McCormick, A. Q., Tze, W. J., & Lapointe, J. (1984). Clinical spectrum of congenital optic nerve hypoplasia: Review of 51 patients. *Developmental Medicine and Child Neurology, 26,* 311–322.

Morishima, A., & Aranoff, G. S. (1986). Syndrome of septo-optic-pituitary dysplasia: The clinical spectrum. *Brain and Development, 70,* 51–53.

Murray, P. G., Patterson, W. F., & Donaldson, M. D. (2005). Maternal age in patients with septo-optic dysplasia. *Journal of Pediatric Endocrinology and Metabolism,* 471–476.

Polizzi, A., Pavone, P. Iannetti, P., Manfre, L., & Ruggieri, M. (2006). Septo-optic dysplasia complex: A heterogeneous malformation syndrome. *Pediatric Neurology, 34,* 66–71.

Saitkowski, R. M., Sanchez, J. C., Andrade, R., & Alvarez, A. (1997). The clinical neuroradiographic and endocrinologic profile of patients with bilateral optic nerve hypoplasia. *Opthalomology, 104,* 493–496.

Skarf, B., & Hoyt, C. S. (1984). Optic nerve hypoplasia in children. Association with anomalies of the endocrine and CNS. *Archives of Ophthalmology, 102,* 62–67.

Ulla, E., Fernell, E., & Jacobson, L. (2004). Cognitive and Behavioural characteristics in blind children with bilateral optic nerve hypoplasia. *Acta Paediatrica, 94,* 1421–1426.

Wales, J. K., & Quarrell, O. W. (1996). Evidence for possible Medelian inheritance of septo-optic dysplasia. *Acta Paediatrica, 85,* 391–392.

Williams, J., Brodsky, M. C., Griebel, M., Glasier, C. M., Caldwell, D., & Thomas, P. (1993). Septo-optic dysplasia: The clinical insignificance of an absent septum pellucidum. *Developmental Medicine and Child Neurology, 35,* 490–501.

DEJERINE–KLUMPKE PALSY

DESCRIPTION

Dejerine–Klumpke palsy (also called Klumpke palsy) was first described in 1885 by Augusta Dejerine–Klumpke as a paralysis of the wrist(s) and hand(s) in infants after birth (Shoja & Tubbs, 2007). She described a disorder involving paralysis of the lower roots of the brachial plexus while noting the role of the sympathetic fibers in this paralysis (Kay, 1998). Neurologists began to explore her discovery further and modern medicine now asserts that lesions to the eighth-cervical (C-8) or first-thoracic (T-1) regions of the spine are responsible for the symptoms of Klumpke palsy (Kay, 1998). This type of brachial plexus palsy is distinguished from other types because only the hand or wrist muscles are paralyzed (Nelson & Tilbor, 1995).

Although Klumpke palsy was much more evident when first observed, it is the least common of the brachial plexus palsies with less than 1 in 1,000 cases reported in the United States each year (Nelson & Tilbor, 1995). This decline is attributed to the vast improvements in modern obstetrics and the rapid decline in the number of breech births (Jennett, Tarby, & Krauss, 2002). There are several modern theories as to how and why lesions to the lower roots of the brachial plexus occur (Kay, 1998). The most widely supported theory is that the lesion or break is caused during birth; however, some neurologists believe that these lesions may be caused during intrauterine life due to the posture and position of the fetus (Kay,

1998). The latter cause is very rare and, thus, is not a widely accepted cause of the disorder (Kay, 1998).

NEUROPATHOLOGY/PATHOPHYSIOLOGY

During childbirth, it is believed that abduction and elevation of the fetal arm and shoulder cause the C-8 and T-1 areas of the spine to stretch and break when force is applied (Jennett et al., 2002). Other, less common reasons for these lesions are compression or traction during birth or an infection or ischemia (Kay, 1998).

There are a number of risk factors and associated medical problems, which make Klumpke palsy more likely to occur. One of the most common risk factors is large birth weight; infants who suffer from Klumpke palsy are much more likely to be over 4,500 grams (Gherman, Ouzounian, Satin, Goodwin, & Phelan, 2003). Other common risk factors include multiparity, more than one birth at a time (Nelson & Tilbor, 1995), and complications during birth, most commonly breech births (Kay, 1998). Other associated disorders and possible risk factors are shoulder dystocia (Gherman et al., 2003) and a fractured clavicle, humerus, or skull (Kay, 1998). Horner syndrome is also associated with Klumpke palsy (Shoja & Tobbs, 2007).

Even though physicians are aware of the possible causes of Klumpke, unfortunately there are no methods for prevention (Kay, 1998). Lesions to the lower roots of the brachial plexus can still occur during a cesarean section, though this is uncommon (Kay, 1998). Although there may not be good prevention techniques, most cases of Klumpke palsy are transient (Gherman et al., 2003; Jannett et al., 2002). The majority of infants with this disorder will spontaneously recover before 1 year of age (Jannett et al., 2002; Kay, 1998). However, research has shown that if the disorder does not spontaneously remit by this time, it will most likely be permanent (Gherman et al., 2003; Jennett et al., 2002).

Klumpke palsy can also occur in adults though much rarer (Jennett et al., 2002). The most common cause of this disorder in adults is trauma to the shoulder and lower area of the brachial plexus (Jennett et al., 2002). Falls in which the shoulder is depressed and improper positioning during surgery are two examples of possible traumas (Jennett et al., 2002). Injuries during sports and traffic accidents are also causes of Klumpke palsy in adults (Jennett et al., 2002). These traumas cause paralysis when the arm is posteriorly forced causing traction on the lower roots (Jennett et al., 2002). Most research on Klumpke palsy, however, focuses on newborns.

NEUROPSYCHOLOGICAL/CLINICAL PRESENTATION

Even in cases with spontaneous recovery, motor function loss can persist (Strombeck, Remahl, Krumlinde-Sundhom, & Sejersen, 2007). Enduring loss of sensory function can also occur although the impairment is less severe than lasting motor impairment (Strombeck et al., 2007). These sensory problems are especially evident in discrimination between hot and cold sensations (Strombeck et al., 2007). Also in infants with Klumpke palsy, as opposed to other types of brachial palsies, peripheral plasticity does not occur, increasing the likelihood of lasting impairments (Strombeck et al., 2007). These preserving impairments have been noted to cause decreases in self-esteem in children who were born with Klumpke palsy (Strombeck & Fernell, 2003). Many of these children reported having strong fears that something will happen to them or they will have problems with affected or unaffected arms (Strombeck & Fernell, 2003). Although Klumpke palsy is generally thought of as an infantile disorder, it can have lasting effects — sensory-motor and emotional — that can persist even when the affected arm has "recovered" (Strombeck & Fernell, 2003).

DIAGNOSIS

The three most employed methods for diagnosis are physical, electrodiagnostic, and radiographic exams (Nelson & Tilbor, 1995), conducted 48 hours postpartum (Kay, 1998). Initially, an X ray of the humerus and clavicle bones will be done to rule out fractures in these areas as possible causes (Nelson & Tilbor, 1995). Electrodiagnostic measures, such as nerve conduction studies of motor and sensory neurons, are performed (Nelson & Tilbor, 1995). Somatosensory evoked potentials are less frequently used but have been found to be helpful in refining clinical evaluations (Kay, 1998; Nelson & Tilbor, 1995). Myelography procedures are more commonly done on adults; however, significant false positives have been obtained using this method (Kay, 1998).

Physical exams involve a neurologist observing spontaneous use and positioning of the insensate hand or wrist in order to determine which parts are not being moved actively and whether the infant's passive range of motion is equal on both sides (Kay, 1998; Nelson & Tilbor, 1995). The infant's primitive reflexes are also tested (Nelson & Tilbor, 1995). Commonly positive/negative stimulus tests are used (Nelson & Tilbor, 1995). For example, the infant may be offered candy or another pleasing stimulus while

D

D

the nonaffected arm is restrained so that the child must reach for the stimulus with the inflicted hand (Nelson & Tilbor, 1995). The child's subsequent behavior is observed (Nelson & Tilbor, 1995). The child is also examined for Horner syndrome, which is often comorbid with Klumpke and affects the T-1 area as well (Kay, 1998). The complication of Horner syndrome is often indicative of a poorer prognosis (Kay, 1998). The infant's other limbs are also examined in order to rule out neonatal tetraplegia and hemiparesis (Kay, 1998).

TREATMENT

Although most cases remit spontaneously, the full recovery rate has been found to be anywhere between 12.9% and 80% (Kay, 1998). Thus, physicians recommend occupational or physiotherapy in order to increase the likelihood of full recovery of the wrist and hand (Kay, 1998; Nelson & Tilbor, 1995). In occupational therapy, range of motion exercises and maximum positioning of the hand and wrist are used in order to maintain the mobility of the joints and avoid contractures (Nelson & Tilbor, 1995). For Klumpke palsy, the emphasis of these exercises is on the wrist and fingers with elbow extensions being included (Nelson & Tilbor, 1995). The goal of therapy is to stimulate and increase awareness of the affected areas (Nelson & Tilbor, 1995). This can be done by attaching bells or toys to a bracelet attached to the affected wrist in order to attract the infant's attention and encourage its use (Nelson & Tilbor, 1995).

Splinting may be used if there is a severe wrist drop (Nelson & Tilbor, 1995). In the past, this method was used much more commonly; however, research has shown that it may actually delay recovery (Kay, 1998). If previously mentioned methods fail, another technique used is nerve repair (Kay, 1998). The earlier this method is employed, the better the infant's chance of recovery. However, some studies have found that nerve repair done as late as 12–24 months can still be helpful (Kay, 1998).

After trying less invasive methods, if the infant has not recovered between 4 and 9 months of age, the option of surgery is explored (Nelson & Tilbor, 1995). More recent research has supported waiting until closer to 9 months of age, as the rate of spontaneous remission is high (Kay, 1998). The abilities of the affected area are measured before the surgery and again after recovery from the surgery (Kay, 1998). Surgery is more likely to be considered earlier in the child's life if Horner syndrome is also present, as this syndrome indicates a poorer prognosis (Kay, 1998). During surgery, electrodiagnostic studies are used as well as neurolysis

(removal of scar tissue) (Nelson & Telbor, 1995). In some cases, a nerve graft may be done (Nelson & Telbor, 1995). Improvement has been noted in cases 6 months after the surgery up to 2 years later; however, if the problem sustains in children over 3 years of age, a tendon and muscle transfer may be done, mostly in the wrist (Nelson & Tilbor, 1995). Although Klumpke palsy can result in pervasive paralysis of the hand and wrist, modern obstetrics and therapy methods have drastically reduced this risk.

Sarah E. West
Charles Golden

Gherman, R. B., Ouzounian, J. G., Satin, A. J., Goodwin, T. M., & Phelan, J. P. (2003). A comparison of shoulder dystocia-associated transient and permanent brachial plexus palsies. *The American College of Obstetricians and Gynecologists, 102,* 544–548.

Jennett, R. J., Tarby, T. J., & Krauss, R. L. (2002). Erb's palsy contrasted with Klumpke's and total palsy: Different mechanisms are involved. *American Journal of Obstetrics and Gynecology, 186,* 1216–1220.

Kay, S. P. J. (1998). Obstetrical brachial palsy. *British Journal of Plastic Surgery, 51,* 43–50.

Nelson, M. R., & Tilbor, A. G. (1995). Birth brachial plexus injury. *The Western Journal of Medicine, 162,* 154.

Shoja, M. M., & Tubbs, R. S. (2007). Augusta Dejerine-Klumpke: The first female neuroanatomist. *Clinical Anatomy, 20,* 585–587.

Strombeck, C., & Fernell, E. (2003). Aspects of activities and participation in daily life related to body structure and function in adolescents with obstetrical brachial plexus palsy: A descriptive follow-up study. *Acta Paediatrica, 92,* 740–746.

Strombeck, C., Remahl, S., Krumlinde-Sundholm, L. K., & Sejersen, T. (2007). Long-term follow-up of children with obstetric brachial plexus palsy II: Neurophysiological aspect. *Developmental Medicine & Child Neurology, 49,* 204–209.

DELIRIUM

DESCRIPTION

Delirium is an acute cerebral state characterized by disturbed consciousness and cognitive dysfunction, including attention and perception. Furthermore, the disorder can affect sleep, psychomotor activity, and emotions. It is important to note that delirium is not categorized as a disease or disorder but rather a manifestation of an array of potential causes that result in a constellation of symptoms. Clinical features typically include decreased attention span and a waxing and waning type of confusion. Delirium is transient and improves quickly with treatment, once precipitating factors have been identified and corrected (Fricchione, Nejad, Esses, & Cummings, 2008), though it is often either misdiagnosed or not diagnosed at all. The main risk factors for developing delirium are old age, cognitive impairment, and other comorbidities. The word *delirium* comes from the Latin word *delirare*, which means "to be out of one's furrow" (Gupta, de Jonghe, Schieveld, Leonard, & Meagher, 2008).

NEUROPATHOLOGY/PATHOPHYSIOLOGY

Little is known about the cause of delirium because the pathophysiology is associated with a wide variety of causal factors, though age does seem to be related, as it is more common among the elderly. Though delirium has some core clinical features, there are a very wide range of precipitating factors, including acute illness, surgery, trauma, and drugs (Sozia et al., 2008). It is considered to be a common acute neuropsychiatric syndrome affecting between 10% and 41% of older medical patients (Siddiqi, House, & Holmes, 2006).

Neuroimaging research for delirium is in its early stages. Because of the practical difficulties and ethical concerns, studies involving serial imaging before, during, and/or after episodes of delirium are scarce. A meta-analysis done by Sozia et al. (2008) of 12 studies yielded consistent findings of an association between delirium and cortical atrophy. The results indicate there is an association between ventricular enlargement and increased white matter lesions. High levels of serum anticholinergic activity, metabolic and structural brain abnormalities, along with decreased acetylcholine activity, may influence the severity of symptoms. Furthermore, acetylcholine insufficiency may lead to disorientation, hallucinations, and memory impairment. Although these findings suggest abnormalities in the brain may play a role in delirium, the data do not necessarily imply a causal relationship in the etiology of delirium (Siddiqi et al., 2006). Hippocampal neurons are affected in the early stages, followed by neurons of the subcortex, brainstem, gray matter, and cerebellum in later stages. Delirium is also known as acute brain syndrome, metabolic encephalopathy, toxic psychosis, and acute brain failure.

NEUROPSYCHOLOGICAL/CLINICAL PRESENTATION

Delirium affects a broad range of functions, including motor behavior, the sleep wake cycle, perception, cognitive thinking, and affective expression. Motor disturbances range from hyperactive to hypoactive, often presented as being agitated and hyperalert to becoming lethargic and hypoalert (America Psychiatric Association, 1999; Gupta et al., 2008). In terms of the sleep wake cycle, disturbances range from unusual daytime napping to severe disruption of night sleep (American Psychiatric Association [APA], 1999; Gupta et al., 2008), and often there is a complete reversal of the night day sleep wake cycle. Disorientation to time, place, and identity of others is not uncommon, but these types of symptoms tend to fluctuate or wax and wane. Cognitive domains affected include attention, alertness, vigilance, and comprehension. Attention is impaired in all aspects, as delirium interferes with the ability to sustain, focus, or shift attention. In fact, inattention is one of the consistent features that is crucial for diagnosis. Short- and long-term memory, orientation, comprehension, and vigilance are impaired, as well as processes related to executive functioning and visuospatial abilities. Speech and language disturbances may present as incoherent semantic content, dysnomia, and paraphasia. All of these symptoms are often taken into account in a clinical setting to help clarify an appropriate diagnosis.

The manifestations of psychotic features complicate approximately 50% of delirium cases. Visual hallucinations are common and delusional content may involve having feelings of imminent danger or feelings of bizarre happenings in the immediate environment. Continually, emotional disturbances such as anxiety, fear, depression, irritability, anger, euphoria, and apathy are also common, with rapid and unpredictable shifts from one emotional state to another often observed (Gupta et al., 2008). Before the symptoms of delirium manifest, there may be hours, days, or weeks of a combination of many of the aforementioned symptoms, with headaches and general uneasiness being the most common (APA, 1999; Gupta et al., 2008).

DIAGNOSIS

Delirium can be difficult to diagnose due to the interaction of multiple factors that creates very different presentations from patient to patient (Fricchione et al., 2008). The most common differential diagnosis is dementia rather than delirium, or a presentation that is superimposed on a preexisting dementia. Therefore, it is critical to ascertain whether the person has dementia rather than delirium or has delirium alone. Cognitive disturbances are common in both delirium and dementia, though the patient with dementia is usually alert without disruptions in consciousness. The severe symptoms associated with delirium usually fluctuate during a 24-hr period, whereas the symptoms for dementia do not and may be long-lasting.

Multiple informants, including family, caregivers, and medical records, are critical when gathering information about the patient with delirium. Determining whether a dementia was present before the onset of a delirium is critical for making a definitive diagnosis of one or both disorders, thus affecting appropriate interventions for treatment. Along with a clinical interview, tests that screen for delirium symptoms, such as delirium diagnostic instruments and symptom severity ratings may help in the clinical evaluation and diagnosis (APA, 1999).

TREATMENT

Several methods may be utilized in the treatment of delirium. Review of current and past medications is essential because delirium may occur when central nervous system drugs reach toxic levels. Discontinuing or reducing the dose of the problematic drug is critical. Delirium is typically considered a medical emergency where immediate intervention involves finding and correcting the current symptoms. Identification and correction of the causal factors require diagnostic tests to identify medical conditions and increased monitoring of the patient's general condition.

The delirium symptoms, mental status, and general medical condition typically require constant monitoring over time. Placing the patient in a supportive environment along with pharmacological intervention are common approaches to treatment, as is educating the patient and his or her family about the illness. Pharmacological interventions may involve the intravenous administration of haloperidol to manage feelings of agitation. The effects of haloperidol on blood pressure, pulmonary artery pressure, heart rate, and respiration are milder than those of intravenous benzodiazepines and other neuroleptics (Fricchione et al., 2008).

Angela Dortch
Raymond S. Dean

American Psychiatric Association. (1999). Practice guidelines for the treatment of patients with delirium. *The American Journal of Psychiatry, 5* (Suppl.), 1–19.

Fricchione, G. L., Nejad, S. H., Esses, J. A., & Cummings, T. J., Jr. (2008). Postoperative Delirium. *The American Journal of Psychiatry, 7,* 803–812.

Gupta, N., de Jonghe, J, Schieveld, J., Leonard, M., & Meagher, D. (2008). Delirium phenomenology: What can we learn from the symptoms of delirium? *Journal of Psychosomatic Research, 3,* 215–222.

Siddiqi, N., House, A. O., & Holmes, J. D. (2006). Occurrence and outcome of delirium in medical in-patients: A systematic literature review. *Age &Ageing, 35,* 350–64.

Sozia, R. L., Sharma, V., Ferguson, K., Shenkin, S. D., Seymour, D. G., & MacLullich, A. M. J. (2008). Neuroimaging studies of dementia: A systematic review. *Journal of Psychosomatic Research, 3,* 239–248.

DEMENTIA PUGILISTICA

DESCRIPTION

Dementia pugilistica (DP) (Millspaugh, 1937), also referred to as chronic traumatic encephalopathy (Parker, 1934), chronic traumatic brain injury (CTBI) (Jordan, 2000), and "punch drunk" (Martland, 1928), refers to a collection of neurological and neuropsychological symptoms believed to be a result of numerous concussive or subconcussive blows to the head (Critchley, 1957; Martland, 1928; Mendez, 1995). Although most commonly reported in boxers, there have been reports of DP in other sports (British Medical Association, 1987).

An early finding was that DP occurred in 17% of retired professional boxers. However, the mean number of years a boxer fights has dropped from 19 years in 1931 to 5 years in 2002, and the mean number of fights has similarly declined from 336 to 13, representing a significant decrease in exposure to head injury in recent years. DP symptoms emerge anywhere from 7 to 35 years after the beginning of a boxer's career, and symptoms usually do not present until after a boxer's career has ended (Clausen, McCrory, & Anderson, 2005; Roberts, 1969).

Chances of developing DP appear to increase with increased exposure to boxing. Specific risk factors include retiring after age 28, boxing more than 10 years, participating in more than 150 bouts (Roberts, 1969), more sparring exposure (Jordan et al., 1996), history of technical knockout or knockout (Jordan et al., 1992), being a "slugger" rather than a "scientific boxer" (Critchley, 1957), and the presence of the apolipoprotein E (APOE) alleles (Jordan et al., 1997). The risk of DP in amateur boxers is substantially lower (Loosemore, Knowles, & Whyte, 2007).

NEUROPATHOLOGY/PATHOPHYSIOLOGY

Neuropathological investigations of DP revealed septa to be wide apart, torn, and fenestrated, whereas ventricles were enlarged and fornices atrophied (Corsellis, Bruton, & Freeman-Browne, 1973). Also observed were cerebellar atrophy (particularly loss of Purkinje cells), glial fibrosis, and a lack of pigmented neurons of the substantia nigra (Corsellis, 1989). Adams and Bruton (1989) reported signs of cerebral, cerebellar, or meningeal hemorrhage. Neurochemically, Uhl, McKinney, and Hedreen (1982) reported atrophy of the nucleus basalis of Meynert and decreased cortical cholinergic activity.

Neurofibrillary tangles have also been observed, particularly deep within the temporal lobe (Constantinidis & Tissot, 1967; Roberts, Allsop, & Bruton, 1990). Furthermore, atrophy of the nucleus basalis of Meynert and decreased cortical cholinergic activity have been noted (Uhl et al., 1982).

NEUROPSYCHOLOGICAL/CLINICAL PRESENTATION

Critchley (1957) described the neuropsychological aspects of DP as insidious in onset and including emotional lability, progressively slower speech and thought, and considerable memory decline. Motor symptoms may include pyramidal, extrapyramidal, and or cerebellar signs (Jordan, 2000). Progression of motor abnormalities may result in ataxia, spasticity, impaired coordination, and parkinsonism. Mendez (1995) reported deficits with processing speed, complex attention, sequencing, memory, executive functions, and finger tapping speed. There have been case reports that failed to display the classic motor dysfunction characteristic of DP (Rochon, 1994).

DIAGNOSIS

Due to the latency of symptom onset in DP, the main question regarding diagnosis revolves around determining whether the neurologic dysfunction can be attributed to boxing. There is often symptom overlap with other dementias and specific neurological disorders (e.g., Alzheimer's disease, Parkinson's disease). Jordan (1993) proposed a classification system of the likelihood of CTBI being caused by boxing (probable, possible, or improbable) based on clinical symptoms. Jordan et al. (1997) also developed a 10-point CTBI rating scale used to assess the severity of injury in boxing, on the basis of cognitive, motor, and behavioral symptoms.

Although no definitive conclusions can be drawn from CT or MRI scans, numerous studies have now documented diffuse atrophy and a cavum septum pellucidum (Bodensteiner & Schaefer, 1997; Cabanis et al., 1986; Casson et al., 1984). EEG results may be normal, or may demonstrate nonspecific slowing (Roberts, 1969).

TREATMENT

DP symptoms may be treated with pharmacologic agents that are used to treat the symptoms of similarly symptomatic neurological disorders. For example, patients experiencing parkinsonian symptoms may be treated with antiparkinsonism medications (Jordan, 2000). The use of cholinergic agents and psychotropic medications are yet to be studied.

Due to the lack of empirical support in treating DP, prevention is of paramount importance. Prevention could be accomplished by closely monitoring those fighters who have risk factors for neurological signs and use of additional protective equipment such as is used by amateur boxers.

Shane S. Bush
Thomas E. Myers

Adams, C. W. M., & Bruton, C. J. (1989). The cerebral vasculature in dementia pugilistica. *Journal of Neurology, Neurosurgery, and Psychiatry, 52*, 600–604.

Bodensteiner, J. B., & Schaefer, G. B. (1997). Dementia pugilistica and cavumsepti pellucidi: Born to box. *Sports Medicine, 24*, 361–365

British Medical Association, Board of Science and Education. (1987). *Boxing*. London, UK: BMA.

Cabanis, E. A., Perez, G., Tamraz, J., Iba Zizen, M., Roger, B., Alfonso, J., et al. (1986). Cephalic magnetic resonance imaging of boxers. Preliminary results. *Acta Radiologica Supplement, 369*, 365–366.

Casson, I. R., Siegel, O., Sham, R., Campbell, E. A., Tarlau, M., & DiDomenico, A. (1984). Brain damage in modern boxers. *Journal of the American Medical Association, 251*, 2663–2667.

Clausen, H., McCrory, P., & Anderson, V. (2005). The risk of chronic traumatic brain injury in professional boxing: Change in exposure variables over the past century. *British Journal of Sports Medicine, 39*, 661–664.

Constantinidis, J., & Tissot, R. (1967). Lesions neurofibrillaires d'Alzheimer genera lisees sans plaques seniles. *Archives Suisse Neurologie Neurochirurgie Psychtatrie, 100*, 117–130.

Corsellis, J. A. (1989). Boxing and the brain. *British Medical Journal, 298*, 105–109.

Corsellis, J. A. N., Bruton, C. J., & Freeman-Browne, D. (1973). The aftermath of boxing. *Psychological Medicine, 3*, 270–303.

Critchley, M. (1957). Medical aspects of boxing, particularly from a neurological standpoint. *British Medical Journal, 1,* 357–362.

Jordan, B. D. (1993). Epidemiology of brain injury in boxing. In B. D. Jordan (Ed.), *Medical aspects of boxing* (pp. 147–168). Boca Raton, FL: CRC Press.

Jordan, B. D. (2000). Chronic traumatic brain injury associated with boxing. *Seminars in Neurology, 20*(2), 179–185.

Jordan, B. D., Matser, J. T., Zimmerman, R. D., & Zazula, T. (1996). Sparring and cognitive function in professional boxers. *Physician and Sports Medicine, 24 (5),* 87–98.

Jordan, B. D., Jahre, C., Hauser, W. A., Zimmerman, R. D., Zarrelli, M., Lipsitz, E. C., et al. (1992). CT of 338 active professional boxers. *Radiology, 2,* 181–185.

Jordan, B. D., Relkin, N. R., Ravdin, L. D., Jacobs, A. R., Bennett, A., & Gandy, S. (1997). Apolipoprotein Ee4 associated with chronic traumatic brain injury in boxing. *Journal of the American Medical Association, 278,* 136–140.

Loosemore, M., Knowles, C. H., & Whyte, G. P. (2007). Amateur boxing and risk of chronic brain injury: Systematic review of observational studies. *British Medical Journal, 335,* 809–817.

Martland, H. S. (1928). Punch drunk. *Journal of the American Medical Association, 91,* 1103–1107.

Mendez, M. F. (1995). The neuropsychiatric aspects of boxing. *International Journal of Psychiatry, 25,* 249–262.

Millspaugh, J. A. (1937). Dementia pugilistica. *United States Naval Bulletin, 35,* 297–302.

Parker, H. (1934). Traumatic encephalopathy of professional pugilists. *Journal of Neurology and Psychopathology, 15,* 20–28.

Roberts, A. H. (1969). *Brain damage in boxers: A study of the prevalence of traumatic encephalopathy among ex-professional boxers.* Pitman Medical & Scientific Publishing.

Roberts, G. W., Allsop, D., & Bruton, C. (1990). The occult aftermath of boxing. *Journal of Neurology, Neurosurgery, and Psychiatry, 53,* 373–378.

Rochon, M. (1994). Présentation d'un cas: L'encephalopathie des boxeurs. *Canadian Journal of Psychiatry, 39,* 211–214.

Uhl, G.R., McKinney, M., & Hedreen, J.C. (1982). Dementia pugilistica: loss of basal forebrain cholinergic neurons and cortical cholinergic markers. *Annals of Neurology, 12,* 99–104.

DERMATOMYOSITIS

DESCRIPTION

Dermatomyositis is an inflammatory muscle disease (myopathy) characterized by proximal muscle weakness and a pathognomonic skin rash (Callen, 2008; Koler & Montemarano, 2001). The muscles most commonly affected are those in the neck, shoulder, and pelvis (Lippincott Williams & Wilkins [LWW], 2008). Muscle tenderness, stiffness, and pain from swelling may be present in some individuals, though the clinical presentation varies (Callen, 2008). Progression and severity of muscle weakness and rash vary from individual to individual; progression is typically slow with multiple flare-ups and remissions (Lippincott Williams & Wilkins [LWW], 2008; Mayo Clinic Staff, 2007). Muscle weakness is symmetrical in nature (LWW, 2008). The first symptom can be either muscle weakness or skin rashes. In some cases, only the characteristic skin rashes are present (Callen, 2008). Over time, distal muscles may become affected in some individuals (LWW, 2008; Myositis Association, 2007). Muscle atrophy leading to deformity, contractures, and tendon damage can occur in later stages or if left untreated, particularly in children. In children, though rarely in adults, calcinosis may occur where calcium deposits form on joints (Callen, 2008).

Rashes characteristic of dermatomyositis include Gottron's papules, a shawl rash, a heliotrope rash, and a V-shaped rash (LWW, 2008). Most of the rashes are symmetrical in nature. Gottron's papules present as violet/red scaly lesions on joints such as knuckles, elbows, and knees (Callen, 2008; Koler & Montemarano, 2001). Heliotrope rash is a purplish rash across an individual's eyelids (Callen, 2008; Koler & Montemarano, 2001). The shawl rash is a diffuse red rash covering the back and shoulder area, whereas the V rash is a diffuse red rash over the collarbone and chest in a V shape (Callen, 2008; Koler & Montemarano, 2001). Both the V and shawl rashes may develop lesions. Other associated skin conditions including a scaly scalp, photosensitivity that exacerbates the rashes, red rashes on exposed skin areas, and cracked and roughened skin on the hands and fingertips are often referred to as "mechanics hands" (Callen, 2008; Koler & Montemarano, 2001). Symptoms common to those in Reynaud's syndrome, such as cold tips of body parts (e.g., fingers and toes), may be present (Callen, 2008). A low-level temperature may be present during flare-ups due to inflammation.

Dermatomyositis occurs twice as often in females as in males (Callen, 2008; LWW, 2008; Mayo Clinic Staff, 2007). Left untreated, there is 50% mortality; with current treatments, this rate decreases to 10% (Dermatomyositis, 2008). Death occurs from associated respiratory failure, heart failure, or malignancy rather than the disease itself (Callen, 2008; LWW, 2008). Although it can occur at any age, there are two peaks of onset: one in childhood and the other between 45 and 65 years of age (Callen, 2008; Mayo Clinic Staff,

2007). Arthritis occurs in up to 35% of cases, and malignant tumors are found in up to 50% of adult cases, though not in children. Prevalence rates range from about 3 to 10 cases in a million (Callen, 2008).

NEUROPATHOLOGY/PATHOPHYSIOLOGY

The etiology of dermatomyositis is unknown, although several causes are suspected, including an autoimmune reaction, viral infection, immunological abnormalities, vascular inflammation, and genetic factors (Callen, 2008; Dermatomyositis, 2008; LWW, 2008; Mayo Clinic Staff, 2007). It is not an infectious disease. In dermatomyositis, an individual's T cells–the cells responsible for coordinating the immune system–mistakenly identify muscle fiber antigens as foreign (LWW, 2008). These fibers are attacked, and a preponderance of T and B cells is present upon muscle biopsy. Elevated levels of creatine kinase and aldolase muscle enzymes are present, which indicate muscle damage (Dermatomyositis, 2008; LWW, 2008; Mayo Clinic Staff, 2007). Creatine kinase is responsible for the production of adenosine-50-triphosphate (ATP) and adenosine diphosphate (ADP) in muscles, which supply energy, and aldolase, which assists in generating ATP. Although other enzymes have been implicated, including rheumatoid factor, erythrocyte sedimentation rate, and certain autoantibodies, they tend to present in less than 50% of cases and cannot be used to diagnose definitively the presence or absence of the disease (Koler & Montemarano, 2001). The presence of these enzymes is confirmed through biopsy and blood work. Physically, there is atrophy of the muscle fiber cells, shrunken polygonal muscle fibers, and groupings of abnormal lymphocytes that have small nuclei (Dermatomyositis, 2008). Complications may occur with dermatomyositis because of weakening muscles, including difficulty swallowing, breathing complications, and gastrointestinal distress (Callen, 2008; Mayo Clinic Staff, 2007). The esophagus may become blocked, necessitating a tracheotomy. A barium swallow can be used to assess the efficacy of pharynx muscles.

NEUROPSYCHOLOGICAL/CLINICAL PRESENTATION

With dermatomyositis, there is impairment in the performance of normal activities (LWW, 2008). Individuals with muscle weakness often first notice signs of fatigue that progresses to difficulty executing basic activities, such as climbing the stairs, walking, and raising their arms above their heads (Callen, 2008;

Myositis Association, 2007). They can develop a slowed gait and have nonfluent production of motor activities. Physical symptoms are often not apparent upon casual observation as individuals may have learned to compensate for and work around affected muscles in many activities of daily living by using alternate muscles (Callen, 2008). Most fine motor skills, such as writing, remain unaffected; in individuals with concurrent arthritis, there is impairment in fine motor production when joints are swollen. On neuropsychological measures, crystallized abilities tend to be stable and do not decrease over the course of the disorder. Except in older individuals with concurrent dementia, memory faculties are intact. Some individuals experience visual impairment as a result of the disease, which affects performance on tasks involving visual scanning and perception. Depression has been reported in related rheumatic diseases, though not specifically in dermatomyositis.

DIAGNOSIS

Dermatomyositis needs to be differentiated from other lymphocyte inflammatory myopathies, polymyositis, muscular dystrophy, psoriasis, dermatitis, and lupus (Koler & Montemarano, 2001). Diagnostic techniques include muscle biopsy, MRI, CT scans, and electromyography (Callen, 2008; Koler & Montemarano, 2001; LWW, 2008). Electromyography is used to establish whether muscle weakness is the result of nerve damage (neuropathy) and can assess whether muscle inflammation is present (Mayo Clinic Staff, 2007). CT scans can be used to assess whether a concurrent malignancy is present that would necessitate treatment. If malignancy is present, other specialists should be called in to determine appropriate treatment. MRI is used to locate muscle inflammation and to choose ideal biopsy sites (Mayo Clinic Staff, 2007). Muscle biopsy is the best way to establish differential diagnosis. Biopsy can confirm the breakdown and rebuilding of muscle tissue, the presence of inflammatory infiltrates (lymphocytes and macrophages), and elevated enzymes (Dermatomyositis, 2008; Mayo Clinic Staff, 2007). Muscle weakness should be symmetrical in nature for dermatomyositis to be diagnosed (Callen, 2008). If only muscle weakness is present without skin rash, polymyositis is suspected (Koler & Montemarano, 2001). If major internal organs are involved, other disorders such as lupus are often suspected. Skin biopsy can be performed to rule out other disorders with similar appearance that can mimic the physical presentation, particularly during early stages (Mayo Clinic Staff, 2007; Koler & Montemarano, 2001).

D

TREATMENT

There is no cure for dermatomyositis; treatment focuses on alleviating the symptoms. For muscle weakness, bed rest can be initially advised to decrease the inflammation (LWW, 2008). In order to decrease muscle weakness and inflammation, the medication of choice is a corticosteroid, specifically prednisone (Callen, 2008; Koler & Montemarano, 2001; LWW, 2008; Mayo Clinic Staff, 2007). Corticosteroids work by suppressing the body's immune system, which inhibits the production of antibodies subsequently decreasing inflammation in an individual's muscle and skin surfaces. The disease typically responds well to corticosteroids and progress is favorable when they are used (Mayo Clinic Staff, 2007). In patients with adverse reactions to the corticosteroids, immunosuppressive agents are used (LWW, 2008). In order to maintain range of motion, prevent muscle atrophy, and prevent muscle contractures, physical therapy is recommended (Koler & Montemarano, 2001; Mayo Clinic Staff, 2007). Physical therapy entails exercises to prevent restriction of muscles, such as stretching or yoga exercises, and gradual strength building once medication has taken effect (Koler & Montemarano, 2001). Overly strenuous physical activities, such as bodybuilding, should be avoided. Sun avoidance techniques are taught, and the use of broad-spectrum sunscreen is strongly encouraged to cope with sun sensitivity (Callen, 2008; Koler & Montemarano, 2001; Mayo Clinic Staff, 2007). Several medications are used to help with the rash component, including antimalarial agents, topical corticosteroids, and intravenous immunoglobin, which is when antibodies are donated from healthy individuals and administered intravenously and used when other treatments fail due to expense (Callen, 2008; Mayo Clinic Staff, 2007).

Christine Corsun-Ascher
Charles Golden

Callen, J. P. (2008). *eMedicine: Dermatomyositis.* Retrieved December 1, 2008, from www.emedicine.com/med/topic2609.htm

Hollister, J. R. (2002). Rheumatic diseases. In W. W. Hay, A. Hayward, M. Levin, & J. M. Sondheimer (Eds.), *Current pediatric diagnosis and treatment* (pp. 833–834). New York: McGraw-Hill Professional.

Koler, R. A., & Montemarano, A. (2001). Dermatomyositis. *American Family Physician, 64*(9), 1565–1572.

Lippincott Williams & Wilkins. (2008). Immune disorders. In Lippincott Williams & Wilkins (Eds.), *Professional guide to diseases* (pp. 293–295). Philadelphia: Lippincott Williams & Wilkins.

Mayo Clinic Staff. (2007). *Dermatomyositis.* Retrieved December 5, 2008, from www.mayoclinic.com/health/dermatomyositis/DS00335

The Myositis Association. (2007). *Dermatomyositis.* Retrieved December 5, 2008, from www.myositis.org/template/page.cfm?id = 183

Winfield, H., & Jaworsky, C. (2008). Connective tissue diseases. In W. F. Lever, D. E. Elder, & R. Elenitsas (Eds.), *Lever's histopathology of the skin* (pp. 293–295). New York: Berghahn Books.

DISORDERS OF WRITTEN LANGUAGE

DESCRIPTION

Disorders of written language (DWL) are also referred to as disorders of written expression. The ability to write develops as part of a complex set of skills involving organization, problem solving, memory retrieval, reading and language abilities, and graphomotor skills. Any delay in these abilities can result in dysfunctional writing skills.

Frank Benson (1979) showed a lot of insight into agraphia. He says, "Agraphia may be defined simply as a loss or impairment of the ability to produce written language, caused by brain damage. There is nothing simple about agraphia, though" (p. 121). Although DWL include disorders caused by brain damage and disorders based on a developmental basis, both are language disorders and, as such, are brain-based disorders. In comparison, writing difficulties based on physical impairments (e.g., various bone disorders) would not be considered to fall under the umbrella of DWL. He notes that all forms of aphasia show agraphia of one sort or another, and the presence of agraphia is one sign of aphasia. However, he is quick to note that agraphia accompanies many disorders other than aphasia. This is best expressed by his comment that, "It would appear that writing is, at best, a tenuous accomplishment for most humans and that almost any brain abnormality can produce considerable disruption of writing skill" (p. 121).

According to Myklebust (1965), written language (visual expressive) is the last language skill we acquire and is dependent upon successful completion of the previous stages (inner, auditory receptive, auditory expressive, visual receptive). Interestingly, written language, the least used and practiced form of language, is 5,000 years old, whereas oral language is over a half million years old (Reed, 1970). According to Gaddes and Edgell (1994), written language is most often the first to show impairment with any type of brain insult. There are three types of DWL: aphasic, apraxic, and mechanical.

NEUROPATHOLOGY/PATHOPHYSIOLOGY

Written language is a very complex function in that its proper functioning depends upon many neuropsychological and other functions working together properly and in concert. If any one of these functions becomes compromised, written language will be adversely affected. For example, written expression in Broca's or Wernicke's aphasia is adversely effected, mostly reflecting the symptoms seen in verbal expression. Congenital deficits in visual and/or auditory perception will adversely affect the development of written expression fairly severely as well. Obviously, trauma to the dominant hand area will have an adverse effect, as will disruptions of manual feedback and severe apraxia.

Hale and Fiorello (2004) say that deficits in handwriting competency are associated with two areas in the brain: the left (dominant) middle frontal gyrus, also known as Exner's area, and the left anterior superior parietal region. The process of writing also involves the frontal regions of the brain in tasks such as organizing ideas into grammatical structure, conveying ideas through words, and editing. However, the posterior regions are also utilized to process somatosensory input used to guide the hand, to visualize the words, and to provide an understanding of the overall writing objective (Hale & Fiorello). Clearly, however, many more areas of the brain are involved in this very complex function.

More specifically, phonological dysgraphia has been associated with damage to the superior temporal lobe, whereas damage to the inferior parietal lobe has been associated with surface (orthographic) dysgraphia. Functional MRI and postmortem studies done on those known to have had lesions have correlated both phonological and surface dysgraphia with lesions of the posterior inferior temporal cortex (Carlson, 2007). Ideomotor dysgraphia is typically associated with lesions or impairment in the left inferior parietal lobe, left supplementary motor cortex, and the corpus callosum (Miller, 2007). Constructional dysgraphia is often a result of lesions of the right parietal lobe (Carlson, 2007). Dysgraphia is also a symptom of the classic Gerstmann's syndrome of the left parietal lobe (angular gyrus, which is also associated with anomia).

NEUROPSYCHOLOGICAL/CLINICAL PRESENTATION

DWL are complex in that they involve many cognitive processes and have a high rate of comorbidity with other language disorders, such as reading and mathematics disorders (Hale & Fiorello, 2004; Sadock & Sadock, 2007). Care should be taken, however, not to jump too quickly to a diagnosis of DWL for someone who is just learning to write, as young children show high variability in their ability to accomplish written language, probably due to the differential development of the requisite areas of the brain.

Teachers may be the first to notice confusion of letters, usage of wrong words chosen to communicate a thought, incorrect or random capitalization within words, incomplete words, or inappropriate spacing between letters. Children may complain of pain when writing or simply refuse to write. When they do write they may present an odd grip of the writing utensil. Illegibility may be present but should not be used as the sole criterion for DWL.

Aphasic dysgraphia is a type of disorder of written language characterized by difficulty with the language-based aspect of writing. Aphasic dysgraphia is further divided into four subtypes: phonological dysgraphia entails impairment in the ability to decode the sounds of phonemes internally and thus difficulty sounding out words and writing them phonetically; surface (orthographic) dysgraphia involves impairment in the ability to hold the visual memory of an entire word; mixed dysgraphia is impairment in the abilities to recall the sequence of letters within words, recall correct letter formations, and inconsistency in correct spelling; finally, semantic (direct) dysgraphia constitutes impairment in understanding the grammatical rules that govern formation of the combination of words and phrases (Miller, 2007). Quite clearly, dysgraphia does occur when there is dyslexia, for the ability to read is essential for the development of writing. However, although there is some controversy over this, dysgraphia of many forms can occur in the absence of any type of dyslexia. Reading ability is necessary but not sufficient for normal writing development.

Apraxic dysgraphia stems from difficulty with the nonlanguage aspects of writing and is divided into three subtypes: ideomotor, ideational, and constructional. Ideomotor dysgraphia is characterized by comprehension of verbal commands but an inability to carry out the command with motor output (writing) (Miller, 2007). Ideational dysgraphia occurs due to an inability to maintain the motor plan of a sequence of gestures needed to write. Difficulty in

D

accessing letters from long-term memory is at the base of this disorder that results in missing and substitution of letters (Zettin, Cubelli, & Rago, 1995). Constructional dysgraphia is the inability to relate geometric locations (Carlson, 2007). Although rare, children with this disorder are incapable of producing written language due to the inability to organize visuospatial input (Miller, 2007). Motor dysgraphia is the only form of mechanical dysgraphia. It is a problem with writing due to motor problems typically related to the hands. It is not due to language or nonlanguage features of writing (Miller, 2007).

Problems that can impede hand skill development also include poor finger movement isolation, decreased timing of movements, graded movement dysfunction, and patterns of movement that are compensatory (Case-Smith, 2001).

DIAGNOSIS

DWL will be diagnosed most often starting in second grade. The following criteria are set forth by the American Psychiatric Association (APA) (2000) to make a diagnosis of disorders of written expression:

1. Writing skills that fall below standardized norms based on age, IQ, and education.
2. The dysfunction described in item 1 results in marked difficulties in school or activities of daily life that require the use of writing.
3. If a sensory deficit exists, the writing dysfunction is below the norm for the disorder.

As a rule, the APA suggests that if the disorder of written language is due to disorders that are neurologically or sensory based, the disorder will be considered an Axis III diagnosis, not Axis I.

Diagnosis must also include the use of tests to assess whether performance is significantly below the average range for a person's age. The Test of Written Language (TOWL) can be helpful in making a diagnosis and should be compared with those of an intellectual evaluation such as the Wechsler Intelligence Scale for Children (WISC-IV) or Wechsler Adult Intelligence Scale (WAIS-IV) to identify overall intellectual functioning. As suggested above, DWL appears to have a high rate of comorbidity with reading and mathematics disorders. There is also limited evidence that language deficits and perceptual motor difficulties tend to co-occur as well (Sadock & Sadock, 2007).

Those with phonological dysgraphia struggle with the spelling of unfamiliar words, phonetically irregular words, and nonwords. However, the skills involving copying and writing from dictation are not impaired. Moreover, familiar words can be written correctly by visualizing the word (Miller, 2007).

People with surface dysgraphia rely solely on their ability to spell words by sounding them out phonetically. Therefore, the skills of spelling regular words and pronounceable nonwords are intact whereas that of phonetically irregular words are difficult (e.g., "said becomes sed") (Miller, 2007, p. 286).

Mixed dysgraphia symptoms include the accurate formation of letters during copying, whereas phonological errors are made when spelling. In addition, often there are errors in the sequencing of letters within words (Miller, 2007).

Words that are dictated to those with direct dysgraphia are reproduced correctly, but the semantic content of what has been written is not understood (Miller, 2007).

Ideomotor dysgraphia can be identified by an inability to perform motor actions to comply with a verbal command (e.g., wave your hand, show a peace sign). Children with ideational dysgraphia have difficulty organizing their thoughts sequentially. They are capable of performing motor tasks in isolation or when given a verbal command but are incapable of stringing together a sequence of actions. For these children, writing is a labor-intensive process characterized by frequent mistakes and erasures (Miller, 2007). This is frustrating for the children because they are able to see the errors they make, but they are unable to prevent them because of their poor written planning ability. This, by the way, is true of most other frontal apraxias as well.

People with (posterior) constructional dysgraphia have the ability to motor plan and carry out motor actions. However, they are impaired in the ability to visualize the spatial arrangements of writing (e.g., staying within the lines, starting at the top left, and writing across to the end of the line, etc.) (Miller, 2007).

Motor dysgraphia is characterized by poor penmanship. There is no cognitive difficulty in processing or writing information, but poor fine motor skills, tremors, or stiffness of the hands impair the ability to hold a writing instrument (Miller, 2007).

Several other conditions need to be ruled out before giving a diagnosis of DWL. It is important to identify whether depression or attention deficit hyperactivity disorder (ADHD) might be causing the difficulty with writing tasks. Both depression and ADHD can interfere with attention and concentration (Sadock & Sadock, 2007). Some other disorders to rule out include impaired vision or hearing, mental retardation, mixed receptive-expressive language disorder, pervasive developmental disorder, developmental coordination disorder, or communication disorders (APA, 2000).

TREATMENT

Accurate assessment of the etiology or basis of the writing difficulty provides important information regarding treatment. Determination of whether the cause is singular or a combination of dysfunction should serve as a guide to the treatment team and as an aid in selecting interventions (Hale & Fiorello, 2004). Providing practice exercises in spelling and writing sentences and reviewing rules of grammar are helpful as remedial treatments. Sadock and Sadock (2007) report that providing continued and consistent one-to-one "expressive and creative writing therapy" (p. 1167) results in positive improvements. They also stress the importance of the interpersonal relationship between the student and the writing specialist to achieve the most effective change. Clearly, maintaining motivation and a positive outlook with appropriate reinforcement positively impacts the overall prospects for long-term change. Careful and clear structure is also very important.

One aspect that is indirectly related to this topic is the emphasis that has been placed on the pencil grip of students learning to write. Although there certainly are grips that can interfere with writing, care should be taken not to force a change in grip from one which, although not normal, is perfectly effective for writing. Most adults can write quite well using many of the seemingly abnormal grips and it may be that, like attempting to change handedness, changing the grip from one that is preferred and effective may have deleterious effects.

DWL involving graphomotor and coordination developmental issues (apraxic and mechanical) may require referral to an occupational therapist for an evaluation and treatment plan. Aphasic and developmental impairments can be addressed utilizing teachers, parents, occupational therapists, and psychologists.

An approach to diagnosis and treatment is the cognitive hypothesis-testing (CHT) model (Hale & Fiorello, 2004). In this regard, the presenting problem is used to develop a working hypothesis about which neuropsychological components may be impaired. Then specific tests are chosen to assess functioning in suspected areas. Once this is done an analysis of how these deficits could impede academic and social functioning is used to determine the best course for treatment. Interested readers are referred to Hale and Fiorello (2004) for a detailed discussion.

Tonya M. Bennett
Teri J. McHale
Henry V. Soper

American Psychiatric Association. (2000). *Diagnostic and statistical manual of mental disorders* (4th ed.). Washington, DC: Author.

Benson, D. F. (1979). *Aphasia, alexia, and agraphia*. New York: Churchill Livingstone.

Carlson, N. R. (2007). *Physiology of behavior* (9th ed.). Boston: Pearson Education.

Case-Smith, J. (2001). *Occupational therapy for children*. Philadelphia: Mosby.

Gaddes, W., & Edgell, D. (1994). *Learning disabilities and brain function*. New York: Springer.

Hale, J. B., & Fiorello, C. A. (2004). *School neuropsychology: A practitioner's handbook*. New York: The Guilford Press.

Sadock, B., & Sadock, V. (2007). *Synopsis of psychiatry* (10th ed.). Philadelphia: Lippincott Williams & Wilkins.

Miller, D. C. (2007). *Essentials of school neuropsychological assessment*. Hoboken, NJ: John Wiley & Son.

Mykelbust, H. (1965). *Development and disorders of written language* (Vol. 1). New York: Grune & Stratton.

Reed, D. (1970). A theory of language, speech, and writing. In H. Singer & R. Ruddell (Eds.), *Theoretical models and processes of reading* (pp. 219–238). Newark: International Reading Association.

Zettin, M., Cubelli, R., & Perino, C. (1995). Impairment of letter formation: The case of "ideomotor" apraxic agraphia. *Aphasiology, 9*(3), 283–294.

DOWN'S SYNDROME

DESCRIPTION

Down's syndrome is a chromosomal disorder that may result from a number of cytogenic variants, resulting in the genetic mutation. Down's syndrome was first recognized as a formal set of physical characteristics in 1866 by Dr. John Langdon Down and later in 1959 was established to be the result of an extra chromosome by Lejeune and his colleagues (Selikowicz, 1997). These physical characteristics, which are commonly observed in the first months of life, often include brachycephaly with a round face, Brushfield's spots, a small mouth with a large protruding tongue, small ears, epicanthal folds with upslanting palpebral fissures, and a flattened or depressed nasal bridge (Berg, 2007). In addition to these physical characteristics, a plethora of neurological complications is also often seen with developmental delay and diffuse muscular hypotonia being the most common. Mental retardation is also quite common with Down's syndrome comprising the majority of children with this degree of cognitive deficiency as it is the most common neurodevelopmental disorder (Nadel, 2003).

NEUROPATHOLOGY/PATHOPHYSIOLOGY

Down's syndrome results from an autosomal chromosome anomaly in which there is the presence, in triplicate, rather than duplicate, of all or part of chromosome 21. In the majority of cases, the extra chromosomal material is present as a separate chromosome. In approximately 5% of the cases, extra chromosomal material on the 21st chromosome is present due to the process of translocation (the transfer of part of one chromosome to another chromosome) (Nadel, 2003).

Individuals with Down's syndrome may present with brachycephalic skulls due to late closure of the anterior fontanelle and metopic suture, calcification of the basal ganglia, delayed myelination, smaller hippocampal formations (Emerson, Kesslak, Chen, & Lott, 1995; Muller & Bussieres, 1996). Around the third to fourth decade of life, parenchymal volume loss, ventricular dilation, and reduced cerebellum size are commonly noted.

NEUROPSYCHOLOGICAL/CLINICAL PRESENTATION

Down's syndrome is characterized by a number of possible physical and neurological features. In regard to the latter, mental retardation is the most commonly associated feature. The degree of mental impairment varies widely and ranges from mild to profound mental retardation with a mean IQ of 40–50. One study found weaker hippocampal functions in children with Down's syndrome, secondary to overall cognitive dysfunction (Pennington, Moon, Edgin, Stedron, & Nadel, 2003). These patients tend to show a decrease in IQ with age. After age 30, these individuals have a very high risk for developing an Alzheimer's type of dementia (Cifra-Bean, 2006). In addition, patients are often delayed in the achievement of developmental milestones and demonstrate deficits in sequential and simultaneous processing.

Sensory and motor issues are also commonly seen. Patients tend to demonstrate fine and gross motor impairments as well as poor balance. Diffuse muscular hypotonia affects most patients. In addition, fine and gross motor impairments, neck pain or discomfort, torticollis, gait impairment, and corticospinal tract dysfunction are common and have been linked with atlantoaxial subluxation and instability resulting in compression of the medulla and spinal cord (Berg, 2007). Increased risk of moyamoya disease has also been seen.

Abnormal physical features such as protruding tongue, prominent epicanthal folds, a round face with flat profile, a short nose with a low bridge, and a simian crease on the hands are common. Many individuals with this disorder have congenital heart defects, thyroid problems, and skeletal problems. Complications such as gastroenterological malformations, hematological anomalies, and upper respiratory infections are also frequently seen in these patients. Life expectancy for patients with this disorder varies. Although some patients survive into their 60s and 70s, the average life expectancy is approximately 40 years due to the high prevalence of heart defects and leukemia among patients with this disorder.

Personality characteristics are highly variable between and within individuals with the syndrome. However, common daily symptoms may include poor frustration tolerance, emotional instability, impulsivity, and attentional difficulties.

DIAGNOSIS

Down's syndrome can be detected prenatally by amniocentesis. Amniocentesis should be considered for mothers who are 35 and older because late maternal age is a major factor in the etiology of Down's syndrome. The National Down Syndrome Society cites that 80% of children with Down's syndrome are born to mothers younger than 35 (www.ndss.org). Mothers who have already had a child with Down's syndrome should consider amniocentesis, especially if chromosome studies revealed that their prior child's Down's syndrome was due to translocation; chromosomal translocation can be transmitted to the child by either parent. Down's syndrome can also be diagnosed at birth by the phenotypic features discussed previously. Usually, diagnosis is not difficult but karyotyping is indicated for confirmation and for determining whether the child has the typical trisomy 21 karyotype or a translocation.

Radiological investigations consisting of skull X-ray, CT, and MRI may be utilized to identify aforementioned neurological abnormalities. Electroencephalogram is sometimes used as patients with Down's syndrome can often present with increased risk of convulsions and seizures. Neuropsychological assessment can prove useful in identifying the nature and extent of any presenting neurocognitive deficits

TREATMENT

No treatment is available to cure or significantly improve the overall functioning of patients with Down's syndrome. Early intervention is most frequently recommended as children with the syndrome are often already at-risk for developmental delays. Current and future treatments involve surgical and/or pharmacological intervention with the medical conditions that are frequently associated with this disorder. Behavioral therapies, including group and family counseling may help to manage behavioral challenges and delays in language if present.

Genetic counseling can help the parents of a Down's syndrome patient assess risk factors involved in having additional children. Supportive counseling can be useful in helping the family deal with their reactions to having a family member with Down's syndrome and can assist parents in dealing with the patient's cognitive deficits and behavior problems.

In order to achieve optimal educational benefits, the patient should receive selective education that is individualized based on each patient's characteristic pattern of cognitive and behavioral limitations.

Matthew Holcombe
Raymond S. Dean
Chad A. Noggle

Berg, B. O. (2007). Chromosomal abnormalities and neurocutaneous disorders. In C. G. Goetz (Ed.), *Textbook of clinical neurology* (pp. 683–697). Philadelphia: Saunders Elsevier.

Citra-Bean, L. (2006). Current research in down syndrome. *Down Syndrome News, 27*, 4.

Emerson, J. F., Kesslak, J. P., Chen, P. C., & Lott, I. T. (1995). Magnetic resonance imaging of the aging brain in Down's syndrome. *Progress in Clinical Biological Research, 393*, 123–138.

Muller, F., & Bussieres, L. (1992). Magnetic resonance imaging of delayed myelination of Down syndrome: A case report and review of the literature. *Journal of Child Neurology, 7*, 417–421.

Nadel, L. (2003). Down syndrome: A genetic disorder in biobehavioral perspective. Retrieved September 13, 2010, from www.u.arizona.edu

National Down Syndrome Society (2010). *Down syndrome fact sheet*. Retrieved September 13, 2010, from www.ndss.org

Pennington, B. F., Moon, J., Edgin, J., Stedron, J., & Nadel, L. (2003). The neuropsychology of Down syndrome: Evidence for hippocampal dysfunction. *Child Development, 74*, 75–93.

Selikowicz, M. (1997). *Down syndrome: The facts* (2nd ed.). Oxford: Oxford University Press.

DRAVET'S SYNDROME

DESCRIPTION

Dravet's syndrome (DS) is a seizure disorder primarily confined to the pediatric population. In adults, prevalence has been reported as less than 1 in 40,000 individuals (Millichap, Koh, Laux, & Nordli, 2009). DS is associated with a mutation of the *SCN1A* gene (Wolff, Cassé-Perrot, & Dravet, 2006) and is even considered diagnostic (Arzimanoglou, 2009). DS often first manifests as frequent febrile seizures in the first year of life. Eventually, febrile seizures subside to myoclonus and status epilepticus. Mental retardation may be seen, and delays in language and motor development are common. Social and behavioral deficits also present with greater frequency in comparison with the normal population.

NEUROPATHOLOGY/PATHOPHYSIOLOGY

Genetically, DS has been associated with mutations to the sodium-channel gene *SCN1A* (Sugawara et al., 2002; Yamakawa, 2002), which may be inherited or acquired de novo (Morimoto et al., 2006). Estimates suggest some 40% to 85% of patients with DS demonstrate mutations in *SCN1A* (Catterall, Dib-Hajj, Meisler, & Pietrobon, 2008; Korff & Nordli, 2006). This gene is responsible for encoding voltage-gated sodium channel Nav1.1, which is one of the most abundant α subunits of sodium channels in the central nervous system, which are essential for action potential generation in excitable cells, including neurons (Brackenbury, Djamgoz, & Isom, 2008; Catterall, Goldin, & Waxman, 2005). Initial seizures may present as normal on electroencephalogram (EEG) but eventually become polymorphic, coinciding with variability in seizure presentation.

Empirical studies have long suggested DS is associated with relatively normal neuroradiological studies in most patients (Guerrini & Dravet, 1997). Nevertheless, some evidence has emerged across the years showing neuroanatomical changes. Most commonly, atrophy of the cerebellum and cerebral cortex have been reported at varying degrees (Dravet, Bureau, Oguni, Fukuyama, & Cokar, 2005). Striano et al. (2007) reviewed neuroimaging and medical history of 58 patients with DS, and they reported findings of focal cortical brain atrophy in eight patients, ventricular abnormalities in six patients (accounting for three of the focal cortical atrophy group), and other brain abnormalities including one with cerebellar atrophy, one with white matter hyperintensity, one with hippocampal sclerosis, and one with focal cortical dysplasia. Of these individuals demonstrating neuroanatomical changes, more individuals did *not* have *SCN1A* mutations. Overall, findings revealed that although neuroanatomical changes can occur with DS, they still are not observed in high numbers.

NEUROPSYCHOLOGICAL/CLINICAL PRESENTATION

Initial seizures are seen within the first year of life and are often triggered by fever. At this point, the presentation is often classified as status epilepticus events. As time goes on, future seizures vary in form with multiple types presenting. They may be focal clonic or generalized. When presenting in a unilateral pattern, it is not uncommon for hemispheric shift to occur within a singular seizure event. Myoclonic, atypical absence, generalized tonic–clonic, and focal or clonic seizures may all present. Episodes of nonconvulsive status epilepticus may also be seen. However, of all these types, myoclonic seizures remain a hallmark characteristic of DS (Arzimanoglou, 2009; Millichap et al., 2009; Zupanc, 2009).

From a neuropsychological standpoint, infants appear to develop normally up to the onset of seizures. As they move into toddlerhood and early childhood, deficits of a cognitive, motor, and behavioral nature emerge. These features manifest in a regressional pattern, beginning between 1 and 3 years of age and stabilizing after 4–5 years of age. During this regressional pattern and thereafter, mental retardation and language delays are observed in a majority of individuals. Psychomotor retardation, ataxia, spasticity, and corticospinal tract signs are also seen. Behaviorally, attention deficit hyperactivity disorder and oppositional defiant disorder present with increased frequency beyond that seen in the normal population (Lordeon, Sitwat, Brehm, & Holder, 2010). These features remain even after the aforementioned stabilization. There is a high risk of death including patients with sudden unexpected death in epilepsy (Dravet et al., 2005).

DIAGNOSIS

EEG is critical to the diagnosis of DS. Although in the initial stages, when symptoms are isolated to frequent febrile seizures, EEG patterns remain largely normal, as the presentation progresses, generalized, polyspikes and multifocal spikes may present. These are often accompanied by focal, slow waves in the vertex and central regions (Arzimanoglou, 2009). Over time, individuals' epileptiform activity decreases and normalizes. CT and MRI should be utilized as part of good practice. However, in the case of DS, neuroimaging is usually normal except for a few cases with dilatation of the cisterna magna or slight diffuse atrophy (Dravet, Bureau, Oguni, Fukuyama, & Cokar, 2002).

Genetic workup is also essential to diagnosis, as the previously noted mutation of the *SCNIA* gene is indicative of the presentation (Arzimanoglou, 2009; Millichap et al., 2009).

Clinical description and differentiation are also essential to diagnosis. Other seizure disorders serve as the main presentations from which DS must be differentiated. Most forms of severe myoclonic epilepsy manifest initial clonic seizures in response to fever; thus, differentiation from febrile convulsions is important. As described by Dravet et al. (2002), seizure onset is often earlier in DS, occurring prior to 1 year of age, whereas febrile convulsions often present between 18 and 24 months. In addition, DS often presents as unilateral clonic seizures that are longer in duration and more frequent. Myoclonic features are not observed in febrile convulsions. Differentiation from other pediatric seizure disorders can be achieved largely by description of the clinical presentation and EEG profiles. The interested reader is recommended to review Lennox–Gastaut's syndrome, West's syndrome, Landau–Kleffner's syndrome, Benign Rolandic epilepsy among others to aid in this differentiation.

TREATMENT

Medicinal intervention serves as the first-line treatment of DS, although response is variable and complete control may not be achieved. Valproate, clonazepam, and lorazepam are the most common and often most effective agents. Diazepam, topiramate, valproate, levetiracetam, and zonisamide have all demonstrated some efficacy in treatment of DS, depending upon the presenting features as well (Arzimanoglou, 2009; Wheless, 2009). Vagus nerve stimulators and utilization of a ketogenic diet have also shown utility in initial reports, although further evaluation is needed (Arzimanoglou, 2009; Wheless, 2009).

Clinical trials have also suggested against certain agents as they demonstrate a tendency to exacerbated seizure activity. Vigabatrin, lamotrigine, carbamazepine, and phenytoin have all demonstrated this tendency (Korff, Laux, Kelley, Goldstein, Koh, & Nordli, 2007; Wheless, 2009).

Even with these interventions, prognosis varies, yet, in general, the outlook is poor. Individuals may continue to experience seizures in the face of medicinal intervention, with fatigue and fever serving as triggers, although the variety of seizure types diminishes (i.e., partial seizures and myoclonus dissipate). Cognitive deficits persist and are often severe to moderate. Emotional and behavioral disorders present at increased rates. Mortality rates may be as high as 15% to 18% (Dravet et al., 2002).

Chad A. Noggle
Javan Horwitz

Arzimanoglou, A. (2009). Dravet syndrome: From electroclinical characteristics to molecular biology. *Epilepsia, 50,* Suppl. 8, 3–9.

Brackenbury, W. J., Djamgoz, M. B., & Isom, L. L. (2008). An emerging role for voltage-gated Na+ channels in cellular migration: Regulation of central nervous system development and potentiation of invasive cancers. *Neuroscientist, 14,* 571–583.

Catterall, W. A., Dib-Hajj, S., Meisler, M. H., & Pietrobon, D. (2008). Inherited neuronal ion channelopathies: New windows on complex neurological diseases. *Journal of Neuroscience, 28,* 11768–11777.

Catterall, W. A., Goldin, A. L., & Waxman, S. G. (2005). International Union of Pharmacology. XLVII. Nomenclature and structure-function relationships of voltage-gated sodium channels. *Pharmacological Reviews, 57,* 397–409.

Dravet, C., Bureau, M., Oguni, H., Fukuyama, Y., & Cokar, O. (2002). Severe myoclonic epilepsy in infancy (Dravet syndrome). In J. Roger, M. Bureau, C. Dravet, P. Genton, C. A. Tassinari, & P. Wolf (Eds.), *Epileptic syndromes in infancy, childhood and adolescence* (3rd ed., pp. 81–103). London: John Libbey.

Dravet, C., Bureau, M., Oguni, H., Fukuyama, Y., & Cokar, O. (2005). Severe myoclonic epilepsy in infancy: Dravet syndrome. *Advanced Neurology, 95,* 71–102.

Guerrini, R., & Dravet, C. (1997). Severe epileptic encephalopathies of infancy, other than West syndrome. In J. Engel Jr. & A. Pedley (Eds.), *Epilepsy: A comprehensive textbook* (pp. 2285–2302). Philadelphia: Lippincott-Raven.

Korff, C., Laux, L., Kelley, K., Goldstein, J., Koh, S., & Nordli, D., Jr. (2007). Dravet syndrome (severe myoclonic epilepsy in infancy): A retrospective study of 16 patients. *Journal of Child Neurology, 22,* 185–194.

Korff, C. M., & Nordli, D. R., Jr. (2006). Epilepsy syndromes in infancy. *Pediatric Neurology, 34,* 253–263.

Lordeon, P., Sitwat, B., Brehm, D., & Holder, D. (2010). Dravet syndrome: A technologist's perspective. *American Journal of Electroneurodiagnostic Technology, 50,* 297–312.

Millichap, J., Koh, S., Laux, L., & Nordli, D., Jr. (2009). Child neurology: Dravet syndrome: When to suspect the diagnosis. *Neurology, 73,* e59–e62.

Morimoto, M., Mazaki, E., Nishimura, A., Chiyonobu, T., Sawai, Y., Murakami, A., et al. (2006). SCN1A mutation mosaicism in a family with severe myoclonic epilepsy in infancy. *Epilepsia, 47,* 1732–1736.

Striano, P., Mancardi, M. M., Biancheri, R., Madia, F., & Gennaro, E. (2007). Brain MRI findings in SMEI and genotype-phenotype correlations. *Epilepsia,* 1–5.

Sugawara, T., Mazaki-Miyazaki, E., Fukushiman, K., Shimomura, J., Fujiwara, T., Hamano, S., et al. (2002). Frequent mutations of SCN1A in severe myoclonic epilepsy in infancy. *Neurology, 58,* 7, 1122–1124.

Wheless, J. W. (2009). Managing severe epilepsy syndromes of early childhood. *Journal of Child Neurology, 24,* 24S–32S.

Wolff, M., Cassé-Perrot, C., & Dravet, C. (2006). Severe myoclonic epilepsy of infants (Dravet syndrome): Natural history and neuropsychological findings. *Epilepsia, 40,* S2, 45–48.

Yamakawa, K. (2002). Mutations of sodium-channels in GEFS+ and SMEI. *Brain Development, 24,* 6, 358.

Zupanc, M. (2009). Clinical evaluation and diagnosis of severe epilepsy syndromes of early childhood. *Journal of Child Neurology, 24,* 6S–14S.

DYSAUTONOMIA

DESCRIPTION

Dysautonomia is characterized by numerous disorders related to dysfunction, either diminished or excessive activity, of the autonomic nervous system or visceral functions. The autonomic nervous system is divided into the sympathetic nervous system (the fight or flight response) and the parasympathetic nervous system (the rest and digest response) (Stewart & Weldon, 2003). The disorder varies from being localized to systemic, to acute and reversible, to chronic and progressive, and may manifest as a primary condition or secondary condition.

Historically, the disease was named neurasthenia and was characterized by acute and enigmatic symptoms including fatigue, weakness, pain, dizziness, and fainting. Prevalence in the distant past was typically confined to females and prognosis was either recovery or terminal (Mathias & Bannister, 1999).

Currently, dysautonomias affect both males and females with over one million individuals in the United States diagnosed with a primary dysautonomia

(Mathias & Bannister, 1999). Ashkenazi Jews tend to be particularly susceptible to familial dysautonomia (FD) with prevalence rates of approximately 1 per 3,600 (Benarroch, Freeman, & Kaufmann, 2007). Some common forms of dysautonomia in the general population include postural orthostatic tachycardia syndrome (POTS) or orthostatic intolerance (OI), neurocardiogenic syncope (NCS), pure autonomic failure (PAF), and multiple systems atrophy (MSA) (Korczyn, 1995). Prognosis for dysautonomias tends to vary based on the specific conditions and may range from transient with full recovery to chronic and progressive.

NEUROPATHOLOGY/PATHOPHYSIOLOGY

The exact pathophysiology and etiology of dysautonomia tends to vary between the subtypes of the condition and is poorly understood. Multiple theories of pathophysiology exist, such as the epitonic or disconnection theories, yet no conclusive understanding has been reached at this time. Perhaps the best explanation at this time is the Excitatory:Inhibitory Ratio (EIR) model, a disconnection model, which purports that when the diencephalon regions of the brain, which tend to be inhibitory, are disrupted by structural or functional means dysautonomias follow particularly in the mesencephalon region of the brain (Baguley, Heriseanu, Cameron, Nott, & Slewa-Younan, 2008). Dysautonomias tend to be exacerbated by environmental factors and minimized by neurotransmitter activity (Baguley et al., 2008). In the case of cognitive impairments in dysautonomias, alpha-synuclein pathology in the neocortical areas of the brain found in Parkinson's disease and dementia with Lewy bodies may play an important role (Poewe, 2007).

What is known is that within the autonomic nervous system, disruption occurs leading to a decline or increase in normal biochemical functions (Mathias & Bannister, 1999). Risk factors for developing dysautonomia are not universal and generally not well known but may include viral illness, brain injury, genetic proclivity, disturbances in posture, toxic exposure to chemicals, autoimmune disorders (i.e., diabetes), physical trauma to the autonomic nervous system, or pregnancy (Mathias & Bannister, 1999).

NEUROPSYCHOLOGICAL/CLINICAL PRESENTATION

Due to the numerous varieties of dysautonomias, clinical presentation tends to differ. Furthermore, the severity of the symptoms may be mild and transient (i.e., reflex sympathetic dystrophy) or severe and

chronic, and successfully treated conditions can recur (i.e., Guillain-Barré syndrome) (Mathias & Bannister, 1999). Common symptoms include excessive fatigue, excessive thirst, dizziness or vertigo, feelings of anxiety or panic, increased or decreased heart rate, and orthostatic hypotension sometimes associated with syncope (Stewart & Weldon, 2003). In addition, individuals may experience constipation or diarrhea, acid reflux, breathing problems, or chest pain (Korczyn, 1995). Other neurologic symptoms may include headaches, facial flushing, nausea, visual disturbances, numbness, nerve pain, loss of consciousness, or seizures (Newby & Jaradeh, 2008). With some variants of dysautonomias, cognitive impairments, such as dementia (i.e., memory loss plus one of the four following conditions: apraxia, aphasia, agnosia, or executive dysfunction), may occur (Newby & Jaradeh, 2008; Poewe, 2007). Sensory dysfunction may also be apparent, specifically related to vibration and thermal appreciation associated with FD (Hilz & Axelrod, 2000). Consequently, dysautonomia may multiply aspects of the individual's quality of life.

DIAGNOSIS

The dysautonomias are divided into two categories: primary dysautonomias, where the autonomic nervous system dysfunction occurs as a primary condition (i.e., familial dysautonomia), or associative or secondary dysautonomias, where the autonomic nervous system dysfunction is secondary to degenerative neurologic disease (i.e., dysautonomia associated with Parkinson's disease) (Low, 1997; Mathias & Bannister, 1999).

In general, dysautonomias are difficult to diagnose due to the fact that reported symptoms tend to be out of proportion to any physical or laboratory findings thus catalyzing skepticism in the medical community. However, for certain subtypes, genetic screening may be useful for differential diagnosis. Diagnosis typically follows the predominant reported symptom. For example, excessive fatigue will be diagnosed as chronic fatigue syndrome (CFS), fainting would be diagnosed as vasovagal or NCS, abnormally high resting pulses would be diagnosed as inappropriate sinus tachycardia (IST), dizziness when standing would be diagnosed as POTS, gastrointestinal complaints would be diagnosed as irritable bowel syndrome (IBS), and pain tends to be diagnosed as fibromyalgia (Korczyn, 1995; Mathias & Bannister, 1999). Other common primary dysautonomias include multiple system atrophy, pure autonomic failure, and familial dysautonomia, whereas common disease-related conditions that can induce autonomic system dysfunction include diabetes, brain injury, or

D

alcohol dependence (Korczyn, 1995; Mathias & Bannister, 1999). In addition, autonomic dysfunction can result in psychiatric conditions like anxiety or panic attacks (Low, 1997; Mathias & Bannister, 1999).

Differential diagnosis for dysautonomias is significant and far supersedes the scope of this entry as many conditions may exhibit similar symptoms (Low, 1997). Thus, specific differential diagnosis for each subtype of dysautonomia should be independently ascertained.

TREATMENT

Medical treatment for dysautonomia tends to be symptomatic and supportive, as there is no cure for this disorder. Due to the relatively unknown etiology and pathophysiology, treatment may be difficult and therapies often tend to be made through trial and error.

Treatment often follows medical and nonmedical therapies. Typical drugs prescribed include tricyclic antidepressants or selective serotonin reuptake inhibitors (SSRIs) that may rebalance the autonomic nervous system; anti-anxiety medications to address anxiety symptoms; medications to address orthostatic hypotension; benzodiazepines to increase inhibitory neurotransmitter availability; alpha-adrenergic agonists to reduce sympathetic nervous system output; and nonsteroidal anti-inflammatory drugs (NSAIDs) to address pain (Axelrod, 2005; Low, 1997). Surgery may be utilized to correct certain conditions associated with the dysautonomia in order to relieve symptoms (Low, 1997).

In addition to the medical therapies, other nonmedical therapies are often recommended including physical activity, physical therapy, alternative therapies (i.e., yoga, massage, stretching, etc.), frequent small meals, a high-salt diet, fluid intake, and compression hose (Korczyn, 1995; Mathias & Bannister, 1999).

Javan Horwitz
Natalie Horwitz
Chad A. Noggle

Axelrod, F. (2005). Familial dysautonomia: A review of the current pharmacological treatments. *Expert Opinion in Pharmacotherapy, 6*(4), 561–567.

Baguley, I., Heriseanu, R., Cameron, I., Nott, M., & Slewa-Younan, S. (2008). A critical review of the pathophysiology of dysautonomia following traumatic brain injury. *Neocritical Care, 8*(2), 293–300.

Benarroch, E., Freeman, R., & Kaufmann, H. (2005). Autonomic nervous system. In C. G. Goetz (Ed.), *Textbook of clinical neurology* (3rd ed., pp. 383–404). Philadelphia: Saunders Elsevier.

Hilz, M., & Axelrod, F. (2000). Quantitative sensory testing of thermal and vibratory perception in familial dysautonomia. *Clinical Autonomic Research, 10*(4), 177–183.

Korczyn, A. (Ed.). (1995). *Handbook of autonomic nervous system dysfunction.* New York: Marcel Dekker.

Low, P. (Ed.). (1997). *Clinical autonomic disorders: Evaluation and management* (2nd ed.). Philadelphia: Lippincott-Raven Publishers.

Mathias, C., & Bannister, R. (Eds.). (1999). *Autonomic failure: A textbook of clinical disorders of the autonomic nervous system* (4th ed.). New York: Oxford University Press.

Newby, R., & Jaradeh, S. (2008). A mystery of perplexing symptoms: Neuropsychological assessment in a case of dysautonomia. In J. Apps, R. Newby, & L. Roberts (Eds.), *Pediatric neuropsychology case studies* (pp. 343–350). New York: Springer Publishing.

Poewe, W. (2007). Dysautonomia and cognitive dysfunction in Parkinson's disease. *Movement Disorders, 22*(17), 374–378.

Stewart, J., & Weldon, A. (2003). Contrasting neurovascular findings in chronic orthostatic intolerance and neurocardiogenic syncope. *Clinical Science, 104,* 329–340.

DYSSYNERGIA CEREBELLARIS MYOCLONICA

DESCRIPTION

Dyssynergia cerebellaris myoclonica, formerly known as Ramsay Hunt's syndrome, represents a syndrome of degenerative and neurological disorders that was first described in 1921 (Berkovic & Andermann, 1990; Marsden & Obeso, 1989). A rare form of progressive cerebellar muscular incoordination, it is more specifically characterized by myoclonus, cognitive impairment, epilepsy, and progressive ataxia. Intention tremor (dyskinetic disorder characterized by wide tremors during voluntary movement) represents one of the hallmark features of the presentation although it is often associated with convulsions and epileptic jerks as well. The tremors are usually found to originate in one extremity and spread gradually, eventually involving the entire voluntary motor system, with the arms usually being more disturbed than the legs. Dyssynergia cerebellaris myoclonica features also include an unsteady gait, loss of muscle tone, physical weakness and loss of strength (asthenia), errors in estimating the range, direction, and force of voluntary movements, and an inability to perform rapidly alternating movements of an extremity (adiadochokinesia), which are all symptoms of cerebellar syndrome. It is suggested that this disorder is genetically inherited with its onset usually in early adulthood, the average age being 30 years (National Institute of Neurologic Disorders and Strokes, 2007).

NEUROPATHOLOGY/PATHOPHYSIOLOGY

Some cases of dyssynergia cerebellaris myoclonica have appeared to be caused by mitochondrial abnormalities within the cells. From a genetic standpoint, the syndrome has been found to be inherited in an autosomal dominant manner, indicating that one parent has the abnormal gene and therefore the children have a 50:50 chance of inheriting the disorder. Other cases have shown the disorder to be inherited in an autosomal recessive manner, indicating that both parents have the defective gene and that the children develop the abnormal genes from both parents. The disease usually progresses over the course of about 10 years and ultimately results in the death of the patient. The specific neurological etiology has been suggested to be impairment in the regulatory mechanism between the nucleus dentatus, nucleus ruber, and the bulbar olive.

NEUROPSYCHOLOGICAL/CLINICAL PRESENTATION

Dyssynergia cerebellaris myoclonica is typically characterized by epilepsy, cognitive impairment, and myoclonus. The symptoms of cognitive impairment are typically mild intellectual deterioration. The patients usually have generalized epileptic seizures that become progressively worse over time. Patients also may have mild symptoms of cerebellar syndrome, but the most common symptom is a progressive ataxia. The syndrome begins with an intention tremor in the limbs, usually in the arms, which constitutes an involuntary shaking or trembling that occurs when an individual is attempting a voluntary movement and does not occur when the individual is at rest. Although the intention tremor typically occurs in one limb, the progression of the syndrome over time will cause the entire muscular system to be affected. Along with a tremor, sudden twitching or contraction of muscle groups can occur, a symptom called myoclonus. Some patients have been noted to experience progressive hearing impairment as well. As the disease progresses, symptoms worsen and begin to include decreased muscle tone, increased weakness and disturbances in fine motor control, difficulty walking, and unsteady gait. Ocular deficits including saccadic velocity reduction, saccadic latency increase, and abnormal smooth pursuit eye movements have also been reported. Structurally, CT scans sometimes show cerebral and cerebellar atrophy.

In addition, EEG studies have demonstrated spontaneous generalized fast-spike and -wave discharges, photosensitivity, and slow background activity.

DIAGNOSIS

The evaluation and diagnosis of dyssynergia cerebellaris myoclonica will typically include a thorough physical examination, neurological workup, neuropsychological evaluation, medical history, and family history (Cleveland Clinic, 2007). Diagnosis is made based on the symptoms that are present, specifically the myoclonus, epilepsy, and symptoms of cerebellar syndrome. Physical examination may reveal intention tremor, myoclonic jerks, convulsions, and/or epileptic jerks. As suggested previously, the tremors usually originate in one extremity and spread gradually, eventually involving the entire voluntary motor system. Furthermore, the patient's arms are usually more disturbed than the legs.

Patients typically exhibit an unsteady gait, loss of muscle tone, physical weakness, loss of strength (asthenia), errors in estimating the range, direction, and force of voluntary movements, and an inability to perform rapidly alternating movements of an extremity (adiadochokinesia), which are all symptoms of cerebellar syndrome. In waking EEG studies, there are spontaneous generalized fast-spike and -wave discharges that are noticeable (Roger, Genton, Bureau, Dravet, & Tassinari, 1989). Results of muscle biopsies in dyssynergia cerebellaris myoclonica are normal; however, some rare cases of "mitochondrial encephalomyopathy" have been reported. Neuropsychological evaluation may be of particular utility to reveal cognitive, visual, or hearing deficits as well as differentiating between other forms of progressive ataxia (Tassinari, Michelucci, Genton, Pellissier, & Roger, 1989). Neuropsychological evaluation can also reveal motor deficits in the upper extremities including muscle weakness and disruption in fine motor control. When done sequentially, neuropsychological assessment may also help to determine the prognosis and progression of the disorder.

TREATMENT

Treatment of dyssynergia cerebellaris myoclonica is symptom based as there is no cure for the disorder. Antiepileptic and neuropathic pain medications are often used to relieve myoclonus and epileptic symptoms. Valproate is a popular drug used to control these symptoms (Somerville & Olanow, 1982). Research has even shown that alcohol consumption can decrease myoclonus (Lu & Chu, 1991). Occupational therapy can be used to accomplish everyday tasks such as mobility, washing, dressing, eating, cooking, and grooming with which patients may have specific problems. There are a variety of assistive devices that can also be utilized to help the patients, including hearing aids if hearing loss is present, walkers or wheelchairs if the lower extremities are affected. Psychosocial interventions may be utilized to help the patient overcome any psychological or social ramifications of the disorder. With treatment, dyssynergia cerebellaris myoclonica syndrome carries a relatively good prognosis with excellent seizure control and very slow progression of the cerebellar syndrome and myoclonus.

Erin L. Tireman
Charles Golden

Berkovic, S. F., & Andermann, F. (1990). Ramsay Hunt syndrome: To bury or to praise. *Journal of Neurology, Neurosurgery, and Psychiatry, 53*, 89–90.

Cleveland Clinic. (2007). *Dyssynergia cerebellaris myoclonica.* Retrieved January 2, 2009, from Cleveland Clinic. Web site: http://my.clevelandclinic.org/disorders/hic_Dyssynergia_Cerebellaris_Myoclonica.aspx

Lu, C., & Chu, N. (1991). Effects of alcohol on myoclonus and somatosensory evoked potentials in dyssynergia cerebellaris myoclonica. *Journal of Neurology, Neurosurgery, and Psychiatry, 54*, 905–908.

Marsden, C. D., & Obeso, J. A. (1989). Viewpoints on the Ramsay Hunt syndrome. The Ramsay Hunt syndrome is a useful clinical entity. *Movement Disorders, 4*, 6–12.

National Institute of Neurologic Disorders and Strokes. (2007). *Dyssynergia Cerebellaris Myoclonus.* Retrieved January 4, 2009, from NINDS. Web site: http://www.ninds.nih.gov/disorders/dyssynergia/dyssynergia.htm

Roger, J., Genton, P., Bureau, M., Dravet, C., & Tassinari, C. A. (1989). Dyssynergia cerebellaris myoclonica (Ramsay Hunt's syndrome) associated with epilepsy: A study of 32 cases. *Neuropediatrics, 18*(1), 17.

Somerville, E. R., & Olanow, C. W. (1982). Valproic acid: Treatment of myoclonus in dyssynergia cerebellaris myoclonica. *Archives of Neurology, 39*(8), 527–552.

Tassinari, C. A., Michelucci, R., Genton, P., Pellissier, J. F., & Roger, J. (1989). Dyssynergia cerebellaris myoclonica (Ramsay Hunt syndrome): A condition unrelated to mitochondrial encephalomyopathies. *Journal of Neurology, Neurosurgery, and Psychiatry, 52*, 262–265.

DYSTONIAS

DESCRIPTIONS

The term "dystonia" was first coined by Hermann Oppenheim in 1911. It is one of the most common movement disorders in humans. Dystonia is a heterogeneous group of disorders characterized by sustained, twisting movements and abnormal postures, which are caused by involuntary, repetitive, and simultaneous contraction (cocontraction) of usually the same groups of opposing muscles (Fahn, 1988).

In one European study, the prevalence was 11.7 per 100,000 for focal dystonia and 3.5 per 100,000 for segmental and generalized dystonia. An earlier Minnesota-based study generated similar results. The frequency is much higher in Ashkenazi Jewish population (about 1/6000–1/2000) and slightly lower in East Asia (Fahn, Jankovic, Hallett, & Jenner, 2007a).

Unlike *chorea*, the abnormal movements in dystonia are usually more sustained and repeatedly involve the same muscle groups (patterned contraction). Contrary to the sinusoidal oscillation of true *tremor*, dystonic tremor is usually directional, that is, jerks in one direction alternate with slower movement in the opposite direction. Unlike *tics*, dystonia is not preceded by an uncomfortable feeling that is relieved by execution of the movement. However, dystonia does associate frequently with tremor and occasionally with myoclonus.

The speed of dystonic movements are determined by the duration of the cocontraction (Fahn et al., 2007a). Very brief (less than a second) cocontractions lead to *dystonic spasms*; several seconds of cocontractions give rise to *dystonic movement*; cocontractions lasting minutes to hours produce *dystonic postures*. When present for weeks, postures transform into permanent fixed *contractures*. Rarely, in children and adolescents with dystonia, sudden marked increase in the intensity of dystonia can lead to a crisis called *dystonia storm*, which can result in acute renal failure secondary to rhabdomyolysis.

NEUROPATHOLOGY/PATHOPHYSIOLOGY

The pathophysiology of primary dystonia is still largely a mystery. With advances in molecular biology, animal models, and neuroimaging, some light has been shed on the mechanism of dystonia.

So far, genetic defects have been identified in more than 10 primary dystonias (Table 1). These genetic disorders are mostly inherited as autosomal dominant conditions with reduced penetrance. The low penetrance indicates that both hereditary vulnerability and environmental insults are required in the manifestation of these primary dystonias.

DYT1, Oppenheim's dystonia, is associated with a three base pair ($\triangle$GAG) deletion in *DYT1* gene (Breakefield et al., 2008). This results in the loss of a glutamic acid residue in the carboxyl-terminal region of torsinA. This mutation leads to a loss of torsinA activity. TorsinA is universally expressed throughout the

Table 1
GENETIC CLASSIFICATION OF PRIMARY DYSTONIA

Locus	Dystonia Type	Protein	Inheritance	Chromosome
DYT1	Oppenheim's torsion dystonia	TorsinA	Autosomal dominant	9q34
DYT2	Autosomal recessive torsion dystonia	Unknown	Autosomal recessive	Unknown
DYT3	Lubag (dystonia-parkinsonism)	Transcription factors	X-linked recessive	Xq13.1
DYT4	Whispering dystonia	Unknown	Autosomal dominant	Unknown
DYT5	Dopa-responsive dystonia (DRD)	GTP-cyclohydrolase1	Autosomal dominant	14q22.1-2
		Tyrosine hydroxylase	Autosomal recessive	11p15.5
DYT6	Adolescent-onset dystonia of mixed type	Unknown	Autosomal dominant	8p21-22
DYT7	Adult-onset focal dystonia	Unknown	Autosomal dominant	18p
DYT8	Paroxysmal nonkinesigenic dyskinesias	Myofibrillogenesis regulator 1	Autosomal dominant	2q33-25
DYT9	Paroxysmal choreoathetosis with episodic ataxia and spasticity	Unknown	Autosomal dominant	1p21
DYT10	Paroxysmal kinesigenic choreoathetosis	Unknown	Autosomal dominant	16p-q
DYT11	Myoclonus dystonia	ϵ-Saroglycan	Autosomal dominant (maternal imprinting)	7q11q25
DYT12	Rapid-onset dystonia-parkinsonism	Na^+/K^+ ATPase $\alpha 3$ subunit	Autosomal dominant	19q
DYT13	Multifocal/segmental dystonia	Unknown	Autosomal dominant	1p
DYT15	Myoclonus dystonia	Unknown	Autosomal dominant	18p

Adapted from Breakefield et al. (2008); Fahn et al. (2007a); Tarsy & Simon (2006).

brain, especially with higher expression level during early brain development. It also presents predominantly in dopamine innervating and cholinergic interneurons in the basal ganglia. Intracellularly, torsinA is located mostly within the lumen of endoplasmic reticulum and nuclear envelope. It belongs to a family of so-called AAA+ (ATPases Associated with diverse cellular Activities) proteins. It has chaperone-like function and likely mediates ATP-dependent folding of substrate proteins.

Neurochemically, there were changes in norepinephrine, serotonin, and dopamine level in various regions of the brain. It is not clear which of these changes are related to the pathophysiology of dystonia. It is possible that failure to maintain an optimal level of activity in the dopamine pathways is pathogenic in dystonia. This hypothesis is supported by the following seemingly contradictory observations: the therapeutic effect of levodopa in dopa-responsive dystonia (DRD), dystonia caused by levodopa and dopamine agonists, dystonia induced by neuroleptics, and the frequent association of dystonia with parkinsonism.

Neuroanatomically, damage to a number of brain regions could produce dystonia – most commonly the basal ganglia, but also the thalamus, brainstem, parietal lobe, and cerebellum.

Theoretically, the patterned cocontraction of agonist and antagonist muscles in dystonia is caused by disturbed "reciprocal inhibition." Overflow dystonia, the contraction of adjacent and distant muscles, is underlined by impaired "surround inhibition." These impairments happen at multiple levels throughout the central nervous system (Fahn et al., 2007a).

NEUROPSYCHOLOGICAL/CLINICAL PRESENTATION

Traditionally, it was believed dystonia patients were relatively free of psychopathology. However, in general, depression is a major comorbidity for dystonia (Heiman et al., 2004). A recent study reports a prevalence of obsessive-compulsive disorder in 20% of patients with primary focal dystonias (Cavallaro et al., 2002). Attention-executive cognitive deficits also have been found in patients with primary dystonia (Scott et al., 2003).

Voluntary movement almost always worsens dystonia (Geyer & Bressman, 2006). When dystonia only presents during voluntary movement, it is called *action dystonia*. In *task-specific dystonia*, dystonic movements present only with particular actions, such as embouchure dystonia of perioral muscles in woodwind musicians. As the disease progresses, actions in remote regions of the body can elicit dystonic movement in the affected regions, so-called *overflow*. Talking is the most common mechanism for producing *overflow dystonia* in other parts of the body. With still further deterioration, *dystonia at rest* ensues. *Paradoxical dystonia*, which is the reverse phenomenon of overflow dystonia, occasionally takes place in dystonia at rest, that is, dystonic movement is abated by voluntary movement. Focal dystonia affecting facial and oromandibular muscles is commonly reduced by voluntary movement. Many patients discover that a tactile or proprioceptive "sensory trick" (*geste antagoniste*), such as touching the involved body part or an adjacent body part, can diminish dystonic activity. Like many movement disorders, dystonia is exacerbated by fatigue, stress, and emotions, and the movements usually subside with relaxation, hypnosis, or sleep.

Classifications of dystonia (Table 2) are based on age of onset, distribution, and cause (Geyer & Bressman, 2006; Tarsy & Simon, 2006).

Age of onset is the single most important factor in predicting the prognosis of primary dystonia. The early-onset dystonias usually first involve limbs. The late-onset ones commonly affect muscles of head and neck. In general, the earlier the age of onset, the more likely it will progress to generalized dystonia. On the contrary, late-onset dystonia tends to remain focal or segmental.

Focal dystonia affects a single body region. For example, *blepharospasm* causes frequent blinking, forced eye closure, or difficulty opening the eyes. *Torticollis* (cervical dystonia) begins as neck stiffness and restricted head mobility, followed by abnormal head posture and irregular head tremor. *Oromandibular dystonia* exhibits involuntary clenching, opening, and lateral shift of the jaw. Severe cases result in jaw pain, dysarthria, dysphagia, and dental trauma. *Spastic dysphonia* is an action dystonia in which talking induces vocal cord adduction (which leads to voice breaks and strain) or abduction (which produces an intermittent, breathy voice). *Writer's cramp* involves involuntary hand postures that interfere with handwriting. Gender appears to play a role in both the prevalence and age at onset of focal dystonia. Women are more at risk and have an earlier age at onset for writer's cramp, but men have an earlier age at onset for cervical dystonia, blepharospasm, and laryngeal dystonia.

Segmental dystonia involves two or more adjacent body regions. *Multifocal dystonia* applies to the involvement of two or more nonadjacent body regions. *Generalized dystonia* is associated with abnormal movements in the legs and at least one part of other areas of the body. *Hemidystonia* affects ipsilateral arm and leg. The anatomical distribution has some prognostic value – complete remissions can occur in patients with cervical dystonia, but remissions occur rarely in generalized dystonia and are usually partial.

Primary dystonias are not accompanied by other neurological comorbidities, except for occasional tremor and myoclonus (Geyer & Bressman, 2006; Tarsy & Simon, 2006). Except for some genetic mutations (see Table 1), no known causes have been identified. In primary dystonia, there are no neuroanatomical abnormalities in imaging studies and no inborn metabolic defects. Most primary dystonias are focal or segmental in distribution, with onset in adulthood. Cervical dystonia is the most common form of primary dystonia.

Secondary dystonia is a large and diverse group of disorders that results from other disease states or exogenous insults; additional neurological deficits are usually present. However, neuroleptics-induced acute dystonia and tardive dystonia usually only consist of dystonic movement. Generalized dystonia of late onset generally indicates secondary dystonia. The causes of secondary dystonia include brain injury, trauma and tumor, medications (levodopa, D2 receptor blockers, anticonvulsants, and ergotism), other toxins, psychogenic factors, and so forth (Geyer & Bressman, 2006).

Dystonia-plus syndrome is a subtype of secondary dystonia associated with parkinsonism or myoclonus, but there is no evidence of neurodegeneration. It is comprised of DRD, myoclonus-dystonia, and rapid-onset dystonia-parkinsonism.

DRD Dopa-responsive dystonia (DYT5) is easily treated and should always be considered in the differential diagnosis of dystonia (Breakefield et al., 2008). This disorder presents in early childhood with features of parkinsonism and abnormal gaits (walking

D

Table 2
CLASSIFICATION OF DYSTONIA

By Age of Onset	By Distribution	By Cause
Early-onset (≤ 26 years)	Focal	Primary
Late-onset (≥ 26 years)	Segmental Multifocal Generalized Hemidystonia	Secondary

From *Principles and practice of movement disorders* (pp. 307–343), by Fahn, S., Jankovic, J., Hallett, M., and Jenner, P. (2007a). Churchill Livingstone Elsevier. Adapted with permission.

on toes), and eventually develops into generalized dystonia. The symptoms usually worsen over the course of the day (diurnal fluctuation). Dramatic and sustained response to low-dose levodopa is the hallmark of this disorder. DRD is inherited in an autosomal-dominant pattern with reduced penetrance. It affects girls more than boys. The mutations severely impair the activity of GTP-cyclohydrolase I, the rate-limiting enzyme in the synthesis of tetrahydrobiopterin, which is a cofactor of monoamine-synthesizing enzyme tyrosine hydroxylase for dopamine and norepinephrine and tryptophan hydroxylase for serotonin. Other variants of DRD result from mutations in genes encoding tyrosine hydroxylase or other enzymes involved in pterin metabolism. All these mutations diminish the activity of tyrosine hydroxylase, which is why low-dose levodopa is efficacious in this disorder since it bypasses this enzymatic defect.

Heredodegenerative dystonia is an inherited disorder with histopathological evidence of brain degeneration. In many of these cases, there are other prominent defects in addition to dystonia, such as mental retardation and neurological deficits. Neuroimaging is usually abnormal. It was thought that the etiology of this type of dystonia is due to disruption in basal ganglia function or dopamine synthesis. Examples for this subtype of dystonia include Wilson's disease, Parkinson's disease, Huntington's disease, lysosomal storage disorders and mitochondrial disorders, and so forth. A more complete list can be found in Geyer and Bressman (2006).

DIAGNOSIS

The diagnosis of dystonia begins with in-depth history taking and physical examination. Special attention needs to be given to birth, developmental stage and history, medication, toxin, trauma, and family history. The goal is to determine whether the dystonia is primary or secondary.

Secondary dystonia commonly has the following features (Geyer & Bressman, 2006): history of exogenous etiology such as trauma or drug exposure; presence of neurological abnormality other than dystonia; onset of dystonia at rest instead of action dystonia; hemidystonia; early onset of speech abnormality; abnormal brain imaging; and abnormal laboratory results. Psychogenic dystonia usually exhibits give-way weakness, false sensory loss, and inconsistent or incongruent movement.

Brain MRI is critical for assessment of secondary dystonia. Imaging studies might reveal a stroke, arteriovenous malformation, or mass lesion such as a tumor or abscess located in the basal ganglia or thalamus or less frequently, in the parietal lobe or cerebellum. If the only neurological deficit is dystonia, searching for rare degenerative or metabolic disorders is unlikely to be productive.

Treatable dystonias need to be aggressively pursued. For example, Wilson's disease should be explored in any patient whose dystonia begins before age 50. Geyer and Bressman (2006) recommended starting with slit-lamp examination to look for Kayser – Fleischer rings and measuring serum ceruloplasmin levels and 24-hr urine copper levels. If these examinations are normal and suspicion remains high, liver biopsy would be the next step to measure hepatic copper content. In Wilson's disease, brain MRI usually shows the face-of-the-giant-panda sign (Geyer & Bressman, 2006) (reflecting hyperintensity in the midbrain tegmentum sparing the red nucleus, preserved signal intensity in the lateral substantia nigra pars reticulate, and hypointensity of the superior colliculus).

TREATMENT

Even though the etiology of primary dystonia is still largely unknown and disease-reversing treatment is still elusive, the current symptomatic treatment of dystonia has greatly improved. It is composed of physical, medical, and surgical therapy (Fahn, Jankovic, Hallett, & Jenner, 2007b; Jankovic, 2006).

Patient education, genetic counseling, and addressing comorbid depression and orthopedic problems are valuable parts of a comprehensive approach to dystonia. Physical therapy and well-fitted braces are used to improve posture and prevent contractures. The brace functions as a substitute to "sensory tricks." For instance, neck and head braces are used to alleviate cervical dystonia, and hand devices are designed to help patients with writer's cramp. It is still controversial whether immobilization with a splint either reduces or exacerbates focal limb dystonia. It was speculated that this type of maneuver results in brain topographic reorganization by removing all motor and sensory input to a limb. Muscle relaxation and biofeedback therapy are useful adjuncts too. It was reported that transcranial magnetic stimulation temporarily improved handwriting in patients with writer's cramp (Siebner et al., 1999).

Except copper chelating treatment in Wilson's disease and levodopa in DRD, there is no specific medication for dystonia. Patients with DRD improve with levodopa, dopamine agonists, anticholinergic drugs, and carbamazepine. DRD may be diagnosed with a trial of levodopa. The starting dose is carbidopa/levodopa 12.5/50 mg a day, which is slowly titrated up to 300–600 mg of levodopa a day over weeks. Generally, lack of response to 300 mg/day excludes the diagnosis of DRD.

Anticholinergic agents, including trihexyphenidyl, benztropine, and diphehydramine, are useful in treating segmental and generalized dystonia. Trihexyphenidyl is started at 1 mg at bedtime and increased to 12 mg a day over 4 weeks. Some patients need up to 60–100 mg a day, which commonly associates with drowsiness, confusion, amnesia, and hallucinations.

Other potentially beneficial medications include benzodiazepins, baclofen, carbamazepine, tetrabenazine, and so forth. One of the most important breakthroughs in the treatment of dystonia is the introduction of botulinum toxin in the 1980s (Jankovic, 2004). At present, the FDA has approved two preparations, botulinum A (Botox) and B (Myobloc) to treat focal dystonia. Botulinum toxin blocks the release of acetylcholine into the neuromuscular junction causing focal temporary chemical-induced denervation and muscle paralysis. In addition to its peripheral effects, this toxin might also change central nervous system abnormalities by suppressing afferent feedback from muscles. Imaging studies indicated that treatment with botulinum toxin normalized the hemispheric asymmetries observed in some dystonia patients (Blood et al., 2006). One possible setback of this treatment is loss of efficacy after long-term use due to development of blocking antibody, though the risk is quite rare with current formulation. Botulinum toxin is not only safe and effective but also leads to meaningful improvements in quality of life, and the benefits are long lasting.

In the past, dystonia patients were treated with pallidotomy or thalamotomy. These procedures have been replaced by deep brain stimulation (DBS) of the globus pallidus (Jankovic, 2006), which mimics the effects of lesions. DBS imposes much lower risk of complications, and its stimulation parameter can be customized individually. This procedure tends to be more effective in early-onset dystonia. It produces a gradual improvement, which maximizes at around 3–6 months.

Haojing Huang

Blood, A. J., Tuch, D. S., Makris, N., Makhlouf, M. L., Sudarsky, L. R., & Sharma, N. (2006). White matter abnormalities in dystonia normalize after botulinum toxin treatment. *Neuroreport, 17,* 1251–1255.

Breakefield, X. O., Blood, A. J., Li, Y., Hallett, M., Hanson, P. I., & Standaert, D. G. (2008). The pathophysiological basis of dystonias. *Nature Reviews Neuroscience, 9,* 222–234.

Cavallaro, R., Galardi, G., Cavallini, M. C., Henin, M., Amodio, S., Bellodi, L., et al. (2002). Obsessive compulsive disorder among idiopathic focal dystonia patients: An epidemiological and family study. *Biological Psychiatry, 52,* 356–361.

Fahn, S. (1988). Concept and classification of dystonia. *Advances in Neurology, 50,* 1–8.

Fahn, S., Jankovic, J., Hallett, M., & Jenner, P. (2007a). Dystonia – phenomenology, classification, etiology, pathology, biochemistry, and genetics. In S. Fahn, J. Jankovic, M. Hallett, & P. Jenner (Eds.), *Principles and practice of movement disorders* (pp. 307–343). Churchill Livingstone Elsevier.

Fahn, S., Jankovic, J., Hallett, M., & Jenner, P. (2007b). Treatment of dystonia. In S. Fahn, J. Jankovic, M. Hallett, & P. Jenner (Eds.), *Principles and practice of movement disorders* (pp. 345–367). Churchill Livingstone Elsevier.

Geyer, H. L., & Bressman, S. B. (2006). The diagnosis of dystonia. *Lancet Neurology, 5,* 780–790.

Heiman, G. A., Ottman, R., Saunders-Pullman, R. J., Ozelius, L. J., Risch, N. J., & Bressman, S. B. (2004). Increased risk for recurrent major depression in DYT1 dystonia mutation carriers. *Neurology, 63,* 631–637.

Jankovic, J. (2004). Botulinum toxin in clinical practice. *Journal of Neurology, Neurosurgery, and Psychiatry, 75,* 951–957.

Jankovic, J. (2006). Treatment of dystonia. *Lancet Neurology, 5,* 864–872.

Scott, R. B., Gregory, R., Wilson, J., Banks, S., Turner, A., Parkin, S., et al. (2003). Executive cognitive deficits in primary dystonia. *Movement Disorders, 18,* 539–550.

Siebner, H. R., Tormos, J. M., Ceballos-Baumann, A. O., Auer, C., Catala, M. D., Conrad, B., et al. (1999). Low-frequency repetitive transcranial magnetic stimulation of the motor cortex in writer's cramp. *Neurology, 52,* 529–537.

Tarsy, D., & Simon, D. K. (2006). Dystonia. *The New England Journal of Medicine, 355,* 818–829.

EATING DISORDERS

DESCRIPTION

Eating disorders (ED) are loosely defined as maladaptive patterns of eating. The disorders involve extreme patterns of eating, including eating too little or too much, in combination with distressing feelings related to self-image and body weight (National Institute of Mental Health [NIMH], 2009a). The two major subtypes of ED as recognized by the *Diagnostic and Statistical Manual of Mental Disorders* (4th ed., text revision) (*DSM IV-TR*) are anorexia nervosa and bulimia nervosa, though the diagnosis of ED not otherwise specified (NOS) is also commonly used in clinical practice to describe a subthreshold clinical presentation of symptoms (American Psychiatric Association [APA], 2000). Anorexia nervosa is characterized by severely disturbed cognitions regarding body image and the associated physiological problems that result; for example, the inability to maintain appropriate body weight because of morbid fear of gaining weight (Striefel-Moore & Smolak, 2001). Bulimia nervosa is also characterized by very poor self-image but is defined by the pattern of binging and an associated compensatory behavior such as fasting, excessive exercise, and/or laxative use (APA, 2000). Within the NOS category is a set of symptoms that have received recent investigation in the literature and are classified as binge eating disorder, with a push to be considered its own formal diagnosis in the future.

Prevalence of ED in the population is approximately 10% (Striefel-Moore & Smolak, 2001); bulimia nervosa is reported with higher incidence at 1% to 3%, and anorexia nervosa 1% (APA, 2000). Generally, prevalence is highest among women and adolescent girls for all types of ED, though it could be conceived that these gender differences may become less disparate in the future with increased societal pressures for male thinness. Caucasian females report higher incidences of ED, with African American and Asian American females reporting the fewest cases. Comorbidity with other psychiatric disorders is very common.

It is important to note the financial costs and societal implications associated with these disorders. In the past decade, an 18% increase in hospital admissions due in part to physical complications of ED has been reported (Agency for Healthcare Research and Quality [AHRQ], 2009). The AHRQ also found a sharp increase in the prevalence of ED among young children (12 years and younger), a particularly important trend since eating disturbances are generally thought to have an onset in adolescence. This report proposed few variations in medical treatment planning and prevention programs. The decrease in costs associated with the disorder and increase of incidence among young people was not addressed.

NEUROPATHOLOGY/PATHOPHYSIOLOGY

The pathophysiology of ED is still unknown, though research in the area is growing. Neuropsychological functioning has been reviewed with varying results within each of the disorders. Psychomotor speed (Jones, Duncan, Brouwers, & Mirsky, 1991; Kingston, Szmukler, Andrewes, Tress, & Desmond, 1996), sustained attention (Laessle, Krieg, Fichter, & Pirke, 1996), selective attention (Jones et al., 1991), and memory (Bayless et al., 2002) have been found to be deficient in patients with anorexia nervosa, though interpretation of these results should be made with caution since other researchers have not consistently found such outcomes. One hypothesis that has been developed to account for these differences relates to the fatigue and lack of energy that is associated with these disorders, which may be manifesting as slower speed, impaired attention, and deficient memory skills (Duchesne et al., 2004). Furthermore, an increase in the ventricular-brain ratio is thought to be present in patients with anorexia nervosa (APA, 2000), as is disturbance of the right parietal lobe (Bradley et al., 1997; Kinsbourne & Bemporad, 1984).

With regard to bulimia nervosa, fewer differences in comparison to normal controls have been reported. Psychomotor retardation (Ferraro, Wonderlich, & Jocic, 1997) and deficits in executive functioning have been noted (Kaye, Bastiani, & Moss, 1995). Specifically related to executive functioning is the inability to inhibit the urge to binge eat and purge. Memory and attention have been studied by several researchers with no significant differences between bulimia nervosa and normals (Duchesne et al., 2004).

E

NEUROPSYCHOLOGICAL/CLINICAL PRESENTATION

Clinical presentation of ED varies according to the type of disorder and severity of symptoms. Symptoms of anorexia nervosa are oftentimes related to the semi-starvation state of the patient. Thus, along with the aforementioned symptoms, patients commonly also report amenorrhea (lack of menstruation), abdominal pain, constipation, fatigue, lack of energy, and cold intolerance (APA, 2000). The most noticeable indicator upon physical examination is the emaciated body of the patient. Mild anemia, hypotension, and dry skin can also be seen (APA, 2000).

Patients with bulimia nervosa may present as seemingly healthy individuals, as the hallmark symptoms of the disorder are often done in isolation when others are not present. Dental decay and cavities are often present as a result of recurrent vomiting. Secondary gastrointestinal and dental disorders have been reported. Furthermore, oftentimes scarring or calluses may develop on the top part of the hand from scraping the teeth when stimulating the gag reflex (APA, 2000). Patients who frequently utilize laxatives may develop constipation upon termination of their use. Amenorrhea can be present in patients with bulimia nervosa, and in rare cases esophageal tears may be present. Excessive exercising is also a symptom of bulimia nervosa but may be present within the NOS category as well.

DIAGNOSIS

Diagnosis of ED is made based on the diagnostic criteria in the *DSM IV-TR*. The most characteristic symptom of anorexia nervosa is the inability or the refusal of the patient to maintain an appropriate body weight for size and age, as determined by body weight less than 85% of which is expected (APA, 2000). The difficulty with this rather arbitrary cutoff weight is that there are often individual differences within this range that are not clinically pathological (Herzog & Delinsky, 2001). Pubertal differences and maturational change are not accounted for in this cutoff definition, and further research in the area is needed to solidify a more precise diagnostic criterion to define expected weight. Nevertheless, intense fears of being fat or gaining weight, maladaptive self-image, and amenorrhea for three consecutive months are also diagnostic criteria for anorexia nervosa (APA, 2000). Specifiers of restricting type and binge eating/purging type can be used to further classify the disorder.

The defining symptom of bulimia nervosa is the cycle of binging and compensatory behaviors. These symptoms are required to be present at least two times a week for 3 months, and disturbance in self-image must also present to warrant the diagnosis. Difficulties with this diagnosis include the lack of empirical support for a clear definition of binge eating. Herzog and Delinsky in their 2001 review of the literature, reported studies that were inconclusive at finding an appropriate "amount" of food required to be considered a "binge." They reported suggestions of using clearer definitions that related to the mood of the patient or the quality rather than quantity of the binge to clarify this issue. Specifiers of purging and nonpurging types are used to further classify the disorder (APA, 2000). Though bulimia nervosa is commonly thought to be related to strictly binging and purging behaviors, patients may also engage in fasting, excessive exercise, or the use of laxatives as compensatory behaviors, thus the nonpurging type specifier. Differential diagnosis between anorexia nervosa, purging type and bulimia nervosa, purging type lies in the refusal to maintain appropriate body weight in anorexia nervosa, whereas patients with bulimia nervosa may be normal weight or even overweight.

Patients presenting with symptoms that are sub-threshold of anorexia nervosa or bulimia nervosa are often diagnosed with ED NOS. This would account for patients with eating disturbances that do not meet all the criteria for either of the aforementioned disorders, but the disturbance created significant difficulties in one or more domains of the patient's life.

TREATMENT

Various psychiatric and pharmacological approaches in the treatment of ED have been reported. Psychotherapy is generally recommended, though typically patients need to be physically and nutritionally stable prior to the onset. Cognitive behavior therapy is cited as the best psychotherapeutic approach (Streigel-Moore & Smolak, 2001), though family therapy with adolescent patients is also advantageous when trying to change maladaptive patterns of eating. Coordination between medical doctors, nutritionists, and mental health therapists is critical in developing treatment planning, as both physical (returning to healthy body weight, eliminating purging behaviors) and emotional facets (body image misperceptions, fear of being fat) need to be addressed. Evidence-based success of pharmacological approaches with anorexia nervosa are sparse within the literature (Berkman et al., 2006) particularly because they often require complex or multiple interventions and dismiss the severity of their illness (Mitchell, 2001). In a literature review of psychopharmacological approaches, Mitchell (2001) reported the efficacy of selective serotonin reuptake inhibitors (SSRIs) with anorexia nervosa patients, in combination with other types of nonpharmocological treatments. At present, fluoxetine is the only FDA-approved drug in the treatment of bulimia nervosa (NIMH, 2009b) and is also generally used in combination with psychotherapy and/or nutritional therapy.

Identifying risk factors associated with all types of ED would be very helpful in the prevention and treatment. Risk factors for ED include careers that require thinness (dancers, gymnasts), extreme levels of stress, history of abuse, or a family history of ED, or other addiction (Garfinkel & Dorian, 2001). Obesity is a risk factor that is specific to bulimia nervosa, though it may contribute to many cases of ED NOS as well. The presence of other psychiatric disorders, such as mood or anxiety disorders, is also considered to be a risk in the development of ED.

Beth Trammell
Raymond S. Dean

Agency for Healthcare Research and Quality. (2009). *Eating disorders sending more Americans to the hospital.* Retrieved September 10, 2009, from http://www.ahrq.gov/news/nn/nn040109.htm

American Psychiatric Association. (2000). *Diagnostic and statistical manual of mental disorders IV-R.* Arlington, VA: Author.

Bayless, J. D., Kanz, J. E., Moser, D. J., McDowell, B. D., Bowers, W. A., Andersen, A. E., et al. (2002). Neuropsychological characteristics of patients in a hospital-based eating disorder program. *Annals of Clinical Psychiatry, 14,* 203–207.

Berkman, N. D., Bulik, C. M., Brownley, K. A., Lohr, K. N., Sedway, J. A., Rooks, A., et al. (2006). *Management of eating disorders* (Evidence Report/Technology Assessment No. 135. AHRQ Publication No. 06-E010). Rockville, MD: Agency for Healthcare Research and Quality.

Bradley, S. J., Taylor, M. J., Rovet, J. F., Goldberg, E., Hood, J., Wachsmuth, R., et al. (1997). Assessment of brain function in adolescent anorexia nervosa before and after weight gain. *Journal of Clinical and Experimental Neuropsychology, 19,* 20–33.

Duchesne, M., Mattos, P., Fontenelle, L. F., Veiga, H., Rizo, L., & Appolinario, J. C. (2004). Neuropsychology of eating disorders: A systematic review of the literature. *Review of Brazil Psychiatry, 26,* 107–117.

Ferraro, F. R., Wonderlich, S., & Jocic, A. (1997). Performance variability as a new theoretical mechanism regarding eating disorders and cognitive processing. *Journal of Clinical Psychology, 53,* 117–121.

Garfinkel, P. E., & Dorian, B. J. (2001). Improving understanding and care for the eating disorders. In R. H. Streigel-Moore & L. Smolak (Eds.), *Eating disorders: Innovative directions in research and practice* (pp. 9–26). Washington DC: American Psychological Association.

Herzog, D. B., & Delinsky, S. S. (2001). Classification of eating disorders. In R. H. Streigel-Moore & L. Smolak (Eds.), *Eating disorders: Innovative directions in research and practice* (pp. 31–50). Washington, DC: American Psychological Association.

Jones, B. P., Duncan, C. C., Brouwers, P., & Mirsky, A. F. (1991). Cognition in eating disorders. *Journal of Clinical and Experimental Neuropsychology, 13,* 711–728.

Kaye, W. H., Bastiani, A. M., & Moss, H. (1995). Cognitive style of patients with anorexia nervosa and bulimia nervosa. *International Journal of Eating Disorders, 18,* 287–290.

Kingston, K., Szmukler, G., Andrewes, D., Tress, B., & Desmond, P. (1996). Neuropsychological and structural brain changes in anorexia nervosa before and after refeeding. *Psychological Medicine, 26,* 15–28.

Kinsbourne, M., & Bemporad, B. (1984). Lateralization of emotion: A model and the evidence. In N. A. Fox & R. J. Davidson (Eds.), *The psychology of affective development* (pp. 259–292). Hillsdale, NJ: Erlbaum.

Laessle, R. G., Krieg, J. C., Fichter, M. M., & Pirke, K. M. (1996). Cerebral atrophy and vigilance performance in patient with anorexia nervosa and bulimia nervosa. *Neuropsychobiology, 21,* 187–191.

Mitchell, J. E. (2001). Psychopharmacology of eating disorders: Current knowledge and future directions. In R. H. Streigel-Moore & L. Smolak (Eds.), *Eating disorders: Innovative directions in research and practice* (pp. 197–212). Washington, DC: American Psychological Association.

National Institute of Mental Health. (2009a). *Anorexia Nervosa.* Retrieved September 6, 2009, from http://www.nimh.nih.gov/health/publications/eating-disorders/anorexia-nervosa.shtml

National Institute of Mental Health. (2009b). *Bulimia Nervosa.* Retrieved September 6, 2009, from http://www.nimh.nih.gov/health/publications/eating-disorders/bulimia-nervosa.shtml

Striefel-Moore, R. H., & Smolak, L. (2001). *Eating Disorders: Innovative directions in research and practice.* Washington, DC: American Psychological Association.

EMPTY SELLA SYNDROME

DESCRIPTION

Empty sella syndrome (ESS) involves a saddle-shaped bony structure called the sella turcica located at the base of the brain and surrounds and protects the pituitary gland. Sella turcica means *Turkish saddle* in Latin. The appearance of an empty sella is seen on neurological imaging when the pituitary gland flattens or shrinks. This phenomenon is referred to as ESS. In the majority of cases, the pituitary gland may be a bit smaller or even of normal size but still functions normally. In other rare cases, the sella turcia may grow larger than normal. A truly empty sella, a missing pituitary gland, is very rare (Bjerre, 1990; Polzin, 2005).

NEUROPATHOLOGY/PATHOPHYSIOLOGY

The pituitary gland, an endocrine gland, secretes several hormones that mediate function of other glands throughout the body, including the thyroid and adrenal glands. It regulates homeostasis, blood pressure, and growth among other important functions (Aron, Findling, & Tyrrell, 2004). The pituitary gland is functionally linked to the hypothalamus by the pituitary stalk. The pituitary gland normally fills the sella turcica. The subarachnoid space surrounds the pituitary stalk, which is filled with cerebrospinal fluid (CSF). The diaphragma sella is a protective barrier formed by the dura mater between the pituitary gland and subarachnoid space (Aron et al., 2004; Polzin, 2005). There are two types of ESS, primary and secondary. Patients with primary ESS have a defect of the diaphragma sella, usually an opening in the membrane causing excessive CSF pressure on the pituitary gland and the walls of the sella turcica. This pressure causes the pituitary gland to flatten (Bjerre, 1990; Kaye, Tress, Brownbill, & King, 1982). Primary ESS is typically seen in women with obesity and hypertension (Jordan, Kendall, & Kerber, 1977). Secondary ESS typically occurs after an injury, surgery, or radiation therapy causing the pituitary gland to regress within the sella turcica. In rare cases, the pituitary gland is completely destroyed (Lee & Adams, 1968).

NEUROPSYCHOLOGICAL/CLINICAL PRESENTATION

Patients with ESS usually present with minimal symptoms or no symptoms at all; however, in rare cases, ESS can produce serious symptoms. Symptoms of primary ESS are often due to excessive build up of CSF causing intracranial pressure contributing to headaches, CSF leakage from the nose, and vision problems (Schlosser & Bolger, 2003). Other symptoms due to pituitary dysfunction may be present, though they are considered rare (e.g., hypertension in women, erectile dysfunction, irregular or absent menstruation, or lowered libido in men, infertility due to increased prolactin levels in women; Jordan et al., 1977). In secondary ESS, patients present with disorders that

reflect the loss or reduction of pituitary function including hypoadrenalism, hypothyroidism, and hypogonadism. Symptoms often include decreased production of sex hormones, decreased libido, impotence in men, amenorrhea in women, infertility in women, low blood pressure, hypoglycemia, diminished metabolism, intolerance of cold temperatures, fatigue, constipation, muscle aches, dry skin, and dry hair (Lee & Adams, 1968). Children with primary ESS are often symptomatic and typically present with growth hormone deficiency. Pituitary tumors, pituitary dysfunction, and early onset puberty is typical seen in children with ESS (Naing & Frohman, 2007; Surtees, Adams, Price, Clayton, & Shalet, 1987). The neuropsychological presentation associated with pituitary dysfunction can include mental slowness and apathy impacting processing speed, working memory, and executive functioning. Given the impact of pituitary dysfunction on patient's lives (e.g., infertility and sexual dysfunction), emotional disturbances including anxiety and depression are often present (Weitzner, Kanfer, & Booth-Jones, 2005).

DIAGNOSIS

Diagnosis is based on specific clinical features and evidence from radiological imaging including CT or MRI (Polzin, 2005). Imaging can be useful in differentiating ESS from other syndromes that produce an enlarged sella. Although in most cases of ESS the pituitary function is normal, other laboratory analysis including blood analysis is usually performed to rule out possible endocrinological abnormalities (Chen, Ying, Yao, Chiu, & Chan, 2008; Gallardo et al., 1992). Occasionally, tests for increased intracranial pressure will be performed, including a lumbar puncture and a retinal examination by an ophthalmologist (Schlosser & Bolger, 2003).

TREATMENT

ESS is not life threatening and usually does not impact life expectancy. In many cases, patients are asymptomatic and do not require any medical intervention. For patients who are symptomatic, treatment for ESS typically involves management of pituitary dysfunction, such as hormone replacement therapy to replace deficient or lacking hormones (Vance, 1994). For patients presenting with increased prolactin levels, bromocriptine may be prescribed to lower prolactin levels to reduce infertility and restore function to the ovaries and testes (De Marinis, Bonadonna, Bianchi, Maira, & Giustina, 2005). All treatments for ESS only manage its symptoms. There is currently no cure for ESS or no procedure to restore the pituitary gland (Polzin, 2005).

Darla J. Lawson

Aron, D. C., Findling, J. W., & Tyrrell, B. (2004). Hypothalamus and pituitary gland. In F. S. Greenspan & D. G. Gardner (Eds.), *Basic and clinical endocrinology* (7th ed., pp. 106–175). Philadelphia, PA: McGraw Hill.

Bjerre, P. (1990). The empty sella. A reappraisal of etiology and pathogenesis. *Acta Neurologica Scandinavica Supplementum, 130,* 1–25.

Chen, C. Y., Ying, S. H., Yao, M. S., Chiu, W. T., & Chan, W. P. (2008). Sphenoid sinus osteoma at the sella turcica associated with empty sella: CT and MR imaging findings. *American Journal of Neuroradiology, 29,* 550–551.

De Marinis, L., Bonadonna, S., Bianchi, A., Maira G., & Giustina, A. (2005). Primary empty sella. *The Journal of Clinical Endocrinology and Metabolism, 90*(9), 5471–5477.

Gallardo, E., Schächter, D., Cáceres, E., Becker, P., Colin, E., Martínez, C., et al. (1992). The empty sella: Results of treatment in 76 successive cases and high frequency of endocrine and neurological disturbances. *Clinical Endocrinology, 37,* 529–533.

Jordan, R. M., Kendall, J. W., & Kerber, C. W. (1977). The primary empty sella syndrome: Analysis of the clinical characteristics, radiographic features, pituitary function and cerebrospinal fluid adenohypophysial hormone concentrations. *American Journal of Medicine, 62*(4), 569–580.

Kaye, A. H., Tress, B. M., Brownbill, D., & King, J. (1982). Intracranial pressure in patients with the empty sella syndrome without benign intracranial hypertension. *Journal of Neurology, Neurosurgery, and Psychiatry, 45,* 209–216.

Lee, W. M., & Adams, J. E. (1968). The empty sella syndrome. *Journal of Neurosurgery, 28*(4), 351–356.

Naing, S., & Frohman, L. A. (2007). The empty sella. *Pediatric Endocrinology Review, 4*(4), 335–342.

Polzin, S. J. (2005). Empty sella syndrome. In S. L. Chamberlin & B. Narins (Eds.), *Gale encyclopedia of neurological disorders.* Detroit, MI: The Gale Group. Retrieved March 17, 2009, from http://www.healthline.com/galecontent/empty-sella-syndrome

Schlosser, R. J., & Bolger, W. E. (2003). Significance of empty sella in cerebrospinal fluid leaks. *Otolaryngology: Head and Neck Surgery, 130*(4), 443–448.

Surtees, R., Adams, J., Price, D., Clayton, P., & Shalet, S. (1987). Association of adverse perinatal events with an empty sella turcica in children with growth hormone deficiency. *Hormone Research, 28,* 5–12.

Vance, M. V. (1994). Hypopituitarism. *New England Journal of Medicine, 330*(23), 1651–1662.

Weitzner, M. A., Kanfer, S., & Booth-Jones, M. (2005). Apathy and pituitary disease: It has nothing to do with depression. *Journal of Neuropsychiatry and Clinical Neurosciences, 17,* 159–166.

ENCEPHALITIS

DESCRIPTION

Encephalitis is an inflammation of the brain, which may be acute or chronic. Although the most frequent cause of acute infectious encephalitis is viral, it may also be mediated by bacterial (i.e., *Mycobacterium tuberculosis*, *M. pneumonia*, and *Bartonella*), fungal (i.e., *Cryptococcus*, Aspergillosis), or parasitic (i.e., *Toxoplasma gondii*, cerebral malaria, human African trypanosomiasis) agents (Kennedy, 2004). Inflammatory encephalopathies include acute disseminated encephalomyelitis (ADEM), which typically follows an infection or vaccination, and acute hemorrhagic leukoencephalopathy (AHLE), a more severe variant of ADEM. Chronic encephalitis includes subacute sclerosing panencephalitis (SSPE), which is preceded by a measles infection; paraneoplastic limbic encephalitis, which is associated with malignancy; and Rasmussen's encephalitis of which the etiology is unknown (for A review, see Stone & Hawkins, 2007). In as many as 62% of cases, the etiology of encephalitis may remain undetermined (Glaser et al., 2003).

NEUROPATHOLOGY/PATHOPHYSIOLOGY

Viruses are the most common agent responsible for known causes of encephalitis, and there are over 100 viruses that have been implicated in the condition. Common viruses include herpes simplex virus (HSV), varicella-zoster virus (VZV), Epstein–Barr virus (EBV), adenoviruses, enteroviruses, and cytomegalovirus (CMV). Encephalitis is most commonly caused by HSV-1 due to primary exposure, reinfection, or reactivation of the virus, which is usually dormant in the cranial nerves and cervical ganglia. The most common neuroradiological finding in HSV encephalitis is enhancement of the medial temporal lobe and orbitofrontal lobe on MRI or CT scans (Stone & Hawkins, 2007), and some research suggests that abnormalities of the temporal lobe may also result from VZV, herpesvirus 6, and EBV (Glaser et al., 2006). Other MRI findings in infectious encephalitis include lesions of the

E

cerebral gray matter and associated white matter, the orbital regions of the frontal lobe, the insular cortex, cerebral convexity and the cingulate gyrus, and more rarely, lesions are found in the basal ganglia, cerebellum, and spinal cord (Davis, 2000). On the other hand, neuroradiological findings suggest that ADEM is associated with MRI hyperintensities in the white matter of both hemispheres and the cerebellum, as well as gray matter of the basal ganglia and thalamus (Davis, 2000; Hynson et al., 2001). Stone and Hawkins (2007) point out that a specific MRI profile for patients with ADEM has not been identified. In AHLE, MRI findings reveal white matter lesions similar to ADEM but with hemorrhages. Further, MRI investigation using FLAIR and T2-weighted sequences of limbic encephalitis reveals hyperintensities of the temporo-mesial structures, indicating unilateral or bilateral swelling at onset and persisting for months or years with eventual atrophy of the temporomesial structures (Urbach et al., 2006). Lesions of the gray matter and subcortical white matter are the most common findings in SSPE.

Functional investigations of infectious encephalitis have indicated interesting findings, although further research is needed and diagnosis should not be based solely on functional evidence. Lee, Newberg, Liebeskind, Kung, and Alivi (2004) examined patients with infectious encephalitis using fluorine-18 fluorodeoxyglucose positron emission tomography and most consistently found hypermetabolism of the medial temporal lobes and suggested that hypermetabolism in this area is associated with inflammation. Furthermore, single photon emission computed tomography (SPECT) investigations of infectious encephalitis found temporal lobe hyperfusion in HSV.

Electroencephalographs often indicate diffuse, nonspecific slowing in both infectious encephalitis and ADEM. Periodic lateralizing epileptiform discharges (PLEDS) may be seen in cases of HSV encephalitis (Kennedy, 2004; McGrath, Anderson, Croxson, & Powell, 1997). The slow waves originate from the temporal lobe and occur at regular intervals, 2–3 Hz/sec (Ch'ien et al., 1977).

Cerebrospinal fluid (CSF) abnormalities are commonly found in many types of encephalitis. Infectious encephalitis, ADEM, and AHLE present with lymphocytic pleocytosis and normal glucose levels. Protein levels in ADEM patients are typically >0.1 mg/L, and CSF protein levels in viral encephalitis may be normal or mildly raised. Red blood cells may be seen in the CSF of patients presenting with AHLE or HSV encephalitis.

NEUROPSYCHOLOGICAL/CLINICAL PRESENTATION

Encephalitis results in multiple systemic symptoms in addition to neurological deficits that may remain severe unless diagnosis and treatment are rapid. Symptoms of encephalitis reported by Glaser et al. (2006) using data collected by the California Encephalitis Project include cerebellar signs such as ataxia and dysmetria. Hydrocephalus was prevalent in a large number of cases involving infection caused by viral, fungal, parasitic, and bacterial agents. Many patients present with seizures. Some display intractable seizures with increased mortality and hospital stay and severe deficits requiring extensive rehabilitation, whereas others demonstrate rapid recovery. Many patients presented with diffuse cerebral edema. Finally, psychosis was present in 51 of the 1,570 patients available for evaluation.

Viral encephalitis typically presents with fever, headache, and muscle rigidity. Neurological symptoms include altered consciousness, stupor, confusion, lethargy, motor weakness, tremor, and motor abnormalities including accentuated deep tendon reflexes. Involvement of the hypothalamic-pituitary-adrenal (HPA) axis may result in complications including hypothermia, poikilothermy, diabetes, and abnormal antidiuretic hormone release; and involvement of the spinal cord may result in flaccid paralysis, loss of reflexes, and paralysis of the bladder and bowel (Johnson, 1996). A study examining the neuropsychological outcome of survivors of HSV encephalitis reported that anterograde memory impairments were most severe and most common and were likely due to impairments in the ability to store new information. Other impairments included deficits in retrograde memory, attention, and concentration, as well as verbal and nonverbal impairments including anomia, and impairments of executive functions. In most cases, impairment was mild to moderate (Utley, Ogden, Gibb, McGrath, & Anderson, 1997). In a longitudinal study examining neurological deficits 6 months to 11 years after infection with HSV, McGrath et al. (1997) found that individuals continued to suffer memory impairment (69%), personality changes (45%) including anxiety, depression, obsessive-compulsive disorder, irritability, insomnia, poor motivation, and attention problems, and some patients exhibited mild motor neuron signs.

Presentation of inflammatory encephalitis is similar to that of multiple sclerosis with multiple neurological symptoms, including altered consciousness, aphasia, ataxia, sensory deficits, motor defects, aphasia, and optic neuritis. Systemic symptoms include fever and headache, and encephalitis is generally preceded by vaccination or infection. In vaccinations, a rash around the injection site may be noticeable. Progressive neurological deterioration is involved in the presentation of AHLE.

Symptoms of paraneoplastic limbic encephalitis include deficits in memory and neuropsychological functioning, personality changes including depression, language disorders, and seizures. Symptoms progress and worsen over weeks or months. Similarly, symptoms of SSPE include personality and behavioral changes followed by symptoms of ataxia, seizures, and myoclonus.

DIAGNOSIS

One of the most important diagnostic tools in differential diagnosis of encephalitis is obtaining a detailed and accurate history, as many agents that cause encephalitis are prevalent in specific geographical locations and/or seasons. Certain occupations may increase exposure to particular agents. For example, arboviruses are transmitted by insects, and the occurrence of encephalitis caused by arboviruses is seasonal. Diagnosis of SSPE may be enhanced by evidence of recent infection or vaccemia.

CSF abnormalities are not conclusive in identifying some agents or infection; however, a definitive diagnosis may be made based on the identification of immunoglobulin M (IgM) antibodies to specific agents, particularly arboviruses and parasites, in the CSF (Davis, 2000). Lymphocytic pleocytosis is 10–200 mm^3 may indicate HSV infection, whereas higher counts implicate other viral agents; in addition, protein levels between 0.6 and 6 g/L may indicate HSV encephalitis (Chaudhuri & Kennedy, 2002). In patients with ADEM, AHLE, and paraneoplastic limbic encephalitis, intrathecal oligoclonal bands may be present indicating localized inflammation in the CNS (Stone & Hawkins, 2007). Although symptoms of inflammatory encephalitis are similar to multiple sclerosis, symptoms of multiple sclerosis are typically unifocal at first (Stone & Hawkins, 2007).

Amplification of viral DNA using polymerase chain reaction (PCR) is a relatively new diagnostic tool for detecting viral agents of encephalitis. Problems of using PCR analyses include having to order tests for specific virus and developing new assays as new viruses emerge (Stone & Hawkins, 2007); however, some researchers suggest the use of "multiplex" PCR assays that test for multiple viruses at once. The accuracy and utility of this approach is reportedly low, but further research is needed (Davies

et al., 2005). Also, type-specific glycoprotein ELISA is used in the identification of infectious agents.

Other diagnostic tools include blood analysis where it is relatively common to find leukocytosis in the blood of patients with some types of viral encephalitis (Kennedy, 2004). Neuroradiological findings previously discussed may be used to aid in the diagnosis but should not be used in isolation. Recent research suggests that diffusion weighted MRI (DW-MRI) may be more sensitive and better able to detect lesions than T2-weighted MRI, resulting in earlier diagnosis (McCabe, Tyler, & Tanabe, 2003). Brain biopsy is also used in diagnosis, though less frequently now than in the past.

Diagnosis of paraneoplastic limbic encephalitis typically precedes the finding of a tumor, most commonly in the lungs. Findings of antibodies anti-HU, Yo, and Ma in the CSF and/or blood may enhance a diagnosis of paraneoplastic LE, as the disease is mediated by antibody response to onconeural antigens (Stone & Hawkins, 2007).

TREATMENT

Treatment of most encephalopathies is primarily supportive and symptom specific, including anticonvulsants for seizures, respirators for respiratory failure, and prophylaxis in cases of deep vein thrombosis and GI ulceration. Acyclovir is a nucleoside analog designed specifically to attack viruses and has made great strides in the treatment of HSV-1 and VZV, reducing mortality rates (from 70% to 30%; Whitley & Lakeman, 1986) and improving cognitive outcome of survivors. The most positive outcomes resulted in treatment latencies in less than 4 days of onset (Hokkanen et al., 1996). Cognitive and neuropsychological outcomes improve with rapidity in treatment (Utley et al., 1997). Treatment with 10 mg/kg/8 hr acyclovir is recommended for 14–21 days with longevity depending primarily upon immunocompetency (Stone & Hawkins, 2008). Intravenous ganciclovir 5 mg/kg in combination with Foscarnet 60 mg/kg/8 hr for duration of 14–21 days is recommended for the treatment of CMV encephalitis.

Immunomodulation is recommended for the treatment of ADEM, AHLE, and Rasmussen's encephalitis. Immunomodulation includes administration of corticosteroids, administration of intravenous immunoglobin, and plasma exchange. Few prospective, controlled studies examining the efficacy of this treatment have been completed, but preliminary reports are favorable. Further research is necessary.

Various strategies have been proposed for the treatment of chronic encephalitis depending upon the etiology. Treatment of SSPE includes administration of interferon alpha and eradication of the measles antigen. Treatment of the malignancy is the typical treatment for paraneoplastic limbic encephalitis, though prognosis is usually poor.

Mandi Musso
Alyse Barker
William Drew Gouvier

Chaudhuri, A., & Kennedy, P. G. E. (2002). Diagnosis and treatment of viral encephalitis. *Post-graduate Medical Journal, 78,* 575–583.

Ch'ien, L. T., Boehm, R. M., Robinson, H., Chien, L., & Frenkel, L. D. (1977). Characteristic early electroencephalographic changes in herpes simplex encephalitis. *Archives of Neurology, 34*(6), 361–364.

Davis, L. E. (2000). Diagnosis and treatment of acute encephalitis. *The Neurologist, 6,* 145–159.

Glaser, C. A., Gilliam, S., Schnurr, D., Forghani, B., Honarmand, S., Khetsuriana, N., et al. (2003). In search of encephalitis etiologies: Diagnostic challenges in the California Encephalitis Project, 1998–2000. *Clinical Infectious Diseases, 36*(6), 731–742.

Glaser, C. A., Honarmand, S., Anderson, L. J., Schnurr, D. P., Forghani, B., Cossen, C. K., et al. (2006). Beyond viruses: Clinical profiles and etiologies associated with encephalitis. *Clinical Infectious Diseases, 43,* 1565–1577.

Hokkanen, L., Poutiainen, E., Valanne, L., Salonen, O., Iivanainen, M., & Launes, J. (1996). Cognitive impairment after acute encephalitis: Comparison of herpes simplex and other aetiologies. *Journal of Neurology, Neurosurgery, and Psychiatry, 61,* 478–484.

Hynson, J. L., Kornberg, A. J., Coleman, L. T., Shield, L., Harvey, A. S., & Kean, M. J. (2001). Clinical and neuroradiologic features of acute disseminated encephalomyelitis in children. *Neurology, 5,* 1308–1312.

Johnson, R. T. (1996). Acute encephalitis. *Clinical Infectious Diseases, 23*(2), 219–224.

Kennedy, P. G. E. (2004). Viral encephalitis: Causes, differential diagnosis, and management. *Journal of Neurology, Neurosurgery, and Psychiatry, 75,* i10–i15.

Lee, B. Y., Newberg, A. B., Liebeskind, D. S., Kung, J., & Alavi, A. (2004). FDG-PET findings in patients with suspected encephalitis. *Clinical Nuclear Medicine, 29*(10), 620–625.

McCabe, K., Tyler, K., & Tanabe, J. (2003). Diffusion-weighted MRI abnormalities as a clue to the diagnosis of herpes simplex encephalitis. *Neurology, 61*(7), 1015–1016.

McGrath, N., Anderson, N. E., Croxson, M. C., & Powell, K. F. (1997). Herpes simplex encephalitis treated with acyclovir: Diagnosis and long term outcome. *Journal of Neurology, Neurosurgery, and Psychiatry, 63,* 321–326.

Stone, M. J., & Hawkins, C. P. (2007). A medical overview of encephalitis. *Neuropsychological Rehabilitation, 17*(4/5), 429–449.

Urbach, H., Soeder, B. M., Jeub, M., Klockgether, T., Meyer, B., & Bien, C. G. (2006). Serial MRI of limbic encephalitis. *Neuroradiology, 48,* 380–386.

Utley, T. F., Ogden, J. A., Gibb, A., McGrath, N., & Anderson, N. E. (1997). The long-term neuropsychological outcome of herpes simplex encephalitis in a series of unselected survivors. *Neuropsychiatry, Neuropsychology, and Behavioral Neurology, 10*(3), 180–189.

Whitley, R. J., & Lakeman, F. (1986). Herpes simplex virus infections of the central nervous system: Therapeutic and diagnostic considerations. *Clinical Infectious Diseases, 20,* 414–420.

ENCEPHALOCELE

DESCRIPTION

Encephalocele is a rare neural tube defect in which the cranial vault fails to close during fetal development. Subsequently, the embryonic ectoderm and neuroectoderm do not separate sufficiently, causing herniation of the meninges and cranial contents (Khan & Turnbull, 2008).

NEUROPATHOLOGY/PATHOPHYSIOLOGY

The defining feature of encephalocele is an opening in the skull, which allows brain tissue to push through. There are two forms of encephalocele: cranial meningocele and cranial encephalocele. The protruding tissue in cranial encephalocele is skin that creates a sack containing meninges, blood vessels, and underlying neural tissue (Shilpakar & Sharma, 2004). In cranial meningocele, the protrusion is a meningeal sac filled with CSF only.

The most prevalent location of encephalocele is the occipital regions; occipital encephalocele accounts for 70% of incidents. Parietal encephalocele is the next most common, accounting for 15% of incidents. In comparison, basal encephalocele is extremely rare, accounting for 10% of incidents (Bozinov, Tirakotai, Sure, & Bertalanffy, 2005; Naidich, Zimmerman, & Bilaniuk, 1996).

The specific etiology of the disorder is not known. It seems that infections, toxins, and genes can all be related to the failure of the closure of the anterior neural tube (Cotran, Kumar, & Robbins, 1994). Folic acid deficiency during pregnancy has also been linked to the occurrence of encephalocele (Singh & Kumar, 2009). Consequently, one study concluded that an estimated 80% reduction in the occurrence of neural tube defects was manifested with the regular consumption of folic acid (Langley-Evans & Langley-Evans, 2002; Reggler, 1995). However, not all studies have confirmed these findings (e.g., Stoll, Alembik, & Dott, 2008).

NEUROPSYCHOLOGICAL/CLINICAL PRESENTATION

Encephalocele occurs in approximately 5% of neural tube disorders, with a significantly higher prevalence in females compared with males (Joó, Papp, Berkes, Papp, & Rigó, 2008). Neurological abnormalities associated with the disorder include hydrocephalus (excessive CSF in the brain), microcephaly (small head), seizures, mental and growth retardation, vision anomalies, spastic quadriplegia, and ataxia.

DIAGNOSIS

Encephalocele is often diagnosed prior to delivery as part of the routine prenatal care. The mainstay diagnostic tool is the use of fetal MRI due to the superior detail obtained of the CNS (Mangels, Tulipan, Tsao, Alarcon, & Bruner, 2000).The median time of ultrasound diagnosis is at 18 weeks after conception (Joó et al., 2008).

Encephalocele patients diagnosed after birth are readily identified by protrusions on the head. The bluish mass is easily compressed and enlarges when the infant cries. Often infants present with meningitis and rhinorrhea of the CSF. A positive Furstenberg's test also helps to confirm the diagnosis. Encephalocele is classified as large, mega, or giant depending upon the size of the protruding sac (Aslan et al., 2007).

Other CNS defects that may be present as comorbid disorders include corpus callosum agenesis or dysgenesis, fusion of thalami, double sagittal sinus, aqueduct stenosis, falx cerebri agenesis, and tentorial dysgenesis (Bozinov et al., 2005). However, hydrocephaly is the most frequent anomaly accompanying encephalocele. In addition, 20% of children with neural tube defects experience coexisting disorders that do not involve the CNS (Stoll, Alembik, & Dott, 2007).

The prognosis is substantially improved if there is an absence of brain tissue in the herniated sac (Banister, Russell, Rimmer, Thorne, & Hellings, 2000). Additional prognostic indicators are contingent upon the size, location, and contents within the sac, and any related genetic abnormalities (Banister et al., 2000).

Encephalocele is delineated from other congenital and neural tube disorders by the presence of herniation in both the meninges and neural components. Still, there are other disorders that present with symptoms similar to encephalocele, which are important to rule out: abscess, benign polyps, malignant neoplasms, branchial cleft cysts, cystic hygroma, hemangioma, teratomas, and myelomeningocele (Khan & Turnbull, 2008). Although the symptoms of these may appear similar, encephalocele is the only disorder that presents with a calvarial defect.

TREATMENT

The most common treatment is surgical excision and repair, most often during infancy. The goals of surgery are to reposition the protruding tissue back into the skull, remove the sac, and correct any craniofacial abnormalities that have occurred (Shilpakar & Sharma, 2004).

If hydrocephalus is present, a shunt may be implanted surgically to allow for drainage. The patient should be provided follow-up support and additional treatment may be required depending on other presenting symptoms (Khan & Turnbull, 2008).

Teri J. McHale
Henry V. Soper
Velisa M. Johnson

Aslan, A., Eser, O., Doğru, O., Aktepe, F., Yurumez, Y., & Fidan, H. (2007). Occipital mega encephalocele associated with acute inflammation. *Pediatric Neurosurgery, 43,* 65–66.

Banister, C. M., Russell, S. A., Rimmer, S., Thorne, J. A., & Hellings, S. (2000). Can prognostic indicators be identified in a fetus with an encephalocele? *European Journal of Pediatric Surgery, 10,* 20–23.

Bozinov, O., Tirakotai, W., Sure, U., & Bertalanffy, H. (2005). Surgical closure and reconstruction of a large occipital encephalocele without parenchymal excision. *Child's Nervous System, 21,* 144–147.

Cotran, R., Kumar, V., & Robbins, S. (1994). *Robbins pathologic basis of disease.* Philadelphia: W.B. Saunders.

Joó, J. G., Papp, Z., Berkes, E., Papp, C., & Rigó, J. (2008). Nonsyndromic encephalocele: A 26-year experience. *Developmental Medicine and Child Neurology, 50*(12), 958–960.

Khan, A., & Turnbull, I. (2008, February 21). *Encephalocele.* Retrieved from http://emedicine.medscape.com/article/403308

Langley-Evans, S. C., & Langley-Evans, A. J. (2002). Use of folic acid supplements in the first trimester of pregnancy. *The Journal of the Royal Society for the Promotion of Health, 122,* 181–186.

Mangels, K., Tulipan, N., Tsao, L. Y., Alarcon, J., & Bruner, J. P. (2000). Fetal MRI in the evaluation of intrauterine myelomeningocele. *Pediatric Neurosurgery, 32*(3), 124–131.

Naidich, T., Zimmerman, R., & Bilaniuk, L. (1996). Midface: Embryology and congenital lesions. In P. Som & H. D. Curtin (Eds.), *Head and neck imaging* (3rd ed.). St Louis, MO: Mosby.

Reggler, J. (1995). Folic acid and the prevention of neural tube defects. *British Medical Journal, 311,* 256.

Shilpakar, S. K., & Sharma, M. R. (2004). Surgical management of encephalocele. *Journal of Neuroscience, 1,* 45–48.

Singh, G., & Kumar, V. (2009, June). Neuroradiology case of the week-case 418: Occipital encephalocele. *Radiology.* Retrieved from http://www.urmc.rochester.edu/smd/Rad/neurocases/Neurocase418.htm

Stoll, C., Alembik, Y., & Dott, B. (2007). Associated malformations in cases with neural tube defects. *Genetic Counseling, 18*(2), 209–215.

Stoll, C., Alembik, Y., & Dott, B. (2008). Are the recommendations on the prevention of neural tube defects working? *European Journal of Medical Genetics, 49,* 461–465.

ENCEPHALOPATHY

DESCRIPTION

Encephalopathy refers to any disease that physically affects the brain. It is often a manifestation of some primary illness. It can cause mood changes, motor dysfunction, disorientation, cognitive deficits, dementia, seizures, involuntary movements, and lethargy (National Institute of Neurological Disorders and Strokes, 2007). There are numerous causes and several types of encephalopathy. The most common types of encephalopathy (hypoxic, hypoxic-ischemic, anoxic, and hepatic) will be covered in detail and other types will be listed briefly. Another not-so-common type is transmissible spongiform encephalopathies (TSE), and this too will be covered in depth.

NEUROPATHOLOGY/PATHOPHYSIOLOGY

Hypoxic encephalopathy is caused by a lack of oxygen to the brain. This can occur through strangulation, drowning, asphyxiation, complications of anesthesia, carbon monoxide poisoning, and high altitudes. Cardiac arrest is the most common cause of hypoxic encephalopathy. Lack of oxygen during birth injuries (e.g., the cord wrapped around the neck) is another cause of hypoxia.

Perinatal asphyxia or hypoxic ischemic encephalopathy is a permanent damage to the brain caused by an inadequate amount of oxygen or blood flow to the brain. The mortality rate in severe cases of hypoxic-ischemic encephalopathy has been reported to be 50% to 75%, 55% of the deaths occurring in the first week of life (Zanelli, Stanley, & Kaufman, 2008). Long-term neurological disabilities are found in those children who survive severe hypoxic-ischemic encephalopathy.

Anoxic encephalopathy is the result of a total lack or absence of oxygen delivery may result in anoxic encephalopathy.

Hepatic encephalopathy occurs when liver (hepatic) failure causes damage to the brain and nervous system. This condition results from improper liver functioning, for example, through hepatitis or cirrhosis, which in turn causes the passage of toxic nitrogenous substances to the blood circulation. Also referred to as portal-systemic encephalopathy, the disorder can lead to coma. Those with hepatic encephalopathy can suffer from alteration in motor coordination and hypokinesia.

In hypoxic-ischemic encephalopathy, neuronal injury at the cellular level is an evolving process. "Following the initial phase of energy failure from the asphyxial injury, cerebral metabolism may recover, only to deteriorate in the secondary phase, or reperfusion. This new phase of neuronal damage, starting at about 6–24 hr after the initial injury, is characterized by cerebral edema and apoptosis" (Zanelli et al., 2008, p. 2).

TSEs are rare disorders seen both in animals and humans. These encephalopathies are not caused by bacteria, virus, or fungi; rather, they are a result of "proteins gone wild," as a resulting of abnormal protein folding, making it a prion disease. Prions are proteins in the brain that lack nucleic acids, such as DNA or RNA, which are compounds that are present in all other living cells. The name is derived based on how the brain tissue appears; it becomes sponge-like in texture and literally has holes in the cortex and cerebellum.

According to the Centers for Disease Control and Prevention (2006), there are three types of inherited TSEs in humans: Gerstmann–Straussler–Scheinker's syndrome, fatal familial insomnia, and other autosomal-dominant families. The five types of human transmissible TSEs are: kuru, Creutzfeldt–Jakob's disease (CJD), sporadic Creutzfeldt–Jakob's disease (sCJD), iatrogenic Creutzfeldt–Jakob's disease (iCJD), and variant Creutzfeldt–Jakob's disease (vCJD).

Other Types of Encephalopathy

Encephalopathy, as mentioned before, refers to a myriad of disorders physically affecting the brain.

■ Ethylmalonic encephalopathy is a rare, inherited condition and is manifested through seizures and abnormal body movements. It may be misdiagnosed as other neurologic disorders (Stedman, 2000).

- Hypertensive encephalopathy is caused by a cerebral edema after an abrupt elevation of blood pressure in someone who suffers hypertension. It may be seen in association with preeclampsia, cyclosporine therapy, and renal disease (Stedman, 2000).
- Septic encephalopathy refers to central nervous dysfunction that occurs in septic patients, and amino acid imbalance is present (Nakamura, Kawagoe, Matsuda, Ebihara, & Koide, 2003).
- Lead encephalopathy is caused by lead ingestion and is characterized by cerebral edema, neurocytosis, status spongiosus, and some reactive inflammation (Stedman, 2000).
- Hypernatremic encephalopathy refers to "subarachnoid and subdural effusions in infants with hypernatremic dehydration" (Stedman, 2000, p. 588).
- Wernicke's encephalopathy is caused by thiamine deficiency; thus, those with a history of alcohol abuse or AIDS could develop this brain disorder (Jasmin, 2008).
- Hashimoto's encephalopathy is a rare condition caused by autoimmune thyroiditis. It is characterized by seizures and stroke-like episodes (Wilcox, To, Koukourou, & Frasca, 2008).
- Mitochondrial encephalopathy is a form of dementia, which is caused by mutations in the genetic material (i.e., DNA) in the mitochondria (Medicine-Net.com, 1999).
- Pancreatic encephalopathy refers to an agitated, confused state, sometimes with hallucinations and limbic rigidity, as a result of a pancreatic disease (Adams & Victor, 1981).

NEUROPSYCHOLOGICAL/CLINICAL PRESENTATION

Changes in daily living should always be noted. Sleep disturbance, decrease in energy, cognitive impairments, and motor dysfunction should be examined. Clumsiness, particularly when there is a rapid shift in movement, impairment of reflexes, slow movement, and tremors can be signs of encephalopathy. Cognitive and sleep disturbances are evident in hepatic encephalopathy.

DIAGNOSIS

EEGs, neuroimaging, blood tests, liver and kidney function tests, and other diagnostic studies may aid in the diagnosis of the causes of the various encephalopathies. A complete neuropsychiatric evaluation, addressing consciousness, orientation, cognitive functioning, sensory and motor functioning, and a thorough history are needed for the diagnosis of hepatic

encephalopathy. An alternate diagnosis should be considered when there is evidence of a focal abnormality. "Concomitant neurologic disease such as subdural hematoma, Wernicke's disease, intercurrent infection (including encephalitis), other metabolic abnormalities (e.g., water, electrolyte, renal function), and drug intoxications (e.g., alcohol, narcotics, sedatives) must be ruled out" (Ferenci et al., 2002, p. 718).

In all TSEs, the gray matter of the CNS of the brain is affected resulting in a spongy appearance with small holes. There is neuronal loss and gliosis (Wisniewski & Sigurdsson, 2006). An interesting feature is the existence of amyloid plaques occurring in an estimated 10% of all CJD cases, with the plaques existing in the cerebellum or the cerebral hemispheres. Amyloid plaques do not react with production of antibodies in response to the prion protein. They also do not produce antibodies to additional amyloidogenic proteins as seen in Alzheimer's disease (Wisniewski & Sigurdsson, 2006).

A person with a TSE commonly presents with behavioral changes, such as impaired judgment and reasoning. Upon conducting a mental status examination and neuropsychological examination, cognitive functioning is markedly decreased. The most common beginning symptoms are cognitive decline and ataxia. Other symptoms include depression, insomnia, poor coordination, memory impairment, dementia, unusual physical sensations, and disturbances in vision (Wisniewski & Sigurdsson, 2006). As the disease progresses, cortical blindness, muscle weakness, and coma are common occurrences. In CJD, myoclonus, rapid, uncontrolled muscle jerking is also a common symptom. All prion diseases have a 100% fatality rate and the average life span ranges from 6 to 18 months. Other symptoms and developments can occur including seizures and extrapyramidal diseases, such as is seen in Parkinson's disease.

The diagnostic criteria for TSEs involve performing a neurological examination and a spinal tap. Administering an EEG can also help see abnormal brain waves that are a result of CJD. To reach a conclusive diagnosis, however, a brain biopsy or autopsy is the definitive diagnostic procedure. The brain biopsy may not always produce infected tissue, so it is most often used as a means to rule out other possible conditions that are treatable (Swierzewski, 2005).

From a differential diagnosis standpoint, it is important to understand the nature of TSEs as the initial symptoms may often be confused with Alzheimer's disease, and it is estimated that the percentage of reported TSE diseases is actually underreported. It is also important to rule out other disorders that present symptoms of dementia such as Alzheimer's disease, encephalitis, chronic meningitis, Pick's disease (frontal and temporal dementias), and lithium poisoning. Additional items to rule out are:

Cortical basal ganglionic degeneration	Motor neuron disease dementia
Frontal and temporal lobe dementia	Herpes simplex encephalitis
HIV-1 encephalopathy/ AIDS dementia	Hydrocephalus
Inherited metabolic disorders	Multi-infarct dementia
Multiple system atrophy	Lewy body disease

Adapted from Wisniewski, T., & Sigurdsson, E. (2006). *Prion related diseases,* by http://www.emedicine.com/neuro/topic662.htm

TREATMENT

Treatment will vary depending on the type, cause, and severity of the encephalopathy. Hepatic encephalopathy should be treated early to prevent long-term damage. Oxygen delivery and circulation should be immediately restored in hypoxic and anoxic encephalopathies to prevent damage, or further damage, to the brain. Permanent and severe brain damage can occur after only a few minutes of oxygen deprivation.

Dietary changes can, in some cases, alleviate symptoms of encephalopathy. Medications, such as anticonvulsants, should usually be prescribed to treat seizures that result from encephalopathy. Cauli et al. (2009) found that decreasing inflammation by giving rats ibuprofen helped to treat the motor deficits caused by hepatic encephalopathy. Jiang, Desjardins, and Butterworth (2009) also found anti-inflammatory benefits in those with hepatic encephalopathy. Researchers gave minocycline to rats, which was shown to prevent microglial activation. In severe cases of hepatic encephalopathy, dialysis or organ replacement may be needed.

As with the treatment, the prognosis may vary depending upon the type, cause, and severity of encephalopathy. Symptoms may be alleviated, but the underlying causes of encephalopathy, in some cases, may not be curable. Death occurs in some cases. Most often, cerebral edema or sepsis may result from a severe form of encephalopathy.

In severe cases of hypoxic-ischemic encephalopathy, mental retardation, epilepsy, and cerebral palsy may occur. Cerebral palsy may occur in the form of hemiplegia, paraplegia, or quadriplegia. These children will need follow-up from specialized clinics. Even in instances where obvious neurological deficits

were not found at birth, when children reached school age, 15% to 20% had significant learning difficulties (Zanelli et al., 2008).

Signorini et al. (2009) injected melatonin in rats and found that levels of free iron, F2-isoprostanes, and F4-neuroprostanes were significantly lower than controls. The researchers found that melatonin played a neuroprotective role in reducing oxidative damage in hypoxic-ischemic encephalopathy. They are hopeful that melatonin could represent a potential safe approach to perinatal brain damage in humans.

Teri J. McHale
Henry V. Soper
Carol Swann

Adams, R., & Victor, M. (1981). *Principles of neurology* (2nd ed.). NewYork: McGraw-Hill.

California Pacific Medical Center. (2004, May). *Learning about your health: Encephalopathy.* Retrieved June 16, 2009, from http://www.cpmc.org/learning/documents/encephalopathy-ws.html

Cauli, O., Rodrigo, R., Piedrafita, B., Llansola, M., Mansouri, M. T., & Felipo, V. (2009). Neuroinflammation contributes to hypokinesia in rats with hepatic encephalopathy: Ibuprofen restores its motor activity. *Journal of Neuroscience Research, 87,* 1369–1374.

Ferenci, P., Lockwood, A., Mullen, K., Tarter, R., Weissenborn, K., Blei, A., et al. (2002). Hepatic encephalopathy – Definition, nomenclature, diagnosis, and quantification: Final report of the working party at the 11th World Congresses of Gastroenterology, Vienna, 1998. *Hepatology, 35*(3), 716–721.

Jasmin, L. (2008, February 13). *Wernicke-Korsakoff syndrome.* Retrieved June 16, 2009, from http://www.nlm.nih.gov/medlineplus/ency/article/000771.htm

Jiang, W., Desjardins, P., & Butterworth, R. (2009). Cerebral inflammation contributes to encephalopathy and brain edema in acute liver failure: Protective effect of minocycline. *Journal of Neurochemistry, 109,* 485–493.

MedicineNet.com. (1999, March 26). *Definition of encephalopathy, mitochondrial (MELAS).* Retrieved June 16, 2009, from http://www.medterms.com/script/main/art.asp?articlekey=8885

Nakamura, T., Kawagoe, Y., Matsuda, T., Ebihara, I., & Koide, H. (2003). Effects of polymyxin B-immobilized fiber hemoperfusion on amino acid imbalance in septic encephalopathy. *Blood Purification, 21*(4–5), 282–286.

National Institute of Neurological Disorders and Stroke. (2007, February 12). *Encephalopathy information page.* Retrieved June 16, 2009, from http://www.ninds.nih.gov/disorders/encephalopathy/encephalopathy.htm

Signorini, C., Ciccoli, L., Leoncini, S., Carloni, S., Perrone, S., Comporti, M., et al. (2009). Free iron, total F2-isoprostanes and total F4-neuroprostanes in a model of neonatal hypoxic ischemic encephalopathy: Neuroprotective effect of melatonin. *Journal of Pineal Research, 46,* 148–154.

Stedman, T. (2000). *Stedman's medical dictionary* (27th ed.). Baltimore Lippincott Williams & Wilkins.

Swierzewski, S. (2005). *Creutzfeldt-Jakob Disease (CJD): Overview, types, incidence, and prevalence.* Retrieved on May 21, 2008, from http://www.neurologychannel.com

Wilcox, R., To, T., Koukourou, A., & Frasca, J. (2008). Hashimoto's encephalopathy masquerading as acute psychosis. *Journal of Clinical Neuroscience, 15*(11), 1301–1304.

Wisniewski, T., & Sigurdsson, E. (2006). *Prion related diseases.* Retrieved on July 15, 2008, from http://www.emedicine.com/neuro/topic662.htm

Zanelli, S., Stanley, D., & Kaufman, D. (2008, December 15). *Hypoxic-ischemic encephalopathy.* Retrieved June 16, 2009, from http://emedicine.medscape.com/article/973501-overview

Epilepsy and Seizures

DESCRIPTION

Epilepsy is a recurrent paroxysmal disorder of cerebral function characterized by sudden brief attacks of altered (or loss of) consciousness, motor activity, sensory phenomena, psychic phenomena, and/or inappropriate behavior as a result of excessive neuronal discharge. A single seizure due to a specific medical difficulty does not fall under this heading. Epilepsy is the most common chronic neurological disease effecting approximately 1% to 4% of the population over the life span (Annegers, 2001). Historically, clinical manifestations of seizures led to names of petite mal, grand mal, or psychomotor. Currently, epileptic seizures are classified by correlation of pathophysiological phenomena with clinical features. There are two major divisions of epileptic seizures: (1) partial or focal seizures and (2) generalized seizures. The major divisions have specific seizure disorders under each classification.

NEUROPATHOLOGY/PATHOPHYSIOLOGY

The neuropathological origin of seizures varies. Along this line, there are two classifications for the causes of epileptic seizures. The classifications are symptomatic and idiopathic. Idiopathic etiology means that no cause can be isolated for the seizure. Symptomatic etiology refers to secondary or acquired seizures. The specific causes may include infection, trauma, tumor vascular malformation, toxic chemicals, or other neurological disorders.

Browne and Holmes (2004) noted that the physiological mechanism of seizures involves disruption of intrinsic membrane stabilizing mechanisms because of the presence of abnormal neuronal membranes or an imbalance of the inhibitory and excitatory neurotransmitter influences. The destabilization and thus excessive discharge are end results of a process that really first arises due to the presence of abnormal neuronal membranes sometimes linked to previous neurological trauma (i.e., symptomatic etiology).

NEUROPSYCHOLOGICAL/CLINICAL PRESENTATION

The neuropsychological and clinical presentation associated with epilepsy include both the features of the seizures themselves as well as associated sequelae of cognitive and behavioral modalities. In regard to the presentation of the seizures, as alluded to earlier, there are various types of seizures. Their preictal, ictal, and postictal patterns depend upon where in the brain the discharge occurs. Table 1 outlines the general aspects of the various seizure types. Again, distinction should be made between the concept of epilepsy, which is a disorder characterized by multiple, recurrent seizures, and seizures themselves, which are singular events.

In terms of the associated neuropsychological and behavioral features, characteristics often coincide with the origin of the seizure. As one would expect, generalized epileptiform activity can often relate to more diffuse cognitive residuals. In terms of partial seizures, that is those of focused origin, the place of origin corresponds largely with the features observed. For example, temporal lobe epilepsy (TLE) has been associated with both attention (Sanchez-Carpintero & Neville, 2003) and memory deficits (Cohen, 1992). Learning disabilities also present in significantly higher frequency. Behaviorally, increased risk of depression and anxiety have not only been associated with TLE but also with the majority of seizure disorders (Ettinger et al., 1998). Still, trends have emerged across the various functional domains including intelligence, attention, and executive functioning, language, and memory. In general, visuospatial functions tend to be relatively spared in most epileptic presentations or only mildly impacted.

Intellectual impairment has been reported in association with the majority of epileptic presentations. However, variability is seen in relation to seizure type, duration and frequency, medicinal treatment, and age of onset (Lee et al., 2003; Meador, 2002). In essence, generalized seizures tend to be

E

Table 1
GENERAL ASPECTS OF THE VARIOUS SEIZURE TYPES IN EPILEPSY

Type of Seizures	Characteristics
Partial or focal seizures	On an EEG, spike discharges are localized within one cerebral hemisphere (cortical or subcortical). These may occur in children, and the incidence rate is likely to increase with age.
Partial seizures with elementary symptomology	Generally, there is no impairment in consciousness and seizures usually involve motor symptoms. These often consist of localized clonic movements involving all or part of the muscles on the side contralateral to the discharging cerebral focus. Aversive seizures are characterized by a turning away from the side of the discharging lesion by the head, eyes, and body. Less common motor seizures are inhibitory in that there is loss of tone, strength, and possibly speech. Jacksonian seizures (i.e., focal motor symptoms begin in one hand or foot and "march" up the extremity or spread similarly from a corner of the mouth) are included. Partial or focal seizures also encompass (1) special sensory or somatosensory symptoms, (2) automatic symptoms, or (3) compound forms.
Partial seizures with complex symptomatology	Generally, some type of impairment in consciousness is associated with these seizures. The seizures usually begin in the temporal or limbic areas. The symptomatology associated with the seizure may be one of the following: (1) impairment in consciousness only, (2) cognitive, (3) affective, (4) psychosensory, (5) psychomotor [automatism], or (6) compound forms. The seizure may begin with somatic sensory phenomena, auras of taste/smell, or lip and tongue movement. Almost invariably, there is alteration of consciousness or mental status and amnesia. These seizures generally involve some time of automatic psychomotor manifestations. Most of the seizures last for 1–2 min and are followed by 1–2 min of confusion.
Partial seizures of the temporal lobe	Behavioral abnormalities and unprovoked aggression can be associated with these seizures. Current information indicates 33% of patients with these seizures experience substantial psychopathology with up to 10% showing signs of depressive psychoses or schizophreniform. Neither surgical treatment nor anticonvulsant medication has exhibited a consistently favorable effect on these psychiatric disorders.
Generalized seizures	These seizures are often subdivided into convulsive (major) and nonconvulsive (minor). Usually affect both consciousness and motor function from the onset. The seizures are presumed to arise in the diencephalon and affect the brain in a symmetric, bilateral, and synchronous manner according to EEG patterns.
Generalized nonconvulsive seizures	Absence seizures (previously called petite mal) attacks are characterized by brief loss or impairment in consciousness, usually 10–30 s with eye or muscle fluttering at a rate of 3 per second and may or may not include a loss of muscle tone. The seizures usually occur in children between the ages of 5 and 10, they rarely begin after the age of 20 and often subside after puberty. Atonic or akinetic seizures occur in young children, e.g., with Lennox–Gastaut syndrome, and are characterized by loss of postural tone and result in falling.
Generalized convulsive seizures	This category includes the following seizures: (1) bilateral massive epileptic myoclonus, (2) clonic, (3) tonic, (4) tonic–clonic (grand mal), and (5) infantile spasms. The most common form of an attack begins with loss of consciousness and motor control and tonic or clonic jerking of all extremities. Bilateral massive epileptic myoclonus are massive seizures that consist of sudden flexion or extension of the body and often begin with a cry.

(cont.)

Table 1
GENERAL ASPECTS OF THE VARIOUS SEIZURE TYPES IN EPILEPSY (Cont.)

Type of Seizures	Characteristics
Generalized convulsive seizures (cont.)	Clonic seizures involve stiffening of muscles and cessation of breathing, whereas tonic seizures involve rhythmic shaking of the muscles.
	Tonic–clonic seizures (grand mal) are characterized by loss of consciousness and stereotyped movement. Stereotyped movement involves tonic then clonic muscle contractions of the extremities, trunk, and head. The seizures are often preceded by an aura. During the seizure, incontinence and tongue biting may occur. The seizures may be followed by a postictal state that may include muscle aches or pains, drowsiness, and/or headaches.
	Infantile spasms are clusters of brief myoclonic jerks. There is a sudden flexion of the arms, forward flexion of the trunk, and extension of the legs in these seizures. High-voltage polyspike- and -slow- wave activity occur in a haphazard fashion in all areas of the head (hypoarrhythmia) on EEGs. Although infantile spasms are usually restricted to the first 3 years of life, the spasms are often replaced by other forms of seizures, and signs of cerebral damage are permanent.

worse than partial seizures, longer duration seizures are worse than shorter seizures, more seizures are worse than less, more medications (polypharmacy) are worse than single-agent control, earlier onset is worse than later onset. Findings have suggested that not only is intellect impacted by epilepsy, but intellectual decline may occur over time, but this seems to be related to generalized seizures and not partial (Dodrill, 2002).

Attention and executive functioning are complex areas within this group as they can be negatively impacted by the epilepsy itself and the medicinal agents used. Inattention has been commonly reported (e.g., Martin et al., 2005). A broad array of executive deficits have been reported, but variability has been seen in terms of frequency. They are most commonly noted in frontal lobe epilepsy, although links have been established with other origin sites, and seem to be more prevalent when seizures originate on the left composed to right. Deficits may be seen in problem solving, abstraction, mental flexibility and shifting, planning, initiation, and self-regulation (Lee & Clason, 2008).

Language deficits are not discussed as frequently as other domains traditionally. There are exceptions in the case where language impairments are characteristic of the presentation (e.g., Landau–Kleffner's syndrome in children [Gordon, 2000]). As with other domains, presentation is related to seizure origin. Left hemisphere origin is far more commonly related to language deficits in epilepsy than right hemisphere origin (e.g., Hermann & Wyler, 1994; Mayeux et al., 1980); however, other studies have found no significant difference (e.g., Hermann & Wyler, 1988; N'Kaoua et al., 2001). In general, differences between hemispheres appear more likely to occur with frontal seizure origin but not necessarily with temporal origin.

Memory deficits in relation to epilepsy have been discussed and have been most related to TLEs (Bornstein et al., 1998). Within this group, discrepancies are noted based on hemispheric origin. Generally speaking, left TLE is linked with verbal memory deficits, whereas right TLE is associated with visual memory deficits (Kim et al., 2003).

DIAGNOSIS

For diagnosis, it is necessary that a careful history be obtained. Critical aspects of this history include an eyewitness account of typical attack, frequency, duration, prior trauma, infection, and toxic episodes. The history will also assist in determining whether the seizures are idiopathic or symptomatic. Diagnosis of epilepsy is usually confirmed by electroencephalograms (EEGs) during normal and/or sleep deprived states. In many ways, video-EEG recording over the course of a few days may be preferred. Intracranial recording may be used prior to resection for more refined localization. Recently, positron emission tomography scans have proven to be very useful in assisting with diagnosis; however, the costs remain prohibitive. In addition to an EEG, several laboratory studies are advisable. A blood count, urinalysis, serological test for syphilis, fasting blood sugar, serum calcium, and glucose may be diagnostic. In the case of seizures with an onset in adulthood and focally abnormal laboratory results, CT or MRI are indicated. Neuropsychological assessment should be used to document neurocognitive deficits.

TREATMENT

The etiology of the seizure determines the approach to treatment. In idiopathic epilepsy, treatment focuses on control of the seizure, usually through medication.

In the case of symptomatic epilepsy, the associated disease is treated and medication is usually continued after the disease is controlled. Dietary and vitamin measures are sometimes recommended. If all conventional methods fail, surgery is considered. Anticonvulsant drugs are the treatment of choice for epilepsy. Drug therapy successfully controls (1) complex partial seizures in 35% of the cases and reduces the frequency of seizures in 50% of cases, (2) 40% of absence seizures and reduces the frequency in 35% of cases, and (3) tonic–clonic seizures in 50% of cases and reduces the frequency in 35% of cases. No anticonvulsant or other drug successfully controls all types of seizures; different drugs are required for each individual patient. More than one drug may be required to successfully control the seizures. Serum concentration and toxicity are important considerations in medication choices. Currently, the most commonly used anticonvulsant drugs are phenytoin (Dilantin), phenobarbital, ethosuximide (Zarontin), carbamazepine (Tegretol), valproic acid (Depakene or Depakote), primidone (Mysolin), clonazepam (Clonopin), and clorazepate (Tranxene). A total of 16 medications have been approved by U.S. Food and Drug Administration and include diazepam (Valium) and mephobarbital (Mebaral).

Sometimes surgical intervention is required to remove the area from which the seizures arise. Again the idea being that the process arises from the presence of abnormal neuronal membranes, thus, removing the problematic area aids in control. This is done only in those instances where medicinal treatment and management have been unsuccessful.

Chad A. Noggle
Raymond S. Dean

Annegers, J. F. (2001). Epidemiology of epilepsy. In E. Wylie (Ed.). The treatment of epilepsy: Principles and practice (3rd ed.). Philadelphia: Lippincott, Williams, & Wilkins.

Bornstein, R. A., Pakalnis, A., Drake, M. E., & Suga, L. J. (1998). Effects of seizure type and waveform abnormality on memory and attention. *Archs Neurol.* 45, 884–887.

Browne, T. R., & Holmes, G. L. (2004). Handbook of epilepsy (3rd ed.). Philadelphia: Lippincott, Williams, & Wilkins.

Cohen, M. (1992). Auditory/verbal and visual/spatial memory in children with complex partial epilepsy of temporal lobe origin. *Brain & Cognition, 20(2)*, 315–326.

Dodrill, C. B. (2002). Progressive cognitive decline in adolescents and adults with epilepsy. *Progress in Brain Research, 135*, 399–407.

Lee, S., Sziklas, V., Andermann, F., Farnham, S., Risse, G., Gustafson, M. et al. (2003). The effects of adjuvant topiramate on cognitive function in patients with epilepsy. *Epilepsia, 44(3)*, 339–347.

Meador, K. J. (2002). Cognitive outcomes and predictive factors in epilepsy. *Neurology, 58 (Suppl 5)*, S21–S26.

Martin, R. C., Griffith, H. R., Faught, E., Gilliam, F., Mackey, M., & Vogtle, L. (2005). Cognitive functioning I community dwelling older adults with chronic partial epilepsy. *Epilepsia, 46*, 298–303.

Gordon, N. (2000). Cognitive functions and epileptic activity. *Seizure, 9*, 184–188.

Hermann, B. P., & Wyler, A. R. (1994). Language function, temporal lobe epilepsy, and anterior temporal lobectomy. In A. R. Wyler, & B. P. Hermann (Eds). *The surgical management of epilepsy*. Boston: Butterworth-Heinemann.

Hermann, B. P., & Wyler, A. R. (1988). Effects of anterior temporal lobectomy on language function: A controlled study. *Annals of Neurology, 23*, 585–588.

Kim, H., Kim., J., Yi, S., & Son, E. I. (2003). Material-specific memory in temporal lobe epilepsy: Effects of seizure laterality and language dominance. *Neuropsychology, 17 (1)*, 59–68.

Mayeux, R., Brandt, J., Rosen J., & Benson D. F. (1980). Interictal memory and language impairment in temporal lobe epilepsy. *Neurology, 30*, 120–125.

N'Kaoua, B., Lespinet, V., Barsse, A., Rougier, A., Claverie, B. (2001). Exploration of hemispheric specialization and lexicosemantic processing in unilateral temporal lobe epilepsy with verbal fluency tasks. *Neuropsychologia, 39*, 635–642.

Lee, P., & Clason, C. (2008).Classification of seizure disorders and syndromes, and neuropsychological impairment in adults with epilepsy. In a Morgan, J., & Ricker, J. (Eds). *Textbook of Clinical Neuropsychology* (pp. 437–465). New York: Taylor & Francis.

Sanchez-Carpintero, R., & Neville, B. G. (2003). Attentional ability in children with epilepsy. *Epilepsia, 44(10)*, 1340–1349.

Ettinger, A. B., Weisbrot, D. M., Nolan, E. E., Gadow, K. D., Vitale, S. A., Andriola, M. R. et al. (1998). Symptoms of depression and anxiety in pediatric epilepsy patients. *Epilepsia, 39 (6)*, 595–599.

ERB'S PALSY

DESCRIPTION

Erb's palsy, also called Erb–Duchenne's palsy or brachial plexus paralysis, is a disorder caused by injury to the arm's main nerves that causes paralysis, stunted growth, and impaired muscular, nervous, and

E

circulatory development in the affected arm. The degree of damage can vary greatly and may result in paralysis that will resolve on its own, require physical therapy, or require surgery, but can be potentially devastating. The damage resulting in Erb's palsy typically occurs due to complications during childbirth but may also occur after birth as a result of trauma in the neck area.

Erb's palsy was first described by British obstetrician William Smellie in 1768 in a case of transient bilateral arm paralysis after a difficult birth. Later, in 1861, Guillaume Benjamin Arnold Duchenne published findings on four infants with identical paralysis of the arm muscles and used the term, "obstetric palsy of the brachial plexus" (Bienstock & Kim, 2009). In 1874, Wilhelm Heinrich Erb, the foremost German neurologist of his time, noted that birth trauma is one of the causes of paralysis following damage to the brachial plexus. Historically, although the physicians disagreed vehemently with each other regarding who first described the disease, both are given credit with the designation of Erb–Duchenne. Due to his prominence in the field of neurology, Erb's name alone is commonly associated with the disorder (Brody & Wilkins, 1969; Sandmire & DeMott, 2002).

NEUROPATHOLOGY/PATHOPHYSIOLOGY

The damage that results in Erb's palsy is typically acquired during birth. A traction injury to the brachial plexus during birth is considered to be the main cause of the disorder, although there are several other potential but less common etiologies of the disorder (Gherman, Ouzounian, Miller, Kwok, & Goodwin, 1998; Peleg, Hasnin, & Shalev, 1997). During birth, the baby's shoulder can get stuck on the mother's pelvic bone, which is called shoulder dystocia. The procedure used to extricate the baby can result in the trauma to the brachial plexus causing Erb's palsy. Recent research has indicated that fewer than half the brachial plexus cases occur during completely normal labor dilation, indicating that the injuries resulting in Erb's palsy are often, but not always, caused solely by a dysfunctional labor, but there are several risk factors for shoulder dystocia (Backe, Magnussen, Johansen, Saellaeg, & Russwurm, 2008).

The damage to the brachial plexus, which is comprised of nerves that travel from the spinal cord into the arms, is typically due to excessive force placed on the neonate's head and neck causing trauma to the nerves. This injury is observed in approximately 1 out of 1,000 births, of which 10% are serious enough to require treatment. The causes of damage to the spinal nerves after birth are varied, but may include injury, tumor, or any trauma to the brachial plexus (Gherman et al., 1998). The brachial plexus nerve bundle comprises five nerves (C5, 6, 7, 8, and T1) that innervate the skin and muscles of the majority of the shoulder, arm, and hand.

There are three types of Erb's palsy that are caused by differing degrees and types of injury to the brachial plexus. Complete brachial plexus palsy is the result of injury to all five of the spinal nerves comprising the brachial plexus resulting in paralysis and sensory loss in the entire arm. Klumpke's palsy involves the C7 and T1 spinal nerves resulting in weakness of the wrist, finger flexors, and small muscles of the hand. Erb's palsy specifically involves C5 and C6 spinal nerves resulting in paralysis of a group of muscles in the shoulder and upper arm.

The injury to the spinal nerves also varies in degree, resulting in avulsion, rupture, neuroma, and/or praxis (Dodds & Wolfe, 2000). Avulsion of the nerves is the most serious injury, in which the nerves are completely torn from the spine. In a rupture of the nerves, the nerves are torn but not completely from the spine. A neuroma of a nerve is formed when scar tissue forms around a nerve after recovery following a trauma. Praxis of the nerves is the least serious injury, in which the nerve does not tear and the nerve heals on its own. The location of the injury and varying degree of severity of the trauma can result in varying clinical presentations from mild and transient to severe and permanently debilitating (Sandmire & DeMott, 2002).

NEUROPSYCHOLOGICAL/CLINICAL PRESENTATION

The neuropsychological and clinical presentation of Erb's palsy depends upon the degree and type of injury to the brachial plexus. In general, the injury can stunt the growth in the affected arm from the shoulder to the fingertips. The patients also have impaired musculature and vasculature development that can lead to additional complications of the disorder. The effects on the muscles of the affected arm leave it smaller, weaker, and less articulate – many patients are unable to lift their arm above the shoulder. The effects on the circulatory system often leave the arm with an inability to regulate body temperature and a reduced ability to heal following an injury.

E

Complete brachial plexus palsy results in paralysis and sensory loss in the entire arm. In addition to the sensory and motor loss, patients with complete brachial plexus palsy may develop Horner's syndrome due to a lack of sympathetic innervation, which cause the affected side of the body to have ptosis (eyelid droop), miosis (constricted pupil), dilation lag, and anhydrosis (decreased sweating) of the face, and blushing of the face (Al-Qattan, 2002). Klumpke's palsy involves the C7 and T1 spinal nerves resulting in weakness of the wrist, finger flexors, and small muscles of the hand. Symptoms of Klumpke's palsy include paralysis of the hand muscles and ulnar nerve numbness. Klumpke's palsy is a rare disease affecting fewer than 200,000 people in the United States.

Erb's palsy specifically involves C5 and C6 spinal nerves resulting in paralysis of a group of muscles in the shoulder and upper arm. In Erb's palsy the arm hangs limp and may rotate inward with the elbow extended. The palm may face up and the flexion of the wrist and hand is preserved. Patients often are unable to lift their arm above the shoulder (Sandmire & DeMott, 2002). Neuropsychological evaluation may reveal deficits on construction or drawing tests if the patient's affected arm is involved in completing the measure.

DIAGNOSIS

The evaluation and diagnosis of Erb's palsy should occur as soon as possible, following the injury. A physical examination of an infant may reveal that the Moro's reflex is absent on the side of the injury. The affected arm may also flop if the baby is rolled from side to side. The examination of the patient will also typically include a thorough physical examination and medical history. X-rays may show damage, but a myelogram using contrast dyes can specifically show damage to the spinal nerves. Electromyogram can also measure nerve conductivity to the muscles by inserting an electrode into the muscle that appears to be affected by the nerve damage. Complete brachial plexus palsy is the result of injury to all five of the spinal nerves comprising the brachial plexus resulting in paralysis and sensory loss in the entire arm. Klumpke's palsy involves the C7 and T1 spinal nerves resulting in weakness of the wrist, finger flexors, and small muscles of the hand. Erb's palsy specifically involves C5 and C6 spinal nerves resulting in paralysis of a group of muscles in the shoulder and upper arm (Dodds & Wolfe, 2000; Sandmire & DeMott, 2002).

TREATMENT

The treatment of Erb's palsy is varied and dependent on the diagnosis of the severity of the disorder (Adler & Patterson, 1967). In mild cases involving praxis with no tearing, the injury may heal on its own shortly after; however, physical therapy and range of motion exercises done as often as possible will help to maintain the range of motion, prevent joint contracture, and to insure optimal recovery. If the injury does not respond, or is more severe, surgery may be required.

The initial surgical interventions for Erb's palsy focus on repairing the damaged nerve tissue. Procedures include neurolysis (clearing the scar tissue from the nerve), nerve grafting (reconnection of the damaged nerve by transplanting a nerve from the leg), and nerve transfer (surgically attaching a functioning adjacent nerve in an attempt to restore functioning). Unfortunately, surgery will not restore normal function, is usually not helpful for older infants, and takes several months, or even years, for the nerves to repair (Dodds & Wolfe, 2000).

Several other surgical options are available that focus on the musculature which, unlike procedures that focus on repairing the nerves, are not time limited and may restore some shoulder, elbow, and hand functioning. The subscapularis muscle can be cut to stretch the muscle, which improves the range of motion. In addition, the latissimus dorsi muscle can be cut in half and rearranged where the muscle is attached, which also improves range of motion (Phippsab & Hoffer, 1995). Several other surgical procedures are available depending upon the presentation of the disorder (Al-Qattan, 2002). Physical and occupational therapy may also be utilized to help the child function as normally as possible in day-to-day life (Sandmire & DeMott, 2002). Psychosocial interventions may also be utilized to help the child overcome any psychological or social ramifications of the disorder.

Eric Silk
Charles Golden

Adler, J. & Patterson, R. (1967). Erb's palsy long-term results of treatments in eighty-eight cases. *Journal of Bone and Joint Surgery, 49*, 1052–1064.

Al-Qattan, M. (2002). Oberlin's ulnar nerve transfer to the biceps nerve in Erb's birth palsy. *Plastic & Reconstructive Surgery, 109*(1), 405–407.

Backe, B., Magnussen, E. B., Johansen, O. J., Saellaeg, G., Russwurm, H. (2008). Obstetric brachial plexus palsy: A birth injury not explained by the known risk factors.

Acta Obstetricia et Gynecologica Scandinavica, 87(10), 1027–1032.

Bienstock, A., & Kim, J. (2009). *Hand, brachial plexus surgery.* Retrieved from http://emedicine.medscape.com/article/1286947-overview

Brody, I. A., & Wilkins, R. H. (1969). Erb's palsy. *Archives of Neurology, 21*(4), 442–449.

Dodds, S., & Wolfe, S. (2000). Perinatalbracial plexus palsy. *Current Opinion in Orthopedics, 11*(3), 202–209.

Gherman, R., Ouzounian, J., Miller, D., Kwok,L.,&Goodwin, T. (1998). Spontaneous vaginal delivery: A risk factor for Erb's palsy? *American Journal of Obstetrics & Gynecology, 178*(3), 423–427.

Peleg, D., Hasnin, J., & Shalev, E. (1997). Fractured clavicle and Erb's palsy unrelated to birth trauma. *American Journal of Obstetrics & Gynecology, 177*(5), 1038–1040.

Phippsab, G.,& Hoffer, M. (1995). Latissimusdorsi and teres major transfer to rotator cuff for Erb's palsy. *Journal of Shoulder and Elbow Surgery, 4*(2), 124–129.

Sandmire, H., & DeMott, R. (2002). Erb's palsy causation: A historical perspective. *Birth, 29*(1), 52–54.

E

F

Fabry's Disease (Anderson-Fabry Disease)

DESCRIPTION

Fabry's disease (FD), also referred to as Anderson-Fabry disease, is a rare progressive X-linked disorder affecting multiple organ systems. FD is characterized by an enzymatic defect resulting in a deficiency of the lysosomal enzyme α-galactosidase A. This deficiency results in the altered metabolism and an accumulation of globotriaosylceramide in various systems throughout the body leading to pathology in multiple organs. FD is an X-linked disorder that manifests in females as well as males. Although symptom presentation in females is variable, some females experience symptoms that are usually characteristic of their male counterparts. FD affects approximately 1 in every 117,000 births and is more prevalent in males (Meikle, Hopwood, Clague, & Carey, 1999). Typical associated symptoms and signs may include neuropathic pain, severe acute pain attacks, acroparesthesia (prickling or burning), tinnitus (ringing sound in the ears) or hearing loss, diarrhea, heart palpitations and pain, various eye disorders or difficulties such as clouding of the cornea, cardiomyopathies, gastrointestinal difficulties, angiokeratoma (appears as skin rash), cerebrovascular accidents, lymphedema, kidney disorders, hypohydrosis, corneal dystrophy, respiratory problems, as well as other symptoms associated with central nervous system pathology (MacDermot, Holmes, & Miners, 2001a, 2001b; Ries et al., 2007). Without treatment, the presence of FD is associated with an average decrease in life span by 15 and 20 years in females and males, respectively (MacDermot et al., 2001a, 2001b). Individuals with FD are at a high risk for renal failure and cardiovascular difficulties.

NEUROPATHOLOGY/PATHOPHYSIOLOGY

FD is an X-linked lipid storage disorder characterized by an enzymatic defect resulting in a deficiency of the lysosomal enzyme α-galactosidase A, also referred to as ceramide trihexosidase. With increasing age, this deficiency results in the altered metabolism and accumulation of globotriaosylceramide in various systems throughout the body leading to dysfunction and pathology in multiple organs. Neurologic complications may be evident in the central and peripheral nervous systems, manifested in areas such as cognitive impairment, autonomic dysfunction, and ischemic or hemorrhagic stroke. Up to 68% of individuals with FD may have either or both white and gray matter lesions, with increased involvement approaching older age. Evidence from MRI has identified the presence of cerebrovascular involvement in some patients by 26 years of age increasing to all patients by 54 years of age, suggesting increased susceptibility to cerebrovascular accidents with increasing age (Crutchfield et al., 1998). Evidence has supported damage to dorsal root ganglia neurons, and axonal degeneration of small fibers as the originator of pain attacks that are often experienced in patients with FD (Gadoth & Sandbank, 1983; Kahn, 1973).

NEUROPSYCHOLOGICAL/CLINICAL PRESENTATION

Overall health-related quality of life in individuals with FD is considerably lower compared with normal individuals (Miners, Holmes, Sherr, Jenkinson, & MacDermot, 2002). More than 70% of individuals present with pain, most often in the hands and feet, and this symptom may be more prevalent in males (Hoffmann et al., 2007). Pain and tingling or numbness (acroparesthesia) of the skin may be induced or exacerbated by external changes in temperature (Hilz, Stemper, & Kolodny, 2000), which may make exercise or movement difficult (MacDermot & MacDermot, 2001). Acroparesthesia may also be elicited by emotional stress and may be present by as early as 3 years of age or younger (Ries et al., 2007). FD was once thought to be asymptomatic in all females due to an unaffected X-chromosome; however, more recent research evinces that symptom presentation may be similar to their male counterparts, such as small fiber neuropathic symptoms (MacDermot et al., 2001b; Mehta et al., 2004). FD results in the accumulation of lipids in multiple organ systems presenting in gastrointestinal problems, ocular difficulties (such as cornea verticillata), tinnitus, heart palpitations and pain, cardiomyopathies, angiokeratoma, lymphedema, kidney disorders, hypohydrosis, respiratory problems, and other symptoms associated with central nervous system pathology. Patients between the ages of 24 and 44 are approximately 12 times more likely to experience a cerebrovascular accident than are individuals from the general population (Mehta & Ginsberg, 2005). With increasing age there is likely to be more cerebral and renal involvement. Onset of cardiomyopathy is up to 10 years earlier and progresses faster in males than in females (Kampmann et al., 2008).

DIAGNOSIS

Due to delayed symptom onset and nonspecific symptomology, it is likely that FD is underdiagnosed (Zarate & Hopkin, 2008). Onset in childhood or early adolescence is most common, but may extend as late as early adulthood, with symptom presentation varying both with age and gender (Hoffmann et al., 2007). However, misdiagnoses are common and an accurate diagnosis may not be established for a 13–16 or more years after the first symptom presentation (Mehta et al., 2004). Hearing loss may be insidious, stretching across all frequency ranges, with the sensory threshold increasing with age (Ries et al., 2007). Secondary to FD, neurologic complications in the form of stroke, for example, may be diagnosed with MRI. Other symptoms indicative of FD include the presence of angiokeratomas, neuropathic pain, tinnitus, proteinuria, corneal lesions, and renal or cerebrovascular difficulties, or cardiomyopathy. Individuals with hypohydrosis may avoid exercise.

Echocardiography may be useful in differential diagnosis between FD cardiomyopathy and hypertrophic cardiomyopathy by the distinct appearance of left ventricular endocardial border (Pieroni et al., 2006). Left ventricular hypertrophy can also be differentiated by features such as acroparesthesia, hypertension, and hypohydrosis (Hoigne et al., 2006).

TREATMENT

Until relatively recently, treatment for FD has been mainly palliative in nature. Recent studies using enzyme replacement therapy (ERT) have been demonstrated to improve the long-term welfare of individuals with FD. ERT reduces the accumulation of globotriaosylceramide attenuating pain associated with FD. ERT has been evinced to improve pain-related quality of life and may also be able to replace neuropathic pain medications (Hoffman et al., 2007; Schiffmann et al., 2001). Some evidence has suggested that the use of ERT may also improve cold and heat thresholds reducing pain, attenuate the frequency of diarrhea, and may help alleviate hypohydrosis (Hilz, Brys, Marthol, Stemper, & Dutsch, 2004). ERT has also been observed to improve cardiac and renal functioning by reducing globotriaosylceramide and other glycolipid deposit levels. Some evidence indicates that improved renal functioning can be sustained with ERT by reducing glycolipid deposits in renal vascular endothelial cells with minimal side effects; however, more evidence is necessitated to establish long-term benefits (Shiffmann et al., 2001; Spinelli et al., 2004). Moderate symptom relief has been achieved through the use of Na^+ channel blocking agents (MacDermot & MacDermot, 2001). Also, due to the fact that cerebrovascular disease is related to morbidity, measures to address related risk factors may be efficacious to the patient's well-being (Mehta & Ginsberg, 2005). At times, ERT may not satisfactorily relieve an individual's discomfort and additional treatment of secondary symptomology is recommended, as well as routine clinical visits.

Anthony P. Odland
Charles Golden

Crutchfield, K. E., Patronas, N. J., Dambrosia, J. M., Frei, K. P., Banerjee, T. K., Barton, N. W., et al. (1998). Quantitative analysis of cerebral vasculopathy in Fabry disease patients. *Neurology, 50*, 1746–1749.

Gadoth, N., & Sandbank, U. (1983). Involvement of dorsal root ganglia in Fabry's disease. *Journal of Medical Genetics, 20*, 309–312.

Hilz, M. J., Brys, M., Marthol, H., Stemper, B., & Dütsch, M. (2004). Enzyme replacement therapy improves function of C-, Aδ-, and Aβ-nerve fibers in Fabry neuropathy. *Neurology, 62*, 1066–1072.

Hilz, M. J., Stemper, B., & Kolodny, E. H. (2000). Lower limb cold exposure induces pain and prolonged small fiber dysfunction in Fabry patients. *Pain, 84*, 361–365.

Hoffmann, B., Beck, M., Sunder-Plassmann, G., Borsini, W., Ricci, R., & Mehta, A. (2007). Nature and prevalence of pain in Fabry disease and its response to enzyme replacement therapy—a retrospective analysis from the Fabry outcome survey. *The Clinical Journal of Pain, 23*(6), 535–542.

Hoigne, P., Attenhofer Jost, C. H., Duru, F., Oechslin, E. N., Seifert, B., Widmer, U., et al. (2006). Simple criteria for differentiation of Fabry disease from amyloid heart disease and other causes of left ventricular hypertrophy. *International Journal of Cardiology, 111*, 413–422.

Kahn, P. (1973). Anderson-Fabry disease: A histopathological study of three cases with observations on the mechanism of production of pain. *Journal of Neurology, Neurosurgery, and Psychiatry, 36*, 1053–1062.

Kampmann, C., Linhart, A., Baehner, F., Palecek, T., Wiethoff, C. M., Miebach, E., et al. (2008). Onset and progression of the Anderson-Fabry disease related cardiomyopathy. *International Journal of Cardiology, 130,* 367–373.

MacDermot, K. D., Holmes, A., & Miners, A. H. (2001a). Anderson-Fabry disease: Clinical manifestations and impact of disease in a cohort of 98 hemizygous males. *Journal of Medical Genetics, 38*(11), 750–760.

MacDermot, K. D., Holmes, A., & Miners, A. H. (2001b). Anderson-Fabry disease: Clinical manifestations and impact of disease in a cohort of 60 obligate carrier females. *Journal of Medical Genetics, 38*(11), 769–775.

MacDermot, J., & MacDermot, K. D. (2001). Neuropathic pain in Anderson-Fabry disease: Pathology and therapeutic options. *European Journal of Pharmacology, 429,* 121–125.

Mehta, A., & Ginsberg, L. (2005). Natural history of the cerebrovascular complications of Fabry disease. *Acta Paediatrica, 94*(Suppl. 447), 24–27.

Mehta, A., Ricci, R., Widmer, U., Dehout, F., Garcia de Lorenzo, A., Kampmann, C., et al. (2004). Fabry disease defined: Baseline clinical manifestations of 366 patients in the Fabry Outcome Survey. *European Journal of Clinical Investigation, 34,* 236–242.

Meikle, P. J., Hopwood, J. J., Clague, A. E., & Carey, W. F. (1999). Prevalence of lysosomal storage disorders. *The Journal of the American Medical Association, 281,* 249–254.

Miners, A. H., Holmes, A., Sherr, L., Jenkinson, C., & MacDermot, K. D. (2002). Assessment of health-related quality-of-life in males in Anderson-Fabry disease before therapeutic intervention. *Quality of Life Research, 11,* 127–133.

Pieroni, M., Chimenti, C., Cobelli, F., Morgante, E., Maschio, A., Gaudio, C., et al. (2006). Fabry's disease cardiomyopathy: Echocardiographic detection of endomyocardial glycosphingolipid compartmentalization. *Journal of the American College of Cardiology, 47*(8), 1663–1671.

Ries, M., Kim, H. J., Zalewski, C. K., Mastroianni, M. A., Moore, D. F., Brady, R. O., et al. (2007). Neuropathic and cerebrovascular correlates of hearing loss in Fabry disease. *Brain, 130,* 143–150.

Schiffmann, R., Kopp, J. B., Austin, H. A., Sabnis, S., Moore, D. F., Weibel, T., et al. (2001). Enzyme replacement therapy in Fabry disease: A randomized controlled trial. *Journal of the American College of Cardiology, 285,* 2743–2749.

Spinelli, L., Pisani, A., Sabbatini, M., Petretta, M., Andreucci, M. V., Procaccini, D., et al. (2004). Enzyme replacement therapy with agalsidase βs disease. *Clinical Genetics, 66,* 158–165.

Zarate, Y. A., & Hopkin, R. J. (2008). Lysosomal storage disease 3: Fabry's disease. *The Lancet, 372,* 1427–1435.

FACTITIOUS DISORDER

DESCRIPTION

Factitious disorder (FD) refers to a psychiatric condition characterized by the deliberate production or feigning of psychological or physical signs or symptoms with the sole intention of assuming the role of a sick person (American Psychiatric Association [APA], 2000). Although early accounts of FD extend back to second-century Rome, the first modern reports of FD describe patients who habitually migrate between hospitals, feigning symptoms, and embellishing their personal histories (Asher, 1951). More recent etiological studies investigating the prevalence of FD have estimated that between 1% and 3% of psychiatric consultation patients qualify for a diagnosis of FD (APA, 2000; Bauer & Boegner, 1996; Sutherland & Rodin, 1990), with rates as high as 6% reported among psychiatric inpatients (Gregory & Jindal, 2006). It is widely believed that the condition is underdiagnosed primarily because one of the hallmarks of FD involves willful deception, which may go undetected by medical staff. However, overdiagnosis may be common in specific cases in which individuals with FD may frequent multiple hospitals using a variety of pseudonyms (APA, 2000).

Characteristically, persons with FD are reported to be three times more likely to be females than males (Frey, 2003). The typical FD patient is 20–40 years of age, is unmarried, and has a history of employment or training in a medical field, such as nursing or medical technology (APA, 2000; Ford, 1983). Such individuals tend to have extensive knowledge of disease and access to equipment needed to fake illnesses. Similarly, FD by proxy typically occurs in mothers who induce illness in their young children, but such abuse may also be perpetrated on older children, adolescents, or other adults in their care (APA, 2000). By contrast, chronic FD, such as Munchausen syndrome (which accounts for approximately 10% of FD cases), tends to affect unmarried, middle-aged males (APA, 2000; Folks, 1995).

Feigned and exaggerated physical signs and symptoms occur much more frequently in patients with FD than do psychological symptoms (APA, 2000). Individuals with FD may be prone to creating actual medical conditions (e.g., raising their own blood sugar, creating scars) as a part of their symptom presentation and may agree to undergo unnecessary procedures to diagnose or treat their "condition."

F

These behaviors can contribute to morbidity and mortality among this population (Folks, 1995; Sutherland & Rodin, 1990). However, the number of deaths per year contributed to by FD is unclear.

Currently, the causes of FD are not well understood or defined. Psychodynamic explanations contend that individuals with FD often have a history of neglect or abandonment, and that the behaviors associated with FD are an attempt to reenact unresolved early issues with parents (Ford, 1983). Other proposed causes include underlying masochistic tendencies, a need to be the center of attention, a need to assume a dependent status, a need to ease feelings of worthlessness or vulnerability, or a need to feel superior to authority figures (Frey, 2003). FD tends to be comorbid with a variety of Axis I and Axis II disorders, including severe personality disorders (most often borderline), mood disorders, anxiety disorders, and substance-related disorders (APA, 2000; Frey, 2003; Gregory & Jindal, 2006). Explanations for FD by proxy mirror those given for FD, differing in that the individual uses another person to satisfy his or her emotional needs.

NEUROPATHOLOGY/PATHOPHYSIOLOGY

The pathophysiology of FD remains unclear. Case reports of abnormalities on EEGs and on brain images of patients with chronic FD suggest that brain morphology may play a role in at least some of the diagnosed cases (Babe, Peterson, Loosen, & Geracioti, 1992; Fenelon, Mahieux, Roullet, & Gullard, 1991; Folks, 1995; Pankratz & Lezak, 1987). However, critics of these findings argue that these studies were small in scale and that the observed abnormalities were nonspecific and rare (Feldman, 2004; Frey, 2003).

NEUROPSYCHOLOGICAL/CLINICAL PRESENTATION

Associated features identified with FD may be detected during clinical intakes and medical interviews. These tendencies may include (1) dramatic or atypical presentation, (2) vague and inconsistent details, (3) an extensive medical record with multiple admissions to various hospitals, (4) familiarity of medical textbook descriptions of illness, (5) an unusual knowledge of medical terminology, (6) pseudologia fantastica (pathological lying regarding history or symptoms), (7) reports of suicidal ideation or attempt, (8) reports of substance abuse or dependence, (9) diagnosis of personality disorder, and (10) reports of trauma or abuse as a child (APA, 2000; Feldman, 2004; Frey, 2003).

Mental status examinations indicate that patients with FD may vary in their presentation, and no established pathognomic signs have been indicated (Frey, 2003). However, frequently documented results include markedly brighter than expected mood, given the patient's medical condition, hallucinations and disturbances of thought process or content, aberrant cognitive functioning and impaired information processing, and approximating answers to questions that are very close to the correct answers (i.e., $1 + 1 = 3$).

Several assessment techniques have been developed to determine the probability of cognitive and neuropsychological symptom exaggeration or feigning in patients. Assessment techniques that are commonly used by neuropsychologists to support suspicions include (1) below chance levels of performance on one or more forced-choice measures of cognitive functioning, (2) significant discrepancy between test data and accepted models of normal and abnormal central nervous system function, and (3) significant discrepancy between test data and levels of observed or reported behavior (for a more in-depth discussion, see Heubrock and Petermann, 1998; Slick, Sherman, and Iverson, 1999). On the Minnesota Multiphasic Personality Inventory-2 (MMPI-2; Butcher, Dahlstrom, Graham, Tellegen, & Kaemmer, 1989), an invalid test profile, elevations of all clinical scales, and specific patterns of elevation on certain validity scales may indicate an attempt to "fake bad" by appearing more psychologically disturbed than is the case (for a more in-depth review, see Greene, 2008 or Rogers, Sewell, Martin, & Vitacco, 2003). Although no assessment instrument or technique can be used in isolation to diagnose factitious symptoms, assessment data can be used in conjunction with information derived from the total clinical context to support suspicions of possible FD diagnosis.

DIAGNOSIS

The *Diagnostic and Statistical Manual of Mental Disorders* (4th ed., text revision) (*DSM-IV-TR*; APA, 2000, p. 517) requires the following three criteria to be met for the diagnosis of FD: (1) intentional production, feigning, or exaggeration of physical and/or psychological signs or symptoms, (2) motivation for the behavior is to assume the sick role, and (3) an absence of external incentives for the behavior (e.g., economic gain, avoiding legal responsibilities). FD can present with predominantly physical, predominantly psychological, or combined psychological and physical symptoms. A fourth type of FD, termed FD not otherwise specified, includes those disorders with factitious symptoms that do not meet the full criteria for FD. The

DSM-IV-TR places FD by proxy (i.e., Munchausen's syndrome by proxy) in this category.

FD appears in the differential diagnosis for many illnesses in which physical symptoms and signs are noted and must be distinguished from a true or real general medical condition or mental disorder. Because FD is characterized as falling on a continuum between somatoform illnesses (e.g., somatization disorder, conversion disorder, hypochondriasis, pain disorder, body dysmorphic disorder) and malingering, careful consideration must be given as to the intent of the patient when diagnosing FD. For example, in somatoform disorders, the production of the symptoms of illness is not intentional, and the motivation for illness is unconscious. However, in FD symptoms are produced intentionally but for unconscious reasons. Conversely, malingering can be differentiated from FD in that symptom production, though intentional and conscious, is linked with an external incentive beyond the sick role (e.g., obtaining compensation, avoiding punishment or duties). Major depression with psychotic features and delusional disorder (somatoform type) can also be present with somatic preoccupations not supported by physical examination, laboratory testing, or imaging. Associated features of these disorders should help to facilitate differential diagnosis. FD by proxy must also be differentiated from overanxious parenting.

TREATMENT

Currently, there is a lack of evidence to support the efficacy of any one single treatment option in regard to FD (Eastwood & Bisson, 2008). Case reports of successfully managed patients with FD tend to use nonconfrontational therapeutic approaches that (1) reinforce positive health behaviors, (2) focus on supportive rather than insight-oriented therapy, (3) address the patient's emotional distress as the source of the illness, (4) emphasize the collaborative role between patient and treatment team, and (5) maintain a consistent relationship with a primary physician regardless of the clinical outcome (Folks, 1995; Frey, 2003; Gregory & Jindal, 2006). Providing medical and psychological support for comorbid conditions may also lead to improvement or resolution of FD behavior. For example, medications to treat the symptoms of personality disorders, such as selective serotonin reuptake inhibitors (SSRIs), have been found to reduce impulsivity, which may lead to some benefits in FD patients (Frey, 2003).

The prognosis for patients with FD is variable. For those individuals with mild FD who actively seek treatment, overcoming their illness is possible and remittance is not uncommon in the fourth decade of life (Frey, 2003). However, chronic FD appears to be more unremitting, and treatment tends to ameliorate symptoms for only short periods of time. In addition, only a small percentage of FD patients will consent to psychiatric treatment upon confrontation (Eastwood & Bisson, 2008; Gregory & Jindahl, 2006). More typically, FD patients tend to deny allegations, with chronic patients typically becoming angry and discharging themselves from the hospital after confrontation. Further, comorbid personality disorders, such as antisocial personality disorder, may prove to limit collaborative relationship building, making cognitive behavioral therapy difficult.

Lisa A. Pass
Andrew S. Davis

American Psychiatric Association. (2000). *Diagnostic and statistical manual of mental disorders* (4th ed., text revision, pp. 513–517; 781–783). Washington, DC: Author.

Asher, R. (1951). Munchausen's syndrome. *Lancet, 1*, 339–341.

Babe, K. S., Jr., Peterson, A. M., Loosen, P. T., & Geracioti, T. D., Jr. (1992). The pathogenesis of Munchausen syndrome: A review and case report. *General Hospital Psychiatry, 14*, 273–276.

Bauer, M., & Boegner, F. (1996). Neurological syndromes in factitious disorder. *Journal of Nervous and Mental Disease, 184*, 281–288.

Butcher, J. N., Dahlstrom, W. G., Graham, J. R., Tellegen, A., & Kaemmer, B. (1989). *Minnesota multiphasic personality inventory-2: Manual for administration and scoring.* Minneapolis, MN: University of Minnesota Press.

Eastwood, S., & Bisson, J. (2008). Management of factitious disorders: A systematic review. *Psychotherapy and Psychosomatics, 77*, 209–218.

Feldman, M. D. (2004). *Playing sick? Untangling the web of Munchausen syndrome, Munchausen by proxy, malingering & factitious disorder.* New York: Routledge.

Fenelon, G., Mahieux, F., Roullet, E., & Guillard, A. (1991). Munchausen's syndrome and abnormalities on magnetic resonance imaging of the brain. *British Medical Journal, 302*(6783), 996–997.

Folks, D. G. (1995). Munchausen's syndrome and other factitious disorders. *Neurologic Clinics, 13*(2), 267–281.

Ford, C. V. (1983). The somatizing disorders: Illness as a way of life. New York: Elsevier Biomedical.

Frey, R. J. (2003). Factitious disorder. In E. Thackery & M. Harris (Eds.), *Gale encyclopedia of mental disorders* (Vol. 1, pp. 389–393). Detroit, MI: Gale.

Greene, R. L. (2008). Malingering and defensiveness on the MMPI-2. In R. Rogers (Ed.), *Clinical assessment of malingering and deception* (pp. 159–181). New York: Guilford Press.

Gregory, R. J., & Jindal, S. (2006). Factitious disorder on an inpatient psychiatry ward. *American Journal of Orthopsychiatry, 76*(1), 31–36.

Heubrock, D., & Petermann, F. (1998). Neuropsychological assessment of suspected malingering: Research results, evaluation techniques, and further directions of research and application. *European Journal of Psychological Assessment, 14*(3), 211–225.

Pankratz, L., & Lezak, M. D. (1987). Cerebral dysfunction in the Munchausen syndrome. *Hillside Journal of Clinical Psychiatry, 9*, 195–206.

Rogers, R., Sewell, K. W., Martin, M. A., & Vitacco, M. J. (2003). Detection of feigned mental disorders: A meta-analysis of the MMPI-2 and malingering. *Assessment, 10*, 160–177.

Slick, D. J., Sherman, E. M. S., & Iverson, G. L. (1999). Diagnostic criteria for malingered neurocognitive dysfunction: Proposed standards for clinical practice and research. *The Clinical Neuropsychologist, 13*(4), 545–561.

Sutherland, A. J., & Rodin, G. M. (1990). Factitious disorder in a general hospital setting: Clinical features, and a review of the literature. *Psychosomatics, 31*, 392–399.

FACTOR V LEIDEN

DESCRIPTION

Factor V Leiden was identified in 1994 by Rogier M. Bertina, in Leiden, Netherlands. Factor V Leiden, a hereditary mutation of the factor V gene, causes a hypercoagulability disorder. The mutation of the factor V gene results in excessive blood clotting and resistance to activated protein C degradation, which, in combination with other risk factors, can cause significant morbidity (Andreoli, 2007). Factor V Leiden is the most common hereditary disorder that predisposes individuals to thrombosis.

NEUROPATHOLOGY/PATHOPHYSIOLOGY

In a healthy individual, the factor V protein functions as a cofactor with factor X, also known as Stuart–Prower factor. Factor X is an enzyme of the coagulation process, which, along with factor V, forms the prothrombinase complex (Andreoli, 2007). The prothrombinase complex catalyzes prothrombin, an inactive zymogen, into thrombin. Thrombin cleaves fibrinogen to fibrin, which polymerizes to form the majority of the meshwork of a thrombus, or blood clot. Protein C, a major physiological anticoagulant, is activated by thrombin into activated protein C (De Stefano & Leone, 1995).

Once activated, protein C regulates blood clot formation by the cleaving and degrading of factor V.

Factor V Leiden is a genetic disorder resulting from a point mutation in the gene encoding of factor V. The mutation, a missense substitution, occurs when factor V protein's amino acid arginine is switched to glutamine. This mutation results in a factor V variant that is resistant to the regulatory work of activated protein C (Bertina et al., 1994). The resistivity of factor V Leiden to activated protein C results in the inability to cleave factor V and a deficiency in the anticoagulation system.

Individuals who are homozygous for the mutated allele are at a higher percentage for risks associated with deep vein thrombosis, than for those who are heterozygous (De Stefano & Leone, 1995).

NEUROPSYCHOLOGICAL/CLINICAL PRESENTATION

The excessive clotting associated with factor V Leiden is mostly restricted to veins, where the clotting may cause deep vein thrombosis. Deep vein thrombosis may occur without symptoms, but typically the affected extremity will be characterized by swelling, pain, redness, warmth of area, and engorging of the superficial veins. Long-term effects that can occur after deep vein thrombosis are edemas, discomfort, and skin complications.

If the venous blood clots break off and travel to the lungs, pulmonary embolism occurs. Symptoms of pulmonary embolism may include difficulty breathing, chest pains, low blood oxygen saturation, cyanosis, rapid breathing, and heart palpitations. Severe cases of pulmonary embolism may involve collapsing, extremely low blood pressure, and sudden death.

It is extremely rare for factor V Leiden to result in blood clots forming in the arteries that may result in a stroke or myocardial infarction. Consequently, minimal research exists on the link between factor V Leiden and neurological complications. Two clinical cases of combined schizencephaly and thrombophilia have been reported in the literature, with both cases caused by mutations to methyltetrahydrofolate reductase and the factor V gene (Goez & Zelnik, 2009). Complications in these cases included both motor and cognitive deficits.

DIAGNOSIS

To diagnose a deep vein thrombosis, an intravenous venography may be performed. Intravenous venography involves injecting a peripheral vein of the affected limb with a contrasting agent and administering X-rays. Physical examinations, imaging of the extremity in question, and a blood test may also be performed in making a diagnosis.

For pulmonary embolisms, diagnosis is based primarily on observed clinical criteria combined with selective testing. Electrocardiogram and electrocardiography findings are used in conjunction with pulmonary angiography, CT scan, and blood test results to formulate a diagnosis.

Diagnosing factor V Leiden as the cause for a thrombotic event should be considered if a family history of venous thrombosis exists or if a Caucasian patient under 45 years of age presents. Methods for diagnosing factor V Leiden include screening with a snake-venom based test, a genetic test, or an Activated Partial Thromboplastin Time test.

TREATMENT

Diagnosing an individual with factor V Leiden occurs following a thrombotic event. Due to the genetic nature of the disorder, a cure does not currently exist. However, knowing your familial medical history may aid in prevention of either deep vein thrombosis or pulmonary embolisms.

Treatment for deep vein thrombosis may require hospitalization. Anticoagulation therapy using heparin is the usual treatment (Snow et al., 2007). Patients who suffer from reoccurring deep vein thrombosis may require life-long anticoagulation therapy. Elastic compression stockings are used in conjunction with anticoagulation therapy as well. If anticoagulation therapy is not successful, an inferior vena cava filter may be used. An inferior vena cava filter prevents new embolisms from entering the pulmonary artery. For extensive blood clots, thrombolysis may be performed.

The most popular treatment option for pulmonary embolisms involves anticoagulation therapy. Heparin or fondaparinux is administered initially, whereas warfarin, acenocoumarol, or phenprocoumon is administered later. If anticoagulation therapy is not successful, an inferior vena cava filter may be used. Both thrombolysis and surgical management are highly debated treatment options that exist as well (Turpie, 2007).

In treating thrombosis or blood clots, drugs such as heparin and warfarin are often used to inhibit the clot's formation and growth. These medications decrease blood coagulation through inhibition of vitamin K, an enzyme needed for forming mature clotting factors.

O. J. Vidal
J. T. Hutton
Antonio E. Puente

Andreoli, T. E. (2007). *Cecil essentials of medicine* (7th ed.). Philadelphia: Saunders, Elsevier.

Bertina, R. M., Koeleman, B. P., & Koster, T. (1994). Mutation in blood coagulation factor V associated with resistance to activated protein C. *Nature, 369*(6475), 64–67.

De Stefano, V., & Leone, G. (1995). Resistance to activated protein C due to mutated factor V as a novel cause of inherited thrombophilia. *Haematologica, 80*(4), 344–356.

Goez, N., & Zelnik, N. (2009). Schizencephaly in infants with thrombophilia. *Journal of Child Neurology, 24*(4), 421–424.

Snow, V., Qaseem, A., & Barry, P. (2007). Management of venous thromboembolism: A clinical practice guideline from the American College of Physicians and the American Academy of Family Physicians. *Annals of Family Medicine, 146*(3), 204–210.

Turpie, A. G. (2007). Oral, direct factor Xa inhibitors in development for the prevention and treatment of thromboembolic diseases. *Arteriosclerosis, Thrombosis, and Vascular Biology, 27*(6), 1238–1247.

FAHR'S SYNDROME

DESCRIPTION

Fahr's syndrome or Fahr's disease refers to a rare neurological condition involving calcification of the basal ganglia, dentate nucleus of the cerebellum, and centrum semiovale (Elshimali, 2005; Manyam, 2005; Modrego, Monjonero, Serrano & Fayed, 2005). The name of the condition originates from a German pathologist named Theodor Fahr, who in 1930 published an article on the topic (Klein, 1998; Manyam, 2005; Ropper & Brown, 2005), although he was not the first to describe calcification in the brain, nor did he contribute much to knowledge of the condition (Manyam, 2005; Ropper & Brown, 2005). However, his name became associated with all forms of bilateral calcifications in the basal ganglia and other parts of the brain (Manyam, 2005). In fact, there is some confusion about the disease because it tends to be used as an umbrella term to describe all forms of bilateral calcification of the basal ganglia and other parts of the brain (Klein, 1998; Manyam, 2005). Furthermore, there have been at least 35 different names over the course of history used to describe the disease, including familial idiopathic brain calcification, bilateral-symmetrical calcification of basal ganglia, and bilateral striopallidodentate calcinosis (Manyam, 2005).

F

NEUROPATHOLOGY/PATHOPHYSIOLOGY

The precise pathological process of this condition is not yet known. Fahr's syndrome is a "neuro-mineral disease" with calcium being the major element present (Manyam, 2005). Other mineral deposits, including arsenic, cobalt, copper, iron, lead, magnesium, phosphorus, silver, zinc, aluminum, are also present (Manyam, 2005). The involvement of the basal ganglia corresponds with the functional picture, but involvement of the basal ganglia themselves is not surprising as numerous disorders have also been associated with such mineralization including, but not limited to, Alzheimer's disease, Down's syndrome, parkinsonism, Alexander's disease, Moebius's syndrome, and so forth (Manyam, 2005). Furthermore, calcification of vessels in the basal ganglia to subtle degrees is seen in many elderly individuals. Fahr's syndrome is clinically relevant as this calcification occurs in higher degrees and may occur earlier in life. This process is of such extensiveness that it may be noted on scans. In general, large deposits are noted in the globus pallidus, putamen, caudate nucleus, internal capsule, dentate nucleus, and the lateral thalamus (Lowe, Lennox, & Leigh, 1997). In addition, small amounts can at times be noted in the cerebellar folia and cerebral cortex, at the junctions between the cortex and white matter (Lowe et al., 1997).

NEUROPSYCHOLOGICAL/CLINICAL PRESENTATION

Fahr's syndrome may present with a mixture of motor and cognitive symptoms (Manyam, 2005; Rosenblatt & Leroi, 2000). The literature most commonly links Fahr's syndrome with choreoathetosis and rigidity although spasticity, other Parkinsonian symptoms (e.g., tremors, muscle rigidity, shuffling gait, etc.), spastic paralysis, and/or bilateral athetosis may also be noted later in the disease course (Ropper & Brown, 2005). Other possible manifestations include cerebellar impairment and speech disorder (i.e., dysarthria). Subcortical dementia and/or focal cortical deficits may also occur as well with the prior more likely than the latter (Manyam, 2005; Rosenblatt & Leroi, 2000). Additional symptoms can include an increased risk of seizures, migraines/headaches, and eye impairments.

DIAGNOSIS

Diagnosing Fahr's syndrome is primarily dependent upon neuroimaging involving CT or MRI scans of the head. These technologies are helpful in not only identifying the calcification but also ruling out other abnormalities of known calcium metabolism as well as developmental defects. Hypoparathyroidism in particular should be ruled out as it is the major differential diagnosis. Differentiating between the two should include examining serum calcium and parathormone levels (Manyam, 2005). Differential diagnosis may also include ruling out other basal ganglia conditions, such as Huntington's disease, Parkinson's disease, and Wilson's disease (Elshimali, 2005; Rosenblatt & Leroi, 2000). Also, the following presentations are all associated with or may be linked with mineralization of the basal ganglia: Alzheimer's disease, Down's syndrome, non-parkinsonian movement disorders, psychosis including schizophrenia, Nasu–Hakola's disease, Moebius's syndrome, neurodegeneration with brain iron accumulation, Alexander's disease, HIV infection and AIDS, meningoencephalitis, lupus cerebritis, chemotherapy and radiotherapy effects, folate deficiency, carbon monoxide poisoning, anoxia, pseudohypoparathyroidism, pseudopseudo-hypoparathyroidism, hyperparathyroidism, and carbonic anhydrase II deficiency (Lowe et al., 1997).

TREATMENT

Research has yet to establish the best method for treating Fahr's syndrome. It has shown that treatment with central nervous system–specific calcium channel blocking agents was unsuccessful. In addition, disodium etidronate treatment resulted in symptomatic benefit in one patient, but there was no reduction in calcification (Manyam, 2005). As a result, treatment is symptom-based as well as supportive.

Amy E. Zimmerman
Chad A. Noggle

Elshimali, Y. I. (2005). The value of differential diagnosis of Fahr's disease by radiology. *The Internet Journal of Radiology, 4*(1), ISSN: 1528–8404.

Klein, C. (1998). Fahr's disease—far from a disease. *Movement Disorders, 13*(3), 620–621.

Lowe, J., Lennox, G., & Leigh, P. N. (1997). Disorders of movement and system degeneration. In D. I. Graham & P. L. Lantos (Eds.), *Greenfield's neuropathology* (6th ed., pp. 281–366). New York: Oxford University Press.

Manyam, B. V. (2005). What is and what is not Fahr's disease? *Parkinsonism and Related Disorders, 11*, 73–80.

Modrego, P. J., Monjonero, J., Serrano, M., & Fayed, N. (2005). Fahr's syndrome presenting with pure and progressive presenile dementia. *Neurological Sciences, 26*, 367–369.

Ropper, A. H., & Brown, R. H. (2005). *Adams and Victor's principles of neurology* (8th ed., pp. 797–849). New York: McGraw-Hill.

Rosenblatt, A., & Leroi, I. (2000). Neuropsychiatry of Huntington's disease and other basal ganglia disorders. *Psychosomatics, 41,* 24–30.

FAMILIAL PERIODIC PARALYSES

DESCRIPTION

Familial periodic paralysis (FPP), also known as periodic paralysis (PP), is a muscular disorder that is autosomal dominant in nature and characterized by periods of flaccid paralysis with failure of deep tendon reflexes and overall failure of muscle to respond to neural stimulation (Holmes, 1941). There are over 30 types of this disorder, but the most common forms are hyperkalemic and hypokalemic.

NEUROPATHOLOGY/PATHOPHYSIOLOGY

The defining feature in all cases of FPP is flaccid weakness of the muscles. In FPP, the muscle membranes do not reach an excitability state following neural stimulation (sarcolemma). There are two primary forms of FPP: hypokalemic and hyperkalemic. All 30 plus types share similar characteristics, but are considered heterogeneous, as there is no single cause for the disorder. In all cases, there is a generalized weakness; most often the muscles of the head and respiratory system are not involved; and during attacks, the stretch reflexes are markedly diminished or completely absent (Sripathi, 2007).

It has been shown that in all cases of FPP the major dysfunction is related to sodium channel depolarization, resulting in inactivity and a lack of excitability in the fibers of the muscles (Sripathi, 2007; Venance et al., 2006). In hypokalemic PP, the serum potassium levels may show a slight decrease, serum creative phosphokinase (CPK) becomes moderately elevated with an attack, and an ECG will show bradycardia, flat T waves, U waves, and ST segment depression (Venance et al., 2006). In hyperkalemic PP, the serum potassium levels will be slightly higher than baseline and will most often not occur beyond the normal range. Serum CPK also becomes mildly elevated during attacks and the ECG will show T waves.

NEUROPSYCHOLOGICAL/CLINICAL PRESENTATION

The defining features in all cases of PP include attacks beginning prior to 25 years of age, fluctuation of potassium levels prior to an attack, one or many groups of muscles are affected, tendon reflexes are poor during an attack, and potassium-level changes during an attack may not be measurable. Once an attack passes, muscle weakness will most often dissipate and return to normal. However, over time and with continued attacks, muscle function may never return to baseline prior to the onset of attacks (Sripathi, 2007; Venance et al., 2006).

The most distinct clinical presentation in the hypokalemic form, which is the most common form of PP, is decreased potassium levels resulting in muscular weakness. Attacks begin most often prior to age 16. Paralysis attacks will most often occur upon waking either during the night or in the morning (Sternberg, Tabti, Hoinque, & Fontaine, 2009).

The second most common form of PP is hyperkalemic paralysis. The most distinct clinical presentation in this form is muscle weakness. Often the onsets of attacks begin after eating, fasting, or vigorous exercise. Unlike hypokalemic attacks, hyperkalemic attacks begin before the age of 10 (Venance et al., 2006).

Another form of FPP is thyrotoxic periodic paralysis (TPP). Interestingly, this type appears to be most common in males of Asian descent, though it can occur in anyone with a history of hyperthyroid disease (Lam, Nair, & Tingle, 2006). Another interesting feature of this disorder is that the attacks most often occur from May to October. Low potassium levels are the hallmark of this disorder, presenting below 2.0 mEq/L during an attack. All other symptoms are similar to hyperkalemic periodic paralysis (HPP). TPP dissipates once euthyroid is established (Levitt, 2007).

A rare form of PP is known as Andersen–Tawil syndrome (ATS). ATS has the characteristic low potassium levels seen in HPP, with the exception that cardiac arrhythmias co-occur (Donaldson, Yoon, Fu, & Ptacek, 2004).

DIAGNOSIS

PP, regardless of the type, is most often diagnosed by a history of paralysis attacks. In addition, blood tests can help to determine whether serum potassium and CPK levels are abnormal (Venance et al., 2006). Sometimes physicians may want to confirm the specific type of FPP a person has by inducing an attack through the use of insulin or dextrose, combined with the use of a treadmill.

HPP symptoms tend to manifest during the first or second decade of life. Individuals with HPP have reported paresthesias, fatigue, and changes in behavior prior to an attack (Venance et al., 2006). Recommended diagnostic tests consist of a complete neurological workup and thyroid function tests (THS,

F

FT4, FT3) (Sternberg, Tabti, Hainque, & Fontaine, 2009).

Hyperkalemic PP usually manifests during the first decade of life and has a high penetrance. The weakness or paralysis will most often last 1–4 hours. Miller et al. (2004) report that myotonia of the eyelid and lid lag may be the only presenting symptoms. They also indicate that proximal myopathy develops over time and with age.

From a differential diagnosis standpoint, it is important to rule out several other medical conditions that can be confused with PP. This includes, but is not limited to, myelopathy, narcolepsy, multiple sclerosis, myasthenia gravis, Guillain–Barré syndrome in childhood, spinal cord hemorrhage or infarction, and chronic inflammatory demyelinating polyradiculoneuropathy.

As previously noted, ATS is a rare form of PP. ATS presents with symptoms similar to other forms of PP, such as increased potassium sensitivity; however, cardiac arrhythmias, ventricular ectopy, and anomalies of the skeleton will also be present (Venance et al., 2006).

TREATMENT

Due to the genetic nature of FPP, it is not a preventable disorder. Hypokalemic paralysis is most often treated by oral or intravenous potassium administration that helps to relieve an attack (Levitt, 2007). Dietary treatment includes eating reduced amounts of carbohydrates and restricting sodium intake. It is also recommended that after periods of rest physical activity and alcohol consumption should be avoided (Venance et al., 2006). Acetazolamide has also been shown to help reduce attacks.

Treatment for hyperkalemic paralysis includes light exercise and a diet that includes increased consumption of carbohydrates. While an attack is occurring, thiazides, acetazolamide, and β-agonists can be helpful in lessening the severity of the attack. The recommended diet requires consistent intake of carbohydrates and decreased consumption of foods that are high in potassium. Fasting and strenuous exercise are also discouraged after a meal, as well as exposure to the cold, for all can set off an attack (Venance et al., 2006).

Teri J. McHale
Henry V. Soper

Donaldson, M., Yoon, G., Fu, Y., & Ptacek, L. (2004). Andersen–Tawil syndrome: A model of clinical variability, pleiotropy, and genetic heterogeneity. *Annals of Medicine, 36*(Supp. 1), 92–97.

Holmes, J. (1941). Familial periodic paralysis. Haemorrhage into lungs in deaths from trauma. *The British Medical Journal,* 80–82.

Lam, L., Nair, R., & Tingle, L. (2006). Thyrotoxic periodic paralysis. *Baylor University Medical Center Proceedings, 19,* 126–129.

Levitt, J. (2007). Practical aspects in the management of hypokalemic periodic paralysis. *Journal of Translational Medicine, 6,* 18.

Miller, T., Dias da Silva, M., Miller, H., Kwiecinski, H., Mendell, J., & Tawil, R., et al. Correlating phenotype and genotype in the periodic paralyses. *Neurology, 63,* 1647–1655.

Sripathi, N. (2007, July 24). *eMedicine.* Periodic paralyses. Retrieved from http://emedicine.medscape.com/article1171678-overview

Sternberg, D., Tabti, N., Hainque, B., & Fontaine, B. (2009, April 28). *Gene reviews.* Retrieved from http://www.ncbi.nim.nih.gov/books/NBK1338/

Venance, S., Cannon, S., Fialho, D., Fontaine, B., Hanna, M., Ptacek, L., et al. (2006). The primary periodic paralyses: Diagnosis, pathogenesis and treatment. *Brain, 129,* 8–17.

FAMILIAL SPASTIC PARAPLEGIA

DESCRIPTION

Familial spastic paraplegia (also called and Strümpell–Lorrain syndrome) is a group of disorders that have a primary clinical feature of progressive, severe, lower extremity spasticity (Fink, 2006). The disease is classified as "uncomplicated" or "pure" when symptoms only include lower extremity weakness, bladder disturbance, and variable impairment of vibratory sensation in the feet. The disease is classified as "complicated" if symptoms include neurologic deficits such as ataxia, mental retardation, dementia, visual or hearing dysfunctions, adrenal insufficiency, extrapyramidal dysfunctions, and ichthyosis (Boustany et al., 1987; Dürr et al., 1994). The age of symptom onset, rate of symptom progression, and extent of disability are variable both within and between the forms of the disorder. Familial spastic paraplegia was first described in 1883, by Strümpell, but later was described in more detail by Lorrain. The disease was discovered to be a genetic disorder and is X-linked, autosomal recessive, or autosomal dominant. Because the clinical presentation of the disorder can vary widely, the classifications of the disease are now based on the mode of inheritance and genetic linkage, although the clinical distinctions between pure and complicated forms of familial spastic paraplegia are also used. The risk of inheriting familial spastic paraplegia depends on particular features of the gene involved. The autosomal-dominant form of familial spastic paraplegia accounts for more than 80% of all familial cases. Currently, several genetic types of familial spastic paraplegia have been identified with the involvement of separate genes (Fink, 2006; Weimer & Wong, 2009).

NEUROPATHOLOGY/PATHOPHYSIOLOGY

Familial spastic paraplegia is typically caused by a mutation in the spastin gene. The mutation in the gene causes an abnormal interaction with microtubules, which disrupts organelle transport on the microtubule cytoskeleton (McDermott, 2003). In either "uncomplicated" or "complicated" forms of familial spastic paraplegia, upper motor neurons involved in voluntary movement degenerate. These upper motor neurons begin in the motor cortex of the brain and extend down the spinal cord and carry signals from the brain to the lower motor neurons. Lower motor neurons send messages to the muscles, telling them to contract or relax. Because of the degeneration, the correct signals do not get to the lower motor neurons, and the muscles do not receive the correct messages causing spasticity and weakness of the affected muscles. The degree of nerve degeneration is directly related to the degree of the disease's symptomatology (Fink, 2006). Typically, the condition principally affects the lower body, but rare forms of the disease can also have upper body or additional neurologic symptoms. The major neuropathologic feature of autosomal-dominant, uncomplicated familial spastic paraplegia is axonal degeneration that is maximal in the terminal portions of the longest descending and ascending tracts. Spinocerebellar fibers are also involved in the disease. In autosomal-dominant, uncomplicated familial spastic paraplegia, different classes of neurons including the corticospinal tract fibers from pyramidal neurons in the motor cortex are involved. All forms of familial spastic paraplegia typically degenerate the longest fibers in the central nervous system (Weimer & Wong, 2009).

NEUROPSYCHOLOGICAL/CLINICAL PRESENTATION

Familial spastic paraplegia is a group of disorders that can have vast differences in clinical presentation; however, all forms of the disorder have a primary clinical feature of progressive, severe, lower extremity spasticity. In "uncomplicated" or "pure" familial spastic paraplegia, symptoms only include lower extremity weakness, bladder disturbance, and variable impairment of vibratory sense in the feet. Patients typically

have normal facial and extraocular movements, no speech disturbance, difficulty swallowing, or evidence of corticobulbar tract dysfunction. The patient's upper extremity muscle tone and strength are normal, but in the lower extremities, muscle tone is increased at the hamstrings, quadriceps, and ankles. The patient's gait typically demonstrates circumduction because of difficulty with hip flexion and ankle dorsiflexion. When present, the impairment of vibratory sense in the feet is a useful diagnostic sign that can help distinguish familial spastic paraplegia from other disorders (Boustany et al., 1987). In "complicated" familial spastic paraplegia, symptoms are similar to the above clinical presentation, but also include neurologic deficits such as ataxia, mental retardation, dementia, visual or hearing dysfunctions, adrenal insufficiency, extrapyramidal dysfunctions, and ichthyosis. The age of symptom onset, rate of symptom progression, and extent of disability are variable both within and between the forms of the disorder. Genetic analysis can further classify familial spastic paraplegia according to the mode of inheritance (autosomal-dominant, autosomal-recessive, and X-linked), and it is preferable to refer to subtypes of the disorder by the mode of inheritance, chromosome involvement, and ultimately the specific genetic mutation (Fink, 1997, 2006; Fink & Heiman-Patterson, 1996; Weimer & Wong, 2009).

DIAGNOSIS

The evaluation and diagnosis of familial spastic paraplegia will typically include a thorough physical examination, medical history, family history, and genetic analysis. X-linked familial spastic paraplegia is rare and genetically heterogeneous, but the autosomal-dominant and autosomal-recessive forms of the disease are more common. Identification of the specific chromosomes involved can help doctors suggest the clinical severity and presentation of symptoms and ultimate prognosis of the disorder (Fink & Heiman-Patterson, 1996). On physical examination, all forms of the disorder have a primary clinical feature of progressive, severe, lower extremity spasticity. In uncomplicated or pure familial spastic paraplegia, symptoms only include lower extremity weakness, bladder disturbance, and variable impairment of vibratory sense in the feet. In complicated familial spastic paraplegia, symptoms are similar, but also include neurologic deficits such as ataxia, mental retardation, dementia, visual or hearing dysfunctions, adrenal insufficiency, extrapyramidal dysfunctions, and ichthyosis (Weimer & Wong, 2009). Neuropsychological evaluation may be of particular use in revealing cognitive, visual, or hearing deficits in complicated familial spastic

F

paraplegia and may be used to differentiate between the two forms of the disorder in diagnosis.

TREATMENT

Although there is currently no way to stop, slow, or reverse the progressive disability of familial spastic paraplegia, there are several different treatments that can help affected individuals (Fink, 2006). Because the disease can affect people in a number of different ways, treatments are varied but include physical therapy, medication, occupational therapy, speech therapy, and psychosocial therapy. Due to the variable degree of deficits in patients, specific individualized treatment plans should be developed to target the patient's specific symptoms. Physical therapy and exercise are considered the most important components of treatment in familial spastic paraplegia. Physical therapy generally focuses on reducing muscle tone, maintaining or improving range of motion and mobility, increasing strength and coordination, and preventing frozen joints, contractures, or bedsores (Weimer & Wong, 2009). The most commonly used medications to help with muscle spasticity include oral and intrathecal baclofen and tizanidine. Diazepam, clonazepam, and dantrolene are also used in treatment. In extreme cases, some individuals may benefit by direct injection of botulinum toxin (Geva-Dayan, Domenievitz, Zahalka, & Fattal-Valevski, 2010; Rousseaux, Launay, Kozolowski, & Daveluy, 2007). Many individuals have urinary or bowel symptoms and a number of medications, techniques, and devices are available for treatment (Fink, 2006; Weimer & Wong, 2009). Occupational therapy focuses on techniques used to accomplish everyday tasks such as mobility, washing, dressing, eating, cooking, and grooming and other activities such as handwriting, driving, housekeeping, or job tasks that patients have specific problems with. There are a variety of assistive devices that can be utilized to help the patient achieve mobility, including walkers or wheelchairs. Speech and swallowing difficulties can be treated by a speech/language pathologist, who can determine appropriate forms of treatment. Psychosocial interventions may also be utilized to help the patient overcome any psychological or social ramifications of the disorder, which are common in familial spastic paraplegia.

Eric Silk
Charles Golden

Boustany, R. N., Fleischnick, E., Alper, C. A., Marazita, M. L., Spense, M. A., Martin, J. B., et al. (1987). The autosomal dominant form of "pure" familial spastic paraplegia. *Neurology, 37,* 910–915.

Dürr, A., Brice, A., Serdaru, M., Rancurel, G., Derouesne, C., Lyon-Caen, O., et al. (1994). The phenotype of "pure" autosomal dominant spastic paraplegia. *Neurology, 44,* 1274–1277.

Fink, J. K. (1997). Advances in hereditary spastic paraplegia. *Current Opinion in Neurology, 10,* 313–318.

Fink, J. K. (2006). Hereditary spastic paraplegia. *Current Neurology and Neuroscience Reports, 6*(1), 65–76.

Fink, J. K., & Heiman-Patterson, T. (1996). Hereditary spastic paraplegia: Advances in genetic research. *Neurology, 46,* 1507–1514.

Geva-Dayan, K., Domenievitz, D., Zahalka, R., & Fattal-Valevski, A. (2010). Botulinum toxin injections for pediatric patients with hereditary spastic paraparesis. *Journal of Child Neurology, 25*(8), 969–975.

McDermott, C. J. (2003). Hereditary spastic paraparesis: Disrupted intracellular transport associated with spastin mutation. *Annals of Neurology, 54*(6), 748–759.

Rousseaux, M., Launay, M. J., Kozolowski, O., & Daveluy, W. (2007). Botulinum toxin injection in patients with hereditary spastic paraparesis. *European Journal of Neurology, 14*(2), 206–212. doi:10.1111/j.1468-1331.2006.01617.x

Weimer, M., & Wong, J. (2009). Lambert-Eaton myasthenic syndrome. *Current Treatment Options in Neurology, 11*(2), 77–84. doi: 10.1007/s11940-009-0010-z

FARBER'S DISEASE

DESCRIPTION

Farber's disease (also known as Farber's lipogranulomatosis and acid ceramidase deficiency) is an inherited, autosomal recessive disorder in which deficiency in acid ceramidase leads to disruptions in storage of lysosomes (Ehlert et al., 2007). Often, symptoms appear within the first few weeks of life, manifesting as a hoarse cry due to fixation of laryngeal cartilage, respiratory distress, and joint sensitivity. These features are followed by the more hallmark symptoms of periarticular and subcutaneous swellings and progressive arthropathy and finally ankylosis (Ropper & Brown, 2007). Death typically occurs by age 2.

NEUROPATHOLOGY/PATHOPHYSIOLOGY

Ceramide is a sphingolipid present in that skin that has been implicated as having important signaling and regulatory roles in cellular differentiation and apoptosis in addition to its structural role (Hannun & Obeid, 2008). Acid ceramidase is an enzyme that is necessary for the catabolism of ceramide. The deficiency of acid ceramidase in Farber's disease leads to excessive accumulation of ceramide in the skin and joints and disruption of its signaling roles. These changes are linked to the development of chronic granulomatous inflammation seen in Farber's disease (Ehlert et al., 2007). Histological examination reveals prominent granulomas comprised of foam cells, which are macrophages that have accumulated lipids, and other immune response cells (e.g., lymphocytes). Widespread lipid storage in neurons is seen.

NEUROPSYCHOLOGICAL/CLINICAL PRESENTATION

Seven phenotypes of Farber's disease have been identified (El-Kamah, El-darouti, Kotoury, & Mostafa, 2009). Type 1 is the classic presentation with skin nodules, joint swelling and deformities, and vocal hoarseness present from the first 2 weeks of life. Types 2 and 3 are intermediate and mild forms, respectively, with longer life expectancies and less neurologic involvement. Type 4 does not manifest joint deformations but involves severe hepatosplenomegaly and death occurs less than a week after birth. Type 5 involves progressive neurologic deterioration and seizures. Type 6 involves a combination of symptoms of Farber's disease and Sandhoff's disease (i.e., exaggerated startle response to sound, blindness, progressive neurologic deterioration, and macrocephaly). Type 7 involves deficiency of ceramidase as well as two other enzymes involved in lipid metabolism.

DIAGNOSIS

In cases involving the classic combination of skin nodules, joint deformities, and vocal hoarseness, Type 1 Farber's disease can be diagnosed by clinical findings. In other cases, diagnosis can be based on results of laboratory assays of enzyme activity and histopathological findings revealing foam cell containing granulomas in subcutaneous nodules (Ehlert et al., 2007).

TREATMENT

Treatment has generally been supportive and aimed at reducing pain. One case study reported reductions in granuloma size, joint pain, and hoarseness following bone marrow transplant (Yeager et al., 2000). A recent study reported promising results from stem cell transplant in four cases involving minimal central nervous system involvement including reductions in subcutaneous nodules and numbers of joints with mobility restrictions (Ehlert et al., 2007).

Jeremy Davis
Chad A. Noggle

Ehlert, K., Frosch, M., Fehse, N., Zander, A., Roth, J., & Vormoor, J. (2007). Farber disease: Clinical presentation, pathogenesis and a new approach to treatment. *Pediatric Rheumatology, 5,* 15–21.

El-Kamah, G., El-darouti, M. A., Kotoury, A. I., & Mostafa, M. I. (2009). Farber disease overlapping with stiff skin syndrome: Expanding the spectrum. *Egyptian Journal of Medical Human Genetics, 10,* 97–104.

Hannun, Y. A., & Obeid, L. M. (2008). Principles of bioactive lipid signalling: Lessons from sphingolipids. *Nature Reviews: Molecular Cell Biology, 9,* 139–150.

Ropper, A. H., & Brown, R. H. (2005). *Adams and Victor's principles of neurology* (8th ed., pp. 797–849). New York: McGraw-Hill.

Yeager, A. M., Uhas, K. A., Coles, C. D., Davis, P. C., Krause, W. L., & Moser, H. W. (2000). Bone marrow transplantation for infantile ceramidase deficiency (Farber disease). *Bone Marrow Transplantation, 26,* 357–363.

FATAL FAMILIAL INSOMNIA

DESCRIPTION

Fatal familial insomnia (FFI) is one of the prion diseases (i.e., transmissible spongiform encephalopathy). FFI is an autosomal-dominant disorder linked to a constellation of mutations at codon 178 coupled with methionine at the polymorphic codon 129 of the prion protein gene (*PRNP*), and aspartic acid to asparagines substitution (Almer et al., 1999; Collinge, 2001; Goldfarb et al., 1992; Lugaresi et al., 1986; Medori et al., 1992).

The clinical features of FFI involve motor abnormalities, dysautonomia, and progressive mental deterioration. The hallmark symptom of FFI, which corresponds with its namesake while distinguishing it from other prion diseases, involves progressive insomnia (Lugaresi et al., 1986).

The FFI genotype has been identified in only 25 families worldwide: five Italian, two French, four American, one Japanese, two Australian, eight German, one Austrian, and two British (Cortelli, Gambetti, Montagna, & Lugaresi, 1999; Gambetti & Lugaresi, 1998). As such, FFI is one of the rarest prion diseases.

F

NEUROPATHOLOGY/PATHOPHYSIOLOGY

Mutations at codon 178 of the *PRNP*, aspartic acid to asparagines substitution (D178N), in conjunction with methionine at the polymorphic position 129 of the mutant allele serves as the genetic basis for FFI. The end result from a neuropathological standpoint is lesioning of the thalamus. Neuronal loss has been further localized to the centromedial, anterior ventral, and dorsomedial nuclei (Manetto et al., 1992). Other nuclei may be inconsistently and less severely affected. This degradation creates a disconnection between thalamolimbic and more caudal structures in the central network that regulates the sleep–wake cycle and body homeostasis in general (Cortelli et al., 1999; Lugaresi, Tobler, Gambetti, & Montagna 1998). Mild spongiosis and gliosis in the orbitofrontal cortex, cingulate gyrus, frontotemporal and parietal lobes, and the inferior olives have all been associated with FFI.

NEUROPSYCHOLOGICAL/CLINICAL PRESENTATION

Clinically, FFI is primarily characterized by progressive insomnia, dysautonomia, and motor signs, with the latter most commonly expressed as cerebellar ataxia (Almer et al., 1999; Goldfarb et al., 1992). Ataxia is often not seen until later stages of the disease and is often accompanied by dysarthria. In those individuals who exhibit greater longevity, these features may actually present as more severe.

Prominent dementia is seen as the disease progresses. Montagna et al. (1998) noted that in the initial stages individuals exhibit increased deficits in sustained attention. This is to some extent related to deficiencies in neurological arousal classified as oneiric stupor. Persistent stupor and eventually a vegetative state manifest prior to death (Gallassi et al., 1996).

Autonomic dysregulation ensues in relation to sleep–wake disturbance as the system becomes overburdened with this lack of recovery. Patients will begin to exhibit tachycardia, increased perspiration, constipation, and dysregulation of respiration and body temperature (Cortelli et al., 1999; Portaluppi, Cortelli, Avoni, Vergnani, Contin, et al., 1994; Portaluppi, Cortelli, Avoni, Vergnani, Maltoni, et al., 1994). This contributes to overactivity of the sympathetic nervous system owing to the development of panic attacks, paranoia, and eventually hallucinations. Death commonly occurs between 6 and 36 months from the time of symptom onset.

DIAGNOSIS

Family history remains the most salient factor in the diagnosis of FFI. As suggested, FFI is an autosomal-dominant disorder linked to a constellation of mutations at codon 178 coupled with methionine at the polymorphic codon 129 of the *PRNP*, and aspartic acid to asparagines substitution (Goldfarb et al., 1992; Lugaresi et al., 1986; Medori et al., 1992). Consequently, genetic analysis is potentially the most powerful diagnostic source.

Beyond genetics, FFI has been associated with characteristic patterns on electroencephalogram marked by continuous oscillations between a diffuse alpha activity typical of relaxed wakefulness and a widespread low amplitude theta activity associated with a condition of drowsiness or subwakefulness. When interspersed with episodes of unresponsiveness during which the patient presents with massive twitches and performs complex purposeful gestures, and that he/she subsequently referred to dreams is considered highly indicative of FFI (Cortelli et al., 1999). However, a fairly definitive pattern arises a few months into the presentation whereby there is a disappearance of sleep spindles and K-complexes.

Although abnormalities can be observed on CT and MRI (e.g., cortical and cerebellar atrophy), these features are not unique to FFI. In comparison, fludeoxyglucose positron emission tomography scans commonly demonstrate hypometabolism in the thalamus with potential involvement of the cingulate gyrus, frontotemporal cortex, and basal ganglia (Cortelli et al., 1997; Montagna et al., 1998).

TREATMENT

FFI is incurable. Furthermore, medicinal interventions to counteract the clinical features of the presentation (e.g., progressive insomnia) has demonstrated little efficacy. As a result, treatment is supportive. Although education for the patient and family is recommended in such cases within other presentations, in many instances they are already well aware of the disease course and prognosis. Seizures may be controlled with anticonvulsant agents.

Chad A. Noggle

Almer, G., Hainfellner, J. A., Brucke, T., Jellinger, K., Kleinert, R., Bayer, G., et al. (1999). Fatal familial insomnia: a new Austrian family. *Brain, 122*, 5–16.

Collinge, J. (2001). Prion diseases of humans and animals: their causes and molecular basis. *Annu Rev Neurosci, 24*, 519–550.

Cortelli, P., Gambetti, P., Montagna, P., & Lugaresi, E. (1999). Fatal familial insomnia: Clinical features and molecular genetics. *Journal of Sleep Research, 8*(Suppl. 1), 23–29.

Cortelli, P., Perani, D., Parchi, P., Grassi, F., Montagna, P., De Martin, M., et al. (1997). Cerebral metabolism in fatal familial insomnia: Relation to duration, neuropathology, and distribution of protease-resistant prion protein. *Neurology, 49*, 126–133.

Gallassi, R., Morreale, A., Montagna, P., Cortelli, P., Avoni, P., Castellani, R., et al. (1996). Fatal familial insomnia: Behavioral and cognitive features. *Neurology, 46*, 935–939.

Gambetti, P., & Lugaresi, E. (1998). Conclusions of the symposium. *Brain Pathology, 8*, 571–575.

Goldfarb, L. G., Petersen, R. B., Tabaton, M., Brown, P., LeBlanc, A. C., Montagna, P., et al. (1992). Fatal familial insomnia and familial Creutzfeldt-Jakob disease: Disease phenotype determined by a DNA polymorphism. *Science, 258*, 806–808.

Lugaresi, E., Medori, R., Montagna, P., Baruzzi, A., Cortelli, P., Lugaresi, A., et al. (1986). Fatal familial insomnia and dysautonomia with selective degeneration of thalamic nuclei. *New England Journal of Medicine, 315*, 997–1003.

Lugaresi, E., Tobler, I., Gambetti, P., & Montagna, P. (1998). The pathophysiology of fatal familial insomnia. *Brain Pathology, 8*, 521–526.

Manetto, V., Medori, R., Cortelli, P., Montagna, P., Tinuper, P., Baruzzi, A., et al. (1992). Fatal familial insomnia: Clinical and pathologic study of five new cases. *Neurology, 42*, 312–319.

Medori, R., Tritschler, H. J., LeBlanc, A., Villare, F., Manetto, V., Chen, H. Y., et al. (1992). Fatal familial insomnia, a prion disease with a mutation at codon 178 of the prion protein gene. *New England Journal of Medicine, 326*, 444–449.

Montagna, P., Cortelli, P., Avoni, P., Tinuper, P., Plazzi, G., Gallassi, R., et al. (1998). Clinical features of fatal familial insomnia: Phenotypic variability in relation to a polymorphism at codon 129 of the prion protein gene. *Brain Pathology, 8*, 515–520.

Portaluppi, F., Cortelli, P., Avoni, P., Vergnani, L., Contin, M., Maltoni, P., et al. (1994). Diurnal blood pressure variation and hormonal correlates in fatal familial insomnia. *Hypertension, 23*, 569–576.

Portaluppi, F., Cortelli, P., Avoni, P., Vergnani, L., Maltoni, P., Pavani, A., et al. (1994). Progressive disruption of the circadian rhythm of melatonin in fatal familial insomnia. *Journal of Clinical Endocrinology & Metabolism, 78*, 1075–1078.

FEBRILE SEIZURES

DESCRIPTION

A febrile seizure is a convulsion associated with fever that occurs during infancy and early childhood. Febrile seizures are distinct from epilepsy as they occur without evidence of underlying neurological etiology or central nervous system infection. However, children with prior neurological impairment can still experience a febrile seizure. Although febrile seizures are typically benign, they cause considerable anxiety in parents (Hirtz, 1997; Shinnar, 2005).

NEUROPATHOLOGY/PATHOPHYSIOLOGY

Febrile seizures occur in infants and young children due to their susceptibility to frequent childhood infections such as otitis media, upper respiratory infection, or a viral infection. To defend against infection, young children respond with considerably higher temperatures than adults (Hirtz, 1997). There are two types of febrile seizures, simple and complex. Simple febrile seizures are a relatively brief generalized event, not exceeding more than 10–15 minutes. They typically do not recur within a 24-hour period or within the same illness. In contrast, complex febrile seizures are prolonged, lasting greater than 15 minutes. They may recur within 24 hours or multiple times during the same illness, or can be focal (Shinnar, 2005). Simple febrile seizures account for approximately 80% to 85% of febrile seizures, whereas complex febrile seizures only account for 15% to 20%. Complex febrile seizures may be indicative of a more serious underlying infection such as encephalitis, meningitis, or an abscess. Viral illnesses are the predominant cause of febrile seizures (Fetveit, 2007). Approximately 20% of children presenting with febrile seizures had a diagnosis of human herpes simplex virus 6 (Yamashita & Morishima, 2005). Shigella gastroenteritis, a bacterial bowel infection, has also been associated with febrile seizures (Hirtz, 1997). Although the exact link to fever and seizures is not known, researchers suspect the role of endogenous pyrogens, such as interleukin-1, which increase neuronal excitability and induce fever. There is also support in the role of cytokines that increase the propensity of seizures (Mazarati, 2005). In addition, there is evidence to support a genetic basis for febrile seizures; however, the exact role of inheritance is uncertain. Concordance rates of siblings are approximately 10%, although if one parent has a history of a febrile seizure, the risk increases to approximately 50% (Hirtz, 1997).

NEUROPSYCHOLOGICAL/CLINICAL PRESENTATION

Febrile seizures are usually benign and most last for less than 2 minutes. The common age of occurrence is between 3 months and 5 years. Approximately 5% of children experience a febrile seizure and about one-third of these children will have additional febrile seizures prior to outgrowing them (Fetveit, 2007).

Febrile seizures are most commonly triggered by a fever greater than 102 °F. The typical presentation of a febrile seizure involves a generalized clonic or tonic–clonic seizure consisting of sudden bilateral muscle contractions of the facial muscles, trunk, arms, and legs. Sudden muscle contractions may cause the child to involuntary cry or moan. Other symptoms include eye rolling, difficulty breathing, urinary incontinence, vomiting, tongue biting, and/or hallucinations. A focal seizure occurs less commonly and the child may present as rigid or exhibit unilateral muscle twitches. Postictally, the child may be confused, be sleepy, or cry (Nelson & Hirtz, 2000). Children with febrile seizures have only a slightly higher incidence of epilepsy compared with the general population, approximately 1% to 2%. However, there is an increased risk of epilepsy developing later in life if the child has had a complex febrile seizure, there is a family history of epilepsy, or if the child has a developmental delay (Fetveit, 2007). There is no evidence that simple febrile seizures cause death or brain damage. However, there is an increased risk of death with complex febrile seizures due to harmful underlying conditions (Hirtz, 1997; Nelson & Hirtz, 2000). There is no risk of mental retardation, reduced performance on intelligence tests, or learning difficulties among children with a history of simple febrile seizures (Camfield, Camfield, & Erikkson, 2007; Nelson & Hirtz, 2000).

DIAGNOSIS

A febrile seizure is diagnosed when a child presents with seizure and a fever, without a history of epilepsy. Ruling out potential causes for a seizure in infants and young children is important, although a full seizure workup including computed tomography (CT) and electroencephalogram (EEG) is typically not warranted with a first-time simple febrile seizure. However, CT and EEG procedures are sometimes utilized with complex febrile seizures. If the child is presenting with persistent fever, petechiae, cyanosis, hypotension, skin rash, repeated seizures, or altered mental status, then a lumbar puncture is used to determine probable infection such as meningitis (Joffe, McCormick, & DeAngelis, 1983).

TREATMENT

Children presenting with active seizures should be treated with airway management and high flow oxygen. Anticonvulsants including benzodiazepines, phenytoin, or phenobarbital may also be necessary. Postictal children should receive supportive care

and antipyretics (e.g., acetaminophen, ibuprofen) as appropriate (Camfield et al., 2007). Although antipyretics are not always effective in preventing recurrence of febrile seizures, they should be used to reduce fever and improve comport. Daily antiepileptic medications for management of simple febrile seizures are usually not necessary; however, some children presenting with complex febrile seizures may require daily antiepileptic medication management. Children with febrile seizures should have frequent neurologic examinations to monitor potential future events and mental status. Parental anxiety needs to be addressed through education and supportive counseling as warranted (Knudsen, 1996).

Darla J. Lawson

Camfield, P. R., Camfield, C. S., & Erikkson, K. J. (2007). Treatment of febrile seizures. In J. Engel, T. A. Pedley, J. Aicardi, M. A. Dichter, & S. L. Moshe (Eds.), *Epilepsy* (pp. 1345–1349). Philadelphia, PA: Lippincott Williams & Wilkins.

Fetveit, A. (2007). Assessment of febrile seizures in children. *European Journal of Pediatrics, 167*(1), 17–27.

Hirtz, D. G. (1997). Febrile seizures. *Pediatric Review, 18*(1), 5–8.

Joffe, A., McCormick, M., & DeAngelis, C. (1983). Which children with febrile seizures need lumbar puncture? A decision analysis approach. *American Journal of Diseases of Children, 137*(12), 1153–1156.

Knudsen, F. U. (1996). Febrile seizures: Treatment and outcome. *Brain Development, 18*(6), 438–449.

Mazarati, A. M. (2005). Cytokines: A link between fever and seizures. *Epilepsy Currents, 5*(5), 169–170.

Nelson, K. B., & Hirtz, D. J. (2000). Febrile seizures. In P. J. Vinken, H. Meinardi, & G. W. Bruyn (Eds.), *Handbook of clinical neurology: The epilepsies part II* (pp. 309–316). Philadelphia, PA: Elsevier Health Sciences.

Shinnar, S. (2005). Febrile seizures. In H. S. Singer, E. H. Kossoff, A. L. Hartman, & T. O. Crawford (Eds.), *Treatment of pediatric neurologic disorders* (pp. 73–78). New York: Informa Health Care.

Yamashita, N., & Morishima, T. (2005). HHV-6 and seizures. *Herpes, 12*(2), 46–49.

FETAL ALCOHOL SYNDROME

DESCRIPTION

Alcohol is a teratogen (toxic to normal fetal development), capable of directly inducing developmental abnormalities in a fetus (Larkby & Day, 1997). In 1981, the U.S. Surgeon General issued the first health advisory recommending that women who are pregnant or planning a pregnancy should refrain from drinking alcohol. In 1996, the Institute of Medicine (IOM) (Stratton, Howe, & Battaglia, 1996) released a report containing broadly defined diagnostic criteria for fetal alcohol syndrome (FAS), partial FAS, alcohol-related birth defects (ARBD), and alcohol-related neurodevelopmental disorders (ARND). These diagnostic categories represent a continuum of effects due to intrauterine alcohol exposure and are subsumed under the rubric of fetal alcohol syndrome deficits (FASD; Schonfeld, Paley, Frankel, & O'Connor, 2006). FAS is seen as the most severe of effects that result from intrauterine alcohol exposure. In 1973, FAS was identified as a birth defect presumed to be caused by prenatal alcohol exposure in utero. Physical findings have been observable at birth to chronic alcoholic mothers of the first children (Jones & Smith, 1973). The incidence of FASD is estimated to affect 1 in 100 children, with full FAS estimated to occur in 0.5 to 2 infants per 1,000 live births in the United States (May & Gossage, 2001). FAS is reported to be the leading known nongenetic cause of mental retardation (National Institute on Alcohol Abuse and Alcoholism [NIAAA], 2000).

NEUROPATHOLOGY/PATHOPHYSIOLOGY

According to O'Leary (2004), the critical period for the damaging effects of teratogens occurs in the first 3–6 weeks of brain development and during that time the brain has its final growth spurt. Therefore, intrauterine alcohol exposure is the most damaging for a developing fetus during the first trimester and the last 2 months of pregnancy. The four primary areas of the brain that are most impacted by intrauterine alcohol exposure include the cerebellum, basal ganglia, corpus callosum, and hippocampus (Wacha & Obrzut, 2004).

The serious consequences of in utero ethanol exposure on the developing brain include: inhibition or retardation of neurogenesis and differentiation, cell death, delayed and aberrant neuronal migration, altered formation of axonal and dendritic projections from the cell body, altered genesis and differentiation of astroglia, altered neuroendocrine function, and abnormal development of several major neurotransmitter systems (Watson, 1992).

NEUROPSYCHOLOGICAL/CLINICAL PRESENTATION

Some of the primary neurobehavioral impairments associated with FASD involve deficits in memory, attention, visual-spatial abilities, declarative learning, planning, cognitive flexibility, processing speed, language, and motor delays (Carmichael Olson, Feldman, Streissguth, Sampson, & Bookstein, 1998). Children with FASD may have deficits in physical, behavioral, emotional, and/or social functioning as a result of prenatal alcohol exposure (Streissguth & O'Malley, 2000). Many children with FASD also have deficits of vision, hearing, speech, and locomotor function, as well as structural and functional brain damage. Furthermore, many secondary disabilities including mental health problems, trouble with law, confinement, alcohol and drug abuse, and dropping out of school are common in children with FASD (Streissguth, 1997). Executive functioning, which has been defined as higher-order psychological abilities involved in goal-oriented behavior under conscious control, is a significant deficit in individuals with FASD (Rasmussen, 2005).

DIAGNOSIS

FAS is primarily diagnosed by the coexistence of three features: prenatal-onset growth deficiency, a characteristic pattern of dysmorphological characteristics read most explicitly in the face, and evidence of central nervous system (CNS) dysfunction (Streissguth et al., 1999). The CNS anomalies can include microcephaly, or other brain structural abnormalities, with no significant catch-up through early childhood, delays in social and motor performance related to mental age, intellectual disability, and neonatal problems including irritability and feeding difficulties (O'Leary, 2004). Characteristic facial features include short palpebral fissures, maxillary hypoplasia, epicanthal folds, thin upper lip, and flattened or elongated philtrum (Wacha & Obrzut, 2007). However, it should be noted that it is not uncommon for children to be exposed to alcohol as a teratogen and not develop these phenotypical features. In such an instance, a diagnostic conclusion of fetal alcohol effects (FAE) is commonly used. Furthermore, in order to be diagnosed with FAS, a child has to have a positive history of maternal alcohol use during pregnancy (O'Leary, 2004). Diagnosis is generally made in infants and young children, age 2 years and older (Wacha & Obrzut, 2004). Diagnosis of FAS is difficult in newborns and adults due to CNS dysfunction being hard to detect in newborns and facial dysmorphology becoming less distinct in adults (O'Leary, 2004).

TREATMENT

Treatment approaches will vary based on each child's specific symptoms. One treatment approach is through prevention programs. The NIAAA (2002) has outlined the various ways in which universal prevention efforts can be implemented such as media attention to drinking during pregnancy, warning posters, evidence that knowledge of FAS has increased over time, and the effectiveness of the alcohol beverage warning label.

Neuropsychological testing is helpful in guiding interventions for children with FASD. Each child diagnosed with FASD has specific strengths and weaknesses, and with a full assessment of these strengths and weaknesses, interventions can be specifically catered to the child's needs. Children exposed to alcohol in utero may need psychiatric help through pharmacological management. Additionally, psychologists to help with behavioral issues and therapists to help their family agree on how to manage and cope with the alcohol-affected individual (Stratton et al., 1996).

Justin J. Boseck
Raymond S. Dean

Carmichael Olson, H., Feldman, J., Streissguth, A. P., Sampson, P. D., & Bookstein, F. L. (1998). Neuropsychological deficits in adolescents with fetal alcohol syndrome: Clinical findings. *Alcoholism: Clinical and Experimental Research, 22*, 1998–2012.

Jones, K. L., & Smith, D. W. (1973). Recognition of the fetal alcohol syndrome in early infancy. *Lancet, 2*, 999–1001.

Larkby, C., & May, N. (1997). The effects of prenatal alcohol exposure. *Alcohol Health and Research World, 21*(3), 192–198.

May, P. A., & Gossage, J. P. (2001). Estimating the prevalence of fetal alcohol syndrome: A summary. *Alcohol Research and Health, 25*, 159–167.

National Institute on Alcohol Abuse and Alcoholism. (2000). *The 10th special report to the U.S. Congress on alcohol and health: Prenatal exposure to alcohol* (Publication No. 00-1583). Washington, DC: Cygnus Corporation.

National Institute on Alcohol Abuse and Alcoholism. (2002). *Fetal alcohol syndrome prevention research.* Retrieved February 28, 2009, from http://pubs.niaaa.nih.gov/publications/arh26-1/58-65.htm

O'Leary, C. M. (2004). Fetal alcohol syndrome: Diagnosis, epidemiology, and developmental outcomes. *Journal of Pediatrics and Child Health, 40*, 2–7.

Rasmussen, C. (2005). Executive functioning and working memory in fetal alcohol spectrum disorder. *Alcohol: Clinical and Experimental Research, 29*, 1359–1367.

Schonfeld, A. M., Paley, B., Frankel, F., & O'Connor, M. J. (2006). Executive functioning predicts social skills following prenatal alcohol exposure. *Child Neuropsychology, 12*, 439–452.

Stratton, K., Howe, C., & Battaglia, F. (Eds.). (1996). *Fetal alcohol syndrome: Diagnosis, epidemiology, prevention, and treatment.* Washington, DC: National Academic press.

Streissguth, A. P. (1997). *Fetal alcohol syndrome: A guide for families and communities.* Baltimore: Paul H. Brookes Publishing.

Streissguth, A. P., Barr, H. M., Bookstein, F. L., Sampson, P. D., & Carmichael Olson, H. (1999). The long-term neurocognitive consequences of prenatal alcohol exposure: A 14-year study. *Psychological Science, 10*(3), 186–190.

Streissguth, A., & O'Malley, K. (2000). Neuropsychiatric implications and long-term consequences of fetal alcohol spectrum disorders. *Seminars in Clinical Neuropsychiatry, 5*, 177–190.

Wacha, V. H., & Obrzut, J. E. (2007). Effects of fetal alcohol syndrome on neuropsychological function. *Journal of Physical and Developmental Disabilities, 19*, 217–226.

Watson, R. (Ed.). (1992). *Alcohol and neurobiology: Brain development and hormone regulation.* Boca Raton, FL: CRC Press.

FIBROMUSCULAR DYSPLASIA

DESCRIPTION

Fibromuscular dysplasia (FMD) is a nonatherosclerotic, noninflammatory vascular disease that affects any and/or all of the three layers in the cephalic, renal, and both extracranial and intracranial arteries (particularly the bilateral internal carotid arteries [ICAs]) (Slovut & Olin, 2004). The exact cause remains unknown although genetic predisposition, trauma, hormonal factors, growth factors, underlying connective tissue disease, skeletal factors, and metabolic and immunological factors have all been proposed as causes of FMD (Camacho et al., 2003; Difazio, Hinds, Depper, Tom, & Davis, 2000; Lindner, 2001; Luscher et al., 1987; Puri & Riggs, 1999). Classification of FMD is further defined by the arterial layer of involvement, including intimal, medial, and/or periadventitial (Harrison & McCormack, 1971).

FMD causes fibrous dysplastic tissue and proliferating smooth muscle cells presenting as constricting bands and a string-of-beads appearance on arteriography (Caplan, 2000). FMD is commonly found in middle-aged women, rarely seen in children, and is most often asymptomatic (Lenzi & Calabresi, 2003). Because of its frequent association with cerebral aneurysms, FMD is often found during the evaluation of subarachnoid hemorrhage (Mettinger, 1982). FMD also causes arterial dissections, producing ischemic stroke syndromes, but it may present as a transient ischemic attack (TIA) or stroke without any evident compromise of the vascular lumen, possibly due to functional constriction (Zurin, Houkin, Asano, Ishikawa, & Abe, 1997). The stroke recurrence rate is quite low, even with no therapy. If the patient is hypertensive, the renal arteries should be studied (Mettinger, 1982). Abdominal angina, claudication, and general vascular insufficiency may also present (Sperati, Aggarwal, Arepally, & Atta, 2009). Involvement of both cervicocranial and renal vessels with FMD carries neurological implications (Dayes & Gardiner, 2005).

NEUROPATHOLOGY/PATHOPHYSIOLOGY

The etiology of the disease is not known, but various opinions have been put forward about the genesis of FMD: genetic predisposition, trauma, hormonal factors, growth factors, underlying connective tissue disease, skeletal factors, and metabolic and immunological factors have all been proposed as causes of FMD, but to date, the etiology remains indefinite (Camacho et al., 2003; Lindner, 2001; Luscher et al., 1987; Sölder, Sterif, Ellemunter, Mayr, & Jaschke, 1997). An alpha-1 antitrypsin deficiency has also been reported (Schievink, Meyer, Parisi, & Wijdicks, 1998; Schievink, Michels, & Piepgras, 1994).

Medial FMD presents with the classical "string of beads" appearance on angiography coupled with a uniform, smooth stenosis (Sperati et al., 2009). Intimal FMD presents with concentric band-like stenoses and smooth tapered lesions (Slovut & Olin, 2004). In rare cases, diffuse, thoracic, and abdominal aortic involvement has been reported (Gatalica, Gibas, & Martinez-Hernandez, 1992; Radhi, McKay, & Tyrrell, 1998).

In terms of neurological correlates, cephalocervical FMD involves the extracranial portion of the ICA (nearly 95%), whereas intracranial FMD is detected primarily in children, causing acute infantile hemiplegia (Emparanza et al., 1989). The carotid arteries often appear elongated and kinked (Kubis et al., 1999). In comparison, the distal ICA is the most frequently involved (Mettinger & Ericson, 1982). This may lead to the development of ipsilateral intracranial aneurysms. Decreased blood flow and/or embolization of platelet aggregates have been correlated with the occurrence of TIAs, cerebrovascular accidents (CVAs), and hemorrhages, in particular, subarachnoid bleeds. Cerebral artery lesions and multiple aneurysms are common, particularly in small and medium-sized arteries (Mettinger & Ericson, 1982).

NEUROPSYCHOLOGICAL/CLINICAL PRESENTATION

No uniform profile is seen in conjunction with FMD. Vertebrobasilar insufficiency, amaurosis fugax, TIA and/or CVAs may present in conjunction with cerebral artery lesions, including carotid and intracranial artery involvement (Schievink et al., 1994; Schievink et al., 1998; Van Damme, Sakalihasan, & Limet, 1999). Although aneurysms and hemorrhage may occur, ischemic stroke is the most common cerebrovascular event (Schievink et al., 1994). The extent of neurological features observed corresponds with the underlying physiology of FMD. Signs and symptoms range from hypertension and dizziness to TIAs, intracerebral hemorrhage, intracranial aneurysm rupture, and/or occlusion of a major cerebral vessel (Dayes & Gardiner, 2005). Focal deficits, including neurological syndromes, occur in relation to the locality of potential infarction in the affected arterial region and distribution. Chronic headaches may also be reported. Increased burden on subcortical areas and white matter is seen over time. Cognitive inefficiency with decreased processing speed may be seen. Individuals are at heightened risk of retrieval-based memory deficits, executive dysfunction, and inattention.

DIAGNOSIS

Angiography is the preferred method of diagnosis of FMD, whether renal or cervicocranial (Camacho et al., 2003; Lenzi & Calabresi, 2003). While the "string of beads" appearance is considered definitive (Wesen & Elliot, 1986), this is primarily associated with medial FMD and thus can preclude recognition of other variants. CT and MRI are used to evaluate for potential CVAs and aneurysms. Neuropsychological assessment becomes essential in the case of intracranial involvement and following neurological events.

TREATMENT

Treatment of FMD varies based on its presentation. Anticoagulation and antiaggregation therapies are the most common forms of treatment (Bhuriya, Arora, & Khosla, 2008; Nomura et al., 2001). Percutaneous transluminal angioplasty may also be used, particularly in those who develop TIAs or stroke (Nomura et al., 2001; Ribi, Mauget, Egger, Khatchatourian, & Villard, 2005). Daily aspirin may be used in cases where FMD has been identified yet the individual remains asymptomatic (Bhuriya et al., 2008). In the case where vasculitis co-occurs, corticosteroids may supplement aforementioned medicinal interventions (Ribi et al., 2005). If aneurysm is present, surgical intervention is required either through clipping or coiling. If renal function becomes compromised, dialysis may be required, but this tends to be rare. Physical and/or neuropsychological rehabilitation is utilized depending on the outcomes of CVAs if they occur or follow neurosurgery if the latter is needed.

Chad A. Noggle
Javan Horwitz

Bhuriya, R., Arora, R., & Khosla, S. (2008). Fibromuscular dysplasia of the internal carotid circulation: An unusual presentation. *Vascular Medicine, 13*, 41–43.

Camacho, A., Villarejo, A., Moreno, T., Simón, R., Muñoz, A., & Mateos, F. (2003). Vertebral artery fibromuscular dysplasia: An unusual cause of stroke in a 3-year-old child. *Development Medicine & Child Neurology, 45*, 709–711.

Caplan, L. R. (2000). *Caplan's stroke: A clinical approach* (3rd ed.). Boston MA: Butterworth-Heinemann.

Dayes, L. A., & Gardiner, N. (2005). The neurological implications of fibromuscular dysplasia. *Mount Sinai Journal of Medicine, 72*(6), 418–420.

Difazio, M., Hinds, S. R., Depper, M., Tom, B., & Davis, R. (2000). Intracranial fibromuscular dysplasia in a six-year-old: A rare cause of childhood stroke. *Journal of Child Neurology, 15*(8), 559–562.

Emparanza, J. I., Aldamiz-Echevarria, L., Perez-Yarza, E., Hernandez, J., Peña, B., & Gaztañaga, R. (1989). Ischemic stroke due to fibromuscular dysplasia. *Neuropediatrics, 20*, 181–182.

Gatalica, Z., Gibas, Z., & Martinez-Hernandez, A. (1992). Dissecting aortic aneurysm as a complication of generalized fibromuscular dysplasia. *Human Pathology, 23*, 586–588.

Harrison, E. G., Jr., & McCormack, L. J. (1971). Pathologic classification of renal arterial disease in renovascular hypertension. *Mayo Clinic Proceedings, 46*, 161–167.

Kubis, N., Von Langsdorff, D., Petitjean, C., Brouland, J. P., Guichard, J. P., Chapot, R., et al. (1999). Thrombotic carotid megabulb: Fibromuscular dysplasia, septae, and ischemic stroke. *Neurology, 52*, 883–886.

Lenzi, G. L., & Calabresi, M. (2003). Fibromuscular dysplasia. *Advance Neurology, 92*, 127–130.

Lindner, V. (2001). Vascular repair processes mediated by transforming growth factor-beta. *Zeitschrift fur Kardiologie, 90*(Suppl. 3), 17–22.

Luscher, T. F., Lie, J. T., Stanson, A. W., Houser, O. W., Hollier, L. H., & Sheps, S. G. (1987). Arterial fibromuscular dysplasia. *Mayo Clinic Proceedings, 62*, 931–952.

Mettinger, K. L. (1982). Fibromuscular dysplasia and the brain. II. Current concept of the disease. *Stroke, 13*, 53–58.

Mettinger, K. L., & Ericson, K. (1982). Fibromuscular dysplasia and the brain. I. Observations of angiographic, clinical and genetic characteristics. *Stroke, 13*, 46–52.

Nomura, S., Yamashita, K., Kato, S., Fujii, Y., Uchida, T., Urakawa, M., et al. (2001). Childhood subarachnoid hemorrhage associated with fibromuscular dysplasia. *Child's Nervous System, 17*, 419–422.

Puri, V., & Riggs, G. (1999). Case report of fibromuscular dysplasia presenting as stroke in a 16-year-old boy. *Journal of Child Neurology, 14*, 233–238.

Radhi, J. M., McKay, R., & Tyrrell, M. J. (1998). Fibromuscular dysplasia of the aorta presenting as multiple recurrent thoracic aneurysms. *International Journal of Angiology, 7*, 215–218.

Ribi, C., Mauget, D., Egger, J. F., Khatchatourian, G., & Villard, J. (2005). Pseudovasculitis and corticosteroid therapy. *Clinical Rheumatology, 24*, 539–543.

Schievink, W. I., Meyer, F. B., Parisi, J. E., & Wijdicks, E. F. (1998). Fibromuscular dysplasia of the internal carotid artery associated with alpha 1-antitrypsin deficiency. *Neurosurgery, 43*, 229–234.

Schievink, W. I., Michels, V. V., & Piepgras, D. G. (1994). Neurovascular manifestations of heritable connective tissue disorders. *Stroke, 25*, 889–903.

Slovut, D. P., & Olin, J. W. (2004). Fibromuscular dysplasia. *New England Journal of Medicine, 350*, 1862–1871.

Sölder, B., Sterif, W., Ellemunter, H., Mayr, U., & Jaschke, W. (1997). Fibromuscular dysplasia of the internal carotid artery in a child with alpha-1-antitrypsin deficiency. *Development Medicine & Child Neurology, 39*, 827–829.

Sperati, J., Aggarwal, N., Arepally, A., & Atta, M. (2009). Fibromuscular dysplasia. *Kidney International, 75*, 333–336.

Van Damme, H., Sakalihasan, N., & Limet, R. (1999). Fibromuscular dysplasia of the internal carotid artery. Personal experience with 13 cases and literature review. *Acta Chirurgica Belgica, 99*, 63–68.

Wesen, C. A., & Elliot, B. M. (1986). Fibromuscular dysplasia of the carotid arteries. *The American Journal of Surgery, 151*, 448–451.

Zurin, A. A., Houkin, K., Asano, T., Ishikawa, T., & Abe, H. (1997). Childhood ischemic stroke caused by fibromuscular dysplasia of the intracranial artery. *Neurologia Medico-Chirurgica (Tokyo), 37*, 542–545.

FRAGILE X SYNDROME

DESCRIPTION

Fragile X syndrome is a genetic disorder, marked by cognitive, behavioral, emotional, and physical symptoms. It is the most common form of inherited mental retardation and affects 1 in 4,000 males and 1 in 8,000 females (Schwarte, 2008).

NEUROPATHOLOGY/PATHOPHYSIOLOGY

Fragile X syndrome results from a repetition of the CGG trinucleotide sequence on the long arm of the X chromosome at location Xq27.3, first identified as a single gene disorder in 1991 (Hall, Burns, Lightbody, & Reiss, 2008). The CGG repetition inactivates the *FMR1* gene, which leads to a decline in production of the fragile X mental retardation protein (FMRP) and prevents the expression of FMRP, which is necessary for normal neuronal development and healthy brain functioning (Huber, 2007; Schwarte, 2008). FMRP functions to regulate various proteins necessary for synaptic development, neuronal maturation, and plasticity (Gothelf et al., 2008; Hall et al., 2008). In fragile X syndrome, the dendritic spines of neurons appear to be longer than in normal controls and are not fully developed (Huber, 2007).

At the Xq27.3 locus, anywhere from 6–50 CGG repeats are considered normal. Individuals with 50–200 repeats are considered premutation carriers, as they may have partial inactivation of the *FMR1* gene, and often show some clinical features of fragile X, although presentation and degree of deficit varies. fragile X syndrome is considered to be present in individuals with greater than 200 CGG repeats, which represents full mutation of the *FMR1* gene.

Recent work has examined the neuroanatomical sequelae associated with fragile X. Gothelf et al. (2008) compared neuroanatomical features in children with fragile X syndrome to age- and sex-matched controls. The investigators found significantly increased size of the caudate nucleus and decreased size of the posterior cerebeller vermis, amygdala, and superior temporal gyrus in those affected with fragile X syndrome.

NEUROPSYCHOLOGICAL/CLINICAL PRESENTATION

The symptoms of fragile X syndrome include moderate to severe mental retardation, attention deficits, and developmental delays (Huber, 2007). The clinical presentation varies greatly among individuals, as fragile X is a disorder with incomplete penetrance, meaning even those with full mutation can remain asymptomatic (Snustad & Simmons, 2003). Although severity of symptoms is somewhat dependent upon the number of CGG repeats, clinical presentation can be vastly different in individuals with the same number of repeats and even in affected individuals within the same family.

Because the syndrome is linked to the X-chromosome, males and females are impacted differently. Males tend to be more severely affected given their possession of only a single X-chromosome, while females with the disorder often have one unaffected X-chromosome, enabling them to potentially maintain some FMRP production, leading to less severe symptoms. Certain neuroanatomical phenotypes may also be associated with more severe cognitive deficits (Gothelf et al., 2008).

Males with fragile X syndrome often have moderate-to-severe mental retardation, with an average full-scale IQ of 40 (Schwarte, 2008). The cognitive profile of females with fragile X is much more variable and can range from normal to moderately impaired intelligence, but often females have low average intelligence. It is also believed that IQ tends to decline over time, but there is debate about whether such decline is due to loss of higher-order abilities, lack of development, or slower learning in affected individuals (Hall et al., 2008; Schwarte, 2008). Persons with the syndrome also typically have better verbal than visuospatial processing abilities. Executive dysfunction, specifically deficits in working memory, is often associated with the syndrome, as is difficulty performing arithmetic (Hall et al., 2008; Schwarte, 2008).

There is a high rate of comorbidity between fragile X syndrome and autism spectrum disorders. Autistic behaviors, such as stereotypies, gaze avoidance, self-injurious behaviors, and social and communication deficits are often apparent in individuals with fragile X syndrome (Schwarte, 2008). In males with fragile X syndrome, 60–90% show autistic features, while in females the rate varies from 25–80% (Gothelf et al., 2008). Further, 15–25% of individuals with fragile X syndrome are believed to meet the diagnostic criteria for autism (Schwarte, 2008). Persons with a comorbid autism diagnosis often have more severe deficits and are associated with poorer functional outcomes, including lower cognitive, language, social, and adaptive development (Fisch et al., 2007).

DIAGNOSIS

Because fragile X syndrome is a genetic disorder, family history plays an important role in suspecting a diagnosis and initiating further testing. Diagnosis of fragile X syndrome is often difficult because of the wide variability of symptoms (Snustad & Simmons, 2003). The diagnosis and severity of symptoms is based on the number of CGG repeats and can be tested with molecular genetic techniques. Clinically, the first

F

F

symptoms of the syndrome are often developmental delays. On average, boys with fragile X syndrome sit unassisted at 10 months, and walk and talk at around 20 months (Schwarte, 2008). Because developmental delays are common in many childhood disorders, without additional suspect of fragile X in the family, children often go misdiagnosed or undiagnosed until much later. The average age of diagnosis of fragile X syndrome is 8 years (Schwarte, 2008).

Fragile X also has characteristic physical symptoms that have diagnostic value, including elongated face, large ears, prominent jaw, macrocephaly, macroorchidism, flat feet, high-arched palate, and joints that are hyperextensive (Schwarte, 2008). However, the physical symptoms of the disorder are not usually apparent at birth or early childhood and do not typically develop until much later, often not until adolescence.

TREATMENT

Because the clinical features of fragile X syndrome are so individualized, treatment must be dependent upon the unique set of physical, cognitive, behavioral, and/or emotional problems. Multidisciplinary approaches are often necessary to address all problem areas. Primary medical doctors are important in the care of persons with fragile X syndrome in order to monitor the presence of common co-occurring medical conditions, such as problems associated with loose connective tissue and seizure disorders (Schwarte, 2008). The efficacy and side effects of medications need to be closely monitored in this population. Behavioral modification plans and medication management are an important component of treatment when behavioral symptoms are present. In children with speech and language difficulties, often a speech-language pathologist will be a part of the treatment team to lessen some of the communication barriers that may be present. Also, to increase likelihood of optimum development, individualized education plans are necessary to help identify strengths and weaknesses and facilitate learning to the individual's greatest capacity.

Shane S. Bush
Kathryn M. Lombardi Mirra

Fisch, G. S., Carpenter, N., Howard-Peebles, P., Holden, J. J., Tarleton, J., Simensen, R., et al. (2007). Studies of age-correlated features of cognitive-behavioral development in children and adolescents with genetic disorders. *American Journal of Medical Genetics Part A, 143A,* 2478–2489.

Gothelf, D., Furfaro, J. A., Hoeft, F., Eckert, M. A., Hall, S. S., O'Hara, R., et al. (2008). Neuroanatomy of fragile X syndrome is associated with aberrant behavior and the fragile X mental retardation protein (FMRP). *Annals of Neurology, 63,* 40–51.

Hall, S. S., Burns, D. D., Lightbody, A. A., & Reiss, A. L. (2008). Longitudinal changes in intellectual development in children with fragile X syndrome. *Journal of Abnormal Child Psychology, 36,* 927–939.

Huber, K. (2007). Fragile X syndrome: Molecular mechanisms of cognitive dysfunction. *American Journal of Psychiatry, 164,* 556.

Schwarte, A. R. (2008). Fragile X syndrome. *School Psychology Quarterly, 23,* 290–300.

Snustad, D. P., & Simmons, M. J. (2003). *Principles of genetics.* New York: John Wiley & Sons.

FRIEDREICH'S ATAXIA

DESCRIPTION

Friedreich's ataxia is an autosomal-recessive disease that causes progressive neurologic disability, cardiomyopathy, and skeletal abnormalities. It was initially described in 1863 by Nicholaus Friedreich, Professor of Medicine in Heidelberg, Germany (Chakravarty, 2003), and it is the most common form of inherited autosomal recessive ataxia. *Ataxia* refers to a lack of coordination with clumsy movements or unsteadiness, and it is present in several diseases and conditions (National Institute of Neurological Disorders and Stroke [NINDS], 2009). The symptoms present in Friedreich's ataxia occur because of degeneration of the nerve tissue in the spinal cord, which results in the loss of position and vibration sense in the legs and arms and diminished reflexes.

NEUROPATHOLOGY/PATHOPHYSIOLOGY

Friedreich's ataxia is an autosomal recessive hereditary disease in which the individual must inherit one affected gene from each parent for the disease to develop. It occurs in about 1 to 2 individuals per 100,000 people, although 1 in 90 Americans of European ancestry carry one affected gene (Chakravarty, 2003). There are no gender differences for this disease, as males and females are affected equally (NINDS, 2009). The mutated gene in Friedreich's ataxia is located on the long arm of chromosome 9 and codes for a protein called frataxin. This protein is responsible for assisting in the production of energy in cells. When it is absent or damaged, the production of energy in mitochondria is impaired, and the cells gradually die. The most common genetic mutation is a GAA trinucleotide repeat, which is a repetition of three nucleotides in the gene that results in reduced or abnormal production of frataxin. Although normal chromosomes may have up to 35 of these trinucleotide repeats, the disease-associated chromosomes contain from 70 to over 1,000 repeats (Pandolfo, 2009). Moreover, researchers have found a correlation between an increased number of trinucleotide repeats and more rapidly progressive disease (Montermini et al., 1997).

Historically, the clinical signs of Friedrich ataxia have been attributed to the effect the disease has on the spinal cord and peripheral sensory nerves (Wollmann, Barroso, Monton, & Nieto, 2002). More recently, neuroimaging studies have revealed more pervasive pathological changes in the CNS with particular emphasis placed upon evidence of cerebellar degeneration (De Michele et al., 1995). Although cerebellar degeneration certainly helps explain the typical motor features of Friedreich's ataxia, given relatively recent advances in the understanding of the relationship between the cerebellum and general cognitive and executive functions, it becomes clear that cerebellar degeneration may also play a significant role in the cognitive deficits associated with the disease.

NEUROPSYCHOLOGICAL/CLINICAL PRESENTATION

Individuals typically present with symptoms of Friedreich's ataxia between the ages of 5 and 15 years. Occasionally, symptoms may emerge as early as 18 months or as late as 50 years. The first symptom that typically appears is gait instability or generalized clumsiness. Eventually, this spreads to the arms and the trunk and affects whole body movement. This results in a swaying, broad-based gait, and poor balance. As ataxia continues to worsen, muscles become weak and atrophic, particularly in the hands, lower legs, and feet. As such, common signs of Friedreich's ataxia are foot deformities such as involuntary bending of the toes (i.e., flexion), turning inward of the foot (i.e., inversion), clubfoot, and hammer toes. Loss of tendon reflex in the knees and ankles are also common, along with a progressive loss of sensation in the extremities. This progressive loss often spreads to other areas of the body. As the disease worsens, the individual may experience slowness or slurring of speech secondary to dysarthria. Nystagmus, or rapid involuntary movements of the eyes, is another common symptom. Scoliosis is one of the most common signs of Friedreich's ataxia, and it may impair breathing if the curving of the spine is severe. In addition, those with Friedreich's ataxia typically report being easily fatigued (Pandolfo, 2009).

Various forms of heart disease are typical. The most common diseases of the heart in Friedreich's ataxia are cardiomyopathy, myocardial fibrosis, and cardiac failure. Also common are heart rate abnormalities like tachycardia and heart block. When these heart diseases are experienced, the individual may present with chest pain, heart palpitations, and shortness of breath. In addition to heart disease, about 10% of those with Friedreich's ataxia develop diabetes mellitus.

The rate of degeneration that occurs in Friedreich's ataxia can vary considerably, likely secondary to the degree of reduction in frataxin. Most commonly, within the first 10–20 years after the first symptom emerges, the person will lose the ability to walk, stand, or sit without support. As the disease progresses into later stages, it is common for individuals to become completely dependent. The most common causes of death in those with Friedreich's ataxia are related to complications of heart disease. Those who are less affected may live into their 60s and 70s, whereas the life span of most individuals with Friedreich's ataxia is reduced with an historical average age of death of 37 years (Harding, 1981).

Flood and Perlman (1987) found that 92% of individuals they tested with Friedreich's ataxia reported mood disturbances. The severity of depression ranged from mild to severe, with a majority of depressive symptoms related to living with a chronic and progressive disease. Other researchers have found evidence of additional emotional disturbances like anxiety and isolation (Giordani et al., 1989).

In addition to mood disturbance, speed of information processing is typically affected as well (Corben et al., 2006). Speed of information processing is commonly measured by reaction time. In two studies, visual and auditory reaction times in those with Friedreich's ataxia were greater compared with those without Friedreich's ataxia (Botez-Marquard & Botez, 1993, 1997). The authors attributed the increase in reaction time to reduced effectiveness of information processing, which could be at least partially related to the cognitive effects of depression or anxiety. However, White, Lalonde, and Botez-Marquard (2000) found evidence of general cognitive slowing in the absence of mood disorder. Other researchers have also found that those with Friedreich's ataxia have difficulty with information processing despite intact executive function (White et al., 2000).

F

Wollmann et al. (2002) found that patients with Friedreich's ataxia demonstrated evidence of significant impairment on verbal fluency tasks that were not secondary to dysarthria or more general cognitive slowing. Rather, the deficit in verbal fluency was believed to be secondary to a verbal retrieval deficit. Consistent with this finding, patients with Friedreich's ataxia also demonstrated evidence of a flat learning curve for rote verbal information, poor performance on measures of immediate and delayed narrative recall, and evidence of proactive interference. However, it is important to note that there was also evidence of impaired delayed cued recall, which suggests that in addition to poor retrieval there may also be diminished verbal consolidation and encoding during new learning activities. There was no evidence of visuospatial memory deficits. However, patients with Friedreich's ataxia did demonstrate evidence of impairment on tasks of complex visuoconstructional and visuoperceptive ability that was independent of motor deficits or general cognitive slowing.

According to Wollmann et al. (2002), measures of general attention were comparable to the matched controls with the exception of verbal span. In addition, visuospatial analysis, mental flexibility, and conceptual organization were well preserved.

DIAGNOSIS

Diagnosis of Friedrich's ataxia is based primarily on clinical presentation. The classic clinical criteria of the disease established in the early 1980s consist of autosomal recessive inheritance, onset before the age of 25 years, absence of lower extremity reflexes, and pyramidal tract involvement (Harding, 1983). Recent advances in genetic testing and further understanding of the role of frataxin have expanded the sensitivity and specificity of diagnosis of Friedrich's ataxia. Currently, genetic testing for the most common genetic markers of the disease can be of benefit in cases where the diagnosis is in question. Neuropsychological testing does not have a large role in the initial diagnosis of this condition but can be used to track the subtle cognitive effects of the disease to assist in treatment planning (Corben et al., 2006).

TREATMENT

Unfortunately, there have been few treatment options available to either reverse or slow the progression of neurological or cardiovascular disease. Most treatment has been supportive and focused on physical or occupational therapeutic techniques and careful monitoring for diabetes and heart disease. Studies of therapies aimed at reducing iron levels seen in the mitochondria of affected cells have been disappointing; however, newer trials evaluating a medication called idebenone have shown some promise (Rustin, Rotig, Munnich, & Sidi, 2002; Wilson & Fishbeck, 1998).

Sarah C. Jenkins
Nick P. Jenkins
Jon C. Thompson

Botez-Marquard, T., & Botez, M. I. (1993). Cognitive behavior in heredodegenerative ataxia. *European Neurology, 33,* 351–357.

Botez-Marquard, T., & Botez, M. I. (1997). Olivopontocerebellar atrophy and Friedreich's ataxia: Neuropsychological consequences of bilateral versus unilateral cerebellar lesion. *International Review of Neurobiology, 41,* 387–410.

Chakravarty, A. (2003). Friedreich's ataxia — Yesterday, today, and tomorrow. *Neurology India, 51,* 176–182.

Corben, L. A., Georgiou-Karistianis, N., Fahey, M. C., Storey, E., Churchyard, A., Home, M., Bradshaw, J. L., & Delatycki, M. B. (1996). Towards an understanding of cognitive function in Friedreich's ataxia. *Brain Research Bulletin, 70*(3), 197–202.

De Michele, G., Di Salle, F., Filla, A., D'Alessio, A., Ambrosio, G., Viscardi, L., et al. (1995). Magnetic resonance imaging in "typical" and "late onset" Friedreich's disease and early onset cerebellar ataxia with retained tendon reflexes. *The Italian Journal of Neurological Sciences, 16,* 303–308.

Flood, M. K., & Perlman, S. L. (1987). The mental status of patients with Friedreich's ataxia. *Journal of Neuroscience Nursing, 19,* 251–255.

Giordani, B., Boivan, M., Berent, S., Gilman, S., Junck, L., Lehtinen, S., et al. (1989). Cognitive and emotional functioning in Friedreich's ataxia. *Journal of Clinical and Experimental Neuropsychology, 11,* 53–54.

Harding, A. E. (1981). Friedreich's ataxia: A clinical and genetic study of 90 families with an analysis of early diagnostic criteria and intrafamilial clustering of clinical features. *Brain, 104,* 589–620.

Harding, A. E. (1983). Classification of the hereditary ataxias and paraplegias. *Lancet, 102,* 1151–1155.

Montermini, L., Richter, A., Morgan, K., Justice, C. M., Julien, D., Castellotti, B., et al. (1997). Phenotypic variability in Friedrich ataxia: Role of the associated GAA triplet repeat expansion. *Annals of Neurology, 41,* 675–682.

National Institute of Neurological Disorders and Stroke. (2009). *Friedreich's ataxia fact sheet.* Retrieved June 25, 2009, from http://www.ninds.nih.gov/disorders/friedreichs_ataxia/detail_friedreichs_ataxia.htm

Pandolfo, M. (2009). Friedreich's ataxia: The clinical picture. *Journal of Neurology, 256,* 3–8.

Rustin, P., Rotig, A., Munnich, A., & Sidi, D. (2002). Heart hypertrophy and function are improved by idebenone in Friedreich's ataxia. *Free Radical Research, 36,* 467–469.

White, M., Lalonde, R., & Botez-Marquard, T. (2000). Neuropsychologic and neuropsychiatric characteristics of patients with Friedreich's ataxia. *Acta Neurologica Scandinavica, 102,* 222–226.

Wilson, R. B., & Fishbeck, K. H. (1998). Normal serum iron and ferritin concentrations in patients with Friedreich's ataxia. *Annals of Neurology, 44,* 132–134.

Wollmann, T., Barroso, J., Fernando, M., & Nieto, A. (2002). Neuropsychological test performance of patients with Friedreich's ataxia. *Journal of Clinical and Experimental Neuropsychology, 24*(5), 677–686.

FRONTOTEMPORAL DEMENTIA

DESCRIPTION

In 1892, Arnold Pick described a patient with a dementing disease who had frontotemporal lobar degeneration and intranuclear inclusions (Pick bodies). He later coined the name of this dementing condition as Pick's disease. Unfortunately, Pick bodies are not the sole cause of this dementing condition described by Arnold Pick, and Pick bodies are found in other types of dementing diseases (Harciarek & Jodzio, 2005). In 1994, the Lund–Manchester group coined frontotemporal dementia (FTD) to alleviate problems that existed with original definition (Tanabe, 2000).

Although many individuals who experience FTD have no family history of dementia, a significant risk factor for developing FTD is a positive family history of dementia. A variety of mutations on several genes have been linked to FTD. Specifically, mutations in encoding the protein tau have been linked to inherited forms of FTD. Other risk factors include thyroid disease and head trauma with a loss of consciousness (Harciarek & Jodzio, 2005).

The onset of FTD is insidious and slow, but life span is dramatically decreased with death typically occurring 10 years from initial onset (Mendonca, Riberio, Guerreiro, & Garcia, 2004). Average age of onset is 52 and is more common in men than women (Harciarek & Jodzi, 2005). FTD is the most commonly diagnosed dementia behind Alzheimer's disease (AD). The prevalence of FTD is 9.4 per 100,000 for ages 60–69, 3.6 per 100,000 for ages 50–59, and 3.8 per 100,00 for ages 70–79 (Freedman, 2007).

Furthermore, unlike AD, the course of FTD severity is not linear (Diehl-Schmid, Pohl, Perneczky, Forstl, & Kurz, 2006). Behavioral disturbances are the most obvious as compared with cognitive abilities during the onset of FTD (Diehl-Schmid et al., 2006; Mendonca et al., 2004). Behavioral symptoms include lack or awareness, poor judgment, and significant personality alterations. Cognitive symptoms include an array of symptoms, but the most prominent is major deficits in language. Most individuals with FTD develop aphasia and move into complete muteness (Harciarek & Jodzio, 2005).

NEUROPATHOLOGY/PATHOPHYSIOLOGY

Functional magnetic resonance imaging has consistently found significant amounts of activity decreased in frontal and parietal regions (Harciarek & Jodzio, 2005). Other types of neuroimaging such as single photon emission computed tomography (SPECT) and positron emission tomography (PET) have found decreased cerebral blood flow and hypometabolism in frontal and anterior temporal lobes (Diehl & Kurz, 2002; Jauss et al., 2001).

Significant structural loss is observed in the frontal lobes, anterior temporal lobes, inferolateral temporal lobe, hippocampus, and in rare cases, this has been found in the basal ganglia as well. Much of the structural atrophy is thought to occur in the left hemisphere. Atrophy in the frontal lobes is associated with decline in social behavior, personal contact, and loss of insight (Diehl et al., 2002; Diehl-Schmid et al., 2006; Harciarek & Jodzio, 2005; Jauss et al., 2001). Atrophy in the anterior temporal lobes (tv-FTD) is associated with the semantic component of FTD (Diehl et al., 2002). FTD patients experience asymmetrical atrophy and decreased neural activity occurring in the left hemisphere approximately 90% of the time (Harciarek et al., 2002).

NEUROPSYCHOLOGICAL/CLINICAL PRESENTATION

The clinical presentation of FTD individuals involves cognitive, achievement, sensory, emotional, and behavioral components. Cognitive deficits involve loss of insight, distractibility, and mental flexibility (Diehl et al., 2002; Jauss et al., 2001). Although individuals with FTD consistently score within normal range on the Mini–Mental State Examination (MMSE), they still experience some memory loss. Their memory loss is attributed to frontal-executive impairment, including deficits in active strategies for learning, planning, and retrieval (Hodges et al., 1999). Overall, most patients with FTD experience decreased verbal output, which could progress to complete mutism (Allain, Bentue-Ferrer, Tribut, Merienne, & Belliard, 2003). Achievement measures show that individuals with FTD experience decreased verbal fluency. Interestingly, written fluency is said to be better than oral naming (Harciarek & Jodzio, 2005). As expected individuals with FTD experience impoverished/spontaneous speech (Diehl et al., 2002; Harciarek & Jodzio, 2005). The emotional presentation of FTD encompasses low levels of depression, but episodes of mania, anger, and irritability are not uncommon. Moreover, individuals affected by FTD are repeatedly unable to show and perceive/interpret basic emotions (Harciarek & Jodzio, 2005). Behavioral presentation of FTD includes a variety of symptoms including aggressiveness, disinhibition, verbal outbursts, impulsivity, compulsivity, preservative behavior, apathy, over activity, and impairment in social and interpersonal skills (Diehl et al., 2002; Diehl-Schmid et al., 2006; Jauss et al., 2001; Harciarek & Jodzio, 2005).

DIAGNOSIS

Similarities exist between AD and FTD, but appropriate assessment of memory, language, attention, and visuospatial abilities can prevent misdiagnoses. Individuals with AD have more overall deficits and acute deficits in episodic memory whereas individuals with FTD experience less overall general memory deficits, and the deficits experienced are attributed to executive impairments (Hodges et al., 1999). Although individuals with AD and FTD are both likely to have aphasia and word-finding problems, individuals with AD are more likely to have severe comprehension problems whereas individuals with FTD display impoverished spontaneous speech (Harciarek et al., 2005). Even though AD causes impairment in attention very early on, FTD elicits severe impairments in executive functioning (Harciarek et al., 2005). A differential diagnosis can also be corroborated by measures of visuospatial abilities. AD individuals experience visuospatial deficits, but individuals with FTD don't commonly experience deficits on measures of visuospatial abilities (Diehl et al., 2002).

FTD is a broad term that encompasses two different subtypes (Allain et al., 2003). The two subtypes that are both diagnosed under FTD can have incredibly different presentations (Hodges et al.,

1999; Tannabe, 2000). The first subtype, a temporal variant of FTD (tv-FTD) is associated with semantic deficits and aphasia (Hodges et al., 1999). Individuals with such a presentation are unable to complete tasks that require new semantic material to be encoded; this loss of "word sense" is caused by not being able to infer semantic representations (Hodges et al., 1999; Tannabe, 2000). In addition, tv-FTD is associated with interpersonal coldness, compulsivity, and rigidity (Harciarek et al., 2005). In comparison, the frontal variant of FTD (fv-FTD) is very similar to the definition coined by the Lund–Manchester groups, where the core symptoms are without the semantic impairments (Tannabe, 2000). Unlike tv-FTD, individuals with fv-FTD are said to have interpersonal openness and impulsive behavior (Harciarek et al., 2005; Hodges et al., 1999). People with fv-FTD show impairments specifically on tasks that assess executive functions (e.g., Rey Complex Figure) (Hodges et al., 1999; Mendonca et al., 2004).

TREATMENT

Unfortunately, the treatment literature is limited to pharmacological interventions. Medications that are beneficial in attenuating some of the symptoms of FTD include trazodone, idazoxan, selective serotonin reuptake inhibitors (SSRIs), amphetamines, selegiline, and neuroleptics. Trazodone is a serotonin reuptake inhibitor that improves behavior at high doses (Lebert & Pasquier, 1999). Idazoxan improves planning abilities, attention, verbal fluency, and episodic memory. SSRIs decrease impulsiveness, depression, and compulsions whereas amphetamines are useful in decreasing apathy, and improving working memory, and executive functioning. Selegiline, a monoamine oxidase inhibitor, improves neuropsychological symptoms. Neuroleptics a type of antipsychotic are beneficial for aggression, and disinhibition (Allain et al., 2003).

Antonio N. Puente

Allain, H., Bentue-Ferrer, D., Tribut, O., Merienne, M., & Belliard, S. (2003). Drug therapy of frontotemporal dementia. *Human Psychopharmacology, 18,* 221–225.

Diehl, J., & Kurz, A. (2002). Frontotemporal dementia: Patient characteristics, cognition, and behavior. *International Journal of Geriatric Psychiatry, 17,* 914–918.

Diehl-Schmid, J., Pohl, C., Perneczky, R., Forstl, H., & Kurz, A. (2006). Behavioral disturbances in the course of frontotemporal dementia. *Dementia and Geriatric Cognitive Disorders, 22,* 352–357.

Freedman, M. (2007). Frontotemporal dementia: Recommendations for therapeutic studies, designs, and approaches. *Le Journal Canadien Des Sciences Neurologiques, 34,* 118–124.

Harciarek, M., & Jodzio, K. (2005). Neuropsychological differences between frontotemporal dementia and Alzheimer's disease: A review. *Neuropsychology Review, 15*(3), 131–141.

Hodges, J. R., Garrad, P., Perry, R., Karalyn, P., Ward, R., Bak, T., et al. (1999). The differentiation of semantic dementia and frontal lobe dementia (temporal and frontal variants of frontotemporal dementia) from early Alzheimer's disease: A comparative neuropsychological study. *Neuropsychology, 13*(1), 31–40.

Jauss, M., Herholz, K., Kracht, L., Pantel, J., Hartmann, T., Jensen, M., et al. (2001). Frontotemporal dementia: Clinical, neuroimaging, and molecular biological findings in 6 patients. *European Archives of Psychiatry and Clinical Neuroscience, 251,* 225–231.

Lebert, F., & Pasquier, F. (1999). Letter to the editor. *Human Psychopharmacology Clinical and Experimental, 14,* 279–281.

Mendonca, A., Ribeiro, F., Guerreiro, M., & Garcia, C. (2004). Frontotemporal mild cognitive impairment. *Journal of Alzheimer's Disease, 6,* 1–9.

Tannabe, H. (2000). Clinical concept of frontotemporal dementia. *Neuropathology, 1,* 65–67.

F

G

GAUCHER'S DISEASE

DESCRIPTION

Gaucher's disease was the first lysosomal storage disorders to be identified. It is an autosomal-recessive disorder caused by a deficiency in the activity of the enzyme beta-glucocerebrosidase, leading to the accumulation of glucocerebroside, a glycolipid, in the lysosomes of macrophages (Brady et al., 1965). It was identified in 1882 by Philippe Gaucher and is the most common of the hereditary lysosomal storage disorders (Barton et al., 1991; Charrow et al., 1998; Zhao & Grabowski, 2002). A considerable amount of the research has been within specific ethnic groups and subtypes as a result of the genetic origin of the disorder (Tylki-Szymanska, Keddache, & Grabowski, 2006).

NEUROPATHOLOGY/PATHOPHYSIOLOGY

There are three clinical phenotypes: Gaucher's disease Type 1 (GD1), nonneuronopathic, and Types 2 and 3 (GD2 and GD3), acute and subacute neuronopathic variations of the disease. GD1 does not affect the central nervous system and accounts for 99% of cases. It occurs most frequently in the Ashkenazi Jewish population, with an incidence of 1 per 450 to 1,000 births. The incidence in the general Caucasian population is 1 per 50,000 (Charrow et al., 1998). Over 200 mutations have been identified (Zhao & Grabowski, 2002).

GD2 is the acute neuronopathic form of Gaucher's disease that is the less common yet most severe type. Patients present with rapidly progressive neurologic symptoms within the first month of life, including trismus, strabismus, retroflection of the head, progressive spasticity, and bulbar signs with dysphagia. Death typically occurs within the first 2 years of life.

GD3 becomes evident in late adolescence or early adulthood. This also being a neuronopathic form of the disease, the clinical manifestations of this variant are believed to be a result of the lipid-laden macrophages that are deposited in tissues including marrow, liver, and spleen. Patients may present with symptoms such as hepatosplenomegaly, anemia, thrombocytopenia, bone involvement (pathologic fractures and bone pain), and occasionally pulmonary, renal, cardiac, and central nervous system involvement.

NEUROPSYCHOLOGICAL/CLINICAL PRESENTATION

Although commonly characterized by lack of central nervous system involvement, Capablo et al. (2008) found significant neurological alterations and subclinical symptoms of peripheral neuropathy in patients with GD1. Patients with GD1 were also found to have elevated somatic complaints, depressed mood, psychological turmoil, and feelings of isolation relative to normals (Packman, Wilson Crosbie, Riesner, Fairley, & Packman, 2006).

Clinical presentation of GD3 shows slowly progressive symptoms, including seizures, horizontal gaze palsy, spasticity, ataxia, cognitive decline, and dementia. As the disease progresses, splenomegaly may occur. Patients generally do not develop all the possible symptoms associated with the disease, and the spectrum of severity is broad.

Neuropsychological studies on patients with GD1 are few, but suggest visuospatial dysfunction. The sequelae of symptoms are generally Parkinsonian in nature. As such, comorbid diagnosis of Parkinson's disease is common (Neudorfer et al., 1996; Tayebi et al., 2003).

DIAGNOSIS

Timely diagnosis and continued monitoring of patients with GD1 is critical given the progressive nature of the disease. Initial diagnosis is clinical and maintained by following symptoms and changes. In addition, the clinical differentiation between GD1 and GD3 is sometimes difficult during the early phase of the disease. Studies have suggested the best method for diagnosis is enzyme assay of beta-glucocerebrosidase activity. Visceral involvement can be assessed at diagnosis using MRI or CT scans (Charrow et al., 1998).

TREATMENT

Previous treatment was limited to symptom management, including splenectomy, blood transfusions, pain medication, surgical repair of fractures and bone necrosis, and bone marrow transplant. Currently, enzyme replacement therapy is being used for GD1. The treatment has been tried in GD3 without success (Goker-Alpan et al., 2008). There is no known effective treatment for Types 2 and 3 (Kingma, 1996). It is suggested that results and effectiveness of treatment depend on complications and overall symptom presentation.

Lindsay J. Hines
Charles Golden

Barton, G. J., Newman, R. H., Freemont, P. F., & Crumpton, M. J. (1991). Amino acid sequence analysis of the annexin super-gene family of proteins. *European Journal of Biochemistry, 198,* 749–760.

Brady, R. O., Kanfer, J. N., & Shapiro, D. (1965). Metabolism of glucocerebrosides. II. Evidence of an enzymatic deficiency In Gaucher's disease. *Biochemistry and Biophysics Research Communications, 18,* 221–225.

Capablo, J. L., Saenz de Cabezon, A., Fraile, J., Alfonso, P., Pocovi, M., & Giraldo, P. (2008). Neurological evaluation of patients with Gaucher disease diagnosed as type 1. *Journal of Neurology, Neurosurgery & Psychiatry, 79*(2), 219–222.

Charrow, J., Esplin, J. A., Gribble, T. J., Kaplan, P., Kolodny, E. H., Pastores, G. M., et al. (1998). Gaucher disease: Recommendations on diagnosis, evaluation, and monitoring. *Archives of Internal Medicine, 158*(16), 1754–1760.

Goker-Alpan, O., Wiggs, E. A., Eblan, M. J., Benko, W., Ziegler, S. G., Sidransky, E., et al. (2008). Cognitive outcome in treated patients with chronic neuronopathic Gaucher disease. *Journal of Pediatrics, 153*(1), 89–94.

Kingma, W. (1996). Gaucher disease: An overview of clinical characteristics and therapy. *Journal of Intravenous Nursing, 19*(2), 79–82.

Neudorfer, O., Giladi, N., Elstein, D., Abrahamov, A., Turezkite, T., Aghai, E., et al. (1996). Occurrence of Parkinson's syndrome in type I Gaucher disease. *Quarterly Journal of Mathematics, 89*(9), 691–694.

Packman, W., Wilson Crosbie, T., Riesner, A., Fairley, C., & Packman, S. (2006). Psychological complications of patients with Gaucher disease. *Journal of Inherited Metabolic Disease, 29*(1), 99–105.

Tayebi, N., Walker, J., Stubblefield, B., Orvisky, E., LaMarca, M. E., Wong, K., et al. (2003). Gaucher disease with parkinsonian manifestations: Does glucocerebrosidase deficiency contribute to a vulnerability to parkinsonism? *Molecular Genetics and Metabolism, 79*(2), 104–109.

Tylki-Szymanska, A., Keddache, M., & Grabowski, G. A. (2006). Characterization of neuronopathic Gaucher disease among ethnic Poles. *Genetics in Medicine, 8*(1), 8–15.

Zhao, H., & Grabowski, G. A. (2002). Gaucher disease: Perspectives on a prototype lysosomal disease. *Cellular and Molecular Life Science, 59*(4), 694–707.

Gerstmann's Syndrome

DESCRIPTION

Gerstmann's syndrome is a constellation of neuropsychological deficits that consists of right/left confusion, finger agnosia (inability to identify fingers), agraphia (inability to write), and acalculia (inability to calculate). Constructional apraxia and mild aphasia can also be present. Despite the relative frequency of the deficits when occurring separately, Gerstmann's syndrome is quite uncommon. True prevalence is unknown due to the difficulties with diagnosis. Patients affected with Gerstmann's syndrome present not only with the core features of the syndrome but also additional neurological difficulties (Miller & Hynd, 2004), which further complicate the condition. In fact, Gerstmann's syndrome is often not clinically "diagnosed" as a stand-alone disorder but rather it is referenced in clinical practice for the purposes of classification of symptoms and treatment planning.

Gerstmann's syndrome is considered to be an acquired condition and almost never described in children, whereas developmental Gerstmann's syndrome is the classification used for children implying a developmental etiology of the deficit. In fact, developmental Gerstmann's syndrome is reported more in the literature, but both are rarely studied and research is sparse. It should not be confused with Gerstmann–Sträussler–Scheinker's disease.

NEUROPATHOLOGY/PATHOPHYSIOLOGY

Deficits related to Gerstmann's syndrome have been localized to the left or dominant parietal lobe, particularly the supramarginal gyrus and the angular and second occipital gyrus (Maeshima, Okumura, Nakai, Itakura, & Komai, 1998; Ropper & Brown, 2005). Other studies have reported bilateral parietal damage (Weinberg & McLean, 1986) and right supramarginal gyrus defect (Weinberg, Harper, & Brumback, 1998), though it seems evident that there is no clear explanation for the cause of the condition, at least neurologically. Other researchers have tried to explain the syndrome's etiology in relation to development, specifically for developmental Gerstmann's syndrome. Some researchers have reported symptoms may be caused by the lack of neurocognitive skills required to master the tasks in the impaired areas (i.e., Semrud-Clikeman & Hynd, 1990), and others have suggested a manifestation of cerebral palsy due to perinatal complications (Kinsbourne, 1968). There does not appear to be a genetic contribution as most

G

individuals come from families not only without the syndrome, but without other learning disabilities (Miller & Hynd, 2004).

NEUROPSYCHOLOGICAL/CLINICAL PRESENTATION

As mentioned, individuals with either type of Gerstmann's syndrome present with a constellation of symptoms including left–right confusion, finger agnosia, dyscalculia, and dysgraphia. Sometimes considered a 5th symptom, constructional dyspraxia is common as well. However, some researchers believe a subthreshold presentation is possible, particularly in children and adolescents, when the individual has learned to compensate for an impaired area (PeBenito, 1987). In developmental Gerstmann's syndrome, patients are characterized by average or better intelligence, elevated verbal scores with lower performance scores, average or better reading scores, age-appropriate language skills, and negative history of traumatic brain injury (Miller & Hynd, 2004). It is not uncommon for individuals' symptoms to diminish over time, particularly in younger children as they learn to adapt to their deficits (National Institute of Neurological Disorders and Stroke [NINDS], 2009).

DIAGNOSIS

Perhaps due to the paucity of literature on Gerstmann's syndrome and the wealth of literature on other types of disorders, a diagnosis of Gerstmann's syndrome or developmental Gerstmann's syndrome is rarely made. Often medical professionals will rely on other diagnoses, which are better known to explain these deficits or serve as the underlying etiology of the symptoms (e.g., cerebrovascular events). Moreover, it is uncommon for individuals to have the syndrome-specific set of deficits without deficits in other areas, which may be better explained by a different diagnostic category. Notable differential diagnoses include fragile X syndrome, Williams's syndrome, Asperger's syndrome, and nonverbal learning disabilities (Miller & Hynd, 2004).

TREATMENT

Currently, there is no evidence-based treatment reported in the literature. Individuals may be referred for behavior therapies or physical therapies to reduce the severity of symptoms, but there is no cure for Gerstmann's syndrome. Continually educating individuals and families of individuals with the syndrome about the disorder can help to minimize any stress or discomfort that may be associated with it. Calculators or computers are also being employed to assist individuals in managing their symptoms (NINDS, 2009).

Beth Trammell
Chad A. Noggle

Kinsbourne, M. (1968). Developmental Gerstmann's syndrome. *Archives of Neurology, 45,* 977–982.

Maeshima, S., Okumura, Y., Nakai, K., Itakura, T., & Komai, N. (1998). Case study Gerstmann's syndrome associated with chronic subdural haematoma: A case report. *Brain Injury, 12,* 697–701.

Miller, C. J., & Hynd, G. W. (2004). What ever happened to developmental Gerstmann's syndrome? Links to other pediatric, genetic and neurodevelopmental syndromes. *Journal of Child Neurology, 19,* 282–289.

National Institute of Neurological Disorders and Stroke (2000). *NINDS Gerstmann syndrome information page.* Retrieved October 28, 2009, from http://www.ninds.nih.gov/disorders/gerstmanns/gerstmanns.htm

PeBenito, R. (1987). Developmental Gerstmann sydrome: Case report and review of the literature. *Developmental Behavior Pediatrics, 8,* 229–232.

Ropper, A. H., & Brown, R. H. (2005). Adams and Victor's principles of neurology (8th ed., pp. 385–412). New York: McGraw-Hill.

Semrud-Clikeman, M., & Hynd, G. W. (1990). Right hemisphere dysfunction in nonverbal learning disabilities: Social, academic, and adaptive functioning in adults and children. *Psychological Bulletin, 107,* 196–209.

Weinberg, W. A., Harper, C. R., & Brumback, R. A. (1998). Examination II: Clinical evaluation of cognitive/behavioral function. In C. E. Coffey & R. A. Brumback (Eds.), *Textbook of pediatric neuropsychiatry* (pp. 171–220). Washington, DC: American Psychiatric Press.

Weinberg, W. A., & McLean, A. (1986). A diagnostic approach to developmental specific learning disabilities. *Journal of Child Neurology, 1,* 158–172.

GERSTMANN–STRÄUSSLER–SCHEINKER DISEASE

DESCRIPTION

Gerstmann–Sträussler–Scheinker (GSS) disease is a rare, inherited prion disease first described in 1936 by Josef Gerstmann (Patel, Thavaseelan, Handel, Wong, & Sigman, 2007; Shevell, 2009). The symptoms and etiology of GSS are similar to other prion diseases,

G

such as Creutzfeldt–Jakob disease (CJD) and fatal familial insomnia (FFI). However, the order of symptom presentation and the morphology of the amyloid plaques distinguish GSS from other prion diseases (World Health Organization [WHO], 2003). GSS is characterized first by progressive limb and truncal ataxia, with cognitive impairments and dementia appearing only in the late stages of the disease (Giovagnoli et al., 2008; Unverzagt et al., 1997, Webb et al., 2008). There is no treatment for GSS, and it is universally fatal (Irisawa, Amanuma, Kozawa, Kimura, & Araki, 2007; Patel et al., 2007).

Prion diseases are a collection of transmissible or heritable disorders that result from the accretion of an abnormal form (PrP^{Sc}) of a normal cellular membrane glycoprotein (PrP^{C}; Liberski, 2008; Tunnell et al., 2008). The accretion of the abnormal protein causes spongiform encephalopathy and cortical atrophy and is assumed to occur via conventional protein replication processes (Liberski, 2008). In GSS, the protein malformation ensues from mutations within the *PrP* gene, typically at or near codon 102. The most common form of GSS occurs when the amino acid leucine is substituted for proline (Yamamoto, Kinoshita, Furukawa, & Kajiyama, 2007; Webb et al., 2008). Alternate substitutions for proline are possible and may account for some of the observed phenotypic variability (Tunnell et al., 2008). GSS is an autosomal dominant disorder, meaning that only one parent must carry the mutated gene for inherited transmission (Shevell, 2009).

NEUROPATHOLOGY/PATHOPHYSIOLOGY

Libersky (2008) reported finding tubovesicular structures in the pre- and postsynaptic terminals of patients with prion diseases, including patients with GSS. He indicated that these structures are unique to prion disorders but are not diagnostic of the variety of disease that will manifest. These structures are spherical or elongated, measuring approximately 27–30 nm in diameter. These filaments or clusters are visible via thin-section electron microscopy, precede the clinical signs of prion diseases, and are present throughout the disease progression, increasing in quantity as symptoms worsen. Lipersky hypothesized that because the tubovesicular structures appear before significant brain damage has occurred and before clinical symptoms are present, the structures themselves may be responsible for the neural damage seen in patients with a prion disease.

NEUROPSYCHOLOGICAL/CLINICAL PRESENTATION

GSS is an unusual prion disorder because it progresses slowly compared with other prion disorders. Continually, it typically presents with motor impairments first, with cognitive symptoms only appearing in later stages of the disease (WHO, 2003). Early motor symptoms are characterized by cerebellar ataxia, with resulting loss of coordination and unsteadiness, impaired motor strength in all limbs (Giovagnoli et al., 2008; Webb et al., 2008), akinesia (Yamomoto, Kinoshita, Furukawa, and Kajiyama, 2007) and in some cases, the return of primitive reflexes, including the Babinski (Irisawa et al., 2007) and tonic neck reflexes (Shevell, 2009). Myoclonic movements have been reported in variant GSS cases but are extremely rare (WHO, 2003). Thus, one can expect patients with the early stages of GSS to have difficulty navigating stairs or cluttered environments. They may also experience difficulty with tasks that require grip strength, such as writing or carrying objects, and may struggle to walk long distances due to their impaired motor strength.

Cognitive impairments appear late in the disease progression (Giovagnoli et al., 2008). The cognitive features include executive function impairment, such as loss of planning ability, disinhibition, loss of initiative, declarative and semantic memory deficits, language deficits, including impaired verbal fluency, slowed processing speed, and impaired intelligence as measured by the standardized intelligence tests (Giovagnoli et al., 2008; Unverzagt et al., 1997). In very late stages of GSS, global dementia and severe personality changes are apparent (WHO, 2003).

DIAGNOSIS

Diagnosis of a prion disease typically begins with diffusion-weighted magnetic resonance (MR) imaging. MR images captured early in the disease progression typically reveal hyperintense signal changes in frontal, temporal, occipital, and parietal cortices (Yamamoto et al., 2007). Unique to the early stages of GSS, however, is an area of low signal intensity in the basal ganglia, centered in the globus pallidus (Irisawa et al., 2007). This area of low signal intensity is probably due to abnormally high iron depositions, common in chronic inflammatory and degenerative disorders. The pattern of signal intensity changes throughout the progression of GSS, with regions becoming visible or obscured as a result of changing patterns of iron deposition masking genuine high-signal intensity areas. In later stages of the disease progression, cortical atrophy and hypodense lesions in the bilateral frontal subcortical region are visible in CT scans (Yamamoto et al., 2007).

The presence of a prion disease is supported by analysis of the patient's cerebrospinal fluid (CSF) (Aksamit, Preissner, & Homburger, 2001; Zerr et al., 2000). Elevated levels of the 14-3-3 protein (>8 ng/mL) in the CSF, as determined by Western Blot technique and elevated neuron-specific enolase (NSE >30 ng/mL), have a positive predictive value of 94.7% and a negative predictive value of 92.4% for the presence of a prion disease. False positives for first analysis may occur in patients with herpes simplex encephalitis, hypoxic brain damage, atypical encephalitis, intracerebral metastases of a bronchial carcinoma, metabolic encephalopathy, and idiopathic progressive dementia. If a second CSF analysis confirms the presence of elevated 14-3-3 protein and NSE levels, a prion protein gene analysis should be conducted as the final confirmatory step.

GSS is distinct from CJD and FFI in the pace of disease progression, the order of clinical symptom presentation, and the morphology of the amyloid plaques that form in the patient's cortex. GSS has a relatively long illness duration compared with CJD (49 months, compared with 4.5–8 months, respectively; Webb et al., 2008; WHO, 2003). In addition, motor symptoms present first in GSS, with cognitive symptoms appearing much later in the illness, whereas CJD first presents as cognitive impairments, followed by motor difficulties. GSS lacks the insomnia component required for a diagnosis of FFI (WHO, 2003). Finally, a histocytological examination of biopsied spongiform brain tissue can confirm the differential diagnosis (Sikorska, Liberski, Sobów, Budka, & Ironside, 2009). GSS amyloid plaques are multicentric, possessing several clusters of dense, interwoven fibrils, with fibrils radiating in a feathered pattern at the periphery. CJD plaques, on the other hand, are organized into thick, tongue-like processes and are often surrounded by vacuoles or vesicles. In comparison with the neuritic plaques and tangle that are hallmarks of Alzheimer's disease, the fibrils in Alzheimer's disease plaques are thinner (4–8 nm diameter) than GSS fibrils (7–9 nm) and organized similar to CJD. FFI lacks amyloid plaques altogether.

TREATMENT

Because GSS is fatal in all cases (Irisawa et al., 2007; Patel et al., 2007), treatment should focus on the comfort and safety of the individual. The patient may receive some benefit from exercise that focuses on balance and coordination. Although these exercises will not cure the motor symptoms, they may ameliorate some of the symptoms' effects by maintaining or developing the patient's proprioceptive ability. The individual's environment should be kept free of clutter to minimize the number of potential hazards, and the individual should be encouraged to avoid stairs and escalators. Wherever possible, rails and ramps should be installed to maximize the individual's safety while navigating the environment. As motor function impairment increases, a walker may become necessary. For ease and safety when sitting down or standing up, the patient should sit only in armchairs that are elevated slightly in the back. This will allow the patient to use his or her arms to aid in sitting and standing, while the tilt of the chair exploits gravity to facilitate the movement.

Individuals with GSS should not drive because of the impairments to executive function. Driving requires concentration, planning, and the ability to shift attention between rapidly changing sets of stimuli — all of which may be impaired in individuals with GSS. Although planning and memory are often impaired, an individual with GSS may be able to maintain some degree of independent living. The patient may find it helpful to have a large whiteboard placed centrally in the home, with a daily to-do list written on it by a caregiver. A timer or alarm clock should be used to cue the individual with GSS to check the board for upcoming tasks. As cognitive impairments become more severe, the individual may require constant supervision, possibly in a hospice setting.

Amanda Ballenger
Raymond S. Dean

Aksamit, A. J., Preissner, C. M., & Homburger, H. A. (2001). Quantitation of 14-3-3 and neuron-specific enolase in CSF in Creutzfeldt-Jakob disease. *Neurology, 57,* 728–730.

Giovagnoli, A. R., Di Fede, G., Aresi, A., Reati, F., Rossi, G., & Tagliavini, F. (2008). Atypical frontotemporal dementia as a new clinical phenotype of Gerstmann-Straussler-Scheinker disease with the PrP-P102L mutation. Description of a previously unreported Italian family. *Neurological Science, 29,* 405–410.

Irisawa, M., Amanuma, M., Kozawa, E., Kimura, F., & Araki, N. (2007). A case of Gerstmann-Sträussler-Scheinker syndrome. *Magnetic Resonance in Medical Sciences, 6*(1), 533–557.

Liberski, P. P. (2008). The tubulovesicular structures — the ultrastructural hallmark for all prion diseases. *Acta Neurobiologiæ Experimentalis, 68,* 113–121.

Patel, S. R., Thavaseelan, S., Handel, L. N., Wong, A., & Sigman, M. (2007). Bilateral manual externalization of testis with self-castration in patient with prion disease. *Urology, 70*, 15–16.

Shevell, M. (2009). The tripartite origins of the tonic neck reflex. *Neurology, 72*, 850–853.

Sikorska, B., Liberski, P. P., Sobów, T., Budka, H., & Ironside, J. W. (2009). Ultrastructural study of florid plaques in variant Creutzfeldt-Jakob disease: A comparison with amyloid plaques in kuru, sporadic Creutzfeldt-Jakob disease and Gerstmann-Sträussler-Scheinker disease. *Neuropathology and Applied Neurobiology, 35*, 46–59.

Tunnell, E., Wollman, R., Mallick, S., Cortes, C. J., DeArmond, S. J., & Mastrianni, J. A. (2008). A novel *PRNP*-P105S mutation associated with atypical prion disease and a rare PrP^{Sc} conformation. *Neurology, 71*, 1431–1438.

Unverzagt, F. W., Farlow, M. R., Norton, J., Dlouhy, S. R., Young, K., & Ghetti, B. (1997). Neuropsychological function in patients with Gerstmann-Sträussler-Scheinker disease from the Indiana Kindred (F198S). *Journal of the International Neuropsychological Society, 3*, 169–178.

Webb, T. E. F., Poulter, M., Beck, J., Uphill, J., Adamson, G., Campbell, T., et al. (2008). Phenotypic heterogeneity and genetic modification of P102L inherited prion disease in an international series. *Brain, 131*, 2632–2646.

World Health Organization. (2003). *WHO manual for surveillance of human transmissible spongiform encephalopathies including variant Creutzfeldt-Jakob disease*. Geneva, Switzerland: WHO.

Yamamoto, S., Kinoshita, M., Furukawa, S., & Kajiyama, K. (2007). Early abnormality of diffusion-weighted magnetic resonance imaging followed by brain atrophy in a case of Gerstmann-Sträussler-Scheinker disease. *Archives of Neurology, 64*, 450–451.

Zerr, I., Bodemer, M., Gefeller, O., Otto, M., Poser, S., Wiltfang, J., et al. (2000). Detection of 14-3-3 protein in the cerebrospinal fluid supports the diagnosis of Creutzfeldt-Jakob disease. *Annals of Neurology, 47*(5), 683–684.

GLOSSOPHARYNGEAL NEURALGIA

DESCRIPTION

Glossopharyngeal neuralgia (GN) is a relatively rare disorder affecting the ninth cranial nerve, with estimations of about 0.8 cases per 100,000 individuals (Katusic, Williams, Beard, Bergstralh, & Kurland, 1991). It shares many features with trigeminal neuralgia. GN is characterized by sharp, typically unilateral, paroxysmal pain in the tonsillar region, pharynx, posterior regions of the tongue, jaw, and/or ear. The painful attacks can be triggered by swallowing, yawning, food contact on the pharynx, talking, chewing, and/or coughing (Biller, 2002; Headache Classification Subcommittee of the International Headache Society, 2004), with some research suggesting that it more commonly affects the left side (Teixeira, de Siqueira, & Bor-Seng-Shu, 2008). The severe pain may last from seconds to minutes (Headache Classification Subcommittee of the International Headache Society, 2004; Rozen, 2004) and the course is usually episodic, with active phases of painful experiences lasting weeks or months, and periods of remission lasting variable lengths of time (De Simone, Ranieri, Bilo, Fiorillo, & Bonavita, 2008).

NEUROPATHOLOGY/PATHOPHYSIOLOGY

GN often appears to be idiopathic in nature. However, vascular compression of the glossopharyngeal nerve has often been reported as a source for GN (Ferroli et al., 2009; Fischbach, Lehmann, Ricke, & Bruhn, 2003; Hiwatashi et al., 2008; Patel, Kassam, Horowitz, & Chang, 2002). A number of other disorders may also be secondary causes for GN. For instance, Eagle's syndrome, which is associated with compression of the glossopharyngeal nerve due to an elongated styloid process, may result in GN (Montalbetti, Ferrandi, Pergami, & Savoldi, 1995; Soh, 1999). McCarron and Bone (1999) reported the case of a patient with "referred" GN arising from a left pontine lesion. A number of other disorders have been reported to cause GN including medullary infarction (Warren, Kotsenas, & Czervionke, 2006), cerebellopontine angle tumor (Phuong, Matsushima, Hisada, & Matsumoto, 2004), adhesive arachnoid (Fukuda, Ishikawa, & Yamazoe, 2002), nasopharyngeal carcinoma (Giorgi & Broggi, 1984), and posterior fossa arteriovenous malformation (Galetta, Raps, Hurst, & Flamm, 1993).

NEUROPSYCHOLOGICAL/CLINICAL PRESENTATION

Regarding the effects of GN on neuropsychological functioning, there have been no published reports investigating the direct effects of GN on memory or cognitive functioning. However, GN may affect neuropsychological functioning from secondary sources, such as the treatment approach. Microvascular decompression is used to treat both GN and trigeminal neuralgia, and both procedures use a lateral suboccipital approach (Hitotsumatsu, Matsushima, & Inoue, 2003). Some investigators have reported the onset of peduncular hallucinosis following microvascular decompression for trigeminal neuralgia (Chen & Lui,

1995; Tsukamoto, Matsushima, Fujiwara, & Fukui, 1993). However, more serious neuropsychological effects may result from the pharmacological treatment of GN.

Anticonvulsant medications are often used to treat GN, and many of these medications may have negative influences on memory and cognitive functioning (Hessen, Lossius, & Gjerstad, 2009). Carbamazepine, in particular, has often been found to negatively affect neuropsychological functioning (Martin et al., 2001; Meador et al., 2007; Salinsky et al., 2002), including information processing speed and attention (Wesnes, Edgar, Dean, & Wroe, 2009) and motor functioning (Mecarelli et al., 2004). These adverse neuropsychological effects may arise partly due to the changes that accompany carbamazepine in neurophysiological functioning. Specifically, carbamazepine is known to increase delta-theta power and reduce alpha frequency rhythm (Mecarelli et al., 2004; Salinsky et al., 2002). Gabapentin has also been found to produce negative effects on neuropsychological functioning (Martin et al., 2001; Salinsky et al., 2002). However, the effects of lamotrigine on neuropsychological functioning are not as severe (Meador et al., 2001, 2005). Indeed, Smith et al. (2006) reported that although lamotrigine was associated with reduced EEG power it was not accompanied by impaired cognitive functioning. Similarly, pregabalin produces relatively minor changes in cognitive and psychomotor functioning (Hindmarch, Trick, & Ridout, 2005).

DIAGNOSIS

The diagnosis of GN is complicated by the fact that it closely resembles trigeminal neuralgia (Soh, 1999; Teixeira, de Siqueira, & Bor-Seng-Shu, 2008). Diagnosis is obtained from the patient's history and by mapping the distribution of pain. The determination of trigger points for pain is important, as injecting the trigger point (often the pharynx) with topical anesthesia may aid in diagnosis if the pain is halted. Further, given the many secondary causes for GN, these additional sources should be evaluated and ruled out. This may involve an otolaryngology consultation and/or imaging of the head using CT or MRI to evaluate for the presence of cerebellopontine angle tumors (Biller, 2002; Rozen, 2004; Soh, 1999). In addition, recent research has supported the use of MRI in visualizing the source of vascular compression that gives rise to GN (Fischbach, Lehmann, Ricke, & Bruhn, 2003). Other investigators have used MRI to specifically evaluate the contribution of the posterior inferior cerebellar artery in causing GN (Boch, Oppenheim,

Biondi, Marsault, & Philippon, 1998; Hiwatashi et al., 2008).

TREATMENT

The treatment of GN may involve both pharmacological and surgical approaches. Regarding pharmacological treatment, anticonvulsants are the medications of choice (De Simone, Ranieri, Bilo, Fiorillo, & Bonavita, 2008; Rozen, 2004; Teixeira, de Siqueira, & Bor-Seng-Shu, 2008). Research has supported a wide range of anticonvulsant medications in effectively treating GN, with some viewing carbamazepine as the favored medication (Rushton, Stevens, & Miller, 1981). Indeed, a number of studies have supported the use of carbamazepine in treating GN (Giza, Kyriakou, Liasides, & Dimakopoulou, 2008; Johnston & Redding, 1990; Saviolo & Fiasconaro, 1987). Other anticonvulsants reported to effectively treat GN include gabapentin (Moretti, Torre, Antonello, Bava, & Cazzato, 2002) and lamotrigine (Titlic, Jukic, Tonkic, Grani, & Jukic, 2006). In addition, pregabalin (Kitchener, 2006) and baclofen (Ringel & Roy, 1987) are reported to be successful in treating GN. However, the benefit from anticonvulsant medication may dissipate with time (Soh, 1999).

With reduced effectiveness of anticonvulsant medications or cases where patients experience medically intractable pain, surgical approaches may then be warranted. The surgical treatment of GN may involve intracranial sectioning of the glossopharyngeal nerve, a procedure resulting in good relief of pain (Ceylan, Karakus, Duru, Baykal, & Koca, 1997; Rushton et al., 1981). Microvascular decompression of the offending artery, however, has received considerable support as an effective treatment approach in appropriate cases. A number of investigators have reported reduced pain following microvascular decompression (Boch et al., 1998; Hitotsumatsu et al., 2003; Patel et al., 2002) as well as long-term benefits (Ferroli et al., 2009; Kondo, 1998; Resnick, Jannetta, Bissonnette, Jho, & Lanzino, 1995; Sampson, Grossi, Asaoka, & Fukushima, 2004). Recently, gamma knife surgery has also been reported to effectively treat GN (Yomo, Arkha, Donnet, & Regis, 2009).

Paul S. Foster
Valeria Drago

Biller, J. (2002). *Practical neurology* (2nd ed.). Philadelphia, PA: Lippincott, Williams, & Wilkins.

Boch, A. L., Oppenheim, C., Biondi, A., Marsault, C., & Philippon, J. (1998). Glossopharyngeal neuralgia associated with vascular loop demonstrated by magnetic resonance imaging. *Acta Neurochirurgica, 140*, 813–818.

Ceylan, S., Karakus, A., Duru, S., Baykal, S., & Koca, O. (1997). Glossopharyngeal neuralgia: A study of 6 cases. *Neurosurgical Review, 20*, 196–200.

Chen, H. J., & Lui, C. C. (1995). Peduncular hallucinosis following microvascular decompression for trigeminal neuralgia: Report of a case. *Journal of the Formosan Medical Association, 94*, 503–505.

De Simone, R., Ranieri, A., Bilo, L., Fiorillo, C., & Bonavita, V. (2008). Cranial neuralgias: From physiopathology to pharmacological treatment. *Neurological Sciences, 29*, S69–S78.

Ferroli, P., Fioravanti, A., Schiariti, M., Tringali, G., Franzini, A., Calbucci, F., et al. (2009). Microvascular decompression for glossopharyngeal neuralgia: A long-term retrospective review of the Milan-Bologna experience in 31 consecutive cases. *Acta Neurochirurgica, 151*, 1245–1250.

Fischbach, F., Lehmann, T. N., Ricke, J., & Bruhn, H. (2003). Vascular compression in glossopharyngeal neuralgia: Demonstration by high-resolution MRI at 3 tesla. *Neuroradiology, 45*, 810–811.

Fukuda, H., Ishikawa, M., & Yamazoe, N. (2002). Glossopharyngeal neuralgia caused by adhesive arachnoid. *Acta Neurochirurgica, 144*, 1057–1058.

Galetta, S. L., Raps, E. C., Hurst, R. W., & Flamm, E. S. (1993). Glossopharyngeal neuralgia from a posterior fossa arteriovenous malformation: Resolution following embolization. *Neurology, 43*, 1854–1855.

Giorgi, C., & Broggi, G. (1984). Surgical treatment of glossopharyngeal neuralgia and pain from cancer of the nasopharynx. A 20-year experience. *Journal of Neurosurgery, 61*, 952–955.

Giza, E., Kyriakou, P., Liasides, C., & Dimakopoulou, A. (2008). Glossopharyngeal neuralgia with cardiac syncope: An idiopathic case treated with carbamazepine and duloxetine. *European Journal of Neurology, 15*, e38–e39.

Headache Classification Subcommittee of the International Headache Society. (2004). *The international classification of headache disorders* (2nd ed.). *Cephalalgia, 24*(Suppl. 1), 9–160.

Hessen, E., Lossius, M. I., & Gjerstad, L. (2009). Antiepileptic monotherapy significantly impairs normative scores on common tests of executive functions. *Acta Neurologica Scandinavica, 119*, 194–198.

Hindmarch, I., Trick, L., & Ridout, F. (2005). A double-blind, placebo- and positive-internal-controlled (alprazolam) investigation of the cognitive and psychomotor profile of pregabalin in healthy volunteers. *Psychopharmacology, 183*, 133–143.

Hitotsumatsu, T., Matsushima, T., & Inoue, T. (2003). Microvascular decompression for treatment of trigeminal neuralgia, hemifacial spasm, and glossopharyngeal neuralgia: Three surgical approach variations: Technical note. *Neurosurgery, 53*, 1436–1443.

Hiwatashi, A., Matsushima, T., Yoshiura, T., Tanaka, A., Noguchi, T., Togao, O., et al. (2008). MRI of glossopharyngeal neuralgia caused by neurovascular compression. *American Journal of Roentgenology, 191*, 578–581.

Johnston, R. T., & Redding, V. J. (1990). Glossopharyngeal neuralgia associated with cardiac syncope: Long term treatment with permanent pacing and carbamazepine. *British Heart Journal, 64*, 403–405.

Katusic, S., Williams, D. B., Beard, C. M., Bergstralh, E. J., & Kurland, L. T. (1991). Epidemiology and clinical features of idiopathic trigeminal neuralgia and glossopharyngeal neuralgia: Similarities and differences, Rochester, Minnesota, 1945–1984. *Neuroepidemiology, 10*, 276–281.

Kondo, A. (1998). Follow-up results of using microvascular decompression for treatment of glossopharyngeal neuralgia. *Journal of Neurosurgery, 88*, 221–225.

Martin, R., Meador, K., Turrentine, L., Faught, E., Sinclair, K., Kuzniecky, R., et al. (2001). Comparative cognitive effects of carbamazepine and gabapentin in healthy senior adults. *Epilepsia, 42*, 764–771.

McCarron, M. O., & Bone, I. (1999). Glossopharyngeal neuralgia referred from a pontine lesion. *Cephalalgia, 19*, 115–117.

Meador, K. J., Gevins, A., Loring, D. W., McEvoy, L. K., Ray, P. G., Smith, M. E., et al. (2007). Neuropsychological and neurophysiologic effects of carbamazepine and levtiracetam. *Neurology, 69*, 2076–2084.

Meador, K. J., Loring, D. W., Ray, P. G., Murro, A. M., King, D. W., Perrine, K. R., et al. (2001). Differential cognitive and behavioral effects of carbamazepine and lamotrigine. *Neurology, 56*, 1177–1182.

Meador, K. J., Loring, D. W., Vahle, V. J., Ray, P. G., Werz, M. A., Fessler, A. J., et al. (2005). Cognitive and behavioral effects of lamotrigine and topiramate in healthy volunteers. *Neurology, 64*, 2108–2114.

Mecarelli, O., Vicenzini, E., Pulitano, P., Vanacore, N., Romolo, F. S., Di Piero, V., et al. (2004). Clinical, cognitive, and neurophysiologic correlates of short-term treatment with carbamazepine, oxcarbazepine, and levetiracetam in healthy volunteers. *Annals of Pharmacotherapy, 38*, 1816–1822.

Montalbetti, L., Ferrandi, D., Pergami, P., & Savoldi, F. (1995). Elongated styloid process and Eagle's syndrome. *Cephalalgia, 15*, 80–93.

Moretti, R., Torre, P., Antonello, R. M., Bava, A., & Cazzato, G. (2002). Gabapentin treatment of glossopharyngeal neuralgia: A follow-up of four years of a single case. *European Journal of Pain, 6*, 403–407.

Patel, A., Kassam, A., Horowitz, M., & Chang, Y. F. (2002). Microvascular decompression in the management of glossopharyngeal neuralgia: Analysis of 217 cases. *Neurosurgery, 50*, 705–710.

Phuong, H. L., Matsushima, T., Hisada, K., & Matsumoto, K. (2004). Glossopharyngeal neuralgia due to an epidermoid tumour in the cerebellopontine angle. *Journal of Clinical Neuroscience, 11*, 758–760.

Resnick, D. K., Jannetta, P. J., Bissonnette, D., Jho, H. D., & Lanzino, G. (1995). Microvascular decompression for glossopharyngeal neuralgia. *Neurosurgery, 36*, 64–68.

Ringel, R. A., & Roy, E. P., III. (1987). Glossopharyngeal neuralgia: Successful treatment with baclofen. *Annals of Neurology, 21*, 514–515.

Rozen, T. D. (2004). Trigeminal neuralgia and glossopharyngeal neuralgia. *Neurologic Clinics, 22*, 185–206.

Rushton, J. G., Stevens, J. C., & Miller, R. H. (1981). Glossopharyngeal (vagoglossopharyngeal) neuralgia: A study of 217 cases. *Archives of Neurology, 38*, 201–205.

Salinsky, M. C., Binder, L. M., Oken, B. S., Storzbach, D., Aron, C. R., & Dodrill, C. B. (2002). Effects of gabapentin and carbamazepine on the EEG and cognition in healthy volunteers. *Epilepsia, 43*, 482–490.

Sampson, J. H., Grossi, P. M., Asaoka, K., & Fukushima, T. (2004). Microvascular decompression for glossopharyngeal neuralgia: Long-term effectiveness and complication avoidance. *Neurosurgery, 54*, 884–889

Saviolo, R., & Fiasconaro, G. (1987). Treatment of glossopharyngeal neuralgia by carbamazepine. *British Heart Journal, 58*, 291–292.

Smith, M. E., Gevins, A., McEvoy, L. K., Meador, K. J., Ray, P. G., & Gilliam, F. (2006). Distinct cognitive neurophysiologic profiles for lamotrigine and topiramate. *Epilepsia, 47*, 695–703.

Soh, K. B. K. (1999). The glossopharyngeal nerve, glossopharyngeal neuralgia and the Eagle's syndrome Current concepts and management. *Singapore Medical Journal, 40*, 659–665.

Teixeira, M. J., de Siqueira, S. R. D. T., & Bor-Seng-Shu, E. (2008). Glossopharyngeal neuralgia: Neurosurgical treatment and differential diagnosis. *Acta Neurochirurgica, 150*, 471–475.

Titlic, M., Jukic, I., Tonkic, A., Grani, P., & Jukic, J. (2006). Use of lamotrigine in glossopharyngeal neuralgia: A case report. *Headache, 46*, 167–169.

Tsukamoto, H., Matsushima, T., Fujiwara, S., & Fukui, M. (1993). Peduncular hallucinosis following microvascular decompression for trigeminal neuralgia: Case report. *Surgical Neurology, 40*, 31–34.

Warren, H. G., Kotsenas, A. L., & Czervionke, L. F. (2006). Trigeminal and concurrent glossopharyngeal neuralgia secondary to lateral medullary infarction. *American Journal of Roentgenology, 27*, 705–707.

Wesnes, K. A., Edgar, C., Dean, A. D., & Wroe, S. J. (2009). The cognitive and psychomotor effects of remacemide and carbamazepine in newly diagnosed epilepsy. *Epilepsy and Behavior, 14*, 522–528.

Yomo, S., Arkha, Y., Donnet, A., & Regis, J. (2009). Gamma knife surgery for glossopharyngeal neuralgia. *Journal of Neurosurgery, 110*, 559–563.

GUILLAIN–BARRÉ SYNDROME

DESCRIPTION

Guillain–Barré syndrome (GBS) is an acute demyelinating inflammatory syndrome involving acute peripheral neuropathy. GBS is a systemic disorder in which the immune system attacks the peripheral nervous system and is often triggered by an acute infectious process, including past surgical infection and vaccinations. Four GBS subtypes have been identified: (1) acute inflammatory demyelinating polyradiculoneuropathy being the most common, (2) acute motor axonal neuropathy, characterized by pure motor involvement, (3) acute motor and sensory axonal neuropathy, a subtype in which both motor and sensory fibers are affected, and (4) Fisher's syndrome in which the hallmark feature is a triad of ophthalmoplegia, ataxia, and areflexia (Hughes & Cornblath, 2005).

Worldwide estimates of GBS suggest an incidence of 1–2 per 100,000 (Pritchard & Hughes, 2004). Men are more often affected than women and the incidence of GBS increases with advancing age (Hughes & Cornblath, 2005). GBS can be debilitating and potentially fatal in 5% of cases, with considerable long-term disability implications. Recovery may take up to 1 or 2 years, though a number of patients continue to experience ongoing complaints (Forsberg, Press, Einarsson, Pedro-Cuesta, & Holmqvist, 2005; Pritchard & Hughes, 2004).

NEUROPATHOLOGY/PATHOPHYSIOLOGY

The pathophysiology of GBS is due to multifocal mononuclear cell infiltration in the peripheral nervous system via activated T lymphocytes and macrophages. Once activated, macrophages invade and denude the axons of the myelin sheaths (Haldeman & Zulkosky, 2005; Pritchard & Hughes, 2004). In particular, demyelination at the nodes of Ranvier has been a major finding. Increased protein is typically evident within the CSF, though it may not be evident during the first few days of illness.

NEUROPSYCHOLOGICAL/CLINICAL PRESENTATION

Many GBS sufferers report acute infection prior to diagnosis of GBS. Often these manifest as flu-like

G

symptoms, including malaise, progressive limb weakness, fatigue, and headache, which quickly progress to ascending paralysis, paresthesia, numbness, and pain (Hughes & Cornblath, 2005). Onset of symptoms usually occurs within 2 weeks, but may go up to 4. Autonomic involvement and respiratory failure requiring assistive ventilation occur in a number of patients, with the latter being associated with poorer prognosis and occasional mortality. Otherwise, neuropsychological data of GBS is sparse to nonexistent.

DIAGNOSIS

Onset of GBS is often sudden and unexpected, but recent infections are present in the majority of cases. Key features include weakness, possible sensory disturbance, and diminished or absent tendon reflexes (hyporeflexia) typically associated with upper motor neuron pathology and the presence of raised protein concentration within the CSF in perhaps 80% of patients, although abnormal CSF findings may not be present initially (Bensa, Hadden, Hahn, Hughes, & Wilson; 2000; Hughes & Cornblath, 2005). Neurophysiological examination may include nerve conduction studies to identify demyelination and slowed conduction velocities (Pritchard & Hughes, 2004). Neurodiagnostic imaging might also be performed but is of limited utility in diagnosing GBS. Finally, GBS exclusion often requires diagnostic testing for the exclusion of other possible syndromes and etiologies.

TREATMENT

Intravenous immunoglobin therapies are the first-line course treatment for GBS. Plasmapheresis (plasma exchange) was the previous primary treatment modality. Continued monitoring in an intensive care-type setting is warranted due to possible complications (e.g., respiratory failure and deep vein thrombosis in nonambulatory individuals). Due to the sudden onset of symptoms, depression and anxiety among patients and family members are to be expected and behavioral health interventions may be warranted. Finally, comprehensive rehabilitation, in addition to immunotherapy, is a primary treatment requirement in patients with GBS to restore premorbid physical and functional status (Hughes & Cornblath, 2005). GBS is potentially fatal, and a number of individuals experience residual effects of the illness lasting up to 2 years, though some reports suggest ongoing disability, including persisting fatigue (Forsberg et al., 2005; Hughes & Cornblath, 2005). Rate of recovery and prognosis are better for younger adults.

Michelle R. Pagoria
Chad A. Noggle

Bensa, S., Hadden. R. D. M., Hahn, A., Hughes, R. A. C., & Wilson, H. J. (2000). Randomized controlled trial of brain-derived neurotrophic factor in Guillain-Barré syndrome: A pilot study. *European Journal of Neurology, 7*, 423–426.

Forsberg, A., Press, R., Einarsson, U., de Pedro-Cuesta, J., Holmqvist, L. W. (2005). Disability and health-related quality of life in Guillain-Barré syndrome during the first two years after onset: A prospective study. *Clinical Rehabilitation, 19*, 900–909.

Haldeman, D., & Zulkosky, K. (2005). Treatment and nursing care for a patient with Guillain-Barré syndrome. *Dimensions of Critical Care Nursing, 24*, 267–272.

Hughes, R. A. C., & Cornblath, D. R. (2005). Guillain-Barré syndrome. *The Lancet, 366*, 1653–1666.

Pritchard, J., & Hughes, R. A. C. (2004). Guillain-Barré syndrome. *The Lancet, 363*, 2186–2188.

HALLERVORDEN–SPATZ DISEASE

DESCRIPTION

Hallervorden–Spatz disease (HSD), more recently termed pantothenate kinase-associated neurodegeneration (PKAN), is a rare, progressive, and fatal autosomal recessive disease affecting both adults and children, though some sporadic cases have been cited within the literature. PKAN is characterized by excessive iron accumulation and discoloration of the medial globus pallidus and substantia nigra. Pathological and clinical features of PKAN include extrapyramidal signs (dystonia, rigidity, parkinsonism, and dysarthria), corticospinal tract involvement, pyramidal motor symptoms, optic atrophy, retinal pigmentation, psychiatric manifestations, cognitive deficits, dementia later in the course of the disease, and eventually death.

PKAN was first identified in 1922 by Julius Hallervorden and Hugo Spatz. The pair witnessed pigmentation of the basal ganglia in five siblings with progressive dysarthria and dementia. The preferred name, PKAN, evolved from moral concerns raised regarding Hallervorden's involvement in euthanasia during World War II (Hinkelbein, Kalenka, & Alb, 2006).

One hallmark feature of PKAN is the "eye of the tiger" sign observed on T2-weighted MRI, due to bilateral low signal intensities within the globus pallidus and hyperintensity within the central or anteriomedial areas of the pallidum associated with iron accumulation (Hinkelbein et al., 2006). These high signal intensities have also been attributed to spongiosis and neuronal vacuolization (Bindu, Desai, Shehanaz, Nethravathy, & Pal, 2006; Hinkelbein et al., 2006).

Worldwide, the incidence of PKAN is estimated to be between 1–3 per million (Freeman et al., 2007; Hinklebein et al., 2006). PKAN appears to affect both genders equally. Although PKAN has been reported in all ethnic groups, the frequency is unknown because it is quite rare (Hinkelbein et al., 2006).

NEUROPATHOLOGY/PATHOPHYSIOLOGY

Mutations in the pantothenate- kinase 2 gene ($PANK_2$) on chromosome 20p13 have been identified (Bindu et al., 2006; Matarin, Singleton & Houlden, 2006). Deficiency of pantothenate kinase may lead to accumulation of cysteine, which in the presence of iron leads to a cytotoxic event causing free radical production (Mendez & Cummings, 2003; Hinkelbein et al., 2006). Postmortem findings reveal cerebral atrophy, pigmentation, and iron accumulation in the globus pallidus and substantia nigra (Freeman et al., 2007). Iron-containing pigment granules, axonal swelling, neuronal loss, gliosis, and demyelination within affected tissues have also been reported (Mendez & Cummings, 2003; Hinkelbein et al., 2006).

NEUROPSYCHOLOGICAL/CLINICAL PRESENTATION

Heterogeneity in clinical presentation has been well established, particularly within same-age subtypes. However, literature involving neuropsychological and clinical features of the disease has been limited as PKAN is extremely rare and small sample sizes and case studies predominate within the literature. Disease onset is typically during the first or second decade, though in rare cases it may occur up to the seventh decade (Freeman et al., 2006; Mendez & Cummings, 2003). Disease course is between 10 and 15 years. Although variations between classification systems exist, three variants of PKAN have been identified: (1) early onset childhood type with onset between 1 and 3 years of age (neuroaxonal dystrophy), (2) classic juvenile type with onset between ages 7 and 12, and (3) the more rare adult type (Mendez & Cummings, 2003). Among the early onset childhood type, a study discovered primary motor developmental delays among all participants (10) followed by cognitive decline. The juvenile type displayed more variability in presentation, including more behavioral features (e.g., verbal aggression and depression) in addition to extrapyramidal motor signs, but without developmental delay (Bindu et al., 2006).

Neuropsychological assessment findings in PKAN are sparse and have revealed a great deal of variability, though age of onset appears to correlate with disease severity, degree of intellectual impairment, and adaptive functioning, with earlier onset having a poorer prognosis (Bindu et al., 2006; Freeman et al., 2007). Furthermore, diversity in symptom expression has made it difficult to capture a clear picture of neuropsychological presentation in patients with PKAN (Freeman et al., 2007). Slow processing speed is common with deficits in visuospatial abilities and memory reported; language may be affected later in the course of the disease (Loring, Sethi, Lee, & Meador, 1990). General intellectual functioning often varies between intact to markedly impaired and is often dependent upon disease progression (Freeman et al., 2007). Within the literature, the presence of dysarthria and neuro-ophthalmologic and motor signs almost universally impact formal neuropsychological assessment procedures making nonstandard administration imperative.

Later in the course of the disease, psychiatric manifestations may develop, though one case study of prodromal behavioral symptoms (e.g., anxiety, depression, irritability, mood lability, and verbal aggression) has been identified. These psychiatric manifestations all occurred before the onset of extrapyramidal and pyramidal motor signs, and behavioral symptoms eventually progressed to paranoid delusions that responded well to antipsychotic medications. (Panas et al., 2007).

DIAGNOSIS

Prior to the advancement of neuroradiologic imaging, confirmation of PKAN was typically given based on autopsy reports indicating aforementioned iron accumulation and discoloration within the brain or based on clinical presentation. Neurodiagnostic imaging with T2 weighted MRI scans may prove useful in the diagnosis of PKAN, although the hallmark "eye of the tiger" sign may be absent in a very small group of PKAN patients. Most recently, identifying the defect on the arm of chromosome 20 has led to positive diagnosis via genetic markers, and diagnosis based on the pathology results of an affected sibling are also possible.

Based on prominent gait disturbance and extrapyramidal signs, differential diagnosis of PKAN includes dementia with Lewy bodies, Parkinson-plus syndromes, progressive supranuclear palsy, Wilson's disease, normal pressure hydrocephalus, and Huntington's disease. As such, clinical features including progressive course and neuro-ophthalmologic findings, molecular testing, and MRI findings all remain important in the diagnosis of PKAN, with genetic markers being the most recent advancement in differential diagnosis.

TREATMENT

There is no cure for PKAN and no specific treatments exist. Current pharmacological treatments include muscle relaxants, spasticity agents, and dopaminergic medications to control motor symptoms. Within the literature, stereotactic procedures of pallidotomy, thalamotomy, and bilateral pallidothalamotomy have been reported, but only in a very small number of patients and relief appears to be temporary in nature (Hinkelbein et al., 2006; Mendez & Cummings, 2003).

Michelle R. Pagoria
Chad A. Noggle

Bindu, P. S., Desai, S., Shehanaz, K. E., Nethravathy, M., & Pal, P. K. (2006). Clinical heterogeneity of Hallervorden-Spatz syndrome: A clinicoradiological study in 13 patients from South India. *Brain and Development, 28,* 343–347.

Freeman, K., Gregory, A., Turner, A., Blasco, P., Hogarth, P., & Hayflick, S. (2007). Intellectual and adaptive behaviour functioning in pantothenate kinase-associated neurodegeneration. *Journal of Intellectual Disability Research, 51,* 417–426.

Hinkelbein, J., Kalenka, A., & Alb, M. (2006). Anesthesia for patients with pantothenate-kinase-associated neurodegeneration (Hallervorden-Spatz disease) — a literature review. *Acta Neuropsychiatrica, 18,* 168–172.

Loring, D. W., Sethi, K. D., Lee, G. P., & Meador, K. J. (1990). Neuropsychological performance in Hallervorden-Spatz syndrome: A report of two cases. *Neuropsychology, 4,* 191–199.

Matarin, M. M., Singleton, A. B., & Houlden, H. (2006). PANK2 gene analysis confirms genetic heterogeneity in neurodegeneration with brain iron accumulation (NBIA) but mutations are rare in other types of adult neurodegenerative disease. *Neuroscience Letters, 407,* 162–165.

Mendez, M. F., & Cummings, J. L. (2003). *Dementia: A clinical approach.* (3rd ed.). Philadelphia: Butterworth-Heinemann.

Panas, M., Spengos, K., Koutsis, G., Tsivgoulis, G., Sfagos, K., Kalfakis, N., et al. (2007). Psychosis as presenting symptom in adult-onset Hallervorden-Spatz syndrome. *Acta Neuropsychiatrica, 19,* 122–124.

HEMICRANIA CONTINUA

DESCRIPTION

Hemicrania continua, also known as chronic paroxysmal hemicrania, is a primary headache disorder that is characterized by continuous pain occurring on one side of the face and varying in severity. Relatively rare, the presentation is marked by a combination of autonomic and migraine-like features. Furthermore, it is categorized by whether the headaches are continuous or remitting. Although the clinical features of hemicrania continua are suggestive of diagnosis, complete response to indomethacin is considered definitive of the presentation in comparison with other primary headache disorders. Women are affected more often than men with a relative ratio of 7:1 (Silberstein & Young, 2007).

NEUROPATHOLOGY/PATHOPHYSIOLOGY

The pathological basis of hemicrania continua remains unknown. Autonomic dysfunction has been proposed as the most likely basis for the presentation (Russell & Vincent, 2000). It has not been associated with characteristic findings on structural imaging (e.g., MRI or CT) or functional techniques (e.g., functional magnetic resonance imaging or positron emission tomography).

NEUROPSYCHOLOGICAL/CLINICAL PRESENTATION

Hemicrania continua is classified as a largely unremitting headache presenting on one side of the face and varying in severity. Although the pain is usually unremitting as patients will report a continuous dull ache between attacks, individuals will commonly have acute episodes of short, stabbing headaches that are in addition to that which is continuously experienced. Some individuals will demonstrate a period of remission in which no headaches are experienced for several weeks or months but upon relapse will manifest persistent headaches in upwards of 6 continuous months.

The features of hemicrania continua are divided into two categories, autonomic and migrainous. In regard to the prior, individuals may develop nose bleeds and/or stuffiness, runny nose, increased perspiration and/or tearfulness, and eye irritation (Silberstein & Young, 2007). In terms of migrainous symptoms, individuals may manifest phonophobia or photophobia in addition to nausea. The symptoms may be exacerbated by, but not limited to, fatigue, physical exertion, stimulants such as caffeine, and/or alcohol. Flexing, rotating, or applying pressure to the upper portion of the neck may serve as a trigger in 10% of patients (Russell & Vincent, 2000).

DIAGNOSIS

Diagnosis is commonly made based on symptom description; however, given that there is considerable clinical overlap with other primary headache syndromes, this is not considered definitive. Rather, full response to indomethacin is considered diagnostic. This helps differentiate hemicrania continua from short-lasting unilateral neuralgiform headache with conjunctival injection and tearing (SUNCT) headaches, which are relatively similar in presentation aside from being shorter in duration and occurring more frequently over the course of an hour (Silberstein & Young, 2007).

As with other primary headache syndromes, diagnostic workup should include neuroimaging to evaluate for and rule out structural anomalies including tumors, aneurysms, or other arteriovenous malformations, as well as other neurological entities.

TREATMENT

Indomethacin is the established treatment for hemicrania continua. In fact, as previously noted, complete response to the agent is itself considered diagnostic. Other commonly used NSAIs may provide some symptom relief but generally not to the same degree as indomethacin. In addition, some patients will demonstrate significant symptom response to tricyclic antidepressants. Beyond these intervention-based methods, preventive measures may also be employed. In particular, "triggers" of headaches should be avoided such as alcohol and particular forms of physical exertion.

Chad A. Noggle
Javan Horwitz

Russell, D., & Vincent, M. (2000). Chronic paroxysmal hemicrania. In J. Olesen, P. Tfelt-Hansen, & K. M. A. Welch (Eds.), *The headaches* (2nd ed., pp. 741–750). Philadelphia, PA: Lippincott Williams & Wilkins.

Silberstein, S. D., & Young, W. B. (2007). Headache and facial pain. In C. G. Goetz (Ed.), *Textbook of clinical neurology* (3rd ed., pp. 1245–1266). Philadelphia, PA: Saunders Elsevier.

HEMIFACIAL SPASM

DESCRIPTION

Hemifacial spasm (HFS) is a movement disorder arising from vascular compression of the seventh cranial facial nerve as it exits the brainstem. Primary HFS involves compression of the facial nerve by an adjacent artery (anterior inferior cerebellar artery, posterior inferior cerebellar artery, or vertebral artery), but in rare instances secondary causes include

H

space-occupying lesion in the cerebellopontine angle, aneurysm, arteriovenous malformations (AVM), tumors within the posterior fossa, and inflammation owing to demyelinating conditions (Colosimo et al., 2006; Glocker, Krauss, Deuschl, Seeger, & Lücking, 1998; Mauriello et al., 1996; Sato, Ezura, Takahashi, & Yoshimoto, 2001).

As the name suggests, HFS presents as unilateral and involuntary tonic–clonic spasms and contractures of the facial nerve (Huh, Han, Moon, Chang, & Chang, 2008).

HFS is a disorder affecting adults and is more common in women, with a prevalence of 14.5 per 100,000 American women and 7.4 per 100,000 American men. Asian populations also appear to have an increased incidence (Tan, Tan, & Khin, 2003). Familial cases of HFS are rare, but do exist (Wilkins, 1991). HFS generally occurs in the fourth or fifth decade with a mean age of onset of 45 years (Mauriello et al., 1996).

NEUROPATHOLOGY/PATHOPHYSIOLOGY

Chronic and focal compression of the facial nerve by an aberrant vessel further causes demyelination of nerve fibers. This causes hyperexcitability of adjacent nerve fibers via ephaptic (false) transmission. It remains controversial as to whether this represents an ephaptic transmission at the nuclear level or at the site of compression (Glocker et al., 1998).

NEUROPSYCHOLOGICAL/CLINICAL PRESENTATION

Neuropsychological data of HFS was not available for review, though HFS is generally considered troubling to those affected due to social embarrassment. In some cases, binocular vision may be affected and interfere with routine tasks such as driving, reading, and writing (Wilkins, 1991).

DIAGNOSIS

Diagnosis of HFS is made via observation of abnormal facial movements. It is important to rule out the following: blepharospasm, facial myokymia, facial tic, facial spasm of a psychogenic etiology, involvement due to lower motor neuron condition (Bell's palsy), focal seizures, and tardive dyskinesia. Secondary causes of HSF, such as space occupying lesions, AVM, and aneurysm, should also be considered and warrant routine CT, MRI, and angiography studies in suspected cases (Wilkins, 1991), particularly when atypical features of facial numbness or weakness are present. Electrophysiological studies are also recommended due to characteristic latency of response witnessed in HFS sufferers (Glocker et al., 1998).

TREATMENT

Spontaneous recovery of HFS is uncommon and surgical intervention via microvascular decompression (MVD) is the most widely accepted treatment. Primary risks include ipsilateral deafness and facial palsy that may be transient but in rare cases permanent (Wilkins, 1991). Recovery of symptoms following MVD may be incomplete with some experiencing a recurrence of symptoms. Recovery from auditory dysfunction appears to be somewhat slower than recovery from facial palsy. Finally, the more immediate and greater severity of facial nerve palsy and auditory dysfunction, the greater the likelihood for persistent and permanent damage. Other cranial nerve damage, including vocal cord paralysis, hoarseness, dysphagia, and surgical complications (e.g., intracranial bleed, wound infection, meningitis, vertebral artery injury) have also been reported (Huh et al., 2008). For patients who suffer postoperative complications of facial muscles, steroid medications and physical therapy may be introduced (Huh et al., 2008; Wilkins, 1991). Pharmacological treatments, such as haloperidol, carbamazepine, baclofen, and clonazepam, have been studied in HFS, but with limited efficacy (Wilkins, 1991). Another researcher also reported successful treatment of HFS owing to rare fusiform aneurysm via intravascular embolization and coiling procedure (Sato et al., 2001). Monitoring auditory evoked potentials during surgery is also suggested for improved outcomes and to minimize postoperative complications of ipsilateral hearing loss.

Michelle R. Pagoria
Chad A. Noggle

Colosimo, C., Bologna, M., Lamberti, S., Avanzino, L., Marinelli, M., Fabbrini, G., et al. (2006). A comparative study of primary and secondary hemifacial spasm. *Archives of Neurology, 63,* 441–444.

Glocker, F. X., Krauss, J. K., Deuschl, G., Seeger, W., & Lücking, C. H. (1998). Hemifacial spasm due to posterior fossa tumors: The impact of tumor location on electrophysiological findings. *Clinical Neurology and Neurosurgery, 100,* 104–111.

Huh, R., Han, I. B., Moon, J. Y., Chang, J. W., & Chung, S. S. (2008). Microvascular decompression for hemifacial spasm: Analysis of operative complications in 1582 consecutive patients. *Surgical Neurology, 69,* 153–157.

Mauriello, J. A., Leonee, T., Dhillon, S., Pakeman, B., Mostafavi, R., & Yepez, M. C. (1996). Treatment choices for 119 patients with hemifacial spasm over 11 years. *Clinical Neurology and Neurosurgery, 98*, 213–216.

Sato, K., Ezura, M., Takahashi, A., & Yoshimoto, T. (2001). Fusiform aneurysm of the vertebral artery presenting hemifacial spasm treated by intravascular embolization: Case report. *Surgical Neurology, 56*, 52–55.

Tan, N. C., Tan, E. K., & Khin, L. W. (2003). Diagnosis and misdiagnosis of hemifacial spasm: A clinical and video study. *Journal of Clinical Neuroscience, 11*, 142–144.

Wilkins, R. H. (1991). Hemifacial spasm: A review. *Surgical Neurology, 36*, 251–277.

HEREDITARY SPASTIC PARAPLEGIA

DESCRIPTION

The hereditary spastic paraplegias (HSPs) encompass a group of neurodegenerative diseases characterized mainly by progressive spasticity and weakness of the lower limbs. The term HSP has been used interchangeably with "Strumpell–Lorrain disease" or "diplegia" in the literature, but these alternatives have become increasingly less common (Ropper & Brown, 2005). A relatively rare disease, its prevalence has been estimated to be between 2 and 9.6 cases per 100,000 individuals (Klebe et al., 2004). The HSPs have been classified into 24 genetically different types, among which there are autosomal-dominant, autosomal-recessive, and X-linked recessive types (Brust, 2006). HSPs are typically classified based on the absence (i.e., uncomplicated or pure HSP) or presence (i.e., complicated) of neurological or clinical features (Cimolin et al., 2007). Most patients with pure HSP are autosomal dominant, whereas complicated forms are autosomal recessive (Salinas, Proukakis, Crosby, & Warner, 2008).

The first clear description of HSP was published by Strumpell in Germany in 1880, though Selligmuller had described a similar disorder 6 years prior (Harding, 1981; Ropper & Brown, 2005). Strumpell reported two brothers similarly affected with HSP at the ages of 37 and 56 years (Harding, 1981; McDermott, White, Bushby, & Shaw, 2000). The brothers' father was suspected to have passed the disorder to his sons, indicating autosomal-dominant transmission (Harding, 1981; McDermott et al., 2000). Although the reflexes in the upper limbs were increased, the most observed abnormality was in their legs (Harding, 1981). Lorrain also made a significant contribution to the early understanding of HSP, documenting pure forms of the disease much like Strumpell (McDermott et al., 2000). However, the definition of pure HSP varied from study to study with some including clinical features, such as pigmentary retinal degeneration and mental retardation, later associated with complicated HSP (Harding, 1981).

It was not until 1981 that is was suggested that the HSPs be divided into complicated and uncomplicated forms (Harding, 1981). Type I was used to refer to those with an age of onset before age 35, exhibiting delays in walking and spasticity of the lower limbs, and Type II was used to describe those with later onset after age 35, who exhibited more marked muscle weakness, urinary difficulties, and sensory loss (Harding, 1981). Type I patients were found to exhibit a slower, more variable course in comparison to more rapidly symptomatic Type II patients (Harding, 1981). Harding's initial classification did not uphold; with many families not meeting his criteria, patients began to be grouped based on presentation in his early work. Harding (1981) also suggested that more than one gene was attributable to HSP, with the core deficit identified as spasticity rather than weakness.

NEUROPATHOLOGY/PATHOPHYSIOLOGY

Although there are autosomal-dominant, autosomal-recessive, and X-linked recessive types of HSP, the most common is autosomal dominant, occurring in about 80% of HSP patients (Klebe et al., 2004). To date, at least 41 spastic paraplegia gene (SPG) loci have been found, with 17 genes associated with HSP (Salinas et al., 2008). The autosomal-dominant type has been linked to chromosomes 2q, 8q, 14q, and 15q, with 2q most common and frequently associated with dementia signs (Ropper & Brown, 2005). Mutations in 10 loci are associated with autosomal-dominant pure HSP: SPG3A, SPAST (formerly SPG4), SPG6, SPG8, SPG10, SPG12, SPG13, SPG19, SPG31, and SPG33 (Depienne, Stevanin, Brice, & Durr, 2007; Salinas et al., 2008). The SPAST gene is most frequently involved, accounting for 40% of cases (Depienne et al., 2007). In autosomal-dominant complicated HSP, alterations in SPG3A, SPAST, SPG9, SPG10, SPG17, and SPG29 have been found (Salinas et al., 2008). The recessive type is associated with chromosomes 8p, 15q, and 16q, 15q being most frequent (Ropper & Brown, 2005). In autosomal-recessive pure HSP, associated loci are SPG5A, SPG7, SPG11, SPG27, and SPG28 (Salinas et al., 2008). Mutation in SPG7, SPG11, SPG14, SPG15, SPG20, SPG21, SPG23, SPG24, SPG25, SPG26, SPG27, SPG28, and SPG30 have been reported relating to autosomal-recessive complicated HSP (Salinas et al., 2008). Loci associated with X-linked transmission include SPG1, SPG2, and SPG16 (Depienne et al., 2007).

The main neurological correlate of HSP is progressive spasticity of the lower limbs attributed to pyramidal tract dysfunction (Depienne et al., 2007). Such dysfunction leads to retrograde degeneration of the corticospinal tracts and posterior columns (Depienne et al., 2007; Ropper & Brown, 2005; Salinas et al., 2008). Axonal degeneration of motor and sensory neurons is most noted at the distal ends of the longest axons within the central nervous system, which innervate the lower extremities (Depienne et al., 2007; McDermott et al., 2000). Patients with pure HSP typically evidence axonal degeneration of the distal portions of the corticospinal tracts, the fasciculus gracilis, and the spinocerebral tracts (Crosby & Proukakis, 2002). Thinning of the columns of Goll, most prominent in the lumbosacral regions and the spinocerebellar tracts, is found (Ropper & Brown, 2005). There is a reduction in the number of Betz and anterior horn cells (Ropper & Brown, 2005). Mitochondrial dysfunction is documented as the second most common cause of HSP (Depienne et al., 2007).

NEUROPSYCHOLOGICAL/CLINICAL PRESENTATION

Presentation of HSP is always subtle but highly variable. The age of onset ranges from infancy to the eighth decade (Brust, 2006). There is gradual development of spastic leg stiffness or weakness, with patients evidencing increasing gait disturbances and trouble walking (Cimolin et al., 2007; Ropper & Brown, 2005). Those with more severe muscle tissue degeneration, particularly in the upper limbs, typically evidence symptoms for more than 15 years (Harding, 1981). Clinical features include hyperreflexia, extensor plantar reflexes, and weakness of pyramidal distribution in the lower limbs (Cimolin et al., 2007; Ropper & Brown, 2005). Children often exhibit delays in walking or "toe-walk," attributed to underdeveloped legs, arched and shortened feet, and a shortening of the calf muscles (Cimolin et al., 2007; Ropper & Brown, 2005). The knees may appear slightly flexed, or adducted and fully extended (Ropper & Brown, 2005). Sensory loss in the feet has been reported (Salinas et al., 2008). Sphincteric function is usually normal but has been linked to HSP (i.e., vesicoureteric reflux, urinary frequency and urgency, bladder sacculation) and correlated with disease duration (Harding, 1981; Ropper & Brown, 2005). Other characteristics can include nystagmus, ocular palsies, optic atrophy, pigmentary macular degeneration, ataxia, sensorimotor

polyneuropathy, ichthyosis, patchy skin pigmentation, epilepsy, and dementia (Ropper & Brown, 2005).

Pure versus complicated forms of HSP is distinguished based on presentation. Among patients who present with pure HSP, symptoms are usually confined to spastic paresis (Cimolin et al., 2007). Other features of pure HSP may include upper limb hyperreflexia, impaired lower limb vibratory sensation, Babinski signs, and urinary urgency and frequency (Brust, 2006; Cimolin et al., 2007). In pure HSP, nervous system and sensory functioning are normal (Ropper & Brown, 2005). Those with pure HSP initially present with upper motor neuron dysfunction, with later stages of the disorder associated with diminished vibration sense, sensory impairment, and urinary sphincter disturbance (Klebe et al., 2004). Complicated HSP has been associated with such co-occurring clinical features as peripheral neuropathy, ataxia, retinal pigmentary degeneration, deafness, optic atrophy, mental retardation, seizures, mental retardation, dementia, and extrapyramidal signs (Brust, 2006; Cimolin et al., 2007).

DIAGNOSIS

A diagnosis of HSP is typically dependent upon family history, the presence or absence of clinical and neurological features, progression of symptoms, and the exclusion of other nongenetic causes of observed spasticity (Depienne et al., 2007). Cerebral and spinal MRI is necessary to rule out other conditions and to determine whether cerebellar or corpus callosum atrophy and/or white matter abnormalities exist, characteristic of HSP (Depienne et al., 2007). MRI of the lumbar or thoracic spinal cord may show thinning, and somatosensory evoked potentials may show delayed conduction when stimulating the legs (Brust, 2006). Magnetostimulation of the corticospinal tract usually shows reduced conduction velocities and evoked potentials in their legs (Brust, 2006). Genetic testing is possible to test in utero or among those suspected, but genetic markers have been found only in less than half of the genetic subtypes (Brust, 2006). Screening regarding SPAST and SPG3A can be used to detect over 50% of autosomal-dominant pure HSP cases (Salina et al., 2008).

Diagnoses to disregard when HSP is suspected can be evaluated based on age of onset. Other diagnoses to consider with a childhood onset include cerebral palsy, Chiari malformation, leucodystrophy, arginase deficiency, abetalipoproteinemia, levadopa-response dystonia, myelitis, and multiple sclerosis (Salinas et al., 2008). If during the 1st year of symptomatology delayed motor milestones present, cerebral palsy may be probable (Salinas et al., 2008). With an adult onset, diagnoses to consider are cervical spine degenerative disease, multiple sclerosis, motor neuron disease, neoplasm, myelitis, dural arteriovenous malformation, Chiari malformation, adrenoleucodystrophy, syphilis, copper deficiency, levadopa-response dystonia, lathyrism, spinocerebellar ataxia, and vitamin deficiency (i.e., B12 and E) (Salinas et al., 2008). If a sporadic case of spastic paraplegia is evidenced after the age of 20 without a family history, HSP should be considered only as a rule out (Salinas et al., 2008). If there is more of an acute onset rather than progressive, as with HSP, vascular or inflammatory causes should be suspected (Salinas et al., 2008). Tests for very long chain fatty acids, white cell enzymes, plasma amino acids, serum lipoprotein analysis, vitamins B12 and E, copper and ceruloplasmin, serum serology, human T-cell leukemia virus 1, and human immunodeficiency virus can be used to indicate causes other than HSP (Salinas et al., 2008).

TREATMENT

No therapy has been found to reduce the progression of HSP (Klebe et al., 2004). However, Harding (1981) found that among HSP patients, only a few had to stop working due to the disorder. HSP did not appear to decrease life expectancy, but quality (Harding, 1981). Drugs suggested to reduce clonus and muscle tightness include benzodiazepines, baclofen, tizanidine, dantrolene, and botulinum toxin type A (Botox) injections (Fink, 2003). To reduce urinary urgency in patients, 5 mg oxybutynin, taken 2–3 times per day, or extended release oxybutynin, taken once per day in a dose varying from 5 to 30 mg, may be used (Brust, 2006). Regular physical therapy is recommended to reduce deconditioning, improve cardiovascular fitness, improve muscle strength and gain, and reduce spasticity. Physical therapy may also be suggested to prevent such complications as contractures and preserve the patient's functioning (Brust, 2006; Klebe et al., 2004). Some patients may qualify for chemodenervation to reduce muscle overactivity (Fink, 2003). Occupational therapy may be necessary, particularly when walking becomes too difficult.

Jessica Holster
Charles Golden

Brust, J. C. (2006). *Current diagnosis and treatment in neurology.* New York: McGraw-Hill.

Cimolin, V., Piccinini, L., D'Angelo, M. G., Turconi, A. C., Berti, M., Crivellini, M., et al. (2007). Are patients with hereditary spastic paraplegia different from patients with spastic diplegia during walking? Gait evaluation using 3D gain analysis. *Functional Neurology, 22,* 23–28.

Crosby, A. H., & Proukakis, C. (2002). Is the transportation highway the right road for hereditary spastic paraplegia? *Am J Hum Genet 71,* 1009–1016.

Depienne, C., Giovanni, S., Brice, A., & Durr, A. (2007). Hereditary spastic paraplegias: An update. *Current Opinion in Neurology, 20,* 674–680.

Fink, J. K. (2003). Advances in the hereditary spastic paraplegias. *Experimental Neurology, 184,* 106–110.

Harding, A. E. (1981). Hereditary pure spastic paraplegia: A clinical and genetic study of 22 families. *Journal of Neurology, Neurosurgery & Psychiatry, 44,* 871–883.

Klebe, S., Stolze, H., Kopper, F., Lorenz, D., Wenzelburger, R., Volkmann, J., et al. (2004). Gain analysis of sporadic and hereditary spastic paraplegia. *Journal of Neurology, 251,* 571–578.

McDermott, C. J., White, K., Bushby, K., & Shaw, P. J. (2000). Hereditary spastic paraparesis: A review of new development. *Journal of Neurology, Neurosurgery & Psychiatry, 69,* 150–160.

Ropper, A. H., & Brown, R. H. (2005). *Adams and Victor's principles of neurology* (8th ed.). New York: McGraw-Hill.

Salinas, S., Proukakis, C., Crosby, A., & Warner, T. T. (2008). Hereditary spastic paraplegia: Clinical features and pathogenetic mechanisms. *The Lancet Neurology, 7,* 1127–1138.

HERPES ZOSTER OTICUS

DESCRIPTION

Herpes zoster (HZ) is a reactivation of a latent chicken pox (varicella) virus. Zoster is a rash, blister, or lesion, usually painful, occurring in older adults (Harpaz, Ortega-Sanchez, & Seward, 2008.) As such, this disease may occur in anyone with a history of the chicken pox infection. HZ oticus is also usually called Ramsay Hunt syndrome. Some feel that only when facial paralysis is also present should the disorder be called Ramsay Hunt syndrome (Harpaz et al., 2008; Sweeney & Gilden, 2001). It develops when there is involvement of the facial and auditory nerves. One usually sees inflammation of the external ear and facial paralysis. These features are usually transitory. There is also involvement of the inner ear, the auditory nerve, the facial nerve, and at times the ninth and tenth cranial nerves. The symptoms can include hearing loss, vertigo, loss of taste, and tongue vesicles (Cunningham et al., 2008).

NEUROPATHOLOGY/PATHOPHYSIOLOGY

The defining feature of HZ oticus is the reactivation of the varicella zoster virus (VZV) within the eighth facial nerve. The VZV will have lain dormant in the sensory or dorsal root ganglion since the initial outbreak of chicken pox, most often during childhood (Harpaz et al., 2008). When the geniculate ganglion is involved, facial paralysis develops (Crabtree, 1974). Hunt (1904) described the geniculate ganglion as comprised of the tympanic membrane, external auditory canal, tragus, antitragus, concha, parts of the helix, and parts of the lobule.

The localization of the zoster eruption is dependent on which sensory afferent fibers flare up. Most often the seventh (facial) and eighth (auditory-vestibular) cranial nerves are involved. As a result, for example, among acute cases sensorineural hearing loss occurs in 10% of individuals and vestibular symptoms occur in 40% of individuals (Syal, Tyagi, & Goyal, 2004).

NEUROPSYCHOLOGICAL/CLINICAL PRESENTATION

The initial presenting symptom is usually otalgia and a burning sensation deep within the ear. In addition, within 1 to 4 days there will be an eruption of painful blisters in or around the external auditory canal. Eruptions can also occur on the face, neck, trunk, in the mouth, or on the tongue. Other reported symptoms include facial drooping, vertigo, decreased or loss of hearing, and tinnitus. At times, pain in the eye and lacrimation may also occur. Because the geniculate ganglion is affected there is also a decrease in taste sensation and decreased salivation.

DIAGNOSIS

Most often, the diagnosis relies on presenting clinical features such as varicelli form rash and otalgia, which must be present in order to make a diagnosis of HZ oticus. The history and neurological examination are of paramount importance. These along with the pain and other clinical features (facial drooping, sores on the tongue, hearing problems, vesicles on the pinna) contribute to the diagnosis. In addition it can be helpful to use the Tzanck preparation that requires a zoster to be scraped for cells. This method is difficult in that it is a struggle to obtain a valid specimen if the outbreak is located in the ear canal. When the preparation is positive the specimen contains multinucleated giant cells.

Also, vesicular fluid can be obtained and combined with human diploid fibroblasts, and after 3–5 days the presence of giant multinucleated cells also support a positive diagnosis.

Several other medical conditions can mimic HZ oticus symptoms, and it is important to rule out the following possible conditions: Bell's palsy, HZ, otitis externa, otitis media, hemorrhagic or ischemic stroke, and cluster, migraine, or tension headaches (Bloem, Doty, & Hirshon, 2008).

TREATMENT

The most common treatment for HZ oticus is the use of antiviral medications that often result in House–Brackmann Grade III recovery (Cunningham et al., 2008). The use of oral steroids has also proven to be effective in reducing posthepatic neuralgia and enhancing facial nerve recovery when combined with antiviral therapy (Murakami et al., 1997). Symptom-related therapy (e.g., analgesic, antibiotics for secondary infection) is also recommended, but if the condition persists care to avoid addiction should be implemented.

Henry V. Soper
Teri J. McHale

Bloem, C., Doty, C., & Hirshon, J. (2008, November 4). *Herpes zoster oticus.* Retrieved from http://emedicine.medscape.com/article/783332

Crabtree, J. (1974). Herpes zoster oticus and facial paralysis. *Otolaryngol Clinics of North America, 7,* 369–373.

Cunningham, A., Breuer, J., Dwyer, D., Gronow, D., Helme, R., Myron, J., et al. (2008). The prevention and management of herpes zoster. *The Medical Journal of Australia, 188*(3), 171–176.

Harpaz, R., Ortega-Sanchez, I., & Seward, J. (2008, June 06). *Prevention of herpes zoster: Recommendations of the advisory committee on immunization practices (ACIP).* Retrieved from http://www.cdc.gov/mmwr/preview/mmwrhtml/rr57e0515al.htm

Hunt, J. (1904). Herpetic inflammation of the geniculate ganglion. A new syndrome and its complication. *Journal of Nervous and Mental Disorder, 34,* 73–96.

Murakami, S., Hato, N., Horiuchi, J., Honda, N., Gyo, K., & Yangihara, N. (1997). Treatment of Ramsay Hunt syndrome with acyclovir-prednisone: Significance of early diagnosis and treatment. *Annals of Neurology, 41,* 353–357.

Sweeney, C., & Gilden, D. (2001). Ramsay Hunt syndrome. *Journal of Neurology, Neurosurgery and Psychiatry, 71,* 149–154.

Syal, R., Tyagi, I., & Goyal, A. (2004). Bilateral Ramsay Hunt syndrome in a diabetic patient. *BMC Ear, Nose and Throat Disorders, 4*, 3.

HIV/AIDS Dementia Complex

DESCRIPTION

Numerous labels have been synonymously applied to the debilitating cognitive, motor, language, and behavioral impairments associated with HIV infection, such as AIDS dementia complex, HIV dementia, and HIV encephalopathy. Recently, the term HIV-associated dementia (HAD) has been employed to characterize the cluster of the most severe symptoms that are to be distinguished from mild cognitive motor disorder (MCMD) (Antinori et al., 2007).

The development of highly active antiretroviral therapy (HAART) changed management of HIV and hence the progression of HAD. Prior to HAART, HAD was typically observed in the late stages of AIDS and was indicative of morbidity and mortality. In some instances, HAD was evidenced in 50% of AIDS patients prior to their death (Ances & Ellis, 2007). The annual incidence of HAD in Western countries prior to HAART was 7%, with a cumulative risk of 5% to 20% (McArthur, 2004). Although the incidence of HAD began declining after HAART, the prevalence rate of individuals with HAD and MCMD has been increasing in some samples, likely due to the increased life span of HIV-infected individuals. In some research, a prevalence rate of 37% for HAD and MCMD was found among individuals even with HAART (Sacktor, 2002; Schifitto et al., 2002). However, rapidly progressive dementia is less commonly observed in the post-HAART era. Instead, chronic and fluctuating forms of HAD are more widespread, and in 4% to 15% of patients, HAD is the presenting clinical manifestation of HIV (McArthur, 2004).

NEUROPATHOLOGY/PATHOPHYSIOLOGY

The development of dementia is typically delayed until severe immunodeficiency develops. After its onset, the progression of HAD is variable (Bouwman et al., 1998). HIV enters the central nervous system (CNS) early by infecting macrophages and monocytes and transporting the virus across the blood brain barrier. The overproduction of various proinflammatory cytokines and chemokines yields neurotoxic agents that create an inflammatory environment by activating uninfected microglia that damage surrounding astrocytes and neurons (Brabers & Nottet, 2006). Although HIV does not directly infect the neuron, the proinflammatory neurotoxins ultimately impair cellular functioning and provoke change in neuronal functioning. Results from immunohistochemistry research have revealed that the virus is most densely located in the basal ganglia (and dopaminergic system), subcortical regions, and frontal cortex. Similarly, pathological changes at autopsy are predominantly subcortical, involving the deep gray and white matter regions.

NEUROPSYCHOLOGICAL/CLINICAL PRESENTATION

Research indicates that the neuropsychological profile of HAD follows the neuropathology and is most consistent with a subcortical process that often involves psychomotor slowing, motor weakness, poor attention and working memory, reduced fluency, executive dysfunction, and decreased learning and memory functioning (Grant, 2008; Nath, Schiess, Rumbaugh, Sacktor, & McArthur, 2008). As such, the most comprehensive neuropsychological test battery for HAD identification would assess all areas of cognitive functioning, including current and premorbid intellectual ability, attention, verbal abilities, visuospatial functions, learning and memory, psychomotor and motor abilities, executive functioning, and personality. However, individual test-taker characteristics must be appreciated, such as sensory limitations, significant fatigue, and/or physical restrictions, any of which may render a lengthy battery impractical, and, thus, warrant modification. Also, as with any assessment, neuropsychological evaluation of HAD requires consideration of factors that can influence test performance, such as age, education, culture, gender, practice effects, and the individual's motivation (Grant, 2008). Neuropsychological tests such as the Trail Making Test — Part B (a measure of speed, attention, and subcortical processing), the California Verbal Learning Test — II (a measure of learning and memory), and the Timed Gate Test are particularly relevant given the indication of preferential impairment of psychomotor speed and memory in HAD (Lopez et al., 1994; Nath et al., 2008; Roos, 2005). For an example of a comprehensive neuropsychological battery to evaluate HIV-related neurocognitive compromise, refer to van Gorp and Root (2008).

Recognizing that early HAD may mimic a variety of psychiatric conditions, particularly major depressive disorder (MDD) (e.g., note the overlapping

H

symptoms such as apathy, forgetfulness, impaired attention), prudent differential diagnostic skills are essential. However, if both HAD and MDD are suspected, an individual should be reevaluated for HAD when his/her depression has remitted. Despite the frequent comorbidity, there is little evidence that pseudodementia in HAD exists, and cognitive deficits generally do not improve with treatment of depression (Antinori et al., 2007).

DIAGNOSIS

HAD is a diagnosis of exclusion that is further complicated by the fact that neurocognitive tests may be nonspecific, and deficits may or may not be present in neurologically asymptomatic patients with HIV. Thus, HAD is particularly difficult to diagnose. In 2007, Antinori et al. proposed that HAD required deficits in two or more cognitive domains, such as attention, memory, and/or abstract reasoning, causing impairment in activities of daily living and an abnormality in either motor or neurobehavioral function. Also, any other etiology of dementia should be ruled out, and there should be an absence of delirium. It is essential to differentiate, as soon as possible, between individuals with HAD and those with MCMD, the latter of whom have decreased function in two cognitive or behavioral domains but are not impaired severely enough to meet the criteria for HAD. Differentiation must also be made between the even less significantly impaired individuals with asymptomatic neurocognitive impairment (ANI).

When evaluating for HAD, any other confounding and/or compounding etiology must be ruled out, such as metabolic and infectious etiologies, psychiatric conditions, substance abuse, opportunistic diseases such as progressive multifocal leukoencephalopathy (PML) or toxoplasmosis, systemic infections, toxic-metabolic states, and adverse medication effects. Although in the early stages of HAD, any or all of the available measures may result in unremarkable findings, there are a variety of methods to assist in the diagnosis of HAD. These include laboratory studies, neuroimaging, EEG, and/or neuropsychological testing. For example, EEG may be used to rule out subclinical seizures that are mimicking dementia. Cerebrospinal fluid (CSF) analyses may be used to exclude CNS infection and to provide useful data regarding potential immunological markers of HAD. Neuroimaging such as positron emission tomography (PET) and functional magnetic resonance imaging (fMRI) may detect decreased metabolism in the thalamus and basal ganglia in the early stages of HAD. CT and MRI scans can reveal brain atrophy, ventricular

enlargement, and increased white matter signal in later stages of the dementia, or assist in identifying other pathology such as that caused by PML. Generally, the degree of cerebral atrophy correlates with the symptoms and progression of HAD.

Neuropsychological testing is particularly valuable in the early screening of asymptomatic high-risk patients (e.g., those with high viral load and low CD4 count) as well as for follow-up evaluations of patients already diagnosed with HAD (Glass & Wesselingh, 1998). One of the most widely accepted and efficient screening tools for HAD is the HIV Dementia Scale, which can yield a total of 12 points—a score less than 6 points is considered abnormal (Power, Selnes, Grim, & McArthur, 1995). The Memorial Sloan–Kettering Rating Scale merges functional ability results with the findings from neuropsychological testing and is helpful for clinical staging of HAD from 0 (normal) to 4 (end stage) (Price & Brew, 1988).

TREATMENT

Several cohort studies have shown that treatment with multiple antiretroviral agents is superior to either no treatment or monotherapy in patients with HAD (McArthur, 2004). Targeting the pathophysiology by using antiretroviral agents with CNS penetration is essential. Some symptoms of HAD may be reversed, and symptom severity may be attenuated by HAART (Nath et al., 2008). Also, cognitive symptoms may be addressed through the use of psychostimulants, which may be particularly effective for early HAD symptoms such as psychomotor slowing and attention deficits (Hinkin et al., 2001). Neuroleptics may be more effective for later-stage HAD. Cognitive skills training and rehabilitation may be employed, and as with any condition, supportive caregivers are vital.

Chriscelyn Tussey
Jason R. Freeman

Ances, B. M., & Ellis, R. J. (2007). Dementia and neurocognitive disorders due to HIV-1 infection. *Seminars in Neurology, 27*(1), 86–92.

Antinori, A., Arendt, G., Becker, J. T., Brew, B. J., Byrd, D. A., & Cherner, M. (2007). Updated research nosology for HIV-associated neurocognitive disorders. *Neurology, 69*(18), 1789–1799.

Bouwman, F. H., Skolasky, R., Hes, D., Selnes, O. A., Glass, J. D., Nance-Sproson, T. E., et al. (1998). Variable progression of HIV-associated dementia. *Neurology, 50,* 1814–1820.

Brabers, N. A., & Nottet, H. S. (2006). Role of the pro-inflammatory cytokines TNF-alpha and IL-1beta in HIV-associated dementia. *European Journal of Clinical Investigation, 36*(7), 447–458.

Glass, J. D., & Wesselingh, S. L. (1998). Viral load in HIV-associated dementia. *Annals of Neurology, 44*(1), 150–151.

Grant, I. (2008). Neurocognitive disturbances in HIV. *International Review of Psychiatry, 20*(1), 33–47.

Hinkin, C. H., Castellon, S. A., Hardy, D. J., Farinpour, R., Newton, T., & Singer, E. (2001). Methylphenidate improves HIV-1-associated cognitive slowing. *Journal of Neuropsychiatry and Clinical Neuroscience, 13,* 248–254.

Lopez, O., Becker, J., Dew, M., Banks, G., Dorst, S., & McNeil, M. (1994). Speech motor control disorder after HIV infection. *Neurology, 44,* 2187–2189.

McArthur, J. C. (2004). HIV dementia: An evolving disease. *Journal of Neuroimmunology, 157*(1–2), 3–10.

Nath, A., Schiess, A. V., Rumbaugh, J., Sacktor, N., & McArthur, J. (2008). Evolution of HIV dementia with HIV infection. *International Review of Psychiatry, 20*(1), 25–31.

Power, C., Selnes, O. A., Grim, J. A., & McArthur, J. C. (1995). The HIV dementia scale: A rapid screening test. *Journal of Acquired Immune Deficiency Syndromes and Human Retrovirology: Official Publication of the International Retrovirology Association, 8*(3), 273–278.

Price, R. W., & Brew, B. J. (1988). The AIDS Dementia complex. *The Journal of Infectious Diseases, 158,* 1079–1083.

Roos, K. (2005). *Principles of neurologic infectious diseases.* New York: McGraw Hill.

Sacktor, N. (2002). The epidemiology of human immunodeficiency virus-associated neurological diseases in the era of highly active antiretroviral therapy. *Journal of Neurovirology, 8*(Suppl. 2), 115–121.

Schifitto, G., McDermott, M. P., McArthur, J. C., Marder, K., Sacktor, N., Epstein, L., et al. (2002). Incidence of and risk factors for HIV-Associated distal sensory polyneuropathy. *Neurology, 58,* 1764–1768.

van Gorp, W. G., & Root, J. (2008). CNS infection: HIV associated neurocognitive compromise. In J. Morgan & J. Ricker (Eds.), *Textbook of clinical neuropsychology.* New York: Taylor & Francis.

HOLMES–ADIE SYNDROME

DESCRIPTION

First described in 1931 (Adie, 1931; Holmes, 1931), Holmes–Adie syndrome (HAS) is a benign condition characterized by tendon areflexia and unilateral pupil dilation. In some instances, the presentation expands bilaterally, affecting both pupils. Delayed responsiveness to near vision effort with delayed redilation is commonly observed (Martinelli et al., 1999). HAS is most commonly spontaneous, although familial or symptomatic forms have been noted (Lowenfield, 1993; Martinelli et al., 1999). Regarding the latter, HAS may present in conjunction with various diseases/disorders affecting the central nervous system, including polyneuropathies (e.g., hereditary, inflammatory, paraneoplastic, diabetic, amyloidotic, and alcohol-related neuropathies), Sjögren syndrome, and both rheumatoid and temporal arthritis (Martinelli et al., 1999).

Epidemiological studies suggest an annual incidence rate of 4–7 per 100,000, with greater prevalence in women compared with men, and a peak incidence rate in the third decade of life, although it is noted across the life span. Onset is gradual in nature, and with time, symptoms often partially recover. In 10% of cases, there is permanent failure of the pupil to react either to light or to near vision (Martinelli et al., 1999).

NEUROPATHOLOGY/PATHOPHYSIOLOGY

The neuropathological literature on HAS is quite sparse, although generally agreeable in that the presentation arises from a partial or total loss of neurons of the ciliary ganglion on the same side as the tonic pupil while peripheral glial cell accumulations are also noted. The basis of this neuronal loss is unknown. Microscopic evaluation has largely ruled-out an infectious process. This has been concluded based on findings demonstrating absence of scarring or inflammatory cells in combination with myelinated fibers passing through the ganglion (Ulrich, 1980). Decreased numbers of nerve cells have been noted in lumbar and thoracic ganglia. Within the posterior roots and medial part of the posterior funiculi of the spinal cord there is nerve-cell destruction with loss of the myelin sheath (Ulrich, 1980). The areflexia that occurs in addition to papillary dilation is associated with impaired spinal monosynaptic connections, particularly afferent projections to motor neuron in their proximal tracts.

NEUROPSYCHOLOGICAL/CLINICAL PRESENTATIONS

HAS is characterized by unilateral pupil dilation and tendon areflexia. Although the pupil dilation starts unilaterally, progression to a bilateral presentation has been noted. This pupil dilation is noted on a continuous basis whereas slit lamp examination

H

demonstrates dysfunction of the papillary sphincter muscle. Consequently, constriction and dilation of the affected pupil is significantly slowed. Beyond unilateral pupil dilation, the absence of deep tendon reflexes is also characteristic of HAS. Multiple tendon reflexes can be affected, although the loss of the Achilles tendon reflex is the most commonly seen. Similar to pupil dilation, though areflexia starts unilaterally, it can become bilateral although at low frequency (i.e., <5%). It is noted that though spontaneous recovery can be observed in regard to pupillary functioning, once areflexia presents, it is permanent. Observing both the tonic pupil and areflexia depends on the timing of assessment, as they often do not present simultaneously until later in the presentation.

Neurocognitive functioning has not been associated with HAS.

DIAGNOSIS

Diagnosis of HAS is presentation based. It should be considered when individuals present with monolateral/unilateral pupil dilation and tendon areflexia. Although most cases are spontaneous, the fact that some are symptom-based emphasizes the importance of considering a primary cause. Particular attention in this regard should be given to polyneuropathies and, to a lesser extent, previously noted forms of arthritis. As recommended by Bremner and Smith (2007), if bilateral tonic pupils, in lieu of unilateral, and tendon areflexia are observed, generalized peripheral or autonomic neuropathy should be considered. If anhydrosis is observed, consideration of Ross's syndrome should be made. Slit lamp examination may be employed to evaluate reactivity of the pupil. In general, the pupil demonstrates both delayed constriction and dilation. Areflexia may be examined through monosynaptic reflex activity assessment. HAS is often associated with an absence of the Achilles' reflex as well as an electrically evoked H reflex of the soleus muscle.

TREATMENT

There is no described treatment for HAS. Medicinal interventions have not demonstrated utility in treating the presentation. Furthermore, there is no surgical intervention that may be employed. In many ways, the symptoms are more bothersome than limiting. For individuals who develop light sensitivity due to the lack of papillary constriction, monolateral patching could be useful.

The sphincter muscle has been found to be absent in some quadrants or thin in others. The cause of the

neuronal degeneration is not known, but the absence of scarring or inflammatory cells and the persistence of myelinated fibers passing through the ganglion, suggests it is unlikely to be the result of infection of conventional bacterial or viral origin or other inflammatory disease. The absence of deep tendon reflexes is also characteristic of HAS, with loss of the Achilles tendon reflex being most frequent.

Monosynaptic reflex activity assessment has shown that the Achilles' reflex is absent in most cases, and the electrically evoked H reflex of the soleus muscle is replaced by an attenuated response. Further, the polysynaptic spinal pathways seem to behave normally in patients with this syndrome. Peripheral motor and sensory nerve conduction velocities are normal and the presence of a tonic vibratory reflex suggests that defective conduction in Ia peripheral afferent fibers does not cause the areflexia. The attenuated response to supramaximal motor nerve stimulation has been considered an indirect index of impaired transmission of Ia afferents to motor neurons in their proximal part. Morphological examination of the lumbar and thoracic ganglia have shown decreased numbers of nerve cells in patients with HAS, and there is evidence of nerve cell destruction, loss of myelin sheaths in the posterior roots and in the medial part of the posterior funiculi of the spinal cord, but without any substantial change in grey or white matter. Thus, electrophysiological and anatomical data suggest that the pathophysiology of areflexia is the result of impaired spinal monosynaptic connections, probably due to structural damage of Ia afferents to motor neurons in their proximal tracts. Histological features common to both affected ciliary and spinal ganglia (spiraling of the stainable part of the proximal axon, neuronophagias, and residual bodies of Nageotte's type) support the concept of HAS as a progressive disease. The association between HAS and more widespread autonomic dysfunction remains controversial. Single case reports or series of HAS have been reported, associated with sweating or cardiovascular dysfunction, diarrhea, and coughing. Tonic pupil, areflexia, and anhydrosis are frequently recognized in published work as Ross's syndrome. In these cases, the tonic pupil is more often bilateral, whereas the loss of flushing and sweating has been detected in a different pattern distribution: segmental, following a dermatomeric distribution, or localized to half of the body. The possible link between HAS and Ross's syndrome remains ill defined, since abnormalities of sweating in a high proportion of HAS patients have been reported. The finding of cholinergic supersensitivity in the iris muscles of patients with Harlequin syndrome (a syndrome of local autonomic failure affecting the face and the arm) may also indicate that Harlequin syndrome is linked with HAS. Cardiovascular system dysfunctions are not always associated with the sweating abnormalities, but they are more prevalent with increasing duration of the condition. HAS may also be detected in a symptomatic form during the course of different diseases of the nervous system, most frequently polyneuropathies. Hereditary, inflammatory, paraneoplastic, diabetic, amyloidotic, and alcohol-related neuropathies can all be complicated by HAS, as can those associated with Sjögren syndrome, rheumatoid arthritis, and temporal arthritis. Sporadic reports have described an association with myopathy, as well as with migraine (Martinelli et al., 1999)

Chad A. Noggle
Michelle R. Pagoria

Adie, W. J. (1931). Pseudo Argyll-Robertson pupils with absent tendon reflexes. *British Medical Journal, 1*, 928–930.

Bremner, F. D., & Smith, S. E. (2007). Bilateral tonic pupils: Holmes–Adie syndrome or generalised neuropathy? *British Journal of Ophthalmology, 91*, 1620–1623.

Holmes, G. M. (1931). Partial iridoplegia associated with symptoms of other diseases in the nervous system. *Transactions of the Ophthalmological Societies of the United Kingdom, 51*, 209–228.

Lowenfield, I. E. (1993). The pupil: Anatomy, physiology, and clinical applications. *Detroit: Wayne State University Press, 1*, 1085–1086.

Martinelli, P., Minardi, C., Ciucci, G., Dalpozzo, F., Giuliani, S., & Scaglione, C. (1999). Neurophysiological evaluation of areflexia in Holmes-Adie syndrome. *Clinical Neurophysiology, 29*, 255–262.

Ulrich, J. (1980). Morphological basis of Adie's syndrome. *European Neurology, 19*, 390–395.

HOLOPROSENCEPHALY

DESCRIPTION

Holoprosencephaly is a cephalic disorder that results from a failure of the forebrain to appropriately divide into the two cerebral hemispheres leading to the formation of a seemingly single-lobed brain. In addition, severe facial and skull defects are noted. Regarding the prior, these phenotypical anomalies vary in presentation in their structural effect of the eyes, nose, and/or upper lip. Prognosis and neurological sequelae is dependent upon the degree of developmental defect as there are three classifications of holoprosencephaly (De Myer & Zeman, 1963). In the most severe form,

alobar holoprosencephaly, there is no hemispheric divide. In most instances these infants die prior to birth or soon after. Semilobar holoprosencephaly represents the median form being characterized by semidivided hemispheres. Finally, lobar holoprosencephaly is the mildest variant with the brain presenting with only very subtle flaws on hemispheric division.

The incidence of holoprosencephaly is approximated to occur in 1 out of 16,000–31,000 births (Cohen, 1989a, b; Frutiger, 1969) and is proposed to be a random genetic anomaly most commonly associated with trisomy 13 although correlations with the presentation and trisomy 18 has also been noted.

NEUROPATHOLOGY/PATHOPHYSIOLOGY

The pathological foundation of holoprosencephaly is not yet known, although there are various defined correlates and proposals. Genetically, it has been most frequently linked to trisomy 13 (Patwl, Dolman, & Bryne, 1972; Patau, Smith, Therman, Inhorn, & Wagner, 1960; Robain & Gorce, 1972; Snodgrass, Butler, France, Crome, & Russell, 1966) although correlations have also been noted with trisomy 18 (Butler, Snodgrass, Sinclair, France, & Russell, 1965; Edwards, Norman, & Roberts, 1961; Robain & Gorce, 1972). Maternal traits have been linked with increased risk of the presentation as well including maternal diabetes, toxoplasmosis, syphilis, and rubella (Barr et al., 1983; Cohen, 1989; Dekaban, 1959; Kalter, 1993).

Developmentally, holoprosencephaly is conceptualized as a disorder of dysfunctional neuronal migration occurring during the 5th and 6th weeks of gestation (Ropper & Brown, 2005). Variation is seen in the degree of structural abnormality owing to a three-tier classification of the presentation. These classifications include alobar, semilobar, and lobar types and are discussed individually. In general, the spectrum is differentiated by how far posterior the lack of hemispheric division extends.

Alobar Holoprosencephaly

Alobar holoprosencephaly represents the most severe form of structural defect. In this variant, the hemispheres are undivided and present with a monoventricular formation coupled with severe hypoplasia of the neopallium. Variation is seen in the surface appearance of the brain including an abnormally thick cortex, polymicrogyria or periventricular and leptomeningeal heterotopias (Jellinger, Gross, Kaltenback, & Grisold, 1981; Mizuguchi & Morimatsu, 1989; Mizuguchi, Maekawa, & Kamoshita, 1994; Probst, 1979). Orientation within the skull itself may also vary (Kitanaka, Iwasaski, &

H

Yamada, 1992). There is no interhemispheric fissure, corpus callosum, or septum, and the frontal lobes are absent (Yakovlev, 1959). The mamillary bodies are often fused and commonly there is only a single cerebral peduncle. The vasculature demonstrates an absence of the anterior and middle cerebral arteries as well as the anterior portion of the circle of Willis whereas the posterior remains largely normal.

Semilobar Holoprosencephaly

Semilobar holoprosencephaly constitutes the median form in terms of the severity of the structural defects present. There is a general continuity of the anterior cortex with no observable hemispheric division. In comparison, more simplistic lobar formation in the posterior regions separated by a relatively shallow interhemispheric fissure is commonly seen. Generally, the more the posterior one travels across the cortex the more prominent the hemispheric divide. Frontal regions remain largely absent, particularly the more anterior they present (Lichtenstein & Maloney, 1954).

Lobar Holoprosencephaly

The mildest form, lobar holoprosencephaly is characterized by nearly normal brain size and hemispheric separation aside from the region on the orbital surface of the frontal pole (Constantinidis, 1969; Fleming & Norman, 1942; Nathan & Smith, 1950). The corpus callosum is commonly absent or hypoplastic, and there is often heterotropic gray matter in the roof of the ventricle.

NEUROPSYCHOLOGICAL/CLINICAL PRESENTATION

The clinical presentation of holoprosencephaly is in many ways dependent upon the degree of developmental disruption. Across all variants, seizures and mental retardation are the most common clinical features. The neurocognitive deficits may be widespread and nonspecific with potential compromise of attention, working memory, language, memory, and visuospatial functioning. Learning deficits are common in children as they progress through schooling. There is no unitary profile. Convulsions, spasticity, quadriplegia, basic motor problems, and speech impairments may all be observed. In rare cases, individuals may develop relatively normal functioning brains with only mild deficits. Consequently, this is often only noted in cases of lobar holoprosencephaly

Midfacial hypoplasia is the most common comorbid feature of holoprosencephaly beyond noted

CNS features. Similar to the subcategories reported to describe the extent of CNS structural disturbance, facial defects are also subdivided consisting of cyclopia, cebocephaly, and ethmocephaly. In cyclopia, the infant develops with a single eye or two eyes close together or even fused. The eye is located where the nose normally develops and a nasal protuberance is instead above the orbits. In these severe deformities, the jaw may be absent and the ears themselves may present under the eyes (Leech, Bowlby, Brumback, & Schaefer, 1988; Pauli, Graham, & Barr, 1981). Cebocephaly presents with a single nostril in the center of a flattened nose. The eyes are underdeveloped and set very close together above the nose. Finally, ethmocephaly presents with a narrow pair of eyes with no nostril. One or both eyes will be abnormally small: this is called microphthalmia. Other possible anomalies include a cleft lip or palate, trigonocephaly, hypertelorism, and hypoplasia of the nasal bones (De Myer, 1967; Roubicek, Spranger, & Wende, 1981).

DIAGNOSIS

Definitive diagnosis is made via neuroradiological examination whereby the lack of hemispheric separation is identified. In more severe forms, intrauterine diagnosis during fetal ultrasound is possible (Twining & Zuccollo, 1993). Consequently, a fair number of these more easily identifiable cases are stillborn. Following birth many infants are recommended for radiological evaluation based on facial dysmorphism. Neuropsychological evaluation may prove useful in milder cases to determine the nature and extent of any presenting neurocognitive deficits, but it is not essential.

TREATMENT

There is no standard treatment for holoprosencephaly, rather it is symptom based. Preventative measures may be taken. As noted previously, maternal diabetes has been suggested as a risk factor; thus, control of such prenatal factors is helpful. Depending upon the nature of facial dysmorphisms, surgical intervention can be undertaken for treatment purposes. This is particularly true in cases such as cleft palates, etc. Special education services can address academic difficulties related to persisting learning or other cognitive deficits associated with the milder forms of the presentation. Physical and occupational therapies may be utilized to address motoric deficits related to the presentation to improve functional outcomes. Anticonvulsants are utilized to manage seizure activity if such symptoms present. Other forms of medicinal intervention may be used to treat endocrine disorders that can commonly occur.

J. Aaron Albritton
Chad A. Noggle

Barr, M., Jr, Hansen, J. W., Currey, K., Sharp, S., Toriello, H., Schmickel, R. D., et al. (1983). Holoprosencephaly in infants of diabetic mothers. *Journal of Pediatrics, 102*, 565–568.

Butler, L. J., Snodgrass, G. J., Sinclair, L., France, N. E., & Russell, A. (1965). E (16-18) trisomy syndrome. Analysis of 13 cases. *Archives of Disease in Childhood, 40*, 600–611.

Cohen, M. M., Jr. (1989a). Perspectives on holoprosencephaly: Part I. Epidemiology, genetics, and syndromology. *Teratology, 40*, 211–235.

Cohen, M. M., Jr. (1989b). Perspectives on holoprosencephaly: Part III. Spectra, distinctions, continuities and discontinuities. *American Journal of Medical Genetics, 34*, 271–288.

Constantinidis, J. (1969). Cingulosynapsis (continuite inter hemispherique du cortex cingulare). *Archives Suisses de Neurologie, Neurochirurgie et de Psychiatrie, 104*, 137–149.

De Myer, W. (1967). The median cleft face syndrome. *Neurology, 17*, 961–971.

De Myer, W., & Zeman, W. (1963). Alobar holoprosencephaly (arhinencephaly) with median cleft lip and palate: Clinical electroencephalographic and nosologic considerations. *Confinia Neurologica Basel, 23*, 1–36.

Dekaban, A. (1959). Arhineencephaly in an infant born to a diabetic mother. *Journal of Neuropathology and Experimental Neurology, 18*, 620–626.

Edwards, J. H., Norman, R. M., & Roberts, J. M. (1961). Sex-linked hydrocephalus: Report of a family with 15 affected members. *Archives of Disease in Childhood, 36*, 481–485.

Fleming, G. W. T. H., & Norman, R. M. (1942). Arhinencephaly with incomplete separation of the cerebral hemispheres. *Journal of Mental Science, 88*, 341–343.

Frutiger, P. (1969). Zur Frage der Arhinecephalie. *Acta Anatomica, 73*, 410–430.

Jellinger, K., Gross, H., Kaltenback, E., & Grisold, W. (1981). Holoprosencephaly and agencies of the corpus callosum; frequency of associated malformations. *Acta Neuropahologica (Berlin), 55*, 1–10.

Kalter, H. (1993). Case reports of malformations associated with maternal diabetes. History and critique. *Clinical Genetics, 43*, 174–179.

Kitanaka, C., Iwasaski, Y., & Yamada, H. (1992). Retroflection of holoprosencephaly: Report of two cases. *Childs Nervous System, 8*, 317–321.

Leech, R. W., Bowlby, L. S., Brumback, R. A., & Schaefer, G. B., Jr. (1988). Agnathia, holoprosencephaly and situs inversus. Report of a case. *American Journal of Medical Genetics, 29*, 483–493.

Lichtenstein, B. W., & Maloney, J. E. (1954). Malformations of the forebrain with comments on the so- called dorsal cyst, the corpus callosum and the hippocampal structures. *Journal of Neuropathology and Experimental Neurology, 13*, 117–128.

Mizuguchi, M., Maekawa, S., & Kamoshita, S. (1994). Distribution of leptomeningeal glioneuronal heterotopia in alobar holoprosencephaly. *Archives of Neurology, 51*, 951–954.

Mizuguchi, M., & Morimatsu, Y. (1989). Histopathological study of alobar holoprosencephaly. 1. Abnormal laminar architecture of the telencephalic cortex. *Acta Neuropathologica (Berlin), 78*, 176–182.

Nathan, P. W., & Smith, M. C. (1950). Normal mentality associated with a maldeveloped "rhinencephalon." *Journal of Neurology, Neurosurgery, and Psychiatry, 13*, 191.

Patau, K., Smith, D. W., Therman, E., Inhorn, S. L., & Wagner, H. P. (1960). Multiple congenital anomoly caused by an extra autosome. *Lancet, 1*, 790–793.

Patwl, H., Dolman, C. L., & Bryne, M. A. (1972). Holoprosencephaly with median cleft lip. *American Journal of Diseases of Children, 124*, 217–221.

Pauli, R. M., Graham, J. M., & Barr, M. (1981). Agnathia, situs inversus, and associated malformations. *Teratology, 23*, 85–93.

Probst, F. P. (1979). *The prosencephalies*. Berlin: Springer Verlag.

Robain, O., & Gorce, F. (1972). Arhinencephalie *Archives Françaises de l'édiatrie, 29*, 861–879.

Ropper, A. H., & Brown, R. H. (2005). *Adams and Victor's principles of neurology* (8th ed.). McGraw-Hill: New York.

Roubicek, M., Spranger, J., & Wende, S. (1981). Frontonasal dysplasia as an expression of holoprosencephaly. *European Journal of Pediatrics, 137*, 229–231.

Snodgrass, G. J., Butler, L. J., France, N. E., Crome, L., & Russell, A. (1966). The "D" (13–15) trisomy syndrome: An analysis of 7 examples. *Archives of Disease in Childhood, 41*, 250–261.

Twining, P., & Zuccollo, J. (1993). The ultrasound markers of chromosomal disease: A retrospective study. *British Journal of Radiology, 66*, 408–414.

Yakovlev, P. I. (1959). Pathoarchitectonics studies of the cerebral malformations. III Arhinencephalies (hototelencephalies). *Journal of Neuropathology and Experimental Neurology, 18*, 22–55.

HOMOCYSTINURIA

DESCRIPTION

Homocystinuria is an autosomal recessive disease that corresponds with a deficiency of cystathione ß-synthase (CBS) resulting in an inability to metabolize methionine. The resulting elevation of homocysteine contributes to a broad array of functional deficits corresponding with abnormalities of the central, vascular, musculoskeletal, and visual systems. Although an array of features may arise secondary to homocystinuria, mental retardation, psychiatric disturbances, dislocation of the optic lens, osteoporosis, thinning and lengthening of long bones, and thromboembolism affecting large and small arteries and veins are the most common (Li & Stewart, 1999). Although the presentation has most commonly been linked to a gene in the subtelomeric area of chromosome 21q22.3, seven different genetic abnormalities are now known to lead to homocystinuria (Mudd, Levy, & Skovby, 1989).

Homocystinuria due to CBS deficiency is a very rare, with a relative prevalence of 1 per 300,000 worldwide, although heightened risk has been reported in Ireland (i.e., 1:65,000 births) (Naughten, Yap, & Mayne, 1998).

NEUROPATHOLOGY/PATHOPHYSIOLOGY

Homocystinuria is an inborn error in the metabolism of sulfur amino acids, most commonly arising from CBS, resulting in an inability to metabolize methionine. CBS condenses homocysteine and serine to produce cystathionine and ultimately cysteine (Miles & Kraus, 2004). This deficiency has been linked with a mutation in the subtelomeric area of chromosome 21q22.3. However, homocystinuria has also been observed secondary to other acquired conditions such as renal impairment or folate deficiency and nitrous oxide oxidation of methylcobalamin (Li & Stewart, 1999). The underlying physiology in these instances is related to ethylenetetrahydrofolate reductase deficiency and various defects in vitamin B metabolism (Engbersen et al., 1995; Ubagai et al., 1995).

Although homocystinuria is not related to primary neuropathological lesions per se, its linkage with thromboembolic disease is associated with heightened rates of central nervous system (CNS) involvement. Infarcts in the cerebrum, cerebellum, midbrain, and thalamus are often seen as a result as are thrombi in the dural sinuses (Cochran, 1992; Mudd et al., 1989). Arterial walls often demonstrate fibrous intimal thickening (White, Rowland, Araki, Thompson, & Cowen, 1965).

NEUROPSYCHOLOGICAL/CLINICAL PRESENTATION

Homocystinuria commonly corresponds with abnormalities of the central, vascular, musculoskeletal, and visual systems. Neuropsychiatric features are among the most common manifestations of homocystinuria. As discussed, homocystinuria relates to the increased risk of thromboembolic disease that can lead to infarctions and, consequently, focal deficits. Mental retardation and tonic–clonic seizures are also common manifestations related to CNS involvement. Approximately 50% of patients present with psychiatric disorders (Abbott, Folstein, Abbey, & Pyeritz, 1987; Omen, 1978), with depression, behavioral disorders, OCD, and personality disorders representing the most common.

Outside of CNS and vascular involvement, patients may demonstrate a combination of visual and musculoskeletal symptoms. Malar flush, hypopigmentation and thinning of hair, and livedo reticularis of the skin may all be seen. In addition, osteoporosis and marfanoid skeletal features present at higher incidence rates (Lee et al., 2005). Ocular features in the form of retina and sclera detachment, myopia, and ectopia lentis are common.

DIAGNOSIS

Diagnosis of homocystinuria can be done through various processes and may include clinical observation as well as analysis at metabolite, enzyme, and DNA levels. Evaluation of homocysteine and sulfur amino acid levels within the plasma is the accepted first-line method of diagnosis (Brattstrom et al., 1988). The cyanide nitroprusside and/or Spaeth–Barber's spot tests can be used to measure the amount of homocysteine in the urine, but they are not as sensitive as plasma analysis (Fowler, 1988; Spaapen, 1996).

Beyond diagnosis of homocystinuria itself, sequelae of the presentation such as seizures or infarcts are diagnosed through standard means. For example, if seizures present, electroencephalography and potentially MRI may be employed as would normally be the case.

TREATMENT

There is no specific cure for homocystinuria. High doses of vitamin B (i.e., pyridoxine) are the most commonly used method of treatment. A methionine diet with supplemental trimethylglycine, folic acid, and cysteine may also be useful. Beyond this, treatment is symptom based. Seizures are treated with standard antiepileptic drugs.

Chad A. Noggle
Javan Horwitz

Abbott, M. H., Folstein, S. E., Abbey, H., & Pyeritz, R. E. (1987). Psychiatric manifestations of homocystinuria due to cystathionine b-synthase deficiency: Prevalence, natural history, and relationship to neurologic impairment and vitamin B$_6$-responsiveness. *American Journal of Medical Genetics, 26,* 959–969.

Bakker, R. C., & Brandjes, D. P. (June 1997). Hyperhomocysteinaemia and associated disease. *Pharmacy World & Science, 19*(3), 126–132.

Brattstrom, L., Israelsson, B., Lindegarde, F., & Hultberg, B. (1988). Higher total plasma homocysteine in vitamin B12 deficiency than in heterozygosity for homocystinuria due to cystathionine b-synthase deficiency. *Metabolism, 37,* 175–178.

Cochran, F. B. (1992). Homocystinuria presenting as sagittal sinus thrombosis. *European Neurology, 32,* 1–3.

Engbersen, A. M., Franken, D. G., Boers, G. H., Stevens, E. M., Trijbels, F. J., & Blom, H. J. (1995). Thermolabile 5,10-methylenetetrahydrofolate reductase as a cause of mild hyperhomocysteinemia. *American Journal of Human Genetics, 56,* 142–150.

Fowler, B. (1988). Amino acids. In: A. H. Gowenlock (Ed.), *Practical clinical biochemistry* (6th edn) (pp. 385–400). London: William Heinmann.

Kraus, J. P., Oliveriusova, J., Sokolova, J., Kraus, E., Vlcek, C., de Franchis, R., et al. (1998). The human cystathionine b-synthase gene: Complete sequence, alternative splicing, and polymorphisms. *Genomics, 52,* 312–324.

Lee, S-J, Lee, D. H., Yoo, H-W, Koo, S. K., Park, E-S, Park, J-W., Lim, H. G., Jung, S-C (2005). Identification and functional analysis of cystathionine beta-synthase gene mutations in patients with homocystinuria. *Journal of Human Genetics, 50,* 648–654.

Li, S. C. & Stewart, P. M. (1999). Homocystinuria and psychiatric disorder: A case report. *Pathology, 31,* 221–224.

Miles, E. W., & Kraus, J. P. (2004). Cystathionine b-synthase: Structure, function, regulation, and location of homocystinuria-causing mutations. *Journal of Biological Chemistry, 279,* 29871–29874.

Mudd, S. H., Levy, H. L., & Skovby, F. (1989). Disorders of transsulfuration. In C. F. Schriver, A. L. Beaudet, W. S. Sly, & D. Valle (Eds.), *The metabolic basis of inherited disease* (pp. 693–734). New York: McGraw-Hill.

Naughten, E., Yap, S., & Mayne, P. D. (1998). Newborn screening for homocystinuria: Irish and world experience. *European Journal of Pediatrics, 157* (Suppl. 2), S84–S87.

Omenn, G. S. (1978). Inborn errors of metabolism: Clues to understanding human behavioural disorders. *Behavior Genetics, 6,* 263–284.

Spaapen, L. (1996). European quality assurance program for the selective screening of inherited disorders of metabolism (ERNDIM). *Journal of Inherited Metabolic Disease, 19*(1), 104.

Ubagai, T., Lei, K. J., Huang, S., Mudd, S. H., Levy, H. L., & Chou, J. Y. (1995). Molecular mechanisms of inborn error of methionine pathway. Methionine adenosyl-transferase deficiency. *Journal of Clinical Investigation, 96,* 1943–1947.

White, H. H., Rowland, L. P., Araki, S., Thompson, H. L., & Cowen, D. (1965). Homocystinuria. *Archives of Neurology, 13,* 455.

HUGHES' SYNDROME

DESCRIPTION

Hughes' syndrome, more commonly known as antiphospholipid syndrome, is an autoimmune disease characterized by the presence of antiphospholipid antibodies (anticardiolipin antibodies, antibodies to B$_2$-glycoprotein I, or lupus anticoagulants). Coagulation occurs as a result of antiphospholipid antibodies that recognize plasma proteins and increase their affinity for anionic phospholipids (Salmon, Guillermina, & Lockshin, 2007; Weiler, 2008). For the diagnosis of Hughes' syndrome, at least one of the following clinical features must be present: (1) one or more thrombotic events in the arteries, veins, or small vessels of any tissue or organ, and (2) recurrent, unexplained fetal losses.

Occlusion of the vascular system at any location throughout the body is a potential consequence of the disease given the increase in coagulation, with the lower limbs, the brain, and the heart being the most at risk (Hanly, 2003). Thrombosis, the most common symptom associated with Hughes' syndrome, may be venous or arterial in nature and may potentially occur in any organ. Venous thrombosis is particularly common in lower limbs and may increase the risk for pulmonary emboli, whereas arterial thrombosis most typically occurs in the brain, potentially causing strokes and ischemic events (Hanly, 2003). Although most patients with Hughes' syndrome present with thrombosis affecting only one organ, rarely a case may be seen wherein thrombosis occurs in at least three organs, known as "catastrophic antiphospholipid syndrome." This severe variation of the disease may onset within days to weeks affecting any organ including the lungs, heart, and brain (Hanly, 2003). Death often results from catastrophic antiphospholipid syndrome due to failure of the affected organs.

NEUROPATHOLOGY/PATHOPHYSIOLOGY

Although the etiology of Hughes' syndrome is unknown, the antiphospholipid antibodies are believed to have a key role in the pathological mechanisms of the disease. It is speculated that anti-phospholipid antibodies are produced in response to viral and bacterial peptides (Hanly, 2003). It has been proposed that the antibodies interfere with coagulation homeostasis by primarily targeting B_2-glycoprotein I, a natural anticoagulant, in addition to prothrombin, protein C, protein S, and annexin V (Roubey, 1996). This interference is suspected to promote thrombosis by creating coagulant states. There is also evidence that the interaction between antiphospholipid antibodies and B_2-glycoprotein I leads to activation of endothelial cells and aggregation of platelets that also promotes coagulation (Hanly, 2003; Levine, Branch, & Ranch, 2002; Salmon et al, 2007). Activation of endothelial cells may also result from B_2-glycoprotein-stimulated interferon-y production. It is suggested that a "second hit" may be necessary for manifestations of the disease to arise, such as neurological trauma, infection, or additive effects of non-immune procoagulant factors (Hanly, 2003).

Fetal loss is common in patients with Hughes' syndrome, particularly after the 10th week of pregnancy. In addition to the laboratory findings, clinical criteria for antiphospholipid syndrome states that one or more unexplained fetal losses after the 10th week (up to the 34th week) of gestation or at least three losses before the 10th week gestation must have occurred (Hanly, 2003). Pregnancy loss is suspected to be induced by antiphospholipid antibodies and results in a complement-driven inflammatory condition that is unable to allow a fetus to thrive. Miscarriages, intrauterine growth restrictions, and fetal death are all consequences potentially triggered by antiphospholipid antibodies (de laat, Mertens, & de Groot, 2008; Weiler, 2008). The pathogenesis of fetal loss in patients with Hughes' syndrome is uncertain, but appears to be associated with an abnormal abundance of complement component C3 in the placenta.

NEUROPSYCHOLOGICAL/CLINICAL PRESENTATION

Neuropsychological aspects of Hughes' syndrome, including cognitive, behavioral, and emotional symptoms have yet to be discussed in the literature, although it can be inferred that injuries resulting from thrombotic events have specific neuropsychological consequences dependent upon the location of the injury in these patients. Male children of women with Hughes' syndrome and comorbid SLE may display a mild verbal processing deficit (Salmon et al., 2007; Neri et al., 2004). Relevant literature has discussed emotional ramifications indicative of depression or bereavement in women who have endured

multiple pregnancy losses (Nemeroff, 1997), and patients with Hughes' syndrome who fit this description should seek psychiatric evaluation for such. Thus, the presentation of the disorder clinically will vary depending upon the location and number of thrombotic events.

DIAGNOSIS

In patients that present with venous or arterial thrombosis, or more than one unexplained pregnancy loss, diagnostic tests should be given to detect anticardiolipin or a positive lupus anticoagulant, both reflecting the presence of antiphospholipid antibodies. Separate from the clinical criteria, Hughes' syndrome may manifest itself less commonly as livedo reticularis, cardiac valve disease, or transient cerebral ischemia (Hanly, 2003). Systemic lupus erythematosus (SLE) has been repeatedly associated with antiphospholipid antibodies and 50% of these patients have a history of thrombotic events (Asherson et al., 1989; Hanly, 2003). In approximately 25% of cases, unexplained pregnancy losses can be attributed to moderate to high levels of antiphospholipid antibodies (Salmon et al., 2007). In addition to the presence of antiphospholipid antibodies, patients who are pregnant or have recently undergone a surgical procedure are at increased risk for developing thrombosis. Other complications seen in pregnant women with Hughes' syndrome are severe preeclampsia and hemolysis, elevated liver enzymes, and low platelets syndrome, which may result in the need to abort the fetus for the mother's safety (Weiler, 2008).

TREATMENT

After the presence of anticardiolipin antibodies or lupus anticoagulant has been detected through laboratory tests such as immunoassays or functional coagulation assays, anticoagulation methods should be adopted for treatment. Methods of immunosuppression have not been proven effective in the treatment of the disease. Pharmacological methods of full anticoagulation are the most supported means of treatment for antiphospholipid syndrome so as to reduce the risk of thrombosis (Hanly, 2003; Petri, 2000; Salmon et al., 2007; Weiler, 2008). For patients with a history of thrombotic events, the preferred therapy is heparin or low-molecular-weight heparin followed by warfarin. Warfarin has been found to reduce the rate of recurrence of thrombosis, but it is not recommended for pregnant patients given its teratogenic effects. Instead, enoxaparin is suggested as a substitute for warfarin during pregnancy (Salmon et al., 2007).

For patients with a history of fetal loss, a regimen of heparin combined with low-dose acetylsalicylic acid (ASA) has been found to be effective in preventing pregnancy loss given the protective effect of ASA on placental function (Salmon et al., 2007; Tincani et al., 2003; Weiler, 2008). This medication regimen has been found to reduce the risk of fetal loss by 54%, although there is still a risk for prematurity and low birth weight in infants born to women with Hughes' syndrome (Salmon et al., 2007). The dose of heparin is typically increased in pregnant women with Hughes' syndrome due to their increased risk of thrombosis in addition to fetal loss. In fact, it is recommended that patients maintain their anticoagulant medication regimen 3 months after pregnancy for continued protection against thromboembolism (Salmon et al., 2007). If treatment is ineffective in women attempting to carry pregnancies to term, there is limited support for intravenous immunoglobulin as a potentially beneficial alternative treatment (Gordon & Kilby, 1998; Hanly, 2003; Salmon et al., 2007).

To determine the efficacy of pharmacological treatments involving heparin, a measure of coagulation (known as the activated partial thromboplastin time) can be used in patients without lupus anticoagulant to detect prolonged activation times. For patients with lupus anticoagulant, antifactor Xa may be measured to infer heparin efficacy.

Although not heavily supported, low-dose ASA has been suggested as an addition to treatment in patients with ischemia related to antiphospholipid antibodies (Hanly, 2003). Hydroychloroquine is an additional recommendation to patients suffering from SLE who also carry antiphospholipid antibodies. The risk of mortality has been found to decrease in patients with catastrophic antiphospholipid syndrome when plasmapheresis is added to the medication regimen (Salmon et al., 2007).

Stephanie Lei Santiso
Charles Golden

Asherson, R., Khamashta, M., Ordi-Ros, J., Derkson, R., Machin, S., Barquinero, J., et al. (1989). The "primary" antiphospholipid syndrome: Major clinical and serological features. *Medicine (Baltimore), 68*, 366–374.

de laat, B., Mertens K., & de Groot, P. (2008). Mechanisms of disease: Antiphospholipid antibodies—from clinical association to pathologic mechanism. *Nature Clinical Practice Rheumatology, 4*, 192–199.

Gordon, C., & Kilby, M. (1998). Use of intravenous immunoglobulin therapy in pregnancy in systemic lupus erythematosus and antiphospholipid antibody syndrome. *Lupus, 7*, 429–433.

Hanly, J. (2003). Antiphospholipid syndrome: An overview. *Canadian Medical Association Journal, Vol 168 (13)*.

Levine, J., Branch, D., & Ranch, J. (2002). The antiphospholipid syndrome. *The New England Journal of Medicine, 346*, 752–763.

Nemeroff, C. (1997). Psychological distress associated with recurrent spontaneous abortion. *Journal Watch Psychiatry, 1997, 1201*, 7–7.

Neri, F., Chimini, L., Bonomi, F., Filippini, E., Motta, M., Faden, D., et al. (2004). Neuropsychological development of children born to patients with systemic lupus erythematosus. *Lupus, 13*, 805–811.

Petri, M. (2000). Treatment of the antiphospholipid antibody syndrome: Progress in the last five years? *Current Rheumatology Reports, 2*, 256–261.

Roubey, R. (1996). Immunology of the antiphospholipid antibody syndrome. *Arthritis Rheumatology, 39*, 1444–1454.

Salmon, J., Guillermina, G., & Lockshin, M. (2007). The antiphospholipid syndrome as a disorder initiated by inflammation: Implications for the therapy of pregnant patients. *Nature Clinical Practice Rheumatology, 3(3)*.

Tincani, A., Branch, W., Levy, R. A., Piette, J. C., Carp, H., Rai, R. S., et al. (2003). Treatment of pregnant patients with antiphospholipid syndrome. *Lupus, 12*, 524–529.

Weiler, H. (2008). Tracing the molecular pathogenesis of antiphospholipid syndrome. *The Journal of Clinical Investigation, 118(10)*.

HUNTINGTON'S DISEASE

DESCRIPTION

Huntington's disease (HD) is an inherited neurodegenerative disorder named after George Huntington, a physician who described the clinical presentation of the disease in his 1872 publication, "On Chorea." The disease results from the mutation of a single gene on chromosome 4. HD is a dominant, autosomal disease; having one parent with HD yields a 50% likelihood of developing the disease. Symptoms of HD typically appear around middle age. Chorea, which refers to excessive, jerky, uncontrolled movements, is a characteristic symptom of HD. Other common symptoms include cognitive decline and emotional disturbance. Though symptomatic treatments are available, the disease is chronic, progressive, and eventually fatal.

NEUROPATHOLOGY/PATHOPHYSIOLOGY

HD is caused by the mutation of a single gene (*IT15*), which is located on chromosome 4 and is responsible for the production of a protein called huntingtin. The mutation of this gene results in an increased number of CAG (cytosine–adenine–guanine) trinucleotide repeats and consequently an expanded polyglutamine sequence. Whereas healthy individuals typically have about 17–20 CAG repeats, individuals with HD have more than 35 CAG repeats (Imarisio et al., 2008). Rosenblatt et al. (2006) found that CAG length was predictive of disease progression, with a more rapidly progressing disease associated with a longer CAG length. The number of CAG repeats is also negatively correlated with the age of onset of HD (Andresen et al., 2006). CAG repeats greater than 50 are associated with juvenile-onset HD, that is, onset before age 20, whereas adult-onset HD is associated with 40–50 CAG repeats (Imarisio et al., 2008).

Neuropathological findings associated with HD include atrophy of neurons in the basal ganglion and cerebral cortex. The disease causes selective neuronal death with the most severe damage in the striatum of the basal ganglion, that is, the caudate nucleus and putamen. Magnetic resonance imaging (MRI) studies of individuals with HD reveal reduced caudate volume, and positron emission tomography (PET) scans show decreases in glucose metabolism and D2 receptor binding (Antonini et al., 1996; Aylward et al., 2000). Presymptomatic individuals within 12 years of onset also display these neurophysiologic characteristics, and caudate volume is negatively correlated with symptom severity (Aylward et al., 2000). MRI studies also reveal there is a reduction of putamen volume in individuals with the HD marker even before they become symptomatic (Harris et al., 1999). Using MRI scans, cognitive dysfunction in individuals with HD, as assessed by the Stroop Test, Trail Making Tests A and B, Benton Visual Retention Test, and CERAD Verbal Learning Test, has been linked to cortical and subcortical atrophy, specifically atrophy of the left sylvian cistern and the caudate (Starkstein et al., 1992). Individuals with HD also display abnormal EEG findings (Bylsma et al., 1994).

The mechanism by which the mutant huntingtin protein in HD causes neuronal destruction is still unclear. One hypothesis suggests that the inappropriate joining of mutant huntingtin proteins with each other and with other proteins may produce toxic aggregates (Scherzinger et al., 1997). Another hypothesis suggests that mutant huntingtin causes mitochondrial impairment in the form of lower calcium membrane potential, which consequently leads to excitotoxicity (Panov et al., 2002).

Huntingin is found in the central nervous system as well as in tissues of the peripheral nervous system; however, neuronal loss is most prominent in the putamen and caudate nucleus. Neurons of the striatum may be most susceptible to HD because these neurons are protected by brain-derived neurotropin factor (BDNF)—a neurotropic factor that is downregulated by the mutant huntingtin gene. As mouse models of HD confirm the influence of BDNF on symptom onset and severity, administration of BDNF may be a possible treatment for HD (Canals et al., 2004).

NEUROPSYCHOLOGICAL/CLINICAL PRESENTATION

The two types of HD, juvenile and adult-onset, have different presentations. Chorea, cognitive deficits, and psychological impairments are the characteristic features of adult-onset HD. In juvenile HD, abnormal voluntary movements, including gait abnormalities and slowed speech, may be present, but chorea is absent. Individuals with juvenile HD are also more likely to suffer from seizures and bradykinesia. The onset of chorea marks the progression of juvenile HD into the adult form of the disease (Kirkwood, Su, Conneally, & Foroud, 2001).

Motor impairment, cognitive deficits, and psychological distress are the classic symptoms of HD. The literature lacks consistent findings regarding the sequence and progression of these symptoms, which appear to be variable across individuals. Generally, symptoms associated with early stages of the disease include abnormalities in gait, mild chorea, slowed eye movements, bradykinesia, and emotional distress, such as sadness and irritability. As the disease progresses, motor impairments become more pronounced, intellectual functioning declines, and more psychological symptoms, such as apathy, depression, and anxiety, may appear. The later stages of the disease are often characterized by more severe language impairments due to motor deficits, rigidity, difficulties chewing and swallowing that may result in weight loss, and incontinence, as well as more severe psychological impairment and cognitive deficits eventually leading to dementia (Kirkwood et al., 2001; Purdon, Mohr, Ilivitsky, & Jones, 1994). Dystonia, sleep disorders, obsessive compulsive symptoms, hallucinations, delusions, and behavioral disorders are other symptoms associated with HD. The cognitive decline related to HD may significantly impact an individual's ability to perform activities of daily living, such as shopping and personal care (Bylsma, Rothlind, Hall, Folstein, & Brandt, 1993). At the later stages of the disease, individuals are often bedridden and need assistance dressing, bathing, and feeding themselves. Death typically results from pneumonia, heart failure, or other complications of the disease about 10–20 years after the onset of symptoms. Individuals with HD also have an increased risk of committing suicide.

Full scale IQ (FSIQ) scores of individuals with HD tend to be significantly lower than the average FSIQ score—even in samples in which the participants with HD had more education than the average population (Wechsler, 1997). The individuals with HD showed the most profound deficits in the processing speed subtests of the WAIS-III (mean PSI = 78.2). Like Alzheimer's disease and Parkinson's disease, HD is characterized by a marked decline in perceptual organizational skills though verbal skills remain relatively intact until the later stages of the disease (Wechsler, 1997). Memory decline in individuals with HD is thought to progress more slowly than memory decline in individuals with Alzheimer's disease but more rapidly than healthy individuals. Individuals with HD show marked impairment in retrieval but do not demonstrate storage deficits as do individuals with Alzheimer's disease. Because of their retrieval deficits, individuals with HD present with greater relative deficits in recall tasks as opposed to recognition tasks (Wechsler, 1997). Also, attention deficits become more pronounced as the disease progresses (Campodonico, Codori, & Brandt, 1996).

DIAGNOSIS

Excessive abnormal movements, cognitive deficits, and emotional impairment are the clinical features most commonly associated with HD. Patients may initially present with any or all of these symptoms. Because HD is an inherited disorder, obtaining a family medical history is an integral part of the diagnostic process. DNA testing, which involves analysis of a blood sample, can be used to confirm a clinical diagnosis of HD and identify individuals with the HD marker, increased CAG repeats, even before they become symptomatic. However, the personal implications of genetic testing should be carefully considered. Though neuroimaging studies have been used to detect brain abnormalities in individuals with HD, these studies by themselves are not diagnostic.

TREATMENT

Currently no treatment is available to reverse or stop the progression of HD; however, symptomatic treatments do exist, and genetic counseling is available. In general, research on the effectiveness of various pharmaceutical agents in the treatment of HD is lacking. Antidopaminergics, including haloperidol,

fluphenazine, and olanzapine, appear to show the most promise in treating chorea; however, research on their effectiveness is limited (Bonelli & Wenning, 2006). Research on the psychiatric treatment of HD is scarce and is largely composed of case studies. Tricyclic antidepressants, SSRIs, MAOI, and electroconvulsive therapy may be effective in the treatment of depressive symptoms associated with HD (Naarding, Kremer, & Zitman, 2001), but more research is needed. Research on the effectiveness of behavioral treatments is also lacking. However, speech therapy may be beneficial in improving the communication abilities of individuals with HD and addressing swallowing difficulties, and physical and occupational therapy may have the potential to prolong mobility and independence (Bilney, Morris, & Perry, 2003).

Alyse Barker
Mandi Musso
William Drew Gouvier

Andresen, J. M., Gayan, J., Djoussc, L., Roberts, S., Brocklebank, D., Cherny, S. S., et al. (2006). The relationship between CAG repeat length and age of onset differs for Huntington's disease patients with juvenile onset or adult onset. *Annals of Human Genetics, 71*, 295–301.

Antonini, A., Leenders, K. L., Siegel, R., Meier, D., Vontobel, P., Weigell-Weber, M., et al. (1996). Striatal glucose metabolism and dopamine D_2 receptor binding in asymptomatic gene carriers and patients with Huntington's disease. *Brain, 119*, 2085–2095.

Aylward, E. H., Codori, A. M., Rosenblatt, A., Sherr, M., Brandt, J., Stine, O. C., et al. (2000). Rate of caudate atrophy in presymptomatic and symptomatic states of Huntington's disease. *Movement Disorders, 15*(3), 552–560.

Bilney, B., Morris, M. E., & Perry, A. (2003). Effectiveness of physiotherapy, occupational therapy, and speech pathology for people with Huntington's disease: A systematic review. *Neurorehabilitation and Neural Repair, 17*(1), 12–24.

Bonelli, R. M., & Wenning, G. K. (2006). Pharmacological management of Huntington's disease: An evidence based review. *Current Pharmaceutical Design, 12*, 2701–2720.

Bylsma, F. W., Peyser, C. E., Folstein, S. E., Folstein, M. F., Ross, C., & Brandt, J. (1994). EEG power spectra in Huntington's disease: Clinical and neuropsychological correlates. *Neuropsychologia, 32*(2), 137–150.

Bylsma, F. W., Rothlind, J., Hall, M. R., Folstein, S. E., & Brandt, J. (1993). Assessment of adaptive functioning in Huntington's Disease. *Movement Disorders, 8*(2), 183–190.

Campodonico, J. R., Codori, A. M., & Brandt, J. (1996). Neuropsychological stability over two years in asymptomatic carriers of the Huntington's disease mutation. *Journal of Neurology, Neurosurgery, and Psychiatry, 61*(6), 621–624.

Canals, J. M., Pineda, J. R., Torres-Peraza, J. F., Bosch, M., Martin-Ibanez, R., Munoz, M. T., et al. (2004). Brain-derived neurotrophic factor regulates the onset and severity of motor dysfunction associated with enkephalinergic neuronal degeneration in Huntington's disease. *The Journal of Neuroscience, 24*(35), 7727–7739.

Harris, G. J., Codori, A. M., Lewis, R. F., Schmidt, E., Bedi, A., & Brandt, J. (1999). Reduced basal ganglia blood flow and volume in pre-symptomatic, gene-tested persons at-risk for Huntington's disease. *Brain, 122,* 1667–1678.

Huntington, G. (1872). On chorea. *Medical and Surgical Reporter, 26,* 317–321.

Imarisio, S., Carmichael, J., Korolchuk, V., Chen, C. W., Saiki, S., Rose, C., et al. (2008). Huntington's disease: From pathology and genetics to potential therapies. *Biochemical Journal, 412*(2), 191–209.

Kirkwood, S. C., Su, J. L., Conneally, P. M., & Foroud, T. (2001). Progression of symptoms in the early and middle stages of Huntington's disease. *Archives of Neurology, 58,* 273–278.

Naarding, P., Kremer, H. P. H., & Zitman, F. G. (2001). Huntington's disease: A review of the literature on prevalence and treatment of neuropsychiatric phenomena. *European Psychiatry, 16,* 439–445.

Panov, A. V., Gutekunst, C. A., Leavitt, B. R., Hayden, M. R., Burke, J. R., Strittmatter, W. J., et al. (2002). Early mitochondrial calcium defects in Huntington's disease are a direct effect of polyglutamines. *Nature Neuroscience, 5*(8), 731–736.

Purdon, S. E., Mohr, E., Ilivitsky, V., & Jones, B. D. W. (1994). Huntington's disease: Pathogenesis, diagnosis and treatment. *Journal of Psychiatry and Neuroscience, 19*(5), 359–367.

Rosenblatt, A., Liang, K. Y., Zhou, H. Abbott, M. H., Gourley, L. M., Margolis, R. L., et al. (2006). The association of CAG repeat length with clinical progression in Huntington disease. *Neurology, 66,* 1016–1020.

Scherzinger, E., Lurz, R., Turmaine, M., Mangiarini, L., Hollenbach, B., Hasenbank, R., et al. (1997). Huntingtin-encoded polyglutamine expansions form amyloid-like protein aggregates in vitro and in vivo. *Cell, 90,* 549–558.

Starkstein, S. E., Brandt, J., Bylsma, F., Peyser, C., Folstein, M., & Folstein, S. E. (1992). Neuropsychological correlates of brain atrophy in Huntington's disease: A magnetic resonance imaging study. *Neuroradiology, 34,* 487–489.

Wechsler, D. (1997). *Wechsler adult intelligence scale–third edition technical manual.* San Antonio, TX: The Psychological Corporation.

HYDRANENCEPHALY

DESCRIPTION

Hydranencephaly is a rare cephalic disorder in which the hemispheres of the brain are replaced with sacs filled with cerebrospinal fluid (CSF). The cerebral hemispheres as a result are completely or almost completely absent, yet the cranium remains relatively normal in size (Stevenson, Hart, & Clericuzio, 2001; Volpe, 2001).

At birth, infants may seem functionally normal as they can reflexively suck, swallow, and cry due to preservation of the brainstem, and sometimes midbrain, diencephalic, and cerebellar regions (Lam & Tang, 2000). However, within the first month or two, deficits become noticeable. These include hypertonia, seizures, and mood instability. Eventually, mental retardation, blindness, deafness, and quadriparesis may become more obvious.

The cause of hydranencephaly remains unclear. To date, it is proposed as a sporadic residual of a destructive process, which some have suggested involves the carotid arteries (Wintour et al., 1996), although others have not supported this, at least as the sole cause of the presentation (Greene, Benacerraf, & Crawford, 1985). Current epidemiological evidence suggests a prevalence of approximately 1 per 5,000 continuing pregnancies (Csabay, Szabó, Papp, Tóth-Pál, & Papp, 1998; Lockshin, 1997).

NEUROPATHOLOGY/PATHOPHYSIOLOGY

In hydranencephaly, all or most of the cerebral hemispheres are replaced by CSF filled sacs (Lange-Cosack, 1944; Watson, 1944). In those instances where both hemispheres are not completely absent, preservation is seen in a posterior to anterior and inferior to superior pattern. For example, although there are cases in which the orbitofrontal cortex is preserved, this is far less likely than preservation of the temporal lobes, which is far less likely than preservation of the occipital lobes. The membranous sac consists of an outer connective tissue layer overlying an irregular patchy layer of glial fibers with occasional residual neurons, mineralized debris, and collections of macrophages (Graham & Lantos, 1997). The brainstem remains preserved. Midbrain, diencephalic, and cerebellar regions are preserved to varying degrees based on the severity of the anatomical disruption.

Although the etiology of hydranencephaly remains unknown, a destructive process is commonly accepted as the basis of the presentation (Heschl, 1859, 1861). More specifically, some have suggested the presentation arises from vascular compromise in the form of ischemia or infarction, whereas hemorrhage is uncommon (Edmondson, Hallak, Carpenter, & Cotton, 1992). This has been suggested given that hydranencephaly commonly originates in the territories fed by the carotid arteries, particularly those fed by the anterior cerebral arteries and middle cerebral arteries (Becker, 1949; Dekaban, 1965; Lange-Cosack, 1944; Myers, 1969). Infectious processes, trauma, irradiation, fetal anoxia, and toxicity have also been linked with cases of hydranencephaly (Duckett, 1995).

NEUROPSYCHOLOGICAL/CLINICAL PRESENTATION

The clinical features of hydranencephaly vary and are largely related to the extent of neuroanatomical disruption. At birth, infants may appear relatively normal. Reflexive crying, sucking, and swallowing may be seen. The head appears of normal size. However, after a few weeks, an array of symptoms may manifest. Thermoregulation and sleep regulation may show disturbance. For infants who survive past the first few weeks, due to preservation of deep nuclei, spasticity, seizures, and minimal psychomotor development is seen (Graham & Lantos, 1997). Infants may appear quite irritable. In the vast majority of cases, blindness and deafness may be observed. There may be slow or halted physical growth. Moderate to profound mental retardation is seen in those infants who live for several years.

DIAGNOSIS

Diagnosis is usually preceded by observation of the aforementioned clinical features, which raises questions of central nervous system involvement. In many instances, diagnosis is made in utero via fetal ultrasound/sonography. The key differential in this case is holoprosencephaly. Identification of the presence of dural attachments and distinctly separate thalami is indicative of hydranencephaly (McGahan, Ellis, Lindfors, Lee, & Arnold, 1988). Following birth, CT or MRI may be utilized.

TREATMENT

There is no cure for hydranencephaly. Treatment is symptom based and supportive. Seizures can be addressed with standard anticonvulsant agents. If hydrocephalus develops, shunting may be considered. In most instances, prognosis is very poor with most children dying prior to their first birthday. In very mild cases, survival for several years may be possible.

Chad A. Noggle
Javan Horwitz

Becker, H. (1949). Uber Hirngefassausschaltungen II. Intrakranielle Gefassverschlussw. *Uber experimentelle Hydranencephalie (Blasenhirn) Dtsch Z Nervenheilkunde, 161,* 446–505.

Csabay, L., Szabó, I., Papp, C., Tóth-Pál, E., & Papp, Z. (1998). Central nervous system anomalies. *Annals of the New York Academy of Sciences, 847,* 21–245.

Dekaban, A. (1965). Large defects in cerebral hemispheres associated with cortical dysgenesis. *Journal of Neuropathology & Experimental Neurology, 24,* 512–530.

Duckett, S. (1995). *Pediatric neuropatholgy.* Malvern, PA: William & Wilkins.

Edmondson, S. R., Hallak, M., Carpenter, R. J., & Cotton, D. B. (1992). Evolution of hydranencephaly following intracerebral hemorrhage. *Obstetrics & Gynecology, 79,* 870–871.

Graham, D. I., & Lantos, P. L. (Eds.). (1997). *Greenfield's neuropathology* (6th ed.). New York: Oxford University Press.

Greene, M. F., Benacerraf, B., & Crawford, J. M. (1985). Hydranencephaly: US appearance during in utero evolution. *Radiology, 156,* 779–780.

Heschl, R. (1859). Gehirndefect und hydrocephalus. *Vierteljahrschrift Fur Praktikale Heilkunde Prague, 61,* 59–74.

Heschl, R. (1861). Ein neuer fall von prencephalie. *Vierteljahrschrift Fur Praktikale Heilkunde, 72,* 102–104.

Lam, Y. H., & Tang, M. H. Y. (2000). Serial sonographic features of a fetus with hydranencephaly from 11 weeks to term. *Ultrasound Obstetrics & Gynecology, 16,* 77–79.

Lange-Cosack, H. (1944). Die Hydranencephalie (Blasenhirn) als Sonderform der Grosshirnlosigkeit. *Archives Psychiatric Nervenkrankheit, 117,* 1–51.

Lockshin, M. D. (1997). Antiphospholipid antibody. Babies, blood clots, biology. *Journal of the American Medical Association, 277,* 1549–1551.

McGahan, J. P., Ellis, W., Lindfors, K. K., Lee, B. C. P., & Arnold, J. P. (1988). Congenital cerebrospinal fluid-containing intracranial abnormalities: A sonographic classification. *Journal of Clinical Ultrasound, 16,* 531–544.

Myers, R. E. (1969). Brain pathology following fetal vascular occlusions: An experimental study. *Investigative Ophthalmology, 8,* 41–50.

Stevenson, D. A., Hart, B. L., & Clericuzio, C. L. (2001). Hydranencephaly in an infant with vascular malformations. *American Journal of Medical Genetics, 104,* 295–298.

H

Volpe, J. J. (Ed.). (2001). *Hypoxic-ischemic encephalopathy, neuropathology, and pathogenesis. Neurology of the newborn* (pp. 296–330). Philadelphia: WB Saunders.

Watson, E. H. (1944). Hydranencephaly. Report of two cases which combine features of hydrocephalus and anencephaly. *American Journal of Disease of Children, 67,* 282–287.

Wintour, E. M., Lewitt, M., McFarlane, A., Moritz, K., Potocnik, S., Rees, S., et al. (1996). Experimental hydranencephaly in the ovine fetus. *Acta Neuropathologica (Berl), 91,* 537–544.

HYDROCEPHALUS

DESCRIPTION

Hydrocephalus is an excessive accumulation of cerebrospinal fluid (CSF) within the cranial cavity — often within the ventricles of the brain — potentially leading to enlarged ventricles, an enlarged skull, cortical flattening, and atrophy of the brain. Hydrocephalus can occur at any age and is related to multiple conditions. As a result of its diverse etiology, the incidence and prevalence of hydrocephalus vary greatly. These figures are most readily available when the condition is present at the time of birth; the majority of studies report a rate of 0.5–0.9 per 1,000 births when there are no other associated defects (Leech, 1991).

The manner in which hydrocephalus arises and its anatomical features coincide with recognized subtypes of the presentation. It may be congenital or acquired in development. Furthermore, it may be described as communicating or noncommunicating (a.k.a. obstructive), which coincides with the nature of CSF flow disturbance. Based on these factors, an array of functional outcomes and deficits may be seen across neurological, cognitive, behavioral, and physical domains as well as others.

NEUROPATHOLOGY/PATHOPHYSIOLOGY

Hydrocephalus has a variety of etiologies. In fact, it is related to many neurologic diseases, and as a result is one of the most common disorders treated by neurosurgeons (Bergsneider, 2001). Hydrocephalus is typically classified by cause (i.e., congenital or acquired); however, the specific cause cannot always be determined (Leech & Goldstein, 1991).

Brain tumors, arachnoid cysts, congenital malformations, trauma, infection, metabolic disease, neoplasms, and vein thrombosis have all been associated with the development of acquired hydrocephalus (Batchelor & Dean, 1996; Leech & Goldstein, 1991). In terms of congenital hydrocephalus, the presentation arises in relation to other structural defects of the central nervous system. Hydrocephalus has been most commonly discussed in relation to spina bifida. In fact, approximately half of the patients with congenital hydrocephalus also present with spina bifida (Leech, 1991). An easy way of suggesting one or the other is that, in most instances, congenital hydrocephalus presents within the first year, and anything after that is far more likely to be acquired.

Regardless of the cause for hydrocephalus, at least one of four general pathophysiologic mechanisms is typically involved. One of these mechanisms is aqueductal stenosis, which entails the aqueduct being too small for the normal passage of CSF (Leech & Goldstein, 1991). Another general mechanism is mechanical blockage. Blockage of the ventricular pathway can occur as the result of tumors, blood, or other materials; in addition, tumors or tumor-like conditions can cause blockage by pressing on this pathway from the outside (Batchelor & Dean, 1996; Leech & Goldstein, 1991). The third general mechanism for hydrocephalus is the obliteration of the subarachnoid space; there is an obstruction to the CSF circulation in this area of the brain (Leech & Goldstein, 1991). Hemodynamic or physiologic causes comprise the fourth general mechanism. The dynamic balance between the production and absorption of CSF is modified by certain conditions, which could then lead to hydrocephalus (Leech & Goldstein, 1991).

Often hydrocephalus is discussed from a pathological standpoint as being either communicating or noncommunicating (a.k.a. obstructive). These terms are used to described whether there is "communication," in other words flow, between the subarachnoid space and the ventricles. However, some have challenged the use of terminology (i.e., Adams & Victor, 1993). The basis of the challenge is that the original conceptualization of communicating hydrocephalus suggests that no blockage of the ventricular system exists and that the hydrocephalus is due to an overproduction of CSF in the choroid plexus, which in reality is quite rare and usually only noted in papillomas. Rather, blockage at some point along the CSF flow pathway, whether it is movement between ventricles, into the subarachnoid space, or at the point of reabsorption, accounts for almost every case (Golden & Bonnemann, 2007). What then becomes of clinical importance is where the blockage occurs and from what, which can delineate treatment approach.

The neuroanatomical presentation of hydrocephalus varies based on the age when the presentation first arises, the basis for its development (e.g., vascular, tumor, etc.), if it is treatable, when it is treated, and the rate and magnitude of ventricular enlargement (Brewer, Fletcher, Hiscock, & Davidson, 2001). In cases of congenital hydrocephalus, cortical gyri appear flattened with shallow and reduced sulci. Microgyria, polygyria, or stenogyria may be noted depending upon when the hydrocephalus began in utero (Golden & Bonnemann, 2007). The features are commonly seen in conjunction with enlarged lateral ventricles regardless of the site of blockage. White matter destruction is commonly noted (Rubin et al., 1976). In the case of blockage preventing CSF moving into the subarachnoid space, this causes enlargement of the lateral ventricles due to the CSF not being able to escape while more CSF is being produced. In the case of reabsorption blockage, this can cause backflow of CSF and eventual buildup in the lateral ventricles. Prior to age 2, when the cranial sutures have yet to begin to fuse, this can lead to an enlarged head with protruding fontanelles as a means of relieving pressure. Often, whether or not the cranial sutures have fused can correspond with the degree of ventricular enlargement. Prior to suture closing, ventricular enlargement can be quite prominent as there is no structural restriction in place as is the case in hydrocephalus developing in a fixed skull. Destruction of nerve fibers, the corpus callosum, and other cerebral commissures may be seen as a result of stretching and breaking (Loveday & Edginton, 2011).

NEUROPSYCHOLOGICAL/CLINICAL PRESENTATION

When the condition is congenital, the main feature is an enlarged head that continues to grow at an abnormally fast rate (Gascon & Leech, 1991a,b). In severe cases, the forehead may bulge and the eyes may appear to have receded into their sockets. Percussion testing of the head can be characterized by a "cracked-pot" sound if the hydrocephalus has developed prior to cranial suture fusion (Golden & Bonnemann, 2007). Prognosis is least favorable when hydrocephalus is present at birth as an isolated condition. Of those infants who do survive, less than half have normal IQs, whereas the rest may exhibit mild to severe mental retardation. Enlargement of the head, greater than two standard deviations above the mean, is the usual presentation of hydrocephalus within the first year of life; however, description is best defined by tracking of head growth over time as opposed to single point measurement. Other symptoms sometimes observed in infants are irritability, lethargy, and delayed motor development (Gascon & Leech, 1991a,b).

Extraocular movements may be impeded causing an upgaze paresis with a "setting sun phenomenon" in infants, whereas unilateral or bilateral abducens and trochlear paresis can also occur (Golden & Bonnemann, 2007). Papilledema can present but over time give way to optic atrophy and further diminished visual acuity, sometimes being bad enough in infants that there is appearance of cortical blindness as the pupil and lens respond properly to visual stimuli, but the information is not "seen" neurologically.

Interestingly, increasing head size is not a part of the clinical presentation of hydrocephalus in childhood and adolescence. For this age group, signs of hydrocephalus may include behavioral changes, decreased school performance, headaches, nausea, vomiting, changes in vision, and poor coordination. Signs of dementia, gait disturbance, and urinary incontinence are possible symptoms for adults with hydrocephalus (Gascon & Leech, 1991a,b). Chronic hydrocephalus may lead to mental retardation and/or optic atrophy with permanent visual loss (Batchelor & Dean, 1996).

Intellectually, low average performance is commonly reported in conjunction with and as a result of slowed development (Jacobs, Northam, & Anderson, 2001; Lindquist, Carlsson, Persson, & Uvebrant, 2005). Domain-specific deficits have been reported in processing speed (Jacobs et al., 2001), cognitive set shifting, and activation–reactivation (Swartout et al., 2008). Visuospatial abilities are often an area of weakness (Baron & Goldberger, 1993) but have been argued as potentially a manifestation of combined visual and motor defects as opposed to a pure visuospatial issue (Baron & Goldberger, 1993; Hetherington & Dennis, 1999; Wills, 1993).

Language is often characterized by dysfluency of speech, "cocktail-party talk/syndrome" (i.e., articulate and coherent expression that is irrelevant and sometimes pointless or without real direction) and preserved syntax and lexicon in the face of disrupted text and discourse (Fletcher et al., 2002).

Memory and learning deficits are fairly prominent. Although some have suggested widespread deficits of this domain characterized by verbal and nonverbal memory deficits, including deficits in both free recall and recognition and memory of both noncontextual and contextual information (Scott et al., 1998), others have suggested a pattern consistent with a prefrontal/subcortical pattern of dysfunction (Yeates et al., 1995). In this regard, cueing and recognition aids performance suggesting retrieval-based and organization deficits.

Finally, executive functioning deficits have been commonly reported with deficits arising in problem solving, planning, abstraction, sequencing, and set shifting in the absence of perseveration, impulsivity, and rule breaking (Fletcher et al., 1995; Snow, 1999).

DIAGNOSIS

Infants with hydrocephalus typically undergo skull radiographs, MRI, or CT scan to determine separation of sutures, areas of thinning of the bones, or intracranial calcifications. A CT scan can show ventricular size and the location and nature of an obstruction if any (Gascon & Leech, 1991a,b); however, MRI is preferred and offers the most refined and accurate evaluation of potential blockage (Golden & Bonnemann, 2007). In cases involving intraventricular hemorrhage, sonography is probably the procedure of choice (Gascon & Leech, 1991a,b). In older patients and even children, in addition to MRI or CT scan, CSF pressure can be monitored by way of a lumbar puncture.

Neuropsychological evaluation should be undertaken in all cases to determine what if any deficits are present. Given the high prevalence of visual deficits, optometry consultation is recommended.

TREATMENT

The primary method of treatment for hydrocephalus is the surgical placement of a shunt, a device that provides drainage of fluid from the brain into the abdominal cavity (Kanev & Park, 1993). Shunting CSF from the dilated ventricles usually results in clinical improvement. Particularly, it can improve potential cognitive development in children (Batchelor & Dean, 1996; Rachel, 1999). However, the longer the disease has been present, the less likely it is that shunting will be curative. Other neurosurgical treatments for hydrocephalus include removal of tumors or cysts, ventricular bypass, ventriculocisternostomy, third ventriculostomy, and coagulation of the choroid plexus (Batchelor & Dean, 1996; Rachel, 1999). In infants where the hydrocephalus appears as a potential acute feature that may resolve over time, such as in the case where it develops in relation to vascular events (e.g., hemorrhage — posthemorrhagic hydrocephalus), permanent shunt placement may not be sought. Rather, temporary treatments such as daily lumbar puncture alone or in combination with CSF-reducing pharmacological practices such as furosemide with acetazolamide may be employed.

For infants and children with hydrocephalus, early intervention or stimulation programs may be helpful when dealing with developmental delays. In older children and adults, when the skull is no longer flexible, treating the underlying cause and

psychological symptoms of hydrocephalus may be most feasible. Supportive or group counseling may be beneficial for treating irritability and changes in mental functioning. For school-aged children, remedial classes and peer support may be beneficial in dealing with academic-related problems.

Matt Holcombe
Raymond S. Dean
Chad A. Noggle

Adams, R., & Victor, M. (1993). *Principals of neurology* (5th ed.). New York: McGraw-Hill

Baron, I.S. & Goldberger, E. (1993). Neuropsychological disturbances of hydrocephalic children with implications for special-education and rehabilitation. Neuropsychological Rehabilitation, 3(4), 389–410.

Batchelor, E. S., Jr., & Dean, R. S. (1996). Pediatric neuropsychology: Interfacing assessment and treatment for rehabilitation. Needham Heights, MA: Allyn & Bacon.

Bergsneider, M. (2001). Evolving concepts of cerebrospinal fluid physiology. *Neurosurgery Clinics of North America, 36*(4), 631–638.

Brewer, V. R., Fletcher, J. M., Hiscock, M., & Davidson, K. C. (2001). Attention processes in children with shunted hydrocephalus versus attention deficit–hyperactivity disorder. *Neuropsychology, 15*(2), 185–198.

Fletcher, J. M., Copeland, K., Frederick, J. A., Blaser, S. E., Kramer, L. A., Northrup, H., et al. (2002). Spinal lesion level in spina bifida: A source of neural and cognitive heterogeneity. *Journal of Neurosurgery, 102*(3), 268–279.

Gascon, G. G., & Leech, R. W. (1991a). Clinical presentation. In R. W. Leech & R. A. Brumback (Eds.), *Hydrocephalus: Current clinical concepts* (pp. 96–104). St. Louis, MO: Mosby Year Book.

Gascon, G. G., & Leech, R. W. (1991b). Medical evaluation. In R. W. Leech & R. A. Brumback (Eds.), *Hydrocephalus: Current clinical concepts* (pp. 105–128). St. Louis, MO: Mosby Year Book.

Golden, J. A., & Bonnemann, C. G. (2007). Developmental structural disorders. In C. G. Goetz (Ed.), *Textbook of clinical neurology* (3rd ed., pp. 561–591). Philadelphia: Saunders Elsevier.

Hetherington, R., & Dennis, M. (1999). Motor function profile in children with early onset hydrocephalus. *Developmental Neuropsychology, 15*(1), 25–51.

Jacobs, R., Northam, E., & Anderson, V. (2001). Cognitive outcome in children with myelomeningocele and perinatal hydrocephalus: A longitudinal perspective. *Journal of Developmental and Physical Disabilities, 13*(4), 389–405.

Kanev, P. M., & Park, T. S. (1993). The treatment of hydrocephalus. *Neurosurgery Clinics of North America, 4*, 611–619.

Leech, R. W. (1991). Epidemiology, risk factors, survival, and quality of life. In R. W. Leech & R. A. Brumback (Eds.),

Hydrocephalus: Current clinical concepts (pp. 79–95). St. Louis, MO: Mosby Year Book.

Leech, R. W., & Goldstein, E. (1991). Classifications and mechanisms. In R. W. Leech, & R. A. Brumback (Eds.), *Hydrocephalus: Current clinical concepts* (pp. 45–70). St. Louis, MO: Mosby Year Book.

Lindquist, B., Carlsson, G., Persson, E. K., & Uvebrant, P. (2005). Learning disabilities in a population-based group of children with hydrocephalus. *Acta Pediatrica, 94(7)*, 878–883.

Loveday, C. & Edginton, T. (2011). Spina bifida and hydrocephalus. In A.S. Davis (Ed.) Handbook of Pediatric Neuropsychology. New York: Springer Publishing Co. (pp. 769–783).

Rachel, R. A. (1999). Surgical treatment of hydrocephalus: A historical perspective. *Pediatric Neurosurgery, 30*, 296–304.

Rubin, R. C., Hochwald, G. M., Tiell, M., Mizutani, H., & Ghatak, N. (1976). Hydrocephalus: Histological and ultrastructural changes in the pre-shunted cortical mantle. *Surgical Neurology, 5(2)*, 109–114.

Scott, M. A., Fletcher, J. M., Brookshire, B. L., Davidson, K. C., Landry, S. H., Bohan, T. C., Kramer, L. A., Brandy, M. E., & Francis, G. A. (1998). Memory functions in children with early hydrocephalus. *Neuropsychology, 12(4)*, 578–589.

Snow, J. H. (1999). Executive processes for children with spina bifida. *Children's Health Care, 28(3)*, 241–253.

Swartout, M. D., Cirino, P. T., Hampson, A. W., Fletcher, J. M., Brandt, M. E., & Dennis, M. (2008). Sustained attention in children with two etiologies of early hydrocephalus. *Neuropsychology, 22(6)*, 765–775.

Wills, K. E. (1993). Neuropsychological functioning in children with spina bifida and or hydrocephalus. *Journal of Clinical Child Psychology, 22(2)*, 247–265.

Yeates, K. O., Enrile, B. G., Loss, N., Blumenstein, E., & Delis, D. C. (1995). Verbal-learning and memory in children with myelomeningocele. *Journal of Pediatric Psychology, 20(6)*, 80–815.

HYDROMYELIA AND SYRINGOMYELIA

DESCRIPTION

Hydromyelia and syringomyelia, sometimes referred to as one and the same, represent two different presentations characterized by abnormalities in or around the central canal in which cavities develop and fill with cerebrospinal fluid (CSF). Syringohydromyelia also falls under this umbrella, representing a more extensive presentation of syringomyelia. In the case of the prior (i.e., hydromyelia), the defect presents in infants and is related to an abnormal widening of the central canal in which the aforementioned cavity arises. This is a developmental defect manifesting, as discussed in the following, in which the primitive large canal of the embryo remains, or due to incomplete fusion of the posterior columns of the spinal cord, most often in the lumbar region (Staemmler, 1942). It may present in isolation or within the context of a more pronounced disorder or anomaly of structural dysfunction such as Arnold–Chiari malformations (MacKenzie & Emery, 1971). In the case of syringomyelia, the accumulation of CSF develops in a cavity causing distension of the central canal of the spinal cord, often due to cavitation secondary to a degenerative or traumatic event (Buettner & Caplan, 1996).

Clinically, both presentations mimic each other, thus the reasons for them often being used interchangeably in name. Individuals may present with pain, motor weakness of the extremities, and sensory loss as the fluid puts increased pressure on nerve cells and their connections. In the case of hydromyelia, it almost always coincides with hydrocephalus or other birth defects such as Chiari malformations.

NEUROPATHOLOGY/PATHOPHYSIOLOGY

Hydromyelia arises from either the primitive large canal of the embryo remaining or due to incomplete fusion of the posterior columns of the spinal cord, most often in the lumbar region (Staemmler, 1942). It may present in isolation or within the context of a more pronounced disorder or anomaly of structural dysfunction such as hydrocephalus, Arnold–Chiari malformations, and Dandy–Walker malformation (MacKenzie & Emery, 1971). Syringomyelia arises from a cavitation of the spinal cord in which the CSF accumulates. It can occur at any age, although it is most commonly noted in middle adulthood. It is associated with a closed cavity and has been noted in relation to spinal cord injuries/trauma and individuals with Chiari II malformation. As time passes, the cavity may remain stable or expand and elongate, increasing the damage to the spinal cord. When there is communication between the cavity and the subarachnoid space, or there is dissection of surrounding white matter, the presentation is termed syringohydromyelia (Buettner & Caplan, 1996; Saremi, 2003). This more expansive involvement also commonly arises from spinal cord injury or Chiari II malformation, although tumors, subarachnoid hemorrhage, and meningitis have also been associated with the presentation (Padmanabhan, Crompton, Burn, & Birchall, 2005; Park, Cail, Broaddus, & Walker, 1989; Saremi, 2003).

H

Both presentations can often be asymptomatic and only identified incidentally. Imaging may not definitively identify the presentations, even though it is considered the definitive diagnostic tool. In lieu of standard imaging approaches, serial slices of the spinal cord may be the only means of identification revealing replacement of normal tissue in the spinal canal with glial tissues although normal ependyma may still line the canal itself.

NEUROPSYCHOLOGICAL/CLINICAL PRESENTATION

Both hydromyelia and syringomyelia patients may present as asymptomatic when the presentations arise in isolation. In cases where they present in conjunction with a more complex presentation such as Arnold–Chiari malformations or hydrocephalus, symptoms are often associated with the broader-based dysfunction and not the hydromyelia itself. The interested reader is recommended to review the entries on Chiari malformations and hydrocephalus in this book. In those patients where symptoms do arise, they may vary and are in many ways related to the locality of the cavity. Pain, motor weakness in the extremities, and sensory loss are the most common features. In addition, affected individuals may manifest chronic headaches, difficulties in ambulation due to spasticity or paralysis of the legs, and/or incontinence of bowel and/or bladder (Steiger, Saccone, & Watson, 2007). In instances where syringohydromyelia manifests, intracranial hypertension (i.e., pseudotumor cerebri) and disrupted flow of cerebrospinal fluid commonly present (Mazzola & Fried, 2003; Owler, Halmagyi, Brennan, & Besser, 2004; Saremi, 2003) (see also the article on Pseudotumor Cerebri).

DIAGNOSIS

MRI is considered as the definitive test for all presentations; however, as discussed previously, serial slices of the spinal cord may be the only means of identification. Again, images should reveal replacement of normal tissue in the spinal canal with glial tissues although normal ependyma may still line the canal itself. CINE MRI may be used to evaluate CSF flow. Lumbar puncture may be used to assess pressure, particularly if there are concerns of intracranial hypertension (Sismanis, 1998). Electromyogram may be useful in determining speed and strength of muscle responsiveness to nerve stimulation. Functional assessment by physical therapy/occupational therapy (PT/OT) may be needed. In all cases, MRI of the brain should also be undertaken, particularly in hydromyelia given relatedness of these presentations to hydrocephalus and other neurological defects such as Arnold–Chiari malformations. Although neurocognitive sequelae are not strongly associated with these presentations, given they co-occur at high rates with other presentations such as hydrocephalus, neuropsychological assessment may be pursued in a manner consistent with the recommendations for those other presentations.

TREATMENT

Surgery remains the hallmark treatment for these presentations. In children with hydromyelia, this is sought once symptoms reach moderate to severe levels. Surgery seeks to correct CSF flow and does so through decompression, laminectomy/syringostomy, percutaneous aspiration, or terminal ventriculostomy (Buettner & Caplan, 1996; Steiger et al., 2007). The pursuit of such treatment depends upon both the cause and duration of the presentation, in addition to severity. Shunting can be useful in relieving intracranial hypertension or increased CSF pressure. Little information was obtained about the utility of diuretics in treatment, although they are effective in cases of intracranial hypertension.

Beyond surgery, physical therapy and occupational therapy are often recommended to regain strength and mobility. Chronic pain may persist depending on the duration of the presentation prior to surgical intervention and its lasting effects on nerves. Standard interventions ranging from physical therapy and occupational therapy, medicinal intervention, and nerve blocks may all be considered.

Chad A. Noggle
Javan Horwitz

Buettner, U. W., & Caplan, L. R. (1996). Syringomyelia and syringobulbia. In T. Brandt, L. R. Caplan, J. Dichgans, H. C. Diener, & C. Kennard (Eds.), *Neurologic disorders* (pp. 653–658). San Diego, CA: Academic Press.

MacKenzie, N. G., & Emery, J. L. (1971). Deformities of the cervical cord in children with neurospinal dysraphism. *Developmental Medicine and Child Neurology, 13*(Suppl. 25), 58–61.

Mazzola, C. A., & Fried, A. H. (2003). Revision surgery for Chiari malformation decompression. *Neurosurgical Focus, 15*(3), Article 3.

Owler, B. K., Halmagyi, G. M., Brennan, J., & Besser, M. (2004). Syringomyelia with Chiari malformation: 3 unusual cases with implications for pathogenesis. *Acta Neurochirurgica (Wein), 146*(10), 1137–1143.

Padmanabhan, R., Crompton, D., Burn, D., & Birchall, D. (2005). Acquired Chiari 1 malformation and syringomyelia following lumboperitoneal shunting for pseudotumour cerebri. *Journal of Neurology Neurosurgery Psychiatry, 76*(2), 298.

Park, T. S., Cail, W. S., Broaddus, W. C., & Walker, M. G. (1989). Lumboperitoneal shunt combined with myelotomy for treatment of syringohydromyelia. *Journal of Neurosurgery, 71*(6), 950–953.

Saremi, F. (2003). *Syringohydromyelia.* eMedicine from WebMD. Retrieved from http://www.emedicine.com/radio/topic670.htm

Sismanis, A. (1998). Pulsatile tinnitus: A 15-year experience. *American Journal of Otolaryngology, 19*(4), 472–477.

Staemmler, M. (1942). *Hydromyelie, syringomyelie und gliose.* Berlin, Germany: Springer Verlag.

Steiger, J., Saccone, P., & Watson, K (2007). Assessment of objective pulsatile tinnitus in a patient with syringohydromyelia. *Journal of the American Academy of Audiology, 18*, 197–205.

HYPERSOMNIA

DESCRIPTION

Hypersomnia is a category of disease marked by frequent drowsiness that is not related to a lack of nighttime sleep. Individuals with hypersomnia often sleep 8–10 hr a night, require frequent naps, and may still feel tired throughout the day. There is an estimated 0.5% to 5% of the population who experience excessive drowsiness without an attributed cause; however, the exact prevalence of those experiencing hypersomnia is unclear. Diagnosis is three times more likely in males, and the age of onset is generally in adolescence. Hypersomnia is fairly rare in individuals over the age of 30 (Sharma, 2007).

NEUROPATHOLOGY/PATHOPHYSIOLOGY

There are two main categories of hypersomnia: idiopathic hypersomnia with long sleep time and without long sleep time. There is no specific area of the brain that can be examined with traditional brain imaging techniques to confirm a diagnosis of idiopathic hypersomnia. However, it has often been identified in individuals who have experienced head trauma. Hypotheses of the causes of hypersomnia due to head trauma include a decrease in blood flow to the thalamus (Nose et.al., 2002) and bilateral lesions to the posterior hypothalamus (Eisehsehr et al., 2003).

Sleep patterns in individuals with idiopathic hypersomnia are generally not significantly different from that of control groups—although some studies have suggested that sleep spindle density is higher in individuals with hypersomnia, and there may be a decrease in slow-wave activity in the early REM episodes of night sleep. Studies of neuropathology of idiopathic hypersomnia have produced hypotheses of alterations in sleep patterns, but no specific indicators are used for diagnosis. Current differences in sleep patterns are generally used to explain individuals' difficulties waking from sleep but do not identify a cause for daytime sleepiness. However, neurophysiologic imaging can be used to rule out differential diagnosis often confused with hypersomnia (Lee-Chiong, 2005), such as responses to medical conditions or certain medications.

NEUROPSYCHOLOGICAL/CLINICAL PRESENTATION

The primary symptoms associated with hypersomnia are daytime drowsiness despite a full night of sleep and frequent naps throughout the day. Although patients are tired most of the day, they will not experience involuntary sleep attacks where they instantly fall asleep without warning, as may be the case with narcolepsy. They may have incidences of difficulties awaking from sleep and often oversleeping alarm clocks or attempts of others to wake them. Psychological presentation may manifest as frequent depressive symptoms. Hallucinations and sleep paralysis can also occur along with symptoms associated with autonomic nervous system dysfunction. Other common presenting symptoms include headache, hypotension, fatigue of muscles, and chronic pain.

Assessing for hypersomnia is most reliably done through self-report of the patient. A number of questionnaires and structured interviews can identify symptoms associated with various sleep disorders. Presentation of symptoms associated with hypersomnia will have an impact on the individual's educational and/or occupational situations. Many individuals first experience symptoms in adolescence when frequent drowsiness can lead to a lack of attention in school, poor grades, or decreased learning ability. Frequent daytime sleepiness can also limit occupational choices because some careers may be dangerous (i.e., those that operate heavy machinery). It can also lead to decreased work productivity and difficulties completing occupational tasks.

H

DIAGNOSIS

The two different types of idiopathic hypersomnia (with and without long sleep time) have similar diagnostic criteria, often assessed during a sleep study. Diagnostic criteria for idiopathic hypersomnia with long sleep time include a complaint of daytime sleepiness on a daily basis for a minimum of 3 months, prolonged nighttime sleep (over 10 hr), difficulty waking at the end of sleep, and exclusion of other sleep disorders using polysomnography and multiple sleep latency test (MLST). Idiopathic hypersomnia without long sleep time is diagnosed if nighttime sleep is experienced for less than 10 but more than 6 hr (Lee-Chiong, 2005). The *DSM-IV-TR* provides specific diagnostic criteria for primary hypersomnia. It states the complaint must be of excessive sleepiness nearly daily for at least 1 month represented by daytime or prolonged sleep that causes distress or impairment in functioning. The *DSM-IV-TR* also requires that the symptoms not be better explained by another sleep disorder, insufficient amounts of sleep, another mental disorder, medical conditions, or substance use (American Psychological Association [APA], 2000).

A major difficulty in differential diagnosis is the identification of sufficient nighttime sleep. If the patient is experiencing difficulty falling asleep or staying asleep, the diagnosis of hypersomnia should not be given. Narcolepsy is a disorder similar to idiopathic hypersomnia with a difference in the absence of cataplexy in hypersomnia. The MSLT can also be used to differentiate by identifying sleep-onset REM periods that are apparent in narcolepsy but not in idiopathic hypersomnia. Circadian rhythm sleep disorders may cause drowsiness, but unlike hypersomnia, the symptoms are apparent early in the morning but diminish later in the day. Daytime drowsiness can also be a symptom of mood disorders including depression and dysthymia. If a diagnosis of a mood disorder is met, it must be considered prior to a diagnosis of hypersomnia. Upper airway resistance syndrome, which causes frequent nighttime arousals due to difficulties in airflow, must be ruled out prior to diagnosis as well. Finally, hypersomnia secondary to general medical conditions such as a brain tumor, chronic pain, obesity, and neurological disorders or as a side effect of a drug or medication must also be ruled out. This can be done by ensuring a thorough medical examination and evaluation of current medical records (APA, 2000; Sharma, 2007).

TREATMENT

Defining the most appropriate course of treatment for hypersomnia can differ from one patient to another, as there is no exact series of treatments or cure for the disorder. Currently, there are treatment modalities using psychopharmacology that can be used to target symptoms associated with hypersomnia. The most common medication used today is modafinil (Provigil). Modafinil is a central nervous system (CNS) stimulant that decreases GABA-mediated neurotransmission to promote wakefulness. Although it has similar effectiveness to other stimulant medications, it has emerged as the most prevalent medication due to the decreased chance of abuse and the minimal side effects. Another CNS stimulant is armodafinil (Nuvigil), which inhibits dopamine reuptake and improves symptoms associated with sleep disorders. Amphetamine sulfate is also a CNS and respiratory stimulant used in cases of primary hypersomnolence. Methylphenidate (Ritalin) can have severe side effects as well as addictive qualities, though it is useful in situations when alertness is needed for safety reasons or when drowsiness could be dangerous to health. Many of these CNS stimulants must be closely monitored for addictive qualities and abuse as well as a series of other side effects such as psychosis, headache, nausea, and dizziness (Sharma, 2007).

In addition to psychopharmacological treatments, a number of therapeutic lifestyle modifications can decrease drowsiness and improve safety. A sleep log can be kept to ensure patients are receiving an appropriate amount of sleep. Individuals may believe they are receiving enough sleep when their sleep patterns are in fact inconsistent or insufficient. A sleep log allows the patient to identify sleep patterns and ensures proper diagnosis. Patients with hypersomnia should also consult with their therapy teams to ensure proper medications in times when drowsiness is dangerous for health, such as driving long distances (Mayo Clinic, 2009). In addition, therapy can be used to address some of the impacts that idiopathic hypersomnia can have on patients' lives. Hypersomnia can often impact individuals' occupational, educational, and social lifestyles. Furthermore, it can result in mood disorders such as depression. Improved lifestyle choices, as well as improved coping skills, can be explored and developed in therapy.

Mindy Scheithauer
Raymond S. Dean

American Psychiatric Association. (2000). *Diagnostic and statistical manual of mental disorders IV-R.* Arlington, VA: American Psychiatric Publishing.

Eisehsehr, I., Noachter, S., von Schlippenbach, C., Uttner, I., Kleine, J., Seelos, K., et al. (2003). Hypersomnia associated with bilateral posterior hypothalamic lesion. *European Neurology, 49,* 169–172.

Lee-Choing, T., (2005). *Sleep: A comprehensive handbook.* Denver, CO: Wiley-IEEE.

Mayo Clinic. (2009). *Idiopathic hypersomnia.* Retrieved March 25, 2009, from http://www.mayoclinic.org/hypersomnia/treatment.html

Nose, I., Ookawa, T., Tanaka, J., Yamamoto, T., Uchimura, N., Maeda, H., et al. (2002). Decreased blood flow of the left thalamus during somnolent episodes in a case of recurrent hypersomnia. *Psychiatry and Clinical Neurosciences, 56,* 277–278.

Sharma, S. (2007). *Primary hypersomnia.* Retrieved March 25, 2009, from http://emedicine.medscape.com/article/291699-overview

HYPERTONIA

DESCRIPTION

Hypertonia is an upper motor neuron condition characterized by abnormally increased muscle tone and resistance to passive movement around joints (Sanger et al., 2003). Highly researched literature referring to the term "hypertonia" can be dated back to the beginning of the 20th century, where early descriptions referenced general stiffening and hardening of the muscles (Mix, Abt, Ridlon, & Parker, 1915). Tension is exhibited throughout the body among those affected, causing difficulty with the execution of smooth, coordinated movements (Cratty, 1995). Hypertonia generally is attributed to motor pathway deficits in the central nervous system, preventing information to be relayed to muscles controlling posture, muscle tone, and reflexes (Sanger et al., 2003).

Four types of hypertonia are used to describe predominant symptoms, including spasticity, paratonia (gegenhalten), dystonia, and rigidity (Lippincott Williams & Wilkins [LWW], 2004). Presentation of hypertonia may include one type or a combination of several features, even within the same limb (Sanger et al., 2003). The resistance to movement observed in hypertonia is attributed to stiffness due to passive muscle properties (e.g., muscle or tendon shortening), muscle fibers that are active before the movement begins (e.g., dystonia), and/or muscle fibers that become active during the movement (e.g., spasticity) (Sanger et al., 2003).

NEUROPATHOLOGY/PATHOPHYSIOLOGY

A shared deficit among those evidencing hypertonic symptoms has been suggested in animal models to include a lower level of γ-aminobutyric acid type A receptors in the central nervous system, most prominent among the lower motor neurons (Gilbert et al., 2002). A mutation in the trafficking protein kinesin binding 1 (*TRAK1*) has been suggested as the primary causative feature, which is associated with elevated baseline firing of lower motor neurons, a predominant feature of hypertonia (Gilbert et al., 2006). Among mice with mutated *TRAK1*, researchers have localized the abnormality to chromosome 9, between markers KIAA1042-intron1 and Cck-3'UTR (Gilbert et al., 2006). A dopamine deficit in the basal ganglia, found among such conditions as dystonia and Parkinson's disease, has also been suggested (Gilbert et al., 2006).

Perinatal causes have been suggested to include meningeal inflammation, hemorrhage, severe bilateral cerebral injury, basal ganglia injury (most prominent with perinatal hypoxic-ischemic insults), and brainstem activation (Volpe, 2008). Myogenic causes in newborns include myotonia, congenital, paramyotonia, and hyperkalemic periodic paralysis (Volpe, 2008). Other ailments associated with hypertonic symptomatology include cerebral palsy, stroke, spinal cord injury, multiple sclerosis, head injury, stiff person syndrome, hereditary spastic paraplegia, Parkinson's disease, and metabolic diseases such as adrenoleukodystrophy and phenylketonuria (Cratty, 1994; Gilbert et al., 2006). The condition may be passed genetically, as with hereditary spastic paraplegia, or an indirect result of injury to the extrapyramidal or corticospinal tracts (e.g., head injury).

Different neurological influences have been associated with the features of hypertonia. Damage to pyramidal and extrapyramidal tracts cause a loss of inhibition and a disruption of the stretch reflex arc, which is important in muscle stretching and contraction (LWW, 2004). With an uninhibited muscle stretch, exaggerated, unmanageable muscle activity occurs, resulting in spasticity (LWW, 2004). The condition of paratonia is attributed to frontal lobe injury, causing a resistance to passive movement (Lippincott Williams & Wilkins, 2004). The cause of dystonia is attributed to a lack of necessary inhibition of the respective muscle (LWW, 2004). Damage to the basal ganglion or loss of cerebral cortex inhibition or control, leading to resistance in flexion as well as extension of a muscle, produces dystonia (LWW, 2004). In comparison, increased activation of alpha lower motor neurons that innervate the extrafusal muscle fibers results in rigidity (Porth, Gaspard, & Matfin, 2006).

NEUROPSYCHOLOGICAL/CLINICAL PRESENTATION

General clinical presentation of hypertonia may include difficulties with the patient's gait, movement,

H

and speech (Sanger at al., 2003). Common deficits incurred by those with hypertonia include being unable to place a flat foot on the floor, extend their big toe, flex their elbow when walking, grasp objects, clean the palm of their hands and finger nails, and extend fingers fully for functional tasks (Richardson et al., 2000). Upper and lower limb presentation is possible (Richardson et al., 2000). Severity varies, but the condition may become so severe that movement may not be possible with respect to a certain joint (Sanger et al., 2003). Among infants, there is a general arching of the back away from the mother (Sanger et al., 2003). Such infants may be described as difficult to comfort, pulling their heads and face away from contact and resisting snuggling into the chest or neck (Sanger et al., 2003). When keeping their head erect when held in a ventral position, these infants will keep their bodies will be almost completely straight (Sanger et al., 2003).

Spasticity, paratonia, dystonia, and rigidity present in different ways clinically. With spasticity, there are hyperactive tendon reflexes and increased resistance to stretching of certain muscles, limiting mobility, daily living, sitting, and sleeping. The "clasp-knife" term is common, referring to rapidly decreasing resistance with flexion (Volpe, 2008). Stiffness is most often observed in the adductors of the arms and legs, flexors of the arms, and extensors of the legs (Harding & Beech, 1996).

Paratonia involves resistance to passive movement that is observed to be proportional to the force applied, so that despite the patient's effort to relax, a limb may be resistant to complying (Good & Couch, 1994). Paratonia is associated with hyperactive tendon reflexes, Babinski's signs, emotional apathy, perseveration, poor attention span, and a reduced avoidance to pain (Good & Couch, 1994). Facial masking, drooling, bradykinesia, lethargy, reduced spontaneous movement, and tremor of the lips, tongue, and fingers may also be present (Good & Couch, 1994). Furthermore, gait may be unstable, and may be characterized by short, shuffling steps (Good & Couch, 1994).

Dystonia characterizes prolonged muscle contractions that cause abnormal movements and posture of the extremities, such as overextension or overflexion of the hand, inversion of the foot, or torsion of the spine or back (Sanger et al., 2003). When limited to specific regions of the body, it may appear as writer's cramp, blepharospasm, torticollis, or opisthotonus (Sanger et al., 2003). Other features presenting with dystonia typically include athetosis, poor dexterity, oromotor abnormalities, and abnormal muscle activation (Sanger et al., 2003). Rigidity refers to the resistance to forced joint movement, inability to return toward a posture or angle, and resistance to reversal in direction of movement by a joint (Sanger et al., 2003). Referred to as "lead-pipe" posture, rigidity may be associated with bradykinesia, tremor, flexed posture, and gait disturbance (Sanger et al., 2003).

DIAGNOSIS

Clinical assessment and neurophysiological evaluation are necessary to make a clear diagnosis. Observation, focusing on posture and range of motion, is essential (Hardong & Beech, 1996). Muscle tone can be clinically assessed with passive movement about a joint, evaluating muscle resistance (Sanger et al., 2003). A palpation of muscles can be used to estimate muscle resting state (Sanger et al., 2003). Electromyography can be used to identify abnormal muscle activity (Richardson et al., 2000). Recordings of muscles at rest with passive stretch can afford information regarding the resting state of the muscles and stretch reflexes (Richardson et al., 2000). By examining agonist and antagonist muscles simultaneously with movement, abnormal cocontraction may be observed as well as the level of voluntary strength of agonist muscles (Richardson et al., 2000). Long-term video recordings may be useful in detecting subtle abnormalities (Volpe, 2008).

When making the diagnosis of hypertonia, or a condition with predominant hypertonic features, further evaluation for other causative factors is necessary. Such attributions may include trauma to the central nervous system (e.g., cervical spinal cord injury, dorsal spine fracture dislocation, spinal compression) and surgical complications (e.g., cordotomy). Other conditions to simultaneously consider include infectious disorders (e.g., syphilis, rabies, tetanus, meningitis), neoplastic disorders (e.g., vertebral metastasis, pheochromocytoma), biochemical disorders (e.g., hypocalcemia, hypoglycemia), deficiency disorders (e.g., pellagra), developmental disorders (e.g., spinal cord angioma), genetic disorders (e.g., infantile neuroaxonal dystrophy, Schwartz–Jampel's syndrome, pseudohypoparathyroidism, Canavan's disease), and age-related disorders (e.g., multiple sclerosis, cerebral cortical atrophy). A psychiatric disorder may be suspected, such as a conversion disorder or anxiety. Sleep deficiency, extreme stress or fear, multi-infarct dementia, hypertension, and hyperventilation all may produce symptoms similar to hypertonia. Drugs (e.g., caffeine, benzodiazepine withdrawal, amphetamine, ephedra) may artificially produce muscle tension.

TREATMENT

Often the treatment for hypertonia is to maintain range of motion and prevent such secondary problems as pain, subluxation, and contracture. Treatment needs are guided by the distribution of spasticity, comorbidity of other conditions, age of the patient, previous treatment attempts, possible side effects, prior reactions to treatments, cost, and dosage needs (Sarnat & Curatolo, 2007). Drugs, including baclofen, diazepam, and dantrolene can be used to reduce spasticity. The dopamine precursor 3,4-dihydroxy-L-phenylalanine can be used in such cases as dystonia and Parkinson's disease to offset dopamine deficits. Botulism toxin can be used with regard to spasticity and other positive features, as it has been found to improve the passive range of movement around the distal limb joint (Richardson et al., 2000). Treatment to help maintain motion typically includes physiotherapy, targeting avoidance of contractures and improvement of strength and body perception, and physical therapy, with active stretching and motion exercises. Daily exercise and stretching is mostly suggested to prevent pain and resistance of movement and can reduce tone for several hours. Splinting may be necessary to prevent certain muscles from tightening. Selective dorsal rhizotomy, a procedure in which the nerves that cause spasticity are cut, can be used in severe cases.

Jessica Holster
Charles Golden

Cratty, B. J. (1994). *Clumsy child syndromes: Descriptions, evaluations, and remediation.* Langhorne, PA: Harwood Academic Publishers.

Gilbert, S. L., Zhang, L., Forster, M. L., Tamaki, I., Soliven, B., Donahue, L. R., et al. (2002). Trak1 mutation disrupts GABA$_A$ receptor homeostasis in hypertonic mice. *Nature Genetics, 38,* 245–250.

Good, D. C., & Couch, J. R. (Eds.). (1994). *Handbook of neurorehabilitation.* New York: Marcel Dekker.

Harding, L., & Beech, J. R. (Eds.). (1996). *Assessment in neuropsychology.* New York: Routledge.

Lippincott Williams & Wilkins. (2004). *Pathophysiology: A 2-in-1 reference for nurses.* Philadelphia: Author.

Mix, C. L., Abt, I. A., Ridlon, J., & Parker, C. A. (Eds.). (1915). *Pediatrics, orthopedic surgery: Vol 5. The practical medicine series.* Chicago: Year Book.

Porth, C., Gaspard, K. J., & Matfin, G. (2006). *Essentials of pathophysiology: Concepts of altered heath states.* Lippincott Williams & Wilkins. 0781770874

Richardson, D., Sheean, G., Werring, D., Desai, M., Edwards, S., Greenwood, R., et al. (2000). Evaluating the role of botulinum toxin in the management of focal hypertonia in adults. *Journal of Neurology, Neurosurgery, & Psychiatry, 69,* 499–506.

Sanger, T. D., Delgado, M. R., Gaebler-Spira, D., Hallett, M., Mink, J. W., & the Task Force on Childhood Motor Disorders. (2003). Classification and definition of disorders causing hypertonia in childhood. *Pediatrics, 112,* 1462–1463.

Sarnat, H. B., & Curatolo, P. (Eds.). (2007). *Handbook of clinical neurology.* San Francisco: Elsevier.

Volpe, J. J. (2008). *Neurology of the newborn* (5th ed.). New York: Elsevier Science.

HYPOTONIA

DESCRIPTION

Hypotonia involves a loss of or abnormally low muscle tone. Tone describes a muscle's tension, whereas strength refers to the ability to modify a muscle's structure. Hypotonia is a symptom of many disorders and can have numerous etiologies—congenital, acquired, or neurological. It can result from congenital disorders such as Tay-Sachs disease, Prader-Willi syndrome, or cerebral palsy. It can be acquired through diseases such as myasthenia gravis, meningitis, encephalitis, infections, and muscular dystrophy. Neurological damage, such as brain trauma, lesions in the cerebellum, and upper or lower motor neuron dysfunction, can also produce hypotonia.

Hypotonia results in a disturbance of voluntary movement as muscles are not under full control. Directed movements may be overly fast or slow in execution. It is characterized by decreased muscle tension, decreased voluntary movements, and hypermotility (appearing double-jointed). Some individuals manifest postural instability. It is most often diagnosed in infancy (infantile hypotonia, "floppy infant syndrome"), and its course varies across the lifetime depending on the etiology. The long-term effects and outcome depend on the nature of the underlying disease and its severity. Hypotonia manifests along a continuum, which ranges from minimal to debilitating impairment. It can involve an individual's entire body or just specific limbs depending upon the underlying cause.

NEUROPATHOLOGY/PATHOPHYSIOLOGY

There is no specific etiology for hypotonia. If it arises from a specific disease, symptoms vary according to

H

the underlying cause. Damage to the peripheral nervous system produces localized hypotonia and muscle weakness, whereas damage to the central nervous system results in low muscle tone with normal muscle strength and tends to affect the entire body. Hypotonia resulting from a stroke is transient and dissipates as the body recovers functioning. It is associated with lesions in the cerebellar pathway, which is responsible for muscle coordination and balance. When a lesion is acute, ipsilateral (same side) hypotonia results. Lesions in the ventral lateral nucleus of the thalamus produce contralateral (opposite side) hypotonia.

Hypotonia can develop due to motor neuron dysfunction. Atrophy of motor neurons in the cerebellum can produce ataxia and hypotonia. Disruption in the flow of information to or from either the lower or upper motor neurons results in hypotonia. Reduced motor neuron activity affects the muscle fibers, leading to ineffective muscle activation that prevents contractures from occurring. In addition, the muscles may become unable to respond to nerve impulses.

NEUROPSYCHOLOGICAL/CLINICAL PRESENTATION

Clinically, individuals with hypotonia evidence motor difficulties. They struggle to initiate movement and follow a movement through to completion. Compound sequences of movements are particularly hard for them to perform, as are rapidly alternating sequences of movements. An individual may be slow in performing movements or performs them in a rapid, jerky fashion. An individual's facial muscles may be affected, which can lead to slurred or poorly pronounced speech and drooling. In addition, postural instabilities often result, leading to a round-shouldered posture and leaning on stationary objects for extra support. Gait disturbances in the form of unsteady pace or weaving may also result. Furthermore, gross and fine motor skills are usually affected, leading to difficulties manipulating objects and writing.

Hypotonia by itself does not affect intellectual or cognitive functioning; however, concurrent disorders can have effects ranging from mental retardation to normal functioning. Individuals may experience difficulties with sensory motor functioning, affecting their performance on educational tasks. The most profoundly affected area is motor performance. Depending on the physical body parts affected, individuals can manifest severe impairment on measures of motor functioning due to difficulties sustaining movement, manipulating objects, and repeating movements.

DIAGNOSIS

Hypotonia needs to be differentiated from muscle weakness, which involves low strength and normal tone. One way in which to establish a diagnosis of hypotonia is through a physical examination in which range of motion of limbs is assessed. Individuals with hypotonia show an extension beyond that which is normal when manipulated. They appear similar to individuals who are double-jointed, but do not display tension when overextended. A pendular reflex is often present upon examination, which is when a reflex is stimulated, and instead of reacting once and returning to the resting position, the limb keeps swinging in the absence of other stimuli.

A thorough examination should be conducted, including assessment of motor and sensory skills, reflexes, and nerve functioning. Diagnosing the underlying cause is difficult, and many tests may be used to assess the concurrent disease process. If brain dysfunction is suspected due to gait disturbance or head trauma, CT scans and MRIs may be used. If motor neuron dysfunction is suspected, electromyogram and nerve conduction studies are used to assess muscle strength and functioning. EMGs can help establish the precise location of hypotonia within the body, thereby assisting in identifying the underlying cause. Genetic testing and blood work can also be used to identify the etiology to provide assistance in determining appropriate interventions.

TREATMENT

There is no cure for hypotonia. If the underlying cause is known, treatment is provided for that specific disorder or condition if available. Once the nature and extent of an individual's hypotonia is established, physical therapy, occupational therapy, speech therapy, and orthopedic devices are provided as necessary. Physical therapy focuses on improving an individual's gross motor skills to compensate for disturbances in daily functioning. Muscle strength is increased if possible, and the individual works on obtaining as much muscle control as possible. In more severe cases, therapy focuses on preventing muscle atrophy. Occupational therapy assists in improving fine motor control, such as handwriting and grasping objects. If an individual experiences breathing, swallowing, or pronunciation difficulties, speech therapy can be used. Orthopedic devices such as braces or splints may be used in more severe cases, as well as surgery.

Christine Corsun-Ascher
Charles Golden

Brazis, P. W., Masdeu, J. C., & Biller, J. (2006). *Localization in clinical neurology.* Philadelphia: Lippincott Williams & Wilkins.

DeMyer, W. (2003). *Technique of the neurologic examination: A programmed text.* New York: McGraw-Hill Professional.

Dow, R. S., & Moruzzi, G. (1958). *The physiology and pathology of the cerebellum.* Minnesota: University of Minnesota.

Farrel, M. H., & Oski, J. A. (2000). *The portable pediatrician.* Philadelphia: Elsevier Health Sciences.

Fletcher-Jansen, E., & Reynolds, C. R. (2004). *Concise encyclopedia of special education: A reference for the education of the handicapped and other exceptional children and adults.* Hoboken, NJ: John Wiley and Sons.

Howle, J. M. (2002). *Neuro-developmental treatment approach: Theoretical foundations and principles of clinical practice.* California: Neuro Developmental Treatment.

National Institute of Neurological Disorders and Stroke. (2007). *Hypotonia information page.* Retrieved December 13, 2008, from http://www.ninds.nih.gov/disorders/hypotonia/hypotonia.htm

Qontro Imprint. (2008). *Hypotonia medical guide: quality guide to understanding and learning about a serious medical disease.* USA: Filiquarian Publishing, LLC.

Sladky, J. T. (2005). Neuromuscular disease in children. In R. B. David (Ed.), *Child and adolescent neurology: Blackwell's neurology and psychiatry access series* (pp. 416–419). Boston: Blackwell Publishing.

H

INCREASED INTRACRANIAL PRESSURE

DESCRIPTION

Increased intracranial pressure (ICP) is a serious medical emergency that is often fatal. Rises in ICP are associated with and can stem from any condition that increases the volume of the intracranial vault, such as brain tumors, subarachnoid hemorrhage, encephalitis, trauma, and brain edema following cerebral infarctions (Ropper, 1998).

In healthy adults, ICP normally falls in the range of 0–15 mmHg, with pressure close to 0 in a standing position and pressure close to 8 in the recumbent position. Pressures between 20 and 40 mmHg are generally considered abnormal and may be associated with increased morbidity, although this depends in part on the specific pathology. In hydrocephalus, for instance, pressures above 15 mmHg can be considered elevated, whereas anything above 20–25 mmHg following head injury is considered abnormal and usually initiates aggressive treatment (Czosnyka & Pickard, 2004). As pressures increase beyond 40 mmHg, there is ischemic damage to neurons and loss of consciousness secondary to diminished cerebral perfusion pressure (CPP) and cerebral blood flow (Ropper & Brown, 2005). Pressures greater than 60 mmHg are imminently fatal due to global ischemia and brain death (Gennarelli & Graham, 2005; Ropper & Brown, 2005).

NEUROPATHOLOGY/PATHOPHYSIOLOGY

The brain, blood, and cerebrospinal fluid (CSF) are contained within the confines of the skull, vertebral canal, and dura mater. Because this container is a closed system that is rigid and relatively inelastic, volumetric increases in any one of these three components must occur at the expense of the other two, a relationship that is known as the "Monroe–Kellie" doctrine (Ropper & Brown, 2005). Thus, raised ICP can result from increases in any one of the intracranial contents. Although there are regulatory mechanisms in place that try to compensate for any increases in volume, they can become exhausted if the volumes (brain, blood, or CSF) continue to increase.

ICP is normally in equilibrium with CSF pressure, and both pressures are largely derived from transmitted vascular pressures (Ropper & Brown, 2005). Therefore, two ways in which ICP can increase are through disturbances of CSF pressure and an increase in venous pressure (Table 1). CPP is the difference between mean ICP measurements and mean arterial blood pressure. CPP is an important variable in that a sufficient level of CPP is required to maintain stable cerebral blood flow (Czosnyka & Pickard, 2004). Increases in ICP, however, cause reductions in CPP and subsequently cerebral blood flow. With severely low CPP/cerebral blood flow, global ischemia can occur, eventually causing brain death.

Following injury to the brain, increased ICP can also occur secondary to mass effects and brain swelling within the confines of the skull (Gennarelli & Graham, 2005). As ICP increases, cerebral circulation and normal cerebral perfusion become compromised, which when unchecked, can ultimately lead to tissue deformation, midline shift, the development of internal hernias, and secondary damage to the upper brainstem (Gennarelli & Graham, 2005).

Table 1
CAUSES OF INCREASED INTRACRANIAL PRESSURE

Causes	Examples
Cerebral or extracerebral mass, which deforms the adjacent brain	Brain tumor, infarction with edema, contusion, hematoma
Generalized brain swelling	Ischemic-anoxic states, hypertensive encephalopathy
Increase in venous pressure	Cerebral venous sinus thrombosis, heart failure, obstruction of the superior mediastinal or jugular veins
Obstruction of CSF flow or absorption	Extensive meningeal disease, hydrocephalus
CSF volume expansion	Meningitis, subarachnoid hemorrhage

IJK

NEUROPSYCHOLOGICAL/CLINICAL PRESENTATION

The primary clinical features of increased ICP include headache, nausea, altered levels of consciousness, papilledema, and vomiting. Clinical assessments cannot accurately quantify increased ICP due to inconsistencies in symptom presentation in addition to the fact that increased ICP may occur in the absence of primary neurologic signs and symptoms (Celis & Robertson, 2008). Indeed, patients can remain normally alert with an ICP of 25–40 mmHg if they have normal blood pressure. Clinical features of increased ICP also differ in infants and small children because their cranial sutures have not yet closed.

DIAGNOSIS

The ventricular catheter connected to an external pressure transducer has been the gold standard for measuring ICP since 1960 (Celis & Robertson, 2008). Diagnosis can also be made through neuroimaging (CT or MRI) or spinal tap, although increased ICP can be present without positive neuroimaging findings such as edema or midline shift. Noninvasive techniques include tympanic membrane displacement, transcranial Doppler's sonography, venous ophthalmodynamometry, tissue resonance analysis, and latency of visual evoked potentials (Celis & Robertson, 2008; Czosnyka & Pickard, 2004).

TREATMENT

The primary treatment goal of increased ICP is to decrease the volume of any one of the three contents within the intracranial vault — blood, brain tissue, or CSF. Ventriculostomy is an effective method of reducing ICP by draining CSF from the frontal horn of the lateral ventricle. With use of ventriculostomy catheters, however, comes the risk of serious complication including ventriculitis and hemorrhage, which are the most common reasons for not monitoring ICP. ICP monitoring is recommended for comatose traumatic brain injury patients with abnormal CT scans and Glasgow Coma Scale scores of 3–8 to assist in the early detection of intracranial mass lesions and to help in informing prognosis (Hartl & Ghajar, 2005).

Ropper (1998) also outlined three medical treatments for raised ICP. The first is hyperosmolar therapy, or the use of osmotic agents, to extract extracelluar water from brain tissue. Mannitol is the most commonly used agent. The second form of medical treatment is to constrict blood vessels via hyperventilation or the use of high-dose barbiturates, thereby reducing cerebral blood volume. Hyperventilation theoretically works by reducing arterial carbon dioxide pressure, which subsequently causes a serum and CSF alkalosis, which in turn leads to cerebral vasoconstriction. Lastly, the third medical treatment is to help prevent reversible causes of edema and avoidable elevations of cerebral blood flow, such as hypertension, fever, and hypoxia.

Anita H. Sim
Maya Yutsis

Celis, R., & Robertson, C. S. (2008). Neuromonitoring in traumatic brain injury. In A. Bhardwaj, D. B. Ellegala, & J. R. Kirsch (Eds.), *Acute brain and spinal cord injury* (pp. 67–80). New York: Informa Healthcare USA.

Czosnyka, M., & Pickard, J. D. (2004). Monitoring and interpretation of intracranial pressure. *Journal of Neurology, Neurosurgery, and Psychiatry, 75,* 813–821.

Gennarelli, T. A., & Graham, D. I. (2005). Neuropathology. In J. M. Silver, T. W. McAllister & S. C. Yudofsky (Eds.), *Textbook of traumatic brain injury* (pp. 27–50). Washington, DC: American Psychiatric Publishing.

Hartl, R., & Ghajar, J. (2005). Neurosurgical interventions. In J. M. Silver, T. W. McAllister & S. C. Yudofsky (Eds.), *Textbook of traumatic brain injury* (pp. 51–58). Washington, DC: American Psychiatric Publishing.

Ropper, A. H. (1998). Principles of coma and neurologic emergencies. In J. H. Stein (Ed.), *Internal medicine* (5th ed., pp. 1081–1085). St. Louis, MO: Mosby.

Ropper, A. H., & Brown, R. H. (2005). *Adam and Victor's principles of neurology* (8th ed.). New York: McGraw-Hill.

INFANTILE HYPOTONIA

DESCRIPTION

Infantile hypotonia is a disease that presents shortly after birth, characterized by a loss or deficiency in muscle tone stemming from a multitude of disorders. Children affected by infantile hypotonia have trouble flexing and utilizing their muscles for extended periods of time and in severe cases, lack the ability to move their muscles at all. The disorder affects males and females equally and can have lifelong consequences on development and learning. In addition to hypotonia, muscle weakness is commonly present although it is not the primary malfunction of the disorder.

Typically, these infants visually present as "floppy" due to muscles being unable to support their limbs and head, which hang loosely off their body. This "floppy" presentation has given rise to the nickname "floppy infant syndrome" for infantile hypotonia. When picking up a normal infant underneath the arms, the muscles will support the child. In a child with hypotonia, the muscles in the arm and shoulders are absent, causing the child to slip through the grasp.

Children struggle to meet developmental milestones such as sitting up, holding themselves up, crawling, and walking due to muscle dysfunction. They are also at risk for respiratory and esophageal complications. The underlying condition is usually one that affects the central nervous system through a congenital disorder or an acquired muscle disorder. However, diagnosing the etiology is a difficult task due to the complexity of causes; there are frequently some clues to narrow down the disorder's origin, but not always.

Infantile hypotonia is most commonly seen as a manifestation of other disorders with Prader–Willi syndrome being the most common, rather than the solitary feature of pathology. Some of the most common disorders which present with infantile hypotonia are Down's syndrome, myasthenia gravis, Prader–Willi syndrome, infant botulism, malnutrition, familial dysautonomia, spinal muscular atrophy (SMA) Type 1, Tay–Sachs' disease, and congenital hypothyroidism.

NEUROPATHOLOGY/PATHOPHYSIOLOGY

The most common neuropathological causes for infantile hypotonia are SMA, congenital muscular dystrophy (CMD), glycogen storage disease, congenital myopathy, and Type II fiber atrophy. SMA is an autosomal recessive hereditary neurodegenerative disease that most commonly results in the degeneration of anterior horn cells in the spinal cord. CMD is a group of autosomal recessive neuromuscular disorders that presents with a degeneration of muscle fibers and a replacement of muscle by adipose connective tissues. Glycogen storage disease is a group of disorders that alter the metabolism of glycogen, which affects the skeletal muscle and leaves the infant susceptible to enlargements of the liver and heart. This form of dysfunction often results in death due to cardiac or respiratory failure. CMD can stem from several sources including centronuclear myopathy, central core myopathy, nemaline myopathy, and congenital fiber type disproportion. Type II fiber atrophy seen in infantile hypotonia results primarily from disuse of the muscle or from a lack of stimulation, which is commonly seen in mental retardation.

NEUROPSYCHOLOGICAL/CLINICAL PRESENTATION

An infant affected by hypotonia will present as if they have no bones in their body with their limbs loosely hanging by their sides and their head "flopping" to the front, back, and sides. A lack of control of muscles in their arms and legs leaves gross motor as well as fine motor control impaired to nonexistent in severe cases. The clinician will also see delays in developmental milestones such as holding themselves up, sitting upright, walking, talking, and feeding themselves. Although children will acquire some of these skills as they grow older, they will do so at a slower rate than other children. Hypotonic children will also be more susceptible to learning problems, language delays, or attentional problems. Not all children will develop significant cognitive difficulties and with early intervention, can reach normal development. The inability to coordinate fine motor skills necessary for grasping, manipulating objects, and speaking will cause impairments on most neuropsychological batteries and can make testing infants with hypotonia difficult.

DIAGNOSIS

Until the recent utilization of DNA-based diagnostic testing, diagnosis rested heavily on clinical presentation or invasive procedures including electrophysiologic studies, muscle biopsy, and spinal tap in order to test for cerebral spinal fluid abnormalities. Infants with hypotonia present a challenge to the clinician due to the disorder having a wide number of possible etiologies. Examining the infant during various stages of arousal is a key element in diagnosis. A physical examination assessing muscle reflexes, tone, and flexibility is still a primary evaluation tool.

More recently, molecular diagnosis through a karyotype test or structural analysis through CT cranial imaging has provided useful information for diagnosis. The karyotype test is a blood test that specifically looks for chromosomal abnormalities that would point to a genetic inheritance. Recent literature has indicated a majority of infants with hypotonia have a genetic defect, structural central nervous system abnormalities, or a cerebral structural abnormality that would cause their muscle dysfunction. Due to the large genetic loading, a thorough family history aiming at maternal neurological disorders, neonatal complications, neuromuscular disorders, or muscle

IJK

weakness and obtaining a medical history of the infant is routine. Connective tissue disorders, neglect, and malnourishment should also be considered as a differential diagnosis. Early diagnosis is essential for effective management and a better prognosis.

TREATMENT

Treatment for infantile hypotonia includes sensory stimulation programs designed to help the child respond to stimuli by sight, sound, touch, smell, and taste. Occupational therapy is recommended for developing fine motor movements of the hands and fingers specially targeted to enable successful daily living skills. Physical therapy is also effective in helping develop motor coordination and muscle strength that helps build muscle tone over time. Dietary restrictions are occasionally needed to control for excessive caloric intake or monitoring comorbid disorders. In severe cases, speech therapy will be needed to assist the child in swallowing, feeding, and communication development. As the child grows older, supportive therapy is also implemented for assistance in dealing with living with this disorder.

David Ritchie
Charles Golden

Birdi, K., Prasad, A., Prasad, C., Chodirker, B., & Chudley, A. (2005). The floppy infant: Retrospective analysis of clinical experience (1990–2000) in a tertiary care facility. *Journal of Child Neurology, 20*(10), 803–808.

Carboni, P., Pisani, F., Crescenzi, A., & Villani, C. (2002). Congenital hypotonia with favorable outcome. *Pediatric Neurology, 26*(5), 383–386.

National Organization for Rare Disorders. (2007). *NORD compendium of rare diseases and disorders.* New Rochelle, NY: Mary Ann Leibert.

Premasiri, M., & Lee, Y. S. (2003). The myopathology of floppy and hypotonic infants in Singapore. *Pathology, 35*(5), 409–413.

Richer, L. P., Shevell, M. I., & Miller, S. P. (2001). Diagnostic profile of neonatal hypotonia: An 11-year study. *Pediatric Neurology, 25*(1), 32–37.

Rowland, L. P. (Ed.). (2005). *Merrit's neurology: Integrating the physical exam and echocardiography.* Baltimore: Lippincott Williams & Wilkins.

Shah, S. M., & Kelly, K. M. (2003). *Principles and practice of emergency neurology: Handbook for emergency physicians.* Cambridge, MA: Cambridge University Press.

Trifirò, G., Livieri, C., Bosio, L., Gargantini, L., Corrias, A., Pozzan, G., et al. (2003). Neonatal hypotonia: Don't forget the Prader-Willi syndrome. *Acta Paediatrica, 92*(9), 1085–1089.

INFANTILE NEUROAXONAL DYSTROPHY

DESCRIPTION

Infantile neuroaxonal dystrophy (INAD), also referred to as Seitelberger's disease, is one of the three neuroaxonal dystrophies, characterized by severe, early-onset degeneration of the axonal bodies. Although the disorder is known to be highly rare, prevalence rates have not been established. The disorder was first described by Seitelberger in 1952 as a possible infantile form of Hallervorden–Spatz disease (Herman, Huttenlocher, & Bensch, 1969). Seitelberger documented four children who exhibited abnormal changes in central nervous system functioning and the development of spheroid bodies, now an acknowledged hallmark of the disorder (Chow & Padfield, 2008; Herman et al., 1969). Cowen and Olmstead in 1963 were the first to use the term INAD, describing the disorder as a unique disease entity (Herman et al., 1969). Children may appear normal at birth but soon develop symptoms between the ages of 6 months and 2 years (Nardocci et al., 1999). Features include initial developmental delays and regression of acquired skills, followed by motor, sensorial, and cognitive impairment (Khateeb et al., 2006; Nardocci et al., 1999). Affected children eventually cannot walk, hear, or see, succumbing to the disease by the age of 10 (Chow & Padfield, 2008; Gordon, 2002; Nardocci et al., 1999).

NEUROPATHOLOGY/PATHOPHYSIOLOGY

The locus for INAD has been mapped to a 1.17-Mb locus on chromosome 22q13.1, with an identified mutation in *PLA2G6* (Chow & Padfield, 2008). Of individuals diagnosed with INAD, 78% exhibit a *PLA2G6* mutation (Kurian et al., 2008). As an autosomal recessive disorder, both parents must be carriers of the mutated *PLA2G6* gene to produce an affected child (Nardocci et al., 1999). With mutation at *PLA2G6*, encoding of isoforms is negatively affected, and an alteration of the shorter enzymatically inactive isoforms occurs, causing inaction (Morgan et al., 2006). Defects in iPLA$_2$ß, a calcium-independent enzyme critical in cell membrane homeostasis, are suspected to underlie the axonal pathology found in INAD (Shinzawa et al., 2008). In mice, deficits in iPLA$_2$ß have been found to lead to motor impairment, spheroids, and vacuoles within the nervous system, suggesting that iPLA$_2$ß dysfunction causes neuroaxonal dystrophy (Shinzawa et al., 2008). These may be a product of changes in membrane permeability, fluidity, and/or ion homeostasis (Shinzawa et al., 2008). Spheroid bodies typically are found in both the central and peripheral nervous systems, found in a rostrocaudal (i.e., anterior to posterior) direction, consisting of proteins but no nucleoproteins (Chow & Padfield, 2008). The spheroid bodies consist of carbohydrate, lipid, and glycogen granules, with a high activity of oxidative enzymes (Chow & Padfield, 2008). The spheroids of the nucleus gracilis demonstrate elevated levels of α-glycero-phosphate dehydrogenase (Chow & Padfield, 2008).

In INAD, axonal changes are present in the tegmentum, thalamus, cerebral and cerebellar cortex, cerebellar nuclei, and posterior columns of the spinal cord (Chow & Padfield, 2008). MRI results show cerebellar atrophy, mainly involving the inferior part of the vermis, and signal hyperintensity of the cerebellar cortex (Nardocci et al., 1999). High iron in the globus pallidus has been reported among 77% of INAD patients using imaging, which can be seen as reduced signal on T2, FLAIR, and T2 gradient and diffusion-weighted MRI sequences or reduced density on a CT scan (Kurian et al., 2008; Morgan et al., 2006). The severity of globus pallidus changes has been correlated with age (Kurian et al., 2008). Iron deposits in the substantia nigra and subthalamic nuclei are present by age 5 (Kurian et al., 2008). Other characteristics on examination include reduced volume in the optic chiasm and optic nerves, suggesting optic pathway atrophy and widespread high amplitude, nonreactive, fast activity at 16–22 Hz with electroencephalogram during both the wake and sleep states, indicating a loss of nerve supply (Aicardi & Castelein, 1979; Kurian et al., 2008). Electromyography also shows chronic denervation, whereas cerebrospinal fluid protein levels are typically normal (Aicardi & Castelein, 1979; Khateeb et al., 2006; Kurian et al., 2008).

NEUROPSYCHOLOGICAL/CLINICAL PRESENTATION

INAD presents in infancy, beginning by age 2 (Nardocci et al., 2008). Symptoms typically initiate after illness, with stress leading to rapid decompensation (Kurian et al., 2008). Appearing in both genders, initial symptoms include slowed psychomotor development and psychomotor regression (Nardocci et al., 1999). Hypotonia, muscle atrophy, pyramidal tract signs with extensor plantar responses, bulbar signs (i.e., difficulty swallowing, dyspnea, and sphincter disturbances), exaggerated deep tendon reflexes, speech deficits, impaired hearing, and spasticity present shortly thereafter (Aicardi & Castelein, 1979; Khateeb et al., 2006; Kurian et al., 2008). Progressive mental

deterioration coincides with the onset of motor difficulties (Kurian et al., 2008). Visual symptoms include nystagmus, strabismus, incoordinate eye movements, optic atrophy, and blindness (Aicardi & Castelein, 1979; Kurian et al., 2008). Sensorial deficits include limited reaction to pinprick and touch (Aicardi & Castelein, 1979).

Mutations in *PLA2G6* also are associated with rapid progression of bulbar dysfunction, spasticity, intentional tremor, dystonia, cerebellar ataxia, contractures, spinal deformity, and dementia (Kurian et al., 2008). Extrapyramidal symptoms, epilepsy, and dysmorphic features are absent (Kurian et al., 2008). Seizures may occur, in partial or generalized convulsive forms, but are rare (Nardocci et al., 1999). Physical features include a prominent forehead, strabismus, small nose, fish mouth, micrognathia, and large and low-set ears. Bedridden by the age of 3, most patients are never able to walk (Nardocci et al., 1999). The ability to sit, stand, and walk in those who learn is lost shortly after the onset of symptoms, often leaving patients blind, tetraplegic, demented, and helpless (Aicardi & Castelein, 1979). Death usually results before the age of 10 (Chow & Padfield, 2008; Gordon, 2002).

DIAGNOSIS

A diagnosis of INAD is made based on a combination of neurological evidence and clinical findings. The presence of axonal bodies, with an onset before the age of 3, a progressive course of spastic tetraplegia, blindness, and dementia presenting by age 4, and psychomotor deterioration including increasing pyramidal tract signs and truncal hypotonia are criteria used to diagnose INAD (Pryse-Phillips, 2003). The presence of abnormal facial features may make the disorder more definitive. Electromyography and MRI results are useful in detecting chronic denervation and cerebellar atrophy (Nardocci et al., 1999). Imaging is needed to detect cerebellar atrophy and the presence of iron within the brain (Morgan et al., 2006). Abnormal electroencephalogram results can be found before age 5 (Niedermeyer & Lopes da Silva, 2004). Histological examination of samples from conjunctiva, skin, rectum, sural nerve, and muscle, supported by electron microscopy, can be utilized to detect spheroid bodies (Chow & Padfield, 2008). Patients with a mutation of *PLA2G6* without the presence of dystrophic axons also can present with a clinical diagnosis of INAD (Morgan et al., 2007). Carrier detection and prenatal diagnosis in affected families are possible with genetic testing.

The most common misdiagnoses of INAD include Hallervorden–Spatz disease, neuroaxonal

IJK

IJK

leucoencephalopathy, spinal muscular atrophy, myopathy, and Schindler disease Type I. In other neuroaxonal dystrophies, including Hallervorden–Spatz disease and neuroaxonal leucoencephalopathy, axonal spheroids are also present (Chow & Padfield, 2008). However, in Hallervorden–Spatz disease cortical involvement is less pronounced, and spheroids are less widespread and most prominent in the basal ganglia, substantia nigra, brainstem, and spinal cord than in INAD (Chow & Padfield, 2008). Neuroaxonal leucoencephalopathy is deciphered from INAD by the presence of severe, subacute dementia, the absence of hyperproteinorrachia, normal nerve conduction velocities, and leucocytes or fibroblasts (Aicardi & Castelein, 1979). Spinal muscular atrophy and myopathy may look like INAD, because of muscle weakness and loss of voluntary movement. With respect to such diagnoses, genetic testing and/or the presence of leucocytes can be used to indicate INAD. Differentiation from Schindler disease Type I can be made through urinary oligosaccharide measurements and enzymatic assays of α-N-acetylgalactosaminidase activity among leukocytes or fibroblasts (Khateeb et al., 2006). Other misdiagnoses include gangliosidosis, metachromatic leukodystrophy, and Leigh's disease.

TREATMENT

At present, there is no known treatment that can stop or reverse the symptoms of INAD. Treatment may focus on individual symptoms and placating the patient, due to the lethality of the disorder. Pain medication is mainly prescribed to eliminate any discomfort. Physical and occupational therapy are recommended to maintain motor functioning and reduce the development of muscle contractures. Feeding tubes are necessary when it becomes too difficult for the patient to eat and swallow due to progressive muscle degeneration and weakness (Nardocci et al., 1999). A review of the literature did not produce any studies evaluating the efficacy or effectiveness of treatment options among patients with INAD.

Jessica Holster
Charles Golden

Aicardi, J., & Castelein, P. (1979). Infantile neuroaxonal dystrophy. *Brain: A Journal of Neurology, 102*, 727–748.

Chow, G., & Padfield, J. H. (2008). A case of infantile neuroaxonal dystrophy-connatal Seitelberger disease. *Journal of Child Neurology, 23*, 418–420.

Gordon, N. (2002). Infantile neuroaxonal dystrophy (Seitelberger's disease). *Developmental Medicine & Child Neurology, 44*, 849–851.

Herman, M. M., Huttenlocher, P. R., & Bensch, K. G. (1969). Electron microscopic observations in infantile neuroaxonal dystrophy. *Archives of Neurology, 20*, 19–34.

Khateeb, S., Flusser, H., Ofir, R., Shelef, I., Narkis, G., Vardi, G., et al. (2006). PLA2G6 mutation underlies infantile neuroaxonal dystrophy. *American Journal of Human Genetics, 79*, 942–948.

Kurian, M. A., Morgan, N. V., MacPherson, L., Foster, K., Peake, D., Gupta, R., et al. (2008). Phenotypic spectrum of neurodegeneration associated with mutations in the PLA2G6 gene. *Neurology, 70*, 1623–1629.

Morgan, N. V., Westaway, S. K., Morton, J. E., Gregory, A., Gissen, P., Sonek, S., et al. (2006). PLA2G6, encoding a phospholipase A2, is mutated in neurodegenerative disorders with high brain iron. *Natural Genetics, 38*, 752–754.

Nardocci, N., Zorzi, G., Farina, L., Binelli, S, Scaioli, W., Ciano, W., et al. (1999). Infantile neuroaxonal dystrophy: Clinical spectrum and diagnostic criteria. *Neurology, 52*, 1472.

Niedermeyer, E., & Lopes da Silva, F. H. (2004). *Electroencephalography: Basic principles, clinical applications, and related fields.* New York: Lippincott Williams & Wilkins.

Pryse-Phillips, W. (2003). *Companion to clinical neurology.* New York: Oxford University Press.

Shinzawa, K., Sumi, H., Ikawa, M., Matsuoka, Y., Okabe, M., Sakoda, S., et al. (2008). Neuroaxonal dystrophy caused by group VIA phospholipase A_2 deficiency in mice: A model of human neurodegenerative disease. *The Journal of Neuroscience, 28*, 2212–2220.

INFANTILE REFSUM DISEASE

DESCRIPTION

Infantile Refsum disease (IRD) is a variant of Refsum disease, a rare, autosomal recessive, peroxisomal disorder that is characterized by the accumulation of phytanic acid in the blood and tissue. IRD differs from Refsum disease in that the peroxisome dysfunction occurs in biogenesis, whereas the structure of the peroxisome is intact in classic Refsum disease (Wills, Manning, & Reilly, 2001). The disorder is characterized by neurological, ocular, and hepatic symptoms. Prognosis is poor with few patients surviving beyond 10 years (van Maldergem et al., 2005).

NEUROPATHOLOGY/PATHOPHYSIOLOGY

In IRD, development of peroxisomes is affected. As a result, a number of enzymes, including the enzyme phytanoyl-CoA hydroxylase, are deficient. The lack of these enzymes leads to a buildup of phytanic acid in the blood and various tissues, especially the liver. Although phytanic acid's role in the development of symptoms is unknown, a number of theories have been proposed.

The leading theory is that high levels of phytanic acid in the tissue lipids impair myelin formation. This malformation of the myelin sheaths is thought to cause the neuropathies and other neurological and neuropsychological symptoms seen in IRD patients (Wills et al., 2001). An alternative hypothesis proposes that increased levels of phytanic acid affect the metabolism of fat-soluble vitamins. With the reduction of their metabolism, vitamin levels become elevated in the tissue leading to the production of toxins. These toxins affect the development of new tissue and cause damage to existing tissue (Levy, 1970).

NEUROPSYCHOLOGICAL/CLINICAL PRESENTATION

IRD is thought to be on the mild spectrum of peroxisomal disorders. As a result, neurological and cognitive symptoms are frequently manifested by developmental delays or partial loss of function but rarely result in total lack of development or loss of function (Wills et al., 2001). Common symptoms of IRD include peripheral neuropathy, sensorineural deafness, visual deficits, mental retardation, and cerebellar ataxia. Postnatal growth can also be retarded resulting in failure to thrive. Motor skills are often deficient as is speech development (Poll-The et al., 2004). Visual problems like night blindness can occur and are usually secondary to retinitis pigmentosa.

DIAGNOSIS

Diagnosis of IRD may be difficult due to the varying symptomatology seen in patients. Four symptoms including peripheral neuropathy, retinitis pigmentosa, cerebellar ataxia, and increased concentration of cerebrospinal fluid (CSF) protein are commonly found in IRD patients. Elevated levels of phytanic acid in the blood and urine are seen. Sensorineuronal deafness, mental retardation, anosmia, distal polyneuropathy, cardiomyopathy, hepatomegaly, facial dysmorphism, and a bilateral shortening of the fourth metatarsal can also be indicators of IRD (Cakirer & Savas, 2005; Ropper & Brown, 2005).

Examination of MRI results reveals signal intensity abnormalities in the dentate nuclei and the periventricular white matter. Abnormal signals have also been seen in the corpus callosum and corticospinal tracts (Choksi, Hoeffner, Karaaslan, Yalcinkaya, & Cakirer, 2003; Dubois, Sebag, Argyropoulou, & Brunelle, 1991). Follow-up MRI scanning is recommended in order to monitor the progression of the disorder (Cakirer & Savas, 2005).

Autopsy findings in patients with IRD have shown fewer axons and a reduction of myelin in the corpus callosum, periventricular white matter, corticospinal tracts, and optic nerves. These results support signal abnormalities seen in MRI scans. Hypoplasia in the granule layer of the cerebellum and Purkinje cells ectopically located in the molecular layer were also seen (Torvik et al., 1988).

Other disorders similar to IRD include Zellweger syndrome, neonatal adrenoleukodystrophy (NALD), and hyperpipecolic acidemia. Chondrodysplasia and renal cysts are commonly seen in patients with Zellweger syndrome but are absent in IRD. In addition, though peroxisomes are dysfunctional in IRD, they are usually completely absent in Zellweger syndrome (Naidu & Moser, 1991). Like IRD, NALD is a disorder caused by an inability to metabolize certain fatty acids. Many of the symptoms are similar across the disorders; however, NALD is seen almost entirely in males (Ropper & Brown, 2005). Hyperpipecolic acidemia shares a peroxisomal defect with IRD. Yet in IRD, phytanic acid is not metabolized whereas metabolization of pipecolic acid is affected in hyperpipecolic acidemia (Tranchant et al., 1993).

TREATMENT

Currently, there is no cure for IRD. Progression of the disease can be slowed by eating a diet low in phytanic acid. Fish, beef, lamb, and dairy products have high levels of phytanic acid and should be avoided. Plasmapheresis should be considered when dietary control of the disorder is ineffective or when rapid reduction of the symptoms is required. Reversal of some of the neurological, cardiac, and dermatological symptoms has been demonstrated with the various treatments, although auditory and visual deficits are frequently less responsive (Wills et al., 2001). Recently, liver transplantation has been shown to be successful in lowering phytanic acid levels and ameliorating symptomatology. This new therapy is promising, yet future research is required to confirm its long-term utility (van Maldergem et al., 2005).

Daniel L. Frisch
Charles Golden

IJK

Cakirer, S., & Savas, M. R. (2005). Infantile Refsum disease: Serial evaluation with MRI. *Pediatric Radiology, 35*(2), 212–215.

Choksi, V., Hoeffner, E., Karaarslan, E., Yalcinkaya, C., & Cakirer, S. (2003). Infantile Refsum disease: Case report. *American Journal of Neuroradiology, 24*(10), 2082–2084.

Dubois, J., Sebag, G., Argyropoulou, M., & Brunelle, F. (1991). MR findings in infantile Refsum disease: Case report of two family members. *American Journal of Neuroradiology, 12*(6), 1159–1160.

Levy, I. S. (1970). Refsum's Syndrome. *Transcripts of the Ophthalmological Society of the UK. 90*, 181–186.

Naidu, S. B., & Moser, H. (1991). Infantile Refsum disease. *American Journal of Neuroradiology, 12*(6), 1161–1163.

Poll-The, B. T., Gootjes, J., Duran, M., De Klerk, J. B., Wenniger-Prick, L. J., Admiraal, R. J., et al. (2004). Peroxisome biogenesis disorders with prolonged survival: Phenotypic expression in a cohort of 31 patients. *American Journal of Medical Genetics Part A, 126A*(4), 333–338.

Ropper, A. H., & Brown, R. H. (2005). *Adams and Victor's principles of neurology* (8th ed.). New York: McGraw-Hill.

Torvik, A., Torp, S., Kase, B. F., Ek, J., Skjeldal, O., & Stokke, O. (1988). Infantile Refsum's disease: A generalized peroxisomal disorder. Case report with postmortem examination. *Journal of the Neurological Sciences, 85*(1), 39–53.

Tranchant, C., Aubourg, P., Mohr, M., Rocchiccioli, F., Zaenker, C., & Warter, J. M. (1993). A new peroxisomal disease with impaired phytanic and pipecolic acid oxidation. *Neurology, 43*(10), 2044–2048.

Van Maldergem, L., Moser, A. B., Vincent, M. F., Roland, D., Reding, R., Otte, J. B., et al. (2005). Orthotopic liver transplantation from a living-related donor in an infant with a peroxisome biogenesis defect of the infantile Refsum disease type. *Journal of Inherited Metabolic Disorders, 28*(4), 593–600.

Wills, A. J., Manning, N. J., & Reilly, M. M. (2001). Refsum's disease. *Quarterly Journal of Mathematics, 94*, 403–406.

INIENCEPHALY

DESCRIPTION

Iniencephaly is a rare neural tube defect arising from a constellation of posterior skull and superior spinal defects. The occipital bone is absent or has a large hole connecting to the foramen magnum. In addition, rachischisis or lordosis of the cervical and thoracic spine is seen due to fusion and disintegration of the vertebrae with extreme retroflexion of the head, presenting in a stargazing position (Halder, Pahi, Pradhan, & Pandey, 1998). First described by Saint-Hilare in 1836 (Stark, 1951), estimates of its incidence range from 1/1,000 to 1/65,000 births (Lewis, 1987; Nishimura & Okamoto, 1976) with a staunch female predominance (Kulaylat & Narchi, 2000).

Iniencephaly may present in two different forms, apertus and clausus, with an encephalocele projection through the occipital bone defect defining the former, whereas the clausus subtype does not present with an encephalocele. The literature has suggested iniencephaly may be a rare and severe form of Klippel–Feil's syndrome, which is discussed in further detail in this text (see Klippel–Feil's syndrome). It has also been commonly linked with Chiari-III defect and has been associated with a number of other central nervous system (CNS) and systemic manifestations discussed in the following.

Prognosis is very poor for infants born with iniencephaly. Many are spontaneously aborted or present as stillborn. Others live for only a short amount of time after birth (i.e., a few hours later). In very mild cases, particularly of the clausus subtype, surgical intervention may be considered but this is very rare and most infants die.

NEUROPATHOLOGY/PATHOPHYSIOLOGY

The pathological basis of iniencephaly is unknown. A few theories have prevailed. Gardner (1967, 1973) has proposed iniencephaly arises from altered growth and altered fluid dynamics of the CNS after the neuropores have closed. This was a modification of suggestions first made by Morgagni (ca. 1760), who suggested that intrauterine hydrocephalus early in prenatal development causes an increased, posterior push of fluid pressure that leads to a separation of the occipital bone region in addition to stemming hydromyelia. Another theory suggests that the entity arises from a failure of the foramen of Magendie to open, thereby causing local hydrocephalus and distension in the region of the fourth ventricle explaining the disruption of the fusion of the cervical neural arches (Nishimura & Okamoto, 1976). Although each theory attempts to explain the mechanism causing the structural defect, none posits a basis for the commencement of this domino effect. In all three instances, however, researchers have agreed that the defect likely arises approximately 47–52 days postgestation. Teratogenic exposure has been associated with iniencephaly including smoking, alcohol use, various illicit drugs, antibiotics including sulfonamide and tetracycline, antihistamines, and antitumor agents as well as infectious processes such as syphilis (Aleksic et al., 1983; Myriantopulos & Melnick, 1987). Still, some have suggested a genetic basis for the presentation arising from deviant gene expression in the embryonic period affecting the dorsoventral orientation of the body axis corresponding with notochordal malpositions (Kjaer, Mygind, & Fischer Hansen, 1999).

As discussed, iniencephaly presents anatomically with absent or incomplete occipital bone at the site of the foramen magnum, in combination with lordosis, rachisis, and variable degrees of fusion of inion with cervicothoracic spine and resultant severe dorsiflexion of head (Tugrul et al., 2007). Microencephaly, polymicrogyria, heterotopic glial tissue in the leptomeninges, atresia of the ventricular system, marked disorganization of the brainstem, vermian agenesis, cerebellar cysts, disorganization of the spinal cord, polyhydramnios, anencephaly, lissencephaly, encephalocele, diaphragmatic hernia, duodenal atresia, and omphalocele have all been associated with iniencephaly as well (Aleksic et al., 1983; Aleksic & Budzilovich, 1987).

NEUROPSYCHOLOGICAL/CLINICAL PRESENTATION

Data regarding neuropsychological/clinical presentation are, in many respects, nonexistent as most infants are stillborn. Those that are born alive often die within a few hours. Although diagnosis is most commonly made on fetal ultrasound, it may be indicated at the time of birth based on the infant's morphological features. They present with the previously discussed retroflexion of the head, in a stargazing position, and severe distortion of the spine. Much of the time the neck is actually absent leading to the skin of the face connecting directly to the skin of the chest and the skin at the back of the head connecting directly to the skin of the back. Additional CNS malformations are as noted previously. Lung hypoplasia, cardiovascular disorders, cleft lip and palate, diaphragmatic hernias, and gastrointestinal malformations may all be seen in those that survive, which, again, is quite rare.

DIAGNOSIS

Diagnosis of iniencephaly is most commonly made via fetal ultrasound. This is best done through sagittal sectioning of the spine to permit accurate evaluation of vertebral anomalies in combination with observation of the occipital bone and foramen magnum (Sahid et al., 2000). Attention should be paid to those hallmark anatomical features as discussed previously. Morphological description in the neonatal period may also be used if ultrasound diagnosis was not made, usually due to lack of availability or non-use. This is not often employed as most infants are stillborn or die within a few hours. It would often only be used

if the case was very mild and survival was possible. This would thus include CT and possibly cranial and spinal X-ray.

TREATMENT

There is no cure for iniencephaly and prognosis is very poor. Infants usually die after only a few hours postdelivery if they are not stillborn (Hammer, Scherrer, Baumann, Briner, & Schinzel, 1990). In cases of such severity that the infant will not live, termination of the pregnancy is sometimes recommended to protect the mother. For mild cases, counseling and thorough discussion with the parent(s) is recommended, both through a supportive and educational modality. In many of the instances, again, termination is often discussed as the distortion of the fetus poses considerable risk to the mother while in the context of the fact that survival is unlikely for the infant. For very mild cases, where survival is possible, neurosurgical intervention can be considered to offer some correction of the cervical deformity (Erdincler et al., 1998; Kulaylat & Narchi, 2000). However, it should be noted that the case reports on this are sparse. Based on a report by Erdincler et al. (1998), at that time only five surviving patients with iniencephaly were known.

Jacob M. Goings
Chad A. Noggle

Aleksic, S., Budzilovich, G., Greco, M. A., Feigin, I., Epstein, F., & Pearson, J. (1983). Iniencephaly: A neuropathologic study. *Clinical Neuropathology, 2,* 55–61.

Aleksic, S., & Budzilovich, G. N. (1987). Iniencephaly. In N. C. Myrianthopoulos (Ed.), *Handbook of clinical neurology* (Vol. 50, pp. 129–136). Amsterdam: Elsevier.

Erdincler, P., Kaynar, M. Y., Canbaz, B., Kocer, N., Kuday, C., & Ciplak, N. (1998). Iniencephaly: Neuroradiological and surgical features. Case report and review of the literature. *Journal of Neurosurgery, 89,* 317–320.

Gardner, W. J. (1967). Myelocele: Rupture of the neural tube? *Clinical Neurosurgery, 15,* 57–79.

Gardner, W. J. (1973). *The dysraphic states. From syringomyelia to anencephaly* (pp. 167–181). Amsterdam: Excerpta Medica.

Halder, A., Pahi, J., Pradhan, M., & Pandey, A. (1998). Iniencephaly—A report of 19 cases. *Indian Pediatrics, 35,* 891–896.

Hammer, F., Scherrer, C., Baumann, H., Briner, J., & Schinzel, A. (1990). Iniencephaly: prenatal and postnatal findings. *Geburtshilfe Frauenheilkd, 50,* 491–494.

Kjaer, I., Mygind, H., & Fischer Hansen, B. (1999). Notochordal remnants in human iniencephaly suggest disturbed dorsoventral axis signaling. *American Journal of Medical Genetics, 84,* 425–432.

Kulaylat, N. A., & Narchi, H. (2000). Iniencephaly: An uncommon neural tube defect. *Journal of Pediatrics, 136,* 414.

Lewis, H. F. (1987). Iniencephalus. *American Journal of Obstetrics and Gynecology, 35,* 11.

Myriantopulos, N. C., & Melnick, M. (1987). Studies in neural tube defects: Epidemiologic and etiologic agents. *American Journal of Medical Genetics, 18,* 404–405.

Nishimura, H., & Okamoto, N. (1976). Iniencephaly. In P. J. Vinken & G. W. Bruyn (Eds.), *Handbook of clinical neurology* (Vol. 30, pp. 257–268). Amsterdam: North Holland.

Sahid, S., Sepulveda, W., Dezerega, V., Gutierrez, J., Rodriguez, L., & Corral, E. (2000). Iniencephaly: Prenatal diagnosis and management. *Prenatal Diagnosis, 20,* 202–205.

Stark, A. M. (1951). A report of two cases of iniencephaly. *The Journal of Obstetrics Gynaecology British Empire, 58,* 462–464.

Tugrul, S., Uludog, M., Pekin, O., Uslu, H., Celik, C., & Ersan, F. (2007). Iniencephaly: Prenatal diagnosis with postmortem findings. *Journal of Obstetrics Gynaecology Research, 33*(4), 566–569.

ISAAC'S SYNDROME

DESCRIPTION

Isaac's syndrome is a disorder of either heritable or, more frequently, acquired origin signified by the continuous signaling of nerves activating muscle activity. It is also referred to as neuromyotonia, quantal squander, Armadillo syndrome, neurotonia, Mertens' syndrome, Isaac-Mertens' syndrome, continuous motor nerve discharges, and generalized myokymia (Hart, Vincent, & Willison, 1999). Maddison (2006) detailed muscle twitching and cramps as the most frequently occurring symptoms. Muscle stiffness, which can result in abnormal posturing, hyperhidrosis (increased sweating), muscle hypertrophy (increase in size of muscle cells), pseudomyotonia (abnormally slow muscle relaxation subsequent to muscle contraction), and muscle weakness are less frequently seen symptoms (Maddison, 2006). Onset includes all ages and can appear spontaneously (Maddison, 2006). Isaacs (1961) first detailed two accounts of the disorder under the name "continuous muscle-fiber activity" and postulated its nerve origin.

NEUROPATHOLOGY/PATHOPHYSIOLOGY

Acquired Isaac's syndrome appears to be primarily autoimmunological, as a result of problems with voltage-gated potassium channels (VGKCs) proper functionality (Hart, Maddison, Newsom-Davis, Vincent, & Mills, 2002). In researching potential causes of peripheral nerve hyperexcitability (PNH), Hart et al. (2002) studied clinical, autoimmune, and electrophysiological presentations of PNH and detected VGKC antibodies, supporting their hypothesis that the antibodies interfere with the proper functionality of the VGKCs, preventing proper neuronal firing. Clinical features included myokymic discharges, patterns of grouped or repetitive discharges of motor unit action potentials, with signature doublet, triplet, or multiplet motor unit discharges.

Viallard et al. (2005) found VGKC antibodies in a patient with acquired Isaac's syndrome, but these antibodies were also found in one case with no apparent neurological disease. These antibodies can also be found in patients with myasthenia gravis and thymoma occasionally (Viallard et al., 2005). In fact, identification of VGKC antibodies and the pattern of neuromyotonic discharge noted in patients with Isaac's syndrome goes beyond those findings of Villard et al. (2005) as this has been noted in previous research as well (Bednarik & Kadanka, 2001). Testing for the antibodies is performed through 125I-alpha-dendrotoxin immunoprecipitation (Bednarik & Kadanka, 2001; Hart et al., 2002).

NEUROPSYCHOLOGICAL/CLINICAL PRESENTATION

Maddison (2006) describes electromyographic (EMG) results as typically including an irregular pattern of activation signals in muscles in Isaac's syndrome, although there are no specific diagnostic criteria currently published. Isaacs (1961) initially described abnormal EMG activity in 1961, following proximal nerve brachial block. He also showed a reduced electrical firing after treatment using the muscle relaxant succinylcholine in conjunction with curare, a neuromuscular blocking agent. In comparison, electroencephalogram (EEG) results are not clinically diagnostic and do not deviate from normal (Maddison, 2006). Many patients report muscle twitching or cramps causing mild to moderate interference with activities of daily living (Hart et al., 2002).

Other potential presenting features may include muscle stiffness, hyperhidrosis, muscle weakness, pseudomyotonia, and sensory symptoms. Sensory symptoms include numbness or a tingling sensation in distal limbs. In addition, muscular hypertrophy, pseudotetany, persistent muscular contractions resembling tetanus in the absence of the bacteria *Clostridium tetani*, central nervous system symptoms, muscle wasting, and autonomic symptoms may also be seen (Hart et al., 2002). Of note, all patients studied by Hart et al. (2002) reported a fluctuation in severity of symptoms over the course of several months, and none experienced a spontaneous remission.

Psychiatric symptoms may include insomnia, irritability, and mild personality change (Hart et al., 2002). The most extreme psychiatric symptoms were seen in those patients with the highest levels of VGKC antibodies (Hart et al., 2002).

DIAGNOSIS

Associated immune-related diseases include neuropathy, myasthenia gravis, thymoma, diabetes mellitus (both insulin dependent and non–insulin-dependent), lung cancer (both small cell and adenocarcinoma, rheumatoid arthritis, amyloidosis, and systemic lupus erythematosus) (Hart et al., 2002).

A differential diagnosis should include stiff-man syndrome, as drugs such as diazepam are beneficial for an individual with stiff-man syndrome, but do not provide relief from Isaac's syndrome (Maddison, 2006). If symptoms of Isaac's syndrome co-occur with hallucinations, Morvan's syndrome may be a more accurate diagnosis (Liguori et al., 2001). As many of the symptoms seen in Isaac's syndrome may also be paraneoplastic, or evidence of cancer at another location, lung cancer and thymus tumors (thymomas) should be considered (Hart et al., 2002).

TREATMENT

Although there is no cure for Isaac's syndrome, palliative care may include treatment with anticonvulsants that work to reduce repetitive neuronal firing (Maddison, 2006). Additional immunosuppression through the additional use of prednisolone and azathioprine has shown promise, but not all patients respond fully to these drugs (Maddison, 2006). Short-term relief from symptoms may also be induced by plasma transfer, which can alleviate symptoms for up to 4 weeks (Liguori et al., 2001). Further research regarding potential treatment is needed.

Maryellen C. Dougherty
Charles Golden

Bednarik, J., & Kadanka, Z. (2001). Volitional and stimulation induced neuromyotonic discharges: Unusual electrophysiological pattern in acquired neuromyotonia. *Journal of Neurology, Neurosurgery and Psychiatry, 70,* 406–407.

Hart, I., Vincent, A., & Willison, H. (1999). Neuromyotonia and antiganglioside-associated neuropathies. In A. G. Engel (Ed.), *Myasthenia gravis and myasthenic disorders.* New York: Oxford University Press.

Hart, I. K., Maddison, P., Newsom-Davis, J., Vincent, A., & Mills, K. R. (2002). Phenotypic variants of autoimmune peripheral nerve hyperexcitability. *Brain, 125,* 1887–1895.

Isaacs, H. (1961). A syndrome of continuous muscle-fibre activity. *Journal of Neurology, Neurosurgery and Psychiatry, 24,* 319–325.

Liguori, R., Vincent, A., Clover, L., Avoni, P., Plazzi, G., Cortelli, P., et al. (2001). Morvan's syndrome: Peripheral and central nervous system and cardiac involvement with antibodies to voltage-gated potassium channels. *Brain, 124,* 2417–2426.

Maddison, P. (2006). Neuromyotonia. *Clinical Neurophysiology, 117,* 2118–2127.

Viallard, J. F., Vincent, A., Moreau, J. F., Parrens, M., Pellegrin, J., & Ellie, E. (2005). Thymoma-associated neuromyotonia with antibodies against voltage-gated potassium channels presenting as chronic intestinal pseudo-obstruction. *European Neurology, 53,* 60–63.

JOUBERT'S SYNDROME

DESCRIPTION

Joubert's syndrome is a genetic disorder with multiple functional impairments secondary to an underdeveloped or absent cerebellar vermis and abnormal brainstem (Joubert, Eisenring, Robb, & Andermann, 1969). In the 1960s, Marie Joubert, a pediatric neurologist, identified an autosomal-recessive syndrome that included ataxia, hyperpnea (abnormal breathing patterns), sleep apnea, abnormal eye movements, and mental retardation (Joubert et al., 1969). Additional features of the syndrome may include abnormal tongue movements, hypotonia, polydactyly (extra fingers and toes), cleft lip or palate, heart defects, and seizures (Saraiva & Baraitser, 1992). Moreover, this syndrome is one of the genetic syndromes correlated with retinitis pigmentosa, a form of retinal degeneration due to progressive loss of photoreceptor cells that may eventually cause blindness (Hartong, Berson, & Dryja, 2006). Prevalence is approximately 1 per 100,000 births, and males and females are equally affected (Hartong et al., 2006). A total of 205 cases have been reported with variable phenotypes (S. Choh, N. Choh, Bhat, & Jehangir, 2009). Prognosis tends to vary based on level of impairment and ranges from mild motor dysfunction and mildly diminished cognitive functions to severe motor dysfunction and moderate mental retardation with 5-year survival rate being 50% (S. Choh et al., 2009; Fennell, Gitten, Dede, & Maria, 1999).

NEUROPATHOLOGY/PATHOPHYSIOLOGY

Several mutations in genes have been identified in those with Joubert's syndrome including AHI1 (a gene whose function has not been identified), NPHP1 (related to nephronophthisis — a disorder of the kidneys involving cysts), and CEP290 (which is also associated with Leber's congenital amaurosis) (Dixon-Salazar et al., 2004; Parisi et al., 2004; Traboulsi, Koenekoop, & Stone, 2006). Genes AHI1 and NPHP1 are respectively correlated to a subset and rare form of Joubert's syndrome.

Neuroanatomical sequelae associated with Joubert's syndrome include abnormalities of the cerebellar vermis and brainstem. Primary findings on imaging include: thinning of the isthmus with widening of the interpeduncular fossa, thickened superior cerebellar peduncles, hypoplasia of the vermis with fourth ventricular deformity, rostral shift of the fastigium, and sagittal vermian cleft due to incomplete fusion of the two halves of the vermis (S. Choh et al., 2009). Cerebellar vermis hypoplasia that is present in Joubert's syndrome is one of the genetic ciliopathies that affects the anchoring basal bodies in cells that are critical in developmental signaling pathways (Adams, Smith, Logan, & Johnson, 2008). Imaging typically reveals a diminished or absent cerebellar vermis, which is involved with stereotypical movements and posture (Gunzler et al., 2007). It is believed that the inability for posterior fossa fiber tracks to cross the midline is significant in this condition (S. Choh et al., 2009).

Joubert's syndrome is also characterized by an abnormal brainstem referred to as a molar tooth sign, or dysplasia of the isthmic portion of the brainstem (Maria et al., 1999). Imaging typically reveals that 85% of patients have the molar tooth sign, which is considered pathognomonic of the disorder (Maria et al., 1999). Additional imaging has revealed "dilation of the cisterna magna, aplasia of the cerebellar vermis with dysplasia of the dentate nucleus, and elongated locus coeruleus, and dysplasia of the caudal medulla" (Maria et al., 1999). Neurochemistry is significant for diminished dopamine processing (Gunzler et al., 2007).

NEUROPSYCHOLOGICAL/CLINICAL PRESENTATION

The clinical presentation of Joubert's syndrome depends upon the development of the brain structures involved, namely the cerebellum and the brainstem. As such, typical symptoms include impairments in voluntary motor coordination (ataxia), periods of rapid abnormal breathing (hyperpnea), abnormal eye movements (nystagmus, strabismus, and ocular motor apraxia), and mental retardation. Neuropsychological findings often demonstrate severe impairments in cognition, verbal memory, visuomotor processing, motor control and speed, and language functioning (Fennell et al., 1999). Patients with mild symptoms tend to functions in the borderline range. Behavioral manifestations typically include a challenging temperament, hyperactivity, aggression, and dependency within the context of delayed physical development (Fennell et al., 1999).

Facial and body morphology for Joubert's syndrome is characterized by microcephaly, ptosis (drooping eyelids) with occasional visual impairments, low-set ears, and open mouth with protruding tongue (Maria, Boltshauser, Palmer, & Tran, 1999). Other possible morphology includes polydactyly (additional fingers and toes), hypotonia, and cleft lip or palate (Maria et al., 1999).

DIAGNOSIS

Diagnosis of Joubert's syndrome currently occurs during the prenatal period at 20–22 weeks of gestation through serial ultrasounds and fetal MRIs (Choh et al., 2009). Following birth, the most evident symptom is hyperpnea and apnea in the absence of lung pathology (Maria et al., 1999). This characteristic often sets Joubert's syndrome apart from other diagnoses. Neurobehavioral evaluation may reveal ataxia and abnormal eye movements among less common symptoms described above, whereas neuropsychological testing may reveal mental retardation.

Head imaging, such as MRI and CT, is utilized to demonstrate structural alterations in the cerebellar vermis and brainstem, specifically the five areas described above that are associated with Joubert's syndrome.

Differential diagnosis includes those other disorders with molar tooth signs including Dekaban–Arima syndrome, severe retinal dysplasia, COACH syndrome (cerebellar vermis hypoplasia, oligophrenia, ataxia, coloboma, and hepatic fibrosis), Senior–Loken's syndrome, Varadi–Papp's syndrome, nephronophthisis, and cogan oculomotor apraxia syndrome (Parisi & Glass, 2009). Joubert-plus syndrome, which accounts for 10% of the diagnoses, is also a consideration but includes the Dandy–Walker malformation (Parisi & Glass, 2009).

TREATMENT

No cure for Joubert's syndrome exists, and treatment is often focused on symptom management and providing support to patients and their families. To address abnormal breathing, infants may be placed on an apnea monitor. Anesthetic agents that may suppress breathing are avoided. Individuals with heart defects, cleft lip or palate, or seizures often require additional medical care and pharmaceutical agents. Due to kidney dysfunction being present, renal functions are monitored regularly. Genetic counseling, prenatal counseling, and screening are also required (Choh et al., 2009). Compensatory therapies, such as physical, occupational, and speech therapy, may also be helpful for some individuals' functional abilities (Maria et al., 1999).

Javan Horwitz
Natalie Horwitz
Chad A. Noggle

Adams, M., Smith, U. M., Logan, C. V., & Johnson, C. A. (2008). Recent advances in the molecular pathology, cell biology and genetics of ciliopathies. *Journal of Medical Genetics, 45*, 257–267.

Choh, S., Choh, N., Bhat, S., & Jehangir, M. (2009). MRI findings in Joubert syndrome. *Indian Journal of Pediatrics, 76*(2), 231–235.

Dixon-Salazar, T., Silhavy, J., Marsh, S., Louie, C., Scott, L., Gururaj, A., et al. (2004). Mutations in the AHI1 gene, encoding jouberin, cause Joubert syndrome with cortical polymicrogyria. *American Journal of Human Genetics, 75*(6), 979–987.

Fennell, E., Gitten, J., Dede, D., & Maria, B. (1999). Cognitive, behavior, and development of Joubert syndrome. *Journal of Child Neurology, 14*(9), 592–596.

Gunzler, S., Stoessl, A., Egan, R., Weleber, R., Wang, P., & Nutt, J. (2007). Joubert syndrome surviving to adulthood associated with a progressive movement disorder. *Movement Disorders, 22*(2), 262–265.

Hartong, D., Berson, E., & Dryja, T. (2006). Retinitis pigmentosa. *Lancet, 368*(9549), 1795–1809.

Joubert, M., Eisenring, J., Robb, J., & Andermann, F. (1969). Familial agenesis of the cerebellar vermis: A syndrome of episodic hyperpnea, abnormal eye movements, ataxia, and retardation. *Neurology, 19*(9), 813–825.

Maria, B., Boltshauser, E., Palmer, S., & Tran, T. (1999). Clinical features and revised diagnostic criteria in Joubert syndrome. *Journal of Child Neurology, 14,* 583–591.

Maria, B., Quisling, R., Rosainz, L., Yachnis, A., Gitten, J., Dede, D., et al. (1999). Molar tooth sign in Joubert syndrome: Clinical, radiologic, and pathologic significance. *Journal of Child Neurology, 14*(6), 368–376.

Parisi, M., Bennett, C., Eckert, M., Dobyns, W., Gleeson, J., Shaw, D., et al. (2004). The *NPHP1* gene deletion associated with juvenile nephronophthisis is present in a subset of individuals with Joubert syndrome. *American Journal of Human Genetics, 75*, 82–91.

Parisi, M., & Glass, I. (2009). *Joubert syndrome*. Retrieved June 2009, from http://www.ncbi.nlm.nih.gov/bookshelf/br.fcgi?book = gene&part = joubert

Saraiva, J., & Baraitser, M. (1992). Joubert syndrome: A review. *American Journal of Medical Genetics, 43*, 726–731.

Traboulsi, E., Koenekoop, R., & Stone, E. (2006). Lumpers or splitters? The role of molecular diagnosis in Leber congenital amaurosis. *Ophthalmic Genetics, 27*(4), 113–115.

IJK

JUVENILE DELINQUENCY

DESCRIPTION

Juvenile delinquency refers to the commission of illegal behaviors by persons under the age of 18, which would be considered criminal if committed by an adult (e.g., murder, assault, theft), as opposed to a specific neuropsychological disorder per se. *Delinquency* is preferred over *criminality* when working with children to emphasize the rehabilitative nature of the juvenile court (see Wynkoop, 2003, 2008). Delinquent behaviors are distinguished from status offenses that are behaviors that are not criminal in nature, but are illegal for children because of their status as children (e.g., running away from home). Status offenses generally do not carry over to become part of one's adult criminal history, whereas adjudications for delinquency generally do. Juvenile courts in the United States process more than 1.5 million cases annually (Grisso, 1998).

NEUROPATHOLOGY/PATHOPHYSIOLOGY

Delinquency is not homogenous in its manifestation or in its causes. Contributing factors include neurodevelopment, general maturational issues, general psychopathology, neuropathology, and social factors (see Wynkoop, 2008). Most nonaggressive/nonviolent delinquent behaviors are best explained by social factors (e.g., upbringing, modeling, being misled) in relation to intellectual and neurocognitive strengths and weaknesses on a developmental continuum, with roughly 60% of the variance in adolescent antisocial behavior accounted for by environmental influences (Reiss et al., 1995). Environmental factors appear to contribute to early nonviolent antisocial behavior, whereas genetic factors appear to contribute to sustained antisocial behavior into adulthood (Lyons et al., 1995; Reiss et al., 1995), although the relationship between genetics and environment is complex.

Aggression and violence in youth are the most troublesome of delinquent behaviors and consequently have received growing attention in recent years. Interestingly, aggression in toddlers appears to be more common than once thought, but tends to dissipate with age in most young children (e.g., Nagin & Tremblay, 1999). Conversely, evidence has accumulated suggesting that prolonged predisposition for aggressive behavior is most likely related to genetic and phenotypic (i.e., environmental influences on the central nervous system and autonomic nervous system) factors (Raine, 2002). For example, malnutrition in the first and/or second gestational trimesters has been linked with antisocial personality in adults (Neugebauer, Hock, & Susser, 1999), and children who are malnourished early in life (compared with controls) demonstrate increased hyperactive and/or aggressive behaviors at age 8, increased externalizing behaviors at 11, and greater conduct difficulties and motor activity at 17 (Liu, Raine, Venables, & Mednick, 2004) in a dose-dependent relationship. Parental substance abuse predicts generally disruptive behavior in children (Loukas, Fitzgerald, Zucker, & von Eye, 2001; Stanger et al., 1999), and maternal smoking during gestation predicts early onset conduct disorder in boys (Weissman, Warner, Wickramaratne, & Kandel, 1999). There is also a strong interaction effect between gestational and/or birth complications and early maternal rejection (i.e., attempted abortion, foster care placement in infancy) in the prediction of aggression and violence among children and adults (Raine, Brennan & Mednick, 1994).

Slow resting heart rate in childhood, suggestive of underlying problems (e.g., reduced noradrenergic function, norepinephrine and/or dopamine dysfunction, low sympathetic nervous system arousal), is "the best-replicated biological correlate of antisocial and aggressive behavior in children" (Raine, 2002, p. 417), and "predicts antisocial and criminal behavior in adulthood" (p. 421). Low salivary cortisol and/or high levels of testosterone have been related to aggression. The relationship between serotonin and aggression has been more complex depending on how serotonin is measured (including precursors and metabolites) and/or manipulated (see Burke, Loeber, and Birmaher, 2004, for a review).

A lack of empathy for the suffering of others has long been postulated as a contributing factor in aggression (Blair, 2002; Decety & Meyer, 2008), and suggestions are that abnormalities in affective processing may contribute as well (Herpertz & Sass, 2000). In fact, one study using fMRI found activation of the amygdala and ventral striatum and underactivation of the paracingulate cortex and temporal–parietal junction in aggressive youth when they witnessed pain inflicted on others, which the researchers interpreted as suggesting that they may have enjoyed watching the pain of others (Decety, Michalska & Akitsuki, 2008; Decety, Michalska, Akitsuki & Lahey, 2009).

Early onset conduct disorder has been associated with reduced right temporal lobe and right temporal gray matter volumes on MRI, more striking than slightly reduced prefrontal volumes, when compared with age-, sex-, and handedness-matched controls (Kruesi, Casanova, Mannheim, & Johnson-Bilder, 2004). Although there is a growing literature on the effects of neuroanatomical dysfunction as a cause or contributing factor to aggression and violence, most studies are conducted on adults and their application to children remains tenuous (see Kruesi & Casanova, 2006; Wynkoop, 2008).

NEUROPSYCHOLOGICAL/CLINICAL PRESENTATION

Juvenile delinquency refers to illicit behaviors that may or may not be related to neurocognitive delay or deficit. Frankly, due to a variety of reasons, including methodological concerns (cf. Burke et al., 2004), our understanding of the relationship between neuropsychological test performance and delinquency is limited (see the article entitled Conduct Disorder and Oppositional Defiant Disorder). Lower IQ assessed by ages 8–10 has been associated with more convictions for violent crimes, a trend that continues well into adulthood (Farrington, 1995) despite race, social class, and motivation to perform on testing (Lynam, Moffitt, & Stouthamer-Loeber, 1993). Spatial difficulties at age 3 that developmentally precede verbal weaknesses by age 11 are often observed in children with a later history of antisocial behavior compared with controls (Raine, 2002). By age 16 or 17, youth with limited, but persistent antisocial behaviors demonstrate impairment in spatial and memory functions relative to controls with no or more limited history of antisocial behaviors (Raine et al., 2005).

DIAGNOSIS

Delinquency is a legal designation, not a clinical diagnosis. Typical associated diagnoses include conduct disorder and child or adolescent antisocial behavior. However, there are other psychological conditions that should be examined via history, neurocognitive, and/or personality assessment (e.g., PIC-R, MMPI-A, PAI-A, APS) when delinquent behaviors are manifest. For example, prevalence data from Otto et al. (1992; unpublished, but recounted in Grisso, 1998) suggest that all forms of psychiatric disturbances among all adolescents range from about 14–22%, but that among delinquents conduct disorder has a base rate of 50–60%, compared with about 1–10% in the general population (American Psychiatric Association [APA], 2000); substance abuse/dependence 25–50%, compared with 5% for cannabis in the general population, with most other prevalence rates for substance abuse/dependence not well characterized (APA, 2000); attention deficit hyperactivity disorder (ADHD) greater than 20%, versus 3–7% among school-aged children in the general population (APA, 2000); affective disorders 30–75%, compared with 0.4–1.6% for bipolar disorders, 6% for dysthymia, 5–12% for men and 10–25% for women who suffer major depression, and lifetime prevalence in the general population (APA, 2000); Posttraumatic Stress Disorder (PTSD) 10–40% versus 8% lifetime prevalence in the general population (APA, 2000); and psychosis 1–6%, compared with roughly 1.5% or less in the general population across the life span (APA, 2000). Prevarication and dissimulation often complicate the clinical picture among youths (cf. Wynkoop & Denney, 2008), including among delinquent youths.

Two diagnostic caveats are in order regarding delinquency data. First, offending youths are often victims of violence themselves (reference their high rate of PTSD). Secondly, while conduct disorder is a prerequisite to antisocial personality disorder in adulthood, most children who meet diagnostic criteria for conduct disorder do not continue to offend in adulthood (Lahey, Pelham, Loncy, Lee, & Willcutt, 2005), thus limiting its predictive utility.

Our understanding of the neuropsychology of delinquency remains incomplete, is based mostly on correlational data, and is sometimes fraught with inconsistent findings, and with the obvious difficulty of applying group data to individual children. Consequently, it is not yet prudent to diagnose a tendency for chronic behavioral disturbance or violence via neurocognitive or physical assessment of a child.

TREATMENT

Treatment/intervention will depend upon target diagnoses and/or symptoms, which places neuropsychologists, as diagnosticians, in a position of value to delinquency service providers. In addition to the treatment of underlying psychological disorders (e.g., medication for psychosis or ADHD), a proclivity toward delinquency is likely best approached behaviorally and/or cognitive-behaviorally (e.g., Rational Behavior Training), sometimes by intervening in the social milieu of the child (e.g., residential or therapeutic foster care placement). However, community safety is often a factor in the court's intervention strategy. A firm grasp of general child development, general child clinical pathology, and the nature of the legal situation (e.g., legal question before the Court or the intervening agency) are required of the competent neuropsychologist serving delinquent youth.

Timothy F. Wynkoop

American Psychiatric Association (APA). (2000). *Diagnostic and statistical manual of mental disorders, fourth edition, text revision.* Washington, DC: Author.

Blair, R. J. R. (2005). Responding to the emotions of others: Dissociating forms of empathy through the study of typical and psychiatric populations. *Consciousness and Cognition, 14,* 698–718.

Burke, J. D., Loeber, R., & Birmaher, B. (2004). Oppositional defiant disorder and conduct disorder: A review of the past 10 years, part II. *Focus: The Journal of Lifelong Learning in Psychiatry, 2,* 558–576.

Decety, J., & Meyer, M. (2008). From emotion resonance to empathic understanding: A social developmental neuroscience account. *Development and Psychopathology, 20,* 1053–1080.

Decety, J., Michalska, K. J., & Akitsuki, Y. (2008). Who caused the pain? A functional MRI investigation of empathy and intentionality in children. *Neuropsychologia, 46,* 2607–2614.

Decety, J., Michalska, K. J., Akitsuki, Y., & Lahey, B. (2009). Atypical empathic responses in adolescents with aggressive conduct disorder: a functional MRI investigation. *Biological Psychology, 80,* 203–211.

Farrington, D. P. (1995). The development of offending and antisocial behavior from childhood: Key findings from the Cambridge study in delinquent development. *Journal of Child Psychology and Psychiatry, 360,* 929–964.

Grisso, T. (1998). *Forensic evaluation of juveniles.* Sarasota, FL: Professional Resource Press.

Herpertz, S. C., & Sass, H. (2000). Emotional deficiency and psychopathy. *Behavioral Science and Law, 18,* 317–323.

Kruesi, M. J. P., & Casanova, M. F. (2006). White matter in liars. *British Journal of Psychiatry, 188,* 293–294.

Kruesi, M. J. P., Casanova, M. F., Mannheim, G., & Johnson-Bilder, A. (2004). Reduced temporal volume in early onset conduct disorder. *Psychiatry Research: Neuroimaging, 132,* 1–11.

IJK

Lahey, B. B., Pelham, W. E., Loney, J., Lee, S. S., & Willcutt, E. (2005). Instability of the DSM-IV subtypes of ADHD from preschool through elementary school. *Archives of General Psychiatry, 62,* 896–902.

Liu, J., Raine, A., Venables, P. H., & Mednick, S.A. (2004). Malnutrition at age 3 years and externalizing behavior problems at ages 8, 11, and 17 years. *The American Journal of Psychiatry, 161,* 2005–2013.

Loukas, A., Fitzgerald, H. E., Zucker, R. A., & von Eye, A. (2001). Parental alcoholism and co-occurring antisocial behavior: Prospective relationships to externalizing behavior problems in their young sons. *Journal of Abnormal Child Psychology, 29,* 91–106.

Lynam, D., Moffitt, T., & Stouthamer-Loeber, M. (1993). Explaining the relation between IQ and delinquency: Class, race, test motivation, school failure, and self-control. *Journal of Abnormal Psychology, 102,* 187–196.

Lyons, M. J., True, W. R., Eisen, S. A., Goldberg, J., Meyer, J. M., Faraone, S. V., et al. (1995). Differential heritability of adult and juvenile antisocial traits. *Archives of General Psychiatry, 52,* 906–915.

Nagin, D., & Trimblay, R. E. (1999). Trajectories of boys' physical aggression, opposition, and hyperactivity on the path to physically violent and nonviolent juvenile delinquency. *Child Development, 70,* 1181–1196.

Neugebauer, R., Hock, H. W., & Susser, E. (1999). Prenatal exposure to wartime famine and development of antisocial personality disorder in early adulthood. *Journal of the American Medical Association, 4,* 479–481.

Otto, R., Greenstein, J., Johnson, M., & Friedman, R. (1992). Prevalence of mental disorders among youth in the juvenile justice system. In J. Cocozza (Ed.), *Responding to the mental health needs of youth in the juvenile justice system* (pp. 7–48). Seattle, WA: National Coalition for the Mentally Ill in the Criminal Justice System.

Raine, A. (2002). Annotation: The role of prefrontal deficits, low autonomic arousal, and early health factors in the development of antisocial and aggressive behavior in children. *Journal of Child Psychology and Psychiatry, 43,* 417–434.

Raine, A., Brennan, P., & Mednick, S. A., (1994). Birth complications combined with early maternal rejection at age 1 year predispose to violent crime at age 18 years. *Archives of General Psychiatry, 51,* 984–988.

Raine, A., Moffitt, T. E., Caspi, A., Loeber, R., Stouthamer-Loeber, M., & Lynam, D. (2005). Neurocognitive impairments in boys on the life-course persistent antisocial path. *Journal of Abnormal Psychology, 114,* 38–49.

Reiss, D., Hetherington, E. M., Plomin, R., Howe, G. W., Simmens, S. J., Henderson, S. H., et al. (1995). Genetic questions for environmental studies: differential parenting and psychopathology in adolescence. *Archives of General Psychiatry, 52,* 925–936.

Stanger, C., Higgins, S. T., Bickel, W. K., Elk, R., Grabowski, J., Schmitz, J., et al. (1999). Behavioral and emotional problems among children of cocaine- and opiate-dependent parents. *Journal of the American Academy of Adolescent Psychiatry, 38,* 421–428.

Weissman, M. M., Warner, V., Wickramaratne, P. J., & Kandel, D. B. (1999). Maternal smoking during pregnancy and psychopathology in offspring followed to adulthood. *Journal of the American Academy of Child and Adolescent Psychiatry, 38,* 892–899.

Wynkoop, T. F. (2003). Neuropsychology of juvenile adjudicative competence. *Journal of Forensic Neuropsychology, 3,* 45–65.

Wynkoop, T. F. (2008). Neuropsychology in the juvenile justice system. In R. Denney & T. Sullivan (Eds.), *Clinical neuropsychology in the criminal forensic setting* (pp. 295–325). New York: Guilford.

Wynkoop, T. F., & Denney, R. L. (2008, January). *Detecting malingered cognitive deficit in children: Underpinnings and state of the current research.* Paper presented at Child Forensic Symposia, University of Toledo School of Medicine, Toledo, OH.

KAWASAKI'S DISEASE

DESCRIPTION

Kawasaki's disease (KD), named after the physician who first reported the illness (Kawasaki, 1967), is an acute febrile vasculitic syndrome of unknown etiology, usually occurring in children under age 5 (Kim, 2006). It is characterized by fever, bilateral nonexudative conjunctivitis, erythema of the lips and oral mucosa, changes in the extremities, rash, and cervical lymphadenopathy (Newburger et al., 2004). Long-term follow-up has shown that approximately 25% of untreated children may develop coronary aneurysm, leading to ischemic heart disease in about 5%, myocardial infarction in about 2%, and death in just under 1% (Kato et al., 1996). KD is also known as acute febrile mucocutaneous lymph node syndrome.

Although the cause of KD is unknown, epidemiological studies have shed light on some of the underlying factors. KD occurs worldwide, although there is markedly greater prevalence in Japan and Korea (Yanagawa & Nakamura, 1986). In the United States, it is most prevalent in Asian Americans, followed by African Americans and Hispanics (Holman, Curns, Belay, Steiner, & Schonberger, 2003). The disease occurs in epidemics, although person-to-person transmission and secondary cases from contact with affected patients are rare (Levin, Tizard, & Dillon, 1991). It occurs more frequently among siblings (2% vs. 0.19% in the general population), with the highest incidence in those under 2 years old (Fujita et al., 1989). These findings are suggestive of an infectious agent as the cause, with a genetic (racial) predisposition, although no known organism has been identified, and the disease is unresponsive to antibiotics.

NEUROPATHOLOGY/PATHOPHYSIOLOGY

KD is associated with severe vasculitis of all blood vessels, affecting predominantly medium-sized coronary arteries. Media of affected vessels show edematous dissociation of the smooth muscle cells. Endothelial cell swelling and subendothelial edema are observed (Kim, 2006). Acute cases of KD often display marked cytokine cascade stimulation (Newburger et al., 2004), with endothelial cell activation, CD68+ monocyte/macrophages, CD8+ (cytotoxic) lymphocytes, and oligoclonal IgA plasma cells being involved in coronary arteritis (Rowley, Shulman, Spike, Mask, & Baker, 2001). Tumor necrosis factor and interleukins 1, 6, 8, 15, 17, and 18 are higher than normal (Kim, 2006).

CNS involvement has not been investigated extensively. However, aseptic meningitis has been documented in 25% of patients who had undergone a lumbar puncture during consultation (Rowley et al., 1988). Furthermore, patients may show localized cerebral hypoperfusion during the acute stage in the absence of abnormal neurological or clinical findings, which normalizes after 1 month (Ichiyama et al., 1998).

NEUROPSYCHOLOGICAL/CLINICAL PRESENTATION

Very little research has examined neuropsychological functioning in persons with KD. King et al. (2000) found that neither cardiac nor CNS findings correlated significantly with any of the cognitive or behavioral measures used in their study. King et al. found that parents rated KD children as having significantly more behavior problems, specifically on scales of internalizing symptoms, somatic complaints, anxious-depressive behavior, and social problems. They were also rated as having significantly more attention problems.

Carlton-Conway et al. (2005) found that 34% of KD children exhibited behavioral changes following recovery. The symptoms included hyperactivity, decreased concentration, increased aggression, and emotional lability, and were reportedly significant enough for parents to seek professional services.

Carlton-Conway et al. then performed PET and MRI scans on seven KD patients who exhibited severe behavioral difficulties. They reported that three showed reduced tracer uptake in the occipital lobes and that "other areas were also affected in two of the cases."

DIAGNOSIS

There are no specific diagnostic tests or pathognomonic features of KD. Diagnosis is based upon an epidemiological case definition that includes: (a) 5 or more days of fever; (b) presence of four of the five following conditions: bilateral conjunctival infection; changes in mucous membranes and upper respiratory tract, such as injected pharynx, dry cracked lips, and strawberry tongue; changes of the peripheral extremities including edema, erythema, desquamation (may occur later); polymorphous rash; cervical lymphadenopathy; and (c) exclusion of staphylococcal and streptococcal infection, measles, leptospirosis, and rickettsial disease (Levin et al., 1991).

TREATMENT

In the acute phase of KD, treatment is directed toward reducing inflammation of the coronary artery wall and preventing coronary thrombosis, while long-term therapy for those who develop coronary aneurysms involves preventing myocardial ischemia or infarction (Kim, 2006). High doses of aspirin are currently used to reduce the inflammatory process in the acute phase. Intravenous immunoglobulin (IVIG) is another established treatment during the acute phase of KD (Durongpisitkul, Gururaj, Park, & Martin, 1995), although the mechanism of action is unknown. Meta-analyses have demonstrated a dose–response effect, with the higher doses of IVIG being more efficacious (Durongpisitkul et al., 1995). The benefit of this therapy is maximal early, preferably within the first 7–10 days. For those 10–15% of KD children who fail to respond to IVIG or aspirin, use of corticosteroids has been suggested (Wright, Newburger, Baker, & Sundel, 1996). For those who develop coronary artery aneurysms, the goal is to prevent thrombosis and myointimal proliferation leading to stenosis (Kim, 2006).

Shane S. Bush
Thomas E. Myers

Carlton-Conway, D., Ahluwalia, R., Henry, L, Michie, C., Wood, L., & Tulloh, R. (2005). Behavior sequelae following acute Kawasaki disease. *BMC Pediatrics, 5,* 14–20.

IJK

Durongpisitkul, K., Gururaj, V. J., Park, J. M., & Martin, C. F. (1995). The prevention of coronary artery aneurysm in Kawasaki disease: A meta-analysis on the efficacy of aspirin and immunoglobulin treatment. *Pediatrics, 96*, 1057–1061.

Fujita, Y., Nakamura, Y., Sakata, K., Hara, N., Kobayashi, M., Nagai, M., et al. (1989). Kawasaki disease in families. *Pediatrics, 61*, 666–669.

Holman, R. C., Curns, A. T., Belay, E. D., Steiner, C. A., & Schonberger, L. B. (2003). Kawasaki syndrome hospitalizations in the United States, 1997 and 2000. *Pediatrics, 112*, 495–501.

Ichiyama, T., Nishikawa, M., Hayashi T., Koga, M., Tashiro, N., & Furukawa, S. (1998). Cerebral hypoperfusion during acute Kawasaki disease. *Stroke, 29*, 1320–1321.

Kato, H., Sugimura, T., Akagi, T., Sato, N., Hashino, K., Maeno, Y., et al. (1996). Long-term consequences of Kawasaki disease. A 10- to 21-year follow-up study of 594 patients. *Circulation, 94*, 1379–1385.

Kawasaki, T. (1967). Acute febrile mucocutaneous syndrome with lymphoid involvement with specific desquamation of the fingers and toes in children. *Japanese Journal of Allergy, 16*, 178–222.

Kim, D. S. (2006). Kawasaki disease. *Yonsei Medical Journal, 47*(6), 759–772.

King, J. W., Schlieper, A., Birdi, N., Cappelli, M., Korneluk, Y., & Rowe, P. C. (2000). The effect of Kawasaki disease on cognition and behavior. *Archives of Pediatric and Adolescent Medicine, 154*, 463–468.

Levin, M., Tizard, J. E., & Dillon, M. J. (1991).Kawasaki disease: recent advances. *Archives of Disease in Childhood, 66*, 1369–1374.

Newburger, J. W., Takahashi, M., Gerber, M., Gewitz, M., Tani, L. Y., Burns, J. C., et al. (2004). Diagnosis, treatment, and long-term management of Kawasaki disease: A statement for health professionals from the Committee on Rheumatic Fever, Endocarditis, and Kawasaki Disease, Council on Cardiovascular Disease in the Young, American Heart Association. *Pediatrics, 114*, 1708–1733.

Rowley, A. H., Gonzalez-Crussi, F., & Shulman, S. T. (1988). Kawasaki syndrome. *Review of Infectious Disease, 10*, 1–15.

Rowley, A. H., Shulman, S. T., Spike, B. T., Mask, C. A., & Baker, S. C. (2001). Oligoclonal IgA response in the vascular wall in acute Kawasaki disease. *Journal of Immunology, 166*, 1334–1343.

Yanagawa, H., & Nakamura, Y. (1986). Nationwide epidemic of Kawasaki disease in Japan during winter of 1985–1986. *Lancet, ii*, 1138–1140.

Wright, D. A., Newburger, J. W., Baker, A., & Sundel, R. P. (1996). Initial intravenous gammaglobulin treatment failure in Kawasaki disease with pulsed doses of corticosteroids. *Journal of Pediatrics, 128*, 146–149.

KEARNS–SAYRE'S SYNDROME

DESCRIPTION

Kearns–Sayre's syndrome (KSS) is a rare mitochondrial disorder, first described by Kearns and Sayre in 1958. The disease is usually dominated by the involvement of skeletal muscles and the nervous system because of mitochondrial dysfunction (hence the term "mitochondrial encephalopathy"). Symptom onset usually occurs before 20 years of age and most commonly presents as progressive external ophthalmoplegia (PEO) with ptosis, pigmentary retinopathy, and one or more of the following: heart block, cerebellar deficits, cerebrospinal fluid (CSF) protein greater than 100 mg/dL, or myopathy affecting facial, cervical, and limb girdle muscles (Anderson et al., 1981; Maceluch & Niedziela, 2006). KSS affects both sexes equally and is characterized by a progressive course leading to premature death in most cases (Maceluch & Niedziela, 2006).

NEUROPATHOLGY/PATHOPHYSIOLOGY

Human mitochondria contain their own DNA (mtDNA) that codes for 13 polypeptides of the respiratory chain subunits, two ribosomal RNAs, and 22 transfer RNAs, in a circular double-stranded genome of approximately 16.5 kb (Anderson et al., 1981). KSS is characterized by sporadically occurring rearrangements (mostly deletion and/or duplications) of mtDNA (Holt, Harding, & Morgan-Hughes, 1988; Moraes et al., 1989; Poulton, Deadman, & Gardiner, 1989; Zeviani et al., 1998). These rearrangements impair oxidative phosphorylation and energy metabolism of mitochondria. The size and site of rearrangements in mtDNA show no consistent pattern or correlation with disease severity. The phenotypic variability in mitochondrial disorders including KSS seems to be influenced by several factors that include age, heteroplasmy (mixture of wild- and mutant-type mtDNA in mitochondria), the type and extent of respiratory chain disruption caused by mutation, and tissue specific for the pathogenic effect. Defects in the electron transport chain can affect any tissue. Tissues requiring the highest levels of energy production are the most severely affected.

The characteristic histological finding is subsarcolemmal accumulation of mitochondria on muscle biopsy, visualized with either a modified Gomori trichrome stain (ragged red fibers) or with a stain for succinate dehydrogenase (ragged blue fibers). Electron microscopic findings include increase in mitochondrial number or size, increased lipid, glycogen droplets, increased mitochondrial matrix, abnormal cristae, and paracrystalline inclusions. The histologic evaluation of muscle may provide evidence to support a diagnosis of KSS, but normal muscle pathology does not exclude KSS, especially in children.

Neuropathologic findings in KSS include spongiform encephalopathy involving both gray and white matter of the cerebrum and cerebellum and primarily gray matter of the brainstem (Sparaco, Bonilla, DiMauro, & Powers, 1993a,b). Extensive neuronal loss is seen throughout the brainstem and cerebellum, and demyelination of white matter possibly secondary to axonal degeneration (Sparaco et al., 1993a,b). Calcium deposits occur in the thalamus and globus pallidus, involving individual mineralized neurons, and also in the parenchyma. Mitochondrial ultrastructural abnormalities are not consistently shown in the brain despite neuropathologic lesions (Sparaco et al., 1993a,b).

NEUROPSYCHOLOGICAL/CLINICAL PRESENTATION

Children with KSS usually appear normal at birth. Similarly, early development is normal. Tissues with high energy demands appear to be more severely affected, and the clinical symptoms depend on the extent to which different organs are affected. Ptosis is usually the first sign of the disease. It is followed by PEO within a few years (Gross-Jendroska, Schatz, McDonald, & Johnson, 1992). PEO affects all the ocular muscles equally and usually begins after the age of 5. Atypical retinitis pigmentosa, with a "salt and pepper–like" appearance is another ocular characteristic of KSS (Isashiki et al., 1998).

The cardiac manifestations occur in more than half (57%) of the patients and usually dominate the later clinical picture of KSS (Berenberg et al., 1977; Young, Shah, Lee, & Hayes, 2005). These conditions include syncopal attacks, dilated cardiomyopathy, congestive heart failure, and cardiac arrest. The cardiac pathology in KSS typically involves the distal bundle of His, bundle branches, and infranodal conductions (Gallastegui, Hariman, Handler, Lev, & Bharti, 1987; Polak, Zijlstra, & Roelandt, 1989). The ECG change typically found in KSS is PR interval prolongation preceding second- or third-degree atrioventricular (AV) block (Clark et al., 1975).

Because brain energetics depends heavily upon oxidative metabolism, the central nervous system (CNS) is particularly susceptible to mitochondrial dysfunction. Furthermore, different CNS regions seem to have different tolerance thresholds for metabolic dysfunction. The most common neurological symptom is cognitive impairment that ranges from mildly delayed development to severe mental retardation (Madsen, Linde, Hasselbalch, Paulson, & Lassen, 1998). Other neurological symptoms include nystagmus, muscle hypotonia, ataxia, dystonic movements, myoclonias, and dementia (Madsen et al., 1998; Sparaco et al., 1993a,b). Cerebellar syndrome also commonly occurs, and CSF analysis demonstrates elevated protein levels (Gascon, Ozand, & Cohen, 2007). Sensorineural hearing loss is a clinically relevant and treatable symptom (Kornblum, Broicher et al., 2005; Zwirner & Wilichowski, 2001). Common findings on brain imaging are intracranial calcification, cerebral and cerebellar atrophy (Valanne, Ketonen, Majander, Suomalainen, & Pinko, 1998). The presence of a combination of high-signal foci on T2-weighted magnetic resonance images in the globus pallidus and subcortical cerebral white matter is characteristic of KSS (Valanne et al., 1998).

Progressive muscle weakness and exercise intolerance appear as common features (Oldfors, Fyhr, Holme, Larsson, & Tulinius, 1990). It usually affects the facial, pharyngeal, trunk, and shoulder muscles, leading to dysarthria and dysphagia in many patients. Sometimes, KSS may first manifest as an endocrinopathy that includes pituitary abnormalities, diabetes mellitus, adrenal insufficiency, growth hormone deficiency, and thyroid dysfunction. Overall, although endocrine abnormalities are common in mitochondrial disorders, in the majority of patients they are masked by encephalomyopathy (Artuch et al., 1998; Schmiedel, Jakson, Schafer, & Reichmenn, 2003).

DIAGNOSIS

As KSS is a multisystemic disorder, a comprehensive clinical investigation must be carried out in order to arrive at a correct diagnosis. The diagnosis is usually based on the clinical picture, family history, and the results of laboratory tests, which may show increased lactate, pyruvate, and creatine kinase levels in the blood; abnormal urine organic and amino acids; elevated lactate and protein levels in CSF. Magnetic resonance spectroscopy may be useful in demonstrating increased lactate levels in the damaged white matter of the brain. MRI or CT of the brain may visualize characteristic CNS changes (Valanne et al., 1998). Electroencephalogram may show evidence of seizure activity or diffuse slow wave suggestive of encephalopathy. Electromyogram may show a myogenic pattern. The only investigations that provide specific evidence of an underlying mtDNA mutation are histochemical staining and electron microscopic studies of muscle biopsy specimens, and genetic analysis of mitochondrial DNA (Maceluch et al., 2006). All cases of KSS should be periodically assessed for cardiac function by ECG and echocardiography. An oral glucose tolerance test should be carried out because of high prevalence of diabetes mellitus.

From a differential diagnosis standpoint, clinical workup must take into consideration and rule out other mitochondrial disease particularly MERRF (myoclonic epilepsy with ragged red fibers) and MELAS (mitochondrial encephalomyopathy, lactic acidosis, and stroke), myasthenia gravis, collagen vascular diseases such as systemic lupus erythematosus, and even presentations such as Lyme disease and Whipple's disease (Gascon et al., 2007).

TREATMENT

No curative treatment is currently available for patients with KSS. Therapy must therefore consist of the prevention and treatment of the typical symptoms and complications associated with the disease. The 2002 American College of Cardiology/American Heart Association guidelines recommend that pacing should be considered in patients with neuromuscular diseases with AV block, such as those with KSS, with or without other symptoms, because there may be an unpredictable progression of AV conduction disease (Gregoratos et al., 2002). Necessary investigations and treatments should be initiated for endocrinopathies. Use of bicarbonates and dialysis may be required for severe episodes of lactic acidosis. Surgical correction of ptosis is possible, but the benefits are usually transient. A moderate degree of exercise has been shown to improve exercise tolerance and muscle metabolism, and this should be recommended to patients with mtDNA disease (Taivassalo et al., 1998). A ketogenic diet may also bring some benefit in restoring proper mitochondrial function, providing energy source through the pathway omitting the deficient enzyme complexes in the energy production chain. Nutritional supplements, such as coenzyme Q10 and ubiquinone, have been tried in an attempt to slow the progression of neurological disease process without proven efficacy (Matthews et al., 1993). Further therapeutic possibilities include the use of creatine because of its potential neuroprotective and antioxidant effects (Kornblum, Schroder et al., 2005). The gene therapy approach includes either increased expression of wild-type copy of the mutated mitochondrial gene in the nucleus or the selective

destruction of mutant mtDNA through importation of restriction enzymes into the mitochondria. But it is not available for clinical use.

Gaurav Jain
Sarita Singhal
Chad A. Noggle

Anderson, S., Bankier, A. T., Barrell, B. G., de Bruijn, M. H. L., Coulson, A. R., & Drouin, J. (1981). Sequence and organization of the human mitochondrial genome. *Nature, 290*, 457–465.

Artuch, R., Pavia, C., Playan, A., Vilaseca, M. A., Colomer, J., Valls, C., et al. (1998). Multiple endocrine involvement in two pediatric patients with Kearns-Sayre syndrome. *Hormone Research, 50*, 99–104.

Berenberg, R. A., Pellock, J. M., Di Mauro, S., Schotland, D. L., Bonilla, E., Eastwood, A., et al. Lumping or splitting? "Ophthalmoplegia plus" or Kearns-Sayre syndrome? *Annals of Neurology, 1*, 37–54.

Clark, D. S., Myerburg, R. G., Morales, A., Befeler, B., Hernandez, F. A., & Gaband, H. (1975). Heart block in Kearns-Sayre syndrome: Electrophysiologic-pathologic correlation. *Chest, 68*, 727–730.

Gallastegui, J., Hariman, R. J., Handler, B., Lev, M., & Bharti, S. (1987). Cardiac involvement in the Kearns-Sayre syndrome. *American Journal of Cardiology, 60*, 385–388.

Gascon, G. G., Ozand, P. T., & Cohen, B. (2007). Aminoacidopathies and organic acidopathies, mitochondrial enzyme defects, and other metabolic errors. In C. G. Goetz (Ed.), *Textbook of clinical neurology* (3rd ed., pp. 641–681). Philadelphia: Saunders Elsevier.

Gregoratos, G., Abrams, J., Epstein, A. E., Freedman, R. A., Hayes, D. L., Hlatky, M. A., et al. (2002). ACC/AHA/NASPE 2002 guideline update for implantation of cardiac pacemakers and antiarrhythmia devices: Summary article. A report of the American College of Cardiology/American Heart Association Task Force on Practice Guidelines (ACC/AHA/NASPE Committee to Update the 1998 Pacemaker Guidelines). *Ciculation, 106*, 2145–2161.

Gross-Jendroska, M., Schatz, H., McDonald, H. R., & Johnson, R. N. (1992). Kearns-Sayre syndrome: A case report and review. *European Journal of Ophthalmology, 2*, 15–20.

Holt, I. J., Harding, A. E., & Morgan-Hughes, J. A. (1988). Deletions of mitochondrial DNA in patients with mitochondrial myopathies. *Nature, 331*, 717–719.

Isashiki, Y., Nakagawa, M., Ohba, N., Kamimura, K., Sakoda, Y., Higuchi, I., et al. (1998). Retinal manifestations in mitochondrial diseases associated with mitochondrial DNA mutation. *Acta Ophthalmologica Scandinavica, 76*, 6–13.

Kornblum, C., Broicher, R., Walther, E., Herberhold, S., Klockgether, T., Herberhold, C., et al. (2005).

Sensorineural hearing loss in patients with chronic progressive ophthalmoplegia or Kearns-Sayre syndrome. *Journal of Neurology, 252,* 1101–1107.

Kornblum, C., Schroder, R., Muller, K., Vorgerd, M., Eggers, J., Bogdanow, M., et al. (2005). Creatine has no beneficial effect on skeletal muscle energy metabolism in patients with single mitochondrial DNA deletions: A placebo controlled, double-blind [31] P-MRS crossover study. *European Journal of Neurology, 12,* 300–309.

Maceluch, J., & Niedziela, M. (2006). The clinical diagnosis and molecular genetics of Kearns-Sayre syndrome: A complex mitochondrial encephalomyopathy. *Pediatric Endocrinology Reviews, 2,* 111–137.

Madsen, P. L., Linde, R., Hasselbalch, S. G., Paulson, O. B., & Lassen, N. A. (1998). Activation/induced resetting of cerebral oxygen and glucose uptake in the rat. *Journal of Cerebral Blood Flow Metabolism, 18,* 742–748.

Matthews, P. M., Ford, B., Dandurand, R. J., Eidelman, D. H., O'Connor, D., Sherwin, A., et al. (1993). Coenzyme Q10 with multiple vitamins is generally ineffective in treatment of mitochondrial diseases. *Neurology, 43,* 884–890.

Moraes, C. T., DiMauro, S., Zeviani, M., Lombes, A., Shanske, S., Miranda, A. F., et al. (1989). Mitochondrial DNA deletions in progressive external ophthalmoplegia and Kearns-Sayre syndrome. *New England Journal of Medicine, 320,* 1293–1299.

Oldfors, A., Fyhr, I. M., Holme, E., Larsson, N. G., & Tulinius, M. (1990). Neuropathology in Kearns-Sayre syndrome. *Acta Neuropathology, 80,* 541–546.

Polak, P. E., Zijlstra, F., & Roelandt, R. T. C. (1989). Indications for pacemaker implantation in the Kearns-Sayre syndrome. *European Heart Journal, 10,* 281–282.

Poulton, J., Deadman, M. E., & Gardiner, R. M. (1989). Duplications of mitochondrial DNA in mitochondrial myopathy. *Lancet, 1,* 236–240.

Schmiedel, J., Jakson, S., Schafer, J., & Reichmann, H. (2003). Mitochondrial cytopathies. *Journal of Neurology, 250,* 267–277.

Sparaco, M., Bonilla, E., DiMauro, S., & Powers, J. M. (1993a). Neuropathology of mitochondrial encephalomyopathies due to mitochondrial DNA defects. *Journal of Neuropathology Experiment Neurology, 52,* 1–10.

Sparaco, M., Bonilla, E., DiMauro, S., & Powers, J. M. (1993b). Neuropathology of mitochondrial encephalomyopathies due to mitochondrial DNA defects. *Journal of Neuropathology Experimental Neurology, 19,* 369–377.

Taivassalo, T., De Stefano, N., Argov, Z., Matthews, P. M., Chen, J., Genge, A., et al. (1998). .Effects of aerobic training in patients with mitochondrial myopathies. *Neurology, 50,* 1055–1060.

Valanne, L., Ketonen, L., Majander, A., Suomalainen, A., & Pihko, H. (1998). Neuroradiologic findings in children with mitochondrial disorders. *American Journal of Neuroradiology, 19,* 369–377.

Young, T. J., Shah, A. K., Lee, M. H., & Hayes, D. L. (2005). Kearns-Sayre syndrome: A case report and review of cardiovascular complications. *Pacing and Clinical Electrophysiology, 28,* 454–457.

Zeviani, M., Moraes, C. T., DiMauro, S., Nakase, H., Bonilla, E., Schon, E. A., et al. (1998). Deletions of mitochondrial DNA in Kearns-Sayre syndrome. *Neurology, 38,* 1339–1346.

Zwirner, P., & Wilichowski, E. (2001). Progressive sensorineural hearing loss in children with mitochondrial encephalomyopathies. *Laryngoscope, 111,* 515–521.

IJK

KENNEDY'S DISEASE

DESCRIPTION

Kennedy's disease (KD), also referred to as "spinal and bulbar muscular atrophy" (SBMA), is a genetic polyglutamine disease characterized by progressive muscle degeneration and androgen insensitivity. The disease is the only polyglutamine triplet-repeat disease that has been discovered, and exclusively affects lower motor neuron functioning (Sinnreich & Klein, 2004). A relatively rare disease, a Scandinavian study estimated prevalence to be 13 occurrences per 85,000 males (Udd et al., 1998). Patients with KD have a normal life expectancy, with death resulting only with complications (e.g., breathing difficulties) (Atsuta et al., 2006).

The first to describe the characteristics of the disease was Kawahara, who in 1897 documented similar features of progressive atrophy of the tongue, dysarthria, dysphagia, and gait disturbance among two brothers and their maternal uncle (Takahashi, 2001). Takikawa later reported of the disease in 1953, being one of the earliest to classify KD as a sex-linked recessive trait (Takahashi, 2001).

Kennedy, who the disease was later named after, published a paper in 1968 documenting the individual familial pattern of KD, implicating it as a sex-linked trait (Kennedy, Alter, & Sung, 1968). Kennedy evaluated two families, in which 11 males exhibited similar features of progressive muscle atrophy (Kennedy et al., 1968). He observed that most patients presented with low backache, muscle cramps, generalized fasciculations, bulbar atrophy, and muscle weakness beginning in the shoulder and pelvic girdle muscles (Kennedy et al., 1968). Kennedy was the first to document the co-occurring presence of diabetes mellitus, tremor, and sensory involvement with KD, which were only later added as characteristics of the disease

(Sinnreich & Klein, 2004). Delwaide, a Belgian neurologist, was the first to refer to the disease as Kennedy's disease, which was later reclassified in 1982 officially as an X-linked bulbospinal neuropathy (Harding et al., 1982).

NEUROPATHOLOGY/PATHOPHYSIOLOGY

The cause for KD has been attributed to mutation of the gene that codes for the androgen receptor (AR) protein, located on chromosome Xq11-12 (Adachi et al., 2007). In 1991, the disease was linked to an abnormal expansion of a trinuceotide CAG repeat in the *AR* gene (La Spada, Wilson, Lubahn, Harding, & Fischbeck, 1991). Polymerase chain reaction (PCR) amplification of DNA segments containing the CAG repeat among KD patients was found to give a band of fragments 75 base pairs larger than controls (La Spada et al., 1991). Using sequence analysis of the *AR* gene, the number of CAG repeats in KD patients ranged from 40 to 52, while ranging from 17 to 26 among controls (La Spada et al., 1991). A longer CAG repeat has been associated with an earlier age of onset and a predominant motor impairment, while a shorter CAG repeat has been associated with a later age of onset and predominant sensory impairment (Ropper & Brown, 2005; Suzuki et al., 2008). Pathogenesis due to this defect has been attributed to diffuse toxic nuclear accumulation of the mutated AR protein and nuclear inclusions of the altered *AR*, with expanded polyglutamine in exon 1, responsible for encoding the N-terminal transactivating domain (Adachi et al., 2007). Other hallmarks include neural and nonneural tissues and residual motor neurons in the brainstem, spinal cord, the skin, testes, and other visceral organs (Adachi et al., 2007). Neurological deficits of KD have been attributed to dysfunction and loss of anterior horn cells and dorsal root ganglion cells (Eisen, 2008).

The genetic basis of KD follows an X-linked recessive pattern of inheritance, with males being the predominant gender to exhibit symptoms (Ropper & Brown, 2005). Females typically serve as carriers, even though they possess the same number of CAG repeats as males with the mutated AR protein (Adachi et al., 2007). Females can present with a mild expression of KD, indicating a less frequent autosomal dominant pattern (Ropper & Brown, 2005). Therefore, the daughter of a female carrier of KD will similarly be a carrier, but the son of a female carrier has a 50% chance of developing active symptomatology. Reduced androgen levels have been suggested to prevent the accumulation of the AR protein in females, preventing symptomatology (Katsuno et al., 2003). Researchers have localized the allele responsible for KD's pattern of inheritance to the long arm of the X-chromosome (Fishbeck et al., 1986).

NEUROPSYCHOLOGICAL/CLINICAL PRESENTATION

The onset of symptoms of KD typically varies but most patients begin to display symptoms in their 30s (Ropper & Brown, 2005). Initial presentation includes muscle cramps and twitching, initiating in the hips, followed by weakness and atrophy of the hip and shoulder musculature (Ropper & Brown, 2005). Muscle weakness and atrophy of the limbs are typically symmetrical, being generalized or most prominent in the proximal muscles (Adachi et al., 2007). Later affecting the bulbar muscles, bilateral facial and masseter muscle weakness, poor uvula and soft palatal movements, and tongue atrophy with fasciculations are evidenced (Adachi et al., 2007). Other symptoms include depressed or absent deep tendon reflexes, mild sensory neuropathy, normal Babinski signs, intention and postural tremor, and a diminished vibration sense in the distal lower extremities (Adachi et al., 2007; Ropper & Brown, 2005).

Androgen insensitivity is occasionally present, associated with gynecomastia, impaired spermatogenesis, testicular atrophy, impotence, reduced fertility, and an increased estrogen effect (Adachi et al., 2007). Normal or elevated testosterone levels are also common (Adachi et al., 2007). The creatine kinase (CK) level is typically elevated (Adachi et al., 2007). Abdominal obesity is typical, but not male pattern baldness (Adachi et al., 2007). Cerebellar symptoms, dysautonomia, and cognitive impairment are absent (Adachi et al., 2007). Physical presentation in the later stages includes difficulty with walking, speech, and swallowing, with some patients eventually being confined to a wheelchair (Adachi et al., 2007).

DIAGNOSIS

Males are most easily diagnosed with KD using genetic testing, assessing for the AR protein mutation. The gene for KD can be found in the blood among both males and females, and used especially with regard to prenatal testing (Roper & Brown, 2005). A biopsy of the scrotal skin can be used to assess AR accumulation, serving as a pathogenic marker of the disease (Banno et al., 2006). Using 1C2 immunostaining, scrotal skin biopsy samples are used to estimate the severity of KD within the nervous system (Banno et al., 2006). This procedure has been suggested to have the potential to predict the course of the disease (Banno et al., 2006). CK and glucose levels may be assessed to confirm the disease (Adachi et al., 2007).

While females are usually asymptomatic, they may present with high amplitude motor unit potentials or an elevated CK level upon evaluation (Schmidt, Greenberg, Allingham-Hawkins, & Spriggs, 2002).

KD may be misdiagnosed with other neuromuscular disorders, with the most common being amyotrophic lateral sclerosis (ALS), commonly referred to as Lou Gehrig's disease. Another late-onset degenerative disease involving the lower motor neurons, patients with ALS may not present with additional pyramidal tract involvement during the early stages of the disorder (Kennedy et al., 1968). Only during the later stage of the disorder will involvement of the lateral columns of the spinal cord and motor cortex be exhibited, with distal distribution of muscle involvement and quick progression occurring (Kennedy et al., 1968). Death results in a few years after the initiation of such symptoms, much in contrast to KD (Kennedy et al., 1968). Other misdiagnoses include spinal muscular atrophy III, glycogen storage disease, Guillian-Barré, myasthenia gravis, and multiple sclerosis. All can be easily differentiated from KD with genetic and biological testing, and the absence of upper motor neuron dysfunction (Adachi et al., 2007).

TREATMENT

Because there is no known cure for KD at present, supportive therapy is most often used to help patients over the course of the disease with lifestyle changes and reducing symptoms (Adachi et al., 2007). Treatment typically involves a combination of physical, occupational, speech, and respiratory therapies. Mobility should be encouraged to maintain range of motion and prevent spinal deformities, with surgery needed on occasion to correct the spine (Adachi et al., 2007). Research is currently underway, with promise relating to androgen deprivation therapy (Banno et al., 2006) and disease-modifying drugs (Katsuno et al., 2005). Banno et al. (2006) found leuprorelin, a gonadotrophin-releasing hormone analogue that decreases the release of gonadotrophins, reduces nuclear accumulations of defective AR, indicating that androgen deprivation may interrupt the progression of KD. Using animal models, geranylgeranylacetone (GGA), a nontoxic anti-ulcer drug which increases heat shock proteins, has been found to inhibit cell death and the accumulation of abnormal AR (Katsuno et al., 2005). Because such research is only preliminary, further research is needed to establish the safety and effectiveness of such treatments before general use among KD patients.

Jessica Holster
Charles Golden

Adachi, J., Waza, M., Katsuno, M., Tanaka, F., Doyu, M., & Sodue, G. (2007). Pathogenesis and molecular targeted therapy of spinal and bulbar muscular atrophy. *Neuropathology & Applied Neurobiology, 33*, 135–151.

Atsuta, N., Watanabe, H., Ito, M., Banno, H., Katsuno, K., Tanaka, F., et al. (2006). Natural history of spinal and bulbar muscular atrophy (SBMA): A case of 223 Japanese patients, *Brain: A Journal of Neurology, 129*, 1446–1455.

Banno, J., Adahi, H., Katsuno, M., Suzuki, K., Atsuta, N., Watanabe, H., et al. (2006). Mutant androgen receptor accumulation in spinal and bulbar muscular atrophy scrotal skin: A pathogenic marker. *Annuals of Neurology, 59*, 520–526.

Eisen, A. (2008). Kennedy's disease: A lower motor neuron model to identify upper motor neuron physiology in ALS. *Clinical Neurophysiology, 119*, 971–972.

Fishbeck, K. H., Lonasescu, V., Ritter, A. W., Lonasescu, R., Davies, K., Ball, S., et al. (1986). Localization of the gene for X-linked spinal muscular atrophy. *Neurology, 36*, 1595–1598.

Harding, A. E., Thomas, P. K., Baraitser, M., Bradbury, P. G., Morgan-Hughes, J. A., & Ponsford, J. R. (1982). X-linked recessive bulbospinal neuronopathy: A report of ten cases. *Journal of Neurology, Neurosurgery & Psychiatry, 45*, 1012–1019.

Katsuno, M., Adachi, H., Doyu, M., Minamiyama, M., Sang, C., Kobayashi, Y., et al. (2003). Leuprorelin rescues polyglutamine-dependent phenotypes in a transgenic mouse model of spinal and bulbar muscular atrophy. *Nature Medicine, 9*, 768–773.

Katsuno, M., Sang, C., Adachi, H., Minamiyama, M., Waza, M., Tanaka, F., et al. (2005). Pharmacological induction of heat-shock proteins alleviates polyglutamine-mediated motor neuron disease. *Proceedings of the National Academy of Sciences of the United States of America, 102*, 16801–16806.

Kennedy, W. R., Alter, M., & Sung, J. H. (1968). Progressive proximal spinal and bulbar muscular atrophy of late onset. A sex-linked recessive trait. *Neurology, 18*, 671–680.

La Spada, A. R., Wilson, E. M., Lubahn, D. B., Harding, A. E., & Fischbeck, K. H. (1991). Androgen receptor gene mutations in X-linked spinal and bulbar muscular atrophy. *Nature, 352*, 77–79.

Ropper, A. H., & Brown, R. H. (2005). *Adams and Victor's principles of neurology* (8th ed.). New York: McGraw-Hill.

Schmidt, B. J., Greenberg, C. R., Allingham-Hawkins, D. J., & Spriggs, E. L. (2002). Expression of X-linked bulbospinal muscular atrophy (Kennedy disease) in two homozygous women. *Neurology, 59*, 770–772.

Sinnreich, M., & Klein, C. J. (2004). Bulbospinal muscular atrophy. *Archives of Neurology, 61*, 1324–1326.

Suzuki, K., Katsuno, M., Banno, H., Takeuchi, Y., Atsuta, N., Ito, M., et al. (2008). CAG repeat size correlates to

IJK

electrophysiological motor and sensory phenotypes in SBMA. *Brain: A Journal of Neurology, 131*, 229–239.

Takahashi, A. (2001). Hiroshi Kawahara (1858–1918). *Journal of Neurology, 248*, 241–242.

Udd, B., Juvonen, V., Hakamies, L., Nieminen, A., Wallgren-Pettersson, C., Cederquist, K., et al. (1998). High prevalence of Kennedy's disease in Western Finland: Is the syndrome underdiagnosed? *Acta Neurologica Scandinavica, 98*, 128–133.

KINSBOURNE'S SYNDROME

DESCRIPTION

Kinsbourne's syndrome is an autoimmune disorder that targets the nervous system. It is a rare condition, with prevalence rates of approximately 1 in 10,000,000 people per year. It typically affects infants and children. The age of onset ranges from 4 months to 6 years, with an average age of 17 to 19 months (Fernandez-Alvarez, Aicardi, Bathien, & International Child Neurology Association [ICNA], 2001; Guerrini, Aicardi, Andermann, & Hallett, 2002). The primary symptoms include sudden onset of irritability or aggression followed by the development of fast, jerking movements of the eyes and the arms, legs, and/or entire body. This may cause the child to have impaired voluntary movement and incoordination. It tends to be recurrent and has residual symptoms of speech and intellectual impairment in about 90% of cases, with 60% of these cases being severe (Bissonnette, Dalens, Luginbuehl, & Marciniak, 2006).

Kinsbourne's syndrome can alternatively be called opsoclonus myoclonus syndrome, opsoclonus myoclonus ataxia, neuroblastoma paraneoplastic syndrome, myoclonic encephalopathy of infants, or opsoclonic encephalopathy dancing eyes syndrome (Bissonnette et al., 2006).

NEUROPATHOLOGY/PATHOPHYSIOLOGY

The condition is associated with a neuroblastoma in 50% of the cases, but it may follow an infection, or be idiopathic (Bissonnette et al., 2006). Neuroblastomas usually originate in the adrenal gland or sympathetic ganglion and are the most common extracranial malignant tumor in children. A number of other tumors may induce the syndrome more rarely, including: ganglioneuroblastoma, ganglioneuroma, medullary thyroid carcinoma, and oat cell carcinoma (Pranzatelli, 1992). Pranzatelli (1992) stated that viral etiologies are the most common type of infection associated with Kinsbourne's syndrome. He reported that

coxsackie B3, Epstein-Barr, *Hemophilus influenzae* meningitis, herpes zoster, immunization, lymphocytic choriomeningitis, mumps, neurosyphilis, polioencephalitis, psittacosis, rubella, *Salmonella typhi* St. Louis encephalitis, tuberculous meningitis, and viral encephalitis have been associated with opsoclonus, myoclonus, or both.

It is hypothesized that the cerebellum or brainstem may be the focus of infarct. However, these hypotheses are based upon as few as 10 patients whom have shown lesions or atrophy in these areas (Zorzi, Nardocci, Erba, & Lanzi, 2002).

NEUROPSYCHOLOGICAL/CLINICAL PRESENTATION

Pranzatelli (1992) described patients with Kinsbourne's syndrome after doing a meta-analysis of the literature. He reported that emotional symptoms of irritability, fatigue, malaise, anxiety, emotional lability, or aggression are often present. Sensory perception is normal. Deep tendon muscle reflexes and muscle strength are usually normal, and the Babinski sign may or may not be present.

Zorzi et al. (2002) completed follow-up analyses on a sample of 16 patients with opsoclonus myoclonus syndrome, or Kinsbourne's syndrome, to evaluate the residual neurological and neuropsychological symptoms. The age of participants at onset ranged from 13 months to 2 years 10 months. Participants received corticosteroid treatment for between 1 month and 18.3 years and follow-up evaluations ranging from 1 month to 18.3 years. Of their sample, nine participants had no residual neurological symptoms. Seven participants had residual motor symptoms such as clumsiness, ataxia or poor coordination, tremor, and dysmetria. Dysmetria refers to the inability to coordinate a movement of a muscle to achieve its desired location, resulting in under or overshooting. One participant showed normal psychological and cognitive functioning. Fifteen participants had emotional, developmental, and cognitive symptoms such as irritability, speech delay, and impaired intelligence (IQs ranging from 31 to 80). Participants with longer duration of treatment showed more severe deficits and a decline in functioning. For example, one participant who was 18 months old at age of onset and received 18.3 years of treatment showed a decline in IQ from 64 at 5.4 years old to 31 at 10 years old. They stated that in all patients with duration of 4 years or longer had functional impairment with cognitive and neurological symptoms. Although the percentages were higher in this study, residual symptoms of motor and mental deficits affect approximately 50% of cases overall (Zorzi et al., 2002).

DIAGNOSIS

Kinsbourne's syndrome occurs approximately equally in males and females (1:1.4) (Pranzatelli, 1992). It appears to have no family inheritance as there have been no reported cases with multiple family members who were affected (Pranzatelli et al., 2005).

The clinical presentation of symptoms reaches its peak 2–7 days after onset. The first symptoms may be changes in emotional features and behavior such as irritability, fatigue, malaise, anxiety, emotional lability, or aggression (Pranzatelli, 1992). Vomiting is often present at onset. Speech may be slurred and become absent over the progression of the illness (Pranzetti, 2005).

Symptoms of myoclonus appear within a few days, involving motor disorders of incoordination, tremor, and flinging movements that may render the child unable to sit, stand, or walk independently. These involuntary movements may affect the face, head, neck, limbs, fingers and hands, legs, and trunk. Facial spasms, particularly of the lips and eyebrows, are apparent even during sleep. Though these motor symptoms occur at rest, they are exacerbated by attempts at voluntary movement, excitement or stress (Pranzatelli, 1992; Zorzi et al., 2002). In addition to myoclonus, resting and intentional tremors have been reported (Pranzatelli, 1992). Resting tremor is a rhythmic tremor that can occur at any time but is exaggerated by stress. Intentional tremor only occurs during exacting, precise fine motor movements. Muscle tone and deep tendon reflexes are usually normal (Pranzatelli, 1992).

Opsoclonus refers to irregular eye movements such as fluttering eyelids or rapid, randomly directed bursts of involuntary movement (Bissonnette et al., 2006). It may be exaggerated by startle, stimulation, or an attempt to fixate the gaze on a specific point. It may persist during sleep and causes sufficient impairment that some patients prefer to keep one eye shut (Pranzatelli, 1992).

The course of Kinsbourne's syndrome may be relapsing or nonrelapsing. The relapsing type is commonly associated with neuroblastoma, which accounts for approximately 50% of cases (Bissonnette et al., 2006). Relapse may be precipitated by infection or change in treatment (Zorzi et al., 2002).

Bissonnette et al. (2006) describe the nonrelapsing type as commonly associated with immunization or viral infections, including coxsackie B3 visu, mumps, togavirus, Epstein-Barr virus, rubella, and poliomyelitis. A direct etiology of infection cannot always be established. Symptoms usually appear within 2 weeks of infection or immunization.

The nonrelapsing type has an average age of onset of 3 years with an average duration of less than 2 weeks.

Because of the high correlation between neuroblastoma and Kinsbourne's syndrome, it is recommended that the patient be investigated through MRI, metaiodobenzylguanidine radionuclide scan, CT Scan, and/or electroencephalogram (EEG) regularly over the course of up to 12 years (Pranzatelli, 1992). The development of symptoms can precede detection of the tumor by several years, so ongoing evaluations are critical (Zorzi et al., 2002).

In cases without a neuroblastoma, the EEG of a patient with Kinsbourne's syndrome is typically normal. The EEG does not demonstrate patterns of spikes and complex wave forms that would be expected due to the motor movements (Zorzi et al., 2002). Cases following viral infection show elevated cerebrospinal fluid (CSF) pleocytosis or immunoglobins. The fourth ventricle may be enlarged, and the patient may have pontine or cerebellar lesions. It is difficult to state whether these infarcts are the result of the premorbid condition or Kinsbourne's syndrome (Fernandez-Alvarez et al., 2001).

Differential diagnosis includes acute cerebellar ataxia syndromes of children that share common motor symptoms. Pranzatelli (1992) suggests diagnosis of acute cerebellar ataxia through urine catecholamine evaluation.

TREATMENT

Treatment often involves excitation of the neuroblastoma or treatment of the precluding infection. Adrenocorticotropic hormone (ACTH) is the most common treatment but may only be maintained for a short period of time due to its side effects of elevated blood pressure, water retention, vomiting, dizziness, potassium and calcium depletion, slowed growth, cardiovascular irregularities, and hyperpigmentation (Pranzatelli, 1992). ACTH is often used to bring about remission of neurological symptoms, before tapering down the dose. This has been found to be effective in 80–90% of cases (Pranzatelli, 1992). Corticosteroids have been used as long-term treatment to address the side effects (Bissonnette et al., 2006). Intravenous immunoglobulins and immunosuppressive drugs have been tried with little success. Specific symptoms may be the target of treatment, such as prescribing a sedative for sleep.

Jessie L. Morrow
Charles Golden

IJK

Bissonnette, B., Dalens, B. J., Luginbuehl, I., & Marciniak, B. (2006). *Syndromes: Rapid recognition and perioperative implications*. New York: McGraw-Hill Professional.

Fernandez-Alvarez, E., Aicardi, J., Bathien, N., & International Child Neurology Association (2001). *Movement disorders in children*. New York: Cambridge University Press.

Guerrini, R., Aicardi, J., Andermann, F., & Hallett, M. (2002). *Epilepsy and movement disorders*. New York: Cambridge University Press.

Pranzatelli, M. R. (1992). The neurobiology of the opsoclonus-myoclonus syndrome. *Clinical Neuropharmacology*, *15*(3), 186–228.

Pranzatelli, M. R., Fernandez-Alvarez, E., Arzimanoglou, A., & Toloso, E. (Eds.). (2005). *Paediatric movement disorders*. Montrouge, France: John Libbey Eurotext.

Zorzi, G., Nardocci, N., Erba, A., & Lanzi, G. (2002). In L. Angelini, M. Bardare, & A. Martini (Eds). *Immune-mediated disorders of the central nervous system in children*. Montrouge, France: John Libbey Eurotext.

KLEINE–LEVIN SYNDROME

DESCRIPTION

Kleine–Levin syndrome (KLS) is a complex and rare neuropsychological disorder, with only 500 cases diagnosed around the world in 2000 (Justo, Calil, Prado-Bolognani, & Muszkat, 2007). The prognosis of KLS is considered benign and not to be life-threatening (Conklin & Taunton, 2005).

KLS predominantly affects adolescent males but it can also occur in females and there have been some reports of onset of the disorder well into adulthood (Arnulf, Zeitzer, File, Farber, & Mignot, 2005; Malomo, Lawal, & Orija, 1998). Onset of symptoms associated with KLS is extremely rapid. Predominant symptoms are characterized by a need for excessive amounts of sleep (hypersomnia), excessive eating (compulsive hyperphagia), and an abnormally high sex drive (Arnulf et al., 2005; Mukaddes, Alyanak, Kora, & Polvan, 1999). In some patients, additional symptoms may also be present. These include cognitive and behavioral disturbances, visual and auditory hallucinations, memory problems, and difficulties with concentration (Wygnamski, Kokia, Barak, Terlo, & Caine, 1996).

KLS episodes are cyclical, lasting days, weeks, and even months, during which all normal patient activities stop. On average, episodes occur twice a year, but can also occur as many as 12 times in a year. Patients can sleep up to 20 hours per day, waking only to eat, urinate, and defecate. Episodes remit spontaneously, leaving the patient in good physical and mental health and sleeping normally in between episodes. Patients may go for a period of weeks, months, or even years without experiencing any symptoms, but symptoms may reappear with little warning (Malomo et al., 1998). Many patients with KLS find that their episodes decrease in intensity and frequency with age, and many experience complete recovery during early adulthood. However, some continue to experience episodes throughout their entire lifetime with no recovery (Conklin & Taunton, 2005).

NEUROPATHOLOGY/PATHOPHYSIOLOGY

As of yet, there are no known causes of KLS and onset appears to be spontaneous. However, research has uncovered some possible precipitating factors that may be associated with the onset of KLS. The most common precipitating factors noted were febrile illness, respiratory infections, and excessive physical and psychological stress. KLS also been observed in association with brain tumors, head injuries, endocrine and metabolic disorders, and encephalitis (Arnulf et al., 2005; Conklin & Taunton, 2005; Ferber & Kryger, 1994; Gua et al., 1996).

Laboratory tests may show slight changes in the EEG during an episode, with minor nonspecific abnormalities. However, physical exams and laboratory tests are normal between episodes (Conklin & Taunton, 2005; Ferber & Kryger, 1994).

It has been hypothesized that KLS symptoms may be related to malfunction of the hypothalamus and hypothalamic-pituitary axis, which helps to regulate sleep, appetite, sex drive, and body temperature (Cheung, 2006). In addition, a focal, transient, and immune-modulated process has been recently suggested (Podesta et al., 2006, p. 649). The frontal and medial temporal lobes have been proposed to be involved in the development of KLS as well (Cheung, 2006), with research indicating that in at least one case of spontaneous recovery, slight hypoperfusion was evident on SPECT in the left temporal lobe 6 years following recovery (Landtblom, Dige, Schwerdt, Safstrom, & Granerus, 2002).

NEUROPSYCHOLOGICAL/CLINICAL PRESENTATION

Although KLS patients may be awakened or awake themselves during episodes, they are likely irritable, lethargic, confused, disoriented, and apathetic at this time. In addition, KLS patients often experience symptoms of depression, disinhibited behaviors (such as aggression, irritability, and hallucinations), as well as compulsive behaviors (such as binge eating and hypersexuality) and anxiety (Malhotra, Das, Gupta, & Muralidharan, 1997; Wygnamski et al., 1996). Residual impairments following remission of KLS can include deficits in both recent visual and verbal memory (Landtblom et al., 2002).

DIAGNOSIS

KLS is often difficult to diagnose initially due to the variability in episodes and the diverse psychiatric symptoms seen among patients. Diagnosis of KLS often begins with a clinical evaluation and a detailed patient history. A complete neurological evaluation, including an EEG, may be performed to rule out any structural brain abnormalities (Malomo et al., 1998).

Symptoms of the following disorders can be seen as similar or related to those of KLS and therefore should be considered during differential diagnosis. Bipolar disorder is often considered due the similarities between KLS symptoms of poor impulse control and those of a manic or hypomanic state. In addition, some of the drug treatments used for KLS, such as lithium, are often used for bipolar disorder (Conklin & Taunton, 2005). Narcolepsy has also been classified as a disorder of excessive somnolence, similar to that of KLS (Visscher, Van Der Horst, & Smit, 1990).

TREATMENT

To date, no effective treatment exists for KLS. Due to spontaneous remission and eventual recovery in many cases, patients with mild forms of KLS may opt for no treatment at all. When treatment is pursued, it is often directed toward the symptoms specific to an individual's case, and treatment often has a supportive and educational focus (Malomo et al., 1998).

The use of medications such as stimulants, anticonvulsants, antidepressants, hormones, lithium, and neuroleptics has been reported in the literature, but these medications have little if any impact on remission of the disorder (Malomo et al., 1998; Mukaddes, Kora, & Bilge, 1999). Amphetamine stimulants were found to improve sleepiness but do not have an effect on the additional symptoms. Results on the use of anticonvulsants were similar to that of no drug treatment. Lithium was found to be successful at treating relapse in a small number of cases. However, when considering the use of this medication, one has to note the small number of cases experiencing a positive

outcome using this drug as well as possible side effects and difficulty of use (Arnulf et. al., 2005). Light therapy has also been suggested in the literature but found to also have little success related to remission (Crumley, 1998). Finally, the majority of reports examining the effectiveness of medications to treat KLS have evaluated outcomes based upon symptom reduction. Moreover, there have been no well controlled research designs that have investigated the long-term treatment safety and effectiveness of the various drugs used to treat symptoms of KLS.

Kelly N. Hutchins
Jon C. Thompson

Arnulf, I., Zeitzer, J. M., File, J., Farber, N., & Mignot, E. (2005). Kleine-Levin Syndrome: A systematic review of 186 cases in the literature. *Brain*, 1–14.

Cheung, G. (2006). Posttraumatic Kleine-Levin syndrome. *General Hospital Psychiatry, 28*, 443–445.

Conklin, C. M. J., & Taunton, J. E. (2005). Kleine-Levin syndrome: A unique cause of fatigue in an athlete. *British Journal of Sports Medicine, 39*(7), 1–2.

Crumley, F. (1998). Light therapy for Kleine-Levin syndrome. *Journal of the American Academy of Child and Adolescent Psychiatry, 37*(12), 1245.

Ferber, R., & Kryger, M. (1994). *Principles and practice of sleep medicine in children.* Philadelphia: W.B. Saunders Company.

Gua, S. F., Soong, W., Liu, H., Hou, J., Tsai, W., Chiu, Y., et al. (1996). Kleine-Levin syndrome in a boy with Prader-Willi syndrome. *American Sleep Disorders Association and Sleep Research Society, 19*(1), 13–17.

Justo, L. P., Calil, H. M., Prado-Bolognani, S. A., & Muszkat, M. (2007). Kleine-Levin syndrome: Interface between neurology and psychiatry. *Arq Neuropsiquiatr, 65*(1), 150–152.

Landtblom, A. M., Dige, N., Schwerdt, K., Safstrom, P., & Granerus, G. (2002). A case of Kleine-Levin syndrome examined with SPECT and neuropsychological testing. *Acta Neurologica Scandinavica, 105*, 318–321.

Malhotra, S., Das, M. K., Gupta, N., & Muralidharan, R. (1997). A clinical study of Kleine-Levin syndrome with evidence for hypothalamic-pituitary axis dysfunction. *Society of Biological Psychiatry, 42*, 299–301.

Malomo, I. O., Lawal, R. A., & Orija, O. B. (1998). Kleine-Levin syndrome: Case report. *East African Medical Journal, 75*(1), 55–56.

Mukaddes, N. M., Alyanak, B., Kora, M. E., & Polvan, O. (1999). The psychiatric symptomology in Kleine-Levin syndrome. *Child Psychiatry and Human Development, 29*(3), 253–258.

Mukaddes, N. M., Kora, M. E., & Bilge, S. (1999). Carbamazepine for Kleine-Levin syndrome. *Journal of the*

IJK

American Academy of Child and Adolescent Psychiatry. 38(7), 791–792.

Podesta, C., Ferreras, M., Mozzi, M., Bassetti, C., Dauvilliers, Y., & Billiard, M. (2006). Kleine-Levin Syndrome in a 14-year-old girl: CSF hypocretin-1 measurements. *Sleep Medicine, 7,* 649–651.

Visscher, F., Van Der Horst, A. R., & Smit, L. M. E. (1990). HLA-DR Antigens in Kleine-Levin syndrome. *Annals of Neurology, 28,* 195.

Wygnamski, T., Kokia, E., Barak, P., Terlo, L., & Caine, Y. G. (1996). The sleeping aviator: Aeromedical disposition of Kleine-Levin syndrome. *Space and Environmental Medicine, 67*(1), 61–62.

KLINEFELTER'S SYNDROME

DESCRIPTION

Klinefelter's syndrome refers to a sex chromosome anomaly characterized by a surplus of X chromosomes in phenotypic males. The 47 XXY type is the most common chromosomal pattern associated with this disorder; however, mosaic patterns such as 46XY/47XXY and, on rare occasions, variants such as 48XXXY are observed. Klinefelter's syndrome occurs in1 in 500 up to 1 in 1,000 live male births.

It was first described by Dr. Henry Klinefelter, who determined that, while all affected males present with the extra X chromosome, physical and neurological presentations may vary. Nevertheless, the typical adult patient with Klinefelter's syndrome is of average or slightly above average height, is sterile, and has small testes, breast development, and a weak growth of facial hair. Cognitively, select deficits in memory, particularly auditory sequential and language development may be noted along with higher rates of learning disabilities.

NEUROPATHOLOGY/PATHOPHYSIOLOGY

Klinefelter syndrome is marked by the XXY chromosomal karotype on the 47th chromosome (i.e., sex chromosome). This aberration is associated with the sex-chromatin-positive form of seminiferous tubular dysgenesis and occurs in 0.9 out of 1000 births, whereas the mosaic form presents in 0.15 out of 1000 births (Berg, 2007). Normal to low testosterone levels are noted and serum levels of follicle-stimulating hormone and luteinizing hormone are elevated in the early second decade (Berg, 2007). It has been positively associated with maternal age.

There appears to be significant differences in brain morphology of individuals with sex chromosome anomalies, such as Klinefelter's syndrome, such that gray matter reduction was observed (Giedd et al., 2007), specifically left temporal lobe gray matter differences (Patwardhan, Eliez, Bender, Linden, & Reiss, 2000). Based on the syndrome's affect on hormone release, many studies have shown that testosterone levels impact spatial performance and functional lateralization in both children (Grimshaw, Sitarenios, & Finegan, 1995) and adults (Hier & Crowley, 1982), as well as verbal intelligence (Netley, 1992). In general, research on this population is difficult due to the lack of consistent manifestation of symptoms and small sample size.

NEUROPSYCHOLOGICAL/CLINICAL PRESENTATION

Intelligence is typically within the normal to low normal range (Stewart, Bailey, Netley, Rovet, & Park, 1986). Patients frequently have delayed speech and language development, poor reading and spelling skills, and often demonstrate poor overall academic performance (Netley & Rovet, 1982). In fact, Graham, Bashir, Stark, Silbert, and Walzer (1988) found that approximately half of boys with XXY were reading one or more grade levels below average compared to their same-aged peers. On neuropsychological tests, patients frequently present with poor gross and fine motor coordination as well as visual-motor and sensory integration difficulties. Deficits in executive functions are common, including difficulties related to planning and inhibition (Temple & Sanfilippo, 2003; Visootsak, Aylstock, & Graham, 2001). Although no specific personality profile typifies this syndrome, there does appear to be a tendency toward introversion, passivity, immaturity, and susceptibility to anxiety.

Physically, children have small firm testes and adults have azoospermia (Ratcliffe, 1982). Primary hypogonadism, infertility, and delayed or poorly developed secondary sex chromosomes are common, whereas gynecomastia, androgen deficiency, and eunuchoid features are also seen but at a lower frequency (Berg, 2007).

DIAGNOSIS

While this disorder can be detected prenatally by amniocentesis or after birth by chromosome analysis and karyotyping, most patients are clinically detected in adolescence or adulthood due to fertility problems, delayed development of secondary sex characteristics, or behavioral/learning difficulties. Later, the diagnosis is confirmed by chromosome studies. Neuropsychological assessment is utilized to identify neuro-cognitive deficits but is not essential to diagnosing the syndrome itself.

TREATMENT

No surgical treatment is currently available to correct the seminiferous tubule dysgenesis that causes sterility in these patients. Enlarged breasts may be surgically reduced and testosterone hormone therapy is frequently used to stimulate growth of facial hair and deepening of the voice (Berg, 2007).

Early identification of patients with Klinefelter's syndrome is recommended so that parents can receive early counseling and information regarding delays in the patient's neuromuscular development, language, and learning. Early identification of the syndrome can also alert parents and school personnel that the patient may require special educational attention given the noted risk of cognitive deficits and learning disabilities. There is also a need for the patient to receive counseling and information during adolescence and adulthood regarding sexuality, gender identification and ability to produce offspring.

Matthew Holcombe
Raymond S. Dean

Berg, B. O. (2007). Chromosomal abnormalities and neuro-cutaneous disorders. In C. G. Goetz (Ed.), *Textbook of clinical neurology* (pp. 683–697). Philadelphia, PA: Saunders Elsevier.

Genetics Home Reference. (2008). *Klinefelter's syndrome.* Retrieved September 19, 2010, from http://ghr.nlm.nih.gov/condition/klinefelter-syndrome

Giedd, J. N., Clasen, L. S., Wallace, G. L., Lenroot, R. K., Lerch, J. P., Wells, E. M., . . . Samango-Sprouse, C. A. (2007). XXY (Klinefelter syndrome): A pediatric quantitative brain magnetic resonance imaging case-control study. *Pediatrics, 119,* 232–240.

Graham, J. M., Jr., Bashir, A. S., Stark, R. E., Silbert, A., & Walzer, S. (1988). Oral and written language abilities of XXY boys: Implications for anticipatory guidance. *Pediatrics, 81,* 795–806.

Grimshaw, G. M., Sitarenios, G., & Finegan, J. A. (1995). Mental rotation at 7 years: Relations with prenatal testosterone levels and spatial play experiences. *Brain Cognition, 29,* 85–100.

Hier, D. B., & Crowley, W. F., Jr. (1982). Spatial ability in androgen-deficient men. *New England Journal of Medicine, 306,* 1202–1205.

National Human Genome Research Institute. (2010). *Learning about Klinefelter's syndrome.* Retrieved September 19, 2010, from http://www.genome.gov/19519068

National Institute of Child Health and Human Development. (2007). *Klinefelter's syndrome.* Retrieved September 19, 2010, from http://www.nichd.nih.gov/health/topics/klinefelter_syndrome.cfm

Netley, C. (1992). Time of pubertal onset, testosterone levels and intelligence in 47,XXY males. *Clinical Genetics, 42,* 31–34.

Netley, C., & Rovet, J. (1982). Verbal deficits in children with 47,XXY and 47,XXX karyotypes: A descriptive and experimental study. *Brain Language, 17,* 58–72.

Patwardhan, A. J., Eliez, S., Bender, B., Linden, M. G., & Reiss, A. L. (2000). Brain morphology in Klinefelter syndrome: Extra X chromosome and testosterone supplementation. *American Academy of Neurology, 54,* 2218–2223.

Ratcliffe, S. G. (1982). Klinefelter's syndrome in adolescence. *Archives of Disorders in Children, 57,* 6–12.

Stewart, D. A., Bailey, J. D., Netley, C. T., Rovet, J., & Park, E. (1986). Growth and development from early to mid-adolescence of children with X and Y chromosome aneuploidy: The Toronto Study. *Birth Defects, 22,* 119–182.

Temple, C. M., & Sanfilippo, P. M. (2003). Executive skills in Klinefelter's syndrome. *Neuropsychologia, 41,* 1547–1559.

Visootsak, J., Aylstock, M., & Graham, J. M., Jr. (2001). Klinefelter syndrome and its variants: An update and review for the primary pediatrician. *Clinical Pediatrics, 40,* 639–651.

KLIPPEL–FEIL'S SYNDROME

DESCRIPTION

Klippel–Feil's syndrome (KFS) is a congenital fusion (failure of segmentation) of the cervical vertebrae that may involve two segments, a congenital block vertebra or the entire cervical spine. Congenital cervical fusion is a result of failure of normal segmentation of the cervical somites during the third to eighth week of life. The skeletal system may not be the only system affected during this time; cardiorespiratory, genitourinary, and auditory systems are frequently involved. The actual incidence of KFS is unknown due to absence

IJK

of population screening studies. However, it has been estimated that it occurs in approximately 1:40,000–42,000 births (Thomsen, Schneider, Weber, Johannisson, & Niethard, 1998; Warmer, 1998). A slight female predominance has been noted (3:2) (Dietz, 2001; Hensinger & MacEwen, 1982).

NEUROPATHOLOGY/PATHOPHYSIOLOGY

The embryonic defect is a failure of segmentation, as opposed to secondary fusion, of the chordamesoderm and its derivative sclerotomes that ultimately go on to form the cervical vertebrae. Although this can go beyond the cervical spine, it is primarily localized to C2, C3, C5, and C6 levels (Golden & Bonnemann, 2007). KFS frequently occurs sporadically, but it can also be inherited as an autosomal-dominant disorder with variable expression and reduced penetrance. It has also been noted in conjunction with specific syndromes including Turner's syndrome, Noonan's syndrome, and Wildervanck's syndrome (Golden & Bonnemann, 2007). In one report, this pattern of inheritance cosegregated with a pericentric inversion involving chromosome 8 (q22.2–q23.3) (Clarke, Kovacic, Yip, & Diwan, 1997). This gene has been labeled the *SGM1* gene and is associated with vertebral fusions and vocal impairment. A balanced translocation between 5q11.2 and 17q23 has also been reported in at least one KFS patient. Familial KFS is heterogeneous with four different genetic classes described, namely KF1, KF2, KF3, and KF4.

Various mouse models for gene identification had particularly focused on *HOX*, *PAX*, and Notch signaling pathways for playing possible roles in vertebral segmental disorders (Chi & Epstein, 2002; Krumlauf, 1994). Although mouse models suggest that *HOX* genes are unlikely to cause extensive cervical spina fusions, promising etiological candidates have been identified in relation to KFS, PAX, and Notch pathway genes (Chi & Epstein, 2002; Krumlauf, 1994; Sarnat, 2006).

NEUROPSYCHOLOGICAL/CLINICAL PRESENTATION

The classic triad of KFS includes a short neck, limitation of neck motion, and a low occipital hairline (Beaty, 2007). However, fewer than half of patients with KFS have all parts of the triad. Limitation of neck motion is the most constant finding (rotation/lateral bending greater than flexion/extension) (Beaty, 2007). If fewer than three vertebrae are fused or if the lower cervical vertebrae are fused, motion is only slightly limited. Webbing of the neck (pterygium colli) is seen in severe involvement. Symptoms usually

are not caused by the fused cervical vertebrae but by open segments adjacent to areas of synostosis that become hypermobile in response to increased stress placed on the area. Symptoms are caused by mechanical or neurological problems, which include local pain due to degenerative arthritis, radicular pain due to nerve root impingement, and spasticity, hyperreflexia, muscle weakness, and paralysis due to spinal cord compression (Beaty, 2007).

Although affected patients have cervical anomalies at birth, KFS usually is diagnosed at a latter age through incidental radiographs. Patients with atlantoaxial fusions found incidentally on radiograph often present at younger ages than patients with more caudal fusion (Tracy, Dromans, & Kusumi, 2004). Patients with extensive fusion also tend to present at a very early age, perhaps because of cosmetic deformity. Some also present with problems related to anomalies in other organ systems that are formed embryologically at the same time as the cervical spine (including the inner ear, heart, and kidneys). Some children exhibit mental retardation or show learning deficits. An association with mirror movements has been reported (Gunderson & Solitare, 1968). It could reflect the soft sign seen in children with mild intellectual deficits or result from an inadequate decussation of the pyramidal tracts or dorsal closure of the cord. Consequently, kyphosis, scoliosis, and spina bifida occulata are often associated with the presentation (Van Kerckhoven & Fabry, 1989). Genitourinary anomalies, hearing impairments, and other skeletal deformities may also present concurrently (Golden & Bonnemann, 2007). In some patients, the congenital synostosis is discovered to be part of a larger, named syndrome such as Wildervanck's syndrome, Mayer–Rokitansky's syndrome, Goldenhar's syndrome, VACTERL syndrome (vertebrae, anus, cardiovascular, tracheoesophageal, renal and limbs), or fetal alcohol syndrome. Table 1 includes associated abnormalities commonly found in KFS.

Table 1
COMMONLY ASSOCIATED ABNORMALITIES FOUND IN KFS

Anomaly	Percentage of Patients
Congenital scoliosis	>50
Rib abnormalities	33
Deafness	30
Genitourinary abnormalities	25–35
Sprengel deformity	20–30
Synkinesia	15–20
Cervical ribs	12–15
Cardiovascular abnormalities	4–29

DIAGNOSIS

Routine radiographs, computed CT scans, and MRI assessments may be useful in the evaluation of KFS. High-quality radiographs of the cervical spine are often the first step to evaluate the nature and extent of fusion (Dietz, 2001). All patients should also have radiographs of thoracic and lumbar spine done to look for any other deformity and to monitor for development of scoliosis (Dietz, 2001). MRI, including flexion and extension MRI, is indicated when preliminary studies suggest instability or stenosis. MRI scans are also helpful in the detection of associated abnormalities like syrinx (i.e., a fluid-filled cavity that develops in either the spinal cord or brainstem) tethered cord (i.e., the presence of an abnormal attachment of the spinal cord to its surrounding tissue), or diastomyelia. CT is helpful in defining bony pathoanatomy but is associated with radiation exposure to the child. Detailed evaluation of all patients is required to rule out other associated anomalies of the cardiovascular, renal, auditory, gastrointestinal, respiratory, and dermatologic systems. Periodic neurologic examination is also necessary to rule out cranial nerve abnormalities, cervical radiculopathy, or myelopathy.

TREATMENT

Traction, cervical collar, and analgesics are useful for mechanical symptoms caused by degenerative joints. Neurological symptoms should be evaluated carefully to locate the exact pathological condition. Three specific patterns of cervical fusion create a high risk for symptomatic instability (Beaty, 2007): C2–C3 fusion with occipitocervical synostosis, extensive fusion over several cervical vertebrae with an abnormal occipitocervical junction, and two fused segments separated by an open joint space. With clinical evidence for compression of the cervical cord, laminectomy is indicated (Sarnat, 2006). Prophylactic fusion of a hypermobile segment remains a doubtful treatment. The risk of neurological compromise must be weighed against further reduction in the neck motion. Cosmetic surgery is quite helpful for Sprengel deformity.

Gaurav Jain
Sarita Singhal
Chad A. Noggle

Beaty, J. H. (2007). Klippel-Feil syndrome. In S. T. Canale & J. H. Beaty (Eds.), *Campbell's operative orthopaedics* (11th ed.). Mosby, MO: Imprint of Elsevier.

Chi, N., & Epstein, J. A. (2002). Getting your Pax straight: Pax proteins in development and disease. *Trends in Genetics, 18,* 41–47.

Clarke, R. A., Kovacic, A., Yip, M. Y., & Diwan, A. (1997). Genetic basis of the Klippel-Feil syndrome. *Journal of Bone and Joint Surgery, 79*-B(4S), 406.

Dietz, F. (2001). Congenital abnormalities of the cervical spine. In S. L. Weinstein (Ed.), *The pediatric spine — principles and practice* (2nd ed., pp. 239–251). Philadelphia: Lippincott Williams & Wilkins.

Golden, J. A., & Bonnemann, C. G. (2007). Developmental structural disorders. In C. G. Goetz (Ed.), *Textbook of clinical neurology* (3rd ed., pp. 561–591). Philadelphia: Saunders Elsevier.

Gunderson, C. H., & Solitare, G. B. (1968). Mirror movements in patients with Klippel-Feil syndrome. *Archives of Neurology, 18,* 675–679.

Hensiger, R. N., & MacEwen, G. D. (1982). Congenital anomalies of the spine. In R. H. Rothman & F. A. Simeone (Eds.), *The spine* (pp. 188–315). Philadelphia: WB Saunders.

Krumlauf, R. (1994). Hox genes in vertebrate development. *Cell, 78,* 191–201.

Sarnat, H. B. (2006). Neuroembryology, genetic programming, and malformations of the nervous system. In J. H. Menkes, H. B. Sarnat, & B. L. Maria (Eds.), *Child neurology* (7th ed., p. 307). Philadelphia: Lippincott Williams & Wilkins.

Thomsen, M. N., Schneider, U., Weber, M., Johannisson, R., & Niethard, F. U. (1997). Scoliosis and congenital anomalies associated with Klippel-Feil syndrome types I-III. *Spine, 22,* 396–401.

Tracy, M. R., Dormans, J. P., & Kusumi, K. (2004). Klippel-Feil syndrome: Clinical features and current understanding of etiology. *Clinical Orthopedics and Related Research, 424,* 183–190.

Van Kerckhoven, M. F., & Fabry, G. (1989). The Klippel-Feil syndrome: A constellation of deformities. *Acta Orthopaedica Belgica, 55,* 107–118.

Warner, W. C. (1998). Pediatric cervical spine. In S. T. Canale (Ed.), *Campbell's operative orthopaedics* (9th ed., pp. 2815–2847). St Louis, MO: Mosby.

KLIPPEL–TRENAUNAY'S SYNDROME

DESCRIPTION

Klippel–Trenaunay's syndrome (KTS) is a rare, congenital disorder that disrupts the normal development of blood and lymph vessels leading to the development of hemangiomas, including port-wine stains

(PWS), and arteriovenous abscesses (Albertini et al., 2008). In addition, asymmetrical hypertrophy of the limbs are often noted, in which one extremity (usually a leg) is significantly larger than its opposite (i.e., the left leg is significantly larger than the right) (Hai & Shrivastava, 2003). Again, the presentation is related to abnormal blood and lymph vessel development; however, the basis for these developmental mishaps remains unknown although some theories have been more favored than others.

KTS is sometimes also referred to as angio-osteohypertrophy syndrome, congenital dysplastic angiectasia, and hemangiectatic hypertrophy. The term Klippel–Trenaunay–Weber's syndrome is also commonly used and has even been adopted as the recognized name by the *International Classification of Diseases-10*.

NEUROPATHOLOGY/PATHOPHYSIOLOGY

The underlying pathophysiology of KTS corresponds with a disruption of the normal development of the peripheral lymph and blood vessels. Although a definitive basis for this disruption has not been agreed upon, dysregulation of angiogenic cells' proliferation and maturation, vasoconstrictor paralysis (Parkes-Weber, 1907), loss of sympathetic tone and resulting dilation of arteriovenous shunting (Bliznak & Staple, 1974), and chronic venous hypertension and venous compression and its resulting alteration of venous pressure have been suggested as contributing factors (Servelle, 1985). Klippel and Trenaunay (1900) actually thought that spinal cord abnormalities may serve as the basis of the presentation.

The presentation is defined by the development of hemangiomas and arteriovenous abscesses. Hemangiomas represent areas on the dermis made up of masses of blood vessels. Port wine stains (PWS) represent specific types of hemangiomas, are most commonly seen on the hypertrophied extremity, and are often the first symptom observed (Jacob et al., 1998; Lambrechts & Carmeliet, 2004). Although the PWS may be relatively shallow in depth and only present slightly above the dermal surface, cases have been noted in which they may have infiltrated the deeper muscle and even bone. The hypertrophied limb presents as significantly larger than its opposite. Although the presentation is traditionally isolated to one limb, multiple extremity, unilateral, and even whole body involvement have been reported (Gloviczki et al., 1983; Samuel & Spitz, 1995). Although most patients with KTS present with no neurological sequelae or underlying neuropathological features, hemangiomas may develop within the brain.

NEUROPSYCHOLOGICAL/CLINICAL PRESENTATION

The clinical features of KTS largely correspond with the morphological characteristics of the presentation: the development of hemangiomas includingPWS and arteriovenous abscesses. In addition, individuals commonly present with a hypertrophied limb. This is more commonly noted to involve the legs although in some instances two limbs present with hypertrophy. This can also be noted in the trunk of the body.

Additional morphological anomalies can include syndactyly, polydactyly, or oligodactyly, more commonly noted in the hypertrophied limb. Varicose veins present at higher rates (i.e., >75%) and are often quite obvious (Gloviczki et al., 1991; Samuel & Spitz, 1995; Servelle, 1985). This also contributes to issues with cellulitis, hemorrhage, paresthesias, and pulmonary emboli (Mikula, Gupta, Miller, & Felder, 1991; Phillips, Gordon, Martin, Haller, & Casarella, 1978). Visual defects related to glaucoma and/or cataracts may develop.

More often than not, neurocognitive functioning is unimpaired in KTS unless hemangiomas develop within the brain raising the potential for focal deficits and seizures. In comparison, Sturge–Weber's syndrome, which demonstrates significant clinical overlap with KTS, is far more commonly linked with seizures and neuropsychological dysfunction due to the neurological involvement noted in association with this presentation.

DIAGNOSIS

Diagnosis is based on the clinical and morphological features of the presentation. It is differentiated from two clinically similar presentations. Sturge–Weber's syndrome is similar to KTS in that it too is a PWS disorder, presents with vascular anomalies, and limb hypertrophy. In comparison, Sturge–Weber's syndrome is far more commonly linked with seizures, neurocognitive dysfunction, and an increased risk of other neurological residuals. Parkes-Weber's syndrome is diagnosed when the individual also develops numerous arteriovenous fistulas in addition to the features commonly noted in KTS.

Imaging is crucial to diagnosis and evaluation of KTS as hemangiomas must be differentiated from vascular malformations, with Doppler ultrasound representing the starting point (Dubois & Garel, 1999; Dubois et al., 1998; Laor & Burrows, 1998). MRI and CT are also useful tools. They can offer refined images of the extent of lesions, including their exact locality and depth of infiltration; however, they cannot differentiate between hemangiomas and vascular malformations like the Doppler can (Kern et al., 2000). Electroencephalogram should be utilized in cases where seizures occur.

TREATMENT

There is no cure for KTS. Treatment is symptom based with focus on relief (Enjolras & Mulliken, 1993). Laser surgery can diminish or erase some skin lesions. Surgery may also be attempted to correct discrepancies in limb size through a method known as debulking, but orthopedic devices may be more appropriate. If seizures present, antiepileptic drugs can be effective in reducing or eliminating symptoms. These coincide with hemangiomas in the brain that may require neurosurgical intervention. Physical therapy is often needed to aid in ambulation issues. KTS is a progressive disorder and complications may be life-threatening, thus continual follow-up and management is required.

Chad A. Noggle

Albertini, G., Onorati, P., De Pandis, F., Giulittle, E., Calcari, L., & Sara, M. (2008). Cognitive level and adaptive behaviour in the Klippel-Trenaunay-Weber syndrome. An example of the potentials of an early intervention model applied to a complex pathology. *Disability and Rehabilitation, 30,* 26, 1999–2000.

Bliznak, J., & Staple, T. W. (1974). Radiology of angiodysplasias of the limb. *Radiology, 110,* 35–44.

Dubois, J., & Garel, L. (1999). Imaging and therapeutic approach of hemangiomas and vascular malformations in the pediatric age group. *Pediatric Radiology, 29,* 879–893.

Dubois, J., Garel, L., Grignon, A., David, M., Laberge, L., Filiatrault, D., et al. (1998). Imaging of hemangiomas and vascular malformations in children. *Academic Radiology, 5,* 390–400.

Enjolras, O., & Mulliken, J. B. (1993). The current management of vascular birthmarks. *Pediatric Dermatology, 10,* 311–313.

Gloviczki, P., Hollier, L. H., Telander, R. L., Kaufman, B., Bianco, A. J., & Stickler, G. B. (1983). Surgical implications of Klippel–Trénaunay syndrome. *Annals of Surgery, 197,* 353–362.

Gloviczki, P., Stanson, A. W., Stickler, G. B., Johnson, C. M., Toomey, B. J., Meland, N. B., et al. (1991). Klippel–Trenaunay syndrome: The risks and benefits of vascular interventions. *Surgery, 110,* 469–479.

Hai, A. A., & Shrivastava, R. B. (2003). *The Association of Surgeons of India: Textbook of surgery* (1st ed.). New Delhi, India: Tata McGraw-Hill.

Jacob, A. G., Driscoll, D. J., Shaughnessy, W. J., Stanson, A. W., Clay, R. P., & Gloviczki, P. (1998). Klippel–Trenaunay syndrome: Spectrum and management. *Mayo Clinic Proceedings, 73,* 28–36.

Kern, S., Niemeyer, C., Darge, K., Merz, C., Laubenberger, J., & Uhl, M. (2000). Differentiation of vascular birthmarks by MR imaging. An investigation of hemangiomas, venous and lymphatic malformations. *Acta Radiologica, 41,* 453–457.

Klippel, M., & Trenaunay, P. (1990). Du naevus variqueux osteohypertrophique. *Archives of General Medicine (Paris), 185,* 641–672.

Lambrechts, D., & Carmeliet, P. (2004). Genetic spotlight on a blood defect. *Nature, 427,* 592–594.

Laor, T., & Burrows, P. E. (1998). Congenital anomalies and vascular birthmarks of the lower extremities. *Magnetic Resonance Imaging Clinics of North America, 6,* 497–495.

Mikula, N., Jr., Gupta, S. M., Miller, M., & Felder, S. (1991). Klippel–Trenaunay syndrome with recurrent pulmonary embolism. *Clinical Nuclear Medicine, 16,* 253–255.

Parkes-Weber, F. (1907). Angioma formation in connection with hypertrophy of limbs and hemi-hypertrophy. *British Journal of Dermatology and Syphilis, 19,* 231–235.

Phillips, G. M., Gordon, D. H., Martin, E. C., Haller, J. O, & Casarella, W. (1978). The Klippel and Trénaunay syndrome: Clinical and radiological aspects. *Radiology, 128,* 429–434.

Samuel, M., & Spitz, L. (1995). Klippel–Trenaunay syndrome: Clinical features, complications and management in children. *British Journal of Surgery, 82,* 757–761.

Servelle, M. (1985). Klippel and Trenaunay's syndrome. 768 operated cases. *Annals of Surgery, 201,* 365–373.

KLUVER–BUCY SYNDROME

DESCRIPTION

Kluver–Bucy syndrome, an extraordinarily rare neurological disorder, was first documented in primates a little more than a century ago. Research by Brown and Shafer (1888) noted unusual behaviors following bilateral damage or removal of large sections of the temporal lobes in primates. The animals no longer expressed fear or aggression, developed voracious appetites for meat, experienced sensory deficits, and would identify all foreign objects orally.

Beginning in the 1930s with Kluver and Bucy, this syndrome resurfaced under the name of temporal lobe syndrome. Although unaware of Brown and Shafer's work, Kluver and Bucy recorded the same behavioral

IJK

changes in primates after severe bilateral temporal lobe damage or removal. Kluver and Bucy did acknowledge they were never interested in deciphering the neural or cortical mechanisms responsible for this syndrome, but instead the general role of the temporal lobe in emotional and sensory functioning.

Why this syndrome has been renamed after Kluver and Bucy remains unclear. Nahm (1997) offers the explanation that Brown and Shafer were ahead of their time and Kluver and Bucy's research happens to coincide with a time period where new and exciting advances were being made in brain research. This timing, in turn, permitted their findings to complement the work of others and be more easily accepted and subsequently frequently cited.

Although human examples of Kluver–Bucy syndrome likely existed throughout history, the first human case was not documented until 1955. An epileptic patient following surgery developed an incomplete case of Kluver–Bucy syndrome, which requires the appearance of only three core symptoms. The first definitive human case came 20 years later in 1975. A 22-year-old man exhibited all six core symptoms following a meningoencephalitis infection, likely herpes simplex encephalitis. Since that time, few cases have been documented, attesting to the unusual nature of the syndrome.

NEUROPATHOLOGY/PATHOPHYSIOLOGY

In humans, the precise lesion locations required for Kluver–Bucy syndrome remain unknown, but disruption in several brain areas, including the limbic system, do result in it. Bilateral temporal ablation, as demonstrated by primate research, remains the principle cause of this syndrome. One case in the literature, however, noted Kluver–Bucy syndrome symptoms after just a left temporal lobe resection (Anson & Kuhlman, 1993).

Temporal lobe damage as the main cause of human Kluver–Bucy syndrome has gained support from autopsy studies. These studies report significant lesions in the medial, inferior, and anterior temporal cortex along with amygdalae and hippocampi impairment, specifically the rhinencephalon regions (Lilly, Cummings, Benson, & Frankel, 1983). Overall, human Kluver–Bucy syndrome may require dual hippocampi damage before it can occur.

An alternative explanation of origin proposes that the connecting fibers leading to and from the temporal lobes are disrupted, essentially isolating them from the rest of the brain. Geschwind (1965) used this to define human Kluver–Bucy syndrome as a disconnection between the visual and limbic system. This may explain the syndrome's associated sensory deficits. Further disruption in the connecting fibers with the frontal cortex and limbic areas can also be used to explain the associated memory, emotional, and sexual behavior problems as well.

Specific damage to the temporal lobe or its connections may be the underlying cause of human Kluver–Bucy syndrome, but a host of medical maladies serve as catalysts for this process. They can be grouped into three categories: pathogen, neurological, or other. The pathogenic causes are bacterial or viral and include herpes simplex encephalitis, mycoplasma bronchitis, anoxic-ischemic encephalopathy, tuberculosis meningitis, and methotrexate leukoencephalopathy. Regarding the neurological causes and deficits, human Kluver–Bucy syndrome is viewed, instead, as comorbid or resulting from a primary neurological disorder. Some of the more common neurological disorders are epilepsy, Pick's disease, Reye's syndrome, Alzheimer's disease, Huntington's chorea, and Parkinson's disease. The last category or "other" is unusual since there seems to be no unifying theme. Among this list, there is head trauma, hypoglycemia, arachnoid cysts, carbon monoxide intoxication, postirradiation, and heat stroke.

NEUROPSYCHOLOGICAL/CLINICAL PRESENTATION

Kluver–Bucy syndrome has six core symptoms. These are visual agnosia, excessive oral tendencies, hypermetamorphosis, placidity, altered sexual behavior, and changes in dietary habits. Although humans and primates will display these symptoms, there may be some differences between species as well as minor variations between subjects.

During visual agnosia or psychic blindness, both humans and primates seem to lose their ability to recognize objects visually despite an intact and functioning system. There is some speculation in the literature that sensory agnosias also appear during auditory and olfactory processing, but research in this area is limited. In humans, the visual agnosia usually becomes prosopagnosia where patients experience difficulty distinguishing among the faces of family, friends, hospital staff, and strangers.

Primates suffering from excessive oral tendencies will attempt to identify all objects (e.g., nonfood and food) by licking, biting, and chewing. Once identified, nonfood items are spit out, whereas the food is eaten. Furthermore, nonhuman primates will not typically use their hands to pick up the items but try to use their mouths in a scooping motion.

The excessive oral tendencies in humans are expressed as hyperphagia and bulimia. Humans will lick, bite, and even engage in self-biting. Caution must be exercised with such patients because they will attempt to taste urine (e.g., urophagia) and fecal matter (e.g., coprophagia).

Hypermetamorphosis, the third core symptom, refers to a compulsive need for humans and primates to examine the minute details of every object they encounter while placid. The fourth symptom is a lack of fear, aggression, or interests. Kluver described hypermetamorphosis in primates as appearing as though they were intoxicated from hallucinogenic drugs. Kluver–Bucy syndrome in humans is unique because some patients will be very aggressive whereas others will not, but almost all will be apathetic.

Altered sexual behavior can be extreme in both primates and humans, but it is reported to be one of the least common core symptoms in humans. Primates will excessively masturbate as well as pursue both hetero- and homosexual relations. Some humans will masturbate compulsively though generally only crude remarks and gestures are made. Their attempts for sexual contact are usually unsuccessful. A few humans have reported changing their sexual preference.

The last core Kluver–Bucy syndrome is a remarkable change in dietary habits. Primates, normally vegetarian, will develop an insatiable hunger for meat. Humans will decrease their intake of meat and vegetables for sweets and nonhealthy foods.

Although human Kluver–Bucy syndrome appears more common in teenagers and adults judging by the literature, it can occur in children. Children are capable of having any of the six core symptoms but will exhibit them in somewhat different ways. For example, instead of making crude sexual remarks, they will thrusts their pelvises or rub their genitals against other objects. Children do seem to recognize their parents and other family members, but direct no attention or attraction toward them. Furthermore, children will not respond to any type of behavioral manipulations from family and hospital staff. As of yet, a complete Kluver–Bucy syndrome case has not been documented in a child.

DIAGNOSIS

Given that Kluver–Bucy is a syndrome, recognition and identification of its symptoms constitutes the primary diagnostic practice. It occurs in relation to infection, trauma, or other acute neurological event; thus, diagnostic workup should also seek to elucidate the pathological correlates. MRI and CT are preferred. Depending on imaging results, lumbar puncture with CSF analysis may be utilized to determine the presence of an infectious process.

TREATMENT

Treatment options, other than those that are pharmacological, for human Kluver–Bucy syndrome are extremely limited. The most effective pharmacological agents appear to be the antipsychotics followed by the selective serotonin reuptake inhibitors (SSRIs). The literature regarding the effectiveness of such agents is mixed, and there appears to be no real cure for Kluver–Bucy syndrome.

The antipsychotic, haloperidol, given frequently (e.g., three times a day) does seem helpful in reducing the altered sexual and excessive oral behaviors while reestablishing normal dietary behaviors. During situations when haloperidol is ineffective, it may be combined with other agents such as risperidone, carbamazepine, and propranolol. The best combinations of these agent types and dosages are usually determined through a trial and error basis with each patient. For nontraumatic Kluver–Bucy syndrome examples, a combination of carbamazepine and leuproline is recommended.

Recently, sertraline and fluoxetine, the SSRIs, have been found to be useful in reducing the altered sexual behaviors in Kluver–Bucy syndrome. In one case, risperidone and carbamazepine were ineffective until fluoxetine was added. Once the patient stopped taking just the fluoxetine, the previous Kluver–Bucy syndrome symptoms returned (Slaughter, Bobo, & Childers, 1999).

Recovery from human Kluver–Bucy syndrome can occur, thus indicating an overall positive prognosis. This is unusual because primate examples rarely improve, even after 2-year follow-ups. Generally, anywhere from 1 month to 1 year after symptoms first appear, patients may experience a return to normal eating, sexual, and emotional behaviors. Hyperorality is often considered the slowest to recover from and may only be partial at best. Human Kluver–Bucy syndrome caused by trauma is generally temporary ranging from 7 days to 1 year after the injury.

Antonio E. Puente

Anson, J. A., & Kuhlman, D. T. (1993). Post-ictal Kluver-Bucy syndrome after temporal lobectomy. *Journal of Neurology, Neurosurgery, and Psychiatry, 56,* 311–313.

Brown, S., & Schafer, E. A. (1888). An investigation into the functions of the occipital and temporal lobes of the monkey's brain. *Philosophical Transactions of the Royal Society of London: Biological Sciences, 179,* 303–327.

IJK

Geschwind, N. (1965). Disconnection syndromes in animals and man. *Brain, 88,* 237–294.

Lilly, R., Cummings, J. L., Benson, F., & Frankel, M. (1983). The human Kluver-Bucy syndrome. *Neurology, 33,* 1141–1145.

Nahm, F. K. D. (1997). Heinrich Kluver and the temporal lobe syndrome. *Journal of the History of the Neurosciences, 6,* 193–208.

Slaughter, J., Bobo, W., & Childers, M. K. (1999). Selective serotonin reuptake inhibitor treatment of post-traumatic Kluver-Bucy syndrome. *Brain Injury, 13,* 59–62.

KRABBE'S DISEASE

DESCRIPTION

Krabbe's disease is an inherited disease that leads to degeneration of the white matter within the central and peripheral nervous systems due to a deficiency of galactocerebrosidase. Classified as a leukodystrophy, the enzyme deficient in the disease is necessary for myelin development and integrity; thus, its deficiency leads to white matter degeneration. Rare in nature, Krabbe's disease occurs in approximately 1 in 100,000 births.

Krabbe's disease is most often diagnosed in infancy, although later-onset cases have been noted, and is terminal in nature. Symptom onset usually occurs at approximately 4–6 months of age, first presenting as a distinct change in temperament in which the infant will cry uncontrollably and exhibit general irritability. As the disease progresses, development halts and eventually reverses, particularly in the realm of motor functioning causing permanent opisthotonic posturing with hypertonic flexion in the extremities. Tonic spasms ensue, particularly in response to sensory stimulation, either visual or auditory (Graham & Lantos, 1997). In the final stages, infants become blind, decerebrate, and die (Graham & Lantos, 1997). There is no cure for Krabbe's disease. Given the presentation is terminal in nature, treatment is supportive, particularly for parents and family.

NEUROPATHOLOGY/PATHOPHYSIOLOGY

Krabbe's disease is defined by widespread white matter degeneration as a result of the system's inability to metabolize galactocerebroside. This is related to deficient activity of lysosomal galactocerebroside-β-galactosidase in the gray and white matter, liver, spleen, serum, leucocytes and fibroblasts (Kolodny, Raghavan, & Krivit, 1991; Suzuki & Suzuki, 1971). Consequently, brain-lipid analysis demonstrates a sever loss of myelin lipids with a significantly elevated concentration of galactocerebroside compared with sulfatide in globoid cells (Austin, 1963a,b).

Neurologically, brains are undersized with smaller gyri and wider sulci and cerebellar folia. There is some loss of differentiation of white matter from gray matter beyond the central white matter pathways (Krabbe, 1916) with occasional segmental demyelination of peripheral nerves (Baram, Goldman, & Percy, 1986). The white matter is decreased in mass and is gliotic, firm, and rubbery to palpation (Maertens & Dyken, 2007). Globoid cells increase in the initial stages of the disease. They are even commonly noted in the pontine tegmentum, medulla, and spinal cords of affected fetuses (Harzer, 1982; Ida, Rennert, Watabe, Eto, & Maekawa, 1994; Martin et al., 1981; Suchlandt, Schlote, & Harzer, 1982). Neuronal degeneration of the thalamus, pons, and dentate nuclei is commonly noted.

By the end-stages of the presentation, microscopic review demonstrates few if any globoid cells (Dunn, 1976) and almost total loss of axons (D' Agostino et al., 1963). Neuronal loss in focal areas including the dentate nucleus and inferior olives have also been noted (Norman et al., 1961; Crome et al., 1973; Shaw et al, 1970). In comparison, when onset is later, the neurological changes are not as prominent. MRI findings may be nearly normal (Graham & Lantos, 1997).

NEUROPSYCHOLOGICAL/CLINICAL PRESENTATION

Irritability and excessive crying are commonly reported as the first symptoms of Krabbe's disease when presenting in infants. Most commonly, onset occurs at 4–6 months of age. Prior to symptom emergence, infants demonstrate a normal developmental period in terms of eye and head control. Soon after these features present, development comes to a halt. Around this same time, infants develop tonic spasms in response to visual or auditory stimulation. Simultaneously, a gradual decline in motor functioning may be noted and feeding difficulties may develop. This motor deterioration leads to a permanent opisthotonic posturing with hypertonic flexion of the extremities (Graham & Lantos, 1997). In the later stages, myoclonic jerking and seizures eventually ensue and blindness develops secondary to optic atrophy. In the final stages, infants become decerebrate (Graham & Lantos, 1997). Infants commonly die between 12 and 18 months of age.

Although the disease most commonly presents in infancy, when onset is later the presentation is more commonly characterized by sensorimotor deficits including gait disturbance, spasticity, neuropathy, and loss of visual acuity. Seizures are not as common and death is not imminent.

DIAGNOSIS

Diagnosis commonly begins with the identification of the clinical symptoms that define Krabbe's disease once development halting is noted. Neuroimaging may be utilized to reveal white matter loss within the cerebrum and cerebellum (Baram et al., 1986). Laboratory diagnosis may be the most accurate; diagnosis is made by enzyme assay of leucocytes or cultured fibroblasts (Graham & Lantos, 1997). Similar capabilities are possible prenatally by assay of chorionic villus samples (Harzer, Hager, & Tariverdian, 1989; Harzer, & Schuster, 1987).

TREATMENT

There is no cure for Krabbe's disease. Given that most infants die prior to 2 years of age, treatment is largely support based. There are some initial findings that suggest benefit of umbilical cord blood stem cells prior to symptom onset in regard to improving neurological outcomes. Bone marrow transplantation has also demonstrated a positive impact in milder cases when used early in the disease process. Nevertheless, treatment remains symptom based.

Chad A. Noggle
Javan Horwitz

Austin, J. H. (1963a). Studies in globoid (Krabbe) leukodystrophy. II. Controlled thin-layer chromatographic studies of globoid body fractions in 7 patients. *Journal of Neurochemistry, 10,* 921–930.

Austin, J. H. (1963b). Studies in globoid (Krabbe) leukodystrophy. I. The significance of lipid abnormalities in white matter in 8 globoid and 13 control patients. *Archives of Neurology, 9,* 207–231.

Baram, T. Z., Goldman, A. M., & Percy, A. K. (1986). Krabbe disease: Specific MRI and CT findings. *Neurology, 36,* 111–115.

Crome, L., Hanefield, F., Patrick, D., & Wilson, J. (1973). Late onset of globoid cell leucodystrophy. *Brain, 96,* 841–848.

D'Agostino, A. N., Sayre, G. P., & Hayles, A. B. (1963). Krabbe's disease. *Archives of Neurology, 8,* 82–96.

Dunn, H. G., Dolman, C. L., Farrell, D. F., Tischler, B., Hasinoff, C., & Woolf, L. I. (1976). Krabbes leukodystrophy without globoid cells. *Neurology, 26,* 1035–1041.

Graham, D. I., & Lantos, P. L. (Eds). (1997). *Greenfield's neuropathology* (6th ed.). New York: Oxford University Press.

Harzer, K. (1982). Prenatal enzymic diagnosis in 24 pregnancies with risk of Krabbe disease. *Clinica Chimica Acta; International Journal of Clinical Chemistry, 122,* 21–28.

Harzer, K., Hager, H. D., & Tariverdian, G. (1987). Prenatal enzymatic diagnosis and exclusion of Krabbe's disease (globoid-cell leukodystrophy) using chorionic villi in five risk pregnancies. *Human Genetics, 77,* 342–344.

Harzer, K., & Schuster, I. (1989). Prenatal enzymatic diagnosis of Krabbe's disease (globoid-cell leukodystrophy) using chorionic villi. Pittfalls in the use of uncultured villi. *Human Genetics, 84,* 83–85.

Ida, H., Rennert, O. M., Watabe, K., Eto, Y., & Maekawa, K. (1994). Pathological and biochemical studies of fetal Krabbe disease. *Brain & Development, 16,* 480–484.

Kolodny, E. H., Raghavan, S., & Krivit, W. (1991). Late-onset Krabbe disease (globoid cell leukodstrophy): Clinical and biochemical features of 15 cases. *Developmental Neuroscience, 13,* 232–239.

Krabbe, K. (1916). A new familial, infantile form of diffuse brain sclerosis. *Brain, 39,* 74–1141.

Maertens, P., & Dyken, R. (2007). Storage diseases: Neuronal ceroid-lipofuscinoses, lipidoses, glycogenoses, and leukodystrophies. In C. Goetz (Ed.), *Textbook of clinical neurology* (pp. 612–639). Philadelphia, PA: Saunders Elsevier.

Martin, J. J., Leroy, J. C., Ceuterick, C., Libert, J., Dodinval, P., & Martin, L. (1981). Fetal Krabbe leukodystrophy. A morphological study of two cases. *Actas Neuropathologica (Berl), 53,* 87–91.

Norman, R. M., Oppenheimer, D. R., & Tingey, A. H. (1961). Histological and chemical findings in Krabbe's leucodystrophy. *Journal of Neurology, Neurosurgery, and Psychiatry, 24,* 223–232.

Shaw, C. M., & Carlson, C. G. (1970). Crystalline structures in globoid-epithelioid cells: An electron microscopic study of globoid leukodystrophy (Krabbe's disease). *Journal of Neuropathology and Experimental Neurology, 29,* 306–319.

Suchlandt, G., Schlote, W., & Harzer, K. (1982). Ultrastrukturelle Befunde bei 9 Feten nach pranataler Diagnose von Neurolipidosen. *Arch Psychiat Nervenkr, 232,* 407–426.

Suzuki, Y., & Suzuki, K. (1971). Krabbe's globoid cell leukodystrophy: Deficiency of glactocerebrosidase in serum, leukocytes and fibroblasts. *Science, 171,* 73–75.

KURU

DESCRIPTION

Kuru is a form of transmissible spongiform encephalopathy (TSE) or prion disease that was identified in the 1950s among the Fore people living in the highlands of Papua New Guinea (Gajdusek & Zigas, 1957). Like other TSEs (e.g., Creutzfeldt–Jakob's disease), kuru is a fatal neurodegenerative disorder thought to be caused by structurally abnormal neuronal proteins (i.e., proteinaceous infectious particles or prions) that have the capability of propagating structural anomalies in neighboring proteins. Kuru was endemic to the Fore people and a few neighboring tribes and was a leading cause of death among Fore women and children in the 1950s. Ingestion of infected brain tissue through the practice of ritual cannibalism of deceased family members was identified as the primary mode of transmission, and the incidence of the disease decreased dramatically after the institution of government prohibitions against cannibalism.

NEUROPATHOLOGY/PATHOPHYSIOLOGY

Early reports of neuropathologic findings in kuru noted neuronal degeneration, demyelination of motor tracts, gliosis, and distinctive round or ovoid amyloid plaques that were observed to have a dark center surrounded by a lighter halo (Fowler & Robertson, 1959; Klatzo, Gajdusek, & Zigas, 1958; Neumann, Gajdusek, & Zigas, 1964). These plaques consequently came to be labeled "kuru plaques" and were noted in approximately 75% of cases (Collins, McLean, & Masters, 2001; Liberski & Brown, 2009). Concentrations were noted in the cerebellum, basal ganglia, thalamus, and cortex; they have been found to contain structurally abnormal prion protein. Subsequent investigations also identified extensive vacuolation or spongiform changes in areas of the cortex, basal ganglia, and cerebellum (Brandner et al., 2008).

NEUROPSYCHOLOGICAL/CLINICAL PRESENTATION

The term *kuru* means shaking or shivering in the Fore language and accurately suggests the predominance of movement disorders in the disease (Liberski & Brown, 2009). The progression of the disease was classified into three stages: ambulatory, sedentary, and terminal (Gajdusek & Zigas, 1959; Kompoliti, Goetz, Gajdusek, & Cubo, 1999). Following a prodromal period involving headache, limb and abdominal pain, and weight loss in the absence of fever, the ambulatory stage was identified by the initial sign of mild locomotor ataxia. Over a period of about 1 month, this progressed to severe astasia, ataxia, and titubation; the patient eventually became unable to walk without a crutch. Horizontal convergent strabismus was observed in some patients during the ambulatory stage. Onset of the sedentary stage was demarcated by the inability to walk without assistance; ataxia, tremor, and postural unsteadiness

continued to progress throughout this stage. The transition to the terminal stage was signaled by the inability to sit without assistance, and the patient became bedridden, mute, and incontinent. Death typically occurred 6–9 months following onset of the disease; common causes of death were starvation, infection from decubitus ulcers, or bronchopneumonia (Gajdusek & Zigas, 1959). Cognitive abilities remain preserved apart from reduced processing speed, but progression to dementia (as in Creutzfeldt–Jakob's disease) was not part of the clinical picture. Mood lability including outbursts of laughter and persistent smiling were often present during the sedentary stage and led to a description of the disease as the laughing death (Liberski & Brown, 2009).

DIAGNOSIS

Given the gradual disappearance of kuru following government prohibitions against ritual cannibalism among the Fore people, diagnosis of the disease is more a matter of historical interest rather than an issue of contemporary clinical relevance (Collins, Lawson, & Masters, 2004; Liberski & Brown, 2009). Diagnosis of kuru was based primarily on clinical features of the disease (Gajdusek & Zigas, 1959). Despite its insidious onset, the progression of kuru was well known among the Fore people and was described in uniform terms across different villages in the endemic area. It came to be readily identified by the physicians who first described it. The initial locomotor ataxia was so subtle that it was often only noticed by the patient, but the rapid progression over the course of several months to severe ataxia and tremor, and the eventual inability to sit upright without assistance were diagnostic.

TREATMENT

No treatment for kuru was identified (Liberski & Brown, 2009). The incidence of the disease declined rapidly once the Fore people stopped practicing ritual cannibalism. The few reported cases in the 21st century have resulted from exceptionally long incubation periods (Collinge et al., 2006).

Jeremy Davis
Chad A. Noggle

Brandner, S., Whitfield, J., Boone, K., Puwa, A., O'Malley, C., Linehan, J. M., et al. (2008). Central and peripheral pathology of Kuru: Pathological analysis of a recent case and comparison with other forms of human prion disease. *Philosophical Transactions of the Royal Society B, 363*, 3755–3763.

Collinge, J., Whitfield, J., McKintosh, E., Beck, J., Mead, S., Thomas, D. J., et al. (2006). Kuru in the 21st century — An acquired human prion disease with very long incubation periods. *Lancet, 367*, 2068–2074.

Collins, S. J., Lawson, V. A., & Masters, C. L. (2004). Transmissible spongiform encephalopathies. *Lancet, 363*, 51–61.

Collins, C., McLean, C. A., & Masters, C. L. (2001). Gerstmann-Sträussler-Scheinker syndrome, fatal familial insomnia, and kuru: A review of these less common human transmissible spongioform encephalopathies. *Journal of Clinical Neuroscience, 8*, 387–397.

Fowler, M., & Robertson, E. G. (1959). Observations on kuru, III: Pathological features in five cases. *Australasian Annals of Medicine, 8*, 16–26.

Gajdusek, D. C., & Zigas, V. (1957). Degenerative disease of the central nervous system in New Guinea: The endemic occurrence of "kuru" in the native population. *The New England Journal of Medicine, 257*, 974–978.

Gajdusek, D. C., & Zigas, V. (1959). Kuru: Clinical, pathological and epidemiological study of an acute progressive degenerative disease of the central nervous system among natives of the eastern highlands of New Guinea. *The American Journal of Medicine, 26*, 442–469.

Klatzo, I., Gajdusek, D. C., & Zigas, V. (1959). Pathology of kuru. *Laboratory Investigation, 8*, 799–847.

Kompoliti, K., Goetz, C. G., Gajdusek, D. C., & Cubo, E. (1999). Movement disorders in kuru. *Movement Disorders, 14*, 800–804.

Liberski, P. P., & Brown, P. (2009). Kuru: Its ramifications after fifty years. *Experimental Gerontology, 44*, 63–69.

Neumann, M. A., Gajdusek, D. C., & Zigas, V. (1964). Neuropathologic findings in exotic neurologic disorders among natives of the highlands of New Guinea. *Journal of Neuropathology and Experimental Neurology, 23*, 486–507.

IJK

LAMBERT–EATON MYASTHENIA SYNDROME

DESCRIPTION

Lambert–Eaton syndrome, also called myasthenic syndrome or Lambert–Eaton myasthenic syndrome, is a rare autoimmune disorder of neuromuscular transmission. Lambert–Eaton syndrome has symptoms that are very similar to myasthenia gravis. Like myasthenia gravis, Lambert–Eaton syndrome involves muscle weakness associated with a disruption in the communication at the neuromuscular junction, but there are clear differences between the disorders (Lang, Newsom-Davis, Wray, Vincent, & Murray, 1981). Lambert–Eaton syndrome affects the presynaptic neuron inhibiting the release of acetylcholine causing muscle weakness, depressed tendon reflexes, posttetanic potentiation, and autonomic changes. It is estimated that 50–70% of patients with Lambert–Eaton syndrome have an identifiable cancer (Chalk, Murray, Newsom-Davis, O'Neill, & Spiro, 1990; Elmqvist & Lambert, 1968).

The disorder was first described by Anderson in 1953 in a patient with lung cancer. However, Lambert, Eaton, and Rooke further published electrophysiological data on six patients with the disorder. Although children, adolescents, and young adults may have Lambert–Eaton syndrome, the disease is usually observed in adults. The incidence of Lambert–Eaton syndrome is difficult to determine due to its low frequency (Sanders, 1995).

NEUROPATHOLOGY/PATHOPHYSIOLOGY

Lambert–Eaton syndrome is an autoimmune disorder of neuromuscular transmission in which the immune system, which normally protects the body, mistakenly attacks the body's voltage-gated calcium channels on the presynaptic motor nerve terminal of sympathetic, parasympathetic, and enteric neurons (Lang, et al., 1981; Lang, Johnston, Leys, Elrington, Marqueze, & Leveque, 1993; Lang, Newsom-Davis, 1995). The disruption of electrical impulses at the voltage-gated calcium channels is a consequence of this autoimmunity

and reduces nerve impulses. The reduction in nerve impulses inhibits the release of acetylcholine from the presynaptic neuron.

Symptoms from the inhibition of activity at the presynaptic neuron include muscle weakness, a tingling sensation in the affected areas, fatigue, and dry mouth (Waterman, Lang, & Newsom-Davis, 1996). The stores of acetylcholine in the presynaptic neuron are normal, so if the neuromuscular transmission can be artificially stimulated, a temporary increase in muscle strength will occur (Sanders, 1995). Lambert–Eaton syndrome is closely associated with cancer, specifically small cell lung cancer. More than half the individuals diagnosed with Lambert–Eaton syndrome eventually develop small cell lung cancer. Lambert–Eaton syndrome may appear up to 3 years before cancer is diagnosed (Chalk et al., 1990).

NEUROPSYCHOLOGICAL/CLINICAL PRESENTATION

The major clinical finding in Lambert–Eaton syndrome is a progressive weakness that does not usually involve the respiratory muscles or the muscles of the face. Typically, the proximal muscles in the lower extremities are affected, although the arms may be affected in some cases. Patients may report difficulty with standing from a sitting position, walking upstairs, or even walking in general. The symptoms may be present for several years before diagnosis is made. Cancer is present or subsequently diagnosed in 50–70% of patients with Lambert–Eaton syndrome (Chalk et al., 1990). Only 25% of patients have ocular or oropharyngeal muscles affected and exhibit symptoms of ptosis, diplopia, and dysarthria. In patients with affected ocular and oropharyngeal muscles, the involvement is not as severe as myasthenia gravis, but it may be difficult to differentiate between the disorders. Research has demonstrated that if a patient's first symptom is ocular weakness, Lambert–Eaton syndrome can be virtually excluded. The respiratory muscles may also be affected, but not as severe as myasthenia gravis. Many patients initially present with autonomic symptoms, specifically dry mouth, but impotence may also be reported. In Lambert–Eaton syndrome reflexes are typically reduced or

L

absent (O'Neil, Murray, & Newsom-Davis, 1988; Sanders, 1995).

DIAGNOSIS

The evaluation and diagnosis of Lambert–Eaton syndrome will typically include a thorough physical examination and medical history. Initially patients may present with autonomic symptoms, specifically dry mouth. Physical examination will typically show muscle atrophy and weakness or even paralysis, but the muscle weakness symptoms will improve with physical activity. The patients may also have decreased or absent reflexes. A Tensilon test, an injection of edrophonium chloride used to block the action of acetylcholinesterase that increases levels of acetylcholine, can be positive in which the patient's muscle strength evaluation is noticeably improved. EMG or nerve conduction velocity tests can also measure nerve conductivity to the muscles by inserting an electrode into the muscle that appears to be affected by the nerve damage (Wirtz et al., 2002).

The above diagnostic measures may not differentiate between myasthenia gravis and Lambert–Eaton syndrome, so the diagnosis of underlying cancer or the detection of acetylcholine antibodies may differentiate between the disorders (Sanders, 1995). Another differentiation between the disorders is that in myasthenia gravis muscle weakness tends to develop in a craniocaudal direction, and in Lambert–Eaton syndrome muscle weakness tends to develop in the opposite direction (Wirtz, Sotodeh, Nijnuis, Van Engelen, Hintzen, de Kort, et al., 2002). The arms may be affected in both disorders, but research has shown that limb weakness specifically confined to the arms is found only in generalized myasthenia gravis and not in Lambert–Eaton syndrome (Sanders, 1995).

TREATMENT

In Lambert–Eaton syndrome, the primary goal of treatment is to treat any tumors or other underlying disorders that are diagnosed during examination. Although rare, respiratory distress or failure is a primary concern in treatment. Plasmapheresis, where blood plasma is removed and replaced with fluid, has been reported to improve symptoms. Pharmacotherapy for Lambert–Eaton syndrome can be initiated only after myasthenia gravis has been excluded. Typical pharmacotherapeutic interventions include the use of cholinesterase inhibitors, immunosuppressants, and/or immunomodulating agents. Physical therapy and exercise are an important component to the treatment of Lambert–Eaton syndrome. Physical therapy

and exercise on an outpatient basis are helpful in maintaining muscle tone and strength (Maddison & Newsom-Davis, 2005; Sanders, 1994, 1995; Verschuuren, Wirtz, Titulaer, Willems, & van Gerven, 2006). Psychosocial interventions may also be utilized to help the patient overcome any psychological or social ramifications of the disorder or an underlying cancer.

Eric Silk
Charles Golden

Chalk, C. H., Murray, N. M., Newsom-Davis, J., O'Neill, J. H., & Spiro, S. G. (1990). Response of the Lambert–Eaton myasthenic syndrome to treatment of associated small-cell lung carcinoma. *Neurology, 40,* 1552–1556.

Elmqvist, D., & Lambert, E. H. (1968). Detailed analysis of neuromuscular transmission in a patient with the myasthenic syndrome sometimes associated with bronchogenic carcinoma. *Mayo Clinic Proceedings, 43,* 689–713.

Lambert, E. H., Eaton, L. M., & Rooke, E. D. (1956). Defect of neuromuscular conduction associated with malignant neoplasma. *American Journal of Physiology, 187,* 612–613.

Lang, B., Newsom-Davis, J., Wray, D., Vincent, A., & Murray, N. M. F. (1981). Autoimmune aetiology for myasthenic (Eaton–Lambert) syndrome. *Lancet, 318*(8240), 224–226.

Lang, B., Johnston, I., Leys, K., Elrington, G., Marqueze, B., & Leveque, C. (1993). Autoantibody specificities in Lambert–Eaton myasthenic syndrome. *Annals of the New York Academy of Science, 681,* 382–393.

Lang, B., & Newsom-Davis, J. (1995). Immunopathology of the Lambert-Eaton myasthenic syndrome. *Springer Seminars in Immunopathology, 17*(1), 3–15.

Maddison, P., & Newsom-Davis, J. (2005). Treatment for Lambert-Eaton myasthenic syndrome. *Cochrane Database of Systematic Reviews,* CD003279.

Sanders, D. B. (1994). Lambert-Eaton myasthenic syndrome: Pathogenesis and treatment. *Seminars in Neurology, 14*(2), 111–117.

Sanders, D. B. (1995). Lambert-Eaton myasthenic syndrome: Clinical diagnosis, immune-mediated mechanisms, and update on therapies. *Annals of Neurology, 37*(1), 63–73.

Verschuuren, J. J., Wirtz, P. W., Titulaer, M. J., Willems, L. N., & van Gerven, J. (2006). Available treatment options for the management of Lambert-Eaton myasthenic syndrome. *Expert Opin Pharmacother, 7*(10), 1323–1336.

Waterman, S. A., Lang, B., & Newsom-Davis, J. (1996). Lambert–Eaton myasthenic syndrome autoantibodies inhibit neurotransmission from postganglionic sympathetic neurons by blocking voltage-gated calcium channels. *Neurology, 46,* 223–224.

Wirtz, P. W., Sotodeh, M., Nijnuis, M., Van Doorn, P. A., Van Engelen, B. G., Hintzen, R. Q., et al. (2002). Difference in distribution of muscle weakness between myasthenia gravis and the Lambert-Eaton myasthenic syndrome. *Journal of Neurology, Neurosurgery & Psychiatry, 73*(6), 766–768.

LANDAU–KLEFFNER SYNDROME

DESCRIPTION

Landau–Kleffner syndrome (LKS) is a rare, childhood neurological disorder characterized by the sudden or gradual development of aphasia (i.e., the inability to understand or express language) and an abnormal EEG. It is also known as *acquired epileptiform aphasia, infantile acquired aphasia, acquired epileptic aphasia*, or *aphasia with convulsive disorder*. The syndrome was first described in 1957 by Dr. William M. Landau and Dr. Frank R. Kleffner, who identified six children with the disorder (Landau & Kleffner, 1957). LKS usually occurs in children between the ages of 3 and 7 years. Typically, children with LKS develop normally but then lose their language skills for no apparent reason. Many affected individuals have seizures but some do not. More than 200 cases have been described in the global literature. A slight predominance in boys has been reported (Sotero de Menezes, 2007).

The cause(s) of LKS remain unknown, and the disorder is not likely to be inherited. Furthermore, the prognosis varies; some affected children have a permanent severe language disorder whereas others regain much of their language abilities over the course of months to years. Remission and relapse may also occur; however, in general, seizures disappear by adulthood (Sotero de Menezes, 2007).

NEUROPATHOLOGY/PATHOPHYSIOLOGY

The pathophysiology of LKS remains poorly understood. Cerebral spinal fluid (CSF), CT, and MRI findings are typically normal (Feekery, Parry-Fielder, & Hopkins, 1993). There may be mild elevations of CSF protein (Pascual-Castroviejo, Lopez-Martín, Martinez-Bermejo, & Perez-Hinojosa, 1992), white matter changes on CT/MRI, or a structural lesion (Otero, Cordova, Diaz, Garcia-Terul, & Del Brutto, 1989).

All children with LKS have abnormal electrical brain waves that can be documented by an EEG. Paroxysmal EEG abnormalities involving the temporal or temporal-parietal-occipital regions are present bilaterally. EEG results usually return to normal by age 15 (Pearl, Carrazana, & Holmes, 2001). Several single-photon emission computed tomography (SPECT) and positron emission tomography (PET) studies on small numbers of patients have shown temporal lobe abnormalities in brain perfusion and glucose metabolism, respectively (Guerreiro et al., 1996; O'Tuama et al., 1992).

NEUROPSYCHOLOGICAL/CLINICAL PRESENTATION

With LKS, normally developing children between the ages of 3 and 7 begin having trouble understanding what is said to them. Doctors often refer to this problem as auditory agnosia or "word deafness." Parents often think that their child is developing a hearing problem or has suddenly become deaf. These children may also appear to be developmentally delayed.

The inability to understand language eventually affects spoken language and may progress to a complete loss of the ability to speak. Children who have learned to read and write before the onset of auditory agnosia can often continue communicating through written language. Nonverbal functions are relatively preserved, and some children develop a type of gestural communication or sign-like language. Intelligence is frequently unaffected. Behavioral disorders such as hyperactivity, aggressiveness, and depression can also accompany this disorder.

DIAGNOSIS

The differential diagnosis of LKS is challenging because of the nonspecific nature of the symptoms. LKS may be misdiagnosed as autism, pervasive developmental disorder, hearing impairment, learning disability, auditory/verbal processing disorder, attention deficit disorder, mental retardation, childhood schizophrenia, or emotional/behavioral problems. Acquired aphasia in children may be secondary to head trauma, brain tumors, stroke, or neurocysticercosis. Like LKS, head injury, brain neoplasms, and cerebrovascular thromboembolism may be associated with an epileptiform EEG and seizures. Other neurologic deficits, such as hemiparesis or signs of increased intracranial pressure, may be a clue of an underlying structural lesion. MRIs, which are typically negative, can clarify the diagnosis. Deaf children may have many of the symptoms of LKS. When in doubt, a sleep EEG is required to rule out LKS (Sotero de Menezes, 2007).

TREATMENT

Pharmacologic treatment includes anticonvulsants and corticosteroids to control seizure activity

(Marescaux et al., 1990; McKinney & McGreal, 1974). Speech and language therapy is indispensable. Surgical therapy including temporal lobectomy has been associated with improvement in both language functioning and seizure control (Cole et al., 1988; Solomon, Parson, Pavlakis, Fraser, & Labar, 1993). Another treatment option is intravenous gamma-globulin (Fayad, Choveiri, & Mikati, 1997). Sign language construction has benefited others. Initiating treatment early improves outcome, although the variable nature of the syndrome renders controlled outcome studies quite difficult.

Some children with long-standing verbal auditory agnosia may successfully be integrated into schools for the deaf, although others continue to have marked deficits in social adaptation, communication, and functioning. Listening can be assisted by increasing speech volume over the ambient noise. Classrooms can be acoustically modified and sound amplification technology can be utilized (Pearl et al., 2001). Introduction of an effective communication system can help alleviate problematic behavior.

Shane S. Bush
George M. Cuesta

Cole, A. J., Andermann, F., Taylor, L., Olivier, A., Rasmussen, T., Robitaille, Y., et al. (1988). The Landau-Kleffner syndrome of acquired epileptic aphasia: Unusual clinical outcome, surgical experience, and absence of encephalitis. *Neurology, 38,* 31–38.

Fayad, M., Choveiri, R., & Mikati, M. (1997). Landau Kleffner syndrome: Consistent response to repeated intravenous gamma-globulin doses: A case report. *Epilepsia, 38,* 489–494.

Feekery, C. J., Parry-Fielder, B., & Hopkins, J. J. (1993). Landau Kleffner syndrome: Six patients including discordant monozygotic twins. *Pediatric Neurology, 9,* 49–53.

Guerreiro, M. M., Camargo, E. E., Kato, M., Menezes Netto, J. R., Silva, E. A., Scotoni, A. E., et al. (1996). Brain single photon emission computed tomography imaging in Landau-Kleffner syndrome. *Epilepsia, 37,* 60–67.

Landau, W. M., & Kleffner, F. R. (1957). Syndrome of acquired aphasia with convulsive disorder in children. *Neurology, 7,* 523–530.

Marescaux, C., Hirsch, E., Finck, P., Maquet, P., Schlumberger, E., Sellal, F., et al. (1990). Landau Kleffner syndrome: A pharmacologic study of five cases. *Epilepsia, 31,* 768–777.

McKinney, W., & McGreal, D. (1974). An aphasic syndrome in children. *Canadian Medical Association Journal, 110,* 637–639.

Otero, E., Cordova, S., Diaz, F., Garcia-Terul, I., & Del Brutto, O. H. (1989). Acquired epileptic aphasia due to neurocysticercosis. *Epilepsia, 30,* 569–572.

O'Tuama, L. A., Urion, D. K., Janicek, M. J., Treves, S. T., Bjornson, B., & Moriarity, J. M. (1992). Regional cerebral perfusion in Landau-Kleffner syndrome and related childhood aphasias. *Journal of Nuclear Medicine, 33,* 1758–1765.

Pascual-Castroviejo, I., Lopez-Martín, V., Martinez-Bermejo, A., & Perez-Hinojosa, A. (1992). Is cerebral arteritis the cause of the Landau Kleffner syndrome? Four cases in childhood with angiographic study. *Canadian Journal of Neurological Science, 19,* 46–52.

Pearl, P. L., Carrazana, E. J., & Holmes, G. L. (2001). The Landau-Kleffner syndrome. *Epilepsy Currents, 1,* 39–45.

Solomon, G. E., Parson, D., Pavlakis, S., Fraser, R., & Labar, D. (1993). Intracranial EEG monitoring in Landau-Kleffner syndrome associated with a left temporal lobe astrocytoma. *Epilepsia, 34,* 557–560.

Sotero de Menezes, M. (2007). *Landau-Kleffner syndrome.* Retrieved November 25, 2008, from www.emedicine.com/neuro/topic182.htm

LEAD INTOXICATION

DESCRIPTION

Lead intoxication, also called plumbism, describes the process by which excessive amounts of lead accumulate within the body, potentially causing harm to multiple organs and systems, including the central nervous system. Although rates of intoxication have dropped as awareness of lead toxicity has increased, including the elimination of known risk factors (e.g., lead-based paint), new cases continue to be documented as routes of exposure vary.

Children remain the most vulnerable to lead intoxication, yet it can be experienced across the life span. Susceptibility in children is due to them absorbing a higher fraction of bioavailable lead in combination with the fact that their system is still developing through growth and cell differentiation and are more vulnerable to inhibition and damage (Holtzman, DeVries, Nguyen, Olson, & Bensch, 1984; Krigman, 1978). Nevertheless, relative consistency is seen in symptoms. Irritability, inattention, memory loss, headaches, impulsivity, lethargy, and general cognitive deterioration may all be seen as a consequence in children and adults (Papanikolaou, Hatzidaki, Belivanis, Tzanakakis, & Tsatsakis, 2005).

NEUROPATHOLOGY/PATHOPHYSIOLOGY

Lead intoxication has various routes but most commonly occurs through respiratory and gastrointestinal (GI) tracts. Phillip and Gerson (1994) noted that approximately 30% to 40% of inhaled lead is absorbed into the bloodstream. In both instances, lead-based paint in homes has been most commonly reported when discussing lead intoxication. For example, children with pica have historically been reported as those with the greatest risk of lead intoxication due to a tendency to eat paint chips among other inedible substances. This risk has dissipated with the reduction of lead-based paint. In terms of respiratory infiltration, this was historically noted in homes that had lead-based paint, poor ventilation, and no air conditioning. In summer months, if the interior became too hot, the lead-based paint could heat to the point that it would give off a vapor that could be inhaled.

Toxicity encephalopathy was traditionally reported to occur when levels exceeded a "clinical" level of 80–100 μg/dL, although milder symptoms have been consistently observed with lesser amounts leading to a reduction of this "clinical" level to 10 μg/dL. Once in the system, the physiological basis of lead's impact is multidimensional. It demonstrates a strong binding capacity for particular proteins in the system that interferes with the production and synthesis of various enzymes and structural protein (Phillip & Gerson, 1994). Because of its dependence upon these various proteins and enzymes, the developing nervous system is particularly vulnerable. Lead is particularly toxic to immature astrocytes and interferes with myelin formation, which may result secondarily in compromise of the blood–brain barrier increasing risk of increased intracranial pressure and encephalopathy (Holtzman et al., 1984). The aforementioned encephalopathy can contribute to global cerebral edema with obliteration of sulci and the lateral ventricles associated with congestion of the meningeal vasculature (Pentshschew, 1965). Synaptogenesis, cell migration, and glial cell growth can also be impeded by lead toxicity (Holtzman et al., 1984). Myelinated axons within white matter are separated by microspongiosis with gliosis and may show variable degeneration (Ohnishi et al., 1977) with variable axonal degeneration.

The cerebellum may be particularly vulnerable due to lead's tendency to compete for binding sites in this region for phosphokinase C, affecting calcium entry into cells, mitochondrial structure, and neuronal function (Bressler & Goldstein, 1991). Consistent with this, petechial hemorrhages are reported at high rates throughout the molecular and Purkinje cell layers of the cerebellum (Verity, 1997). In rodent models, reduction in the thickness of the cerebellar molecular layer and stunted Purkinje cell dendrite arborization have been reported in addition to reduced cortical synaptogenesis and complexity (McCauley et al., 1979).

Aside from the cerebellum, the hippocampus has also demonstrated relative susceptibility to lead intoxication. In their studies, Valpey et al. (1978) found cortical and cerebellar atrophy with selective neuronal loss in the hippocampus and cerebellum and neuronal chromatolysis in the reticular formation (Verity, 1997). Extensive neuronalnecrosis of hippocampal neurons as well as neurons of the fascia dentate has been reportedly observed (81–84-GL). Additional studies of the hippocampus revealed a decrease in the density of mossy fiber boutons in combination with hypertrophy of granule cells (Slomianka et al., 1989).

Finally, neurotransmitter disruption has been commonly associated with lead intoxication. Spontaneous neurotransmitter release and an inhibition of what would otherwise be controlled stimulated release of neurotransmitters have been reported. Dopaminergic, cholinergic, and glutamatergic systems have all been found to be affected by lead intoxication (Cory-Slechta, 1997; Davis, 1990). Inhibition of GABA uptake has also been reported (Seidman et al., 1987)

NEUROPSYCHOLOGICAL/CLINICAL PRESENTATION

Variability is seen clinically from person to person when it comes to lead intoxication. Mediating factors include age and toxicity levels. Although greater levels are associated with greater toxicity, as suggested, residuals can be seen even with small amounts of lead. In a meta-analysis by Davis (1990) of four key studies on lead and behavior, they found that lead can cause impaired neurobehavioral activity at a level of 10–15 μg/dL. Initial or early symptomology in both adults and children include headache, potentially photophobia, irritability, inattention and feeling cognitively "foggy" or "sluggish," memory loss (mainly retrieval based), and low-level cognitive impairment (Papanikolaou et al., 2005). In children, as elevated levels persist or increase, behavioral symptoms of impulsiveness, inability to follow sequences or directions, decreased play activity, lowered IQ, learning deficits, and increased inattentiveness are commonly seen (Papanikolaou et al., 2005). Infants and toddlers may demonstrate delays in normal physical and mental development. Adults commonly report peripheral neuropathy of extensor muscle groups and mild sensory loss. Wrist drop and foot drop have been commonly documented.

In regard to neurocognitive functioning, no unitary profile exists, with diverse domains being indicted (Bellinger, 2011). Executive functions have demonstrated greatest susceptibility in children

L

(Bellinger, Hu, Titlebaum, & Needleman, 1994) but also have been reported in adults (Schwartz & Otto, 2000). In this latter study, Schwartz and Otto (2000) also noted deficits in verbal memory, learning, and visuoconstructional abilities in a sample of 535 adult patients with lead intoxication compared with controls. Similar findings have been noted in pediatric populations. Drops in verbal IQ of roughly five points have been noted in children with lead burdens between 25 and 55 µg/dL (Needleman et al., 1990). Fine motor dysfunction has been reported (Ris et al., 2004) as have visuoconstructional abilities (Baghurst et al., 1995).

DIAGNOSIS

Diagnosis of lead intoxication is laboratory based. Both blood lead level and zinc protoporphyria should be obtained through diagnostic chelation following infusion of 1 g of calcium ethylenediaminetetra-acetic acid (EDTA) with more than 600 grams of lead over a 72-hour period indicating elevation (Bolla & Cadet, 2007). Excessive levels are determined through blood analysis with comparisons made based on age and gender as children have lower tolerance than adults and thus toxicity is reached at lower levels. Furthermore, unborn fetuses of pregnant women are also vulnerable; thus, the limits for women of childbearing age are set in accordance with accepted pediatric levels. Currently, greater than 10 µg/dL is considered excessive for infants, children, and women of childbearing age. In adults, levels greater than 30 µg/dL are considered elevated. However, as noted by Papanikolaou et al. (2005), there is no measurable level of lead in the body below which no harm occurs, so the less the better. Research has consistently demonstrated deficits in children and adults below these thresholds.

Beyond the aforementioned analyses, MRI and CT are beneficial given the potential for neurological deterioration. White matter tracts should be carefully evaluated, thus also potentially suggesting the role of diffusion tensor imaging in diagnostic workup. Hippocampal and cerebellar regions should be closely evaluated.

Neuropsychological assessment should be comprehensive in its approach. Although particular attention should be placed on executive functions, domains of attention, verbal learning and memory, and visuoconstructional and visuospatial skills, other domains may still be impacted on a case-by-case basis.

TREATMENT

Treatment of lead intoxication understandably is directed at reducing levels of lead in the system. Chelation therapy is the standard method of removing lead from the system and is also a key tool in diagnosis. Calcium disodium EDTA and dimercaptosuccinic acid (DMSA) have both been used in chelation therapy to remove lead from the system as part of treatment as well as for diagnostic purposes (Lee et al., 2000; Wedeen, 1992). Dietary supplementation has also been effective.

Increased dietary calcium has been found to reduce the absorption of lead in infants and children (Bogden et al., 1992; Mahaffey, Gartside, & Glueck, 1986). Increased intakes of magnesium, phosphate, alcohol, and dietary fat have demonstrated similar benefits in terms of their reduction of gastrointestinal absorption of lead (Barltrop & Meek, 1979).

Although chelation therapy controls further toxicity secondary to increased lead levels, in many ways the consequences of the initial level elevations are irreversible. This is particularly true when it comes to neuropsychological outcomes. Although chelation therapy has been shown to decrease blood lead levels appropriately in children with concentrations as high as 20–45 µg/dL, the cognitive impairments presenting at that point in time cannot be reversed (Lee et al., 2000; Wedeen, 1992). Given this, appropriate services should be initiated based on findings of neuropsychological assessment such as special education services, cognitive rehabilitation, and training. If mood or behavioral issues remain prevalent, therapy, behavioral modification, and, if need be, pharmacological intervention may be utilized as deemed appropriate.

Jacob M. Goings
Chad A. Noggle

Baghurst, P. A., McMichael, A. J., Tong, S., Wigg, N. R., Vimpani, G. V., & Robertson, E. F. (1995). Exposure to environmental lead and visual-motor integration at age 7 years: The Port Pirie Cohort Study. *Epidemiology, 6,* 2, 104–109.

Barltrop, D., & Meek F. (1979). Effect of particle size on lead absorption from the gut. *Archives of Environmental Health, 34,* 280–285.

Bellinger, D. (2011). Toxic Effects. In: Davis, A. Handbook of Pediatric Neuropsychology (955–962). New York, NY: Springer Publishing.

Bellinger, D., Hu, H., Titlebaum, L., & Needleman, H. (1994). Attentional correlates of dentin and bone lead levels in adolescents. Archives of Environmental Health, *49,* 98–105.

Bogden, J. D., Gertner, S. B., Christakos, S., Kemp, F. W., Yang, Z., Katz, S. R., et al. (1992). Dietary calcium modifies concentrations of lead and other metals and renal calbindin in rats. *The Journal of Nutrition, 122,* 1351–1360.

Bolla, A., & Cadet, J. (2007). Exogenous Acquired Metabolic Disorders of the Nervous System: Toxins and Illicit Drugs. In: Goetz C. Textbook of Clinical Neurology. Philadelphia: Saunders.

Bressler, J. P., & Goldstein, G. W. (1991). Mechanisms of lead neurotoxicity. *Biochemical Pharmacology, 41*, 4, 479–484.

Cory-Slechta, D. A. (1997). Relationships between Pb-induced changes in neurotransmitter system function and behavioral toxicity. *Neurotoxicology, 18*, 3, 673–688.

Davis, J. M. (1990). Risk assessment of the developmental neurotoxicity of lead. *Neurotoxicology, 11*, 2, 285–291.

Holtzman, D., DeVries, C., Nguyen, H., Olson, J., & Bensch, K. (1984, Fall). Maturation of resistance to lead encephalopathy: Cellular and subcellular mechanisms. *Neurotoxicology, 5*, 3, 97–124.

Krigman, M. R. (1978, October). Neuropathology of heavy metal intoxication. *Environmental Health Perspectives, 26*, 117–120.

Lee, B., Ahn, K. D., Lee, S. S., Lee, G. S., Kim, Y. B., & Schwartz, B. S. (2000). A comparison of different lead biomarkers in their associations with lead-related symptoms. *International Archives of Occupational and Environmental Health, 73*, 5, 298–304.

Mahaffey, K. R., Gartside, P. S., & Glueck, C. J. (1986). Blood lead levels and dietary calcium intake in 1- to 11-year-old children. The Second National Health and Nutrition Examination Survey, 1976 to 1980. *Pediatrics, 78*, 2, 257–262.

Needleman, H.L, Schell, A., Bellinger, D., et al. (1990). The long-term effects of exposure to low dose of lead in childhood: An 11 year follow-up report. *The New England Journal of Medicine, 322*, 83–88.

Ohnishi, A., Schilling, W.S., Brimijoin, W.S. et al. (1997). Lead neuropathy. 1. Morphometry, nerve conduction ad choline acetyltransferase transport: New finding of endoneurial oedema associated with segmental demyelination. *Journal of Neuropathology & Experimental Neurology, 36*, 499–518.

Papanikolaou, N. C., Hatzidaki, E. G., Belivanis, S., Tzanakakis, G. N., & Tsatsakis, A. M. (2005). Lead toxicity update. A brief review. *Medical Science Monitor: International Medical Journal of Experimental and Clinical Research, 11*, 10, RA329–RA336.

Pentschew A. (1965). Morphology and morphogenesis of lead encephalopathy. *Acta Neuropathol (Berl), 5*, 133–160.

Phillip, A. T., & Gerson, B. (1994). Lead poisoning—Part I. Incidence, etiology, and toxicokinetics. *Clinics in Laboratory Medicine, 14*, 2, 423–444.

Ris, M. D., Dietrich, K. N., Succop, P.A., & Berger, O.G (2004). Early exposure to lead and neuropsychological outcome in adolescence. *Journal of International Neuropsychological Society, 10 (2)*, 261–270.

Schwartz, B. S., Stewart, W. F., Bolla, K. I., et al. (2000). Past adult lead exposure is associated with longitudinal decline in cognitive function. *Neurology, 55*, 1144–1150.

Seidman, B.C., Olsen, A. W., Verity, M. A. (1987). Triethyl lead inhibits Y-aminobutyric acid binding to uptake sites in synaptosomal membranes. *Journal of Neurochemistry, 49*, 415–420.

Slomianka, L., Rungby, J., West, M. J. et al. (1989). Dosedependent bimodel effect of low-level lead exposure on the developing hippocampal region of the rat: A volumetric study. *Neurotoxicology, 10*, 177–190.

Valpey, R., Sumi, M., Copss, MK, Goble, G.J. (1978). Acute and chronic progressive encephalopathy due to gasoline sniffing. *Neurology, 28*, 507–510.

Verity, M.A. (1997). Toxic disorders. In D.I. Graham & P.L. Lantos (Eds.) *Greenfield's Pathology* (6th Ed.). London: Arnold (pp. 755–811).

Wedeen, R. (1992). Removing lead from bone: Clinical implications of bone lead stores. *Neurotoxicology, 13*, 4, 843–852.

LEIGH'S SYNDROME

DESCRIPTION

Leigh's syndrome, also called subacute necrotizing encephalomyelopathy, is a rare neurometabolic disorder that is characterized by an acute degeneration of the brain, spinal cord, and optic nerve. It was first described in 1951 in a 7-month-old infant who showed severe nerve damage that resulted in lesions in the brainstem. The disorder is characterized by a rapid degeneration of the central nervous system and the development of symmetrical patches of demyelinated nerves. Leigh's syndrome is most commonly diagnosed in infancy or early childhood; however, there are a limited number of adult cases reported. Research pertaining to adult onset Leigh's syndrome does not currently exist and the cause is unknown.

Characteristically the individual will develop normally until approximately 1 year of age, at which time a gradual reduction of development may be seen; previously learned skills such as walking, sucking, and crawling show a significant regression. Throughout the progression of the disease, these developmental changes will continue to regress to previous states. Prognosis for the disease is poor and death usually occurs within 1–2 years after symptoms first appear. In some rare cases, individuals have reportedly lived to early adolescence.

NEUROPATHOLOGY/PATHOPHYSIOLOGY

Leigh's syndrome has been shown to be associated with a thiamine deficiency. This deficiency appears

L

to result from an inhibitor that is present in body fluids that prevents the formation of the thiamine (Pincus et al., 1973). Due to the disturbance of thiamine metabolism, paralysis of the motor nerves in the eye (ophthalmoplegia), rapid involuntary movement of the eye (nystagmus), and disordered gaze, Leigh's syndrome is said to resemble Wernicke's disease; however, the hypothalamus and mammillary bodies are not affected in Leigh (Dale & Federman, 2008; De Vivo & Hirano, 2005; Murphy, 1973; Murphy, Isohashi, Weinberg, & Utter, 1981; Ropper & Brown, 2005). Lesions are noted to be quite extensive and very distinctive and consist of a combination of cell necrosis, demyelination, and vascular proliferation that can be found in the midbrain, pons, medulla, spinal cord, thalamus, basal ganglia, and cerebellum, and in the optic nerve and tracts. Cranial nerve abnormalities have also been observed. (Dale & Federman, 2005; De Vivo & Hirano, 2005; De Vivo & Hirano, 2008; Ropper & Brown, 2005; Williams et al., 1977). In the majority of cases the cerebral spinal fluid is normal; however, the levels of protein may be increased. Pyruvate and lactate levels have been found to be elevated in the blood and urine and indicate a potential disorder of mitochondrial oxidation (Atalar, Egilmez, Bulut, & Icagasioglu, 2005; Williams et al., 1977).

The most commonly identified biochemical abnormalities that lead to Leigh's syndrome have been found to exist in pyruvate dehydrogenase metabolism and oxidative phosphorylation (OXPHOS) defects (Complexes 1 and IV) (Murphy et al., 1981). All gene mutations are said to be transmitted in an autosomal recessive fashion. In the event that the deficiency occurs in the enzyme pyruvate dehydrogenase, the variation of the disease is said to be X-linked and for this reason shows a greater occurrence in boys, where girls are likely to be the carriers (De Vivo & Hirano, 2005; Macnair, 2006).

There are four types of mutations in the nuclear-encoded respiratory chain subunits that have been identified in Leigh's syndrome patients. One mutation exists in the gene coding for the flavoprotein subunit of Complex II (Shoffner, 2003). The other three mutations exist in Complex I subunits, specifically 18-KDa that maps to chromosome 5, NDUSF9, and 51-kDa. However, it is noted that these deficits do not produce the metabolic abnormalities that are known to occur in Leigh's syndrome.

Complex IV deficits are frequently observed and may be the result of a mutation in the *SURF1* gene, which causes poor assembly of cytochrome-c-oxidase. When both parents carry the mutated gene, their children have a 25% chance of having a child that is affected (Macnair, 2006; Shoffner, 2003). A final defect that can lead to Leigh's syndrome may be the result of a mutation of the mitochondrial DNA that may also lead to the deficiency of cytochrome-c-oxidase. Oxygen respiration is essential to the functioning of the mitochondria. Thus, when cellular respiration is dysfunctional, a deficit of supply to the mitochondria occurs, ultimately preventing the mitochondria from operating properly. This type of defect is one of the rarest causes of Leigh's syndrome (Pecina, Gnaiger, Zeman, Pronicka, & Houstek, 2004).

NEUROPSYCHOLOGICAL/CLINICAL PRESENTATION

Infants with this disease develop normally for up to 2 years prior to developing the first symptoms. In infants, the first symptoms include poor sucking, loss of head control, poor appetite, vomiting, irritability, and weight loss. If the onset occurs within the second year, a delay in walking, ataxia, psychomotor regression, respiration disturbance, and abnormal movement of limbs can be seen. Disorders of gaze may also occur when the degeneration begins to affect the optic nerve. Cognitive and intellectual deterioration may also begin to develop, specifically loss of previous ability for speech. The onset is very swift as is the deterioration. In some cases, heart difficulties have been noted. In the case of adult onset, the regression of previously developed skills, ataxia, respiration disturbance, vision difficulties, limb weakness, and hearing difficulties can also be seen; however, the progression of the disease is slower.

The course of Leigh's syndrome is characterized by remissions and exacerbations. The frequency and intensity is varied among individuals depending on the acuteness of the disease. Exacerbations may be associated with a high fever, or a high carbohydrate diet. The prognosis is poor for individuals diagnosed with Leigh's syndrome—most do not live more than 2 years—although there have been a couple of cases reported of individuals who live into adolescence and adulthood.

DIAGNOSIS

Leigh's syndrome is difficult to diagnose due to the broad variability in symptoms and the many genetic causes of the disease. Characteristically the individual will develop normally until approximately 1 year of age, at which time a gradual reduction of development may be seen; previously learned skills such as walking, sucking, and crawling show a significant regression. Throughout the progression of the disease, there will be continued degeneration. This marked decline in function is the first clinical sign for diagnosis. Thereafter, Leigh's syndrome is typically detected through blood and urine screening followed by genetic tests that are performed to confirm the presence or absence of the abnormal gene. In addition, evidence of brain lesions may be seen in CT scans and in MRIs. Electron microscopy may also show an increase of mitochondria in rare cases. As these symptoms overlap with many other degenerative diseases of childhood, modern diagnosis depends on genetic analysis.

TREATMENT

There are little to no successful treatments for Leigh's syndrome. In some cases, thiamine and vitamin B1 supplements are given as an attempt to decrease the rate of deterioration (Rocco, Lamba, Minniti, Caruso, & Naito, 2000). Over time, however, the effectiveness of these treatments plateau and deterioration continues. In some cases, a high fat, low carbohydrate diet may be prescribed. Similar to thiamine treatment, the benefits of this type of treatment are short-lived and degeneration continues.

Danielle S. Dance
Charles Golden

Altalar, M. H., Egilmez, H., Bulut, S., & Icagasioglu, D. (2005). Magnetic resonance spectroscopy and diffusion-weighted imaging findings in a child with Leigh's disease. *Pediatrics International, 47,* 601–603.

Dale, D. C., & Federman, D. D. (2008). *ACP Medicine.* New York: Web MD..

De Vivo, D. C., & Hirano, M. (2005). Mitochondrial diseases with mutations of nuclear DNA. In L. P. Rowland (Ed.), *Merritt's neurology.* Philadelphia: Lippincott Williams & Wilkins.

McCandless, D. W., & Hodgkin, W. E. (1977). Subacute necrotizing Encephalomyelopathy (Leigh's disease). *Pediatrics, 60*(6), 935–937.

Mcnair, T. (2006). *Leigh's disease. BBC health.* Retrieved January 7, 2009.

Murphy, J. V. (1973). Subacute necrotizing encephalomyelopathy (Leigh's disease): Detection on the heterozygous carrier state. *Pediatrics, 51*(4), 710–715.

Murphy, J. V., Isohashi, F., Weinberg, M. B., & Utter, M. F. (1981). Pyruvate carboxylase deficiency: An alleged biochemical cause of Leigh's disease. *Pediatrics, 68*(3), 401–404.

Pecina, P., Gnaiger, E., Zeman, J., Pronicka, E., & Houstek, J. (2004). Decreased affinity for oxygen of cytochrome-c oxidase in Leigh syndrome caused by SURF1 mutations. *American Journal of Physiology, 287,* 1384–1388.

Pincus, J. H., Cooper, J. R., Murphy, J. V., Rabe, E. F., Lonsdale, D., & Dun, H. G. (1973). Thiamine derivatives in sub acute necrotizing encephalomyelopathy. *Pediatrics, 51*(4), 716–721.

Rocco, M. D., Lamba, L. D., Minniti, G., Caruso, U., & Naito, E. (2000). Outcome of thiamine treatment in a child with Leigh disease due to thiamine-responsive pyruvate dehydrogenase deficiency. *European Journal of Paediatric Neurology, 4*(3), 115–117.

Ropper AH, Brown RJ: Adams and Victor's principles of neurology, 8th edn.. New York, McGraw-Hill, 2005.

Shoffner, J. M. (2003). Oxidative phosphorylation diseases and disorders of pyruvate oxidation. In C. D. Rudolph, A. M. Rudolph, M. K. Hostetter, G. Lister, & N. J. Siegel (Eds.), *Rudolph's pediatrics.* McGraw-Hill.

Williams, J. L., Monnens, L. A. H., Trijbels, J. M. F., Veerkamp, J. H., Meyer, A. E. F. H., Van Dam, K., et al. (1977). Leigh's encephalomyelopahty in a patient with cytochrome c oxidase deficiency in muscle tissue. *Pediatrics, 60*(6), 850–857.

LENNOX–GASTAUT'S SYNDROME

DESCRIPTION

Lennox–Gastaut's syndrome (LGS) is a form of childhood epilepsy primarily characterized by tonic seizures during sleep or at times of awakening. Symptoms onset fairly early and may have been preceded historically by infantile spasms/West's syndrome. Atonic, atypical absence, myoclonic seizures, and/or status epilepticus are also common manifestations (Foldvary-Schaefer & Wyllie, 2007). Clinical manifestations may vary. Mental retardation of moderate to severe degrees is seen. In fact, the latter is noted in a majority of cases and may be noted even prior to seizure activity.

LGS accounts for approximately 2% to 3% of all cases of childhood epilepsy (Farrell & Tatum, 2006). Symptoms most commonly onset between 1 and 8 years of age. The presentation is often noted in relation to other central nervous system (CNS) manifestations.

NEUROPATHOLOGY/PATHOPHYSIOLOGY

Generalized cerebral atrophy is often observed. The etiological basis is often determined in approximately 70% of cases (Arzimanoglou, Guerrini, & Aicardi, 2004). As suggested, LGS is usually seen in conjunction with other CNS malformations of either a genetic or acquired basis. CNS infections, tuberous sclerosis, and other noncutaneous disorders, CNS development disorders, and hypoxic events have been associated with LGS. LGS is preceded by West's syndrome in approximately 20% to 30% of children and is related to poorer outcomes (Gastaut et al., 1966; Genton, Guerrini, & Dravet, 2000).

NEUROPSYCHOLOGICAL/CLINICAL PRESENTATION

As suggested, LGS is a seizure disorder characterized by a mixture of seizure types, with an onset in childhood, usually between 1 and 8 years of age, and potentially preceded historically by infantile spasms. Atypical absence seizures can present, which are longer in duration or more complicated than traditional or typical absence seizures. Generalized tonic–clonic seizures are also associated with the presentation as are atonic seizures. Regarding the latter, this leads to an acute loss of muscle tone, leading to these sometimes being referred to as drop seizures. This constitutes a risk for children, as they may hit their head when falling. As a result, children often wear protective helmets to reduce risk of serious injury.

From a neuropsychological standpoint, a unitary profile is not really seen. Rather, individuals demonstrate generalized and global deficits in cognition (Besag, 2006). More than half of all children demonstrate severe mental retardation, with 20% to 60% arising even prior to seizure onset (Foldvary-Schaefer & Wyllie, 2007). Mild to moderate mental retardation is noted in the remaining children. Normal functioning is rarely ever noted and, again, the pattern is fairly generalized without sparing or more prominent dysfunctions noted in particular areas. Coinciding with this general dysfunction, learning deficits are prominent.

Behaviorally, children exhibit tendencies toward irritability, increased anger, and impulsivity. They can demonstrate tendencies toward explosiveness and destructive behavior at times of agitation.

DIAGNOSIS

Diagnosis is made through a combination of clinical features and electroencephalogram, which is essential to diagnosis. The pattern commonly reveals diffuse slow spike-wave complexes or polyspike-wave discharges during wakefulness and bursts of diffuse fast rhythms at 10–20 Hz during sleep (Beaumanoir & Blume, 2005; Dulac & N'Guyen, 1993; Gastaut et al., 1966). This pattern is noted in conjunction with the clinical features of mental deterioration, behavioral disturbance, and drug-resistant epilepsy marked by atonic and atypical absence seizures during the day and largely nocturnal tonic seizures.

TREATMENT

LGS responds poorly to standard anticonvulsant treatment. Polytherapy is often needed. Rufinamide, lamotrigine, and topiramate have all been approved by the U.S. FDA for the treatment of LGS. However, empirical reviews have still suggested that these are not highly effective (Hancock & Cross, 2003). Clonazepam and valproic acid have also demonstrated utility (Foldvary-Schaefer & Wyllie, 2007). Phenytoin and rectal diazepam are useful in the treatment of serial tonic seizures and status epilepticus with refractory cases potentially benefitting from felbamate or a ketogenic diet (Foldvary-Schaefer & Wyllie, 2007). In highly refractory cases, particularly a lack of response of atonic seizures, neurosurgical intervention may be required in the form of a corpus callosotomy. Implantation of vagus nerve stimulators have also shown some efficacy.

As previously suggested, children should wear protective helmets to avoid secondary injury resulting from atonic (a.k.a. drop) seizures. For children who can function in a school setting, multiple services are often required by way of individualized education programs and special education services.

Chad A. Noggle

Arzimanoglou, A., Guerrini, R., & Aicardi, J. (2004). Lennox-Gastaut syndrome. In *Aicardi's epilepsy in children* (3rd ed., pp. 38–50). Philadelphia: Lippincott Williams and Wilkins.

Beaumanoir, A., & Blume, W. (2005). The Lennox-Gastaut syndrome. In J. Roger, M. Bureau, C. Dravet, P. Genton, C. A. Tassinari, & P. Wolf (Eds.), *Epileptic syndromes in infancy, childhood and adolescence* (4th ed., pp. 125–148). Paris: John Libbey Eurotext.

Besag, F.M. (2006). Cognitive and behavioral outcomes of epileptic syndromes: Implications for education and clinical practice. *Epilepsia, 47* (Suppl. 2), 119–125.

Dulac, O., & N'Guyen, T. (1993). The Lennox-Gastaut syndrome. *Epilepsia, 34* (Suppl. 7), 7–17.

Farrell, K., Tatum, W.O. IV (2006). Encephalopathic generalized epilepsy and Lennox-Gastaut syndrome. In E. Wyllie, A. Gupta, D.K. Lachhwani (Eds.) *The treatment of epilepsy: Principles and practice* (4th ed., pp. 429–440). Philadelphia: Lippincott, Williams, & Wilkins.

Foldvary-Schaefer, N., & Wyllie, E. (2007). Epilepsy. In C. G. Goetz (Ed.), *Textbook of clinical neurology* (3rd ed., pp. 1213–1244). Philadelphia: Saunders Elsevier.

Gastaut, H., Roger, J., Soulayrol, R., Tassinari, C.A., Regis, H., Dravet, C. (1966). Childhood epileptic encephalopathy with diffuse slow spikes and waves (otherwise known as "petit mal variant") or Lennox syndrome. *Epilepsia, 7*, 139–179.

Genton, P., Guerrini, R., & Dravet, C. (2000). The Lennox-Gastaut syndrome. In H. Meinardi (Ed.), *Handbook of clinical neurology: The epilepsies, part II* (pp. 211–222). Amsterdam: Elsevier.

Hancock, E., & Cross, H. (2003). Treatment of Lennox-Gastaut syndrome. *Cochrane Database of Systematic Reviews, (3)*, CD0P3277.

LESCH–NYHAN SYNDROME

DESCRIPTION

Medical student Michael Lesch and Dr. William Nyhan published a 1964 paper in which they described two brothers presenting with delayed motor development, increased muscle tone, positive Babinski signs, involuntary movements, self-injurious behavior (SIB), mental retardation, and crystals of uric acid in the urine. Now known as Lesch–Nyhan syndrome (LNS), it results from a recessive X-linked chromosomal abnormality that leads to a deficiency of the hypoguanine phosphoribosyltransferase (HPRT) enzyme that leads to increased purine production. LNS occurs in approximately 1:100,000–1:380,000 births and most frequently occurs in boys (Sikora et al., 2006). A milder variant (Lesch–Nyhan variant, LNV) is also known, defined by increased HPRT activity 1.5% to 50% of normal levels and hyperuricemia, but milder cognitive and motor symptoms and the absence of SIB characteristic of LNS.

NEUROPATHOLOGY/PATHOPHYSIOLOGY

LNS is caused by a mutation on the X chromosome, *HPRT1* gene, located at q26-q27 causing a deficiency in the HPRT enzyme that is part of the purine salvage pathway. Hypoguanine phosphoribosyltransferase catalyzes the conversion of purine bases to nucleic acids (hypoxanthine to inosinic acid guanidine to guanylic acid). Hypoxanthine is converted to uric acid by xanthine oxidase, and increased levels of hypoxanthine due to defects in the HPRT enzyme result in increased uric acid production and hyperuricemia. In infants, uric acid crystals can sometimes be seen in the diaper and patients may present with renal stones, neuropathy, manifestation of gout, and if untreated, renal failure (Nyhan, 1976). No specific locations on the *HPRT* gene have been implicated in LNS; however, several sites have been deemed "mutational hotspots," and it is suggested that less severe LNVs may result from mutations that allow partial HPRT enzyme activity (Jinnah et al., 2000). Mutations of HPRT can affect intracellular concentrations of the HPRT enzyme, most likely due to enzyme instability, or can impair catalytic activity of HPRT (Eads et al., 1994).

It is likely that many features of LNS may be attributed to dysfunction of dopamine and the basal ganglia, including motor abnormalities and SIB (Visser, Bar, & Jinnah, 2000). Reduction in size and volume of the caudate have been noted in LNS patients compared to controls (Harris et al., 1998; Wong et al., 1996). A positron emission tomography study found a reduction in dopamine binding in the caudate and putamen in LNS patients compared to controls and patients with Rett's syndrome. In addition, reduced total brain volume, atrophy of the brainstem, thickening of the skull marrow, and pneumatization of the sinuses were found in five of the seven patients with LNS (Harris et al., 1998).

NEUROPSYCHOLOGICAL/CLINICAL PRESENTATION

Motor impairments are severe in classic is brain-derived neurotrophic growth factor LNS, and most patients never achieve independence in unsupported sitting or walking. Hypotonia develops at approximately 3–6 months of age. At 6–12 months, infants demonstrate an inability to sit up and involuntary movements which progress in severity through the fourth year or life. Then motor abnormalities become static, neither worsening nor improving in most cases. Dystonia is the most prominent motor feature of LNS and is present in the upper body, mandible, and lower body causing difficulty or inability in grasping, speaking, and walking, respectively. Choreoathetosis (spastic movements of the limbs and face), dysarthia (slurred speech), difficulty swallowing and frequent vomiting, and ballism (abnormal swinging, hurling, or jerking movements) were also reported in patients with LNS (Jinnah et al., 2006; Olson & Houlihan, 2000).

The first descriptions of LNS included mental retardation with IQ scores less than 50. However, it has been recognized that motor and speech deficits may limit testing and individuals with LNS may have intellectual functioning higher than suggested by their measured IQ scores. There are published case reports of LNS patients with average intelligence; however, in these patients sustained attention remained impaired

(Scherzer & Ilson, 1969). In a survey designed specifically to assess cognitive ability in LNS patients, caretakers reported that all subjects over 5 years of age were alert and oriented to date, location, and identity of caregivers; 97% of the patients reportedly showed appropriate affect and an understanding of events and environment. In that same study, anecdotes provided by caretakers alluded to memory abilities. Parents also indicated that LNS patients over the age of 5 were capable of inductive and deductive reasoning, as they were able to understand the plots of movies and keep up with sports programs. Though speech is difficult for LNS patients, parents report the ability to improve communication skills with training. In most children, academic ability was impaired and found to be below grade level and cognitive ability (Anderson, Ernst, & Davis, 1992). Research using standardized measures has shown that over 70% of LNS patients obtain IQ scores in the ranges associated with mental retardation (Jinnah, DeGregorio, Harris, Nyhan, & O'Neill, 2000; Matthews, Solan, & Barabas, 1995). Individuals with LNV typically obtain scores lower than normals, but higher than typical LNS patients (Schretlen, Harris, Park, Jinnah, & Del Pozo, 2001).

The hallmark of LNS is SIB that begins at approximately 2 years of age; however, the range of age at onset varies from 5 months to 10 years. Self-injury is related to stressful situations and worsens in aversive situations. Patients' sensory modalities are intact and they are capable of feeling pain; however, they are compulsively driven to injure themselves, and though they are conscious of their behavior, it is apparently beyond their volitional control. In a survey of 40 parents of patients with LNS, approximately 50% reported that their children were able to predict activities that precipitate SIB (Anderson & Ernst, 1994). Patients often show remorse afterwards. Biting is the most prevalent form of self-injury often causing loss of tissue around the mouth and amputation of fingers. Other forms of SIB include head banging, arching of the spine, throwing limbs or head out when passing by a doorway when in wheelchair, and snapping the head back. After approximately 5 years of age, new forms of SIB rapidly evolve (Anderson & Ernst, 1994; Robey, Reck, Giacomini, Barabas, & Eddey, 2003). Aggression toward others has also been reported in patients with LNS and, like self-injury, appears to be beyond the patient's control. Individuals with LNV typically do not self-injure, but often have difficulty with attention (Schretlen et al., 2005).

DIAGNOSIS

Developmental delay, motor abnormalities, and uric acid crystals may be seen in infancy. Definitive diagnoses may be made by examining erythrocyte HPRT enzyme concentrations (less than 1.5% of normal concentrations in classic LNS) and alternatively, screening for the HPRT gene mutation. Levart (2007) presented a case report in which diagnosis of LNS was not straightforward and was made only through examination of serum uric acid and subsequent mutation screening of the HPRT1 gene. He concluded that a diagnosis of LNS must be ruled out in every boy with supposed cerebral palsy with no history of perinatal illness by carefully examining the patient for hyperuricosuria.

Nyhan (1976) defined a spectrum of HPRT deficiency. He defined full-blown LNS as showing virtually no HPRT enzyme activity under any conditions, whereas those with partial variant LNV showed some HPRT activity, but still less than 50% of the normal values. Alternatively, Levart (2007) suggests that patients be diagnosed with LNS if HPRT enzyme activity is less than 1.5% under all conditions, and those with levels between 1.5% and 10% may be diagnosed as "neurologic variants."

TREATMENT

Presently, there is no remedy for HPRT deficiency; however, patients with LNS are treated with medication to lessen uric acid production, motor abnormalities, and SIB. Allopurinol is an inhibitor of xanthine oxidase and may be used to lower blood levels of uric acid, preventing kidney stones and gout manifestations; however, doses should be carefully monitored as too much allopurinol may cause increased excretions of uric acid. In addition, a potassium citrate mixture may be used to increase the solubility of uric acid. Baclofen and diazepam are used to lessen muscle spasms. Diazepam has the additional benefit of reducing anxiety but also presents a risk for developing dependency. Tetrabenzine and L-dopa have proven successful in ameliorating some movement disabilities (McCarthy, 2004). Pharmacologic treatments of SIB with agents such as benzodiazepines, neuroleptics, chloral hydrates, anticonvulsives, and antidepressants have shown variable success with parental reports indicating that anticonvulsives and benzodiazepines being the most effective (Anderson & Ernst, 1994).

Behavior therapy is pallative, but not curative, and in many cases of LNS, individuals must be restrained in order to prevent injury. Most patients are at ease in restraints and may show terror when they are not restrained (Anderson & Ernst, 1994; Nyhan, 1976). Affected individuals often participate in decisions regarding restraints. Another technique used in the management of SIB is dental extraction. In Anderson and Ernst's (1994) survey, 60% of patients with LNS had teeth extracted to prevent injurious side effects of biting, and all of the parents reported no regrets.

Some researchers suggest that there may be a gene by environment interaction involved in SIB. Such as changes in the brain resulting from for example, HPRT deficiency may cause changes in the brain lead to the expression of certain behaviors which are subsequently reinforced by parents' actions. In Anderson and Ernst's (1994) survey, over 42% of parents indicated that their child occasionally used SIB to obtain a desired goal. Psychosocial therapy has variable success in the LNS population. Behavior modification alleviated SIB to some degree in 70% of patients surveyed (Anderson & Ernst, 1994). Reports indicate variable success with combinations of play therapy, extinction, desensitization, and reinforcement (Olson & Houligan, 2000).

LNS is a recessive, X-linked, genetic disorder resulting in disruption of the purine salvage pathway via the HPRT enzyme. The disorder manifests in hyperuricemia, and disorders in motor, neurological, cognitive, and behavioral functions — the hallmark of LNS being the severity of self-injury that individuals are compulsively driven to engage in. Although there is no remedy for HPRT deficiency, treatments of hyperuricemia and motor disorders have proven highly successful. The efficacy of treatments of SIB has been variable and entirely pallative.

Mandi Musso
Alyse Barker
William Drew Gouvier

Anderson, L. T., & Ernst, M. (1994). Self-injury in Lesch-Nyhan disease. *Journal of Autism and Developmental Disorders*, 24(1), 67–81.

Anderson, L. T., Ernst, M., & Davis, S. V. (1992). Cognitive abilities of patients with Lesch-Nyhan disease. *Journal of Autism and Developmental Disorders*, 22(2), 189–203.

Eads, J. C., Scapin, G., Xu, Y., Grubmeyer, C., & Sacchettini, J. C. (1994). The crystal structure of human hypoxanthine-guanine phosphoribosyltransferase with bound GMP. *Cell, 78*, 325–334.

Harris, J. C., Lee, R. R., Jinnah, H. A., Wong, D. F., Yaster, M., & Bryan, R. N. (1998). Craniocerebral magnetic resonance imaging measurement and findings in Lesch-Nyhan syndrome. *Archives or Neurology, 55*, 547–553.

Jinnah, H. A., De Gregorio, L., Harris, J. C., Nyhan, W. L., & O'Neill., J. P. (2000). The spectrum of inherited mutations causing HPRT deficiency: 75 new cases and a review of 196 previously reported cases. *Mutation Research, 463*, 309–326.

Jinnah, H. A., Visser, J. E., Harris, J. C., Verdu, A., Larovere, L., Ceballos-Picot, I., et al.; Lesch-Nyhan Disease International Study Group. (2006). Delineation of the motor disorder of Lesch-Nyhan disease. *Brain, 12*(9, Pt. 5), 1201–1217.

Levart, T. K. (2007). Rare variant of Lesch-Nyhan syndrome without self-mutilation or nephrolithiasis. *Pediatric Nephrology, 22*, 1975–1978.

Matthews, W. S., Solan, A., & Barabas, G. (1995). Cognitive functioning in Lesch-Nyhan syndrome. *Developmental Medicine and Child Neurology, 37*, 715–722.

McCarthy, G. (2004). Medical diagnosis, management, and treatment of Lesch-Nyhan disease. *Nucleosides, Nucleotides, & Nucleic Acids, 23*(8 & 9), 1147–1152.

Nyhan, W. L. (1976). Behavior in the Lesch-Nyhan syndrome. *Journal of Autism and Childhood Schizophrenia, 6*(3), 235–252.

Olson, L., & Houlihan, D. (2000). A review of behavioral treatments used for Lesch-Nyhan syndrome. *Behavior Modification, 24*(2), 202–222.

Robey, K. L., Reck, J. F., Giacomini, K. D., Barabas, G., & Eddey, G. E. (2003). Modes and patterns of self-mutilation in person with Lesch-Nyhan disease. *Developmental Medicine and Child Neurology, 45*(3), 167–171.

Schretlen, D. J., Harris, J. C., Park, K. S., Jinnah, H. A., & Del Pozo, N. O. (2001). Neurocognitive functioning in Lesch-Nyhan disease and partial hypoxanthine-guanine phosphoribosyltransferase deficiency. *Journal of the International Neuropsychological Society, 7*, 805–812.

Schretlen, D. J., Ward, J., Meyer, S. M., Yun, J., Puig, J. G., Nyhan, W. L., et al. (2005). Behavioral aspects of Lesch-Nyhan disease and its variants. *Developmental Medicine and Child Neurology, 47*(10), 673–677.

Sherzer, A. L., & Ilson, J. B. (1969). Normal intelligence in the Lesch-Nyhan syndrome. *Pediatrics, 44*(1), 116–120.

Sikora, P., Pijanowska, M., Majewski, M., Bienias, B., Borzecka, H., & Zajaczkowska, M. (2006). Acute renal failure due to bilateral xanthine urolithiasis in a boy with Lesch-Nyhan syndrome. *Pediatric Nephrology, 21*, 1045–1047.

Visser, J. E., Bar, P. R., & Jinnah, H. A. (2000). Lesch-Nyhan disease and the basal ganglia. *Brain Research Reviews, 32*, 449–475.

Wong, D. F., Harris, J. C., Naidu, S., Yokoi, F., Marenco, S., Dannals, R. F., et al. (1996). Dopamine transporters are markedly reduced in Lesch-Nyhan disease *in vivo*. *Proceedings of the National Academy of Sciences, 93*, 5539–5543.

LEWY BODY DEMENTIA

DESCRIPTION

Lewy body dementia (LBD) and its underlying pathology of Lewy bodies with diffuse cortical distribution was first described by Friedrich Heinrich Lewy in 1923 (Holdorff, 2002). However, the inclusionary bodies named after him were first identified and described in 1913. Since then, neuropathological and

L

clinical criteria have been outlined — and currently, it is well accepted that the main clinical symptoms essential for diagnosis involve a progressive cognitive decline, with pronounced cognitive fluctuations, especially related to alertness and attention, such as frequent drowsiness, lethargy, lengthy periods of time spent staring into space, or disorganized speech, and is frequently associated with recurrent visual hallucinations, visuospatial dysfunction, and early parkinsonian motor symptoms, such as rigidity and the loss of spontaneous movement. The constellation of symptoms is such that LBD has been conceptualized as bridging the gap between Alzheimer's disease and Parkinson's disease.

Onset generally occurs toward the end of an individual's fifth decade of life and progresses until death, which often comes after 10–15 years (Louis, Gaoldman, Powers, & Fahn, 1995).

NEUROPATHOLOGY/PATHOPHYSIOLOGY

The defining neuropathology of this disease is a cortical accumulation of Lewy bodies — an eosinophilic (hematoxylin and eosin staining), round inclusion found in the cytoplasm. Cortical amyloid plaques similar to those seen in Alzheimer's disease can also co-occur with the cortical Lewy bodies. If the Lewy bodies are noted in cortical regions, they are also commonly seen in brainstem regions. Also implicated in LBD is alpha-synuclein protein — a presynaptic protein. Multiple neurotransmitters, including acetylcholine and dopamine, are diminished. The apolipoprotein E subtype four (ApoE4) genotype is overrepresented in LBD but only when it occurs with concomitant Alzheimer's disease.

Pathologically, the brain appears largely to slightly atrophic. The cingulate gyrus, insular cortex, and parahippocampal gyrus often demonstrate the greatest proliferation of cortical Lewy bodies (Caselli & Boeve, 2007). Unlike other primary neurodegenerative diseases, LBD pathology spreads relatively early to the occipital lobes. Degeneration of basal ganglion regions including substantia nigra decay eventually occur and correspond with the parkinsonian features that present clinically. Likewise, atrophy of the nucleus basalis similar to that which is seen in Alzheimer's disease is commonly noted.

NEUROPSYCHOLOGICAL/CLINICAL PRESENTATION

Clinically, patients present with a chronic complaint of dementia in combination with the proposed core features of cognitive fluctuation, visual hallucinations, and parkinsonism (McKeith et al., 2005). Fluctuations in cognitive function occur with varying levels of alertness and attention. Visual hallucinations are seen and very commonly are in the shape of animals, insects, and persons. Parkinsonian motor features appear relatively early in LBD with dementia preceding or occurring simultaneously with the features of parkinsonism and add to the severity (Lopez et al., 2000).

Executive function deficits and visuospatial impairment may be more prominent in persons with LBD than in those with Alzheimer's disease (e.g., outcomes on the Stroop, digit span backwards). In addition, in comparison to patients with Alzheimer's disease, LBD has been associated with significantly worse processing speed, sequencing, and letter fluency but significantly better performance in naming and verbal memory (Ferman et al., 1999). Memory dysfunction may not be present at the initial evaluation, but it certainly will develop later in the course of the disease. Suggestive and supportive features can include nonvisual hallucinations, delusions, syncope, rapid eye movement (REM) sleep disorder, neuroleptic sensitivity, depression, apathy, autonomic impairment, and brief episodes of loss of consciousness. On neurological examination, patients may show some parkinsonian motor signs and gait impairment. Myoclonus may precede severe dementia. Resting tremor occurs less frequently than in Parkinson's disease.

DIAGNOSIS

A diagnosis of probable LBD requires the presence of dementia and at least two of the three core features of fluctuating level of attention, recurrent visual hallucinations, or parkinsonism. Additional suggestive features include REM sleep disorder, neuroleptic sensitivity, low dopamine transporter uptake in basal ganglia on SPECT or PET. One of these suggestive features can be substituted for a core feature. Possible LBD is diagnosed when only one core or suggestive feature accompanies the dementia.

Primary diagnosis remains clinical and is based on the clinical presentation as listed above. Diagnoses with overlapping symptomatology include Parkinson's disease dementia, Alzheimer's disease, cortical basal ganglionic degeneration, progressive supranuclear palsy, and frontotemporal lobar degeneration. Reversible causes of dementia should be ruled out by laboratory studies. Structural neuroimaging is required to rule out other etiologies. MRI findings in LBD typically show less hippocampal atrophy than patients with Alzheimer's disease. SPECT scanning or PET scanning may show decreased occipital lobe blood flow or metabolism in LBD but not in Alzheimer's disease. Reduced dopamine transporter activity in the basal ganglia is seen with PET scanning or SPECT scanning. If there is concern that the fluctuating mentation and hallucinations may represent temporal lobe epilepsy, an electroencephalogram should be considered.

TREATMENT

There are no curative or disease-modifying treatments available for LBD. Symptomatic treatment consists of controlling the cognitive, psychiatric, and motor symptoms of the disorder. Acetylcholinesterase inhibitors can be tried to treat the cognitive symptoms of LBD, and they may also be of some benefit in reducing the psychiatric and motor symptoms (McKeith, 2002). A trial of treatment with levodopa/carbidopa can be considered as it may improve motor function in some patients; however, this can serve to exacerbate the neuropsychiatric features. Hallucinations are not always bothersome to this patient group and should only be treated if they are disturbing or dangerous to the patient. Consequently, medicinal treatment of neuropsychiatric features, based on the type of agent used, can promote an exacerbation of parkinsonian symptoms. As a result, standard neuroleptics such as Haldol and so forth due to neuroleptic sensitivity that could worsen the motor symptoms should be avoided. Rather, agitation could be treated with atypical neuroleptics such as clozapine, quetiapine, or aripiprazole when cholinesterase inhibitors are ineffective (Miyasaki et al., 2006).

Glen R. Finney
Daniela Rusovici

Caselli, R. J., & Boeve, B. F. (2007). The degenerative dementias. In C. G. Goetz (Ed.), *Textbook of clinical neurology* (3rd ed., pp. 699–733). Philadelphia: Saunders Elsevier.

Ferman, T. J., Boeve, B. G., Smith, G. E., Silber, M. H., Kokmen, E., Petersen, R. C., et al. (1999). REM sleep behavior disorder and dementia: Cognitive differences when compared with AD. *Neurology, 52*, 951–957.

Holdorff, B. (2002). Friedrich Heinrich Lewy (1885–1950) and his work. *Journal of the History of the Neurosciences, 11*, 1, 19–28.

Lopez, O. L., Wisniewski, S., Hamilton, R. L., Becker, J. T., Kaufer, D. I., & DeKosky, S. T. (2000). Predictors of progression in patients with AD and Lewy bodies. *Neurology, 54*, 1774–1779.

Louis, E. D., Goldman, J. E., Powers, J. M., & Fahn, S. (1995). Parkinsonian features of eight pathologically diagnosed cases of diffuse Lewy body disease. *Movement Disorders, 10*, 188–194.

McKeith, I.G. (2002). Dementia with Lewy bodies. *The British Journal of Psychiatry, 180*, 144–147.

McKeith, I. G., Dickson, D. W., Lowe, J., Emre, M., O'Brien, J. T., Feldman, H., et al., (2005). Consortium on DLB. Diagnosis and management of dementia with Lewy bodies: Third report of the DLB Consortium. *Neurology, 65*, 12, 1863–1872.

Miyasaki, J. M., Shannon, K., Voon, V., Ravina, B., Kleiner-Fisman, G., Anderson, K., et al. (2006). Practice parameter: Evaluation and treatment of depression, psychosis, and dementia in Parkinson disease (an evidence-based review): Report of the Quality Standards Subcommittee of the American Academy of Neurology. *Neurology, 66*, 7, 996–1002.

L

LIPOID PROTEINOSIS

DESCRIPTION

Lipoid proteinosis, also known as Urbach–Wiethe's disease or *hyalinosis cutis et mucosae*, is a very rare hereditary disorder transmitted by an autosomal recessive gene. The most striking and common features are hoarseness in speech and pox-like acneiform and thickening of the skin and mucous membrane of the pharynx and larynx. This often leads to restricted movement of the tongue and visible skin thickening around the eyes and areas of mechanical friction (e.g., elbows, hands, knees). The disorder usually manifests with vocal symptoms soon after birth to within the first year, whereas skin complications usually develops in the first few years of life. Damage to the medial temporal lobe of the brain has also been documented in a larger percent of cases, with incidents of epilepsy also common in such cases. Difficulties in emotional regulation and memory, executive processing, and comorbidity with certain Axis I disorders have also been documented. The disorder was first described by a Viennese dermatologist and an otorhinolaryngologist, Urbach and Wiethe, in 1929 with 300 plus cases reported since such time.

NEUROPATHOLOGY/PATHOPHYSIOLOGY

Lipoid proteinosis is a recessive inherited gene disorder that has been linked to the mutation of the extracellular protein 1 gene classified as *ECM1*, with over 20 pathogenic mutations classified (Hamada et al., 2002). *ECM1* in humans encodes glycoprotein that is believed to have key roles in bone mineralization and epidermal differentiation. It has been hypothesized as a "biological glue" that acts as a homeostasis for the skin, used in roles such as regulation of basement membrane and growth factor binding (Chan, 2004). The disease is characterized by rings of excessive basement membrane surrounding blood vessels and irregular reduplication of lamina densa at the dermal-epidermal junction. These mutations most often lead to invasion of the mucosa of the pharynx, tongue, soft palate, and lips. Hoarseness in vocal projection is the most common result from such development following birth, though more severe cases can lead to a restricted tongue and respiratory difficulty. Often the most visible symptom is beaded eye papules. There are often noticeable, waxy yellow papules and nodules with skin thickening in other areas. This often occurs in areas such as the hands, elbows, buttocks, and knees where friction is encountered (Nanda, Alsaleh, & Al-Sabah, 2001).

Beyond dermatological symptoms, a significant number of documented cases (approximately 50% to 75%) also have shown bilateral, circumscribed, and symmetrical damage to the medial temporal region of the brain. This is an area containing both the amygdala and hippocampus. In this region calcium minerals find their way to the tissue and harden (i.e., calcification). The disorder has been documented to show strong and prevalent calcification in the amygdaloid complex. However, case studies suggest that the age of onset, severity of calcification, and the spreading to surrounding areas such as the uncinate and para-hippocampal gyri can vary greatly (Emsley & Paster, 1985; Siebert, Hans, & Bartel, 2003). It is also common for epilepsy (specifically in the temporal lobe) to occur when such calcification is noted. These seizures can often be visual or olfactory in nature, and often have loss of consciousness with or without automatisms and behavioral disturbances (Claeys et al., 2007).

NEUROPSYCHOLOGICAL/CLINICAL PRESENTATION

The main body of research concerning neuropsychological issues with lipoid proteinosis is based on the study of the amygdala. This is due to the disorders unique feature of often having calcification damage specific to this location. General research on the amygdala has been shown to be involved in the regulation of emotions, specifically fear, as well as aspects of episodic memory, and executive functioning (Tranel & Hyman, 1990). The body of studies on lipoid proteinosis patients with medial temporal lobe damage varies greatly in their supportive findings of the functions

of the amygdala. There is also a wide range of case studies that document varying levels of intelligence and comorbid Axis I disorders associated with the disorder. In the largest known sample study of patients with lipoid proteinosis (Thornton et al., 2008) a statistically significant number of comorbid disorders were found including anxiety disorders (33%), mood disorders (33%), psychosis (22%), and schizophrenia (15%). Furthermore, the study found that these patients were significantly less likely to identify both positive and negative emotions, showed impairment in memory, and lowered executive functioning. The study also showed that these patients performed significantly worse on assessments that dealt with identity of emotional expressions such as the Ekman facial emotional recognition test. They also performed worse on assessments testing the memory and executive functioning—specifically tests of visual organization, design initiative, dual sequencing, and abstract thinking (Thornton et al., 2008). These results have also been supported by other studies that showed poor performance with measure of executive functioning, implying symptoms of reduced decision making under both conditions of ambiguity and risk (Brand, Grabenhorst, Starcke, Vandekerckhove, & Markowitsch, 2007).

Other studies have not found such strong results for emotional regulation, executive functioning, and memory problems. Various subject groups have shown different ranges of intelligence from the above average to borderline range or lower. In one study of nine lipoid proteinosis patients (Sibert et al., 2003), they found that patients were able to identify different emotional faces despite amygdala damage. They did find, however, that differentiation of emotional expression does appear to suffer with damage to the amygdala as well as emotional memory, though there was no specific preference to negative emotions or fear. A majority of these cases also had a high school or college education and showed far less cognitive problems in comparison to other studies (Sibert et al., 2003). Although there is no clear understanding for such variation, both timing of symptom onset and rate of degeneration play a role in terms of cognitive functioning and emotional regulation. There is also a difference in what specific areas of the brain beyond the amygdala are affected in each case, which may also factor into the severity of symptoms (Papps, Calder, Young, & O'Carroll, 2003).

DIAGNOSIS

The disorder usually manifests its first symptom within a year or so after birth. This is most often the hoarseness in voice quality due to infiltration of the lungs and vocal cords. In more severe cases the infiltration may cause respiratory problems or a stiffening of the tongue. Visible papules and nodules along with generalized skin thickening usually occur within the next several years. Most noticeably these can be found around the eyes, elbows, hands, and buttocks (Nanda, Alsaleh, & Al-Sabah, 2001). CT scans or MRIs often show degeneration and calcification in the medial temporal lobes, often in the amygdale region (Siebert et al., 2003). Such brain degeneration has been linked to seizures and migraines also specific to this area. There is also evidence that with more severe degeneration and early onset, paranoia and psychotic features may manifest (Claeys et al., 2007). It may also be a biological root for anxiety disorders and mental retardation (Thornton et al., 2008)

In the past, the disorder was also believed to have features similar to porphyria and cutaneous amyloidosis. There was also some former similarities found with diabetic microangiopathy. Today, however, the most definitive way to diagnose lipoid proteinosis is through gene analysis for mutations in gene *ECM1*. To date, there are over 20 different mutations documented for the gene. The gene is recessive and there are believed to be several identified families, most notably in the Northern Cape Province of South Africa (Hamada et al., 2002).

TREATMENT

There is no known cure for lipoid proteinosis to date, though discovery of the *ECM1* gene does provide hope. In the past oral steroids and oral dimethyl sulphoxides have been used with lackluster results. Carbon dioxide laser surgery to the vocal cords and eyelids of thickened skin regions has been shown to have some success with dermatological issues (Hamada, 2005).

Peyton Groff
Raymond S. Dean

Brand, M., Grabenhorst, F., Starcke, K., Vandekerckhove, M., & Markowitsch, H. J. (2007). Role of the amygdale in decisions under ambiguity and decisions under risk: Evidence from patients with Urbach-Wiethe disease. *Neuropsychologia, 45*(9), 1305–1317.

Claeys, K. G., Claes, L. R., Van Goethem, J. W., Sercu, S., Merregaert, J., Lambert, J., et al. (2007). Epilepsy and migraine in patient with Urbach-Wiethe disease. *Seizure, 16*(4), 465–468.

Chan, I. (2004). The role of extracellular matrix protein 1 in human skin. *Clinical Experimental Dermatology, 29*(1), 52–56.

Emsley, R. A., & Paster, L. (1985). Lipoid proteinosis presenting with neuropsychiatric manifestations. *Journal of Neurology, Neurosurgery, and Psychiatry, 48*(12), 1290–1292.

Hamada, T. (2005). *Lipoid Proteinosis*. Retrieved March 10, 2009, from Orphanet Encyclopedia. Web site: http://www.orpha.net/data/patho/GB/uk-lipoidproteinosis.pdf

Hamada, T., McLean, W. H., Ramsay, M., Ashton, G. H., Nanda, A., Jenkins, T., et al. (2002). Lipoid proteinosis maps to 1q21 and is caused by mutations in the extracellular matrix protein 1 gene (ECM1). *Human Molecular Genetics, 11*(7), 833–840.

Nanda, A., Alsaleh, Q. A., & Al-Sabah, H. (2001). Lipoid proteinosis: Report of four siblings and brief review of the literature. *Pediatric Dermatology, 18*(1), 21–26.

Papps, B. P., Calder, A. J., Young, A. W., & O'Carroll, R. E. (2003). Dissociation of affective modulation of recollective and perceptual experience following amygdale damage. *Journal of Neurology, Neurosurgery, and Psychiatry, 74*, 253–254.

Siebert, M., Hans, J. M., & Bartel, P. (2003). Amygdala, affect and cognition: Evidence from 10 patients with Urbach-Wiethe disease. *Brain, 126*(12), 2627–2637.

Thornton, H. B., Nel, D., Thornton, D., Honk, J. V., Baker, G. A., & Stein, D. J. (2008). The neuropsychiatry and neuropsychology of Lipoid Proteinosis. *Journal of Neuropsychiatry Clinical Neuroscience, 20*(1), 86–92.

Tranel, D., & Hyman, B. T. (1990). Neuropsychological correlates of bilateral amygdale damage. *Neurology, 47*(3), 349–355.

LISSENCEPHALY

DESCRIPTION

Lissencephaly is a cerebral developmental disorder characterized by a smooth cortical surface following defective neuronal migration during the first trimester of pregnancy (Cardoso et al., 2000; Dobyns, 1987; Verloes, Elmaleh, Gonzales, Laquerrière, & Gressens, 2007). Neuronal migration is a brain development process in which nerve cells move from their place of origin to their ultimate location during fetal development. Lissencephaly is a type of neural migration disorder; it occurs because the process of developing neurons proceeding to their permanent place is disrupted, leading to an arrest of the ordered migration of neurons to the cortex (Dobyns, 1987; Verrotti et al., 2009). The surface of a normally developed brain is formed by a complex series of folds (also called gyri or convolutions) and grooves (also called sulci).

L

In individuals with lissencephaly, the normal convolutions are absent or only partly formed, making the surface of the brain appear smooth (Verloes et al., 2007); thus, the term "lissencephaly," from the Greek words "lissos" (smooth) and "encephalus" (brain), was used to describe the broad feature of an agyric or pachygyric brain (Walker, 1942). In addition, a normally developed cerebral cortex has six distinct cellular layers, but the brains of individuals with lissencephaly have only four. With such disturbances of brain maturation, individuals with lissencephaly are often profoundly retarded from birth and often develop seizure disorders (Reiner & Lombroso, 1998; Reiner & Sapir, 1998; Wynshaw-Boris, 2007).

The range of disorders associated with lissencephaly has become more defined as neuroimaging and knowledge of genetics has provided more insights into the causes of migration disorders. Possible causes of lissencephaly include inherited genetic conditions, new random genetic mutations, intrauterine viral infections, viral infections of the fetus during pregnancy, or interruptions of the blood supply to the fetus's brain during the first trimester of pregnancy (Dobyns & Truwit, 1995; Dorovini-Zis & Dolman, 1977). Communities with a high rate of parental consanguinity have much greater incidence of individuals with lissencephaly than other forms of noninherited neuronal migration disorders (Al-Qudah, 1998). Lissencephaly may occur as an isolated birth defect or may be associated with other birth abnormalities occurring together in a specific inherited syndrome. Some cases of lissencephaly result from deletions of certain identified genes involving neuronal migration (Pilz et al., 1998; Wynshaw-Boris, 2007).

NEUROPATHOLOGY/PATHOPHYSIOLOGY

To date, mutations of five different genes have been known to cause different types of lissencephaly in humans. Each of these genes has been shown to play a role in normal cell migration (Forman, Squier, Dobyns, & Golden, 2005; Koul, Jain, & Chacko, 2005). Subtypes of lissencephaly are generally divided into two distinct pathologic forms based on differences in the physical structure of the brain — Type I (classical) lissencephaly and Type II lissencephaly (cobblestone dysplasia) (Verloes et al., 2007; Verrotti et al., 2009). Type I lissencephaly results in four, rather than six, layers in the cortex and shows a smooth brain surface with relatively few broad gyri. The cortex is markedly thicker with larger than normal posterior ventricles. The corpus callosum is often small and sometimes absent (Forman et al., 2005; Koul et al., 2005).

Type I lissencephaly can be seen in a number of genetic syndromes or can occur by itself in a condition called isolated lissencephaly sequence (ILS). The majority of ILS is a result of mutations or deletions in one of two identified genes involved in brain development, namely *LIS1* and *XLIS* (or Doublecortin/DCX). *LIS1* is a gene located on the short arm of chromosome 17, identified as the first lissencephaly gene, and the first gene recognized to be part of an intracellular signaling pathway involved in neuronal migration (Reiner & Sapir, 1998; Wynshaw-Boris, 2007). Most deletions and mutations in the *LIS1* gene are sporadic and are not present in other family members. *XLIS* (or *DCX*) is a gene located on the long arm of the X chromosome. Mutations in *XLIS* cause X-linked lissencephaly in males; mothers who carry the mutation may or may not display the symptoms. Subcortical band heterotopia (SBH) is a milder form of lissencephaly, often seen in female carriers of *XLIS*. Studies show that *LIS1* mutations affect mainly the parietal and occipital regions, whereas the frontal cortex is more affected in individuals with mutated *XLIS* (Pilz et al., 1998; Reiner & Sapir, 1998).

Miller–Dieker syndrome (MDS) is a commonly seen genetic syndrome involving Type I lissencephaly. In MDS, the effect of the deletions of the *LIS1* gene extends to nearby genes required for normal development of other organ systems. Thus, individuals with MDS often produce more severe disorders than individuals with ILS, in which the mutations are constrained within single genes (Cardoso et al., 2000; Reiner & Lombroso, 1998). As a result, in addition to the features associated with lissencephaly, children with MDS also have distinct facial features, including a high forehead, a small jaw, a short upturned nose, thin lips, and narrowing at the temples. Calcium deposits in the midline of the brain are common in MDS, but not in ILS or other syndromes.

Type II lissencephaly is also called cobblestone dysplasia because of the pebbled appearance of the surface of the cerebral cortex. Unlike Type I lissencephaly, in which the abnormally thick cortex has a smooth interface with the underlying white matter, brains of individuals with cobblestone dysplasia often show abnormalities of the white matter, enlarged ventricles, underdeveloped brainstem and cerebellum, and absence of the corpus callosum. Examples of disorders associated with Type II lissencephaly include cobblestone lissencephaly without other birth defects, Fukuyama congenital muscular dystrophy, muscle-eye-brain disease, and Walker–Warburg syndrome (Dobyns, Kirkpatrick, Hittner, Roberts, & Kretzer, 1985).

NEUROPSYCHOLOGICAL/CLINICAL PRESENTATION

Individuals with lissencephaly often experience seizures/infantile spasms, mental retardation, psychomotor developmental delay, failure to thrive, muscle spasticity (hypotonia), microcephaly (a smaller than normal head), dysmorphism, and poor scholastic performance. Other symptoms may include craniofacial anomalies, difficulty swallowing and eating, and anomalies of the hands, fingers, or toes (Günör et al., 2007; Verloes et al., 2007). Epilepsy is associated with lissencephaly and is often resistant to conventional treatment (Koul et al., 2005). Respiratory illnesses and recurrent aspiration are common. In particular, individuals with Type I lissencephaly usually have severe mental retardation. Babies with ILS often have small jaws and hollowing at the temporal region (Koul et al., 2005).

Many infants with lissencephaly appear normal at birth, although some may have immediate respiratory problems. Head size is usually within normal limits at birth; however, as the baby grows, the growth slows down, resulting in a small head (microcephaly) (Günör et al., 2007). Following the initial few months after birth, parents may begin to notice lessened activity, inability to visually track objects, and feeding problems in the baby. Feeding difficulty may include choking, gagging, or regurgitating food or liquid. Apnea and muscle weakness are also common. Over time, muscle weakness may change to excessive muscle tension (spasticity). Seizures occur in most children with lissencephaly and frequently begin within the first year of life. These are usually severe and difficult to control with medication. Repeated bouts of pneumonia from swallowing food down an airway and into the lungs also are common.

DIAGNOSIS

The diagnosis of lissencephaly is usually made through neuroimaging at or soon after birth with the help of CT and/or MRI. Diagnosis by ultrasound cannot be reliably made until 26–28 weeks' gestation when the normal gyri and sulci become well defined (Dorovini-Zis & Dolman, 1977; Kojima et al., 2002). When lissencephaly is suspected, chorionic villus sampling, a screening technique for genetic defects, can test for some lissencephaly with a known genetic mutation (Miny, Wolfgang, & Jürgen, 1993).

MRI findings can be used to help diagnose Type I lissencephaly through detecting the absence of, or very shallow, convolutions on the surface of a markedly thick cerebral cortex and sometimes enlargement of the ventricles (Ghai et al., 2006). Individuals with MDS have more severe MRI findings than individuals with ILS. The smooth brain appearance is more striking in the back portion of the brain in individuals with chromosome 17 *LIS1* deletions and mutations, whereas it is more obvious in the front part of the brain in individuals with *XLIS* mutations. In addition, underdevelopment of a part of the cerebellum on MRI also helps identify individuals with *XLIS* mutations (Dorovini-Zis & Dolman, 1977). A CT scan can be done to look for calcium deposits in the midline of the brain in individuals with MDS, which is not seen in other lissencephaly syndromes (Cibis & Fitzgerald, 1995). Individuals with SBH often have minor changes in the gyri, shallow sulci, and ribbons of white and gray matter beneath the cortex that show up on MRI. Likewise, signs of Type II lissencephaly also can be detected through MRI, including a cobblestone appearance of the cortex, enlarged ventricles, abnormalities of the white matter, and changes in the cerebellum, corpus callosum, and brainstem (Kojima et al., 2002).

To confirm the diagnosis of MDS or ILS, high resolution chromosome testing and other specialized genetic tests are often helpful in determining whether a deletion is sporadic or due to an inherited chromosome rearrangement. If necessary, mutation analysis can be performed to look for specific errors in the sequence of *LIS1* and *XLIS* genes (Cibis & Fitzgerald, 1995).

In addition to MRI and CT testing, a careful clinical evaluation and examination by a medical geneticist is necessary to confirm the diagnosis and evaluate the child for the presence of a syndrome. After a precise diagnosis is made, genetic counselors should be able to give the family accurate information about the inheritance pattern and describe the likelihood of the condition recurring in future births (Cibis & Fitzgerald, 1995).

TREATMENT

There are no cures to reverse the effects of lissencephaly; treatment for those with lissencephaly is symptomatic and depends on the severity and locations of the brain malformations. Although medical management of seizures is available, most seizures associated with lissencephaly are resistant to conventional treatment (Gurrrini, Sicca, & Parmeggiani, 2003). Infantile spasms may be treated with adrenocorticotropic hormones, though they are not always effective. Shunting can be required for hydrocephalus.

For children who continue to have serious feeding difficulty, a gastrostomy feeding tube placement can be considered to ensure adequate nutrition.

Liquids and thin foods can be thickened to make swallowing easier and avoid aspiration problems. Reflux can be managed with medications. Physical and occupational therapy can help prevent or reduce tightening of the joints and help normalize muscle tone; however, the improvements are often limited and temporal. Medical management is available for recurrent infections. However, the progress and average life expectancy for individuals with lissencephaly vary depending on the type of lissencephaly, the particular syndromes involved, and the degree of brain malformation. Many individuals with lissencephaly show no significant development beyond a 3–5-month-old level (Dobyns & Truwit, 1995). Life span can be significantly shortened by recurrent aspiration and pneumonia (Reiner & Lombroso, 1998). Individuals with Type I lissencephaly usually need lifelong care for all basic needs. Infants and toddlers with MDS usually die by 2 years of age, but the majority of babies with ILS live into childhood. Many infants with Type II lissencephaly die in infancy, whereas individuals with SBH may have near-normal or normal development and life span. As such, supportive care is likely needed to help with comfort and nursing needs for children affected and their family.

Mei Chang
Andrew S. Davis

Al-Qudah, A. A. (1998). Clinical patterns of neuronal migrational disorders and parental consanguinity. *Journal of Tropical Pediatrics, 44,* 351–354.

Cardoso, C., Leventer, R. J., Matsumoto, N., Kuc, J. A., Ramocki, M. B., Mewborn, S. K., et al. (2000). The location and type of mutation predict malformation severity in isolated lissencephaly caused by abnormalities within the LIS1 gene. *Human Molecular Genetics, 9*(20), 3019–3028.

Cibis, G. W., & Fitzgerald, K. M. (1995). Abnormal electroretinogram associated with developmental brain anomalies. *Transactions of the American Ophthalmological Society, 93,* 147–158.

Dobyns, W. B. (1987). Developmental aspects of lissencephaly and the lissencephaly syndromes. *Birth Defects Original Article Series, 23*(1), 225–241.

Dobyns, W. B., Kirkpatrick, J. B., Hittner, H. M., Roberts, R. M., & Kretzer, F. L. (1985). Syndromes with lissencephaly. II. Walker-Warburg and Cerebro-oculo-muscular syndromes and a new syndrome with Type II lissencephaly. *American Journal of Medical Genetics, 22,* 157–195.

Dobyns, W. B., Stratton, R. F., & Greenberg, F. (1984). Syndromes with lissencephaly. I. Miller-Dieker and Norman-Roberts syndromes and isolated lissencephaly. *American Journal of Medical Genetics, 18,* 509–526.

Dobyns, W. B., & Truwit, C. L. (1995). Lissencephaly and other malformations of cortical development: 1995 update. *Neuropediatrics, 26,* 132–147.

Dorovini-Zis, K., & Dolman, C. L. (1977). Gestational development of brain. *Archives of Pathologic Laboratory Medicine, 101*(4), 192–195.

Forman, M. S., Squier, W., Dobyns, W. B., & Golden, J. A. (2005). Genotypically defined lissencephalies show distinct pathologies. *Journal of Neuropathology and Experimental Neurology, 64*(10), 847–857.

Ghai, S., Fong, K. W., Toi, A., Chitayat, D., Pantazi, S., & Blaser, S. (2006). Prenatal US and MR imaging findings of lissencephaly: Review of fetal cerebral sulcal development. *RadioGraphics, 26,* 389–405.

Guerrini, R., Sicca, F., & Parmeggiani, L. (2003). Epilepsy and malformations of the cerebral cortex. *Epileptic Disorders, 5,* 9–26.

Günör, S., Yalnizoğlu, D., Turanli, G., Saatçi, I., Erdogan-Bakar, E., & Topcu, M. (2007). Malformations of cortical development: Clinical spectrum in a series of 101 patients and review of the literature. *The Turkish Journal of Pediatrics, 49,* 120–130.

Kojima, K., Suzuki, Y., Seki, K., Yamamoto, T., Sato, T., Tanaka, T., et al. (2002). Prenatal diagnosis of lissencephaly (Type II) by ultrasound and fast magnetic resonance imaging. *Fetal Diagnosis and Therapy, 17,* 34–36.

Koul, R., Jain, R., & Chacko, A. (2005). Pattern of childhood epilepsies with neuronal migrational disorders in Oman. *Journal of Child Neurology, 21*(11), 945–949.

Miny, P., Wolfgang, H., & Jürgen, H. (1993). Genetic factors in lissencephaly syndromes: A review. *Child's Nervous System, 9*(7), 413–417.

Pilz, D. T., Matsumoto, N., Minnerath, S., Mills, P., Gleeson, J. G., Allen, K. M., et al. (1998). LIS1 and XLIS (DCX) mutations cause most classical lissencephaly, but different patterns of malformation. *Human Molecular Genetics, 7*(13), 2029–2037.

Reiner, O., & Lombroso, P. J. (1998). Development of the cerebral cortex: II. Lissencephaly. *Journal of the American Academy of Child and Adolescent Psychiatry, 37*(2), 231–232.

Reiner, O., & Sapir, T. (1998). Abnormal cortical development; towards elucidation of the LIS1 gene product function. *International Journal of Molecular Medicine, 1*(5), 849–853.

Verloes, A., Elmaleh, M., Gonzales, M., Laquerrière, A., & Gressens, P. (2007). Genetic and clinical aspects of lissencephaly. *Revue Neurologique, 163*(5), 533–547.

Verrotti, A., Spalice, A., Ursitti, F., Papetti, L., Mariani, R., Castronovo, A., et al. (2009, March 3). New trends in neuronal migration disorders. *European Journal of Pediatric Neurology,* Mar 3.

Walker, A. E. (1942). Lissencephaly. *Archives of Neurological Psychology, 48,* 13–29.

Wynshaw-Boris, A. (2007). Lissencephaly and LIS1: Insights into the molecular mechanisms of neuronal migration and development. *Clinical Genetics, 72*(4), 296–304.

LOCKED-IN SYNDROME

DESCRIPTION

Locked-in syndrome is a rare neurological presentation in which individuals present with complete paralysis of all the voluntary muscles of the body leading to quadriplegia and mutism. In essence, the only voluntary movements that remain possible are eye movements and eye blinking. The presentation is acquired, most commonly occurring as a result of a cerebrovascular accident although traumatic brain injury, degenerative processes, and neurotoxicity can serve as causes. Regardless of the underlying etiology, the pathological basis of the presentation corresponds with lesioning of the ventral pons. The presentation has also been called cerebromedullospinal disconnection, de-efferented state, pseudocoma, and ventral pontine syndrome.

NEUROPATHOLOGY/PATHOPHYSIOLOGY

Locked-in syndrome is most commonly associated with a lesion of the ventral pons. Although this lesion impairs global motor functioning by way of corticospinal and corticobulbar pathway disruption, somatosensory pathways and the ascending systems essential to arousal and wakefulness remain spared (Ropper & Brown, 2005). Eyelid control remains intact as well due to sparing of particular midbrain areas (Ropper & Brown, 2005).

The most prevalent etiology of locked-in syndrome is an occlusion of the basilar artery leading to the aforementioned ventral pons. This more often than not is related to cerebrovascular trauma due to a thrombus. Infarction, traumatic brain injury, and medicinal overdose have also all been associated with the presentation by way of lesioning the ventral pons.

NEUROPSYCHOLOGICAL/CLINICAL PRESENTATION

Locked-in syndrome presents as quadriplegia and mutism in conjunction with preserved neurocognitive functioning. In some instances, when symptoms first present they manifest as hemiparesis, but within a few hours symptoms progress to bilateral hemiplegia and finally classic features of locked-in syndrome (Fisher, 1988). Communication remains possible via eye movements and blinking as the supranuclear ocular motor pathways are spared (Hammerstad, 2007; Love & Biller, 2007). Consciousness and awareness remain unimpaired.

DIAGNOSIS

Locked-in syndrome is diagnosed based on a combination of the clinical presentation and neuroimaging findings. Initial workup is commonly undertaken with CT as is standard practice in the acute phase following a potential cerebrovascular or traumatic event. Eventually, if not contraindicated, MRI is utilized to offer a more detailed view of the anatomical area of interest. Differential diagnosis must rule out severe motor neuropathy (e.g., Guillain-Barré syndrome), pontine myelinolysis, and/or periodic paralysis as they may all have a similar effect (Ropper & Brown, 2005). Differentiation from a state of coma is made by bedside examination to determine whether the patient is conscious and alert. To make this determination efficiently, evaluation over a longer period of time is often required (Ropper & Brown, 2005).

TREATMENT

The lesion(s) associated with locked-in syndrome is permanent and incurable although a very small portion of patients will regain minimal and specific functions. In many respects, treatment is simply supportive and educational. A substantially high percentage of patients with locked-in syndrome die within approximately 6 months following the trauma.

Chad A. Noggle

Fisher, C. M. (1988). "The herald hemiparesis" of basilar artery occlusion. *Archives of Neurology, 45*, 1301–1303.

Hammerstad, J. P. (2007). Strength and reflexes. In C. G. Goetz (Ed.), *Textbook of clinical neurology* (3rd ed., pp. 243–288). Philadelphia, PA: Saunders Elsevier.

Love, B. B., & Biller, J. (2007). Neurovascular system. In C. G. Goetz (Ed.), *Textbook of clinical neurology* (3rd ed., pp. 405–434). Philadelphia, PA: Saunders Elsevier.

Ropper, A. H., & Brown, R. J. (2005). *Adams and Victor's principles of neurology* (8th ed.). New York: McGraw-Hill.

LYME DISEASE

DESCRIPTION

Lyme disease is a tick-borne disease caused by a spirochete transmitted to humans through bites of blacklegged (or deer) ticks. The disease was identified after a number of children living near Lyme, Connecticut, presented with a unique symptom cluster in the 1970s. Although the disease has been reported in all 50 states, the incidence is highest in New England and Mid-Atlantic states, Minnesota, Wisconsin, and northwestern California. Initial symptoms often include a rash at the site of the bite, malaise, and fatigue; later manifestations may include neurologic, cardiovascular, and musculoskeletal symptoms (Bratton, Whiteside, Hovan, Engle, & Edwards, 2008; Centers for Disease Control and Prevention, 2008).

NEUROPATHOLOGY/PATHOPHYSIOLOGY

Lyme disease is transmitted to humans by blacklegged ticks (*Ixodes scapularis*) in New England and the Great Lakes regions, and western blacklegged ticks (*Ixodes pacificus*) in the West (Bratton et al., 2008). In larval and nymphal stages of the life cycle, *Ixodes* ticks feed on the white-footed mouse, which is the primary host for the spirochete (*Borrelia burgdorferi*) responsible for Lyme disease. Adult *Ixodes* ticks feed on deer, which do not carry *B. burgdorferi*. Infection with *B. burgdorferi* initially occurs at the site of the tick bite, and the most common initial symptom is a distinctive rash (erythema migrans) that gradually expands over the course of several days. Transmission occurs only after prolonged attachment and feeding (greater than 24 hours).

Histologic examination of erythema migrans lesions reveals immune response to the infectious spirochete including increased lymphocytes, macrophages, proinflammatory cytokines, and antibody production (Steere, Coburn, & Glickstein, 2004). After an interval (ranging from 3 to 30 days), the organism may spread through the lymph system and bloodstream with a propensity for the central nervous system (CNS), joints, heart, and eyes. In many ways it mimics syphilis in that after inoculation, spirochetemia transpires with widespread dissemination, which when involving the CNS, presents as meningitis (Roos, 2007).

NEUROPSYCHOLOGICAL/CLINICAL PRESENTATION

The course of Lyme disease has been classified into three stages (Steere et al., 2004). During the first stage, the most common sign of infection is the development of a spreading skin lesion (erythema migrans) at the site of the tick bite within 1–2 weeks. The characteristic presentation of erythema migrans is a bull's-eye or target-shaped rash that is not painful but may itch. Additional symptoms of fatigue, malaise, elevated temperature, and joint pain are also found in one-third of cases or fewer. After the initial localized infection, the second stage is generalized infection in which *B. burgdorferi* is found in the cerebrospinal fluid (CSF) and blood as well as spread through organs including the heart, retina, liver, spleen, meninges, and brain. During the second stage, additional erythema migrans lesions may develop, joint or muscle pain may be present, and neurological signs may occur. Neurologic symptoms of disseminated infection can include meningitis, neuropathy (especially, facial nerve palsy), radiculopathy, and subtle encephalopathy with memory and concentration difficulties and changes in mood and sleep. Elevated protein levels in CSF differentiate disseminated infection from viral infection. In children, the primary neurologic symptom is acute facial paralysis. If left untreated, transition to a third stage will occur 6 months to several years after infection and includes primarily rheumatologic (chronic arthritis, especially in the knees) or neurologic symptoms. Third-stage neurologic manifestations may include chronic meningitis resulting in narrowing of leptomeningeal arteries and subsequent infarction (Miklossy, Kuntzer, Bogousslavsky, Regli, & Janzer, 1990).

A minority of patients who have been treated for Lyme disease continue to report neurocognitive and musculoskeletal symptoms in a syndrome referred to as *posttreatment chronic Lyme disease* (PCLD; Radolf, 2005). PCLD is controversial due to differences of opinion on whether it represents persistent infection or a noninfectious condition akin to chronic fatigue syndrome (Halperin et al., 2007; Radolf, 2005). The neurocognitive features of Lyme encephalopathy may include difficulty with verbal memory, naming, and attention in addition to changes in mood and sleep patterns (Bratton et al., 2008). Although these symptoms persist in a number of patients, studies have failed to consistently evidence objective neurocognitive deficits despite lowered positive affect (Elkins, Pollina, Scheffer, & Krupp, 1999) and subjective memory complaints (Kaplan et al., 2003). In a comparison of patients with PCLD and patients with abnormal findings in CSF, patients with CSF abnormalities demonstrated objective memory deficits, and both groups of patients reported greater memory complaints than controls (Kaplan et al., 1999). At long-term follow-up, patients previously diagnosed with Lyme disease scored within normal limits on measures of attention, processing speed, verbal memory, and verbal fluency (Kalish et al., 2001). Neuropsychological outcomes in children treated for Lyme disease consistently demonstrate a good prognosis with no neurocognitive differences found between children treated for Lyme disease and controls at 2- and 4-year follow-up (Adams, Rose, Eppes, & Klein, 1994, 1999) and across a range of follow-up intervals from 7 to 161 months (Vázquez, Sparrow, & Shapiro, 2003).

DIAGNOSIS

Diagnosis of Lyme disease relies heavily on clinical features and is supported when the presentation includes an erythema migrans lesion and history of living or traveling in an endemic region (Bratton et al., 2008; Wormser et al., 2006). History of a tick bite can be helpful to ascertain, but patients frequently do not recall a tick bite. Typical laboratory tests (e.g., blood counts) are nonspecific for Lyme disease, and serologic tests (e.g., antibody titers) are often inconclusive as seroconversion may occur late, be absent, or indicate prior exposure rather than recent infection.

TREATMENT

Treatment of Lyme disease may include oral or parenteral antimicrobial regimens (for medications and dosages see Halperin et al., 2007). Adjustments in the pharmacotherapeutic regimen are made when neurologic symptoms are present. Treatment guidelines for PCLD are variable, and there is no strong evidence for continued antimicrobial therapy in those patients. Oral doxycycline (100 mg twice daily for 2 weeks) is useful in addressing the facial palsy that may occur in the absence of CSF abnormalities whereas intravenous ceftriaxone for 4 weeks is preferred for other neurological features related to Lyme disease (Roos, 2007). As suggested, transmission is usually dependent upon prolonged attachment and feeding over a 24 hour period. Consequently, prevention becomes an essential intervention. When going into areas that are more likely to have ticks, individuals may use repellants. In addition, clothing that reduces the chances of ticks getting on the person or into hidden areas is recommended. Carefully checking one self for ticks after leaving such higher-risk areas is recommended.

Jeremy Davis
Chad A. Noggle

Adams, W. V., Rose, C. D., Eppes, S. C., & Klein, J. D. (1994). Cognitive effects of Lyme disease in children. *Pediatrics, 94,* 185–189.

Adams, W. V., Rose, C. D., Eppes, S. C., & Klein, J. D. (1999). Long-term cognitive effects of Lyme disease in children. *Applied Neuropsychology, 6,* 39–45.

Bratton, R. L., Whiteside, J. W., Hovan, M. J., Engle, R. L., & Edwards, F. D. (2008). Diagnosis and treatment of Lyme disease. *Mayo Clinic Proceedings, 83,* 566–571.

Centers for Disease Control and Prevention. (2008). *Surveillance for Lyme disease—United States, 1992–1996* (Surveillance Summaries, Morbidity and Mortality Weekly Report, Vol. 57, SS-10). Atlanta, GA: Author.

Elkins, L. E., Pollina, D. A., Scheffer, S. R., & Krupp, L. B. (1999). Psychological states and neuropsychological performances in chronic Lyme disease. *Applied Neuropsychology, 6,* 19–26.

Halperin, J. J., Shapiro, E. D., Logigian, E., Belman, A. L., Dotevall, L., Wormser, G. P., et al. (2007). Practice parameter: Treatment of nervous system Lyme disease (an evidence-based review). *Neurology, 69,* 91–102.

Kalish, R. A., Kaplan, R. F., Taylor, E., Jones-Woodward, L., Workman, K., & Steere, A. C. (2001). Evaluation of study patients with Lyme disease, 10–20 year follow-up. *The Journal of Infectious Diseases, 183,* 453–460.

Kaplan, R. F., Jones-Woodward, L., Workman, K., Steere, A. C., Logigian, E. L., & Meadows, M. E. (1999). Neuropsychological deficits in Lyme disease patients with and without other evidence of central nervous system pathology. *Applied Neuropsychology, 6,* 3–11.

Kaplan, R. F., Trevino, R. P., Johnson, G. M., Levy, L., Dornbush, R., Hu, L. T., et al. (2003). Cognitive function in post-treatment Lyme disease: Do additional antibiotics help? *Neurology, 60,* 1916–1922.

Miklossy, J., Kuntzer, T., Bogousslavsky, J., Regli, F., & Janzer, R. C. (1990). Meningovascular form of neuroborreliosis: Similarities between neuropathological findings in a case of Lyme disease and those occurring in tertiary neurosyphilis. *Acta Neuropathologica, 80,* 568–572.

Radolf, J. (2005). Posttreatment chronic Lyme disease—What it is not. *The Journal of Infectious Diseases, 192,* 948–949.

Roos, K. L. (2007). Viral infections. In C. G. Goetz (Ed.), *Textbook of clinical neurology* (3rd ed., pp. 919–968). Philadelphia, PA: Saunders Elsevier.

Steere, A. C., Coburn, J., & Glickstein, L. (2004). The emergence of Lyme disease. *The Journal of Clinical Investigation, 113,* 1093–1101.

Vázquez, M., Sparrow, S. S., & Shapiro, E. D. (2003). Long-term neuropsychologic and health outcomes of children with facial nerve palsy attributable to Lyme disease. *Pediatrics, 112,* e93–e97.

Wormser, G. P., Dattwyler, R. J., Shapiro, E. D., Halperin, J. J., Steere, A. C., Klempner, M. S., et al. (2006). The clinical assessment, treatment, and prevention of Lyme disease, human granulocytic anaplasmosis, and babesiosis: Clinical practice guidelines by the Infectious Diseases Society of America. *Clinical Infectious Diseases, 43,* 1089–1134.

L

M

MACHADO–JOSEPH'S DISEASE

DESCRIPTION

Machado–Joseph's disease (MJD) is a slow, progressive neurodegenerative disease. It is one of 28 spinocerebellar ataxias (SCA type 3) that are dominantly inherited. It is caused by an unstable and expanded CAG trinucleotide repeat in the *MJD1* gene on chromosome 14q32.1 (Onodera et al., 1998). First reported in North American families of Portuguese-Azorean ancestry, and now found throughout the world, MJD is the most prevalent autosomal-dominant cerebellar ataxia in North America, Europe, and much of Asia. As a result of the significant familial patterns, there have been a number of studies examining the disease in specific ethnic groups (Burk, 2007).

NEUROPATHOLOGY/PATHOPHYSIOLOGY

MJD belongs to a class of genetic disorders called triplet repeat diseases. These disorders are characterized by the frequent and abnormal repetition of the "CAG" sequence on a gene located on chromosome 14q32.1. This results in the production of a mutated protein that is called ataxin-3. Ataxin-3 accumulates in the cells of the body producing inclusion bodies that interfere with the normal operation of the nucleus. This in turn causes the cell to die, as the nucleus is unable to maintain the health of the cell. Disorders like MJD generally show more severe symptoms in children of parents with MJD disease, with the disease starting earlier and progressing faster in the children.

The disease causes central nervous degeneration, producing a widespread pattern of lesions in the brain. The progression is suggested to primarily involve the cerebellar dentate nucleus, pallidum, substantia nigra, subthalamic, red and pontine nuclei, select cranial nerve nuclei, and the anterior horn and Clarke's column of the spinal cord. Central nervous white matter lesions are confined to the medial lemniscus, spinocerebellar tracts, and dorsal columns. Involvement of the cerebellar Purkinje cell layer and the inferior olive is disputed (for a review, see Rub, Brunt, & Deller, 2008). MRI findings have suggested severe atrophy of the pons, globus pallidus, and middle and superior cerebellar peduncles as well as a degree of atrophy of the frontal and temporal lobes (Murata et al., 1998). This pattern affects many functional systems, resulting in an array of clinical presentations.

NEUROPSYCHOLOGICAL/CLINICAL PRESENTATION

The pattern of central nervous neurodegeneration includes the visual, auditory, vestibular, somatosensory, ingestion-related, dopaminergic, and cholinergic systems (Rub et al., 2008). The earliest and most common symptom is gait ataxia (Spinella & Sheridan, 1992). Additional symptoms include dysarthria, dysphagia, dystonia, bradykinesia, intentional tremor, oculomotor disorders, exophthalmos, sensory deficits (peripheral neuropathy), pyramidal, and extrapyramidal dysfunctions, autonomic dysfunctions, sleep disturbances, and muscle wasting (Sudarsky, Corwin, & Dawson, 1992).

Individuals with the disease have been found to have a number of functional difficulties as a result of central nervous system dysfunction. Performance on neuropsychological assessment most commonly indicates deficits in memory and executive functioning, specifically attention, verbal fluency, and cognitive flexibility (Burk et al., 2003; Garrard, Martin, Giunti, & Cipolotti, 2008; Kawai et al., 2004; Radvany, Camargo, Costa, Fonseca, & Nascimento, 1993). Poor performance on Theory of Mind tasks has also been found (Garrard et al., 2008). Many studies suggest slowed processing on visual measures, as well as visuospatial and constructional deficits (Maruff et al., 1996; Zawacki, Grace, Friedman, & Sudarsky, 2002). The presence of depression and anxiety is also common in individuals with the disease (Kawai et al., 2004; Zawacki et al., 2002). A number of studies have also emphasized an absence of cognitive impairment (Burk, 2007), including studies focused on executive dysfunction (Sequeiros & Coutinho, 1993; Spinella & Sheridan, 1992). Some studies have suggested the cognitive profile is unrelated to age of onset, age at time of evaluation, and/or education (Maruff et al., 1996). However, symptoms of dementia

M

and delirium have been found in late stages of patients with history of a relatively young onset age and long clinical course (Ishikawa et al., 2002).

DIAGNOSIS

MJD is clinically diagnosed and genetically confirmed (Maciel et al., 2001). Early diagnosis can be made by recognizing symptoms or by presymptomatic genetic testing. Family history is important in prognosis and defining symptomatology. Prenatal diagnosis of MJD has been found to be successful (Sequeiros et al., 1998; Tsai et al., 2003).

TREATMENT

An effective treatment has not yet been established, and thus treatment is focused on symptom management and support. Patients usually become wheel-chair bound approximately 15 years after symptom onset; thus, environmental manipulations eventually become warranted to aid in home living and mobility (e.g., ramps, chair lifts, etc.). With a median survival of 20–30 years (Klockgether, 2007), patients and family members may benefit from supportive services to aid in adjustment to continued deterioration and eventually end-of-life issues.

Lindsay J. Hines
Charles Golden

Burk, K. (2007). Cognition in hereditary ataxia. *Cerebellum, 6*(3), 280–286.

Burk, K., Globas, C., Bosch, S., Klockgether, T., Zuhlke, C., Daum, I., et al. (2003). Cognitive deficits in spinocerebellar ataxia type 1, 2, and 3. *Journal of Neurology, 250*(2), 207–211.

Garrard, P., Martin, N. H., Giunti, P., & Cipolotti, L. (2008). Cognitive and social cognitive functioning in spinocerebellar ataxia: A preliminary characterization. *Journal of Neurology, 255*(3), 398–405.

Ishikawa, A., Yamada, M., Makino, K., Aida, I., Idezuka, J., Ikeuchi, T., et al. (2002). Dementia and delirium in 4 patients with Machado-Joseph disease. *Archives of Neurology, 59*(11), 1804–1808.

Kawai, Y., Takeda, A., Abe, Y., Washimi, Y., Tanaka, F., & Sobue, G. (2004). Cognitive impairments in Machado-Joseph disease. *Archives of Neurology, 61*(11), 1757–1760.

Klockgether, T. (2007). Ataxias. In C. G. Goetz (Ed.), *Textbook of clinical neurology*. Philadelphia: Saunders, Elsevier.

Maciel, P., Costa, M. C., Ferro, A., Rousseau, M., Santos, C. S., Gaspar, C., et al. (2001). Improvement in the molecular diagnosis of Machado-Joseph disease. *Archives of Neurology, 58*(11), 1821–1827.

Maruff, P., Tyler, P., Burt, T., Currie, B., Burns, C., & Currie, J. (1996). Cognitive deficits in Machado-Joseph disease. *Annals of Neurology, 40*(3), 421–427.

Murata, Y., Yamaguchi, S., Kawakami, H., Imon, Y., Maruyama, H., Sakai, T., et al. (1998). Characteristic magnetic resonance imaging findings in Machado-Joseph disease. *Archives of Neurology, 55*(1), 33–37.

Onodera, O., Idezuka, J., Igarashi, S., Takiyama, Y., Endo, K., Takano, H., et al. (1998). Progressive atrophy of cerebellum and brainstem as a function of age and the size of the expanded CAG repeats in the MJD1 gene in Machado-Joseph disease. *Annals of Neurology, 43*(3), 288–296.

Radvany, J., Camargo, C. H., Costa, Z. M., Fonseca, N. C., & Nascimento, E. D. (1993). Machado-Joseph disease of Azorean ancestry in Brazil: The Catarina kindred. Neurological, neuroimaging, psychiatric and neuropsychological findings in the largest known family, the "Catarina" kindred. *Arq Neuropsiquiatr, 51*(1), 21–30.

Rub, U., Brunt, E. R., & Deller, T. (2008). New insights into the pathoanatomy of spinocerebellar ataxia type 3 (Machado-Joseph disease). *Current Opinion Neurology, 21*(2), 111–116.

Sequeiros, J., & Coutinho, P. (1993). Epidemiology and clinical aspects of Machado-Joseph disease. *Advances in Neurology, 61*, 139–153.

Sequeiros, J., Maciel, P., Taborda, F., Ledo, S., Rocha, J. C., Lopes, A., et al. (1998). Prenatal diagnosis of Machado-Joseph disease by direct mutation analysis. *Prenatal Diagnosis, 18*(6), 611–617.

Spinella, G. M., & Sheridan, P. H. (1992). Research initiatives on Machado-Joseph disease: National Institute of Neurological Disorders and Stroke Workshop summary. *Neurology, 42*(10), 2048–2051.

Sudarsky, L., Corwin, L., & Dawson, D. M. (1992). Machado-Joseph disease in New England: Clinical description and distinction from the olivopontocerebellar atrophies. *Movement Disorders, 7*(3), 204–208.

Tsai, H. F., Liu, C. S., Chen, G. D., Lin, M. L., Li, C., Chen, Y. Y., et al. (2003). Prenatal diagnosis of Machado-Joseph disease/spinocerebellar ataxia type 3 in Taiwan: Early detection of expanded ataxin-3. *Journal of Clinical Laboratory Analysis, 17*(5), 195–200.

Zawacki, T. M., Grace, J., Friedman, J. H., & Sudarsky, L. (2002). Executive and emotional dysfunction in Machado-Joseph disease. *Movement Disorders, 17*(5), 1004–1010.

MACRENCEPHALY

DESCRIPTION

Macrencephaly, also called megalencephaly, refers to the presentation of an abnormally large brain for an infant or child's age and gender. It is the third most common central nervous system malformation behind micrencephaly and hydrocephalus. The term is often used interchangeably with macrocephaly but this is inaccurate. Although macrencephaly refers to an abnormally large brain, macrocephaly simply refers to an abnormally large head. This categorical error originates from the fact that brain and skull growth usually present in parallel with one another thus both terms are often accepted as describing the same morphological feature (Harding & Copp, 1997). Deviations from this principle are more often seen on the micrencephalic side, whereby the skull plates fuse prematurely while the brain attempts to grow normally.

Macrencephaly is classified by a brain size that is two or more standard deviations above the average and originates from an overactivity in the process of neuron proliferation. Although the process ceases once the appropriate number of cells are produced within a layer or area, in macrencephaly an overabundance of cells are produced causing a general disruption and disorganization of the system. Similar to microcephaly, macrencephaly's morphological opposite, the term is purely descriptive and not suggestive of an underlying etiology. As such, it can occur developmentally or secondary to another primary presentation such as Alexander's disease and neurofibromatosis. The overproduction of cells in various areas and layers most prominently disrupts the electrical and neuronal integrity of the system, increasing risk of seizures, sensorimotor deficits, and diffuse neurocognitive deficits including mental retardation. It is differentiated from hemimegalencephaly in which only one hemisphere is enlarged.

NEUROPATHOLOGY/PATHOPHYSIOLOGY

Macrencephaly arises from excessive brain growth. As previously suggested, it often represents a feature of another primary manifestation. Alexander's disease, Canavan's disease, and Tay–Sachs's disease are the most common causes of macrencephaly. The mechanism by which the presentations cause macrencephaly varies yet can be linked to their advancing metabolic dysfunctions. The interested reader is recommended to review these individual entries within this text. Anatomically, it presents with diffuse increase in brain volume in the presence of normal or only slightly enlarged ventricles. The cortex is often disorganized owning to part of the volumetric increase. Cellular and neuronal swelling and effacement of cortex lamination also serve as root causes (Ropper & Brown, 2005). This disruption occurs at the point of neuroblast formation during embryogenesis (Ropper & Brown, 2005). When this is isolated to only one of the hemispheres, it is termed hemimegalencephaly.

NEUROPSYCHOLOGICAL/CLINICAL PRESENTATION

Few empirical studies have sought to outline the neuropsychological consequences of macrencephaly itself given it is often a manifestation of another underlying etiology. Again, the reader is referred to the articles on the most common underlying causes and their specific sequelae (e.g., Alexander's Disease, Canavan's Disease, Tay-Sachs' Disease, Neurofibromatosis). In general, individuals often present with mental retardation. Furthermore, increased prevalence of seizures and epilepsy is also reported.

DIAGNOSIS

Fetal ultrasound can often first identify the presentation within the womb. MRI and/or CT scan are recommended in the neonatal period and are most accurate. Electroencephalogram best identifies seizure activity and should always be done when macrencephaly is noted. Neuropsychological testing should be undertaken to identify neurocognitive functioning. Beyond this, standard diagnostic practices recommended for those entities most likely to serve as the underlying basis of macrencephaly should be employed and are discussed elsewhere.

TREATMENT

Given macrencephaly constitutes a structural abnormality and is often associated with another primary presentation, there is no cure. Treatment is focused on symptom resolution or treatment of the primary etiology. In regard to the latter, readers are encouraged to see these specific diseases/disorders in regard to their method of treatment. Consequently, prognosis is directly related to the underlying etiology. Therapeutic support should be with a multidimensional focus. Given that a variety of symptoms may be observed in relation to macrencephaly, interventional services ranging from physical and occupational therapy, speech therapy, and special education may all be relevant depending upon the functional profile. In some instances where the presentation is related to a terminal primary diagnosis (e.g., Tay–Sachs' disease), supportive therapy for the family is warranted.

Chad A. Noggle

M

Harding, B., & Copp, A. J. (1997). Malformations. In D. L. Graham & P. L. Lantos (Eds.), *Greenfield's neuropathology* (6th ed., pp. 397–533). New York: Oxford.

Ropper, A. H., & Brown, R. H. (2005). *Adams and Victor's principles of neurology. Developmental diseases of the nervous system* (8th ed., pp. 850–894). New York: McGraw-Hill.

MAPLE SYRUP URINE DISEASE

DESCRIPTION

Maple syrup urine disease (MSUD) is an inherited metabolic dysfunction that leads to an accumulation of the branched-chain amino acids (BCAAs) and the corresponding branched-chain 2-keto acids (BCKAs) (Chuang & Shih, 2001). This occurs due to a deficiency of branched-chain l-2-keto acid dehydrogenase complex (BCKD) activity. To a lesser extent, specific hydroxyl derivatives also accumulate (Treacy et al., 1992). The buildup of these compounds within the central nervous system (CNS) results in pronounced neurological dysfunction that may include manifestation of convulsions, seizures, ataxia, psychomotor delay, mental retardation, and, in some instances, coma. Rare in prevalence, MSUD has an occurrence of 1 in 185,000 worldwide (Chuang & Shih, 2001). However, higher incidence rates of roughly 1 in 200 births have been noted in Mennonite settlements throughout the Midwest purportedly due to a founder effect (Mitsubuchi et al., 1992).

There is no cure for the disorder. Treatment is commonly focused on dietary/nutritional management in combination with more targeted interventions to further regulate the accumulative compounds. To this end, peritoneal dialysis, exchange transfusion, hemodialysis, hemofiltration, hemodiafiltration, and/or administration of a large dose of thiamine are all options for treatment. Beyond this, treatment is focused on addressing the residuals of neurological dysfunction.

NEUROPATHOLOGY/PATHOPHYSIOLOGY

MSUD is an inherited disorder. It represents a metabolic flaw that results from a severe deficiency of BCKD activity (Bridi, 2003). The by-product of this dysfunction is system-based accumulation of the BCAAs leucine, isoleucine, and valine, and the corresponding BCKAs l-2-ketoisocaproic, l-2-ketoisovaleric, and l-2-keto-3-methylvaleric acids (Chuang & Shih, 2001; Yeman, 1986). The hydroxyl derivatives l-2-hydroxyisocaproic, l-2-hydroxyisovaleric, and l-2-hydroxy-3 methylvaleric acids, produced by the reduction of their respective l-2-keto acids, also accumulate but to a lesser degree (Treacy et al., 1992). Ketoacidosis manifests and represents a clinical feature of MSUD (Nyhan, 1984).

From a neuropathological standpoint, MSUD impact is multifaceted and generally diffuse. In the initial stages, the cerebral peduncles and the dorsal part of the brainstem are primarily involved. The discussed accumulation contributes to demyelination, edema, reduced brain uptake of essential amino acids, brain energy deficiency, and neuronal apoptosis (Aráujo et al., 2001; Jouvet et al., 2000; Pilla et al., 2003). In patients who die, generalized spongy CNS degeneration is noted (Gascon, Ozand, & Cohen, 2007).

Neurotransmitter disturbance is also a common outcome of the presentation (Tavares et al., 2000). In animal models, specific disturbances are in the form of reduced brain tissue concentrations of glutamate, aspartate, and GABA (Dodd et al., 1992). Cerebral edema is also commonly noted with preferential targeting of the pyramidal tracts of the spinal cord and the white matter of the cerebral hemispheres, corpus callosum, and dentate nuclei (Chuang & Shih, 2001).

NEUROPSYCHOLOGICAL/CLINICAL PRESENTATION

Beyond aforementioned metabolic features, MSUD is manifested as heterogeneous clinical phenotypes, ranging from classical to mild variants (Schadewaldt & Wendel, 1997). Although the features may vary from person to person, the salient features that have been most commonly noted in classical MSUD include ketoacidosis, failure to thrive, poor feeding, apnea, ataxia, seizures, coma, psychomotor delay, and mental retardation presenting in the neonatal period (Nyhan, 1984). Variability across other forms has been proposed as being possibly due to the distinct residual enzyme activity that itself may vary. In fact, MSUD patients can be divided into five different clinical and biochemical phenotypes (Chuang & Shih, 2001).

Acutely sick children or adults with MSUD first present with muscle fatigue, epigastric pain, vomiting, and increased confusion (Korein, Sansaricq, Kalmijn, Honig, & Lange, 1994; Riviello, Rezvani, DiGeorge, & Foley, 1991). Neurological sequelae are present in most patients having been linked to both white matter demyelination and diffuse subcortical gray matter edema (Korein et al., 1994; Riviello et al., 1991). Dystonia, stupor, hallucination, and sleep disturbances may present. There is a high prevalence of ataxia and psychomotor delay (Nyhan, 1984). Cognitively, mental retardation is commonly seen over the long term. Even in those who have milder neurological involvement, learning disabilities are seen at higher rates of incidence (Chuang & Shih, 2001). Death during acute metabolic decompensation results from central transtentorial herniation.

DIAGNOSIS

MSUD must be ruled out in any case of neonatal lethargy progressing to coma; with altering tone changes; in the absence of changes in blood pH, glucose, and ammonia; and regardless of the presence of an infection (Gascon et al., 2007). Definitive diagnosis is accomplished through urinalysis or evaluation of the plasma. Diagnostic findings are that of elevated L-leucine, isoleucine, and valine.

Electroencephalogram (EEG) and neuroimaging can also have a role in diagnostics in terms of identifying CNS involvement as opposed to confirming MSUD. EEG often presents with a characteristic sharp wave pattern described as comb-like. It is an essential tool given the relative prevalence of seizures in this population, even when the disorder is controlled.

On MRI, white matter attenuation may be seen fairly early on. Edema may be observed in the deep cerebellum, the dorsal part of the brainstem, the cerebral peduncles, and the dorsal limb of the internal capsule initially and then spreads to include the central white matter, particularly of the frontal lobes (Gascon et al., 2007).

Neuropsychological assessment is essential once children come of age to determine the nature and extent of any presenting neurocognitive deficits. Domains of impairment may vary. Assessment should also seek to evaluate academic domains as children would naturally be at greater risk for learning disabilities.

TREATMENT

Treatment begins with identification of the presentation. Given classical MSUD presents in the neonatal period with metabolic decompensation that may prove fatal or contribute to various neurological sequelae and psychomotor retardation, management of this decompensation as early as possible is essential. This is attempted by suppressing catabolism and facilitating the incorporation of free amino acids in body protein by drip infusion of balanced electrolytes and hypertonic glucose solution in combination with nutritional management and nasogastric feeding with or without insulin administration (Berry et al., 1991; Parini et al., 1991; Townsend & Kerr, 1982; Wendel, Langenbeck, Lombeck, & Bremer, 1982). Peritoneal dialysis, hemodialysis, exchange transfusion, hemodiafiltration, and/or administration of a large dose of thiamine to enhance the residual activity of branched-chain ketoacid dehydrogenase complex may be utilized in an attempt to remove the accumulating toxic metabolites (Rutledge et al., 1990; Thompson, Butt, Shann et al., 1991; Thompson, Francis, & Halliday, 1991). Beyond management of the biochemical components of the presentation, treatment is symptom based and related to standard practices of addressing those residuals. For example, learning disabilities may be addressed through special education services or other classroom or educational adaptations.

Jacob M. Goings
Chad A. Noggle

Araújo, P., Wassermann, G. F., Tallini, K., Furlanetto, V., Vargas, C. R., Wannmacher, C. M. D., et al. (2001). Reduction of large neutral amino acid levels in plasma and brain of hyperleucinemic rats. *Neurochemistry International, 38*, 529–537.

Berry, G. T., Heidenreich, R., Kaplan, P., Levine, F., Mazur, A., Palmieri, M. J., et al. (1991). Branched-chain amino acid free parenteral nutrition in the treatment of acute metabolic decompensation in patients with maple syrup urine disease. *The New England Journal of Medicine, 324*, 175–179.

Bridi, R., Araldi, J., Sgarbi, M. B., Testa, C. G., Durigon, K., Wajner, M., et al. (2003). Induction of oxidative stress in rat brain by the metabolites accumulating in maple syrup urine disease. *International Journal of Developmental Neuroscience: The Official Journal of the International Society for Developmental Neuroscience, 21*(6), 327–332.

Chuang, D. T., & Shih, V. E. (2001). Maple syrup urine disease (branched-chain ketoaciduria). In C. R. Scriver, A. L. Beaudet, W. L. Sly, & D. Valle (Eds.), *The metabolic and molecular bases of inherited disease* (8th ed., pp. 1971–2005). New York: McGraw-Hill.

Dodd, P. R., Williams, A. L., Gundlach, A. L., Harper, P. A. W., Healy, P. J., Dennis, J. A., et al. (1992). Glutamate and gamma-aminobutyric acid neurotransmitter systems in the acute phase of maple syrup urine disease and citrullinemia encephalopathies in newborn calves. *Journal of Neurochemistry, 59*, 582–590.

Gascon, G. G., Ozand, P. T., & Cohen, B. (2007). Aminoacidopathies and organic acidopathies, mitochondrial enzyme defects, and other metabolic errors. In C. G. Goetz (Ed.), *Textbook of clinical neurology* (3rd ed., pp. 641–681). Philadelphia, PA: Saunders Elsevier.

Jouvet, P., Rustin, P., Taylor, D. L., Pocock, J. M., Felderhoff-Mueser, U., Mazarakis, N. D., et al. (2000). Branched chain amino acids induce apoptosis in neural cells without mitochondrial membrane despolarization or cytochrome *c* release: Implications for neurological impairment associated with maple syrup urine disease. *Molecular Biology of the Cell, 11,* 1919–1932.

Korein, J., Sansaricq, C., Kalmijn, M., Honig, J., & Lange, B. (1994). Maple syrup urine disease: Clinical, EEG, and plasma amino acid correlations with a theoretical mechanism of acute neurotoxicity. *International Journal of Neuroscience, 79,* 21–45.

Mitsubuchi, H., Matsuda, I., Nobukuni, Y., Heidenreich, R., Indo, Y., Endo, F., et al. (1992). Gene analysis of Mennonite maple syrup urine disease kindred using primer-specified restriction map modification. *Journal of Inherited Metabolic Disease, 15,* 181–187.

Nyhan, W. L. (1984). *Abnormalities in amino acid metabolism in clinical medicine* (pp. 21–35). Norwalk, CT: Appleton-Century-Crofts.

Parini, R., Sereni, L. P., Bagozzi, D. C., Corbetta, C., Rabier, D., Narcy, C., et al. (1991). Nasogastric drip feeding as the only treatment of neonatal maple syrup urine disease. *Pediatrics, 92*(2), 280–283.

Pilla, C., Cardozo, R. F. D., Dutra, C. S., Wyze, A. T. S., Wajner, M., & Wannmacher, C. M. D. (2003). Effect of leucine administration on creatine kinase activity in rat brain. *Metabolic Brain Disease, 18,* 17–25.

Riviello, J. J. Jr., Rezvani, I., DiGeorge, A. M., & Foley, C. M. (1991). Cerebral edema causing death in children with maple syrup urine disease. *Journal of Pediatrics, 119,* 42–45.

Rutledge, S. L., Havens, P. L., Haymond, M. W., McLean, R. H., Kan, J. S., & Brusilow, S. W. (1990). Neonatal hemodialysis: Effective therapy for the encephalopathy of inborn errors of metabolism. *Journal of Pediatrics, 116,* 125–180.

Schadewaldt, P., & Wendel, U. (1997). Metabolism of branched-chain amino acids in maple syrup urine disease. *European Journal of Pediatrics, 156*(Suppl. 1), S62–S66.

Tavares, R. G., Santos, C. E. S., Tasca, C., Wajner, M., Souza, D. O., & Dutra-Filho, C. S. (2000). Inhibition of glutamate uptake into synaptic vesicles of rat brain by the metabolites accumulating in maple syrup urine disease. *Journal of Neurological Science, 181,* 44–49.

Thompson, G. N., Butt, W. W., Shann, F. A., Kirby, D. M., Henning, R. D., Howells, D. W., et al. (1991). Continuous venovenous hemofiltration in the management of acute decompensation in inborn errors of metabolism. *Journal of Pediatrics, 118,* 879–884.

Thompson, G. N., Francis, D. E., & Halliday, D. (1991). Acute illness in maple syrup urine disease: Dynamics of protein metabolism and implications for management. *Journal of Pediatrics, 119,* 35–41.

Townsend, I., & Kerr, D. S. (1982). Total parenteral nutrition therapy of toxic maple syrup urine disease. *The American Journal of Clinical Nutrition, 36*(2), 359–365.

Treacy, E., Clow, C. L., Reade, T. R., Chitayat, D., Mamer, O. A., & Scriver, C. R. (1992). Maple syrup urine disease: Interrelationship between branched chain amino-, oxo-, and hydroxyacids implications for treatment association with CNS dysmelination. *Journal of Inherited Metabolic Disease, 15,* 121–135.

Wendel, U., Langenbeck, U., Lombeck, I., & Bremer, H. J. (1982). Maple syrup urine disease—therapeutic use of insulin in catabolic states. *European Journal of Pediatrics, 139*(3), 172–175.

Yeman, S. J. (1986). The mammalian 2-oxoacid dehydrogenase: A complex family. *Trends in Biochemical Science, 11,* 293–296.

MATHEMATICS DISORDERS

DESCRIPTION

To meet criteria for mathematics disorder, an individual's mathematics ability must be substantially below that expected given the person's measured intelligence, age, and age-appropriate education (American Psychiatric Association [APA], 2000). Mathematics ability must be assessed via individually administered standardized tests, and the impairment must show significant interference with academic achievement or daily activities that require math skills. It is estimated that one in every five learning disorder cases is mathematics disorder, and approximately 1% of school-age children have mathematics disorder (APA, 2000). Some studies estimate that the prevalence rate of mathematics disorder is as much as 4.6% (Lewis, Hitch, & Walker, 1994) or 5% to 6% (Shalev, Auerback, Manor, & Gross-Tsur, 2000). Mathematics deficits are often associated with other learning disabilities (Fleishner, 1994; L. S. Fuchs, D. Fuchs, & Prentice, 2004). Shalev, Manor, and Gross-Tsur (1997) found that nearly 17% of children with mathematics disorder also have dyslexia, and an additional 26% have attention deficit hyperactivity disorder. Dyscalculia is a term often used in mathematics disorder research and is defined by both the inability to demonstrate appropriate mathematics competence (Butterworth, 2003) and the inability to successfully create mathematical relationships (Beachman & Trott, 2005).

The APA (2000) notes that in mathematics disorder, impairment may present amidst a number of skills including perceptual skills (e.g., reading or recognizing arithmetic signs or numerical symbols, and grouping objects), linguistic skills (e.g., naming or understanding mathematical operations or terms, and decoding problems into mathematical symbols), attention skills (e.g., remembering to add carried numbers, observing operational signs, and copying figures or numbers correctly), and mathematical skills (e.g., counting objects, learning multiplication tables, and following mathematical sequences). Mathematics disorder typically becomes apparent in the second or third grade, as formal mathematics instruction is typically not administered until this point. Among children with high IQ, mathematics disorder may not appear until fifth grade or later, as the child may be able to function near grade level in earlier grades (APA, 2000).

Lyon, Fletcher, and Barnes (2003) note several recent studies that point to heritable factors in math disabilities. Gross-Tsur, Manor, and Shalev (1996) examined children with a specific math disability and 10% reported having at least one family member who also had difficulties with math. Shalev et al. (2001) report that the prevalence of math disabilities is about 10 times greater among individuals with family members who also have math disorders when compared with the general population. Finally, Alarcon, DeFries, Light, and Pennington (1997) found that 58% of monozygotic twins shared a math disability, versus only 39% among dizygotic twins.

NEUROPATHOLOGY/PATHOPHYSIOLOGY

Lyon et al. (2003) note that neither studies of brain structure nor brain function have been conducted in children with mathematics disorder, though studies of brain lesions in adults have shown that fairly specific math skills can be preserved or lost, depending upon brain injury patterns. Dehaene and Cohen (1997) found that dissociable neural networks comprise mathematical knowledge. One network in the left hemisphere is involved in storage and retrieval of arithmetic fact. Another parietal network is involved in manipulation of numerical quantities. Lyon et al. note that similar findings have been demonstrated in other studies (Chochon, Cohen, van de Moortele, & Dehaene, 1999).

PET and fMRI studies have examined math processes in normal adults (Lyon et al., 2003). Precise calculation and estimation have demonstrated different neural correlates (Dehaene, Spelke, Pinel, Stanescu, & Tsivkin, 1999). The left hemisphere's inferior prefrontal cortex and the left angular gyrus are involved in precise calculation. Bilateral activation among the inferior parietal lobes is involved in estimation.

Regarding nonphysiological causes of mathematics disorder, Michaelson (2007) notes several potential culprits in the literature. Miller and Mercer (1997) believed that low intelligence is a contributor to the development of dyscalculia. Ashcraft (1995) believed that mathematical anxiety plays a part in the development of symptoms even after some remediation following the implementation of psychological intervention. Two other studies cite ineffective teaching strategies as a culprit, emphasizing the early childhood years as a particularly sensitive time frame that may impact vulnerable students (Butterworth, 2003; Shalev et al., 2001).

NEUROPSYCHOLOGICAL/CLINICAL PRESENTATION

Young children experiencing mathematical impairments often have problems with both procedural knowledge and math facts (Geary, Hamson, & Hoard, 1999). Although these difficulties persist in some children, other children develop an ability to retrieve math facts, though subsequent procedural knowledge difficulties persist (Lyon et al., 2003).

Lyon et al. (2003) note differences between individuals with both reading and mathematics deficits and individuals with mathematics deficits alone. Children demonstrating mathematical impairments without reading deficits show difficulties with several aspects of nonverbal processing, such as somatosensory and motor skills, visuospatial skills, and problem-solving abilities (Rourke, 1993). Further, they are more likely to show procedural problems related to math. Alternatively, children with both reading and math impairments demonstrate pervasive problems with concept formation and language formation skills (Rourk, 1993). These dually diagnosed comorbid children are more likely to show difficulties with fact representation and retrieval.

Lyon et al. (2003) reviewed a study by Geary, Hamson, and Hoard (2000) that is in line with the above findings. It was found that children with comorbid reading and math disabilities struggled with number comprehension tasks and counting. Children with math disability alone did not struggle with number comprehension tasks, although they did struggle with counting in both the first and second grades. In the first grade, both groups struggled with fact retrieval. Retrieval errors decreased among children with math disability alone, though continued among children with comorbid math and reading disabilities. Indeed, math difficulties among children with comorbid mathematics and reading disabilities are typically different from math difficulties among children with mathematics disabilities in isolation.

Research with brain-injured children provides some evidence for the hypothesis that children with poor math skills but adequate reading skills have procedural deficits that involve trying to solve written computations with inadequate, developmentally immature algorithms (Lyon et al., 2003). Children with brain injury as well as developmental disability often experience math difficulties (Shalev et al., 2000). Children with hydrocephalus or spina bifida who demonstrate good word recognition and poor math skills have shown more frequent procedural errors when compared with age-matched controls (Barnes et al., 2002). In this study, both groups made similar errors in visuospatial processing and math fact retrieval. Notably, the procedural errors made by the brain-injured children were similar to those made by younger, math ability-matched controls. Therefore, the children with brain injury made written computation errors that were developmentally immature, as they were similar to younger children with their same level of ability (Lyon et al., 2003).

Regarding social and occupational functioning deficits, Bynner and Parsons (1997) found that inadequate numeracy skills are more harmful to an individual's employability versus inadequate literacy skills. Beachman and Trott (2005) note that general life skills involve a certain level of numerical aptitude, and children with dyscalculia develop into adults who are impaired by their inadequate quantitative reasoning skills, which in turn affects their understanding of money, time, space, and direction. Indeed, mathematics disorder is significant as it can impair functioning not only in the child as a student, but in the adult as a functioning member of society.

DIAGNOSIS

Michaelson (2007) notes three well-documented methods of diagnosing dyscalculia. The first is measurement of the child's attainment of age-appropriate mathematical skills. This can be achieved through administration of standardized assessments that measure such skills (Shalev et al., 2001). Diagnosis can be reached if there is an inconsistency between intellectual capability and assessment results (Geary, 2004) or if there is a disparity, typically of about 2 year levels, between the child's performance and age-expected performance (Semrud-Clikeman et al.,

1992). The second method is a direct observation of several mathematical behaviors such as underdeveloped problem-solving strategies (Geary, 1990), errors due to poor working memory span (Siegel & Ryan, 1989), deficient long-term recall of arithmetic facts (Geary et al., 2000), or overall high error rates (Geary, 1993). Finally, the third method is a software program developed by Butterworth (2003) called the dyscalculia screener. This program assesses numerical proficiency in children between ages 6 and 14. This program calculates a standardized score based on median reaction time and accuracy in three categories: number comparison, dot enumeration, and arithmetic achievement (based on addition and multiplication).

Traditional assessment of learning disabilities involves a model focused on problems within the individual. Diagnostic assessment is determined through an ability-achievement discrepancy in which achievement test(s) and ability test(s) are given, and discrepancies between one and two standard deviation warrant diagnosis. Further, "severe" discrepancies allow access to special education services (Shinn, 2005). Shinn (2005) criticizes this method as 19 states require a severe ability-achievement discrepancy; however, they do not define "severe" and therefore schools and local education agencies create their own criteria. Further, students often must fail for a considerable period of time before becoming eligible for formal assessment and services. Shinn notes that if all students in a school or school district demonstrate severe academic deficits, the problem is not within the student but within the system; therefore, it is also important to assess the system.

In line with the criticisms above, Peterson and Shinn (2002) recommend that students be identified based on their achievement discrepancies within a particular context such as school or school district. In this problem-solving model, it is important to assess the level of performance of typical students, and a local achievement norm must be created. Curriculum-based measurement (CBM) involves the use of validated and standardized short-duration tests (Fuchs & Deno, 1991) that assess basic skills in mathematics computation as well as reading, spelling, and written expression (Deno, 1985, 1986, 1989, 2003; Shinn, 1989, 1998). Mathematics computation CBMs involve 2–5 mintue probes in which students write answers to computational problems. CBMs are time-efficient, reasonably inexpensive, and easy to learn (Shinn, 2005). They may be used to identify at-risk students (Shinn & Marston, 1985), aid in progress monitoring (Marston & Magnusson, 1985), and develop local norms (Shinn, 1988).

In 2004, the Individuals with Disabilities Education Act enabled schools to use response to intervention (RTI) to determine learning disability status (Daly, Martens, Barnett, Witt, & Olson, 2007). RTI models involve continuous assessment of student response to evidence-based interventions and consist of a three-tier, fixed sequence delivery of strength and type of intervention (Daly et al., 2007). Tier 1 involves universal screening and intervention, delivered on both the class and school-wide levels, ruling out inadequate instruction as a source of low performance (Gresham, 2004). Tier 2 involves administering select interventions to children that do not adequately respond to Tier 1. Tier 3 provides more intensive intervention to children that do not respond to the first two tiers.

Notably, teacher estimates of student academic skill can be utilized to identify target skills for academic intervention and assess whether intervention is effective (Eckert & Arbolino, 2005). Several standardized measures are available for this purpose. Eckert and Arbolino (2005) note that only three standardized measures currently exist that assess teacher perception of student academic skill in the classroom. These include the Academic Competence Evaluation Scales (ACES; DiPerna & Elliott, 2000), the Academic Performance Rating Scale (APRS; DuPaul, Rapport, & Perriello, 1991), and the Teacher Rating of Academic Performance (TRAP; Gresham, Reschly, & Carey, 1987). The ACES assesses children in kindergarten through grade 12. This measure contains two scales that assess academic skill in areas such as reading and mathematics, and academic enablers, such as study skills, engagement, and motivation. Item number ranges from 66 to 73, depending upon student grade level. The APRS assesses academic skills and work performance in the areas of reading, mathematics, spelling, and written language based on 19 questions on a 5-point Likert-type scale. The TRAP consists of 5 items that measure overall academic achievement, as well as items that assess reading and mathematics. This TRAP has shown a 91% accuracy rate when differentiating students with specific learning disabilities from students without academic difficulties.

TREATMENT

Lyon, Fletcher, Fuchs, and Chhabra (2006) summarized three studies that examined instructional components that enhance student math competence in grades 2–6 (L. S. Fuchs, D. Fuchs, Hamlett, Phillips, & Bentz, 1994; Fuchs et al., 1997; L. S. Fuchs, D. Fuchs, Phillips, Hamlett, & Karns, 1995)—one that did so in kindergarten (L. S. Fuchs, D. Fuchs, & Karns, 2001), and one in first grade (L. S. Fuchs, D. Fuchs, Yazdian, & Powell, 2002). A combination of five components were found to yield significant improvement in children with mathematics disorder as well as those with low-, average-, and high-achievement: (1) clear, procedurally explicit, concept-based explanations, (2) pictorial representations, (3) gradually faded verbal rehearsal, (4) timed practice with mixed problem sets, and (5) cumulative review with previously mastered problem types.

Regarding mathematics problem solving, it has been demonstrated that a framework of teaching methods (which specifically helps students find connections between familiar and novel tasks and broadens student schemas) is more effective than teacher instruction in word problem solution rules alone (Fuchs et al., 2003a, 2003b). This framework includes (1) teaching students to explore novel-looking problems by recognizing irrelevant problem components and thus indentifying familiar problem components for which solutions are known, (2) teaching students to create schemas by demonstrating how irrelevant problem components can change without altering problem-solving rules, and (3) familiarizing students with the idea of transfer in the context of learning to solve problems never before seen.

Trott (2003) noted several strategies that have brought improvements in students with dyscalculia. Among them he reports the importance of breaking multistep problems into small, manageable parts. Further, colored pens and markers can be used to highlight question parts. Regarding teacher instruction, Trott recommends using large posters to serve as a memory trigger of basic concepts, which are not easily retained in short-term memory. He also recommends the use of flow diagrams to clarify procedures, flash cards for memorization, and giving guidance to students regarding the basic study skills of time management, organization, and studying. Michaelson (2007) notes that these tips would facilitate learning in all students, not only those with a learning disorder.

Cognitive-behavioral intervention models have resulted in self-instruction strategy techniques (Hallahan, Kauffman, & Lloyd, 1996) that have proven effective (Seabaugh & Schumaker, 1993). A main component of this approach involves teaching students to verbalize the steps that must be used to solve a particular problem. After the student has mastered application of the problem-solving method, he or she is taught to utilize subvocal self-instruction.

Provision of feedback to the student has proven a useful tool in improving mathematics skills in individuals afflicted with mathematics disorder. For 20

M

weeks, L. S. Fuchs, D. Fuchs, Hamlett, and Whinnery (1991) administered math tests twice per week to students via computers that provided immediate feedback. Forty students with mathematics disorder were identified prior to the study. Half of these students were given a performance feedback graph with a goal line superimposed over the graph throughout the study. The other half of the students were shown the graph without the goal line. Greater performance stability was found among students who were provided a goal line on their feedback graph. Lyon et al. (2006) highlight the benefits that can be found through engaging students in performance monitoring when learning both math fact retrieval skills and procedural math skills.

Lyon et al. (2006) described several specific programs that have been effectively used with students with mathematics disorder. Connecting math concepts (S. Engelmann, Carnine, O. Engelmann, & Kelly, 1991) utilizes highly structured lessons that involve frequent teacher questions and student answers. This program was developed out of the DISTAR arithmetic program (Engelman & Carnine, 1975) and several studies have documented the efficacy of both programs among children with mathematics disorder (Carnine, 1991). Lyon et al. further note that research regarding math peer-assisted learning strategies (PALS) has documented the importance of instruction that targets both procedural skill and conceptual knowledge along with the use of guided peer-mediated practice. Such approaches have been found to improve performance in kindergarten through 6th grade, not only for students with mathematics disorder, but also low-, average-, and high-achieving peers (Fuchs et al., 2001; Fuchs et al., 2002).

Audrey L. Baumeister
William Drew Gouvier

Alarcon, M., DeFries, J. C., Light, J. C., & Pennington, B. F. (1997). A twin study of mathematics disability. *Journal of Learning Disabilities, 30,* 617–623.

American Psychiatric Association. (2000). *Diagnostic and statistical manual of mental disorders (DSM-IV-TR).* Washington, DC: Author

Ashcraft, M. H. (1995). Cognitive psychology and simple arithmetic: A review and summary of new directions. *Mathematical Cognition, 1,* 3–34.

Barnes, M. A., Pengelly, S., Dennis, M., Wilkinson, M., Rogers, T., & Faulkner, H. (2002). Mathematics skills in good readers with hydrocephalus. *Journal of the International Neuropsychological Society, 8,* 72–82.

Beachman, N., & Trott, C. (2005). Screening for dyscalculia within HE (Higher Education). *MSOR Connections, 5*(1), 1–4.

Butterworth, B. (2003). *Dyscalculia screener: Highlighting pupils with specific learning difficulties in math.* London: Nelson Publishing Company.

Bynner, J., & Parsons, S. (1997). *Does numeracy matter?* London: The Basic Skills Agency.

Carnine, D. W. (1991). Increasing the amount and quality of learning through direct instruction: Implications for mathematics. In J. W. Lloyd, N. N. Singh, & A. C. Repp (Eds.), *The regular education initiative: Alternative perspectives on concepts, issues, and models* (pp. 163–175). Sycamore, IL: Sycamore.

Chochon, F., Cohen, L., van de Moortele, P. F., & Dehaene, S. (1999). Differential contributions of the left and right inferior parietal lobules to number processing. *Journal of Cognitive Neuroscience, 11,* 617–630.

Daly, E. J., Martens, B. K., Barnett, D., Witt, J. C., & Olson, S. C. (2007). Varying intervention delivery in response to intervention: Confronting and resolving challenges with measurement, instruction, and intensity. *School Psychology Review, 36*(4), 562–581.

Dehaene, S., & Cohen, L. (1997). Cerebral pathways for calculation: Double dissociation between rote verbal and quantitative knowledge of arithmetic. *Cortex, 33,* 219–250.

Dehaene, S., Spelke, E., Pinel, P., Stanescu, R., & Tsivkin, S. (1999). Sources of mathematical thinking: Behavioral and brain-injury evidence. *Science, 284,* 970–974.

Deno, S. L. (1985). Curriculum-based measurement: The emerging alternative. *Exceptional Children, 52,* 219–232.

Deno, S. L. (1986). Formative evaluation of individual student programs: A new rule for school psychologists. *School Psychology Review, 15,* 358–374.

Deno, S. L. (1989). Curriculum-based measurement and alternative special education services: A fundamental and direct relationship. In M. R. Shinn (Ed.), *Curriculum-based measurement: Assessing special children* (pp. 1–17). New York: Guilford Press.

Deno, S. L. (2003). Developments in curriculum-based measurement. *Journal of Special Education, 37,* 184–192.

DiPerna, J. C., & Elliott, S. N. (2000). *Academic competence evaluation scales.* San Antonio, TX: Psychological Corporation.

DuPaul, G. J., Rapport, M. D., & Perriello, L. M. (1991). Teacher ratings of academic skills: The development of the Academic Performance Rating Scale. *School Psychology Review, 20,* 284–300.

Eckert, T. L., & Arbolino, L. A. (2005). The role of teacher perspectives in diagnostic and program evaluation decision making. In R. Brown-Chidsey (Ed.), *Assessment for intervention: A problem-solving approach* (pp. 65–81). New York: Guilford.

Engelman, S., & Carnine, D. W. (1975). *DISTAR arithmetic I* (2nd ed.). Chicago: Science Research Associates.

M

M

Engelmann, S., Carnine, D. W., Engelmann, O., & Kelly, B. (1991). *Connecting math concepts*. Chicago: Science Research Associates.

Fleishner, J. E. (1994). Diagnosis and assessment of mathematics learning disabilities. In G. R. Lyon (Ed.), *Frames of reference for the assessment of learning disabilities: New views on measurement issues* (pp. 441–458). Baltimore: Brookes.

Fuchs, L. S., & Deno, S. L. (1991). Paradigmatic distinctions between instructionally relevant measurement models. *Exceptional Children, 57*(6), 488–500.

Fuchs, L. S., Fuchs, D., Hamlett, C. L., Phillips, N. B., & Bentz, J. (1994). Class wide curriculum-based measurement: Helping general educators meet the challenge of student diversity. *Exceptional Children, 60*, 518–537.

Fuchs, L. S., Fuchs, D., Hamlett, C. L., Phillips, N. B., Karns, K., & Dutka, S. (1997). Enhancing students' helping behavior during peer-mediated instruction with conceptual mathematical explanations. *Elementary School Journal, 97*, 223–250.

Fuchs, L. S., Fuchs, D., Hamlett, C. L., & Whinnery, K. (1991). Effects of goal line feedback on level, slope, and stability of performance within curriculum based measurement. *Learning Disabilities Research and Practice, 6*, 65–73.

Fuchs, L. S., Fuchs, D., & Karns, K. (2001). Enhancing kindergartners' mathematical development: Effects of peer-assisted learning strategies. *Elementary School Journal, 101*, 495–510.

Fuchs, L. S., Fuchs, D., Phillips, N. B., Hamlett, C. L., & Karns, K. (1995). Acquisition and transfer effects of class wide peer-assisted learning strategies in mathematics for students with varying learning histories. *School Psychology Review, 24*, 604–620.

Fuchs, L. S., Fuchs, D., & Prentice, K. (2004). Responsiveness to mathematical problem-solving instruction: Comparing students at risk of mathematics disability with and without risk of reading disability. *Journal of Learning Disabilities, 37*(4), 293–306.

Fuchs, L. S., Fuchs, D., Prentice, K., Burch, M., Hamlett, C. L., Owen, R., et al. (2003a). Explicitly teaching for transfer: Effects on third-grade students' mathematical problem solving. *Journal of Educational Psychology, 95*(2), 293–305.

Fuchs, L. S., Fuchs, D., Prentice, K., Burch, M., Hamlett, C. L., Owen, R., et al. (2003b). Enhancing third-grade students' mathematical problem solving with self-regulated learning strategies. *Journal of Educational Psychology, 95*(2), 306–315.

Fuchs, L. S., Fuchs, D., Yazdian, L., & Powell, S. R. (2002). Enhancing first-grade children's mathematical development with peer-assisted learning strategies. *School Psychology Review, 31*, 569–584.

Geary, D. C. (1990). A componential analysis of an early learning deficits in mathematics. *Journal of Experimental Child Psychology, 498*, 363–383.

Geary, D. C. (1993). Mathematical disabilities: Cognitive, neuropsychological and genetic components. *Psychological Bulletin, 114*, 345–362.

Geary, D. C. (2004). Mathematics and learning disabilities. *Journal of Learning Disabilities, 37*(1), 4–15.

Geary, D. C., Hamson, C. O., & Hoard, M. K. (2000). Numerical and arithmetical cognition: A longitudinal study of process and concept deficits in children with learning disability. *Journal of Experimental Child Psychology, 77*, 236–263.

Geary, D. C., Hoard, M. K., & Hamson, C. O. (1999). Numerical and arithmetical cognition: Patterns of functions and deficits in children at risk for a mathematical disability. *Journal of Experimental Child Psychology, 74*, 213–239.

Gresham, F. M. (2004). Current status and future directions of school-based behavioral interventions. *School Psychology Review, 33*, 326–343.

Gresham, F. M., Reschly, D., & Carey, M. P. (1987). Teachers as "tests": Classification accuracy and concurrent validation in the identification of learning disabled children. *School Psychology Review, 26*, 543–553.

Gross-Tsur, V., Manor, O., & Shalev, R. S. (1996). Developmental dyscalculia: Prevalence and demographic features. *Developmental Medicine and Child Neurology, 38*, 25–33.

Hallahan, D. P., Kauffman, J. M., & Lloyd, J. (1996). *Introduction to learning disabilities*. Needham Heights, MA: Allyn & Bacon.

Lewis, C., Hitch, G. J., & Walker, P. (1994). The prevalence of specific arithmetic difficulties and specific reading difficulties in 9- to 10-year-old boys and girls. *Journal of Child Psychology and Psychiatry, 35*, 283–292.

Lyon, G. R., Fletcher, J. M., & Barnes, M. C. (2003). Learning disabilities. In E. J. Mash & R. A. Barkley (Eds.), *Child psychopathology* (pp. 520–586). New York: Guilford.

Lyon, G. R., Fletcher, J. M., Fuchs, L. S., & Chhabra, V. (2006). Learning disabilities. In E. J. Mash & R. A. Barkley (Eds.), *Treatment of childhood disorders* (3rd ed., pp. 512–591). New York: Guilford.

Marston, D., & Magnusson, D. (1985). Implementing curriculum-based measurement in special and regular education settings. *Exceptional Children, 52*, 266–276.

Michaelson, M. T. (2007). An overview of dyscalculia: Methods for ascertaining and accommodating dyscalculic children in the classroom. *The Australian Mathematics Teacher, 63*(3), 17–22.

Miller, S. P., & Mercer, C. D. (1997). Educational aspects of mathematics disabilities. *Journal of Learning Disabilities, 30*, 47–56.

Peterson, K. M., & Shinn, M. R. (2002). Severe discrepancy models: Which best explains school identification practices for learning disabilities? *School Psychology Review, 31*, 459–476.

Rourke, B. P. (1993). Arithmetic disabilities specific and otherwise: A neuropsychological perspective. *Journal of Learning Disabilities, 26,* 214–226.

Seabaugh, G. O., & Schumaker, J. B. (1993). The effects of self-regulation training on the academic productivity of secondary students with learning problems. *Journal of Behavioral Education, 4,* 109–133.

Semrud-Clikeman, M., Biederman, J., Sprich-Buckminster, S., Krifcher-Lehman, B., Faraone, S. V., & Norman, D. (1992). Comorbidity between ADHD and learning disability: A review and report in a clinically referred sample. *Journal of the American Academy of Child and Adolescent Psychiatry, 31,* 439–448.

Shalev, R. S., Auerbach, J., Manor, O., & Gross-Tsur, V. (2000). Developmental dyscalculia: Prevalence and prognosis. *European Child and Adolescent Psychiatry, 9,* 58–64.

Shalev, R. S., Manor, O., & Gross-Tsur, V. (1997). Neuropsychological aspects of developmental dyscalculia. *Mathematical Cognition, 33,* 105–120.

Shalev, R. S., Manor, O., Kerem, B., Ayali, M., Badichi, N., Friedlander, Y., et al. (2001). Developmental dyscalculia is a familial learning disability. *Journal of Learning Disabilities, 34,* 59–65.

Shinn, M. R. (1988). Development of curriculum-based local norms for use in special education decision making. *School Psychology Review, 17,* 61–80.

Shinn, M. R. (Ed.). (1989). *Curriculum-based measurement: Assessing special children.* New York: Guilford Press.

Shinn, M. R. (Ed.). (1998). *Advanced applications of curriculum-based measurement.* New York: Guilford Press.

Shinn, M. R. (2005). Identifying and validating academic problems in a problem-solving model. In R. Brown-Chidsey (Ed.), *Assessment for intervention: A problem-solving approach* (pp. 219–246). New York: Guilford.

Shinn, M. R., & Marston, D. (1985). Differentiating mildly handicapped, low-achieving and regular education students: A curriculum-based approach. *Remedial and Special Education, 6,* 31–45.

Siegel, L. S., & Ryan, E. B. (1989). The development of working memory in normally achieving and subtypes of learning disabled children. *Child Development, 60,* 973–980.

Trott, C. (2003). Mathematics support for dyslexic students. *MSOR Connections, 3*(4), 17–20.

MELKERSSON–ROSENTHAL'S SYNDROME

DESCRIPTION

Melkersson–Rosenthal's syndrome (MRS) is a systemic neurological disorder characterized by recurring facial paralysis, swelling of the face and lips (usually the upper lip), and the development of folds and grooves on the tongue. After recurrent attacks (ranging from days to years in between), swelling may persist and increase, eventually becoming permanent. The lip may become hard, cracked, and fissured with a reddish-brown discoloration. Swellings may occur on extra-facial regions, such as the lumbar region and the dorsal aspect of the hands and feet (Odom, James, & Berger, 2000). Although early manifestations of the syndrome can start at any age, onset usually is in young adulthood, and it affects females two to three times as often as males (Greene & Rogers, 1989; Hornstein, Stosiek, Schönberger, & Meisel-Stosiek, 1987). The disorder is named after Ernst Melkersson and Curt Rosenthal. Prevalence of this syndrome is about 0.08%. The typical course is chronic recurrent or progressive involvement over decades (Aliağoğlu et al., 2008; Minor, Fox, Bukantz, & Lockey, 1987; Stein & Mancini, 1999).

NEUROPATHOLOGY/PATHOPHYSIOLOGY

MRS is characterized by oral noncaseating granulomatous lesions, similar to those associated with Crohn's disease, sarcoidosis, food allergies, contact allergies, and focal dental sepsis. MRS is also reported to occur in childhood. The etiology and the mechanism of the disease are still not known, although genetic factors, infectious agents, allergic reactions to various foods and food additives, and autoimmune diseases have all been considered in the etiology of MRS (Ozgursoy et al., 2009; Pisanty & Sharav, 1969). It can be symptomatic of Crohn's disease or sarcoidosis; temporal MRI revealed no pathological finding in patients with recurrent PFP, and chest X-ray was normal in all patients. Although there is no specific radiological finding for MRS, chest X-ray and temporal and cranial CT or MRI can be used to exclude other diseases (Ozgursoy et al., 2009).

NEUROPSYCHOLOGICAL/CLINICAL PRESENTATION

The disorder is characterized by recurring facial paralysis, swelling of the face and lips (usually the upper lip), and the development of folds and grooves on the tongue. After recurrent attacks (ranging from days to years in between), swelling may persist and increase, eventually becoming permanent. The lip may become hard, cracked, and fissured with a reddish-brown discoloration. Swellings may occur on extrafacial regions, such as the lumbar region and the dorsal aspect of the hands and feet (Odom et al., 2000). Facial palsy occurs in 30–50% of cases. The paralyzed side is generally the side with swelling (Stein & Mancini, 1999). There has been no report of any cognitive or psychological impairment directly associated with MRS in the literature.

DIAGNOSIS

MRS is a rare disorder characterized by a triad of recurrent orofacial swelling and recurrent paralysis of the facial nerve and lingua plicata. The complete triad only occurs in 25% of MRS cases. Other symptoms may include granulomas in other facial sites, regional lymphadenopathy, fever, psychotic disorders, and hyperplastic gingivitis are associated with MRS (Nagel & Foelster-Holst, 2006). The most dominant manifestation of the syndrome is facial edema, which is acute, diffuse, painless, nonpitting, and mostly confined to the lips (Zimmer, Rogers, Reeve, & Sheridan, 1992). Ozgursoy et al. (2009) reported that the clinical picture of MRS can vary according to the department specialty where the patient was treated.

TREATMENT

Corticosteroids or clofazimine appear to be the best therapeutic options (Nagel & Foelster-Holst, 2006). Decompression of facial nerve throughout its bony canal may be indicated for patients with recurrent or persistent attacks of facial paralysis despite medical treatment (Dutt, Mirza, Irving, & Donaldson, 2000). Surgical procedures such as mucosa, submucosa and tangential muscle resection, crescent-shaped commissuroplasty, and facial liposuction have been deemed effective when orofacial swelling becomes unrelenting (Tan, Atik, & Calka, 2006). Reported successfully treating two patients with infliximab, which has strong anti-inflammatory properties and has been used successfully in Crohn's disease, rheumatoid arthritis, or psoriasis.

MRS may recur intermittently after its first appearance. It can become a chronic disorder. Intravenous high dosage of methylprednisolone has also shown some relief of symptoms (Kesler, Vainstein, & Gadoth, 1998). Spontaneous recovery of the majority of symptoms occurs in some cases, although reoccurrence is common with repeated episodes resulting in progressively worse recovery (Samuels & Feske, 2003).

Issac Tourgeman
Charles Golden

Aliağoğlu, C., Yildirim, U., Albayrak, H., Gosugur, N., Memişoğullari, R., & Kavak, A. (2008). Melkersson-Rosenthal syndrome associated with ipsilateral facial, hand, and foot swelling. *Dermatology Online Journal*, *14*(1), 7.

Dutt, S. N., Mirza, S., Irving, R. M., & Donaldson, I. (2000). Total decompression of facial nerve for Melkersson-Rosenthal syndrome. *The Journal of Laryngology and Otology, 114*, 870–873.

Greene, R. M., & Rogers, R. S. (1989). Melkersson-Rosenthal syndrome: A review of 36 patients. *Journal of American Academy of Dermatology, 2*, 1263–1270.

Hornstein, O. P., Stosiek, N., Schönberger, A., & Meisel-Stosiek, M. (1987). Classification and scope of clinical variations of Melkersson-Rosenthal syndrome. *Zeitschrift Für Hautkrankheiten, 62*, 1453–1466.

Kesler, A., Vainstein, G., & Gadoth, N. (1998). Melkersson-Rosenthal syndrome treated by methylprednisolone. *Neurology, 51*(5), 1440–1441.

Minor, M. W., Fox, R. W., Bukantz, S. C., & Lockey, R. F. (1987). Melkersson-Rosenthal syndrome. *Journal of Allergy and Clinical Immunology, 80*, 64–67.

Nagel, F., & Foelster-Holst, R. (2006). Cheilitis granulomatosa Melkersson-Rosenthal syndrome. *Der Hautarzt; Zeitschrift für Dermatologie, Venerologie, und verwandte Gebiete, 57*(2), 121–126.

Odom, R. B., James, W. D., & Berger, T. G. (2000). *Diseases of the skin: Clinical dermatology* (9th ed.). Philadelphia: W. B. Saunders Company.

Ozgursoy, O. B., Karatayli Ozgursoy, S., Tulunay, O., Kemal, O., Akyol, A., & Dursun, G. (2009). The etiology of MRS is still unknown Melkersson-Rosenthal syndrome revisited as a misdiagnosed disease. *American Journal of Otolaryngology, 30*(1), 33–37.

Pisanty, S., & Sharav, Y. (1969). The Melkersson-Rosenthal syndrome. *Oral Surgery, Oral Medicine, and Oral Pathology, 27*, 729–733.

Samuels, M., & Feske, S. K. (2003). *Office practice of neurology* (2nd ed.). New York: Churchill Livingstone.

Stein, S. L., & Mancini, A. J.,(1999). Melkersson-Rosenthal syndrome in childhood: Successful management with combination steroid and minocycline therapy. *Journal of American Academy of Dermatology, 41*, 746–748.

Tan, O., Atik, B., & Calka, O. (2006). Plastic surgical solutions for Melkersson-Rosenthal syndrome: Facial liposuction and cheiloplasty procedures. *Annals of Plastic Surgery, 56*(3), 268–273.

Zimmer, W. M., Rogers, R. S., Reeve, C. M., & Sheridan, P. J. (1992). Orofacial manifestations of Melkersson-Rosenthal syndrome: A study of 42 patients and review of 220 cases from the literature. *Oral Surgery, Oral Medicine, and Oral Pathology, 76*, 610–619.

M

MENINGITIS

DESCRIPTION

Meningitis refers to a potentially lethal medical condition characterized by inflammation of the meninges. Common symptoms of meningitis include headache, fever, nuchal rigidity, photophobia, and altered level of consciousness. A variety of pathogens can cause meningitis, including viruses, bacteria, and fungi, as well as ingested agents such as drugs or chemicals. The condition is often categorized by its etiology. Viral meningitis is the most common type of meningitis and is typically not life-threatening. A wide variety of viral agents, including enteroviruses, herpes simplex virus, West Nile virus, varicella zoster virus (VSV), mumps, polio, and HIV, can cause viral meningitis. Bacterial meningitis is less common than viral meningitis, but more often results in residual neurological impairments or death. Pathogens responsible for the most common types of bacterial meningitis include *Streptococcus pneumoniae*, *Neisseria meningitidis*, group B streptococcus, *Listeria*, *monocytogenes*, *Haemophilus influenzae*, and group B streptococcus. Fungal meningitis can be caused by a wide variety of pathogens, including *Cryptococcus*, *Blastomyces*, *Histoplasma*, *Coccidioides*, *Aspergillus*, *Candida*, and other molds (Gottfredsson & Perfect, 2000). An assortment of drugs and chemicals has also been implicated as causal agents of meningitis. These include nonsteroidal anti-inflammatory drugs (NSAIDs) (e.g., ibuprofen, sulindac, tolmetin, naproxen), antimicrobial drugs (e.g., sulfonamindes, trimethoprim), radiographic agents, chemotherapeutic drugs, and corticosteroids (Marinac, 1992).

NEUROPATHOLOGY/PATHOPHYSIOLOGY

Viruses can enter the central nervous system (CNS) and cause inflammation of the meninges through many different mechanisms. Some viral agents that cause meningitis infect leukocytes, multiply in the bloodstream, and enter the brain via the vascular system. Viral pathogens can also bypass the blood–brain barrier via transport through neural tissue. After infiltrating the CNS, the viral agents may travel through the cerebrospinal fluid (CSF). When CSF containing viral pathogens enters the subarachnoid space, inflammation of the meninges can result (Chadwick, 2005).

Bacterial meningitis typically initiates from colonization of a pathogen on the nasopharynx of the host organism. The bacteria may enter the bloodstream and then the CSF through the choroid plexus. After bacterial pathogens infiltrate the blood–brain barrier, the host's defense system is activated, and cytokines, chemokines, and proteolytic enzymes are released. These defenses are usually insufficient in managing the resultant inflammation. Increased permeability of the blood–brain barrier, increased intracranial pressure, and cerebral edema often result. Cell wall slough and excretia byproducts of the pathogen may increase the host's immune response to such a degree that neuronal injury results from the host's own immune response (Tunkel & Scheld, 1993).

NEUROPSYCHOLOGICAL/CLINICAL PRESENTATION

Fever, neck stiffness, and altered mental status are the classic triad of meningitis symptoms. However, research has shown that many individuals do not display all of these symptoms (van de Beek et al., 2004). Along with the classic triad, headache is another common symptom of meningitis. Individuals with meningitis may also experience photophobia, vomiting, chills, seizures, and/or papilledema. Depending upon the type of meningitis, a petechial or purpuric rash may also be present. The Kernig and Brudzinski signs have also been used as clinical indicators of meningeal inflammation.

The clinical presentation of meningitis varies depending upon the etiology and age of the individual. Viral meningitis usually runs a benign course. Children with viral meningitis may present with meningism (neck stiffness, photophobia, and headache), fever, vomiting, respiratory problems, lethargy, irritability, poor appetite, and/or a rash (Chadwick, 1995; Dagan, Jenista, & Menegus, 1988). Infants with viral meningitis are more likely to suffer from seizures and present with focal neurological signs than older patients. Headache, fever, photophobia, and neck stiffness are common symptoms seen in adults with viral meningitis as well.

The presentation of bacterial meningitis is very similar to that of viral meningitis; however, bacterial meningitis typically runs a longer and more complicated course. Research has shown that most adults with acute community-acquired bacterial meningitis present with two or more of the following symptoms: headache, fever, neck stiffness, or a compromised mental state (van de Beek et al., 2004). Young children with bacterial meningitis are more likely than older children and adults to present with nonspecific symptoms, including fever, lethargy, anorexia, vomiting, and irritability (Stechenberg, 2008).

The prevalence of residual neurological deficits resulting from meningitis varies depending upon the age of the individual and etiology of the inflammation. Young children, immunocompromised adults, the elderly, and bacterial meningitis survivors are more likely to suffer from neurological sequelae. Grimwood et al. (1995) found that 26.9% of individuals who survive school-age bacterial meningitis suffer from functional impairments. Hearing disabilities are a common residual of bacterial meningitis. Other less common sequelae include mental retardation, spasticity, paresis, and seizure disorders (Baraff, Lee, & Schriger, 1993).

A childhood history of bacterial meningitis is associated with a variety of cognitive, educational, and behavioral deficits. Bacterial meningitis survivors often exhibit IQ deficits as well as memory and learning deficits (Anderson, Anderson, Grimwood, & Nolan, 2004; Grimwood et al., 1995). Bacterial meningitis survivors also display executive control deficits and are poorer readers than controls (Anderson et al., 2004; Grimwood et al., 1995). Parent and teacher ratings indicate bacterial meningitis survivors have more behavioral problems than controls and show poorer psychological adjustment (Grimwood et al., 1995).

Schmidt et al. (2006) found that survivors of bacterial meningitis reported significantly more difficulties performing daily activities than survivors of viral meningitis and controls. In the same study, both survivors of bacterial meningitis and viral meningitis showed deficits in executive functions and visuoconstructive functions when compared with healthy controls. Survivors of bacterial meningitis also performed significantly poorer on measures of working memory than survivors of viral meningitis and healthy controls. Occupational impairment led to retirement in a small minority (0.07%) of bacterial meningitis survivors and none of the viral meningitis survivors. MRI findings revealed lower brain volume and higher ventricular volume in survivors of bacterial meningitis compared with survivors of viral meningitis (Schmidt et al., 2006).

DIAGNOSIS

An analysis of CSF extracted through a lumbar puncture is important in diagnosing meningitis. Biochemical markers of meningitis include reduced glucose concentration in CSF, increased CSF white blood cell counts, and elevated protein levels. In the case of bacterial meningitis, the results of CSF Gram stains can be helpful in identifying the causal agent and appropriate antibiotic treatments. If a Gram stain is negative, CSF biochemical markers are sometimes helpful in differentiating viral meningitis from bacterial meningitis. Normal CSF glucose concentration is common in viral meningitis. Also, very seldom are leukocyte counts greater than 1,000 leukocytes/mm^3 in individuals with viral meningitis (Marinac, 1992).

Extraction of CSF through a lumbar puncture is contraindicated when brain abnormalities that could lead to herniation are suspected. Clinicians may order a computed tomography (CT) scan before a lumbar puncture is performed in order to assess for brain abnormalities predisposing the individual to brain herniation. Because ordering a CT scan often delays treatment, the scan may not be ordered unless the patient presents with neurological deficits, a compromised state of consciousness, papilledema, previous brain pathology, or a suppressed immune system. Even if a lumbar puncture cannot be performed, it is recommended that antibiotic therapy be given promptly if bacterial meningitis is suspected. For individuals with bacterial meningitis, early diagnosis and antibiotic treatment greatly improve prognosis.

TREATMENT

Treatment of meningitis depends upon the causal agent. Bacterial meningitis warrants antibiotic treatment. A positive Gram stain can be used to identify the pathogen that should be targeted and guide antibiotic treatment. Drugs used to treat bacterial meningitis include ampicillin, chloramphenicol, ceftriaxone, cefotaxime, and vancomycin (Quagliarello & Scheld, 1997). Corticosteroids, such as dexamethasone, may also be used to reduce the often injurious immune response of the host organism (de Gans & van de Beek, 2002). Viral meningitis typically improves on its own without specific treatment. Aciclovir, an antiviral drug, may be given if meningitis is caused by the herpes simplex virus or VSV (Chadwick, 2005). However, in general, viral meningitis only warrants palliative care. With regard to prophylactic treatment of meningitis, vaccines are now available for meningitis caused by meningococci, *H. influenzae* type B, pneumococci, and the mumps virus. Antifungal drugs, including amphotericin B, flucytosine, and fluconazole, have been used to treat fungal meningitis (Bicanic & Harrison, 2004). Individuals with drug- or chemical-induced aseptic meningitis should receive symptomatic treatment, and, if possible, administration of the drug or chemical exposure believed to be causing the inflammation should be discontinued.

Alyse Barker
Mandi Musso
William Drew Gouvier

Anderson, V., Anderson, P., Grimwood, K., & Nolan, T. (2004). Cognitive and executive function 12 years after childhood bacterial meningitis: Effect of acute neurologic complications and age of onset. *Journal of Pediatric Psychology, 29*(2), 67–81.

Baraff, L. J., Lee, S. I., & Schriger, D. L. (1993). Outcomes of bacterial meningitis in children — A meta-analysis. *Pediatric Infectious Disease Journal, 12*(5), 389–394.

Bicanic, T., & Harrison, T. S. (2004). Cryptococcal meningitis. *British Medical Bulletin, 72,* 99–118.

Chadwick, D. R. (2005). Viral Meningitis. *British Medical Bulletin, 75,* 1–14.

Dagan, R., Jenista, J. A., & Menegus, M. A. (1988). Association of clinical presentation, laboratory findings, and virus serotypes with the presence of meningitis in hospitalized infants with enterovirus infection. *The Journal of Pediatrics, 113,* 975–978.

de Gans, J., & van de Beek, D. (2002). Dexamethasone in adults with bacterial meningitis. *The New England Journal of Medicine. 347*(20), 1549–1556.

Gottfredsson, M., & Perfect, J. R. (2000). Fungal meningitis. *Seminars in Neurology, 20*(3), 307–322.

Grimwood, K., Anderson, V. A., Bond, L., Catroppa, C., Hore, R. L., Keir, E. H., et al. (1995). Adverse outcomes of bacterial meningitis in school-age survivors. *Pediatrics, 95*(5), 646–656.

Marinac, J. S. (1992). Drug- and chemical-induced aseptic meningitis: A review of the literature. *The Annals of Pharmacotherapy, 26,* 813–822.

Quagliarello, V. J., & Scheld, W. M. (1997). Treatment of bacterial meningitis. *The New England Journal of Medicine, 336*(10), 708–717.

Schmidt, H., Heimann, B., Djukic, M., Mazurek, C., Fels, C., Wallesch, C. W., et al. (2006). Neuropsychological sequelae of bacterial and viral meningitis. *Brain, 129,* 333–345.

Stechenberg, B. (2008). Bacterial meningitis. In L. L. Barton & N. R. Friedman (Eds.), *The neurological manifestations of pediatric infectious diseases and immunodeficiency syndromes* (pp. 193–198). Totowa, NJ: Humana Press.

Tunkel, A. R., & Scheld, W. M. (1993). Pathogenesis and pathophysiology of bacterial meningitis. *Annual Review of Medicine, 44,* 103–120.

van de Beek, D., de Gans, J., Spanjaard, L., Weisfelt, M., Reitsma, J. B., & Vermeulen, M. (2004). *The New England Journal of Medicine, 351*(18), 1849–1859.

MENKES'S DISEASE

DESCRIPTION

Menkes's disease (MD) or kinky hair syndrome is a rare X-linked neurodegenerative disorder of infancy caused by a defect in copper transport (Barnerias et al., 2008; Buisson et al., 2006; Danks et al, 1973; Menkes et al., 1962; Robertson, 2004). It is characterized by progressive cerebral degeneration with psychomotor deterioration and seizures, connective tissue alteration with hypopigmentation of skin and hair, and recurrent episodes of hypothermia with failure to thrive. MD has an incidence ranging from 1 of 100,000 to 1 to 250,000 live births (Kaler, 1994).

An estimated 15–30 affected babies are expected to be born in the United States each year (Robertson, 2004). One-third of these cases are predicted to be nonfamilial cases, representing new mutations. About one-third of cases result from new mutations in the gene and occur in people with no history of the disorder in their family. Affected infants may be born prematurely. Symptoms appear during infancy and are largely a result of abnormal intestinal copper absorption with secondary deficiency in copper-dependent mitochondrial enzymes. Normal or slightly slowed development may proceed for 2–3 months, and then there will be severe developmental delay and a loss of early developmental skills. Death usually occurs by 3 years of age.

MD is related to the loss of a copper transporting adenosine triphosphatase (ATPase; ATP7A) involved in the export of dietary copper from the gastrointestinal tract and its transport into organelles (Buisson et al, 2006; Chelly et al., 1993; Tumer, Moller, & Horn, 1999). As a result of a mutation in the *ATP7A* gene, copper is poorly distributed to cells in the body. Copper accumulates in some tissues, such as the small intestine and kidneys, while the brain and other tissues have unusually low levels. The decreased supply of copper can reduce the activity of numerous copper-containing enzymes that are necessary for the structure and function of bone, skin, hair, blood vessels, and the nervous system. It is caused by defects in an X-chromosome gene that encodes an intracellular copper transporting adenosine phosphatase. This gene product is localized to the trans-Golgi network and normally governs incorporation of copper into secreted copper enzymes (Robertson, 2004). MD affects all tissues and organs in the body, except for the liver where *ATP7A* is not expressed. The copper transport across the blood–brain barrier is also defective resulting in severe brain copper deficiency, which leads to mental retardation (de Bie, Wijmenga & Klomp, 2007).

NEUROPATHOLOGY/PATHOPHYSIOLOGY

MD presents with low levels of copper in plasma, liver, and brain because of impaired intestinal absorption. There is reduced activity of numerous copper-dependent enzymes and paradoxic accumulation of copper in certain tissues, kidney, spleen, skeletal muscle, and pancreas. Cultured fibroblasts in which reduced egress of radiolabeled copper is demonstrated in pulse chase experiments. Levels of plasma and cerebrospinal fluid catechols influenced by dopamine beta hydroxylase (DBH) activity are distinctly abnormal and provide a highly sensitive and specific diagnostic marker for this disorder. Plasma catechol analysis is arguably the best diagnostic test for at-risk newborns during the first month of life because other biochemical parameters are unreliable in this period and molecular analysis is less rapid. Early identification of affected infants is a fundamental requirement for successful intervention, underscoring the assay's importance (Kaler et al., 2008; Robertson, 2004). There can be extensive neurodegeneration in the gray matter of the brain. Arteries in the brain can also be twisted with frayed and split inner walls. This can lead to rupture or blockage of the arteries and weakened bones (i.e., osteoporosis) may result in fractures.

Barnerias et al. (2008) demonstrated the possible coexistence of cytotoxic oedema of the putamen and head of caudate nuclei with white matter vasogenic oedema of the temporal lobes in MD. Acute cerebral damage observed on MRI might result from the combined effects of acute metabolic stress due to infectious disease and prolonged status epilepticus, acting on a highly susceptible developing brain. Moreover, vascular dysfunction and defect of energy production, due to superoxide dismutase and COX deficiencies, strongly increase the damage observed. In MD, this vasogenic oedema observed during status epilepticus, not only results from thrombotic occlusion but also from deficiency of blood supply to the developing brain, induced by progressive vasculopathy secondary to impairment of lysyl oxidase (Danks, Cartwright, Stevens, & Townley, 1973). In MD, secondary mitochondrial energy failure is also observed and results from dysfunction of cytochrome oxidase and superoxide dismutase. Neuronal damage is caused by the dysfunction of oxidative phosphorylation and the increased mitochondrial production of free radicals (Barkovich et al., 1993).

CT and MRI reveal progressive cerebral atrophy with a subdural hematoma or effusion in the neocortex, cerebellum, basal ganglia, and thalami (Robain, Aubourg, Routon, Dulac, & Ponsot, 1988; Takahashi et al., 1993). Neuronal degeneration predominates in cerebral and cerebellar cortices and in the basal ganglia (Buisson, 2008; Robain et al., 1988; Uno & Arya, 1987). Hsich, Robertson, Irons, Soul, and du Plessis (2000) reported bilateral infarctions of deep gray matter nuclei,

a finding not previously described in MD. Potential mechanisms for these cerebrovascular lesions in MD include the susceptibility to free radical attack and inadequate energy supply from oxidative phosphorylation. Hypopigmentation results from deficiency of tyrosinase, low lysyl oxidase activity causes numerous connective tissue disturbances, deficient DBH results in faulty catecholamine production, and poor cross linking of keratin with resulting steely hair is secondary to inadequate sulfhydryl oxidase activity. In the brain, lack of cytochrome *c*-oxidase, superoxide dismutase, and peptidyl alpha amidating activity in combination with aneurysm due to deficient lysyl oxidase will lead to severe dysfunction with progressive mental retardation (Barnerias et al., 2008; de Bie et al., 2007).

NEUROPSYCHOLOGICAL/CLINICAL PRESENTATION

The disease is characterized by severe mental retardation and progressive deterioration that develops at an early stage. Patients also fail to achieve developmental milestones. Spontaneous movement is limited. Drowsiness and lethargy are also present (Danks, 1972; Menkes, 1962; Robertson, 2004). It is characterized by progressive cerebral degeneration with psychomotor deterioration and seizures, connective tissue alteration with hypopigmentation of skin and hair, and recurrent episodes of hypothermia with failure to thrive; so symptoms exist across all neurological and cognitive functions.

DIAGNOSIS

The hallmark feature of MD is kinky hair, eyebrows, and eyelashes that are colorless or steel-colored and easily broken. In ethnic groups with black hair, the hair can also be blonde or brown. Onset of MD typically begins during infancy. Signs and symptoms of this disorder include depressed nasal bridge, sagging facial features, mental retardation, and developmental delay. At 2–3 months, there is a loss of previously obtained developmental milestones and the onset of hypotonia, failure to thrive, and seizures. In rare cases, symptoms begin later in childhood and are less severe. Patients may also present with temperature instability, hypoglycemia, and eyelid ptosis. Autonomic abnormalities may also result from selective loss of sympathetic adrenergic function (Barnerias et al., 2008; Buisson et al., 2006; Danks, 1972; Kaler, 1994; Menkes, 1962; Robertson, 2004).

MD should be differentiated from other diagnoses that have an onset in infancy and present with similar symptoms. Leigh's disease is a neurometabolic disorder characterized by loss of motor ability, hypotonia, and seizures with a rapidly progressing onset between the ages of 3 months and 2 years. Phenylketonuria, an autosomal recessive genetic disorder, also presents with seizures and mental retardation. Laboratory screening can be used to differentiate these diseases from MD. Also, both of the diseases do not present with the short and brittle hair as seen in MD. Pollitt's syndrome, biotin deficiency, and argininosuccinic aciduria also present with similar symptoms and should be ruled out in diagnosis (Beers & Berkow, 1999). Occipital horn syndrome is a milder form of MD in which the overall neurologic function is great with complaints of orthostatic hypotension and chronic diarrhea (Robertson, 2004).

TREATMENT

Early diagnosis and institution of subcutaneous copper injections have been successful in about 20% of infants treated within 2 weeks of life ($n = 18$). The type and severity of the underlying mutation appear to be an important factor in response to early treatment (Robertson, 2004). Early treatment with subcutaneous (under the skin) or intravenous (in a vein) injections of copper supplements (in the form of acetate salts) may be of some benefit. Neonatal diagnosis of MD by plasma neurochemical measurements and early treatment with copper may improve clinical outcomes. Affected newborns who have mutations that do not completely abrogate *ATP7A* function may be especially responsive to early copper treatment (Kaler et al., 2008).

Isaac Tourgeman
Charles Golden

Barkovich, A. J., Good, W. V., Koch, T. K., & Berg, B. O. (1993). Mitochondrial disorders: Analysis of their clinical and imaging characteristics. *AJNR American Journal of Neuroradiology, 14*, 1119–1137.

Barnerias, C., Boddart, N., Pascale, G., Isabelle, D., Pannier, L. H., Dulac, O., et al. (2008). Unusual magnetic resonance imaging features in Menkes disease. *Brain & Development, 30*, 489–492.

Beers, M. H., & Berkow, R. (1999). *The Merck manual of diagnosis and therapy* (17th ed.). Rathway, NJ: Merck Research Laboratories.

Buisson, N. B., Kaminska, A., Nabbout, R., Barnerias, C., Isabelle, D., de Lonlay, P., et al. (2006). Epilepsy in Menkes disease: Analysis of clinical stages. *Epilepsia, 47*, 380–386.

Chelly, J., Tumer, Z., Tonnesen, T., Petterson, A., Ishikawa-Brush, Y., Tommerup, N., et al. (1993). Isolation of a candidate gene for Menkes disease that encodes a potential heavy metal binding protein. *Nature Genetics, 3*, 14–19.

Danks, D. M., Campbell, P. E., Stevens, B. J., Mayne, V., & Cartwright, E. (1973). Menkes's kinky hair syndrome: An inherited defect in copper absorption with widespread effects. *Pediatrics, 50*, 188–201.

Danks, D. M., Cartwright, E., Stevens, B. J., & Townley, R. R. (1973). Menkes' kinky hair disease: Further definition of the defect in copper transport, *Science, 179*, 1140–1142.

Hsich, G. E., Robertson, R. L., Irons, M., Soul, J. S., & du Plessis, A. J. (2000) Cerebral infarction in Menkes' disease. *Pediatric Neurology, 23*, 425–428.

Kaler, S. G. (1994). Menkes disease. *Advances in Pediatrics, 41*, 263–304.

Kaler, S. G., Holmes, C. S., Goldstein, D. S., Tang, J., Godwin, S. C., Donsante, A., et al. (2008). Neonatal diagnosis and treatment of Menkes disease. *The New England Journal of Medicine. 358*(6), 605.

Menkes, J. H., Alter, M., Steigleder, G. K., Weakley, D. R., & Sung, J. H. (1962). A sex-linked recessive disorder with retardation of growth, peculiar hair, and focal cerebral and cerebellar degeneration. *Pediatrics, 29*, 764–779.

Robain, O., Aubourg, P., Routon, M. C., Dulac, O., & Ponsot, G. (1988). Menkes disease: A golgi and electron microscopic study of the cerebellar cortex. *Clinical Neuropathology, 7*, 47–52.

Robertson, D. (2004). *Primer on the autonomic nervous system*. American Press.

Takahashi, S. Ishii, K., Matsumoto, K., Higano, S., Ishibashi, T., Zuguchi, M., et al. (1993). Cranial MRI and MR angiography in Menkes' syndrome. *Neuroradiology, 35*, 556–558.

Tumer, Z., Moller, L. B., & Horn, N. (1999). Mutation spectrum of ATP7A, the gene defective in Menkes disease. *Advances in Experimental Medicine and Biology, 448*, 83–95.

Uno, H., & Arya, S. (1987). Neuronal and vascular disorders of the brain and spinal cord in Menkes kinky hair disease. *American Journal of Medical Genetics*, (Suppl. 3), 367–377.

MENTAL RETARDATION

DESCRIPTION

Mental retardation has been recognized through history as an abnormality. In 1799, French physician Marc Itard worked with a child, known as the "wild boy of Aveyron," with the goal of adapting him to society. Although Dr. Itard failed to cure the boy, who he named "Victor," it was one of the first attempts to treat an individual with mental retardation (Lane, 1976). During the summer of 1846, Dr. Buckminster Brown visited the Hospital for the Cure and Education of Cretins on the Abendberg, canton of Berne, Switzerland. According to Dr. Brown, cretins and idiots were isolated from the population of the institution, which was located on the Swiss Alps, with the hope that they could be treated using treatments such as gymnastic exercise. At that time, individuals with mental retardation were known as innocents, simpletons, cretins, or idiots (Brown, 1847). In fact, derogatory terms such as idiot, fool, moron, and imbecile were applied in diagnostic and legal terminology to refer to individuals with mental retardation (Volkmar & Dykens, 2002).

Today, individuals with mental retardation are still associated with their deficits such as lack of intelligence (IQ test scores of 70 or less) or lack of adaptive social skills. However, there has been a change in the focus on mental retardation from what a person cannot do to what a person can do. In addition, there is greater emphasis on inclusion rather than exclusion. With treatment and assistance, some individuals with mental retardation have overcome their condition in order to function in society with relative normality. For instance, consider the case of Christopher Burke (1995) who suffers from Down's syndrome (a form of mental retardation), yet he became an actor who starred in the TV show *Life Goes On*, despite his condition. The purpose of this chapter is to present a detailed coverage of the essential neurological, neuropsychological, and other aspects of mental retardation.

NEUROPATHOLOGY/PATHOPHYSIOLOGY

In many ways, it is futile to attempt to discuss the neuropathological underpinnings of mental retardation. In essence, it is best conceptualized as a symptom as opposed to a disorder in and of itself. Mental retardation has been seen as a consequence of genetic/chromosomal abnormalities, disrupted neurological development, and perinatal factors. Genetic/chromosomal abnormalities constitute the most common basis for mental retardation. Trisomy 21 (i.e., Down's syndrome), Trisomy 18 (Edward's syndrome), Trisomy 13 (Pautau's syndrome), Trisomy 8, Trisomy 5 (Cri-du-chat syndrome), Fragile X syndrome, Klinefelter's syndrome, Turner's syndrome, and phenylketonuria are just a few of the genetic chromosomal disorders in which mental retardation commonly presents as a symptom.

All cephalic disorders, when children survive, have shown a substantial risk of mental retardation in addition to an array of other neurological symptoms. These include colpocephaly, holoprosencephaly, hydranencephaly, lissencephaly, porencephaly, and schizencephaly. This list obviously does not include cephalic presentations such as anencephaly as death often occurs prior to or immediately following birth. For some of these more severe forms, infants may live for up to a year or slightly more, but this is quite rare.

Perinatal factors linked with increased risk of mental retardation, among other neurological defects, include infectious processes, drug or toxic substance exposure, and trauma. Infectious processes include cytomegalovirus, herpes simplex, and rubella. Drug and toxic substance exposure include alcohol, cocaine, and the array of other illicit substances. Finally, maternal trauma can include irradiation, maternal suffocation, or physical injury among other things.

By all means, the presentations reported are not all inclusive. Rather, the emphasis is on the broad correlates of genetic/chromosomal abnormalities, infectious processes, and prenatal trauma. The interested reader is encouraged to read the literature on these individual presentations in regard to their pathological link to mental retardation. Many of which are included in this text. Beyond these, there is literature demonstrating links between gestational time, birth weight, and neonatal and early childhood environment and intellectual capacities.

NEUROPSYCHOLOGICAL/CLINICAL PRESENTATION

The clinical presentation of mental retardation remains consistent with its diagnostic criteria. Mental retardation is marked by significant limitations in both intellectual functioning and adaptive functioning, occurring prior to age 18. In regard to intellectual functioning, this corresponds with abilities two standard deviations or more below the population mean. Given mental retardation itself is best conceptualized as a symptom, it commonly coincides with other neuropsychological, academic, behavioral, emotional, and/or social deficits that may be specific to an underlying disease or disorder but not specific to mental retardation.

DIAGNOSIS

There are multiple definitions of mental retardation, which share common points. The American Association on Mental Retardation (Luckasson et al., 2002) provides the following definition:

> Mental retardation is a disability characterized by significant limitations both in intellectual functioning and in adaptive behavior as expressed in

conceptual, social, practical adaptive skills. This disability originates before age 18. (p. 8)

The *Diagnostic and Statistical Manual of Mental Disorders*, fourth edition, text revision *(DSM-IV-TR)* (American Psychiatric Association [APA], 2000) defines mental retardation similarly. It states that the disorder is characterized by intellectual functioning that is significantly subaverage (that is, an IQ of approximately 70 or below) with onset before 18 years of age and concurrent deficits or impairments in adaptive functioning. The *DSM-IV-TR* provides separate codes for Mild, Moderate, Severe, and Profound Mental Retardation and for Mental Retardation, Severity Unspecified (APA, 2000).

Both definitions focus on deficits on intellectual and adaptive functioning and they agree that the mental retardation symptoms must appear before the age of 18. Through time, the primary tool to assess mental retardation, intellectual deficits, has been the use of IQ (intelligence quotient) tests such as the Wechsler Intelligence Scales for Children, 3rd Edition (WISC-III; Wechsler, 1991) Stanford-Binet Intelligence Scales, 4th Edition (Thorndike, Hagen, & Sattler, 1986a, 1986b), and Kaufman Assessment Battery for Children (K-ABC; Kaufman & Kaufman, 1983). Recently, adaptive skills have been incorporated in the definition of mental retardation; thus, adaptive tests are used in the assessment of mental retardation including the Vineland Adaptive Behavior Scales (Sparrow, Balla, & Cicchetti, 1984) and the Adaptive Behavior Assessment System (Harrison & Oakland, 2000). Today, the combination of intelligence and social adaptive measures of functioning are applied in the diagnosis of mental retardation.

Neuropsychological testing has been used to distinguish among individuals with mental retardation that might have another disorder. For instance, Palmer (2006) compared performances in neuropsychological testing among 10 individuals with comorbid mental retardation and dementia with 12 individuals with only mental retardation. The comparison was based on measures of attention, executive functions, language, dementia screening, as well as memory and learning. Palmer's results indicated that there are significant differences in neurocognitive measures between the two groups. Although participants from the dementia group showed more severe defects in memory and learning, agnosia, semantic verbal fluency as well as attention and executive functions, both groups did show significant neuropsychological deficits.

In another study, Shultz et al. (2004) evaluated screening tools for dementia in 38 older adults with mental retardation. The instruments used included the dementia scale for Down's syndrome (Gedye, 1995), the Dementia Questionnaire for Mentally Retarded Persons, and the Reiss Screen for Maladaptive Behavior. It was found that the dementia scale for Down's syndrome and the Dementia Questionnaire were accurate in assessing dementia. However, a slight difference in effectiveness from the Dementia Questionnaire might be because mentally retarded individuals show less cognitive symptoms of dementia, which puts the dementia scale for Down's syndrome at a disadvantage against the Dementia Questionnaire.

Neuropsychological tests have also been used in the assessment of cognitive deficits in individuals with mental retardation. Vicari, Albertini, and Caltagirone (1992) identified cognitive profiles of 32 adolescents with mental retardation using neuropsychological assessment, which included measures of verbal functions, memory, visuoconstructive and visuospatial skills. Results from Vicari et al. indicated that the neuropsychological test battery distinguished cognitive profiles of participants with mental retardation. Furthermore, findings suggest that (a) since cognitive deficits of mental retardation vary depending on the skills impaired and the severity of the deficits, then mental retardation impairment is heterogeneous across all skills; and (b) a set of neuropsychological assessments exploring single cognitive functions is necessary to accurately identify and understand cognitive profiles from individuals with mental retardation.

Assessment of mental retardation has been a complicated issue for educators, psychologists, and mental health professionals particularly because the cognitive and language skills of individuals with mental retardation make the assessment difficult (Smith, 2005). For instance, Flynn (2000) suggested a change to adaptive behavior tests instead of intelligence tests because of the lack of justification of an IQ criterion as related with impaired adaptive behavior. Similarly, Graue et al. (2007) compared Wechsler Adult Intelligence Scale, 3rd Edition (WAIS III) scores among 26 participants with mild mental retardation and 25 community volunteers who feigned mental retardation. Consistent with criticisms toward intelligence measures, Graue et al. found no significant difference between IQ scores, thus the scores from WAIS III did not distinguish individuals who feigned from individuals with genuine mental retardation.

Despite the social and professional criticisms, intelligence measures are supported as the primary tool in the diagnosis of mental retardation. Umphress (2008) compared IQ test scores from the Reynolds Intellectual Assessment Scales (RIAS; Reynolds &

Kamphaus, 1998) and the WAIS III to investigate whether results are comparable when measures are given by a same tester on the same day. Umphress found similar IQ scores in general, but significant difference between RIAS and WAIS III scores less than 80 was present. Similarly, Watkins and Campbell (1992) found the WAIS-R to be stable and reliable in a sample of 50 adults with mental retardation during 2–5 years, which was consistent with results from Rosen, Stallings, Floor, and Nowakiwska (1968).

Neuropsychological testing has also been applied to identify individuals who might be feigning mental retardation. For example, Marshall and Happe (2007) studied which neuropsychological tests of effort and motivation would be appropriate if feigning of cognitive deficits might be present. They administered a comprehensive neuropsychological battery to 100 mentally retarded participants including the WAIS III (Wechsler, 1997), the Wechsler Memory Scale (WMS) III (Wechsler, 1997), the forced choice recognition portion of the California Verbal Learning Test II (CVLT-II; Delis, Kramer, Kaplan, & Ober, 2000), and Vocabulary Digit Span Test from the WAIS III Digit Span Test (Mittenberg, Theroux-Fichera, Zilinski, & Heibronner, 1995). It was found by Marshall and Happe that the scores from the forced portion of the CVLT-II, WMS III, and V-DS difference score are appropriate to distinguish individuals who might be feigning mental retardation.

TREATMENT

John F. Kennedy's administration proposed a new approach toward mental retardation in the 1960s with a focus on prevention, treatment, and rehabilitation (Kennedy, 1963). Such a policy marked a shift in terms of the importance of mental retardation as a relevant issue in society. Thus, an emphasis has been placed not only on the treatment of mental retardation as a disorder but also efforts have been directed toward finding ways to promote increased social engagement of individuals with mental retardation. Dykens (2006) supported the application of positive psychology on mental retardation with a focus on positive mental states such as happiness, contentment, hope, engagement, and strengths. Similarly, Favell, Realon, and Sutton (1996) examined individuals with severe and profound mental retardation from two intermediate care facilities. According to Favell et al. facial expressions could be applied as a practical method of measuring happiness in individuals with mental retardation.

Other treatments of mental retardation have the objective of integrating individuals with mental retardation to relatively normal life. For instance, LeBlanc, Hagopian, and Maglieri (2000) found that token economy with response cost procedure is effective in eliminating inappropriate social interaction, verbal aggression, and inappropriate sexual behavior in 26-year-old mentally retarded males. In another study, it was found that interactions between peer buddies improved communication behaviors, reciprocity of interactions, and enhanced range of communication behaviors in five high school students with mental retardation (Hughes et al., 2002).

Carlos Ojeda
Antonio E. Puente

American Psychiatric Association. (2000). *Diagnostic and statistical manual of mental disorders* (4th ed., text revision). Washington, DC: Author.

Brown, B. (1847). *The treatment and cure of cretins and idiots: With an account of a visit to the institution on the Abendberg, canton of Berne, Switzerland, during the summer of 1846.* Boston: William D. Ticknor & Co.

Burke, C. (1995). Foreword. In L. Nadel & D. Rosenthal (Eds.), *Down syndrome: Living and learning in the community* (p. ix). New York: Willey.

Delis, D. C., Kramer, J. H., Kaplan, E., & Ober, B. A. (2000). *California Verbal Learning Test* (2nd ed.). San Antonio, TX: The Psychological Corporation, Harcourt Assessment Company.

Dykens, E. M. (2006). Toward a positive psychology of mental retardation. *American Journal of Orthopsychiatry, 76,* 185–193.

Favell, J., Realon, R., & Sutton, K. (1996). Measuring and increasing the happiness of people with profound mental retardation and physical handicaps. *Behavioral Interventions, 11,* 47–58.

Flynn, J. (2000). The hidden history of IQ and special education: Can the problems be solved? *Psychology, Public Policy, and Law, 6,* 191–198.

Gedye, A. (1995). *Dementia Scale for Down Syndrome. Manual.* Vancouver, BC: Gedye Research and Consulting.

Graue, L. O., Berry, D. T., Clark, J. A., Sollman, M. J., Cardi, M., Hopkins, J., et al. (2007). Identification of feigned mental retardation using the new generation of malingering detection instruments: Preliminary findings. *Clinical Neuropsychologist, 21,* 929–942.

Harrison, P. L., & Oakland, T. (2000). *Adaptive behavior assessment system.* San Antonio, TX: The Psychological Corporation.

Hughes, C., Copeland, S. R., Wehmeyer, M. L., Agran, M., Cai, X., & Hwang, B. (2002). Increasing social interaction between general education high school students and their peers with mental retardation. *Journal of Developmental and Physical Disabilities, 14,* 387–402.

Kaufman, A. S., & Kaufman, N. L. (1983). *K-ABC; Kaufman Assessment Battery for Children*. Circles Pines, MN: American Guidance Service.

Kennedy, J. (1963). Mental illness and mental retardation. Message from the president of the United States relative to mental illness and mental retardation. *American Psychologist, 18,* 280–289.

Lane, H. L. (1976). *The wild boy of Aveyron*. Cambridge: Harvard University Press.

LeBlanc, L., Hagopian, L., & Maglieri, K. (2000). Use of a token economy to eliminate excessive inappropriate social behavior in an adult with developmental disabilities. *Behavioral Interventions, 15,* 135–143.

Luckasson, R., Borthwick-Duffy, S., Buntinx, W., Coulter, D., Craig, E., Reeve, A., et al. (2002). *Mental retardation: Definition, classification, and systems of supports* (10th ed.). Washington, DC: American Association on Mental Retardation.

Marshall, P., & Happe, M. (2007). The performance of individuals with mental retardation on cognitive tests assessing effort and motivation. *The Clinical Neuropsychologist, 21,* 826–840.

Mittenberg, W., Theroux-Fichera, S., Zilinski, R., & Heibronner, R. (1995). Identification of malingered head injury on the Wechsler Adult Intelligence Scale-Revised. *Professional Psychology: Research and Practice, 26,* 491–498.

Palmer, G. A. (2006). Neuropsychological profiles of persons with mental retardation and dementia. *Research in Developmental Disabilities, 27,* 299–308.

Reynolds, C. R., & Kamphaus, R. W. (2003). *Manual for the Reynolds Intellectual Assessment Scales and the Reynolds Intellectual Screening Test*. Lutz, FL: Psychological Assessment Resources.

Rosen, M., Stallings, L., Floor, L., & Nowakiwska, M. (1968). Reliability and stability of Wechsler IQ scores for institutionalized mental subnormals. *American Journal of Mental Deficiency, 73,* 218–225.

Shultz, J., Aman, M., Kelbey, T., Wallace, C. L., Burt, D. B., Primeaux-Hart, S., et al. (2004). Evaluation of screening tools for dementia in older adults with mental retardation. *American Journal of Mental Retardation, 109*(2), 98–110.

Smith, T. C. (2005). Assessment of individuals with mental retardation: Introduction to special issue. *Assessment for Effective Intervention, 30*(4), 1–4.

Sparrow, S., Balla, D. A., & Cicchetti, D. V. (1984). *Vineland Adaptive Behavior Scales*. Circle Pines, MN: American Guidance Service.

Thorndike, R. L., Hagen, E. P., & Sattler, J. M. (1986a) *Stanford-Binet Intelligence Scale* (4th ed.). Chicago: Riverside.

Thorndike, R. L., Hagen, E. P., & Sattler, J. M. (1986b). *Technical manual for the Stanford-Binet Intelligence Scale* (4th ed.). Chicago: Riverside.

Umphress, T. B. (2008). A comparison of low IQ scores from the Reynolds Intellectual Assessment Scales and the

Wechsler Adult Intelligence Scale—Third Edition. *Intellectual and Developmental Disabilities, 46,* 229–233.

Vicari, S., Albertini, G., & Caltagirone, C. (1992). Cognitive profiles in adolescents with mental retardation. *Journal of Intellectual Disability Research, 36,* 415–423.

Volkmar, F., & Dykens, E. (2002). Mental retardation. In M. Rutter & E. Taylor (Eds.). *Child and adolescent psychiatry* (4th ed., pp. 697–710). Oxford: Blackwell.

Watkins, C. Jr., & Campbell, V. (1992). The test-retest reliability and stability of the WAIS-R in a sample of mentally retarded adults. *Journal of Intellectual Disability Research, 36,* 265–268.

Wechsler, D. (1991). *Wechsler Intelligence Scale for Children* (3rd ed.). New York: Psychological Corporation.

Wechsler, D. (1997). *Manual for Wechsler Adult Intelligence Scale* (3rd ed.). San Antonio, TX: The Psychological Corporation.

METACHROMATIC LEUKODYSTROPHY

DESCRIPTION

Metachromatic leukodystrophy (MLD) is a lysosomal storage disorder marked by the accumulation of cerebroside sulfate (sulfatide) within the nervous system and other tissue (Austin, 1959, 1973). Although first described in 1910 by Alzheimer (Austin, 1959), the condition was not fully delineated until 1933 when Greenfield (1933) noted it to be a form of diffuse sclerosis in which oligodendroglial degeneration (Kolodny, 1997) was characteristic. So far, three different clinical subtypes have been described for this disorder—a late infantile form (the most common), a juvenile form (may be subdivided into early and late juvenile forms), and an adult form (Polten et al., 1991). All forms of the disease involve a progressive deterioration of motor and neurocognitive function. The typing is somewhat arbitrary because the types overlap and some cases do not fall neatly within a single type. MLD actually describes a continuum of clinical severity. However, mortality and morbidity rates do vary with earlier onset being associated with a more rapid progression. Collectively, an approximate incidence of 1 out 40,000 births has been suggested with no discrepancies among racial/ethnic groups or sexes.

NEUROPATHOLOGY/PATHOPHYSIOLOGY

Mitochondrial leukodystrophy represents an autosomal-recessive disorder localized to chromosome 22 q13.31 (Moraes et al., 1989). To date more than 60 mutations have been identified (Polten et al., 1991). It results from a deficiency of the lysosomal enzyme arylsulfatase A (ARSA). This deficiency leads to an accumulation of the sulfatides within the central nervous system (CNS) and peripheral nervous system (PNS), especially cerebroside sulfate. This is due to the fact that the sulfatides are stored in the lysosomes of miroglia and neuronal cells within the CNS and Schwann cells of the PNS. The overabundance of the sulfatides (as much as 4–8 times normal amounts) leads to a breakdown of the myelin within these systems. Less commonly, MLD may stem from a deficient cerebroside sulfatase activator protein, saposin B (Kolodny, 1997; Polten et al., 1991). This results in near normal ARSA activity, yet individuals excrete globotriaosylceramide and digalactosylceramide in addition to sulfatides (Wallace et al., 1988) owing to the clinical and pathological overlap. Variations in the allele mutation have been linked with subtype expression.

One variation is pathologically characterized by a G to A transition that eliminates the splice donor site at the start of intron 2, with the resultant total loss of enzyme activity. Homozygosity for this allele and compound heterozygotes (with other unknown allele) are usually associated with late infantile onset. The second pathological variation is characterized by a C to T transition that results in the substitution of leucine for proline at amino acid 426 producing an enzyme with 3% residual activity. It is most commonly associated with the adult onset forms for both homozygous and compound heterozygotes forms. The presence of both alleles is associated with juvenile onset.

A reduction in ARSA activity from 5% to 10% of control values is seen in up to 20% of the healthy population. This nonpathogenic reduction in enzyme activity is caused by homozygosity for a pseudodeficiency allele (Harvey, Carey, & Morris, 1998; Penzien et al., 1993). Individuals who are homozygous for this allele are asymptomatic, although in some, MRI shows lesions of white matter (McFaul, 1982; Zhang et al., 1991).

Histopathological evaluation commonly demonstrates demyelination, gliosis, and macrophages with vacuolated cytoplasm throughout the white matter (Harvey et al., 1998; Kolodny, 1997; Polten et al., 1991, pp. 4–6). The membrane-bound sulfatide containing vacuoles exhibit "metachromasia" when toluidine blue staining is employed presenting as brown or with a golden hue as opposed to the usual blue of myelin. All the involved areas have loss of oligodendroglia. Metachromatic bodies stain strongly positive with periodic acid–Schiff (PAS) and alcian blue in white matter of the brain. Metachromatic granules also are found in the renal tubules, bile duct epithelium, gallbladder, islet cell and ductal epithelium of the pancreas, reticular zone of the adrenal cortex, and liver (Iizuka et al., 2003). Similar changes in peripheral nerves are observed and can be detected in urine also.

NEUROPSYCHOLOGICAL/CLINICAL PRESENTATION

The clinical presentations are discussed separately in relation to the three disease subtype forms.

Late Infantile Subtype

In the late infantile variant, the typical age of onset is between 12 and 18 months. It is characterized by a gait disorder, strabismus, impairment of speech, spasticity, intellectual deterioration that appears gradually, and coarse tremors or athetoid movements of the extremities develop later. Reduced or even absent deep tendon reflexes are also seen. Unexplained bouts of fever, severe abdominal pain, optic atrophy, and seizures are seen as the disease progresses. Death occurs within 6 months to 4 years after the onset of symptoms (Brown et al., 1981). Elevated cerebrospinal fluid (CSF) protein, decreased conduction velocity in the peripheral nerves, and normal electroretinograms are seen (Kim et al., 1997). On MRI, the areas of demyelination are marked by high signal intensity on T2-weighted images seen in the periventricular regions, the centrum semiovale, the splenium, the genu of the corpus callosum, the internal capsule, and the pyramidal tracts. Characteristically, the subcortical white matter, including the arcuate fibers, is spared until late in the disease.

Juvenile Subtype

The juvenile subtype MLD is the most rare in comparison with the infantile (most common) and adult variants (Austin et al., 1968) with neurologic symptoms becoming evident at around 5 years of age, characterized by loss of motor developmental milestones, decreased attention span, speech disturbances, decline in school performance, gait disturbances, tremors, clumsiness, loss of previously achieved skills, intellectual decline, behavioral changes (Alves, Pires, Guimarães, & Miranda, 1986). Older patients develop an organic mental syndrome and progressive corticospinal, corticobulbar, cerebellar, or, rarely, extrapyramidal signs.

M

Adult Subtype

The adult subtype has been observed as early as 15 years of age (Black, Taber, & Hurley, 2003). Clinically, it often first presents with dementia or psychiatric manifestations (Bagary et al., 2003; Denier et al., 2007; Hagberg, Sourander, & Thoren, 1962) — features similar to schizophrenia, post partum psychosis or any nonspecific psychoses. Rarely, the disease begins as a peripheral neuropathy. The variant forms with arylsulfatase-activator deficiency present a clinical picture of late infantile or juvenile MLD.

DIAGNOSIS

The time of onset of neurological symptoms, the presence of ataxia, spasticity, and depressed deep tendon reflexes with elevated CSF protein content and reduced nerve conduction velocity suggest the diagnosis (Maertens & Dyken, 2007). Marked reduction in or absent urinary or leukocyte ARSA activity is seen. Brain MRI shows white matter lesions and atrophy characteristic of MLD but nonspecific. Other nonspecific abnormal laboratory test results include slowed motor nerve conduction velocities, a reduced auditory-evoked brainstem response, and a nonfunctioning gallbladder. Brown metachromatic bodies can be found on biopsy of various peripheral nerves as early as 15 months after the onset of symptoms. Segmental demyelination of peripheral nerves is also seen (Barth, Ward, Harris, Saad, & Fensom, 1994). The confirmation of diagnosis is based on the demonstration of reduced action of ARSA activity in the leucocytes or cultured skin fibroblast (Eto, Tahara, Tokoro, & Maekawa, 1983).

From a differential diagnosis standpoint, in general, ARSA pseudodeficiency, attention deficit hyper-kinetic disorder, Kabre's disease, schizophrenia and other psychoses, antisocial personality disorder, X-linked adrenoleukodystrophy and multiple sulfatase deficiency must all be considered.

TREATMENT

The treatment for this disease requires a multidisciplinary approach. No effective treatment is present to reverse the disease so far. Pharmacological intervention varies and is employed as a means of controlling symptoms. This includes treatment of behavioral problems, feeding difficulties, and for controlling seizures. Bone marrow transplantation (Kapaun et al., 1999; Kidd et al., 1998) may slow the progression of the disease. Recombinant human arylsulfatase A (rhARSA) enzyme (Sevin, Aubourg, & Cartier, 2007)

and gene therapy (Biffi et al., 2006) have shown some efficacy in treatment although these remain experimental. Rehabilitative efforts also play a role in ongoing care. This is often multidisciplinary in approach and involves or may involve occupational therapists, physical therapists, neurologists, ophthalmologists, pediatricians, orthopedists, genetic counselors, psychologists, bone marrow transplant physicians, and metabolic disease specialists. Patient and family education is available from numerous sources and is strongly recommended. In general, prognosis is very poor. In infants, as suggested, progression is relatively rapid. In adults, progression is slower yet insidious.

Gaurav Jain
Sarita Singhal
Chad A. Noggle

Alves, D., Pires, M. M., Guimarães, A., & Miranda, M. C. (1986). Four cases of late onset metachromatic leucodystrophy in a family: Clinical, biochemical and neuropathological studies. *Journal of Neurology, Neurosurgery, & Psychiatry, 49,* 1417–1422.

Austin, J. (1959). Metachromatic sulfatides in cerebral white matter and kidney. *Proceedings of the Society for Experimental Biology and Medicine, 100,* 361–364.

Austin, J. H. (1973). Studies in metachromatic leukodystrophy. *Archives of Neurology, 28,* 258–264.

Austin, J., Armstrong, D., Fouch, S., Mitchell, C., Stumpf, D., Shearer, L., et al. (1968). Metachromatic leukodystrophy (MLD): VIII. MLD in adults: Diagnosis and pathogenesis. *Archives of Neurology, 18,* 225–240.

Bagary, M. S., Symms, M. R., Barker, G. J., Mutsatsa, S. H., Joyce, E. M., & Ron, M. A. (2003). Gray and white matter brain abnormalities in first-episode schizophrenia inferred from magnetization transfer imaging. *Archives of General Psychiatry, 60,* 779–788.

Barth, M. L., Ward, C., Harris, A., Saad, A., & Fensom, A. (1994). Frequency of arylsulphatase A pseudodeficiency associated mutations in a healthy population. *Journal of Medical Genetics, 31,* 667–671.

Biffi, A., Capotondo, A., Fasano, S., del Carro, U., Marchesini, S., Azuma, H., et al. (2006). Gene therapy of metachromatic leukodystrophy reverses neurological damage and deficits in mice. *The Journal of Clinical Investigation, 116*(11), 3070–3082.

Black, D. N., Taber, K. H., & Hurley, R. A. (2003). Metachromatic leukodystrophy: A model for the study of psychosis. *The Journal of Neuropsychiatry and Clinical Neurosciences, 15,* 289–293.

Brown, F. R., III, Shimizu, H., McDonald, J. M., Moser, A. B., Marquis, P., Chen, W. W., et al. (1981). Auditory evoked brainstem response and high-performance liquid chromatography sulfatide assay as early indices of metachromatic leukodystrophy. *Neurology, 31,* 980–985.

Denier, C., Orgibet, A., Roffi, F., Jouvent, E., Buhl, C., Niel, F., et al. (2007). Adult-onset vanishing white matter leukoencephalopathy presenting as psychosis. *Neurology, 68,* 1538–1539.

Eto, Y., Tahara, T., Tokoro, T., & Maekawa, K. (1983). Various sulfatase activities in leukocytes and cultured skin fibroblasts from heterozygotes for the multiple sulfatase deficiency (Mukosulfatidosis). *Pediatric Research, 17,* 97–100.

Greenfield, J. G. (1933). A form of progressive cerebral sclerosis in infants associated with primary degeneration of the interfascicular glia. *The Journal of Neurology and Psychopathology, 13,* 289–302.

Hagberg, B., Sourander, P., & Thoren, L. (1962). Peripheral nerve changes in the diagnosis of metachromatic leucodystrophy. *Acta Paediatrica Scandinavica, 51*(Suppl. 13S), 63–71.

Harvey, J. S., Carey, W. F., & Morris, C. P. (1998). Importance of the glycosylation and polyadenylation variants in metachromatic leukodystrophy pseudodeficiency phenotype. *Human Molecular Genetics, 7,* 1215–1219.

Kapaun, P., Dittmann, R. W., Granitzny, B., Eickhoff, W., Wulbrand, H., & Neumaier-Probst, E. (1999). Slow progression of juvenile metachromatic leukodystrophy 6 years after bone marrow transplantation. *Journal of Child Neurology, 14,* 222–228.

Kidd, D., Nelson, J., Jones, F., Dusoir, H., Wallace, I., McKinstry, S., et al. (1998). Long-term stabilization after bone marrow transplantation in juvenile metachromatic leukodystrophy. *Archives of Neurology, 55,* 98–99.

Kim, T. S., Kim, I. O., Kim, W. S., Choi, Y. S., Lee, J. Y., Kim, O. W., et al. (1997). MR of childhood metachromatic leukodystrophy. *AJNR. American Journal of Neuroradiology, 18,* 733–738.

Kolodny, E. H. (1997). Metachromatic leukodystrophy and multiple sulfatase deficiency: Sulfatide lipidosis. In R. N. Rosenberg, et al. (Ed.), *The molecular and genetic basis of neurological disease* (2nd ed., pp. 433–442). Boston: Butterworth–Heinemann.

Martens, P., & Dyken, R. (2007). Storage diseases: Neuronal ceroid-lipofuscinoses, lipidoses, glycogenoses, and leukodystrophies. In C. Goetz (Ed.), *Textbook of clinical neurology* (pp. 612–639). Philadelphia, PA: Saunders Elsevier.

McFaul, R. (1982). Metachromatic leucodystrophy: Review of 38 cases. *Archives of Disease in Childhood, 57,* 168–175.

Menkes, J. H. (1966). Chemical studies of two cerebral biopsies in juvenile metachromatic leukodystrophy: The molecular composition of cerebroside and sulfatides. *Journal of Pediatrics, 69,* 422–431.

Penzien, J. M., Kappler, J., Herschkowitz, N., Schuknecht, B., Leinekugel, P., Propping, P., et al. (1993). Compound heterozygosity for metachromatic leukodystrophy and arylsulfatase: A pseudodeficiency allele is not associated with progressive neurological disease. *American Journal of Human Genetics, 52,* 557–564.

Polten, A., Fluharty, A. L., Fluharty, C. B., Kappler, J., von Figura, K., & Gieselmann, V. (1991). Molecular basis of different forms of metachromatic leukodystrophy. *The New England Journal of Medicine, 324,* 18–22.

Sevin, C., Aubourg, P., & Cartier, N. (2007). Enzyme, cell and gene-based therapies for metachromatic leukodystrophy. *Journal of Inherited Metabolic Disease, 30*(2), 175–183.

Zhang, X. L., Rafi, M. A., DeGala, G., & Wenger, D. A. (1991). The mechanism for a 33 nucleotide insertion in mRNA causing sphingolipid activator protein (SAP1) deficient metachromatic leukodystrophy. *Human Genetics, 87,* 211–215.

MICROCEPHALY

DESCRIPTION

Microcephaly is a neurodevelopment disorder describing a patient with an abnormally smaller head circumference than others. Head measurements tend to be smaller by more than two standard deviations compared with average size for the age, sex, race, and period of gestation of the individual. Development of the disorder may occur congenitally, being present at birth, or over the first few years of life. The comparison is normally obvious when comparing the head size to the rest of the body. The smaller head is normally a result of an underdeveloped brain (Dekaban & Sadowsky, 1978), which indicates high propensities toward mental retardation.

The presentation is largely descriptive in nature representing a feature/symptom of a primary presentation. Specifically, microcephaly is associated with a number of presentations including but not limited to certain cephalic, genetic/chromosomal disorders, neurometabolic syndromes, and prenatal teratogenic processes. In many respects, the degree of growth impairment (i.e., how small the head is) demonstrates a negative linear relationship with the severity of functional impairments such that the smaller the head is the greater the deficits. These deficits may present as general mental retardation or as domain-specific abnormalities such as speech and language delays or sensorimotor deficits. There is also increased

M

prevalence of other neurological issues such as seizures as well as additional morphological anomalies such as facial-structural anomalies and widespread musculoskeletal dwarfism.

NEUROPATHOLOGY/PATHOPHYSIOLOGY

Microcephaly presents secondary to either halted growth of the cortex or premature closure and fusion of cranial plates. In both instances, microcephaly is best categorized as a symptom of a large-scale presentation that constitutes the underlying pathology. Ross and colleagues (1977) classified microcephaly dichotomously based on whether there is or is no associated malformations. Microcephaly vera represents a primary hereditary form of microcephaly in which by adulthood the skull is as much as 3–5 standard deviations below the mean for circumference (Golden & Bonnemann, 2007). The presentation is associated with other morphological traits including normal facial size but with a narrow and sharply receding forehead, and globally reduced stature. At birth infants present with an anthropoid appearance (Ropper & Brown, 2005). As would be expected, the staunch reduction in head circumference corresponds with prominent functional impairments including moderate to severe mental retardation and motor limitations. Two genes have been identified thus far in relation to this presentation including microcephalin (*MCPH1*) and *ASPM* (Bond et al., 2002)

In regard to microcephaly occurring secondary to disrupted brain growth, this has been noted in association with genetic/chromosomal disorders, neurometabolic disorders, and neurodevelopmental/neuromigrational disorders that have their own pathological bases. Some examples include lissencephaly, Down's syndrome, and phenylketonuria (PKU) (untreated). To date, microcephaly has been associated with 176 different syndromes in which at least one case of microcephaly has been reported (Van Allen et al., 1993). A more refined synthesis of the literature by Jones and colleagues (MRC, 1991) demonstrated that 39 syndromes have been identified in which microcephaly is seen as a primary characteristic whereas 21 others are occasionally associated with resulting microcephaly.

Sporadic microcephaly that seems unassociated with other structural anomalies often suggests a teratogenic (e.g., infectious or toxic) basis (Hanshaw et al., 1985). These include maternal substance use/abuse such as alcohol or cocaine and diseases such as cytomegalovirus, measles, and/or chickenpox. Other developments of microcephaly may be due to instances of trauma particularly in the third trimester of pregnancy.

The brain is characterized by a general reduction in the number of primary and secondary sulci. The cortex oftentimes is thicker than usual with diminished numbers of neurons, and there are higher rates of associated cerebellar hypoplasia and degeneration of the substantia nigra (Golden & Bonnemann, 2007; Ropper & Brown, 2005).

NEUROPSYCHOLOGICAL/CLINICAL PRESENTATION

As noted, microcephaly commonly manifests secondary to other primary presentations (e.g., Down's syndrome). Consequently, these presentations correspond with their own clinical picture that goes beyond the functional afflictions purely associated with microcephaly itself. Still, particular features have been correlated with microcephaly. Morphologically, patients with microcephaly are often easy to notice because of their narrow, receded forehead, pointed vortex, and flattened occiput. However, they generally have normal facial features. This is a result of the face growing at normal rates despite the lack of head growth.

Depending on brain development, patients may present with hyperactivity and mental retardation, varying in degree based on severity of cognitive deficit. Increased prevalence of seizures and convulsions has been associated with the presentation, and varying degrees of motor impairments are observed.

DIAGNOSIS

Diagnosis of microcephaly is purely morphologically based. Current guidelines stipulate a threshold of head circumference of approximately two standard deviations below the mean in comparison with normative data based on sex, body size, and developmental stage (Droghari et al., 1987). X-ray may be utilized to evaluate cranial sutures and plates whereas MRI and CT may be employed to evaluate brain integrity. Genetic testing and metabolic evaluations may be utilized to evaluate for potential underlying causes. Neuropsychological evaluation, physical and occupational therapy evaluations, and speech evaluations are useful in identifying potential underlying impairments.

TREATMENT

There is no standard treatment for microcephaly. Treatment is symptom based, corresponding with the functional deficits associated with the microcephaly itself or in relation to the underlying pathology.

Consequently, treatment may include speech, occupational, or physical therapy. Special education services may be required to address academic deficits if they exist. If neurological symptoms such as seizures or convulsions present, medicinal intervention may be used. In instances where the presentation occurs secondary to premature fusion of cranial plates, surgical intervention may be used. Although such interventions can be employed to promote a normal lifestyle as much as possible, microcephaly is still associated with a reduced life expectancy compared with normal healthy persons.

J. Aaron Albritton
Chad A. Noggle

Bond, J., Roberts, E., Mochida, G. H., Hampshire, D. J., Scott, S., Askham, J. M., et al. (2002). ASPM is a major determinant of cerebral cortical size. *Nature Genetics, 32*, 316–320.

Dekaban, A. S., & Sadowsky, D. (1978). Changes in brain weights during the span of human life: Relation of brain weights to body heights and body weights. *Annals of Neurology, 4*, 345–356.

Droghari, E., Smith, I., Beasley, M., & Lloyd, J. K. (1987). Timing of strict diet in relation to fetal damage in maternal phenylketonuria. *Lancet, ii*, 927–930.

Eichorn, D. H., & Bayley, N. (1962). Growth in head circumference from birth through adulthood. *Child Development, 33*, 257–271.

Golden, J., & Bonnemann, C. (2007). Developmental structural disorders. In C. Goetz (Ed), *Textbook of clinical neurology* (pp. 562–591). Philadelphia, PA: Saunders Elsevier.

Gruenwald, P., & Minh, H. (1960). Evaluation of body and organ weights in perinatal pathology. I. Normal standard derived from autopsies. *American Journal of Clinical Pathology, 39*, 247–253.

Hanshaw, J. B., Dudgeon, J. A., & Marshall, W. C. (1985). *Viral diseases of the fetus and newborn* (2nd ed.). Philadelphia, PA: W. B. Saunders.

Larroche, J. C., & Maunoury, T. (1973). Analyse statistique de la croissance ponderale des foetus et des visceres pendant la vie intrauterine. *Archives Francaises de Pediatrie, 30*, 927–949.

MRC Vitamin Study Research Group. (1991). Prevention of neural tube defects: Results of the Medical Research Council Vitamin Study. *Lancet, 338*, 131–137.

Nellhaus, G. (1968). Head circumference from birth to eighteen years. Practical composite international and interracial graphs. *Pediatrics, 41*, 106–119.

Potter, E. L., & Craig, J. M. (Eds.) (1976). *Pathology of the fetus and infant* (3rd ed.). Chicago, IL: Year Book Publishers.

Remington, J. S., & Klein, J. O. (1976). *Infectious disease of the fetus and newborn infant.* Philadelphia, PA: W. B. Saunders.

Ropper, A. H., & Brown, R. H. (2005). *Adams and Victor's principles of neurology* (8th ed.). New York, NY: McGraw-Hill.

Ross, J. J., Frias, J. L., Vinken, P. J., & Bruyn, G. W. (Eds.) (1977). Microcephaly. In *Handbook of clinical neurology* (pp. 507–524). Amsterdam, The Netherlands: North-Holland Publishing Co.

Van Allen, M. I., Kalousek, D. K., Chernoff, G. F., Jurilloff, D., Harris, M., McGillivray, B. C., et al. (1993). Evidence for multisite closure of the neural tube in humans. *American Journal of Medical Genetics, 47*, 723–743.

MIGRAINES

DESCRIPTION

A survey of neurologists found that patients seek consultation for headaches more than any other complaint and represent up to one-third of total patients in their care (World Health Organization [WHO], 2004). Migraines constitute a common primary headache disorder that are marked by severe pain on one or both sides of the head, nausea or upset stomach, and hypersensitivity to sound or light (International Headache Society, 2004). The pain is often described as pulsating and of moderate to severe intensity. A majority of patients experience pain localized to one side of the head, though this pain may eventually spread to the other side. A subset of migraine sufferers experience neurological symptoms that may include sensory, perceptual, motor, and/or cognitive disturbances; these symptoms are known as the migraine aura (Hooker & Raskin, 1986). These symptoms tend to resolve within 1 hour but lead to the onset of a migraine. Migraine attacks can last from 4 to 72 hours and most commonly affect adults between the ages of 35 and 45 years. It is estimated that approximately 6–8% of men and 15–18% of women experience some form of migraine each year. Further, migraines have been identified as one of the top 20 causes of disability among adults of all ages; as a result, estimates of their financial cost to society are high (WHO, 2004).

NEUROPATHOLOGY/PATHOPHYSIOLOGY

As a primary headache disorder, migraines are believed to have a genetic basis, though exact etiology remains largely unknown (Gardner, 2006). A vascular theory of migraine was widely accepted for many years, wherein it was thought that the pain associated with migraine headaches was the result of dilated cranial vessels (Wolff, 1948). This model has been criticized due to recent research suggesting that cranial vessel dilation is not necessary for migraine pain to occur (e.g., Schoonman et al., 2008).

A more recent theory of migraine pathophysiology points to a neurogenic origin and classifies migraine as a CNS disorder (Agnoli & De Marinis, 1985; Cutrer & Charles, 2008). Headache pain is believed to be generated centrally and to involve the serotonergic system (Goadsby, 2000; Hamel, 2007; Hargreaves & Shepheard, 1999; Silberstein, 2004). A range of evidence implicating serotonin in the experience and prevention of acute attacks supports this theory (e.g., Ferrari, Roon, Lipton, & Goadsby, 2001; Silberstein, 2005).

Today clinicians widely agree that migraine is a neurovascular disorder, though recent evidence from human imaging studies suggests that vasodilation may not play an important role in headache pathophysiology (Schoonman et al., 2008). Future research utilizing technological advancements will likely elucidate the neuropathological mechanisms of migraine.

NEUROPSYCHOLOGICAL/CLINICAL PRESENTATION

Neuropsychological testing may play a role in determining the impact of migraines on an individual's cognitive functioning, but evidence of cognitive declines in migraine sufferers is presently inconclusive (O'Bryant, Marcus, Rains, & Penzien, 2006). In reality, research on neuropsychological profiles associated with migraine is limited despite the prevalence and severity of migraine headaches. Even those studies examining relationships between cognitive performance and migraines have led to conflicting findings. Although some studies suggest that there are no significant differences in cognitive functioning between migraine sufferers and healthy controls (e.g., Bell, Primeau, Sweet, & Lofland, 1999), other studies indicate that migraine patients show deficits across a number of neuropsychological domains (e.g., Hooker & Raskin, 1986).

In a study by Bell et al. (1999), cognitive performance of patients with chronic migraines, patients with nonheadache chronic pain, and patients with mild traumatic brain injury (TBI) were compared. Across domains of cognitive efficiency, memory, and visuoperceptual ability, no differences between chronic pain and migraine patients were found,

though the mild TBI patients performed significantly worse. Notably, this study did not include a control group of healthy subjects. However, a large community study suggests that these findings hold across the life span among people with and without migraine; though age is predictive of cognitive functioning, migraine diagnosis is not (Jelicic, van Boxtel, Houx, & Jolles, 2000).

That being said, a body of literature suggests that the cognitive abilities of migraine sufferers versus healthy controls do indeed differ, especially across memory and attention domains. There is some evidence suggesting that cognitive functioning is impaired among migraine sufferers only when they are experiencing an acute attack (Meyer, Thornby, Crawford, & Rauch, 2000). Other investigations suggest more lasting impairment in cognitive functioning.

For example, Hooker and Raskin (1986) compared migraine patients with and without aura to healthy controls, finding that both migraine groups obtained significantly lower scores than the control group on a tactual learning task and delayed story recall. Furthermore, migraine without aura patients significantly outperformed migraine with aura patients on the grooved pegboard and aphasia screening tasks. These results led Hooker and Raskin to conclude that migraine sufferers experience greater impairment on a neuropsychological battery than those without migraines. In addition, they argue that migraine with aura may lead to greater functional impairment than migraine without aura, though other evidence suggests that impairments are greater for those with migraine without aura across verbal memory domains (Le Pira et al., 2000). Another line of research suggests that the length of headache history and frequency of attacks may predict level of impairment (Calandre, Bembibre, Arnedo, & Becerra, 2002). Clearly, additional research is necessary to elucidate the relationships between migraine and neuropsychological functioning.

Associations between migraine and psychological functioning are more straightforward. For example, the experience of migraines increases a person's likelihood of experiencing depression (and vice versa; see Breslau, Lipton, Stewart, Schultz, & Welch, 2003). Relationships between migraine and anxiety have also been uncovered; migraine sufferers are more likely to develop panic disorder than individuals without migraine, and associations between migraine and other anxiety disorders are currently being researched (Silberstein, 2001; Smitherman, Penzien, & Maizels, 2008). Due to the well-established effects of anxiety and depression on cognitive functioning, it is important to consider possible psychiatric comorbidities when evaluating the emotional and cognitive functioning of migraine patients.

DIAGNOSIS

Diagnosis of migraines is largely based on clinical presentation and symptom report. As suggested earlier, migraines are divided into two major subtypes: migraine with aura and migraine without aura (International Headache Society, 2004). To meet criteria for migraine without aura, a patient must have experienced five or more headache attacks lasting anywhere from 4 to 72 hours. The headaches must be characterized by two or more of the following symptoms: moderate to severe pain, pulsating quality, unilateralization, and exacerbation by routine physical activity. Furthermore, at least one of the following symptoms should accompany the attack: nausea or vomiting, sensitivity to light, and/or sensitivity to sound.

Migraine with aura was previously identified as "classic" migraine. To meet criteria for migraine with aura, the patient must have experienced neurological symptoms that last for less than 60 minutes; these neurological symptoms must occur either before, during, or after a headache with symptoms similar to those of migraine without aura.

Although this offers some distinction between migraine types from a descriptor standpoint, diagnosis must more specifically attempt to determine the underlying etiology as they may result from a variety of structural anomalies including tumors, infections, and vascular malformations. Cerebrovascular presentation must also be considered as should metabolic issues, hypoxia, hypoglycemia, as well as various other presentations. Differential diagnosis must consider other primary headache disorders such as cluster headaches, hypnic headaches, short-lasting, unilateral, neuralgiform headache attacks with conjunctival injection and tearing headaches, and tension-type headaches (Siloberstein & Young, 1995).

TREATMENT

Treatment for migraines typically involves some form of pharmacological intervention. Serotonin agonists have been shown to be successful in the treatment of acute headache attacks and several preventive forms of pharmacotherapy are effective, including GABA inhibitors, beta-adrenergic blocking agents, and tricyclic antidepressants (Goadsby, 2000). Analgesics and anti-inflammatory medications have also been shown to successfully treat acute attacks (Lipton et al., 1998).

Biofeedback and relaxation training are also sometimes used to provide relief from migraine pain. Research suggests that such techniques are effective, with comparable effectiveness to prophylactic medication (Andrasik, 2004).

Amy R. Steiner
Chad A. Noggle
Amanda R. W. Steiner

Agnoli, A., & De Marinis, M. (1985). Vascular headaches and cerebral circulation: An overview. *Cephalagia, 5,* 9–15.

Andrasik, F. (2004). Behavioral treatment of migraine: Current status and future directions. *Expert Review of Neurotherapeutics, 4,* 403–413.

Bell, B. D., Primeau, M., Sweet, J. J., & Lofland, K. R. (1999). Neuropsychological functioning in migraine headache, nonheadache chronic pain, and mild traumatic brain injury patients. *Archives of Clinical Neuropsychology, 14,* 389–399.

Breslau, N., Lipton, R. B., Stewart, W. F., Schultz, L. R., & Welch, K. M. (2003). Comorbidity of migraine and depression: Investigating potential etiology and prognosis. *Neurology, 60,* 1308–1312.

Calandre, E. P., Bembibre, J., Arnedo, M. L., & Becerra, D. (2002). Cognitive disturbances and regional cerebral blood flow abnormalities in migraine patients: Their relationship with the clinical manifestations of the illness. *Cephalalgia, 22,* 291–302.

Cutrer, F. M., & Charles, A. (2008). The neurogenic basis of migraine. *Headache, 48,* 1411–1414.

Ferrari, M. D., Roon, K. I., Lipton, R. B., & Goadsby, P. J. (2001). Oral triptans (serotonin 5-HT(1B/1D) agonists) in acute migraine treatment: A meta-analysis of 53 trials. *Lancet, 42,* 1668–1675.

Gardner, K. L. (2006). Genetics of migraine: An update. *Headache, 46,* S19–S24.

Goadsby, P. J. (2000). The pharmacology of headache. *Progress in Neurobiology, 62,* 509–525.

Hamel, E. (2007). Serotonin and migraine: Biology and clinical implications. *Cephalalgia, 27,* 1293–1300.

Hargreaves, R. J., & Shepheard, S. L. (1999). Pathophysiology of migraine: New insights. *Canadian Journal of Neurological Sciences, 26,* 12–19.

Hooker, W. D., & Raskin, N. H. (1986). Neuropsychologic alterations in classic and common migraine. *Archives of Neurology, 43,* 709–712.

International Headache Society (2004). Migraine. *Cephalalgia: An International Journal of Headache, 24,* 24–36.

Jelicic, M., van Boxtel, M. P., Houx, P. J., & Jolles, J. (2000). Does migraine headache affect cognitive function in the elderly? Report from the Maastricht Aging Study (MAAS). *Headache, 40,* 715–719.

Le Pira, F., Zappala, G., Guiffrida, S., Lo Batolo, M. L., Reggio, E., Morana, R., et al. (2000). Memory disturbances

M

in migraine with and without aura: A strategy problem? *Cephalalgia, 20,* 475–478.

Lipton, R. B., Stewart, W. F., Ryan, R. E., Saper, J., Silberstein, S., & Sheftell, F. (1998). Efficacy and safety of acetaminophen, aspirin, and caffeine in alleviating migraine headache pain. *Archives of Neurology, 55,* 210–217.

Meyer, J. S., Thornby, J., Crawford, K., & Rauch, G. M. (2000). Reversible cognitive decline accompanies migraine and cluster headaches. *Headache, 40,* 638–646.

O'Bryant, S. E., Marcus, D. A., Rains, J. C., & Penzien, D. B. (2006). The neuropsychology of recurrent headache. *Headache, 46,* 1364–1376.

Schoonman, G. G., van der Ground, J., Kortmann, C., van der Geest, R. J., Terwindt, G. M., & Ferrari, M. D. (2008). Migraine headache is not associated with cerebral or meningeal vasodilation: A 3T magnetic resonance angiography study. *Brain, 131,* 2192–2200.

Silberstein, S. D. (2001). Shared mechanisms and comorbidities in neurologic and psychiatric disorders. *Headache, 41,* 11–17.

Silberstein, S. D. (2004). Migraine pathophysiology and its clinical implications. *Cephalalgia, 24,* 2–7.

Silberstein, S. D. (2005). Preventive treatment of migraine. *Review of Neurological Diseases, 2,* 167–175.

Silberstein, S. D., & Young, W. B. (1995). Migraine aura and prodrome. *Seminal Neurology, 45,* 175–182.

Smitherman, T. A., Penzien, D. B., & Maizels, M. (2008). Anxiety disorders and migraine intractability and progression. *Current Pain and Headache Reports, 12,* 224–229.

Wolff, H. G. (1948). *Headache and other head pain.* New York: Oxford University Press.

World Health Organization. (2004, March). Headache disorders. *Fact Sheet, 277.*

MILLER FISHER SYNDROME

DESCRIPTION

Miller Fisher syndrome (MFS) is a rare variant of Guillain–Barré syndrome (GBS) (also known as acute inflammatory demyelinating polyneuropathy, acute idiopathic polyradiculoneuritis, acute idiopathic polyneuritis, French polio, Landry's ascending paralysis, and Landry–Guillain–Barré syndrome), which is an acquired nerve disease that is characterized by abnormal muscle coordination, paralysis of the eye muscles, and absence of the tendon reflexes. Several variants of GBS exist, but MFS is relatively common, representing approximately 5% of GBS cases.

The key symptoms of the disorder involve a triad of ataxia (gross lack of coordination of muscle movements), areflexia (complete loss of deep tendon reflexes), and ophthalmoplegia (paralysis of the extraocular muscles). The major difference in the presentation of MFS is that the disease causes a descending paralysis that begins in the upper body and gradually spreads downward, whereas GBS cases tend to cause an ascending paralysis, starting in the legs and moving upward. MFS symptoms typically start in the eye muscles, then slowly descend to the neck and arms. (Mori, Kuwabara, Fukutake, Yuki, & Hattori, 2001). The disease is considered an acute inflammatory demyelinating polyneuropathy (Scelsa & Herskovitz, 2000).

MFS is not typically life-threatening like GBS, but its symptoms can include respiratory failure and are very debilitating. Similar to GBS, MFS may be preceded by a viral illness (Guarino, Stracciari, Cirignotta, D'Alessandro, & Pazzaglia, 1995; Roos, 2007). The majority of individuals with MFS have a unique antibody that characterizes the disorder (Plomp, Molenaar, O'Hanlon, Jacobs, Veitch, Daha, et al., 1999). The disease is considered an acute inflammatory demyelinating polyneuropathy.

GBS was first described by the French physician Jean Landry in 1859. Then, in 1916, Georges Guillain, Jean Alexandre Barré, and Andre Strohl diagnosed two soldiers with the syndrome, but also discovered the key diagnostic abnormalities of the disorder. In 1956, C. Miller Fisher was the first to describe the classic triad of ophthalmoplegia, ataxia, and areflexia as being the hallmark pathology of the disorder (Fisher, 1956).

NEUROPATHOLOGY/PATHOPHYSIOLOGY

All forms of GBS constitute acute inflammatory demyelinating polyneuropathies that are caused by an immune response to a foreign antigen that is mistargeted to nerve tissues. Gangliosides are the faulty targets of the immune system, which are composed of glycosphingolipids and are components of the cell plasma membrane that modulates cell signal transduction events. Gangliosides are present especially in the nodes of Ranvier of nerve tissue (Mori, et al., 2001). Specifically, the GQ1b ganglioside is the target in the MFS. Elevated antibodies to GQ1b are found in MFS and suggest an immune attack against GQ1b gangliosides that are concentrated in the paranodal regions of extraocular nerves (Willison, Veitch, Paterson, & Kennedy, 1993). GBS patients who present with ophthalmoplegia as a symptom also display elevated antibodies to GQ1b (Plomp, et al., 1999). The symptoms of generalized weakness in MFS may be due to motor nerve terminal blockade (Halstead, Humphreys, Goodfellow, Wagner, Smith, & Willison,

2005). The autoimmune attack on the peripheral nerves causes inflammation of the myelin and nerve conduction block, which leads to the symptoms of muscle paralysis, sensory, and/or autonomic disturbances (Mori, et al., 2001).

NEUROPSYCHOLOGICAL/CLINICAL PRESENTATION

MFS typically presents with the classic triad of ataxia (gross lack of coordination of muscle movements), areflexia (complete loss of deep tendon reflexes), and ophthalmoplegia (paralysis of the extraocular muscles). The differentiation from GBS is that MFS symptoms present as a descending paralysis, proceeding in the reverse order of GBS. The acute onset of paralysis of the extraocular muscles is a cardinal feature of MFS. The degree of ataxia in patients tends to be more debilitating than the accompanying sensory loss and is primarily noted during gait and in the trunk, with lesser involvement of the limbs. MFS patient's symptoms may also include ptosis, facial palsy, or bulbar palsy. Symptoms may include mild limb weakness, but motor strength is typically spared (Mori, et al., 2001). Anti-GQ1b antibodies are prominent in MFS, and dense concentrations of GQ1b ganglioside are found in the oculomotor, trochlear, and abducens nerves, which may explain the relationship between anti-GQ1b antibodies and ophthalmoplegia found in the disorder (Plomp, et al., 1999; Willison, et al., 1993). Patients may have reduced or absent sensory nerve action potentials and an absent tibial H reflex. Neuropsychological findings are dependent upon the severity and nature of the deficits found, but may include visual and motor disturbances. Recovery from MFS typically occurs within 1–3 months of the onset of the disorder, so clinical symptoms of the disorder are time limited (Mori, et al., 2001).

DIAGNOSIS

The evaluation and diagnosis of MFS will typically include a thorough physical examination and medical history. The acute onset of the classic triad of ataxia (gross lack of coordination of muscle movements), areflexia (complete loss of deep tendon reflexes), and ophthalmoplegia (paralysis of the extraocular muscles) are typically the presenting symptoms of the disorder. The diagnosis typically also includes the development of descending muscle paralysis, absence of fever, and a likely inciting event. Patients may report problems with coordination, walking, standing, vision problems, tingling, numbness, dizziness, and/or nausea. A spinal tap is typically performed in order to assess the cerebral spinal fluid for elevations in protein levels without an accompanying increase in cell count. Electromyography (EMG) and/or nerve conduction velocity (NCV) tests can also measure nerve conductivity to the muscles by inserting an electrode into the muscle that appears to be affected by the nerve damage. Electrodiagnostic testing is almost always used to diagnose conduction abnormalities and verify the symptoms of the disorder. Neuropsychological findings may include visual and motor disturbances. Unfortunately, due to the acute nature of the disorder, clinical findings may not become abnormal until after the onset symptoms or may be limited to 1–3 months due to recovery from the disorder (Mori, et al., 2001).

TREATMENT

The treatment for MFS is intravenous immunoglobulin (IVIg) or plasmapheresis and supportive care, which is identical to the treatment for GBS (Hughes, Raphael, Swan, & van Doorn, 2006). The immediate concern in treatment is the potential for respiratory failure. Once the patient's vital signs are stabilized and the diagnosis is confirmed, treatment should be initiated immediately because treatment is no longer effective after 2 weeks of the onset of symptoms. Both plasmapheresis and immunoglobulin have been shown to be equally effective and a combination of the two is not significantly better than either alone in treatment. Plasmapheresis, where blood plasma is removed and replaced with fluid, is a procedure in which antibodies are removed from the blood. IVIg is considered an immunomodulator and is beneficial in treating autoimmune disorders (Hughes, et al., 2006). Physical therapy and occupational therapy may be utilized depending on the nature of the patient's deficits. Psychosocial interventions may also be utilized to help the patient overcome any psychological or social ramifications of the disorder.

Eric Silk
Charles Golden

Fisher, M. (1956). An unusual variant of acute idiopathic polyneuritis (syndrome of ophthalmoplegia, ataxia and areflexia). *New England Journal of Medicine, 1956*(255), 57-65.

Guarino, M., Stracciari, A., Cirignotta, F., D'Alessandro, R., & Pazzaglia, P. (1995). Neoplastic meningitis presenting with ophthalmoplegia, ataxia, and areflexia (Miller Fisher syndrome). *Archieves of Neurology, 52*, 443-444.

Halstead, S., Humphreys, P. D., Goodfellow, J. A., Wagner, E. R., Smith, R. A. G., & Willison, H. J. (2005).

Complement inhibition abrogates nerve terminal injury in Miller Fisher syndrome. *Annals of Neurology, 58*, 203-210.

Hughes, R. A., Raphael, J. C., Swan, A. V., & van Doorn, P. A. (2006). Intravenous immunoglobulin of Guillian-Barre syndrome. *Cochrane Database of Systematic Reviews, 25*(1).

Mori, M., Kuwabara, S., Fukutake, T., Yuki, N., & Hattori, T. (2001). Clinical features and prognosis of Miller Fisher syndrome. *Neurology, 56*, 1104-1106.

Plomp, J. J., Molenaar, P. C., O'Hanlon, G. M., Jacobs, B. C., Veitch, J., Daha, et al. (1999). Miller Fisher anti-GQ1b antibodies: Alpha-latrotoxin-like effects on motor end plates. *Annals of Neurology, 45*(6), 189-199.

Roos, K. L. (2007). Viral infections. In C. G. Goetz (Ed.), *Textbook of clinical neurology* (3rd ed., chap. 41). Philadelphia: Saunders Elsevier.

Scelsa, S. N., & Herskovitz, S. (2000). Miller Fisher syndrome: Axonal, demyelinating or both? *Electromyography and Clinical Neurophysiology, 40*, 497-502.

Sharar, E. (2006). Current therapeutic techniques in severe Guillain-Barre syndrome. *Clinical Neuropharmacology, 29*(1), 45–51.

Willison, H. J., Veitch, J., Paterson, G., & Kennedy, P. G. E. (1993). Miller Fisher syndrome is associated with serum antibodies to GQlb ganglioside. *Journal of Neurology, Neurosurgery, and Psychiatry, 56*, 204-206.

Mitochondrial Cardiomyopathy

DESCRIPTION

Since discovery of the first pathogenic mutation of mitochondrial DNA (mtDNA) in 1988, more than 150 distinct mutations of mtDNA have been identified (Ruiz-Pesini et al., 2007). These mutations are associated with a number of different disorders, as nearly all tissues of the body rely upon mitochondrial oxidative phosphorylation for production of adenosine triphosphate. Many of these disorders affect the myocardium because this tissue relies heavily upon oxidative metabolism.

mtDNA is a 16.5-kb circular molecule of double-stranded DNA. Cardiomyopathy is one such manifestation of mitochondrial cytopathies. It rarely constitutes the dominant feature, especially in adults, but case reports have demonstrated that this can be seen (Azevedo et al., 2010). However, epidemiological evidence suggests a relative occurrence in approximately 20% of cases of mitochondrial diseases (Darin et al., 2001). Cardiomyopathy, along with myopathy with encephalopathy, lactic acidosis and stroke-like episodes, chronic progressive external ophthalmoplegia (PEO), deafness, pure myopathy, maternal inherited diabetes, and kidney disease, may all present as phenotypical by-products of these mitochondrial cytopathies inherited from the mother (Chinnery, Howell, Andrews, & Turnbunll, 1999; Donovan & Severin, 2006; Guillausseau et al., 2001; Vilarinho et al., 1999). The presentations manifest as weakness due to defects in energy metabolism and thus muscular weakness. With cardiomyopathy (i.e., weakness of the heart muscles), this can contribute to depleted oxidation and blood flow, most commonly diagnosed with echo Doppler and echocardiogram.

NEUROPATHOLOGY/PATHOPHYSIOLOGY

Mitochondrial cardiomyopathy may result from mutations in nuclear- or mitochondrial-encoded genes and this conveys the complexity of the potential inheritance patterns (e.g., maternal, autosomal recessive). mtDNA is transmitted vertically in a nonmendelian manner from the mother to both male and female progeny due to the fact that during formation of the zygote, the mtDNA is derived exclusively from the oocyte (Hirano, Davidson, & DiMauro, 2001). Thus, it is important to recognize this pattern of inheritance when determining whether a particular family may possess an mtDNA mutation. A problem arises, however, in that maternal relatives with a lower percentage of an mtDNA mutation may possess fewer symptoms (oligosymptomatic) or even be asymptomatic as compared with the proband. Thus, it is important for clinicians to inquire as to the presence of the more subtle symptoms or signs in maternally related members of the family when noting the history of the patient (Hirano et al., 2001).

Polyplasmy is an important principle to consider with regard to mtDNA genetics (Fadic & Johns, 2000). Essentially, each mitochondrian contains several copies of mtDNA and each cell contains multiple mitochondria. As a result, there are potentially many thousands of copies of mtDNA in each cell and alteration of mtDNA may be present in some of the mtDNA molecules (heteroplasmy) or in all of them (homoplasmy). Clinical severity is dependent upon the proportion of mutant mtDNA (Hirano et al., 2001). Mitotic segregation may also influence the expression of mtDNA. As heteroplasmic cells divide, the proportion of mutant mtDNA allocated to daughter cells may shift and vary, altering the degree of heteroplasmy in subsequent generations of cells. This mitotic segregation may partially explain the different phenotypic expressions in patients with mtDNA mutations (Fadic & Johns, 2000; Hirano et al., 2001). Another factor that can influence clinical manifestations of mtDNA mutation is related to the tissue threshold effect, which refers to the balance between energy supply and the oxidative demands of various organs (Fadic & Johns, 2000). Organs and tissues that are metabolically active and more dependent on oxidative metabolism, such as the heart, will be more vulnerable and more frequently affected by mtDNA mutations (Fadic & Johns, 2000; Hirano et al., 2001). Thus, the critical threshold will vary in different tissues and organs (Hirano et al., 2001).

A number of investigations have also examined structural brain changes associated with mitochondrial cardiomyopathy. Mitochondrial diseases may result in structural changes in deep gray matter structures and stroke-like lesions that do not necessarily conform to vascular territories (Saneto, Friedman, & Shaw, 2008). Several case reports have been published detailing MRI findings in patients with Kearns–Sayres syndrome (KSS). These studies have reported that KSS is associated with high-intensity foci (Kamata et al., 1998) and changes in deep gray matter nuclei, (Sacher, Fatterpekar, Edelstein, Sansaricq, & Naidich, 2005) as well as white matter hyperintensities (Hourani, Barada, Al-Kutoubi, & Hourani, 2006; Sacher et al., 2005). Wray, Provenzale, Johns, and Thulborn (1995) examined structural changes based on MRI in a group of patients with mitochondrial myopathy (three with KSS and five with chronic PEO). A variety of abnormal MRI findings were reported, including cerebral cortical and cerebellar atrophy, as well as hyperintensities in the cerebral and cerebellar white matter, basal ganglia, brainstem, and thalamus. It was also noted that the MRI findings did not always conform to specific neurological signs and symptoms.

NEUROPSYCHOLOGICAL/CLINICAL PRESENTATION

Three major clinical entities are associated with sporadic mtDNA deletions and duplications, including KSS, Pearson bone marrow/pancreas syndrome, and sporadic PEO with ragged red fibers (DiMauro et al., 2003). Of these three clinical disorders, cardiac involvement is most prominent in KSS, a multisystem disease defined by an onset before age 20, PEO, and pigmentary retinopathy, in addition to at least one of the following: cardiac conduction block, cerebellar syndrome, and CSF protein greater than 100 mg/dl (Gallastegui, Hariman, Handler, Lev, & Bharati, 1987; Rowland, Hays, DiMauro, DeVivo, & Behrens, 1983).

Cardiac conduction abnormalities often appear years after the development of ptosis and ophthalmoplegia (Channer, Channer, Campbell, & Rees, 1988; Charles, Holt, Kay, Epstein, & Rees, 1981; Marin-Garcia, Goldenthal, Flores-Sarnat, & Sarnat, 2002; Roberts, Perloff, & Kark, 1979) and may include prolonged intraventricular conduction time, bundle-branch block, and atrioventricular block (Hirano et al., 2001). Many patients experience a third-degree atrioventricular block, which is a complete blockage of the electrical conduction from the atrium to the ventricle (Lee et al., 2001; Welzing et al., 2009) and placement of a pacemaker may be a lifesaver for these patients and patients with bifascicular block (Anan et al., 1995; Rheuban, Ayres, Sellers, & DiMarco, 1983). Cardiomyopathy seems to be a less frequent condition and appears much later in the course of illness (Hirano & DiMauro, 1996). Because cardiomyopathy can be fatal (Hubner, Gokel, Pongratz, Johannes, & Park, 1986) and cardioembolic strokes have been reported (Kosinski, Mull, Lethen, & Topper, 1995; Provenzale & VanLandingham, 1996), cardiac transplant may be warranted for some KSS patients (Hirano et al., 2001).

Although primarily considered a disorder of cardiac functioning, recent research has demonstrated that mitochondrial cardiomyopathy can affect cerebral functioning. The cardiogenic embolisms that may arise from mitochondrial cardiomyopathy are thought to be a source of ischemic strokes in this patient population. Provenzale and VanLangingham (1996) reported the case of an individual with KSS who experienced a stroke in the territory of the left middle cerebral artery that was thought to arise from a cardiogenic embolism. Kosinski, Mull, Lethen, and Topper (1995) also reported the case of a patient with KSS who experienced sudden onset of left-sided hemiparesis and was found to have experienced a stroke in the right striatocapsular region. A recent review of the literature suggests that episodes of stroke are a dominant feature of some mitochondrial disorders, including KSS (Finsterer, 2009).

Given the effect of mitochondrial cardiomyopathy on the brain, it is reasonable to conclude that this condition may affect memory and cognitive functioning. However, to date there have been very few studies reported that sought to examine the relationship between mitochondrial cardiomyopathy and neuropsychological functioning. Indeed, a review of the literature found only one such investigation. Bosbach, Kornblum, Schroder, and Wagner (2003) examined neuropsychological functioning in a group of patients with chronic PEO and KSS. They reported a range of neuropsychological deficits within the sample, including visuoconstructional abilities, attention, and cognitive flexibility. Certainly, more research needs to be

M

conducted to further explore the types of neuropsychological deficits seen in patients with mitochondrial cardiomyopathy, including cognitive and memory functioning. Given that stroke is common in these patients and that this disease is associated with diabetes, the possibility also seems to exist that they are at increased risk for vascular dementia as these symptoms are risk factors. Future research will need to explore the validity of this proposition.

DIAGNOSIS

Diagnosis is multifaceted. Given that cardiomyopathy often presents as a secondary manifestation, diagnosis of the broader presentation is also a common part of diagnostic workup. Diagnosis of cardiomyopathy commonly entails a combination of echo Doppler and echocardiogram investigations. The prior allows for evaluation of possible hypertrophic and obstructive properties. Maximal flow velocities permit determination of hypertensive properties and locality. Echocardiogram should be performed to evaluate for features of pericardial effusion, while also giving readings on heart rate as well as QTc and PR intervals (Davignon et al., 1979). Chest X-ray may also be employed.

For consideration of underlying mitochondrial pathology, oximetric measurements and spectrophotometric enzyme analyses on mitochondria, and ultrastructural and enzyme histochemical analyses on muscle biopsies are commonly employed (Tiranti et al., 1999; Tulinius, Holme, Kristiansson, Larsson, & Oldfors, 1991). mtDNA investigation may be undertaken by way of Southern blotting with point mutation investigations (Manouvrier et al., 1995).

TREATMENT

Treatment is symptom based. Some patients require oxygen to counteract deoxygenation. With hypertensive effects, medicinal intervention may be employed; however, this is only used on a case-by-case basis given the risk of cerebrovascular events. Heart transplantation has been employed in instances where patients are deemed viable candidates. Given cardiomyopathy may be seen in conjunction with other phenotypical manifestation such as diabetes and kidney failure, these entities often require medical intervention ranging from medicinal treatment to dialysis. Prognosis can be poor depending on the severity of the constellation of symptoms; interventions can take on a supportive mind-set. Genetic counseling may also be recommended for mothers.

Paul S. Foster
Valeria Drago

Anan, R., Nakagawa, M., Miyata, M., Higuchi, I., Nakao, S., Suehara, M., et al. (1995). Cardiac involvement in mitochondrial diseases: A study on 17 patients with documented mitochondrial DNA defects. *Circulation, 91,* 955–961.

Azevedo, O., Vilarinho, L., Almeida, F., Ferreira, F., Guardado, J., Ferreira, M., et al. (2010). Cardiomyopathy and kidney disease in a patient with maternally inherited diabetes and deafness caused by the 3243A 1 G mutation of mitochondrial DNA. *Cardiology, 115,* 71–74.

Bosbach, S., Kornblum, C., Schroder, R., & Wagner, M. (2003). Executive and visuospatial deficits in patients with chronic progressive external ophthalmoplegia and Kearns-Sayre syndrome. *Brain, 126,* 1231–1240.

Channer, K. S., Channer, J. L., Campbell, M. J., & Rees, J. R. (1988). Cardiomyopathy in the Kearns-Sayre syndrome. *British Heart Journal, 59,* 486–490.

Charles, R., Holt, S., Kay, J. M., Epstein, E. J., & Rees, J. R. (1981). Myocardial ultrastructure and the development of atrioventricular block in Kearns-Sayre syndrome. *Circulation, 63,* 214–219.

Chinnery, P. F., Howell, N., Andrews, R. M., & Turnbull, D. M. (1999). Clinical mitochondrial genetics. *Journal of Medical Genetics, 36,* 425–436.

Darin, N., Oldfors, A., Moslemi, A. R., Holme, E., & Tulinius, M. (2001). The incidence of mitochondrial encephalomyopathies in childhood: Clinical features, morphological, biochemical, and DNA abnormalities. *Annals of Neurology, 49,* 377–383.

Davignon, A., Rautaharju, P., Boisselle, E., Soumis, F., Megelas, M., & Choquette, A. (1979). Percentile charts: ECG standards for children. *Pediatric Cardiology, 1,* 133–152.

DiMauro, S., Bonilla, E., Mancuso, M., Filosto, M., Sacconi, S., Salviati, L., et al. (2003). Mitochondrial myopathies. *Basic and Applied Myology, 13,* 145–155.

DiMauro, S., & Hirano, M. (1998). Mitochondria and heart disease. *Current Opinion in Cardiology, 13,* 190–197.

Donovan, L. E., & Severin, N. E. (2006). Maternally inherited diabetes and deafness in a North American kindred: Tips for making the diagnosis and review of unique management issues. *Journal of Clinical Endocrinology & Metabolism, 91,* 4737–4742.

Fadic, R., & Johns, D. R. (2000). Mitochondrial DNA and the genetics of mitochondrial disease. In S. M. Pulst (Ed.), *Neurogenetics* (pp. 293–315). New York: Oxford University Press.

Finsterer, J. (2009). Management of mitochondrial stroke-like-episodes. *European Journal of Neurology, 16,* 1178–1184.

Gallastegui, J., Hariman, R. J., Handler, B., Lev, M., & Bharati, S. (1987). Cardiac involvement in the Kearns-Sayre syndrome. *American Journal of Cardiology, 60,* 385–388.

Guillausseau, P. J., Massin, P., Dubois-La-Forgue, D., Timsit, J., Virally, M., Gin, H., et al. (2001). Maternally inherited diabetes and deafness: A multicenter study. *Annals of Internal Medicine, 134,* 721–728.

Hirano, M., Davidson, M., & DiMauro, S. (2001). Mitochondria and the heart. *Current Opinion in Cardiology, 16,* 201–210.

Hirano, M., & DiMauro, S. (1996). Clinical features of mitochondrial myopathies and encephalomyopathies. In R. J. M. Lane (Ed.), *Handbook of muscle disease* (pp. 479–504). New York: Marcel Dekker.

Hourani, R. G., Barada, W. M., Al-Kutoubi, A. M., & Hourani, M. H. (2006). Atypical MRI findings in Kearns-Sayre syndrome: T2 radial stripes. *Neuropediatrics, 37,* 110–113.

Hubner, G., Gokel, J. M., Pongratz, D., Johannes, A., & Park, J. W. (1986). Fatal mitochondrial cardiomyopathy in Kearns-Sayre syndrome. *Virchows Archiv: A, Pathological Anatomy and Histopathology, 408,* 611–621.

Kamata, Y., Mashima, Y., Yokoyama, M., Tanaka, K., Goto, Y., & Oguchi, Y. (1998). Patient with Kearns-Sayre syndrome exhibiting abnormal magnetic resonance image of the brain. *Journal of Neuro-ophthalmology, 18,* 284–288.

Kosinski, C., Mull, M., Lethen, H., & Topper, R. (1995). Evidence for cardioembolic stroke in a case of Kearns-Sayre syndrome. *Stroke, 26,* 1950–1952.

Lee, K. T., Lai, W. T., Lu, Y. H., Hwang, C. H., Yen, H. W., Voon, W. C., & Sheu, S. H. (2001). Atrioventricular block in Kearns-Sayre syndrome: A case report. *Kaohsiung Journal of Medical Sciences, 17,* 336–229.

Manouvrier, S., Rötig, A., Hannebique, G., Gheerbrandt, J. D., Royer-Legrain, G., Munnich, A., (1995). Point mutation of the mitochondrial tRNA (Leu) gene (A 3243 G) in maternally inherited hypertrophic cardiomyopathy, diabetes mellitus, renal failure, and sensorineural deafness. *Journal of Medical Genetics, 32,* 654–656.

Marin-Garcia, J., Goldenthal, M. J., Flores-Sarnat, L., & Sarnat, H. B. (2002). Severe mitochondrial cytopathy with complete A-V block, PEO, and mtDNA deletions. *Pediatric Neurology, 27,* 213–216.

Provenzale, J. M., & VanLandingham, K. (1996). Cerebral infarction associated with Kearns-Sayre syndrome-related cardiomyopathy. *Neurology, 46,* 826–828.

Rheuban, K. S., Ayres, N. A., Sellers, T. D., & DiMarco, J. P. (1983). Near-fatal Kearns-Sayre syndrome: A case report and review of clinical manifestations. *Clinical Pediatrics, 22,* 822–825.

Roberts, N. K., Perloff, J. K., & Kark, R. A. P. (1979). Cardiac conduction in the Kearns-Sayre syndrome (A neuromuscular disorder associated with progressive external ophthalmoplegia and pigmentary retinopathy): Report of 2 cases and review of 17 published cases. *American Journal of Cardiology, 44,* 1396–1400.

Rowland, L. P., Hays, A. P., DiMauro, S., DeVivo, D. C., & Behrens, M. (1983). Diverse clinical disorders associated with morphological abnormalities of mitochondria. In C. Cerri & G. Scarlato (Eds.), *Mitochondrial pathology in muscle diseases* (pp. 141–158). Padua: Piccin Medical Publishers.

Ruiz-Pesini, E., Lott, M. T., Procaccio, V., Poole, J. C., Brandon, M. C., Mishmar, D., et al. (2007). An enhanced MITOMAP with a global mtDNA mutational phylogeny. *Nucleic Acids Research, 235*(database issue), D823–D828.

Sacher, M., Fatterpekar, G. M., Edelstein, S., Sansaricq, C., & Naidich, T. P. (2005). MRI findings in an atypical case of Kearns-Sayre syndrome: A case report. *Neuroradiology, 47,* 241–244.

Saneto, R. P., Friedman, S. D., & Shaw, D. W. (2008). Neuroimaging of mitochondrial disease. *Mitochondrion, 8,* 396–413.

Tiranti, V., Jaksch, M., Hofmann, S., Galimberti, C., Hoertnagel, K., Lulli, L., et al. (1999). Loss-of-function mutations of SURF-1 are specifically associated with Leigh syndrome with cytochrome C oxidase deficiency. *Annals of Neurology, 46,* 161–166.

Tulinius, M. H., Holme, E., Kristiansson, B., Larsson, N. G., & Oldfors, A. (1991). Mitochondrial encephalomyopathies in childhood: I. Biochemical and morphological investigations. *The Journal of Pediatrics, 119,* 242–250.

Vilarinho, L., Santorelli, F. M., Coelho, I., Rodrigues, L., Maia, M., Barata, I., et al. (1999). The mitochondrial DNA A3243G mutation in Portugal: Clinical and molecular studies in 5 families. *Journal of the Neurological Sciences, 163,* 168–174.

Welzing, L., von Kleist-Retzow, J. C., Kribs, A., Eifinger, F., Huenseler, C., & Sreeram, N. (2009). Rapid development of life-threatening complete atrioventricular block in Kearns-Sayre syndrome. *European Journal of Pediatrics, 168,* 757–759.

Wray, S. H., Provenzale, J. M., Johns, D. R., & Thulborn, K. R. (1995). MR of the brain in mitochondrial myopathy. *American Journal of Neuroradiology, 16,* 1167–1173.

MITOCHONDRIAL MYOPATHIES

DESCRIPTION

Mitochondrial myopathies and mitochondrial encephalomyopathies (collectively, MMPs) are a heterogenous group of disorders characterized by muscle weakness,

M

often presenting as progressive external ophthalmoplegia (PEO) (Fitzsimons, 1981), and neurological symptoms due to inefficient mitochondria. Mitochondria are responsible for metabolizing nutrients, such as fat, protein, and sugar, into energy for use by the cell. Inefficient mitochondria cannot convert these nutrients, which may result in a lack of energy for cellular processes and an accumulation of nutrient molecules that are toxic to the cell and its organelles. Cells with high energy demands, such as neurons and muscle cells, are most strongly affected by MMP.

Over 40 types of mitochondrial diseases have been identified (Neargarder, Murtagh, Wong, & Hill, 2007), each with its own unique cluster of symptoms, ranging in severity from mild to life threatening. Neurological symptoms may include seizures, stroke-like episodes, migraines, ataxia, and deafness (Finsterer, 2006; Kelly, 2008).

NEUROPATHOLOGY/PATHOPHYSIOLOGY

MMP is typically a matrilineal hereditary disease; however, some adult-onset cases may be the result of a point mutation or deletion within the mitochondrial DNA (Taivassalo, Fu, et al., 1999; Wallace, Lott, Shoffner, & Ballinger, 1994). The severity of the symptoms' expression depends largely upon the percentage of mutant mitochondria inherited from the mother (Kelly, 2008; Wallace et al., 1994). In general, mitochondrial abnormalities occur in skeletal muscle fibers in aged humans. These deficits occur secondary to defects in the respiratory chain enzymes and abnormalities of preoxidation associated with mitochondrial DNA deletions (Hruszkewcyz, 1992; Weller, Cumming, & Mahon, 1997).

NEUROPSYCHOLOGICAL/CLINICAL PRESENTATION

Ataxia and muscle weakness, two of the most common symptoms in MMPs (Kelly, 2008), may present in any muscle tissue—skeletal, cardiac, or smooth—depending upon the specific syndrome. PEO (progressive paralysis of the external ocular muscles) and ptosis (drooping of the eyelid) may cause vision problems that are especially serious in children, due to children's sensitivity to sensory input during certain critical periods. Weakness of the head, neck, mouth, or throat may cause postural difficulties, articulation problems, or difficulty in eating and swallowing. Focal limb paralysis and flaccid paralysis may inhibit an individual's ability to perform daily living tasks and may impair or slow the fine motor control required for many academic tasks, such as writing and

typing. Young children with MMP may have delays in achieving developmental motor milestones such as sitting up, crawling, standing, and walking without support (Kelly, 2008). Conduction block, an abnormality in the heart's ability to maintain a steady pulse, is the result of mitochondrial dysfunction and muscle weakness at the heart's nodes (Kelly, 2008). This may present as either tachycardia (Kitagawa, Odachi, Taniguchi, & Kuzuhara, 2000) or bradycardia (Finsterer, Stöllberger, Steger, & Cozzarini, 2007) and can result in sudden death. Gastrointestinal problems are also common, resulting from dysfunction of the smooth muscle tissue in the digestive tract. Painful gastrointestinal cramping, feelings of fullness, diarrhea, and vomiting are common symptoms (Kelly, 2008) that may affect a patient's vigor and involvement in daily living, social, or academic activities.

Seizures, stroke-like symptoms, and cognitive delays may result from insufficient ATP to fuel neuronal processes. Impairment of executive function, attention, language, memory, and visuospatial functioning has been demonstrated (Neargarder et al., 2007). The stroke-like events commonly seen in mitochondrial myopathy, encephalopathy, lactic acidosis, and stroke-like episodes (MELAS) increase neuronal excitability, creating greater energy demands, and initiate cascades of seizures. If left unchecked, these seizures can create additional stroke-like lesions, beginning the cycle again (Iizuka, 2008). This cycle may lead to permanent, global neural deterioration and dementia. Diabetes is another common symptom of MMPs that impairs blood flow and significantly increases the patient's risk of developing peripheral neuropathy (Fitzsimons, 1981; Kelly, 2008). Peripheral neuropathy impairs the individual's sensorimotor ability, creating difficulties with coordination and pain perception in distal limb areas. Thus, mild injuries may be common and may become severe infections due to poor circulation and lack of awareness of the presence of the injuries.

DIAGNOSIS

Patients who present with PEO, ptosis (drooping eyelid), progressive muscle weakness, exercise intolerance (unusually intense feelings of exhaustion following physical exertion), stroke-like episodes, epilepsy, diabetes mellitus, ataxia, wasting of the neck and shoulder muscles, difficulty swallowing, or a combination of these symptoms affecting multiple organ systems should be screened for the presence of MMP (Kelly, 2008). A thorough family history that reveals matrilineal soft signs, such as deafness, short stature, migraine headaches, and PEO, may indicate the presence of MMP. If MMP is present, lactate acid stress test (LST) and muscle biopsy should reveal the presence of ragged red fibers, abnormal proliferation of mitochondria, and cytochrome *c* oxidase (COX) deficiencies (Finsterer & Milvay, 2004; Matsuoka, Goto, Yoneda, & Nonaka, 1991; Melone et al., 2004), while blood enzyme tests should show elevated lactate and pyruvate levels. Elevated levels of serum creatine kinase may indicate mitochondrial DNA depletion syndrome, a specific MMP (Kelly, 2008). Genetic tests of mitochondria from blood or muscle samples will indicate the particular nature of the mitochondrial mutation, and pinpoint the specific syndrome.

A simple yet effective screening method for MMP is the lactate stress test (LST). In this test, patients perform an aerobic exercise under a continuous, unadjusted, low workload. Serum levels of lactic acid, a by-product of anaerobic metabolism, are measured before, during, and after exercise. Patients with MMP show abnormally high levels of lactic acid following exercise compared with their resting state or non-MMP controls. Thus, LST is an effective, inexpensive diagnostic method for identifying the impaired oxidative process in patients with MMP (Finsterer & Milvay, 2004). Furthermore, comparing the ratio of lactate versus pyruvate may help indicate which part of the electron transport chain is blocked (Kelly, 2008).

Patients with stroke-like symptoms should be examined using both conventional MRI and diffusion-weighted MRI (dwMRI) to determine whether the lesion is related to an ischemic event or MMP. Patients with MELAS, a specific MMP syndrome, often present with stroke-like symptoms. Conventional MRI may reveal infarct-like lesions, which should be further examined with dwMRI. Normal or increased apparent diffusion coefficient values indicate the probable presence of MELAS (Kolb et al., 2003; Oppenheim et al., 2000). In addition, dynamic computerized tomography, serial cerebral angiography, and xenon-enhanced computed tomography for some patients has revealed vasodilation and normal blood flow within the affected regions, precluding the probability of ischemic stroke (Ooiwa et al., 1993).

Modified Gomori trichrome staining sometimes reveals clusters of diseased mitochondria accumulated in the subsarcolemmal region of the muscle fiber, making the fiber appear ragged red. Ragged red fibers are a hallmark of myoclonic epilepsy and ragged red fiber disease (MERRF, myoclonic epilepsy with ragged red fibers). In addition, histocytological studies have revealed that the mitochondria in ragged red fibers is frequently COX deficient, often lacking the COX-I, COX-II, or COX-IV complexes (Matsuoka et al., 1991; Melone et al., 2004; Rifai, Welle, Kamp, & Thornton, 2005; Shoffner et al., 1990).

Differential diagnosis of patients presenting with PEO or ptosis should rule out myasthenia gravis, ocular myositis, oculopharyngeal muscular dystrophy, thyroid associated orbitopathy, and congenital fibrosis of the extraocular muscles. Serum creatine kinase and lactate levels should be investigated, while electromyography, nerve conduction studies, and MRI of the orbits should be performed. The presence of multiple-organ symptoms in conjunction with the imaging and conduction studies supports the diagnosis of MMP (Schoser & Pongratz, 2006). When patients' muscle weakness presents in the neck and shoulder region, polymyositis and amyotrophic lateral sclerosis (ALS) should be considered the differential diagnoses (Rahim, Gupta, Bertorini, & Ledoux, 2003). The early stages of MMP closely mimic the clinical and electrophysiological symptoms of ALS. LST and muscle biopsy should indicate the presence of mitochondrial proliferation, if MMP is present (Finsterer, 2002).

TREATMENT

Treatment of MMP is symptom oriented. Patients with motor deficits or dystonia may require the support of a wheelchair or a walker for locomotion. If the diaphragm is affected by muscle weakness, a respirator will facilitate breathing. If neck or throat weakness creates significant impairment in swallowing, a feeding tube may be necessary, and individuals with heart block may benefit from the use of a pacemaker (Finsterer, 2006; Finsterer et al., 2007; Kelly, 2008). Diabetic symptoms can be managed with insulin and diet monitoring, and seizures can be controlled with medication (Kelly, 2008). Hearing and vision impairments can be corrected or partially corrected with hearing aids and glasses (Kelly, 2008; Zwirner & Wilichowski, 2001). For patients with ptosis there are specially modified glasses with "ptosis props," small bars that help support the upper eyelids.

Physical therapy may improve the overall strength, motility, and endurance of individuals with MMP (Kelly, 2008). Research indicates improvements in both human (Taivassalo, DeStefano et al., 1999; Taivassalo, Fu et al. 1999) and animal (Wenz, Diaz, Hernandez, & Moraes, 2009) models. It appears that resistance exercise and short-term endurance exercise at low intensities can delay MMP onset, induce antioxidant enzymes, increase the ratio of wild-type to mutant mitochondria, and prolong the life span of affected individuals.

Amanda Ballenger
Raymond S. Dean

M

Finsterer, J. (2002). Mitochondriopathy as a differential diagnosis of amyotrophic lateral sclerosis. *Amyotrophic Lateral Sclerosis and Other Motor Neuron Disorders, 3,* 4, 219–224.

Finsterer, J. (2006). Central nervous system manifestations of mitochondrial disorders. *Acta Neurologica Scandinavica, 114,* 4, 217–238.

Finsterer, J., & Milvay, E. (2004). Stress lactate in mitochondrial myopathy under constant, unadjusted workload. *European Journal of Neurology, 11,* 12, 811–816.

Finsterer, J., Stöllberger, C., Steger, C., & Cozzarini, W. (2007). Complete heart block associated with noncompaction, nail-patella syndrome, and mitochondrial myopathy. *Journal of Electrocardiology, 40,* 4, 352–354.

Fitzsimons, R. B. (1981). The mitochondrial myopathies: 9 case reports and a literature review. *Clinical and Experimental Neurology, 17,* 185–210.

Hruszkewcyz, A. M. (1992). Lipid preoxidation and mtDNA degeneration. A hypothesis. *Mutational Research, 275,* 243–248.

Iizuka, T. (2008). Pathogenesis and treatment of stroke-like episodes in MELAS. *Rinsho Shinkeigaku, 48,* 11, 1006–1009.

Kelly, R. (2008). Facts about mitochondrial myopathies. *MDA Publications.* Retrieved April 29, 2009, from http://mda.org/Publications/mitochondrial_myopathies.html

Kitagawa, T., Odachi, K., Taniguchi, A., & Kuzuhara, S. (2000). Sudden death due to ventricular tachycardia in a case of mitochondrial myopathy, encephalopathy, lactic acidosis, and stroke-like episodes (MELAS). *Neurological Medicine, 53,* 1, 45–50.

Kolb, S. J., Costello, F., Lee, A. G., White, M., Wong, S., Schwartz, E. D., et al. (2003). Distinguishing ischemic stroke from the stroke-like lesions of MELAS using apparent diffusion coefficient mapping. *Journal of Neurological Science, 216,* 1, 11–15.

Matsuoka, T., Goto, Y., Yoneda, M., & Nonaka, I. (1991). Muscle histopathology in myoclonus epilepsy with ragged-red fibers (MERRF). *Journal of Neurological Science, 106,* 2, 193–198.

Melone, M. A., Tessa, A., Petrini, S., Lus, G., Sampaolo, S., di Fede, G., et al. (2004). Revelation of a new mitochondrial DNA mutation (G12147A) in a MELAS/MERRF phenotype. *Archives of Neurology, 61,* 2, 269–272.

Neargarder, S. A, Murtagh, M. P., Wong, B., & Hill, E. K. (2007). The neuropsychologic deficits of MELAS: Evidence of global impairment. *Cognitive and Behavioral Neurology, 20,* 2, 83–92.

Ooiwa, Y., Uematsu, Y., Terada, T., Nakai, K., Itakura, T., Komai, N., et al. (1993). Cerebral blood flow in mitochondrial myopathy, encephalopathy, lactic acidosis, and stroke-like episodes. *Stroke, 24,* 2, 304–309.

Oppenheim, C., Galanaud, D., Samson, Y., Sahel, M., Dormont, D., Wechsler, B., et al. (2000). Can diffusion-weighted magnetic resonance imaging help differentiate stroke from stroke-like events in MELAS? *Journal of Neurology, Neurosurgery, and Psychiatry, 69,* 2, 248–250.

Rahim, F., Gupta, D., Bertorini, T. E., & Ledoux, M. S. (2003). Dropped head presentation of mitochondrial myopathy. *Journal of Clinical Neuromuscular Disorders, 5,* 2, 108–114.

Rifai, Z., Welle, S., Kamp, C., & Thornton, C. A. (2005). Ragged red fibers in normal aging and inflammatory myopathy. *Annals of Neurology, 37,* 1, 24–29.

Schoser, B. G., & Pongratz, D. (2006). Extraocular mitochondrial myopathies and their differential diagnoses. *Strabismus, 14,* 2, 107–113.

Shoffner, J. M., Lott, M. T., Lezza, A. M., Seibel, P., Ballinger, S. W., & Wallace, D. C. (1990). Myoclonic epilepsy and ragged-red fiber disease (MERRF) is associated with a mitochondrial DNA tRNA(Lys) mutation. *Cell, 61,* 6, 931–937.

Taivassalo, T., DeStefano, N., Chen, J., Karpati, G., Arnold, D. L., & Argov, Z. (1999). Short-term aerobic training response in chronic myopathies. *Muscle and Nerves, 22,* 9, 1239–1243.

Taivassalo, T., Fu, K., Johns, T., Arnold, D., Karpati, G., & Shoubridge, E. A. (1999). Gene shifting: A novel therapy for mitochondrial myopathy. *Human Molecular Genetics, 8,* 6, 1047–1052.

Wallace, D. C., Lott, M. T., Shoffner, J. M., & Ballinger, S. (1994). Mitochondrial DNA mutations in epilepsy and neurological disease. *Epilepsia, 35,* Suppl. 1, 43–50.

Weller, R. O., Cumming, W. J. K., & Mahon, M. (1997). Diseases of muscle. In D. I. Graham & P. L. Lantos (Eds.), *Greenfield's neuropathology* (6th ed.). New York: Oxford University Press.

Wenz, T., Diaz, F., Hernandez, D., & Moraes, C. T. (2009). Endurance exercise is protective for mice with mitochondrial myopathy. *Journal of Applied Physiology, 106,* 5, 1712–1719.

Zwirner, P., & Wilichowski, E. (2001). Progressive sensorineural hearing loss in children with mitochondrial encephalomyopathies. *Laryngoscope, 111,* 3, 515–521.

MOEBIUS SYNDROME

DESCRIPTION

Moebius syndrome is a rare congenital disorder characterized by congenital facial diplegia with convergent strabismus due to absence or underdevelopment of the 6th and 7th cranial nerves. In some instances, the facial paralysis is complete with individuals not being able to even close their eyes.

Furthermore, though structural degradation of the 6th and 7th cranial nerves define Moebius syndrome, the 3rd, 5th, 8th, 9th, 11th, and/or 12th cranial nerves may also be affected. Facial weakness is often noted soon after birth due to infants exhibiting an inability to suck in combination with an inability to move their eyes back and forth. Additional symptoms may also be seen and are discussed below.

To date the pathophysiological basis of Moebius syndrome remains unclear. Both ischemic and hypoxic theories remain the most prevalent. Furthermore, though there is no cure for Moebius syndrome, symptom-based treatment and support can promote a normal life.

NEUROPATHOLOGY/PATHOPHYSIOLOGY

Absence or underdevelopment of the 6th and 7th cranial nerves produces a mask-like expressionless face in neonates characterized by internal strabismus, facial diplegia, and bilateral abducens palsies (Mobius, 1888). The cause of these cranial nerve anomalies is unknown. Some have suggested a vascular etiology for the structural decay, either by way of intrauterine hypoxic or ischemic trauma (Briegel, 2006). However, teratogenic exposure has also been suggested. For example, cocaine usage by the mother has been associated with increased risks of Moebius syndrome (Puvabanditsin, Garrow, Augustin, Titapiwatanakul, & Kuniyoshi, 2005).

The morphological anomalies noted on the 6th and 7th cranial nerves in combination with other pathological features have been utilized to suggest multiple classifications, some supporting a vascular- or trauma-based etiology and others not (Towfight, Marks, Palmer, & Vannucci, 1979). In some instances, there is a relative lack of necrosis or degenerative change. In combination with brainstem anomalies such as olivary dysplasia, this would suggest against an acquired defect pointing more toward a primary malformation (Richter, 1960). Still, focal necrosis and calcification in brainstem nuclei supporting an infectious or hypoxic basis has also been noted as has aplasia and/or hypoplasia of cranial nerve nuclei (Sudarshan & Goldie, 1985).

Beyond the 6th and 7th cranial nerves, other oculomotor and lower cranial nerves including the 3rd, 5th, 8th, 9th, 11th, and 12th cranial nerves may also be involved. Cerebellar hypoplasia has also been noted in isolated incidence presumed to be also explained by ischemia occurring between 5th and 6th weeks of gestation (Harbord, Finn, Hall-Craggs, Brett, & Baraitser, 1989). Children with Moebius syndrome are at higher risk for mental retardation and autism suggesting the potential for involvement of the cerebral cortex in addition to brainstem regions. Peripherally, musculoskeletal abnormalities may present.

NEUROPSYCHOLOGICAL/CLINICAL PRESENTATION

The hallmark feature of Moebius syndrome is congenital facial diplegia with convergent strabismus. At birth, infants are often unable to suck and may also have difficulties swallowing, which together or even singularly impede their ability to feed. Simultaneously, infants are often unable to close their eyes completely. Facial diplegia may present as mask-like expressions. Difficulties in smiling are common. In addition, speech may be disturbed secondary to motoric limitations. Furthermore, it can be complicated by congenital deafness of a neurosensory origin (Golden & Bonnemann, 2007).

Abducens palsy, complete external ophthalmoplegia, lingual palsy, clubfeet, brachial disorder, and/or an absent pectoral muscle may all be seen as they have been noted in higher rates in children with Moebius syndrome (Henderson, 1939). Neurocognitive deficits are varied with no unitary profile emerging. Mild mental retardation is seen in approximately 10% to 15% of cases (Golden & Bonnemann, 2007).

DIAGNOSIS

Diagnosis is commonly symptom based. Given it is observed soon after birth, the most common differential is from the facial palsy associated with forceps or other birth injury. Oftentimes this differential is easy as Moebius syndrome presents bilaterally and often has other associated weaknesses. Centronuclear myopathy, mitochondrial myopathies, myasthenic syndromes, myotonic dystrophy, facioscapulohumeral dystrophy, structural congenital myopathies, inflammation, infection, and neoplasms must all be considered as well.

Aside from clinical evaluation of the functional impairments, diagnostic workup includes MRI and skeletal X-ray to evaluate for the various aforementioned presentations that must be ruled out.

TREATMENT

There is no cure for Moebius syndrome; rather, treatment is symptom based. Because affected infants commonly have difficulties sucking and swallowing, feeding tubes may be required. Speech therapy is commonly required to improve oral-motor functioning to improve pronunciation capabilities while also seeking to improve potential eating and/or swallowing difficulties. Surgical intervention may be attempted in some instances to offer some increased movement of facial muscles.

Chad A. Noggle
Amy R. Steiner

Briegel, W. (2006). Neuropsychiatric findings of Möbius sequence: a review. *Clinical Genetics, 70,* 91–97.

Golden, J., & Bonnemann, C. (2007). Developmental structures disorders. In C. Goetz (Ed.), *Textbook of clinical neurology* (pp. 561–591). Philadelphia, PA: Saunders Elsevier.

Harbord, M. G., Finn, J. P., Hall-Craggs, M. A., Brett, E. M., & Baraitser, M. (1989). Moebius' syndrome with unilateral cerebellar hypoplasia. *Journal of Medical Genetics, 26,* 579–582.

Henderson, J. L. (1939). The congenital facial diplegia syndrome: Clinical features, pathology and etiology. *Brain, 62,* 381.

Heubner, O. (1900). Ueber angeborene Kernmangel (infantiler Kernschwund, Moebius). *Charite-annalen, 25,* 211–243.

Mobius, P. J. (1888). Ueber angeborene doppelseitige Abducens-Facialis-Lahmung. *Munchner Med Wochenschr, 35,* 108–111.

Puvabanditsin, S., Garrow, E., Augustin, G., Titapiwatanakul, R., & Kuniyoshi, K. M. (2005). Poland-Mobius syndrome and cocaine abuse: A relook at vascular etiology. *Pediatric Neurology, 32(4),* 285–287.

Richter, R. B. (1960). Unilateral congenital hypoplasia of the facial nucleus. *Journal of Neuropathology & Experimental Neurology, 19,* 33–41.

Ropper, A. H., & Brown, R. H. (2005). *Adams and Victor's principles of neurology* (8th ed.). New York: McGraw-Hill.

Sudarshan, A., & Goldie, W. D. (1985). The spectrum of congenital facial diplegia (Moebius syndrome). *Pediatric Neurology, 1,* 180–184.

Towfight, J., Marks, K., Palmer, E., & Vannucci, R. (1979). Moebius syndrome. Neuropathological observations. *Acta Neuropathologica (Berlin), 48,* 11–17.

MONOMELIC AMYOTROPHY

DESCRIPTION

Monomelic amyotrophy (MMA), also known as Hirayama's disease, is a disease characterized by progressive loss of lower motor neurons, leading to muscular atrophy in a single limb (usually an arm). It was first described by Hirayama in 1959. Regionally based, MMA has primarily been reported in Asian countries, including Japan, India, and Korea among others. It is extremely rare in the Western hemisphere (de Visser, de Visser, & Verbeeten, 1988; Serratrice, Pellissier, & Pouget, 1987).

The presentation often first arises in the late teens and early 20s in males. As lower motor neurons deteriorate, muscular wasting takes place in the affected limb. The progression is insidious, spanning 2–5 years after which time the degeneration ceases. To date, the underlying cause remains unknown and no cure or treatment has proven very effective. Although muscular wasting, and consequently strength and coordination of voluntary movement, in the affected limb is a hallmark of the presentation, pain or sensory loss often do not occur. Although the upper extremities are most commonly affected, it can present in the lower extremities. When an upper limb is involved, it is referred to as brachial MMA (BMMA) or classic Hirayama's disease (Hirayama, Toyukura, & Tsubaki, 1959), whereas, in the rare instance where a lower limb is affected, it is termed crural MMA (Gourie-Devi & Nalini, 2003).

O'Sullivan–McLeod syndrome is a variant of MMA. In this presentation, progression is particularly slow and results in wasting of only the hand and forearm as opposed to the whole arm.

NEUROPATHOLOGY/PATHOPHYSIOLOGY

The pathological basis of MMA remains unknown. Viral infections (Kao, Liu, Wang, & Chern, 1993; Kao, Wu, & Chern, 1993), vascular insufficiency of the spinal cord (Hirayama et al., 1987), heavy physical activity (Gourie-Devi, Gururaj, Vasisth, & Subbakrishna, 1993) and focal cord atrophy as a result of stretching of the cord during flexion of the neck (Gourie-Devi, Rao, & Suresh, 1992; Metcalf, Wood, & Bertorini, 1987; Mukai, Matsuo, Muto, Takahashi, & Sobue, 1987), and microcirculatory disturbances in the territory of the anterior spinal artery territory (Hirayama, 1991; Sethi et al., 2006) have all been suggested as potential bases, though none can explain the geographical predominance in Asia (Gourie-Devi, 2007). From a neuropathological standpoint, the presentation is characterized by segmental anterior horn cell involvement causing wasting and weakness of predominantly one upper or lower limb, without evidence of sensory dysfunction (Hirayama et al., 1959). Forward displacement of the lower dural sac and flattening of the lower cervical spinal cord during flexion movements are common and related to transient cord compression (Fu et al., 2007; Hirayama & Tokumaru, 2000). This flattening presents more prominently on the side of the affected limb. Over time, the cervical spin may demonstrate relative atrophy and increased signal intensity (Pradhan & Gupta, 1997). MRI showing signal void in posterior epidural space pulsating synchronously with cardiac beat suggesting passive dilatation of the epidural venous plexus has been reported (Pal et al., 2008).

NEUROPSYCHOLOGICAL/CLINICAL PRESENTATION

The prototypical feature of MMA is an atrophied limb, usually an upper extremity, although involvement of lower extremities has been noted. Reduced strength, coordination, and absence of stretch reflexes are noted in the affected limb. However, hyporeflexia may also be present in other limbs, suggesting a more diffuse pathology (Pal et al., 2008). Coldness of hands, hyperhidrosis, and aggravation of motor symptoms on exposure to cold and abnormalities of sympathetic skin response are also sometimes noted (Gourie-Devi & Nalini, 2001).

The presentation is marked purely by lower motor neuron features, whereas upper motor neuron signs are not seen in conjunction with the presentation (Gourie-Devi & Nalini, 2003). Furthermore, MMA presents without involvement of cranial nerves, pyramidal tracts, sensory, cerebellar, or extrapyramidal systems and cortical functions (Gourie-Devi & Nalini, 2003). Neurocognitive deficits are not associated with the presentation as the cortex is spared.

DIAGNOSIS

Diagnosis is based on clinical presentation and taking of a thorough history. Particularly, the focal wasting of a limb in conjunction with those features previously described, as well as the absence of those features not associated with the presentation (e.g., upper motor neuron signs).

Beyond description and assessment of the clinical features, diagnosis is often aided by MRI and EMG. Hirayama and colleagues (Hirayama & Tokumaru, 2000) demonstrated cinematographic MRI patterns involving signal void in the posterior epidural space with synchrony with cardiac pulse. This was related to passive dilatation of the epidural venous plexus. EMG can be used to demonstrate denervation in the affected limb. MRI as well as CT can also be useful in demonstrating muscular atrophy. Sequential clinical assessment is essential to ensure that more expansive clinical features do not emerge suggesting another motor

neuron disease. Measurement of central motor conduction time may also be a useful tool to determine the prevalence of subclinical involvement of motor pathways (Pal et al., 2008). MRI and CT of the entire CNS should be employed to rule out more expansive presentations. Neuropsychological testing often does not aid in diagnosis as MMA does not involve the cortex.

TREATMENT

There is no cure or standard treatment for MMA. As previously noted, an insidious progression of muscular wasting takes place over the course of 2–5 years, reaching a plateau where further deterioration is not seen. Although interventions may be offered during this progression, particularly after the wasting stabilizes, muscle strengthening exercises and training in hand coordination through physical therapy/occupational therapy is most useful.

Michelle R. Pagoria
Chad A. Noggle

de Visser, M., de Visser, B. W. O., & Verbeeten, B. (1988). Electromyographic and computed tomographic findings in five patients with monomelic spinal muscular atrophy. *European Neurology, 28,* 135–138.

Fu, Y., Fan, D. S., Zhang, J., Pei, X. L., Han, H. B., & Kang, D. X. (2007). Clinical features and dynamics of cervical magnetic resonance imaging in Hirayama disease. *Beijing Da Xue Xue Bao, 39,* 189–192.

Gourie-Devi, M. (2007). Monomelic amyotrophy of upper or lower limbs. In A. A. Eisen, P. J. Shaw (Eds.), *Handbook of clinical neurology* (pp. 207–227). Amsterdam, Netherlands: Elsevier, BV.

Gourie-Devi, M., Gururaj, G., Vasisth, S., & Subbakrishna, D. K. (1993). Risk factors in monomelic amyotrophy — a case control study. *NIMHANS Journal, 11,* 79–87.

Gourie-Devi, M., & Nalini A. (2001). Sympathetic skin response in monomelic amyotrophy. *Acta Neurologica Scandinavica, 104,* 162–166.

Gourie-Devi, M., & Nalini, A. (2003). Long-term follow-up of 44 patients with brachial monomelic amyotrophy. *Acta Neurologica Scandinavica, 107,* 215–220.

Gourie-Devi, M., Rao, C. J., & Suresh, T. G. (1992). Computed tomographic myelography in monomelic amyotrophy. *Journal of Tropical and Geographical Neurology, 2,* 32–37.

Hirayama, K. (1991). Non-progressive juvenile spinal muscular atrophy of the distal upper limb (Hirayama disease). In J. M. de Jong (Ed.), *Diseases of the motor system* (pp. 107–120). Amsterdam, Netherlands: Elsevier Science Publishers BV.

M

M

Hirayama, K., & Tokumaru, Y. (2000). Cervical dural sac and spinal cord in juvenile muscular atrophy of distal upper extremity. *Neurology, 54,* 1922–1926.

Hirayama, K., Tomonaga, M., Kitano, K., Yamada, T., Kojima, S., & Arai, K. (1987). Focal cervical poliopathy causing juvenile muscular atrophy of distal upper extremity: A pathological study. *Journal of Neurology, Neurosurgery, & Psychiatry, 50,* 285–290.

Hirayama, K., Toyukura, Y., & Tsubaki, T. (1959). Juvenile muscular atrophy of unilateral upper extremity: A new clinical entity. *Psychiatry Neurology Japan, 61,* 2190–2197.

Kao, K. P., Liu, W. T., Wang, S. J., & Chern, C. M. (1993). Lack of serum neutralizing antibody against poliovirus in patients with juvenile distal spinal muscular atrophy of upper extremities. *Brain & Development, 15,* 219–221.

Kao, K. P., Wu, Z. A., & Chern, C. M. (1993). Juvenile lower cervical spinal muscular atrophy in Taiwan: Report of 27 Chinese cases. *Neuroepidemiology, 12,* 331–335.

Metcalf, J. C., Wood, J. B., & Bertorini, T. E. (1987). Benign focal amyotrophy: Metrizamide CT evidence of cord atrophy. Case report. *Muscle Nerve, 10,* 338–345.

Mukai, E., Matsuo, T., Muto, T., Takahashi, A., & Sobue, I. (1987). Magnetic resonance imaging of juvenile–type distal and segmental muscular atrophy of upper extremities. *Clinical Neurology (Japan), 27,* 99–107.

Pal, P. K., Atchayaram, N., Goel, G., Geulah, E. (2008). Central motor conduction in brachial monomelic amyotrophy. *Neurology India, 56*(4), 438–443.

Pradhan, S., & Gupta, R. K. (1997). Magnetic resonance imaging in juvenile asymmetric segmental spinal muscular atrophy. *Journal of the Neurological Sciences, 146,* 133–138.

Serratrice, G., Pellissier, J. P., & Pouget, J. (1987). Etude nosologique de 25 cas d'amyotrophie monomelique chronique. *Revue Neurologique (Paris), 143,* 201–210.

Sethi, P. K., Khandelwal, D., Thukral, R., Torgovnick, J. (2006). Neuroimage: Monomelic amyotrophy. *European Neurology, 56*(4), 261

MOYAMOYA'S DISEASE

DESCRIPTION

Moyamoya's disease (MD) is a rare cerebrovascular disease of unknown etiology; it was given this name because moyamoya, a Japanese word that means "puff of smoke," accurately describes the characteristic feature of the vascular network that is seen on cerebral angiograms in the diagnosis of the disease (Suzuki & Takaku, 1969). The highest prevalence rates are found in Asia, with an 8:1 male-to-female ratio. Age of onset tends to be around age 5 or in the 40s (Wakai et al., 1997). Although no specific infectious pathogens have been identified, infection of the head and neck has been implicated (Yamada et al., 1997). An inherited polygenic or autosomal dominant role with low penetrance has also been suggested (Mineharu et al., 2008).

NEUROPATHOLOGY/PATHOPHYSIOLOGY

Progressive occlusion of the internal carotid arteries, along with its main branches in the circle of Willis, leads to the formation of a fine vascular network (moyamoya vessels) that functions as collateral pathways for blood supply (Fukui, 1997). Childhood onset typically leads to transient ischemic attacks (TIA) or cerebral infarction, while adult patients are more likely to develop intracranial bleeding in addition to TIA and cerebral infarction (Fukui et al., 2000). Familial occurrences account for about 15% of cases (Yamauchi, Houkin, Tada, & Abe, 1997) and are characterized by a higher female to male ratio, younger age of onset, and earlier presentation of symptoms (Nanba et al., 2006).

NEUROPSYCHOLOGICAL/CLINICAL PRESENTATION

Preoperative IQ is strongly correlated with patient's age and cerebral blood flow, with older patients displaying significantly lower IQ (Ishii, Takeuchi, Ibayashi, & Tanaka, 1984). Performance IQ increased the most postoperatively. Neuropsychological findings, based on small samples, include decreases in IQ and motor functions over the course of 15 years (Kurokawa et al., 1985), and widespread neurocognitive and motor impairment preoperatively, with improvements noted at 1 and 3 years postoperatively (Bowen, Marks, & Steinberg, 1998). Matsushima, Aoyagi, Nariai, Takada, and Hirakawa (1997) found 80% of patients' IQ scores remained in the average range at 9.5 years postsurgical intervention. MD-related cerebrovascular accidents tend to result in deficits characteristic of the site of the cerebrovascular accident (CVA) (Jefferson, Glosser, Detre, Sinson, & Liebeskind, 2006).

DIAGNOSIS

Cerebral angiography is considered the gold standard of diagnosis (Kuroda & Houkin, 2008). Diagnostic criteria include: (1) stenosis or occlusion of the terminal portions of the internal carotid arteries and proximal portions of the anterior and/or middle cerebral arteries; (2) abnormal vascular networks in the arterial phase in the vicinity of arterial occlusion; and (3) bilateral involvement (Fukui et al., 2000). Unilateral involvement is termed a "probable case," which tends to progress to bilateral involvement in children but not in adults (Fukui et al., 2000).

Six stages of angiographic changes have been described (Kuroda & Houkin, 2008; Suzuki & Kodama, 1983): (1) narrowing of the carotid fork; (2) initiation of basal moyamoya; (3) intensification of moyamoya along with defects of the middle and anterior cerebral arteries; (4) moyamoya minimizes, while posterior cerebral arteries become defective; (5) further reduction in moyamoya; (6) disappearance of moyamoya, with cerebral blood flow supplied only from the external carotid artery. CSF abnormalities have also been described, including increased concentrations of certain growth factors and cytokines (Malek, Connors, Robertson, Folkman, & Scott, 1997).

TREATMENT

Surgical revascularization is the only effective treatment for MD. Direct bypass methods are effective for improving brain hemodynamics and resolving ischemic attacks immediately after surgery, and involve anastomosis of the superior temporal artery and the middle cerebral artery (Karasawa, Kikuchi, Furuse, Kawamura, & Sakaki, 1978). Indirect methods induce spontaneous angiogenesis between the brain surface and vascularized donor tissue (Ishii, 1986; Karasawa, Kikuchi, Furuse, Sakaki, & Yoshida, 1977; Kawaguchi et al., 1996; Kinugasa, Mandai, Kamata, Sugiu, & Ohmoto, 1993). Following treatment with encephaloduroarteriosynangiosis, cognitive outcome has been shown to be very poor in those younger than 2 years of age, with a more positive outcome if the operation is performed within 3 months of MD onset (Matsushima et al., 1992).

Shane S. Bush
Thomas E. Myers

Bowen, M., Marks, M. P., & Steinberg, G. K. (1998). Neuropsychological recovery from childhood moyamoya disease. *Brain and Development, 20*, 119–123.

Fukui, M. (1997). Guidelines for the diagnosis and treatment of spontaneous occlusion of the circle of Willis ("moyamoya" disease). Research Committee on Spontaneous Occlusion of the Circle of Willis (Moyamoya disease) of the Ministry of Health and Welfare, Japan. *Clinical Neurology and Neurosurgery, 99*, S238–S240.

Fukui, M., Kono, S., Sueishi, K., & Ikezaki, K. (2000). Moyamoya disease. *Neuropathology, 20*, S61–S64.

Ishii, R. (1986). Surgical treatment of moyamoya disease. *No Shinkei Geka, 14*, 1059–68 (in Japanese).

Ishii, R., Takeuchi, S., Ibayashi, K., & Tanaka, R. (1984). Intelligence in children with moyamoya disease: Evaluation after surgical treatments with special reference to changes in cerebral blood flow. *Stroke, 15*, 873–877.

Jefferson, A. L., Glosser, G., Detre, J. A., Sinson, G., & Liebeskind, D. S. (2006). Neuropsychological and perfusion MR imaging correlates of revascularization in a case of moyamoya syndrome. *American Journal of Neuroradiology, 27*, 98–100.

Karasawa, J., Kikuchi, H., Furuse, S., Kawamura, J., & Sakaki, T. (1978). Treatment of moyamoya disease with STA-MCA anastomosis. *Journal of Neurosurgery, 49*, 679–88.

Karasawa, J., Kikuchi, H., Furuse, S., Sakaki, T., & Yoshida, Y. (1977). A surgical treatment of "moyamoya" disease "encephalo-myo-synangiosis". *Neurologia Medico-Chirurfica (Tokyo), 17*, 29–37.

Kawaguchi, T., Fujita, S., Hosoda, K., Shibata, Y., Komatsu, H., & Tamaki, N. (1996). Multiple burr-hole operation for adult moyamoya disease. *Journal of Neurosurgery, 84*, 468–476.

Kinugasa, K., Mandai, S., Kamata, I., Sugiu, K., & Ohmoto, T. (1993). Surgical treatment of moyamoya disease: Operative technique for encephalo-duro-arterio-myo-synangiosis, its follow-up, clinical results, and angiograms. *Neurosurgery, 32*, 527–531.

Kurokawa, T., Tomita, S., Ueda, K., Narazaki, O., Hanai, T., Hasuo, K., et al. (1985). Prognosis of occlusive disease of the circle of Willis (Moyamoya disease) in children. *Pediatric Neurology, 1*, 274–277.

Kuroda, S., & Houkin, K. (2008). Moyamoya disease: Current concepts and future perspectives. *Lancet Neurology, 7*, 1056–1066.

Malek, A. M., Connors, S., Robertson, R. L., Folkman, J., & Scott, R. M. (1997). Elevation of cerebrospinal fluid levels of basic fibroblast growth factor in moyamoya and central nervous system disorders. *Pediatric Neurosurgery, 27*, 182–189.

Matsushima, Y., Aoyagi, M., Nariai, T., Takada, Y., & Hirakawa, K. (1997). Long-term intelligence outcome of post-encephalo-duro-arterio-synangiosis childhood Moyamoya patients. *Clinical Neurology and Neurosurgery, 99*(S2), S147–S150.

Matsushima, T., Inoue, T., Suzuki, S. O., Fujii, K., Fukui, M., & Hasuo, K. (1992). Surgical treatment of moyamoya disease in pediatric patients-comparison between the results of indirect and direct revascularization procedures. *Neurosurgery, 31*, 401–405.

M

Mineharu, Y., Liu, W., Inoue, K., Matsuura, N., Inoue, S., Takenaka, K., et al. (2008). Autosomal dominant moyamoya disease maps to chromosome 17q25.3 *Neurology, 70*, 2357–2363.

Nanba, R, Kuroda, S., Tada, M., Ishikawa, T., Houkin, K., & Iwasaki, Y. (2006). Clinical features of familial moyamoya disease. *Child's Nervous System 22(3)*, 258–262.

Suzuki, J., & Takaku, A. (1969). Cerebrovascular "moyamoya" disease. Disease showing abnormal net-like vessels in base of brain. *Archives of Neurology, 20*, 288–299.

Suzuki, J., & Kodama, N. (1983) Moyamoya disease—A review. *Stroke, 14*, 104–109.

Wakai, K., Tamakoshi, A., Ikezaki, K., Fukui, M., Kawamura, T., Aoki, R., et al. (1997). Epidemiological features of moyamoya disease in Japan: Findings from a nationwide survey. *Clinical Neurology and Neurosurgery, 99*, S1–S5.

Yamada, H., Deguchi, K., Tanigawara, T., Takenaka, K., Nishimura, Y., Shinoda, J., et al. (1997). The relationship between moyamoya disease and bacterial infection. *Clinical Neurology and Neurosurgery, 99*, S221–S224.

Yamauchi, T., Houkin, K., Tada, M., & Abe, H. (1997). Familial occurrence of moyamoya disease. *Neurology and Neurosurgery, 99*, S162–S167.

Mucopolysaccharidoses

DESCRIPTION

Mucopolysaccharidoses (MPS) are a family of seven inherited metabolic disorders characterized by lysosomal enzyme deficiencies. Impaired or absent production of these enzymes leads to decreased degradation of glycosaminoglycans (GAGs). Intralysosomal GAG accumulations occur and interfere with normal cellular functioning. These diseases cause various forms of progressive neurologic and somatic dysfunction. Their manifestations vary based on the type and extent of enzyme dysfunction. The overall frequency of MPS is between 1.5 and 3.5 per 100,000 live births (Spranger, 2006).

MPS I is classified into three separate disorders based on the severity of the clinical manifestations. Pfaundler–Hurler disease, or simply Hurler's disease (MPS I-H), is the most severe disease process, whereas Schiene's disease (MPS I-S) has a milder clinical presentation. Hurler–Schiene's disease (MPS I-H/S) falls somewhere in the middle. The incidence of MPS I is 1:100,000 (Orchard et al., 2007).

MPS II, or Hunter's disease, is the only nonautosomal-recessive MPS disorder. It has an X-linked recessive inheritance pattern. As a result, this is an almost exclusively male disease. However, it can be seen in certain females with skewed inactivation of X chromosomes (Pyeritz, 2007).

MPS III, also known as Sanfilippo's disease, is a category of four separate lysosomal enzyme deficiencies, designated A–D that all result in the buildup of heparan sulfate (Fraser et al., 2005).

MPS IV, known as Moquiro's disease, is divided into two categories, MPS IVA and MPS IVB, which designate two different enzyme defects. However, both diseases cause an increased accumulation of both keratan sulfate and chondroitin sulfate. MPS IVA typically presents as a more severe disease than MPS IVB (Spranger, 2007).

MPS VI, referred to as Maroteaux–Lamy disease, is a rare disease with an incidence of 1:235,000 (Orchard et al., 2007).

MPS VII, also known as Sly syndrome, is caused by a defect in beta-galactosidase, which causes pathologic accumulation of dermatan sulfate and heparan sulfate. The accumulated storage products are dermatan sulfate and heparan sulfate (Maertens & Dyken, 2007).

MPS IX, known as hyaluronidase deficiency, or Natowicz syndrome, is a defect in hyaluronidase 1. There is only one reported case of MPS IX (Spranger, 2006).

Multiple sulfatase deficiency is also a recognized rare form of MPS. This occurs with defective arylsulfatase A, B, and C enzymes and leads to the storage of dermatan sulfate and heparan sulfate. (Maertens & Dyken, 2007).

NEUROPATHOLOGY/PATHOPHYSIOLOGY

The pathophysiology and neuropathology of the MPS disorders relates to the specific type of enzyme deficiency.

MPS I is characterized by a deficiency in alpha-L-iduronidase that results from a mutation of the *IUA* gene

In MPS I, radiological studies show a characteristic skeletal dysplasia, diosmosis multiplex. This is often seen on X-rays as thickened ribs and ovoid vertebral bodies. Enlarged, coarsely trabeculated diaphyses and irregular epiphysis and metaphysis can also be seen. Thickened calvarium, premature closure of the lamboid and sagittal sutures, shallow orbits and enlarged J-shaped sellas are often seen as well. In Hurler's syndrome, macrocephaly, communicating hydrocephalus with progressive ventricular enlargement and increased intracranial pressure (ICP) are common findings on MRI. White matter lesions are more prominent in MPS I-H than MPS I-H/S or MPS I-S (Vedolin et al., 2007).

MPS II (Hunter's disease) results from a mutation involving iduronate sulfate sulfatase, which is encoded on chromosome Xq28. Point mutations are the most common type and appear in over 80% of MPS II patients. However, major deletions or rearrangements have also been detected and result in more severe pathology. The accumulated proteins are dermatan sulfate and heparan sulfate (Spranger, 2006). Brain MRI demonstrates decreased cerebral volume, brain atrophy, and white matter lesions (Vedolin et al., 2007). The four enzymes deficient in MPS III are heparan-N-sulfatase (Type A), alpha-N-glucosaminidase (Type B), acetyl-coenzyme A, alpha-glucosaminide acetyltransferase (Type C), and N-acetyl glucosamine 6-sulfase (Type D), result in slowly progressive central nervous system (CNS) degeneration with mild somatic disease (Fraser et al., 2005). Disproportionate neurological involvement compared with somatic symptoms is unique to MPS III (Spranger, 2006).

In MPS IVA, the gene encoding N-acetylgalacto-samine-6-sulfatase has been mapped to chromosome 16q24.3. A W273L mutation of the *GLB1* gene at 3p21.33 causes MSIVB. *GLB1* encodes for beta-galactosidase. In both MSIVA and MSIVB, the product of accumulation is keratan sulfate (Wraith, 1995).

MPS VI is caused by mutations of the *ARB* gene on chromosome 5q11-13. This gene encodes N-acetylgalactosamine-4-sulfatase, also called arylsulfatase B (Spranger, 2006). Brain MRI demonstrates white matter lesions and hydrocephaly to the same degree as is found in other MPS disorders. This is unexpected, as clinical findings typically show little neurological compromise (Vedolin et al., 2007).

MP VII is caused by the mutation of the *GUSB* gene, located on chromosome 7q21.11. This results in a deficiency of beta-glucuronide and intracellular storage of GAG fragments. Ultrasound can be used to detect lethal nonimmune hydrops fetalis in utero. Peripheral blood smear demonstrates coarse granulocytic inclusions. Occasionally, the less severe disease presentations can be discovered incidentally based on the peripheral blood smear findings (Spranger, 2006).

The mutation of the *HYAL1* gene on chromosome 3p21.2-21.2 causes MPS IX. This gene is responsible for encoding 1 of 3 hyaluronidase. Radiographic studies show small erosions in both acetabulae.

NEUROPSYCHOLOGICAL/CLINICAL PRESENTATION

Although variability may be seen across presentations in terms of their specific enzyme deficiency, as a group

there is considerable overlap in the resulting sequelae of each subtype. All subtypes of MPS result in a build-up of mucopolysaccharides in cellular lysosomes making the brain a primary storage site. As a consequence, CNS involvement is seen in all forms as the most common functional outcome. Somatic dysplasia, insidious decline of mentation, and a progressive decline in motor control are all commonly observed (Maertens & Dykens, 2007). Mental retardation is a prominent feature in all subtypes.

In MPS I, although infants may appear to develop normally, by 6 months of age facial abnormalities, hepatosplenomegaly, and umbilical and inguinal hernias become apparent. Otis media and visual defects are also commonly seen. Developmentally, though initial motor development may seem on time, these skills are soon lost and severe mental retardation develops. Type 2 of this variant is associated with less severe symptoms. Individuals are generally undersized and have severe joint defects. Hepatosplenomegaly is often observed. While mental deficits are observed, they are less severe, commonly presenting as just mild mental retardation. Finally, Type 3 may present with any of the features observed in MPS I and MPS II, but in milder forms.

In MPS II, two variants are described. Both may demonstrate facial anomalies similar to those observed in MPS I variants. Types 1 and 2 are both associated with a skin rash, commonly presenting on the extremities. The primary differences functionally between the two types of MPS II is that Type 1 is associated with severe mental retardation whereas Type 2 is not.

MPS III has four variants. All are associated with manifestation of clinical symptoms developing around 2 years of age after an apparent period of normal development. At that point in time, an array of cognitive and behavioral symptoms may develop including aggression, hyperactivity, and speech deficits. Mental retardation is seen with progressive deterioration. Motor dysfunction also presents in relation to a progressive deterioration impeding children's ability to walk. Physical features may be similar to those observed in MPS I and MPS II.

MPS IV has two variants. As with the other subtypes, the first type is more severe than the second. Compression of the spinal cord and brainstem may result in neurological features. The majority of other features are muscoskeletal based.

DIAGNOSIS

All MPS disorders can be diagnosed using enzyme assays. Enzyme levels can be measured via serum leukocytes or cultured fibroblasts using commercially available or radio-labeled substrate.

Semiquantitative spot test for increased urinary GAG excretion are quick and inexpensive initial evaluation methods. However, they are limited by false positive and negative rates. Quantifying total urinary excretion of GAGs can be done via chemical quantification of uronic acid containing substances. Though this will demonstrate the mucopolysacchariduria, tandem mass spectrometry is necessary to determine type-specific profiles. Patients with Moquiro's syndrome can be diagnosed by urine reactive to monoclonal antibodies. Radiographs of the chest, spine, pelvis, and hands may demonstrate signs of dystosis multiplex (Spranger, 2006).

Prenatal diagnosis is available for all MPS diseases and can be undertaken using cell cultures from amniocentesis or chorionic villus biopsy or enzyme assay. Directly measuring GAGs in amniotic fluid is unreliable. There are currently no neonatal screening tests for MPS (Spranger, 2006).

TREATMENT

Hematopoetic cell therapy (HCT), including bone marrow or umbilical cord blood transplantation demonstrates clinical improvement in children with MPS I, MPS II, and MPS VI. Significant improvements in somatic disease and increased life expectancy have been reported. Improvement or resolution of growth failure, hepatosplenomegaly, joint stiffness, facial appearance, sleep apnea, heart disease, communicating hydrocephalus, and hearing loss have also been documented. Enzyme activity in serum and urinary GAG excretion may normalize. In general, anticipated decline in cognitive function arrests with HCT. However, if patients with baseline mental development index greater than 70 receive transplants before 2 years of age, they have improved long-term neurological outcomes. Though storage material diminishes in the myocardium and coronary arteries, valvular thickening has not been shown to resolve with treatment. In addition, evidence is still unclear as to the efficacy of HCT in improving orthopedic complications (Orchard et al., 2007). Overall results of HCT are more promising when using related, rather than random HLA matched donors. Major limiting factors include, graft failure, which occurs in up to 30% of patients, and transplant-related deaths (Spranger, 2006).

Enzyme replacement therapy for patients is now available for patients with MPS I, MPS VI, and in clinical trials for treatment of MPS II, MPS IVB, and MPS VII (Wenger, Coppola, & Liu, 2003 and Spranger, 2007). For MPS I, laronidase (Aldurazyme) infusions every 2 weeks for 1 year in adolescent and adult patients reduced hepatosplenomegaly and improved pulmonary function, sleep apnea, and joint mobility. For MPS VI, galsulfase (Naglazyme) has been approved to reduce somatic manifestations of disease (Pyertiz, 2007). Since these enzymes do not cross the blood–brain barrier, they do not prevent neurocognitive or CNS complications. Enzyme replacement is recommended in young patients to stabilize somatic disease manifestations prior to transplant therapy (Spranger, 2006).

Care for medical complications of MPS is also necessary. This typically involves assembling a multidisciplinary team. For patients with hydrocephalus, ventricular-peritoneal shunting may be necessary. Behavioral disturbances can be managed with behavioral or medication therapy. Disturbed sleep-wake cycles most commonly seen in MPS III best respond to melatonin therapy (Fraser et al., 2005). Patients with atlanto-axial instability benefit from upper cervical fusion. Anticonvulsants have been effective in treating MPS-related seizures. Ophthalmologic surgery can improve corneal opacities and retinal degeneration (Spranger, 2006).

Rebecca Durkin
Chad A. Noggle

Fraser, A., Gason, A., Wraith, J. E., & Delatycki, M. B. (2005). Sleep disturbance in Sanfilippo syndrome: A parental questionnaire study. *Archives of Disease in Childhood, 90,* 1239–1242.

Maertens, P., & Dyken, R. (2007). Lipoidoses. In C. G. Goetz (Ed.), *Textbook of clinical neurology* (pp. 616–625). Philadelphia, PA: Saunders.

Orchard, P. J., Blazar, B. R., Wagner, J., Charnas, L., Kivit, W., & Tolar, J. (2007). Hematopoetic cell therapy for metabolic disease. *Journal of Pediatrics, 151,* 340–346.

Pycritz, R. E. (2007). Inherited diseases of connective tissue. In L. Goldman & D. Ausiello (Eds.), *Cecil medicine* (23rd ed.). Philadelphia, PA: Elsevier.

Spranger, J. (2006). The mucopolysaccharidoses. In D. L. Rimoin, J.M. Connor, R. E. Pyeritz, & B. R. Korf (Eds.) *Emery and Rimoin's principles and practice of medical genetics* (5th ed., pp. 1797–1806). New York: Churchill Livingstone.

Vedolin, L., Schwartz, I. V. D., Komlos, M., Schuch, A., Azevedo, A. C., Viera, T., et al. (2007). Brain MRI in mucopolysaccharidosis: Effect of aging and correlation with biochemical findings. *Neurology, 69,* 917–924.

Wenger, D. A., Coppola, S., & Liu, S. (2003). Insight into the diagnosis and treatment of lysosomal storage diseases. *Archives of Neurology, 60,* 322–328.

Wraith, J. E. (1995). The mucopolysaccharidoses: A clinical review and guide to management. *Archives of Disease in Childhood, 72*, 263–267.

MULTIFOCAL MOTOR NEUROPATHY

DESCRIPTION

Multifocal motor neuropathy (MMN) is a progressive neurological disorder that affects primarily motor neurons. It is rare, affecting approximately 1–2 per 100,000 individuals (Misulis & Head, 2007). It is an incurable, but treatable, disease that is more prevalent in men than women (approximately a 3:1 ratio). Furthermore, MMN most commonly affects young adults with approximately two-thirds of individuals suffering from MMN being less than 45 years of age. Consequently, the mean age of onset is approximately 40. However, it is rare in children. It is often mistaken for other neurological disorders, such as amyotrophic demyelinating polyneuropathy lateral sclerosis (ALS) and chronic inflammatory demyelinating polyneuropathy (CIDP).

NEUROPATHOLOGY/PATHOPHYSIOLOGY

Although the exact cause of MMN is unknown, it is believed that the etiology involves an autoimmune cell-mediated process. Immunoglobulin M antibodies are believed to erroneously target ganglioside GM1 cells of affected individual's nerve cells as foreign: GM1, GM2, and possibly glycolipids (Nobile-Orazio, Cappellari, & Priori, 2006). This immune response destroys neuronal tissue, including the myelin sheath, which encapsulates nerve cells. This destruction causes nerve cells to undergo demyelination, which invariably causes conduction deceleration, leading ultimately to partial or complete motor nerve blockade, termed as conduction block (CB; Bradley, Daroff, Fenichel, & Jankovic, 2008; Delmont et al., 2008; Filo, Szodkowska, Hosiec, & Bogucki, 2008; Lewis, 2007). This demyelination occurs predominantly in motor nerves. Focal motor CB ultimately causes denervation of motor neurons. Due to denervation of motor neurons, individuals who suffer from MMN commonly suffer from progressive paresis and muscle weakness across common terminal motor neurons (Nobile-Orazio, 2008). Sensory nerves are commonly spared; however, some studies suggest that some sensory involvement may occur (Filo et al., 2008). However, this sensory demyelination occurs in the absence of significant clinical findings.

NEUROPSYCHOLOGICAL/CLINICAL PRESENTATION

The Joint Task Force of the European Federation of Neurological Societies and the Peripheral Nerve Society define MMN as a "slowly progressive or stepwise progressive, asymmetrical limb weakness, or motor involvement having a motor nerve distribution in at least two nerves, for more than 1 month and no objective sensory abnormalities except for minor vibration sense abnormalities in the lower extremities" (van Schaik et al., 2006).

A common initial clinical presentation is an inability or weakness in extending fingers (Donaghy, 1999; Misulis & Head, 2007). This is a common early first sign. It is hypothesized that one of the early nerves implicated in this disorder is the posterior interosseous nerve. The onset is usually insidious; however, once muscle weakness begins, it is progressive. Individuals may also complain of muscle cramps, as well as fasciculations. Common sites include a peripheral nerve distribution in areas such as the radial nerve in the upper extremity and the peroneal nerve, resulting in wrist drop and foot drop, respectively (Misulis & Head, 2007). This is usually an asymmetric presentation. Reflexes are usually normal initially; however, there may be a slight reduction or slowing in distal reflexes initially. As the disease process progresses, reflexes may diminish completely and individuals develop muscle wasting. In addition, individuals often complain of paresthesias, numbness, or tingling in the affected areas.

DIAGNOSIS

Nerve conduction studies are essential in diagnosing MMN. EMG studies demonstrate focal motor conduction blockade. In greater than 50% of the cases, you would observe a reduction in amplitude of muscle-evoked response (Olney, Lewis, Putnam, & Campellone, 2003). Some conduction studies and electromyography show diffuse innervation without significant conduction abnormalities.

Anti-GM ganglioside antibodies are measured using ELISA. This is considered to be elevated with IgM titer of greater than 1:400. Although nonspecific, assays for antiganglioside antibodies are positive in 25% to 80% of the cases. However, individuals who suffer from ALS also have elevated immunoglobulin M antiganglioside antibodies in 15% of the cases.

M

A comprehensive physical examination is also important. Physical examination findings include weakness and decreased muscle size as a result of muscle wasting. Usually, upper extremities are affected greater than lower extremities. You will also notice muscle twitching. Deep tendon reflexes are often decreased. Cranial nerve involvement is usually rare; if present, it usually involves areas on the face or tongue, including the ocular, fascicular, and hypoglossal nerves.

Although the cerebral spinal fluid is commonly unaffected, up to one-third of individuals who suffer from MMN have elevated proteins in their cerebral spinal fluids.

In differentiating MMN, it is important to include in the differential diagnosis CIDP and ALS. CIDP is another autoimmune disease that has a similar presentation to Guillain–Barré. This is also a cell-mediated immune response affecting myelin, causing demyelination. In this condition, decreased motor nerve conduction is common. This may progress to complete CBs. You would also have elevated cerebral spinal fluid protein, as well as muscle weakness; however, muscle weakness is often symmetrical in CIDP (asymmetrical in MMN). Nerve damage is usually proximal (versus distal in MMN) and sensory deficits are common. With CIDP, it is common to have sural nerve demyelination with a characteristic onion-bulb formation and inflammatory infiltrates histologically. Eighty percent of individuals who suffer from CIDP fully recover from this illness.

Another disorder to consider in the differential diagnosis is ALS. This disorder is common in the central nervous system as well as the peripheral nervous system. This disorder is progressive and invariably fatal. It affects the anterior horn cells of the spinal cord and cranial nerve nuclei, with a propensity toward the brainstem. This causes muscle atrophy, fasciculation, and spasticity. The cause of this disorder is unknown, but we do know that it has a familial predisposition and occurs in 5% to 10% of individuals with similarly affected family members. Age of onset is in the 50s–60s.

TREATMENT

Historically, the treatment of MMN has been wrought with controversy (Nobile-Orazio et al., 2006). Initially it was believed that treatments such as prednisone and plasma exchange are efficacious in treating other neurological disorders like CIDP. However, it was discovered that these treatments are ineffective in the treatment of MMN and, in some instances, potentially exacerbate progressive muscle weakness and CB.

At the present time the standard treatment of choice for MMN is the use of intravenous immunoglobulin (IVIg; Harbo et al., 2009; Nobile-Orazio et al., 2002; van Schaik et al., 2006). It is believed that this treatment helps to attenuate the cell-mediated autoimmune response caused by anti-GM antibodies. The impact of IVIg is ultimately to counteract the overactive immune response and to increase muscle strength and conduction velocity. The usual dosage is 2 g/kg per day for 2–5 days followed by maintenance treatment (Terenghi et al., 2004). Maintenance treatment may entail weekly to monthly injections. Early in course of illness, in which muscle weakness is present in the absence of CB, treatment may be plausible. However, with the progression of the disorder usually comes varying levels of disability. It is during this course of the illness that IVIg is indicated. In some instances, if individuals are refractory to IVIg, other immunosuppressant drugs may be beneficial, such as cyclophosphamide, interferon, or azathioprine (van Schaik et al., 2006) Due to risk of toxicity, cyclophosphamide is a suboptimal alternative.

With progression of MMN, individuals may develop physical disability and comorbid psychological/psychiatric disorders. This includes clinical depression, anxiety, substance use, and other compromised coping behaviors. Standard treatments of these disorders, including biological modalities and therapy, are indicated.

Stephen Robinson

Bradley, W., Daroff, R., Fenichel, G., & Jankovic, J. (2008). Multifocal motor neuropathy with conduction block. In *Neurology in clinical practice* (5th ed., Vol. 2, pp. 2300–2302). Amsterdam: Elsevier.

Delmont, E., Azulay, J., Giorgi, R., Attarian, S., Verschueren, A., Uzenot, D., et al. (2008). Multifocal motor neuropathy with and without conduction block a single entity? *Neurology, 67*, 592–596.

Donaghy, M. (1999). Classification and clinical features of motor neuron diseases and motor neuropathies in adults. *Journal of Neurology, 246*, 331–333.

Filo, M., Szodkowska I., Hosiec, T., & Bogucki, A. (2008). Multifocal motor neuropathy with conduction block with sensory fibre involvement in a diabentic patient. Case report. *Neurologia I Neurochirurgia Polska, 42*(3), 267–273.

Harbo, T., Andersen, H., Hess, A., Hansen, K., Sindrup, S., & Jakobsen, J. (2009). Subcutaneous versus intravenous immunoglobulin in multifocal motor neuropathy: A randomized, single-blinded cross-over trial. *European Journal of Neurology, 16*, 631–638.

Lewis, R. (2007). Neuropathies associated with conduction block. *Current Opinion in Neurology, 20*, 525–530.

Misulis, K., & Head, T. (2007). Multifocal motor neuropathy. *Netter's Concise Neurology, 340–341.*

Nobile-Orazio, E. (2008). What's new in multifocal motor neuropathy in 2007–2008? *Journal of the Peripheral Nervous System, 13,* 261–263.

Nobile-Orazio, E., Cappellari, A., Meucci, N., Carpo, M., Terenghi, F., Bersano, A., et al. (2002). Multifocal motor neuropathy: Clinical and immunological features and response to IVIg in relation to the presence and degree of motor conduction block. *Journal of Neurology Neurosurgery & Psychiatry, 72,* 761–766.

Nobile-Orazio, E., Cappellari, A., & Priori, A. (2006). Multifocal motor neuropathy: Current concepts and controversies. *Muscle and Nerve, 31,* 663–680.

Olney, R., Lewis, R., Putnam, T., & Campellone, J., Jr. (2003). Consensus criteria for the diagnosis of multifocal motor neuropathy. *Muscle & Nerve, 27,* 117–121.

Terenghi, F., Cappellari, A., Bersano, A., Carpo, M., Barbieri, S., & Nobile-Orazio, E. (2004). How long is IVIg effective in multifocal motor neuropathy? *Neurology, 62,* 666–668.

van Schaik, I. N., Bouche, P., Illa, I., Leger, J.-M., Van den Bergh, P., Cornblath, D. R., et al. (2006). European Federation of Neurological Societies/Peripheral Nerve Society guideline on management of multifocal motor neuropathy. *Journal of the Peripheral Nervous System, 11,* 1–8.

Multi-Infarct Dementia

DESCRIPTION

Multi-infarct dementia (MID) is a disorder characterized by a stepwise deterioration of cognitive functioning associated with strokes or accumulated transient ischemic attacks. The term "multi-infarct dementia" was coined by Hachinski, Lassen, and Marshall (1974) when they described the relationship between atherosclerosis and mental deterioration. They explained that dementia is not directly caused by atherosclerosis, rather it may lead to recurring small infarcts which can cause mental deterioration. Additional risk factors for MID include hypertension, cardiovascular disease, high cholesterol, diabetes mellitus, and cigarette smoking. The disease is more prevalent in males than females. Along with cognitive deficits, individuals with MID may suffer from psychological symptoms and motor impairments. The disorder is irreversible, though pharmacological treatment and management of risk factors may be helpful in preventing further progression.

NEUROPATHOLOGY/PATHOPHYSIOLOGY

Computed tomography (CT) and magnetic resonance imaging (MRI) can be used to identify infarcts in individuals with suspected MID. Infarcts may occur in cortical or subcortical structures. Affected brain functions may vary among individuals with MID depending on the site, size, and number of lesions; however, some widespread pathological radiographic findings have been generally observed. For example, MRI scans have shown that individuals with MID have a smaller genu area of the corpus callosum than healthy controls (Lyoo, Satlin, Lee, & Renshaw, 1997). PET findings reveal individuals with MID have lower cerebral glucose metabolism rates in gray matter compared to healthy controls, and lower cerebral metabolic rates in gray matter are associated with more severe intellectual impairment (Meguro et al., 1991). PET scans of persons with MID demonstrate decreased cerebral blood flow and lower cerebral oxygen metabolism in the cerebral cortex, basal ganglia, and thalamus (De Reuck et al., 1998). Also, longer P300 latencies of event-related potentials have been associated with MID and decreased cognitive functioning, as assessed by WAIS scores (Neshige, Barrett, & Shibasaki, 1988).

NEUROPSYCHOLOGICAL/CLINICAL PRESENTATION

Symptoms of MID include confusion, memory deficits, motor impairments, hemiparesis, sleep disturbances, gait abnormalities, speech impairments, somatic complaints, and psychological symptoms, including depression and anxiety as well as psychosis. Speech deficits in individuals with MID are typically characterized by impairment in speech mechanics, including articulation, prosody, pitch, and rate. Individuals with MID may also display deficits in narrative writing and writing to dictation. Furthermore, failure to follow complex instructions, reduced phrase length, and poorer performance on word list generation tasks are also associated with more severe cognitive impairments (Powell, Cummings, Hill, & Benson, 1988). "Extensor plantar response, pseudobulbar palsy, gait abnormalities, exaggeration of deep tendon reflexes, or weakness of an extremity" (p.158) may be displayed by individuals with MID (American Psychiatric Association [APA], 2000). Within each

M

M

individual, MID differentially affects various neuro-psychological functions. The presence and severity of deficits depend on a variety of factors including the location, magnitude, and number of infarctions.

DIAGNOSIS

MID was included in the *Diagnostic and Statistical Manual of Mental Disorders-Third Edition, Revised (DSM-III-R)*. Criteria for MID included stepwise progression of cognitive decline with acquired differential deficits among various functions; focal neurological deficits; and evidence of an association between cerebrovascular disease and the dementia (APA, 1987). In the *DSM-IV* (APA, 1994), the term "multi-infarct dementia" was replaced with "vascular dementia." Diagnostic criteria for vascular dementia, as defined in the current *DSM-IV-TR*, include memory impairments and aphasia, apraxia, agnosia, and/or executive functioning deficits that result in social or occupational impairments as well as focal neurological signs and symptoms or laboratory findings of cerebrovascular disease, the cause of the dementia (APA, 2000). More recently "vascular cognitive impairment" has been proposed to replace the term "vascular dementia" (Bowler, 2007), to allow the inclusion of persons with symptomatic vascular disease that have not yet crossed the threshold for a dementia diagnosis. Vascular dementia and vascular cognitive impairment are more comprehensive concepts than MID because they include dementias resulting from various other circulatory etiologies in addition to multiple cerebral infarctions.

MID and Alzheimer disease (AD) are often difficult to differentiate. Accurate diagnosis is even more challenging because these disorders are not mutually exclusive. Generally, AD is associated with a more gradual course than MID. Like AD, memory impairment is associated with MID; however, memory deficits resulting from MID are typically not as severe as deficits resulting from AD. For example, a comparison of neuropsychological performance between individuals with AD to individuals with MID found that while individuals in both groups showed broad impairments, those with AD obtained significantly lower overall mean scores on the neuropsychological battery. The largest differences between the groups were on measures of memory and learning, including orientation, paragraph recall, picture recognition memory, and face-name learning, on which individuals with AD performed more poorly. Psychomotor deficits, however, may be more pronounced in individuals with MID (Taylor, Gilleard, & McGuire, 1996), and individuals with MID may also demonstrate

poorer performance on measures of executive function and speech mechanics than individuals with AD (Looi & Sachdev, 1999; Powell et al., 1998). While individuals with AD show poverty of content of speech, individuals with MID produce shorter utterances with less grammatical complexity.

Sultzer, Levin, Mahler, High, and Cummings (1993) found that individuals with MID displayed greater levels of psychopathology than individuals with AD. In the same study, psychopathology was not correlated with cognitive impairments in individuals with MID, but more severe psychiatric symptoms have been associated with greater dementia severity in individuals with AD (Sultzer et al., 1993; Sultzer, Levin, Mahler, High, & Cummings, 1992). Overall neuropsychological presentation is not very useful in distinguishing between individuals with MID and AD, as variability among individuals within these groups is more salient than differences between groups.

The Ischemic Score, developed by Hachinski et al. (1975), has demonstrated utility in differentiating individuals with MID and AD. The scale is comprised 13 features characteristic of MID. Abrupt onset, fluctuating course, history of stroke, focal neurological symptoms, and focal neurological signs have a point value of 2, and stepwise deterioration, nocturnal confusion, relative preservation of personality, depression, somatic complaints, emotional incontinence, history or presence of hypertension, and evidence of associated atherosclerosis have a point value of 1. Total scores range from 0 to 18. Scores above 6 are indicative of MID, while scores below 5 are indicative of AD. Rosen, Terry, Fuld, Katzman, and Peck (1980) confirmed the utility of the Ischemic Score in differentiating individuals with AD from individuals with MID or both MID and AD; however, they suggested an abbreviated revision of scale that would only include eight features, namely, abrupt onset, stepwise deterioration, somatic complaints, emotional incontinence, history or presence of hypertension, history of strokes, and focal neurological signs and symptoms.

TREATMENT

Generally, MID is chronic and irreversible. However, pharmacological approaches are available to treat symptomology and prevent further decline. Heparin-induced extracorporeal LDL/fibrinogen precipitation (HELP) has been found to ameliorate the pathologic hemorheologic state associated with MID (Walzl, 2000). Also, rivastigmine has been shown to be more effective than nimodipine in improving behavioral symptoms associated with MID, including hallucinations, aberrant behavior, sleep disturbances, and anxiety disorders. Individuals with MID who are treated with rivastigmine also show a reduced reliance on other medications, including neuroleptics and benzodiazepines (Moretti, Torre, Antonello, Cazzato, & Pizzolato, 2008). The effectiveness of vinpocetine has also been investigated. In a clinical trial, individuals who received this medication demonstrated preserved scores on the digit span backward test after 3 months (Kemeny, Molnar, Andrejkovics, Makai, & Csiba, 2005). When five individuals with MID were treated with physostigmine, results revealed reduced P300 latencies and significant increases in the WAIS scores of four of the participants (Neshige et al., 1988). Treatment of MID also involves the management of various risk factors, including cardiovascular disease, high cholesterol, diabetes mellitus, and hypertension.

Alyse Barker
Mandi Musso
William Drew Gouvier

American Psychiatric Association. (1987). *Diagnostic and statistical manual of mental disorders* (3rd ed., rev.). Washington, DC: Author.

American Psychiatric Association. (1994). *Diagnostic and statistical manual of mental disorders* (4th ed.). Washington, DC: Author.

American Psychiatric Association. (2000). *Diagnostic and statistical manual of mental disorders* (4th ed., text rev.). Washington, DC: Author.

Bowler, J. V. (2007). Modern concept of vascular cognitive impairment. *British Medical Bulletin, 83,* 291–305.

De Reuck, J., Decoo, D., Marchau, M., Santens, P., Lemahieu, I., & Strijckmans, K. (1998). Positron emission tomography in vascular dementia. *Journal of Neurological Sciences, 154,* 55–61.

Hachinski, V. C., Iliff, L. D., Zilhka, E., Duboulay, G. H., McAllister, V. L., Marshall, J., et al. (1975). Cerebral blood-flow in dementia. *Archives of Neurology, 32*(9), 632–637.

Hachinski, V. C., Lassen, N. A., & Marshall, J. (1974). Multi-infarct dementia: A cause of mental deterioration in the elderly. *The Lancet, 304*(7874), 207–209.

Kemeny, V., Molnar, S., Andrejkovics, M., Makai, A., & Csiba, L. (2005). Acute and chronic effects of vinpocetine on cerebral hemodynamics and neuropsychological performance in multi-infarct patients. *Journal of Clinical Pharmacology, 45,* 1048–1054.

Looi, J. C. L., & Sachdev, P. S. (1999). Differentiation of vascular dementia from AD on neuropsychological tests. *Neurology, 53,* 670–678.

Lyoo, I. K., Satlin, A., Lee, C. K., & Renshaw, P. F. (1997). Regional atrophy of the corpus callosum in subjects with Alzheimer's disease and multi-infarct dementia. *Psychiatric Research: Neuroimaging Section, 74,* 63–72.

Meguro, K., Doi, C., Ueda, M., Yamaguchi, T., Matsui, H., Kinomura, S., et al. (1991). Decreased cerebral glucose metabolism associated with mental deterioration in multi-infarct dementia. *Neuroradiology, 33,* 305–309.

Moretti, R., Torre, P., Antonello, R. M., Cazzato, G., & Pizzolato, G. (2008). Different responses to rivastigmine in subcortical dementia and multi-infarct dementia. *American Journal of Alzheimer's Disease & Other Dementias, 23*(2), 167–176.

Neshige, R., Barrett, G., & Shibasaki, H. (1988). Auditory long latency event-related potentials in Alzheimer's disease and multi-infarct dementia. *Journal of Neurology, Neurosurgery, and Psychiatry, 51,* 1120–1125.

Powell, A. L., Cummings, J. L., Hill, M. A., & Benson, D. F. (1988). Speech and language alterations in multi-infarct dementia. *Neurology, 38,* 717–719.

Rosen, W. G., Terry, R. D., Fuld, P. A., Katzman, R., & Peck, A. (1980). Pathological verification of ischemic score in differentiation of dementias. *Annals of Neurology, 7,* 486–488.

Sultzer, D. L., Levin, H. S., Mahler, M. E., High, W. M., & Cummings, J. L. (1992). Assessment of cognitive, psychiatric, and behavioral disturbances in patients with dementia: the Neurobehavioral Rating Scale. *Journal of the American Geriatrics Society, 40*(6), 549–555.

Sultzer, D. L., Levin, H. S., Mahler, M. E., High, W. M., & Cummings, J. L. (1993). A comparison of psychiatric symptoms in vascular dementia and Alzheimer's disease. *American Journal of Psychiatry, 150*(12), 1806–1812.

Taylor, R., Gilleard, C. J., & McGuire, R. J. (1996). Patterns of neuropsychological impairment in dementia of the Alzheimer type and multi-infarct dementia. *Archives of Gerontology and Geriatrics, 23,* 13–26.

Walzl, M. (2000). A promising approach to the treatment of multi-infarct dementia. *Neurobiology of Aging, 21,* 283–287.

MULTIPLE SCLEROSIS

DESCRIPTION

Multiple sclerosis (MS) is a degenerative and autoimmune condition that affects 100–130 per 100,000 people in the United States (Kurtzke & Wallin, 2000). Currently, MS is considered one of the most prevalent chronic neurological disorders in young and middle adulthood, with a peak incidence in the third decade and the highest prevalence within 40–59 years of age. Women present a higher tendency to develop MS with an average ratio of 2.6:1. The clinical presentation of MS is caused primarily by demyelination (destruction of the myelin sheath), with associated inflammation and visible white matter lesions in magnetic resonance studies being a prominent feature. Etiological causes of MS are still unknown; however, the interaction of genetic and environmental factors has been postulated as most important susceptibility agents (Ebers, 2008). There is a latitudinal variation in the prevalence of MS, being reportedly more frequent in areas more distant from the Equator and mounting evidence between the inverse relation between sun exposure and the development of MS (MacLean & Freedman, 2009). MS presentation is characterized by episodes of focal deficits of the optic nerves, and spinal cord and brain injury that usually require medical attention and that might remit and recur sporadically for years. Clinical symptoms in MS include motor weakness, paraparesis (motor weakness on lower extremities), vision changes, diplopia, nystagmus, dysarthria, intention tremor, ataxia, somatosensory changes (paresthesias), and bladder dysfunction. Other important and common, but sometimes underreported, symptoms include cognitive and affective changes (Haase, Tinnefeld, Lieneman, Ganz, & Faustmann, 2003). Diagnosis in MS is difficult due to the relapsing and remitting pattern, the subtle nature of symptoms and the apparent similarity with other diseases especially autoimmune ones. MS subtypes have been identified as relapsing–remitting MS (RRMS), progressive relapsing, primary progressive, and secondary progressive. The most aggressive and likely type to produce morbidity is primary progressive. Another important clinical category within the MS spectrum is the clinically isolated syndrome (CIS) an isolated CNS syndrome (optic neuritis, incomplete transverse myelitis, brainstem or cerebellar lesion), which is often the first MS attack (Thrower, 2007). The use of MRI has enlightened our knowledge of this disease and has replaced other studies used in the past to aid in the diagnosis of MS. Earlier diagnosis is now possible with its routine use (Bakshi, Hutton, Miller, & Radue, 2004).

Treatment methods in MS aim to decrease the possibility of new clinical relapses or slowing of the progression of the disease by MRI. The first method of treatment is through interferons, which are naturally occurring antiviral proteins. Glatiramer acetate, which acts in the immune system to spare myelin from further attack, has shown to alter the natural history of RRMS. Natalizumab, and chemotherapeutic agents are used in secondary progressive MS, and other less conventional therapies are intravenous corticosteroids

intravenous immunoglobulin or plasma exchange. In MS, neuropsychology presents an important bridge between the physical (e.g., brain lesions) and cognitive and emotional (e.g., memory and depression) areas. In doing so, the Cartesian dualism is hinged to form one continuum. The end result of neuropsychological assessment is heightened understanding and advanced treatment of the patient with MS.

NEUROPATHOLOGY/PATHOPHYSIOLOGY

MS is largely an inflammatory demyelinating autoimmune disease that is thought to develop by a combination of genetic and environmental factors. Pathologic damage is caused by T lymphocytes that become activated and gain entrance to the blood–brain barrier. This entrance causes an inflammatory response that in turn attacks the myelin. During the disease process, only central myelin produced by oligodendrocytes is affected, which causes astrocytes to respond by forming a glial scar. These patches of demyelination in the white matter of the brain or spinal cord disrupt central nerve transmission. Pathologic studies along with more advanced neuroimaging techniques indicate axonal damage and neuronal loss that eventually lead to brain atrophy. Axon loss is the major cause of irreversible disability in patients with MS (Dutta & Trapp, 2007). Antibody- and complement-mediated myelin phagocytosis (macrophages engulfing cellular debris), in this case myelin, is also a pathophysiological process occurring later in the degenerative process of this disease (Dhib-Jalbut, 2007). These disease processes have been well documented in postmortem specimens of MS patients.

Neurobiological Markers

Many biological markers have been studied in MS, and the most widely used markers are those obtained through a spinal tap from the CSF like myelin basic protein (MBP), immunoglobulin (IgG) index, and oligoclonal bands (OGCB). The genetic region most clearly associated with MS susceptibility is the human leukocyte antigen (HLA) locus on the short arm of chromosome 6 (6p21) (De Jager et al., 2008). In various studies, the HLA region has been estimated to confer somewhere between 10% and 50% of the inheritability of MS. In Caucasian MS populations of northern European descent, the critical MS-associated genetic region is thought to reside near the class II *locus and is comprised of a group of genes with specific alleles that tend to occur in certain fixed combinations termed haplotypes. In molecular terms, the

"DR2" haplotype is designated as HLA-DRB1*1501, DQA1*0102, and DQB1*0602. These DR molecules are comprised of alpha and beta chains (encoded by A and B genes, respectively), and the polymorphisms are predominantly present in the beta chain. Of the more than 100 beta-chain sequence variations identified in humans, only one (1501, also designated as DR2) is associated with MS, and the DR2 gene is the most important genetic contributor to MS susceptibility identified to date.

Neuroimaging Techniques

MRI can be used to demonstrate dissemination in space and time within the brain and spinal cord, which has led to its common use as a paraclinical measure for diagnosis of MS including diagnosing patients with CIS. In addition, MRI is used to monitor the progress of disease in patients with clinically definite MS, including assessment of lesions and atrophy (Bakshi et al., 2004). Several MRI techniques can be used to study MS (Table 1). The most important ones, required for diagnosis are T2-weighted images (showing areas of demyelination and edema) and gadolinium-enhanced (T1) images (indicating the presence of acute inflammation). T1 images also help to determine the presence of "black holes" or axonal damage. On T2 and FLAIR, MS lesions are seen as hyperintense, ovoid-shaped, periventricular white matter lesions oriented perpendicular to the ventricular surface (known as Dawson's fingers). They also commonly appear as corpus callosal, juxtacortical, and infratentorial lesions involving the posterior fossa and spinal cord.

Not widely available but useful in the evaluation of MS patients is the functional MRI that helps to evaluate neuronal circuits needed for diverse brain functions. It measures critical circuitry involved in response to injury, activation, loss of function, and recovery of function. Magnetic resonance spectroscopy (MRS) is another MRI technique that has gained much interest in recent years because it can be used to detect early abnormalities even in otherwise normal-appearing brain tissue. Studies have shown that decreased N-acetyl aspartate (NAA) levels reflect axon damage that is an important cause of disability. NAA is a biochemical found in neurons considered an index of axonal integrity and functional activity. In 2003, Cristodoulou et al. found a correlation between neuropsychological symptoms and NAA/Cr ratios on the brain central ventricular areas, with a higher correlation on the right hemisphere. Some researchers hypothesize that the cognitive and emotional symptoms observed at early stages of the disease could be

Table 1
INFORMATION PROVIDED BY MRI

Techniques	Importance
T1	Gadolinium-enhancing lesions detect blood–brain barrier leakage, inflammatory disturbances, and recent (≤ 6 weeks) activity, with lesion formation.
	Hypointense lesions (black holes) reflect more severe tissue pathology, including axon loss and correlates with disability.
T2	Hyperintense lesions provide total burden of disease measure, including reversible and irreversible pathologies. Most predictive of disease course in early MS. Hyperintense T2 lesions can reflect a variety of pathologic processes in addition to demyelination, such as inflammation, edema, axonal loss, and remyelination
Diffusion weighted	Detects abnormalities in both lesions and normal-appearing CNS tissue. Detects white matter changes.
Flair (fluid attenuated inversion recovery)	Hyperintense lesions

more related to early biochemical changes than to structural damage caused by lesions and inflammation (Benedict, Weinstock-Guttman, Fishman, Sharma, & Tjoa, 2004).

Magnetic Resonance Spectroscopy in MS

MRS is a noninvasive neuroimaging technique that allows the in vivo quantification of brain neurochemistry by measuring concentration of key metabolites (Stanley, 2002) like NAA, mio-inositol, choline, and Cr. Over the past 20 years, MRS has been used to study the pathological mechanisms of neurological and psychiatric disorders, monitor long-term changes, identify differences among diagnostic groups, and study cognitive dysfunction on these disorders (Ross & Sachdev, 2004). The relative quantity or amount of these metabolites is usually determined by comparing their resonance peaks. Other methods like event-related potentials, brain size volume, cerebral metabolic rate, and cerebral blood flow have not been

M

found to be strongly associated with cognitive functions, and due to cerebral plasticity measures of neural integrity such as MRS, should be the most sensitive to the neuropathology that leads to cognitive decline (Zivadinoff & Bakshi, 2004). Interestingly, in MS these lowered levels of NAA do not correlate with the total amount of lesions (Fillipi et al., 2003), which are critical in the diagnosis of MS criteria (Mc-Donald, Compston, & Edan, 2001). This represents an important finding and might support the cognitive/ neuropsychological deficits that have been observed in MS patients in early stages of the disease.

Diffusion Weighted Imaging and Diffusion-Tensor Imaging in MS

The magnetic resonance signal is intrinsically sensitive to motion at the molecular level. Two complementing MRI techniques known as diffusion-weighted and diffusion tensor-imaging (DWI and DTI) are capable of measuring water diffusion[1] and diffusion anisotropy[2]. Of particular relevance for the study of MS neuropathology is the fact that these diffusion-based MRI techniques are capable of characterizing white matter integrity and the orientation of white matter fiber bundles.

Increased water diffusion serves as a marker for cell membrane disruption. Moderate correlations have been found for DTI diffusivity and fractional anisotropy (FA) and cognitive functions on normal appearing gray matter and normal appearing white matter (Rovaris et al., 2002). Moreover, longitudinal studies using DTI[3] and mean diffusivity have found progressive microstructural changes after 18 months in the normal appearing matter that do not correlate with lesions and atrophy (Ojera et al., 2005). Water diffusion is restricted within intact white matter fibers. It is inferred that the more anisotropic the water diffusion is in a particular region of the brain, the more restricted it is and the higher the probability that it is constrained within intact tissue. By measuring the degree of directional anisotropy of diffusion, the DTI technique probes tissue integrity on a microscopic scale that is not possible to achieve using conventional anatomical MRI techniques such as those used for clinical diagnosis of MS.

The most recent DTI data on MS patients have shown that normal appearing white matter showed

significant increased diffusivity as measured by the Apparent Diffusion Coefficient (ADC) and reduced FA compared with controls, whereas ADC had a stronger association to clinical disability than lesion load (Vrenken et al., 2006). Another recent study, with 23 early onset MS patients, showed decreased FA on normal-appearing white matter, which confirms occult tissue damage (Tortorella et al., 2006). In view of the most recent studies and metabolite quantification with MRS, DTI seems to be, for the moment, one of the most promising neuroimaging techniques available for the study of diffuse white matter degeneration. DTI is susceptible to subtle global tissue degeneration at a microscopic scale in otherwise normal appearing white matter using conventional anatomical MRI techniques, and it could become a potential diagnostic marker for MS at preclinical or early clinical stages (Table 1).

Spinal Tap

Spinal tap is a relatively easy procedure that can be done in MS patients to exclude any other infectious or inflammatory process that could mimic MS. CSF is taken for analysis that includes markers that aid in the diagnosis of the disease (Table 2).

Evoked Potentials

Evoked potentials (EPs) are electrodiagnostic studies that aid in the diagnosis of MS when history, clinical findings, or imaging studies do not confirm it and more evidence is needed. EPs evaluate processing pathways of sensory nerve tracts in the spinal cord,

---

[1] Diffusion with tissue integrity in a microscopic scale.
[2] Diffusion anisotropy, associated with restricted diffusion.
[3] DTI, using directionally selective diffusion measurements, is used to determine the degree of anisotropy in the diffusion of water.

Table 2
CSF DISEASE MARKERS IN MS

Marker	Description
Oligoclonal bands (OGCB)	OGCB are produced by the over-representation of particular antibodies. They are *typical* of the CSF of MS patients, but not *exclusive* to it.
Intrathecal immunoglobulin production (IgG, IgM)	Immunoglobulins are produced by plasma cells and are integral in adaptive immune responses. Polyclonal increases of IgG occur in chronic infection and inflammation.
Myelin basic protein (MBP)	A major component of myelin, MBP is increased in the CSF of some, but not all, MS patients following a demyelinating episode.

thalamus, and sensory cortex, auditory pathways in the brainstem and optic nerve function. These studies help to determine whether there has been an otherwise silent demyelinating lesion to the CNS. Among the evoked potential studies, the highest yield for diagnosis in people with probable M S are the somato-sensory EPs, followed by the visual EPs. As a group, their use has declined due to the advent of MRI as a tool for diagnosis.

NEUROPSYCHOLOGICAL/CLINICAL
PRESENTATION

MS is a chronic recurrent inflammatory neurological disease in which immune-mediated events contribute to subsequent neurologic impairment and disability. It is a complex and frequently active disease process that involves diverse pathological and clinical features. Based mostly in studies of the natural history of the MS disease, some clinical subtypes have been defined (Table 3). It is known that the majority of individuals followed in natural history studies develop progressive disability over long periods of time. Also later stages of the disease are marked by reduced relapses but continued worsening and progressive deterioration.

The clinical presentation and course of MS is variable and sometimes unpredictable as it is influenced by brain pathology and the individual disease course in each patient. Similarly, the neuropsychological symptoms can vary within subtypes at different stages of the disease (Patti, Amato, Trojano, Lijoi, & Bastianello, 2008). Although MS subtypes have been identified based on severity and progression, the clinical neuropsychological presentation within subtypes is quite unpredictable and overlaps with motor/neuromuscular and affective domains. However, despite the difficulties in establishing a neuropsychological profile in MS, some variables including the area of the lesions, progression of disease, number of years from initial diagnosis, mood/depression, and fatigue mediate the neuropsychological symptoms in each patient (Amato, Zipoli, & Portaccio, 2006). Recently, some researchers have established that neuropsychological symptoms are one of the most disabling yet poorly understood and measured features of the disease and have been documented in 40% to 60% of the patients (Huijbregts et al., 2004; Rao et al., 1991). Also, these symptoms can predict performance on simple and complex activities of daily living (Gaudino et al., 2006) needed for occupational tasks and independent living.

Comprehensive neuropsychological assessments evidence that in MS these symptoms may be broadly subdivided into two broad categories that include mood and cognitive functioning difficulties (Feinstein, 2004). Although they vary in severity, cognitive symptoms in MS involve deficits on visuospatial skills, memory, speed of processing, visuospatial abilities, sensorimotor functions, executive functions, concept formation, abstract reasoning, and verbal fluency

Table 3
CLINICAL SUBTYPES OF MULTIPLE SCLEROSIS (MS)

Relapsing-remitting MS	This is the major MS subtype. Approximately 66–85% of patients with a diagnosis of MS start out with relapsing MS, but after 10 years, only half are still relapsing. Relapsing MS patients show a high rate of inflammatory lesion activity (gadolinium-enhancing lesions).
Primary progressive MS	This subtype accounts for 10–15% of MS. Patients show gradual worsening from onset, without disease attacks. These patients tend to be older and often present with a spinal cord dysfunction without obvious brain involvement. This subtype is the least likely to show inflammatory lesion activity on MRI (gadolinium-enhancing). Unlike the other subtypes of MS, men are as likely as women to develop primary progressive MS.
Progressive relapsing MS	This subtype accounts for about 5% of MS. Patients show slow worsening from onset, with superimposed attacks. Recent studies suggest these patients are similar to primary progressive patients.
Secondary progressive MS	This is the major progressive subtype and accounts for approximately 30% of MS. About half of the relapsing MS patients usually transition to secondary progressive disease. They show gradual worsening, with or without superimposed relapses. Natural history studies of untreated relapsing MS indicate 50% of patients will be secondary progressive at 10 years and almost 90% by 25 years. This form of MS shows a lower rate of inflammatory lesion activity than relapsing MS, yet the total burden of disease continues to increase. This most likely reflects ongoing axonal loss.

M

(Schulthesis, Garay, & DeLuca, 2001). Cognitive symptoms have been found to be a good predictor of distress and disability (Rao et al., 1991), as well as occupational, social, and overall impairment (Bagert, Camplair, & Bourdette, 2002; Rao et al., 1991). Although no consensus has been established neuropsychological impairment in MS seems to increase and overlap with physical disability and progression (Bobholz & Rao, 2003).

Cognitive deficiencies tend to be more prevalent in the later stages (Beatty, Goodkin, Monson, Beatty, & Hertsgaard, 1998; Heaton, Nelson, Thompson, Burks, & Franklin, 1985), although in some cases they may be detectable at an early phase of the disease (Bagert et al., 2002; Grant, McDonald, Trimble, Smith, & Reed, 1984; Lyon-Caen et al., 1986). Earlier symptoms can involve information processing speed and verbal fluency (Arango-Laspirilla, DeLuca, & Chiaravalloti, 2007). The later symptoms may involve deficits in memory, conceptual/abstract reasoning, attention, moderate to severe decrease in the speed of information processing, and visuospatial functions (Bagert et al., 2002; Rao, 1986; Ron, Callanan, & Warrington, 1991). A recent study with 416 relapsing–remitting patients found that processing speed seems to be the most significant cognitive symptom in RRMS (Nocentini et al., 2006).

Sensorimotor Functions

As discussed earlier, MS primary symptoms involve sensorimotor dysfunction; however, presentations are different and therefore the severity and the pattern of dysfunction may vary in each case. Visual impairment is a cardinal symptom in optic neuritis. Motor output sequences become slower due to demyelization and the degeneration characteristic of MS. In MS, motor impairment can be evident with tests that involve different aspects of gross and fine motor output, motor speed, and perceptual skills. In fact, many of the most current cognitive batteries recommended for MS have tried to control for sensory motor effects like the Paced Auditory Serial Addition Test (PASAT), the oral Symbol Digit Modalities Test (SDMT), the Rao's Brief Repeatable Battery (BRB), and the Stroop Color Word Task in order to assess more complex cognitive skills.

Visuospatial Skills, Visuoconstructive Abilities

Visuospatial and visuoperceptual abilities are complex procedures that include sensorimotor, executive, and perceptual abilities. In general, these appear to be impaired in approximately 20% of patients with MS (Prakash, Snoook, Lewis, Motl, & Kramer, 2008).

Taking into consideration that patients might experience significant visuospatial, visuoperceptual, and visuoconstructive abilities, cognitive evaluation should be specific and take into account the perceptual deficits that might interfere with other cognitive domains. The Benton Visual Orientation Tests are helpful in determining visuospatial and visuoperceptual difficulties. Clinical treatment and recommendations for MS patients should be supported with a minimal screening of visual functions since the quality of life and safety of a patient might change (e.g., driving) as a direct consequence of visuospatial impairment.

Memory

Performance in memory measures of MS might be in part influenced by the attention and psychomotor speed difficulties that these patients experience; therefore, measures used to evaluate different aspects of a patient's memory should control for the above, for example, visuoperceptual deficits and processing speed. Short-term memory and working memory (WM) studies in MS have found that arithmetic seems to be more impaired in patients with MS suggesting that WM deficits tend to be more pervasive as they involve processing simultaneous information. In addition to evaluating processing speed, the PASAT evaluates verbal WM. Consistently, studies have found that 20% to 25% of MS patients tend to present significant impairment on the PASAT as compared with controls (Demaree, DeLuca, Gaudino, & Diamond, 1999; Rao, Leo, Bernardin, & Unverzagt, 1991). Other studies using newer experimental procedures such as the N-back Test that RRMS patients present impairment relative to complexity after taking simple motor speed into account (Parmenter, Shucard, Benedict, & Shucard, 2006; Parmenter, Shucard, & Shucard, 2007). WM deficits seem to be directly related to the course and severity of the disease and primary progressive patients seemed to be more impaired in WM (Zakanis, 2000). Similarly, De Luca establishes that the fundamental difficulties in WM are directly related to processing speed. (DeLuca et al., 2004).

Long-term memory performance seems to be associated with WM and processing speed; however, MS patients tend to maintain an adequate capacity to learn new information (DeLuca, Barbieri-Berger, & Johnson, 1994) and learning trials of lists evidence that the learning slope remains intact (DeLuca et al., 2004; Prakash et al., 2008). Long-term declarative memory impairment also seems to be mediated by impairment in retrieval of information, whereas storage and consolidation of memory seem to be relatively preserved where recognition trials seem to improve retrieval and represent the learning and consolidation processes (Randolph, Arnett, & Higginson, 2001). Difficulties in long-term memory in MS seem to be related to poor encoding, semantic clustering, reduction of semantic categorization, and interference (Arnett et al., 1997).

Speed of Processing

Processing speed deficits seem to be the most evident and fundamental deficit in MS (DeLuca et al., 2004; Parmenter et al., 2007). Due to the white matter abnormalities of MS and lack of myelin in nerve conduction, processing speed difficulties are identified in many patients with MS (DeLuca et al., 2004). However, the differences in the Trail Making Test are not that evident (Arnett et al., 1997). Understanding the challenges of conducting assessments accurately, Rao (1990) developed the PASAT to specifically evaluate the processing capacities without the visual and motor interference that might be present in the disease. The PASAT has been translated and adapted to many languages and has become part of the official National Multiple Sclerosis Society recommended cognitive screening.

Executive Functions

The Wisconsin Card Sorting Test (WCST) and the Halstead Category Test (HCT) are the most commonly used assessments for evaluating executive functions in terms of planning, flexibility, and inhibition. On both measures, MS patients seem to present moderate to severe deficits that are in part mediated by processing speed difficulties (Arnett et al., 1997). Executive deficits in MS have been associated with depressed mood. However, it seems that nonspeeded tax index using the Tower of London (TOL) (as measured by the TOL-moves per trial) indicated a deficient nonspeeded central executive skill secondary to the slow information processing deficits (Arnett, Higginson, & Randolph, 2001). Also, deficits in executive functions may be evident in clinical observations and everyday quality of life questionnaires.

Language/Verbal Fluency

Studies of neuropsychological measures of language functioning in MS have found that verbal fluency tends to be affected even at early stages of the disease (Beatty, 2002; Prakash et al., 2008). In contrast, confrontational naming seems to be more preserved (Vlaar & Wade, 2003). However, in the areas of verbal comprehension and overall verbal IQ (Wechsler Adult Intelligence Scale [WAIS]), MS patients have exhibited

mild difficulties (Matotek, Saling, Gates, & Sedal, 2001; Prakash et al., 2008), although deficits seem to be associated with time and severity of the disease (Drake, Allegri, & Carrá, 2002).

Intellectual Abilities

As a consequence of sensory motor difficulties observed in MS, general intelligence measures like the Wechsler's Intelligence Scale reveal that MS patients tend to have difficulties in performance subtests and perceptual reasoning indexes (Prakash et al., 2008). However, when comparing performance within the MS samples, performance IQ seems to be more impaired than verbal IQ even in patients with no physical disability as measured with Expanded Disability Status Scale (EDSS) (Prakash et al., 2008). Nonetheless, intelligence as a general measure depends on lower hierarchy functions like speed of processing, sensory, and motor functions, which are all consistently negatively affected in patients with MS. In conclusion, neuropsychological assessments adapted for MS should always be considered as alternate and supplemental instruments rather than the traditional batteries of intelligence.

Affective and Emotional Symptoms

Cognitive difficulties can be confounded by the emotional symptoms and psychiatric manifestations that accompany this disorder. In contrast, some researchers support that the cognitive symptoms observed in MS patients lack motor and physical impairment, whereas others observe a connection between physical disability and cognitive symptoms (Van Den Burg et al., 1987).

The emotional disturbances most commonly associated with MS are depression and anxiety (Randolph, Arnett, & Freeske, 2004). However, findings support that depression is the most prominent emotional disturbance identified in MS (Arnett, 2005). Proper identification of depression in MS might be difficult since the cardinal symptoms of MS are very similar and overlap with the fiscal disability. Further, in some tests such as the Beck Depression Inventory, many items such as the ones involving fatigue could be specific symptoms more associated with MS than symptoms of depression. For example, concentration difficulties, psychomotor retardation, and sexual dysfunction in MS patients can be considered symptoms of depression, but they can also be a pathophysiological manifestation of MS (Voss et al., 2001). In 2001, Voss and colleagues discovered that physical

M

disability and fatigue were indirectly predictive of depressed mood via recreational functioning. However, fatigue was directly related to depressed mood in MS. Another study conducted by Arnett and Randolph in 2006 using the Beck Depression Inventory and the Chicago Multiscale Depression Inventory (CMDI) Evaluative Symptoms and the CMDI-Vegetative Symptoms assessed different symptom clusters of mood (negative evaluative and neurovegetative) and its relation to active coping strategies in MS. Interestingly, they found that although the lifetime prevalence of depression seems to be very high, the mood symptoms tend to be more variable over long periods of time than negative or neurovegetative symptoms, and increased use of active coping strategies tended to decrease depressed mood longitudinally (Arnett & Randolph, 2006). Also, they found that MS patients that use Beta interferon tended to present a higher risk for depression. Other studies of MS and depression have focused on exploring what affective and cognitive factors contribute to the presence of depression symptoms. One of these studies found that objective executive difficulties contributed to depression; however, the authors found depressive attitudes and depression treatment also mediated memory complaints (Memory Functioning Questionnaire [MFQ]). The authors concluded that interventions for depression might improve the patient's self-perceptions and quality of life (Randolph et al., 2004).

Fatigue in MS

In MS patients experience unpredictable fluctuations in their energy and mood that result in physical, psychological, and social deficits. Some research has shown that in MS patients, fatigue was a direct effect of a patient's mood state (Voss et al., 2001). Nevertheless, fatigue in MS can be distinguished from fatigue related to traditional symptoms of depression, based on the fact that fatigue in MS is aggravated by heat, is often alleviated by sleep, and lasts for only a few hours compared with the more persistent fatigue associated with depression (Patten & Metz, 2002). Alternative treatments such as yoga have been reported to improve fatigue symptoms; other pharmacological treatments such as modafinil have presented mixed results. Assessing each patient's individual symptoms of fatigue is crucial in determining best treatment options.

DIAGNOSIS

Current diagnosis of MS requires a more specific set of criteria requiring the evidence of recurrent

neurological deficits, which typically consist of sensory disturbances, optic neuritis, diplopia, limb weakness, clumsiness, and gait ataxia. The diagnosis of MS since its original descriptions has been one based mostly on history and clinical findings. Recurrent neurological deficits disseminated in space and time are basic requirements for diagnosis. These deficits can include sensory disturbances, optic neuritis, diplopia, limb weakness, clumsiness, and gait ataxia. Different diagnostic criteria have been developed over time, and currently MRI has been recognized as an essential tool to exclude other possible diagnosis, to give uniformity to a disease that has such variable presentations, and to account that there was progression of disease. In 2001, the McDonald International Panel proposed a new diagnostic scheme for diagnosis, which replaced previous criteria, incorporated MRI findings (Table 4) and paraclinical studies such as CSF and visual EPs with neurological history and examination. These criteria were revised in 2005. Diagnosis of MS according to McDonald criteria requires either clinical or radiographic evidence of one or more "attacks" with dissemination in time in conjunction with objective evidence by clinical examination or MRI of lesions with dissemination in space. Revised MRI criteria for dissemination in time requires either gadolinium-enhancing lesion(s) at least 3 months after onset of a clinical event but not corresponding to the site associated with the event or detection at any time of a new T2 lesion that was not present on a reference scan performed at least 30 days after an initial event. Despite evolving MS diagnostic criteria, for an accurate diagnosis, there is no substitute for careful consideration of the patient's history, neurological examination, imaging results, laboratory tests, CSF analysis, EPs, and testing that excludes other possible diagnosis.

Clinically Isolated Syndrome

This refers to patients who present with an isolated CNS syndrome (optic neuritis, incomplete transverse myelitis, brainstem or cerebellar lesion), which is often the first MS attack. Clinical, MRI, and CSF studies indicate that such patients with normal brain MRI and CSF have a low risk of developing MS. In contrast, those with abnormal MRI have a high risk of developing MS (Tintoré et al., 2003).

In patients with CIS suggestive of demyelination, evidence for dissemination in time and space could be provided by MRI alone. Dissemination in space can be identified by meeting three of four MRI criteria, or, alternatively, by showing at least two lesions plus the presence of OGCB (or elevated IgG index) in

Table 4
MRI EVIDENCE OF DISSEMINATION IN SPACE BY McDONALD CRITERIA

		Disease Categories	Examples
3 of the following (one spinal cord lesion can be substituted for one brain lesion):		Vascular diseases	Vasculitis, antiphospholipid antibody syndrome, CADASIL, cerebrovascular disease, Susac syndrome
■ One gadolinium-enhancing lesion or 9 T2 hyperintense lesions		Infectious diseases	Bacterial (Lyme disease, syphilis, Whipple's disease), viral (HIV infection, human T-lymphotrophic virus Type-1 infection, herpes viruses, progressive multifocal leukoencephalopathy, JC virus)
■ One or more juxtacortical lesions			
■ One or more infratentorial lesions			
■ Three or more periventricular lesions			

Common	Uncommon		
■ Sensory problems (numbness or tingling of a body part)	■ Bladder problems	Neoplastic diseases	Primary brain tumor (i.e., CNS lymphoma), metastatic tumors, paraneoplastic syndromes
	■ Bowel problems		
■ Weakness	■ Sexual dysfunction	Structural or compressive conditions	Cervical spondylosis, degenerative disc disease, Chiari malformation, dural arteriovenous fistulas, syrinx
■ Difficulty walking	■ Cognitive difficulties		
■ Monocular decreased vision	■ Pain		
■ Poor coordination		Inflammatory diseases	Collagen vascular diseases (SLE, Sjogren's syndrome), neurosarcoidosis, Bechet's disease

Brain Lesions	Spinal Cord Lesions		
High signal on T2-weighted and FLAIR MRI sequences	1 or 2 vertebral segments in length	Genetic conditions	Leukodystrophies (adrenoleukodystrophy, adrenomyeloneuropathy), lysosomal storage diseases, Fabry's disease, mitochondrial diseases
When actively inflamed, often enhanced with gadolinium contrast	Generally incomplete cross-sectional involvement (dorsolateral common)		
Position abutting ventricles (often perpendicular)	Less likely to enhance with gadolinium contrast	Metabolic diseases	Vitamin B12 deficiency, acquired copper deficiency, folate deficiency, hyperhomocysteinemia, vitamin E deficiency
Juxtacortical position (gray–white junction)	No cord swelling		
Involvement of brainstem, cerebellum, or corpus callosum	Better seen with STIR MRI sequences	Psychogenic conditions	Conversion disorder, depression, anxiety

CSF. In a multicenter study, it was shown that if Barkhof/Tintoré criteria are fulfilled the likelihood for conversion to clinically definite MS is much higher and the time much shorter than if criteria are not fulfilled (Korteweg et al., 2006).

Early, routine, and yearly assessment of neurological symptoms in MS patients is a critical aspect required in the careful monitoring of a patient's disease progression, response to treatment, and overall quality of life. Despite the evidence that cognitive and emotional symptoms have a significant impact on the patient's quality of life, a study revealed that in 2002, MS clinics and neurological practices did not routinely conduct neuropsychological assessments. This may have been attributed to a lack of consensus in the field about the right way to evaluate MS (Benedict et al., 2002). As a result of the discrepancy, a group of neurologists and neuropsychologists from the United States, Canada, the United Kingdom, and Australia met together and agreed that the new standard for diagnosing MS would require a minimal neuropsychological assessment. These experts developed the Minimal Assessment of Cognitive Function in MS (MACFIMS). The MACFIMS is a 90 min battery composed of seven neuropsychological tests that evaluate the domains of processing speed, WM, learning and memory, executive function, visuospatial processing, word retrieval, and provides recommendations for evaluation of sensorimotor functions, fatigue, and depression (Benedict et al.,

M

2002). Some of the tests that have proven to be effective with MS patients are Rao's BRB, MS Neuropsychological Screening Questionnaire, PASAT, SMDT (Smith, 1982), California Verbal Learning Test, and the Brief Visuospatial Memory Test.

TREATMENT

Today there are many innovative disease-modifying treatments for MS that aim to decrease the possibility of new clinical relapses or slow the progression of the disease by MRI. The first method of treatment is through interferons, which are naturally occurring antiviral proteins. Interferon beta-1a low dose (Avonex) and high dose (Rebif) as well as interferon beta-1b (Betaseron) have been shown to alter the natural history of RRMS. The interferon treatments have been shown to decrease the number of exacerbations and may slow the progression of the physical disability. These medications vary in their dose and frequency and are thought to work by modifying the effects of endogenous interferons on the immune system. Other treatment available is glatiramer acetate (Copaxone), which consists of a mixture of peptide fragments thought to act as a decoy for the immune system to spare myelin from further attack. All of the above treatments are injected subcutaneously with the exception of interferon beta-1a low dose which is injected intramuscularly. Current therapeutic treatments have been shown to work best in the more active inflammatory phases early in the disease. Natalizumab is a monoclonal antibody given intravenously once per month for patients who have been on the above medications with poor response or have eventually failed treatment. Chemotherapeutic agents such as mitoxantrone are being used as an alternative form of treatment for more aggressive progression like in the case of secondary progressive MS. The chemotherapeutic form of treatment is more a last resort because of the amount of undesirable side effects it causes. Newer therapies are currently under study including oral medications to avoid relapses. Unfortunately, none of the existing pharmaceutical interventions "cure" the disease. In addition, the markers for success are typically MRI lesions, which, as indicated earlier, do not appear to have a strong correlation with functional and cognitive limitations.

For acute exacerbations, intravenous corticosteroids are the treatment of choice that is frequently used for the purpose of hastening recovery in a patient who has already had a relapse. These anti-inflammatory agents suppress cell migration into the CNS, reducing inflammation around active plaques. They are usually administered for 3–5 days and then rapidly tapered down or discontinued. Less conventional therapies that can be used at times, in more aggressive cases, are intravenous immunoglobulin or plasma exchange. Symptomatic therapy includes treatment for associated spasticity, pain, bladder dysfunction, tremors, or fatigue. It is very important for the clinician to assess symptoms that can be secondary to fatigue, heat, lack of rest, or inadequate diet since these can mimic an acute relapse associated with a worsening of previous deficits. The addition of nonmedical interventions may be as critical, if not more, than the previously discussed interventions. These would include but not be limited to temperature regulation, fatigue control, massage, controlled exercise, vocational intervention, and psychotherapy.

The course of this disease is quite variable in each patient. Relapses may have measurable and lasting impact causing disability at a later time. Subtle clinical symptoms can be related to active inflammatory activity that can go unnoticed in the absence of careful evaluation. It is thought that roughly 15% of MS patients will never have a relapse and that most MS patients will eventually develop the secondary progressive form of MS. Factors that have been associated with poorer prognosis are frequent relapses in the first 2 years, primary progressive onset, male sex, the presence of multiple MRI lesions, and early motor or cerebellar findings.

EDSS is the most widely used scale for assessing level of disability in MS patients (Kurtzke, 1983). This rating system is frequently used for classifying and standardizing the condition of people with MS; it is also an important tool in clinical trials (can be used as inclusion/exclusion criteria and to compare results). The score is based on a clinical neurological examination and consists of a number scale from 0 to 10 where the range from 0.0 to 4.5 includes patients who are ambulatory and the range from 5.0 to 9.5 is defined by impairment of ambulation. Although it provides an objective measure, there is an apparent discrepancy between conventional lesions in MRI and clinical disability as measured by this scale (Li et al., 2006) since it places emphasis on the ability to walk and it may not be able to detect the extensive clinical changes that patients can experience.

In general, the course and manifestation of symptoms in MS are quite variable in each patient. Relapses may have measurable and lasting impact causing disability at a later time. Subtle clinical symptoms can be related to active inflammatory activity that can go unnoticed in the absence of careful evaluation. It is thought that roughly 10% of patients have benign MS and that 70% will become secondary progressive.

Liza San Miguel-Montes
Brenda Deliz-Roldán
Kriste Treftz-Puente

Amato, M. P., Zipoli, V., & Portaccio, E. (2006). Multiple sclerosis related cognitive changes: A review of cross-sectional and longitudinal studies. *Journal of Neurology Science, 245,* 41–46.

Arango-Laspirilla, J. C., DeLuca, J., & Chiaravalloti, N. (2007). Neuropsychological profile of multiple sclerosis. *Psicothema, 19*(1), 1–6.

Arnett, P. A. (2005). Longitudinal consistency of the relationship between depression symptoms and cognitive functioning in multiple sclerosis. *Central Nervous System Spectrums, 10*(5), 372–382.

Arnett, P. A., Higginson, C. I., & Randolph, J. J. (2001). Depression in multiple sclerosis: Relationship to planning ability. *Journal of the International Neuropsychological Society, 7*(6), 665–674.

Arnett, P. A., Higginson, C. I., Voss, W. D., Wright, B., Bender, W. I., & Wurst, J., et al. (1999). Depressed mood in multiple sclerosis: Relationship to capacity demanding memory and attentional functioning. *Neuropsychology, 13*(3), 434–446.

Arnett, P. A., & Randolph, J. J. (2006). Longitudinal course of depression symptoms in MS. *Journal of Neurology, Neurosurgery, & Psychiatry, 77,* 606–610.

Arnett, P. A., Rao, S., Graffman, J., Bernardin, L., Luchetta, T., Binder, J., et al. (1997). Executive functions in multiple sclerosis: An analysis of temporal ordering, semantic encoding, and planning abilities. *Neuropsychology, 11*(4), 535–544.

Bagert, B., Camplair, P., & Bourdette, D. (2002). Cognitive dysfunction in multiple sclerosis: Natural history, pathophysiology and management. *Central Nervous System Drugs, 16*(7), 445–455.

Bakshi, R., Hutton, G. J., Miller, J. R., & Radue, E. W. (2004). The use of magnetic resonance imaging in the diagnosis and long-term management of multiple sclerosis. *Neurology, 63*(Suppl. 5), S3–S11.

Beatty, W. W. (2002). Fluency in multiple sclerosis: Which measure is best? *Multiple Sclerosis, 8,* 261–264.

Beatty, W. W., Goodkin, D. E., Monson, N., Beatty, P. A., & Hertsgaard, D. (1998). Anterograde and retrograde amnesia in patients with chronic progressive multiple sclerosis. *Archives of Neurology, 45,* 611–619.

Benedict, R. H., Fisher, J. S., Archibald, C. J., Arnett, P. A., Beatty, W. W., Bobholz, J., et al. (2002). Minimal neuropsychological assessment in multiple sclerosis patients: A consensus approach. *Clinical Neuropsychology, 16*(3), 381–397.

Benedict, R. H., Weinstock–Guttman, B., Fishman, I., Sharma, J., & Tjoa, C. W. (2004). Prediction of neuropsychological impairment in multiple sclerosis: Comparison of conventional magnetic resonance imaging measure atrophy and lesion burden. *Archives of Neurology, 61*(2), 226–230.

Bobholz, J. A., & Rao, S. M. (2003). Cognitive dysfunction in multiple sclerosis: A review of recent developments. *Current Opinion in Neurology, 16,* 283–288.

Cristodoulou, C., Krupp, L. B., Liang, Z., Huang, W., Melville, P., Roque, C., et al. (2003). Cognitive performance and MR markers of cerebral injury in cognitively impaired MS patients. *Neurology, 60*(11), 1793–1798.

DeLuca, J., Barbieri-Berger, S., & Johnson, S. K. (1994). The nature of memory impairments in multiple sclerosis: acquisition versus retrieval. *Journal of Clinical & Experimental Neuropsychology, 16*(2), 183–189.

DeLuca, J., Christodoulou, C., Diamond, B. J., Rosenstein, E. D., Kramer, N., Ricker, J. H., et al. (2004). The nature of memory impairment in chronic fatigue syndrome. *Rehabilitation Psychology, 49*(1), 62–70.

De Jager, P. L., Simon, K. C., Munger, K. L., Rioux, J. D., Hafler, D. A., & Ascherio, A. (2008). Integrating risk factors: HLA-DRB1*1501 and Epstein–Barr virus in multiple sclerosis. *Neurology, 70*(13, Pt. 2), 1113–1118.

Demaree, H. A., DeLuca, J., Gaudino, E. A., & Diamond, B. J. (1999). Speed of information processing as a key deficit in multiple sclerosis: Implications for rehabilitation. *Journal of Neurology, Neurosurgery & Psychiatry, 67*(5), 661–663.

Dhib-Jalbut, S. (2007). Pathogenesis of myelin/oligodendrocyte damage in multiple sclerosis. *Neurology, 68*(22, Suppl. 3), S13–S21; discussion S43–S54.

Drake, M., Allegri, R. F., & Carrá, A. (2002). Alteraciones del Lenguaje en Pacientes con Esclerosis Múltilpe. *Neurología, 17*(1), 12–16.

Dutta, R., & Trapp, B. D. (2007). Pathogenesis of axonal and neuronal damage in multiple sclerosis. *Neurology, 68*(22, Suppl. 3), S22–S31; discussion S43–S54.

Ebers, G. C. (2008). Environmental factors and multiple sclerosis. *Lancet Neurology, 7*(3), 268–277.

Feinstein, A. (2004). The neuropsychiatry of multiple sclerosis. *Canadian Journal of Psychiatry, 49*(3), 157–163.

Fillipi, M., Bozzali, M., Rovaris, M., Gonen, O., Kesavadas, C., Ghezzi, A., et al. (2003). Evidence for widespread axonal damage at the earliest clinical stages of multiple sclerosis. *Brain, 126,* 433–437.

Gaudino, E., DeLuca, J., Voebel, G., Goverover, Y., Moore, N., & Halper, J. (2006). Using the MSFC to predict performance on complex activities of daily living in MS. Paper presented at the Annual Meeting of the International Neuropsychological Society, Boston, MA. 2006.

M

Grant, I., McDonald, W. I., Trimble, M. R., Smith, E., & Reed, R. (1984). Deficient learning and memory in early and middle phases of multiple sclerosis. *Journal of Neurology, Neurosurgery & Psychiatry, 47*, 250–255.

Haase, C. G., Tinnefeld, M., Lieneman, M., Ganz, R. E., & Faustmann, P. M. (2003). Depression and cognitive impairment in disability free early multiple sclerosis. *Behavioral Neurology, 14*, 39–45.

Heaton, R. K., Nelson, L. M., Thompson, D. S., Burks, J. S., & Franklin, G. M. (1985). Neuropsychological findings in relapsing-remitting and chronic-progressive multiple sclerosis. *Journal of Consulting and Clinical Psychology, 53*, 103–110.

Huijbregts, S. C., Kalkers, N. F., de Sonneville, L. M., de Groot, V., Reuling, I. E., & Polman, C. H. (2004). Differences in cognitive impairment of relapsing remitting, secondary, and primary progressive MS. *Neurology, 63*, 335–339.

Korteweg, T., Tintoré, M., Uitdehaag, B., Rovira, A., Frederiksen, J., Miller, D., et al. (2006). MRI criteria for dissemination in space in patients with clinically isolated syndromes: A multicentre follow-up study. *Lancet Neurology, 5*(3), 211–217.

Kurtzke, J. F. (1983). Rating neurologic impairment in multiple sclerosis: An expanded disability status scale (EDSS). *Neurology, 33*(11), 1444–1452.

Kurtzke, J. F. & Wallin, M. T. (2000). Epidemiology. In J. S. Burks & K. P. Johnson (Eds.), *Multiple sclerosis: Diagnosis, medical management, and rehabilitation* (pp. 49–71). New York, NY: Demos Medical Publishing, Inc.

Li, D., Held, U., Petkau, J., Daumaer, M., Barkhof, F., Fazekas, F., et al. (2006). MRI T2 lesion burden in multiple sclerosis: A plateauing relationship with clinical disability. *Neurology, 66*(9), 1384–1389.

Lyon-Caen, O., Jouvent, R., Hauser, S., Chaunu, M. P., Benoit, N., & Widlöcher, D. (1986). Cognitive function in recent-onset demyelinating diseases. *Archives of Neurology, 43*, 1138–1141.

MacLean, H., & Freedman, M. (2009). Multiple sclerosis: Following clues from cause to cure. *Lancet Neurology, 8*(1), 6–8.

Matotek, K., Saling, M. M., Gates, P., & Sedal, L. (2001). Subjective complaints, verbal fluency, and working memory in mild multiple sclerosis. *Applied Neuropsychology, 8*(4), 204–210.

McDonald, W. I., Compston, A., & Edan, G. (2001). Recommended diagnostic criteria for multiple sclerosis: Guidelines from the International Panel on the diagnosis of multiple sclerosis. *Annals of Neurology, 50*, 121–127.

Nocentini, U., Pasqualetti, P., Bonavita, S., Buccafusca, M., DeCaro, M., Farina, D., et al. (2006). Cognitive dysfunction in patients with relapsing remitting multiple sclerosis. *Multiple Sclerosis, 12*(1), 77–78.

Ojera, C., Rovaris, M., Inanucci, G., Valasina, P., Caputo, D., Cavarretta, R., et al. (2005). Progressive grey matter damage in patients with relapsing remitting multiple sclerosis: A longitudinal diffusion tensor magnetic resonance imaging study. *Archives of Neurology, 62*(4), 578–584.

Parmenter, B. A., Shucard, J. L., Benedict, R. H., & Shucard, D. W. (2006). Working memory deficits in multiple sclerosis: comparison between the n-back task and the Paced Auditory Serial Addition Test. *Journal of the International Neuropsychological Society, 12*(5), 677–687.

Parmenter, B. A., Shucard, J. L., & Shucard, D. W. (2007). Information processing deficits in multiple sclerosis: A matter of complexity. *Journal of the International Neuropsychological Society, 13*(3), 417–423.

Patten, S., & Metz, L. (2002). Interferon ß1a and depression in secondary progressive MS: Data from the SPECTRIMS trial. *Neurology, 59*(5), 744–746.

Patti, F., Amato, M. P., Trojano, M., Lijoi, A., & Bastianello, S. (2008). Relationship between cognitive impairment and magnetic resonance imaging parameters in patients with early relapsing remitting multiple sclerosis: Results from the Multicenter COGIMUS 2008 (COGnitionImpairment in Multiple Sclerosis Study). *Neurology, 70*(Suppl. D1), P04. 170.

Prakash, R., Snoook, E., Lewis, J., Motl, R., & Kramer, A. F. (2008). Cognitive impairments in multiple sclerosis: A meta-analysis. *Multiple Sclerosis, 1*(9), 1250–1261.

Randolph, J. J., Arnett, P. A., & Freeske, P. (2004). Metamemory in multiple sclerosis: Exploring affective and executive contributions. *Archives of Clinical Neuropsychology, 19*(2), 259–279.

Randolph, J. J., Arnett, P. A., & Higginson, C. I. (2001). Metamemory and tested cognitive functioning in multiple sclerosis. *The Clinical Neuropsychologist, 15*(3), 357–368.

Rao, S. M. (1986). Neuropsychology of multiple sclerosis: A critical review. *Journal of Clinical Experimental Neuropsychology, 8*, 503–542.

Rao, S. M. (1990). Cognitive Function Study Group, NMSS. *A manual for the brief repeatable battery of neuropsychological tests in multiple sclerosis.* New York: National Multiple Sclerosis Society.

Rao, S. M., Leo, G. J., Bernardin, L., & Unverzagt, F. (1991). Cognitive dysfunction in multiple sclerosis I: Frequency patterns & prediction. *Neurology, 41*(5), 685–691.

Rao, S., Leo, G. J., Ellington, L., Nauertz, T., Bernardin, L., & Unverzagt, F. (1991). Cognitive dysfunction on multiple sclerosis II: Impact on employment and social functioning. *Neurology, 41*(5), 692–696.

Ron, M. A., Callanan, M. M., & Warrington, E. K. (1991). Cognitive abnormalities in multiple sclerosis: A psychometric and MRI study. *Psychological Medicine, 21*, 59–68.

Ross, A. J., & Sachdev, P. (2004). Magnetic resonance spectroscopy in cognitive research. *Brain Research Reviews, 44,* 83–102.

Rovaris, M., Inannucci, G., Falautano, M., Possa, F., Martinelli, V., Comi, G., & Fillipi, M. (2002). Cognitive dysfunction in patients with mildly disabling relapsing–remitting multiple sclerosis: an exploratory study with diffusion tensor MR imaging. *Journal of the Neurological Sciences,* 195(2), 103–109.

Schulthesis, M. T., Garay, E., & DeLuca, J. (2001). The influence of cognitive impairment on driving performance in multiple sclerosis. *Neurology, 56,* 1089–1094.

Smith, A. (1982). *The symbol digit modalities test manual: Revised.* Los Angeles: Western Psychological Services.

Stanley, J. A. (2002). In vivo magnetic resonance spectroscopy and its implications to neuropsychiatric disorder. *Canadian Journal of Psychiatry, 47,* 315–326.

Thrower, B. W. (2007). Clinically isolated syndromes: Predicting and delaying multiple sclerosis. *Neurology,* 68(24, Suppl. 4), S12–S15.

Tintoré, M., Rovira, A., Río, M., Nos, C., Grivé, E., Sastre-Garriga, J., et al. (2003). New diagnostic criteria for multiple sclerosis: Application in first demyelinating episode. *Neurology,* 60(1), 27–30.

Tong, B., Yip, J., Mc Lee, T., & Li, L. (2002). Frontal fluency and memory functioning among multiple sclerosis patients in Hong Kong. *Brain Injury,* 16(11), 987–995.

Tortorella, P., Rocca, M. A., Mezzapesa, D., Ghezzi, A., Lamanthia, L., Comi, G., et al. (2006). MRI quantification of gray and white matter damage in patients with early onset multiple sclerosis. *Journal of Neurology,* 253(7), 903–907.

Van den Burg, W., van Zomeren, A. H., Minderhoud, J. M., Prange, A. J., & Meijer, N. S. (1987). Cognitive impairment in patients with multiple sclerosis and mild physical disability. *Archives of Neurology, 44,* 49–501.

Vlaar, A. M., & Wade, D. T. (2003). Verbal fluency assessment of patients with multiple sclerosis: Test–retest and inter-observer reliability. *Clinical Rehabilitation, 17,* 756–764.

Voss, W. D., Arnett, P. A., Higginson, C. I., Randolph, J. J., Campos, M. D., & Dyck, D. G. (2001). Contributing factors to depressed mood in multiple sclerosis. *Archives of Clinical Neuropsychology, 17,* 113–115.

Vrenken, H., Pouwels, P. J., Geurts, J. J., Knol, D. L., Polman, C. H., Barkhof, F., et al. (2006). Altered diffusion tensor in multiple sclerosis normal-appearing brain tissue: Cortical diffusion changes seem related to clinical deterioration. *Journal of Magnetic Resonance Imaging,* 23(5), 628–636.

Zakanis, K. K. (2000). Distinct neurocognitive profiles in multiple sclerosis subtypes. *Archives of Clinical Neuropsychology,* 15(2), 115–136.

Zivadinoff, R., & Bakshi, R. (2004). Role of MRI in multiple sclerosis: Inflammation and lesions. *Frontiers in Bioscience, 9,* 665–683.

MULTI-SYSTEM ATROPHY

DESCRIPTION

In 1960, Dr. Milton Shy at the National Institutes of Health and Dr. Glen Drager at Baylor College of Medicine first identified and named Shy-Drager syndrome, currently known as multi-system atrophy with orthostatic hypotension (Shy & Drager, 1960). Other terms used for this syndrome include livopontocerebellar atrophy, striatonagral degeneration, and Parkinson's plus (Bannister & Oppenheimer, 1972). The etiology remains unknown, yet autoimmune dysfunction or neurotoxins have been proposed to play some role in its composition (Bensimon, Ludolph, Agid, Vidailhet, Payan, & Leigh, 2008).

The disorder is progressive and is characterized by an excessive drop in blood pressure when standing, also referred to as supine hypotension, that often leads to sensations of dizziness or fainting. Not all cases of multi-system atrophy exhibit hypotension; however, such cases are rare. Still, as a result, multi-system atrophy is often classified as with or without orthostatic hypotension. Other symptoms of multi-system atrophy with orthostatic hypotension include urinary incontinence, constipation, sexual impotence in men, generalized weakness, visual disturbances (i.e., diplopia), difficulty breathing and swallowing, sleep disturbances, decreased sweating, and movement symptoms (Watanabe et al., 2002). These generalized symptoms may often be misdiagnosed as other disorders with similar presentations (i.e., autoimmune disorders, movement disorders, autonomic dysfunction disorders, etc.), especially in the formative stages of the disease process and considering how blood pressure is often monitored in a seated position.

Prevalence of multi-system atrophy is approximately 46 per 1,000,000 with typical age of onset in the late 50s early 60s with 55% of cases being male (Bensimon et al., 2008). The course of the disease is 7 to 10 years with respiratory failure as the primary cause of mortality (Watanabe et al., 2002).

NEUROPATHOLOGY/PATHOPHYSIOLOGY

Regarding the pathophysiology, initially it was believed that damage to gray matter was paramount;

however, with understanding of glial cells, it became apparent that white matter involvement is actually more important (Burn & Jaros, 2001). Thus, the glial involvement and accompanying demyelination play a distinct role in the pathogenesis of multi-system atrophy with orthostatic hypotension.

The etiology for the cell loss is unknown and there is little evidence to confirm autoimmune and toxic (i.e., saxitoxin) agents as contributory; neither is there evidence to suggest a genetic cause (Daniel, 1992).

The pathophysiology of multi-system atrophy with orthostatic hypotension is attributed to progressive neuronal and oligodendroglial loss in various neuroanatomic regions with symptoms correlating to the areas involved (Wenning, Colosimo, Geser, & Poewe, 2004). For example, orthostatic hypotension and urinary incontinence are the result of preganglionic damage of the intermediolateral cell columns; cerebellar ataxia, nystagmus, and dysarthria are due to damage in the cerebellar cortex, pontine nuclei, and inferior olives, respectively and motor abnormalities, akinesia, and rigidity are secondary to cortical motor areas and basal ganglia, globus pallidus, and putamen, respectively (Wenning et al., 2004). The degeneration of Onuf's nucleus that is the sacral anterior horn cells is associated with urinary, sexual, and anorectal impairments (Vodusek, 2001).

NEUROPSYCHOLOGICAL/CLINICAL PRESENTATION

The clinical presentation of multi-system atrophy with orthostatic hypotension is characterized by autonomic dysfunction, parkinsonian symptoms, and ataxia (Bannister & Oppenheimer, 1972). Common preliminary symptoms includes an "akinetic-rigid syndrome" (characterized by diminished initiation speed and bradykinetic movements), with less common symptoms including balance problems often with falls, genitourinary problems (including incontinence and retention), and erectile dysfunction (Geser & Wenning, 2006).

Progression of the disease is marked by increased parkinsonism, cerebellar dysfunction, and autonomic dysfunction. Clinical evaluation will reveal bradykinesia and rigidity, poor balance (i.e., dizziness or fainting when standing up) and coordination, and impaired parasympathetic body functions (Watanabe et al., 2002). The latter consists of urinary incontinence, impotence, constipation, dry mouth or skin, difficulties with regulating body temperature, and abnormal breathing especially during sleep. Cognitive functions are generally normal, yet confusion and dysarthria

may also be present especially later in the disease progression (Watanabe et al., 2002).

DIAGNOSIS

Multi-system atrophy with orthostatic hypotension was classically divided into three types; however, recent changes have elucidated a four-domain classification system: autonomic failure/urinary dysfunction, parkinsonism, cerebellar ataxia, and corticalspinal dysfunction (Gilman et al., 1998).

Diagnosis is confirmed upon autopsy; however, certain tests exist that inform the differential. Brain imaging may be normal or demonstrate cerebellar atrophy and striatonigral degeneration (i.e.. putaminal lesions) (Burn & Jaros, 2001). Other tests include scintigraphy, positron emission tomography (PET), autonomic function test, and sphincter electromyography (Colosimo, Tiple, & Wenning, 2005).

Differential diagnoses are numerous and include chorea, cortical basal ganglionic degeneration, Hallervorden-Spatz disease, idiopathic orthostatic hypotension, mitochondrial cytopathies, multiple sclerosis, neuroacanthocytosis, neurosarcoidosis, neurosyphillis, olivopontocerebellar atrophy, Parkinson's disease, Parkinson plus syndromes, and Pelizaeus-Merzbacher disease (Geser & Wenning, 2006). Differentiation of Parkinson's from multi-system atrophy tends to be difficult, yet is possible when impairments are rapid, there is a poor response to levadopa (i.e., confusion), autonomic dysfunction (i.e., urinary problems or orthostatic hypotension) is prominent, rigidity and bradykinesia are more pronounced than tremor, speech is dysarthric, there are falls and an absence of dementia, and abnormal breathing patterns are noted (Burn, Sawle, & Brooks, 1994).

Another common differential with multi-system atrophy is pure autonomic failure, which may be difficult to differentially diagnose in the early stages. Unlike pure autonomic failure, which is a result of peripheral impairments, multi-system atrophy is secondary to central impairments (Geser & Wenning, 2006). Additionally, the progression of pure autonomic failure is slower than multi-system atrophy, and pure autonomic failure has low plasma norepinepherine levels (Geser & Wenning, 2006).

Multi-system atrophy may be differentially diagnosed from progressive supranuclear palsy by analysis of horizontal and vertical ocularmotor movements that demonstrate that the latter maintain slowing of the saccades (Burn et al., 1994). Those with progressive supranuclear palsy often demonstrate different physiologic responses to autonomic function tests, and cardiovascular dysfunction is exclusionary to this diagnosis (Burn et al., 1994). Multi-system atrophy may be differentially diagnosed from cortico-basal ganglionic degeneration in that the onset of the former is typically characterized by unilateral rigidity and dystonia. Unlike multi-system atrophy, apraxia is focused in the cortex (Geser & Wenning, 2006). Cerebrovascular etiologies are ruled out through imaging.

TREATMENT

There is no cure for multiple system atrophy with orthostatic hypotension, and the goal of interventions is to control symptoms. Anti-Parkinson medication, such as carbidopa-levodopa (Sinemet), may be utilized, as well as pharmaceutical agents to manipulate blood pressure (Colosimo et al., 2005). As the disease progresses, artificial feeding tubes, breathing assistance, and/or surgery may all be required to address more severe problems such as bradycardia and dysphagia among others (Colosimo et al., 2005).

In addition to the multiple pharmacological treatments for multi-system atrophy, nonpharmacologic treatments may include specific mechanical maneuvers and clothing to address orthostatic hypotension, diet alteration, catheterization, speech therapy for improvements in dysphagia and communication, and physical therapy to prevent deconditioning (Colosimo et al., 2005).

Javan Horwitz
Natalie Horwitz
Chad A. Noggle

Bannister, R., & Oppenheimer, D. (1972). Degenerative diseases of the nervous system associated with autonomic failure. *Brain, 95*(3), 457–474.

Bensimon, G., Ludolph, A., Agid, Y., Vidailhet, M., Payan, C., & Leigh, P. (2008). Riluzole treatment, survival and diagnostic criteria in Parkinson plus disorders: The NNIPPS Study. *Brain, 132*, 156.

Burn, D., & Jaros, E. (2001). Multiple system atrophy: Cellular and molecular pathology. *Molecular Pathology, 54*(6), 419–426.

Burn, D., Sawle, G., & Brooks, D. (1994). Differential diagnosis of Parkinson's disease, multiple system atrophy, and Steele-Richardson-Olszewski syndrome: Discriminant analysis of striatal 18F-dopa PET data. *Journal of Neurology, Neurosurgery and Psychiatry, 57*(3), 278–284.

Colosimo, C., Tiple, D., & Wenning, G. (2005). Management of multiple system atrophy: State of the art. *Journal of Neural Transmission, 112*(12), 1695–1704.

Daniel, S. (1992). The neuropathology and neurochemistry of multiple system atrophy. In R. Bannister & C. Mathias (Eds.), *Autonomic failure: A textbook of clinical disorders* (3rd ed., pp. 564–585). Oxford, England: Oxford University Press.

Geser, F., & Wenning, G. (2006). The diagnosis of multiple system atrophy. *Journal of Neurology, 253*, 3–15.

Gilman, S., Low, P., Quinn, N., Albanese, A., Ben-Shlomo, Y., Fowler, C., . . . Wenning, G. (1998). Consensus statement on the diagnosis of multiple system atrophy. American Autonomic Society and American Academy of Neurology. *Clinical Autonomic Research, 8*(6), 359–362.

Shy, G., & Drager, G. (1960). A neurological syndrome associated with orthostatic hypotension: A clinical-pathologic study. *Archives of Neurology, 2*, 511–527.

Vodusek, D. (2001). Sphincter electromyography and differential diagnosis of multiple system atrophy. *Movement Disorders, 16*, 600–607.

Watanabe, H., Saito, Y., Terao, S., Ando, T., Kachi, T., Mukai, E., . . . Sobue, G. (2002). Progression and prognosis in multiple system atrophy: An analysis of 230 Japanese patients. *Brain, 125*, 1070–1083.

Wenning, G., Colosimo, C., Geser, F., & Poewe, W. (2004). Multiple system atrophy. *Lancet Neurology, 3*, 93–103.

MUSCULAR DYSTROPHY

DESCRIPTION

The muscular dystrophies (MDs) describe a group of genetic and inherited diseases in which specific genes that control muscle function are found to be defective (Emery, 2008). This group of genetic diseases is marked by the progressive and increasing weakness and degeneration of the skeletal or voluntary muscles, which control movement. In general, incorrect and missing genetic information in patients with MD prevents their bodies from correctly producing proteins that are used in building and maintaining muscles. Although such characteristics may appear to be pervasive in all patients with MD, it is important to recognize that over 30 subtypes of MD have been identified.

Characteristics of MDs that are not specific to a particular subtype include the effects of the disease on striated, voluntary muscles. In many subtypes of MD, the disease affects both sides of the body in a symmetrical manner, from the bottom up (i.e., loss of lower extremity or torso control precedes loss of hand function), and maturation of MD occurs before deterioration (flaccid paralysis), although the individual does not always appear to be getting worse. For many subtypes of MD, the disease further affects the body and the related cause of death includes respiratory infection (problems immobilizing secretions) or

M

M

heart attack, which typically occurs in the late teens or early 20s. Still, other MDs do not become evident until adulthood (i.e., oculopharyngeal muscular dystrophy) (Emery, 2008).

The most common MD in children is Duchenne's muscular dystrophy (DMD), which occurs in 1 in every 3,300 live male births (Iannacome, 1992). The diagnosis for DMD is based on physical characteristics, as well as medical history and testing results. Typically, children with DMD present motor delays such as abnormal walking patterns, waddling, and frequent falling (Iannacome, 1992). Another physical indication of this disorder is the decreased muscle size in the calves or any muscle group. A deficiency of the membrane protein, dystrophin, causes the progressive deterioration of muscle fibers (Van Deutekom, 2005). Mutations in the DMD gene cause the disorder (Lalic et al., 2005).

Becker's muscular dystrophy (BMD) is another more common subtype that often resembles DMD. BMD is caused by the same gene mutations that also cause DMD, but in individuals with BMD, protein produced is abnormal despite the mutant gene's normal synthesis of dystrophin (Emery, 2008). Though individuals with BMD display similar symptoms to those with DMD (i.e., symmetrical weakness — weakness in lower limbs, followed by upper limb weakness), these individuals tend to have a later onset (in their teens and 20s), and may have relatively mild weakness compared with those with DMD.

Although MDs are, in general, fairly rare, specific subtypes of the disease appear to occur at higher incidences than others. Besides DMD and BMD (which are considered higher incidence MD subtypes), some of the more common forms of MD include Emery–Dreifuss' muscular dystrophy, limb-girdle muscular dystrophy, facioscapulohumeral muscular dystrophy, distal muscular dystrophy, oculopharyngeal muscular dystrophy, congenital muscular dystrophies, and myotonic dystrophy.

NEUROPATHOLOGY/PATHOPHYSIOLOGY

Because MD is a genetic disorder, a primary pathological characteristic is defects in the gene's ability to produce or contain a specific protein. Gene abnormalities differ based on the specific diagnosed subtype of MD (Emery, 2008). As mentioned previously, DMD is the most commonly occurring form of MD. Symptoms associated with DMD (the weakening of muscles) can be explained by the absence of the dystrophin protein within the gene. Mutations in the dystrophin gene are identified in more than 75% of patients with DMD or BMD. Along with other related proteins,

dystrophin retains the structure of a muscle fiber membrane. Mutations in mRNA produce a truncated dystrophin molecule in which carboxy terminus is missing thereby inhibiting proper binding with dystrophin-associated proteins at the point of the cell membrane and thus resulting in the dystrophin deficiency in the DMD type (Siddique, Sufit, & Siddique, 2007). Because individuals with DMD lack this protein, the membrane breaks down and allows leakage, thus allowing substances and molecules within the fiber to leak into the blood stream. One particular substance that leaks from the fiber is creatine kinase (CK), a muscle enzyme that is necessary for muscle contractions (Iannacome, 1992). BMD is characterized by preserved carboxy terminus, producing milder symptoms associated with this type (Matsumura et al., 1993).

Besides genetic mutations present in patients with MD, some hypotheses exist regarding the effects of such deficiencies (i.e., the absence of dystrophin) on the brain. In addition to motor impairment, differences in intellectual functioning (slightly lower IQ) may be present in patients with MD. Specifically, children with DMD appear to have more difficulties in verbal IQ in comparison with performance IQ (Yiu & Kornberg, 2008). For impairments in verbal IQ, such as problems with poor long-term and working verbal memory or poor reading and expressive skills, it has been hypothesized that such difficulties are not due to structure abnormalities within the brain, but cellular abnormalities as a result of the lack of dystrophin in the brain (Hinton, De Vivo, Nereo, Goldstein, & Stern, 2001).

NEUROPSYCHOLOGICAL/CLINICAL PRESENTATION

The primary clinical features of MD include motor delays, impairments, and/or abnormal gait. In those with DMD, children present with difficulties getting up from the ground (i.e., using hands to "crawl" up their legs), running, and jumping, or may display frequent falling or toe-walking, which is typically observed between 3 and 5 years (Yiu & Kornberg, 2008). Further motor impairments may be observed through proximal muscle weakness, in which the lower extremities are affected prior to the upper extremities. Patients with MD may be described as having a "waddling" gait, enlarged calves, and are often wheelchairbound during early adolescence (Siddique et al., 2007).

Besides motor deficits evident in patients with MD, cardiovascular and respiratory complications may occur. For example, atrial and ventrical arrhythmias and ventricular dysfunction may develop in later childhood due to lack of physical activity, despite a high frequency of cardiac involvement (Yiu & Kornberg, 2008). Furthermore, chronic respiratory complications are typically present in patients with MD. Such individuals may develop restrictive lung disease, in which respiratory vital capacity increases, followed by an increased risk of death.

In addition to the aforementioned complications associated with MD, some impairments in intellectual functioning may occur at a rate higher than that of the general population. For example, intellectual disability is observed in 30% of males with DMD, with a mean IQ of 85 (Yiu & Kornberg, 2008). Such individuals also display a higher incidence of attention deficit hyperactivity disorder.

DIAGNOSIS

When developing an understanding of MD, it is imperative for individuals to consider the diagnostic measures that are taken. The diagnosis for MD is based on physical characteristics as well as medical history and testing results. Again, physical indications as mentioned in the description of the clinical presentation are useful in diagnosing MD. For example, children with DMD present with motor delays such as abnormal walking patterns, waddling, and frequent falling (Iannacome, 1992). Another physical indication of this disorder is the decreased muscle size in the calves or any muscle group. In addition to the observation of physical characteristics associated with MD, several genetic analyses are likely to be employed, including genetic counseling, prognostications, and antenatal diagnostics (Kakulas, 2008). As mentioned, patients with DMD have abnormally high levels of CK, approximately 10 times higher than normal. By examining both the physical symptoms and the CK levels, physicians have a fair indication for the diagnosis of DMD.

Three diagnostic tests typically used to identify MD include blood tests, electromyography, and a muscle biopsy. Two blood tests are conducted in order to measure the levels of CK and to examine DNA mutations. An electromyography is a test that is conducted in order to measure the electrical activity of a muscle fiber, also known as an action potential. Patients with MD tend to have small measures of action potentials. The third diagnostic test, a muscle biopsy, is a crucial aspect in the diagnosis because it allows direct examination of muscle tissue. In a muscle biopsy, one must search for the dystrophin content. If dystrophin is absent from the patient's

muscle, a diagnosis of DMD is typically appropriate. If dystrophin is present in abnormal amounts, the individual may have BMD.

When interpreting the prognosis for DMD, the mean age at which the patient is no longer ambulatory is 11 years (Iannacome, 1992). Common complications of DMD include orthopedic deformities, respiratory problems, heart failure, as well as psychological needs (academic, emotional, and behavioral needs). In other subtypes of MD, however, symptoms do not appear until adulthood (i.e., oculopharyngeal muscular dystrophy).

TREATMENT

While the disease progresses, it is important that physicians implement strategies to manage the complications of MD. When considering management of the disorder, the patient's mobility and quality of life should remain the most important goal (Iannacome, 1992; Siddique, Sufit, & Siddique, 2007). In order to assist in orthopedic insufficiencies, physical therapists may work with patients and their families by introducing motion exercises that can be performed at home. Occasionally, surgical procedures are considered to correct deformities. One example of an orthopedic deformity is the presence of scoliosis, which progresses once the patient becomes wheelchair bound.

Another obstacle to which an individual with MD is bound is the respiratory deficiency due to weakness in truncal muscles. Although the immune system and lung tissue is normal in MD patients, they may lack the ability to clear the airway and improve ventilation. To prevent pneumonia and respiratory failure, physicians may recommend pressure ventilation during sleep to improve oxygenation and endurance during the day. In later stages of the disease, the individual and the family may be required to decide whether they want to use artificial ventilation as a means of prolonging the life of the patient with MD.

During examination of management strategies for patients with MD, physicians often consider the emotional aspects of the patients' disorder. Families often benefit from some form of counseling during a grieving phase after a diagnosis is made. Clinical depression in patients usually results from family discord, loss of function, and fear of dying (Iannacome, 1992). Specialists may assist in dealing with the coming to terms with these aspects of MD.

Although there is, unfortunately, no cure for MD, there are a variety of treatments. However, many of these treatments continue to be experimental procedures. Corticosteroids are the most commonly employed form of treatment, showing some efficacy in delaying motor deterioration (Siddique, Sufit, & Siddique, 2007). Although this is the most common treatment, it involves side effects that cause controversy. For example, the side effects of prednisone do not enable the trial to be truly double blind. Also, it is safer for lower doses of prednisone to be dispersed due to the side effects of steroids. Physicians must consider the fact that once an individual is nonambulatory, prednisone is no longer effective.

Another treatment for MD is myoblast transfer therapy, most commonly applied to the Duchenne subtype. Here, normal muscle precursor cells (myoblasts) are introduced to muscles that are deficient of the dystrophin gene. Ideally, cells derived from other skeletal muscles will be used to genetically correct these cells and be used as a source of replacement myoblasts (Lee-Pullen & Grounds, 2005). Unfortunately, myoblast transfer may be painful due to several myoblast injections as well as repeated biopsies that evaluate the results of the treatment. An additional proposed treatment is gene therapy. For gene therapy to be effective, genetic material must somehow enter every muscle fiber in order to reverse the dystrophic process. Although these treatments have been helpful in prolonging the lives of MD patients, research continues to be done to further the potential of finding a cure.

Sarah C. Connolly
Chad A. Noggle

Emery, A. E. H. (2008). *Muscular dystrophy* (3rd ed.). New York: Oxford University Press.

Hinton, V. J., De Vivo, D. C., Nereo, N. E., Goldstein, E., & Stern, Y. (2001). Selective deficits in verbal working memory associated with a known genetic etiology: The neuropsychological profile of Duchenne muscular dystrophy. *Journal of the International Neuropsychological Society, 7*, 45–54.

Iannacome, S. T. (1992). Current status of Duchenne muscular dystrophy. In J. B. Bodensteiner (Ed.), *The pediatric clinics of North America—pediatric neurology* (39th ed., Vol. 4, pp. 879–894). Philadelphia: W.B. Saunders Company.

Kakulas, B. A. (2008). A brief history of muscular dystrophy research: A personal perspective. *Neurology India, 3*(56), 231–235.

Lalic, T., Vossen, R. H., Coffa, J., Schouten, J. P., Guc-Scekic, M., & Radivojevic, D. (2005). Deletion and duplication screening in the DMD gene. *European Journal of Human Genetics, 13*, 1231–1234.

Lee-Pullen, T. F., & Grounds, M. D. (2005). Muscle-derived stem cells: Implications for effective myoblast. *Life, 57*(11), 731–736.

Matsumara, K., Tome, F. M., Ianaescu, V., Ervasti, J. M., Anderson, R. D., Romero, N. B., et al., (1993). Deficiency of dystrophin-associated proteins in Duchenne muscular dystrophy patients lacking the COOH-terminal domains of dystrophin. *Journal of Clinical Investigation, 92*, 866–871.

Siddique, N., Sufit, R., & Siddique, T. (2007). In C.G. Goetz (Ed.) *Textbook of clinical neurology* (3rd ed. pp. 781–812) Philadelphia: Saunders Elsevier.

Van Deutekom, J. C. (2005). The 'Pro-sense' approach to Duchenne muscular dystrophy. *Journal of Human Genetics, 13*, 518–519.

Yiu, E. M., & Kornberg, A. J. (2008). Duchenne muscular dystrophy. *Neurology India, 56*(3), 236–247.

MYASTHENIA GRAVIS

DESCRIPTION

Myasthenia gravis (MG) is a chronic autoimmune disease that demonstrates preferential targeting and impairment of neuromuscular functioning leading to fluctuating degrees of muscle weakness and fatigability. Current estimates suggest MG has a relative prevalence of 1 out of 2,500–5,000 (Mantegazza, Baggi, Antozzi, et al., 2003; Vincent, Palace, & Hilton-Jones, 2001). It is most commonly seen in women under 40 years of age as well as men and women between the age of 50 and 70. The presentation originates from an altering, blockade, and/or destruction of acetylcholine receptors by antibodies. Clinically, weakness of eye and facial muscles are often the first symptoms. Dysphagia and dysarthria may also manifest. Peripheral involvement of the extremities may also be observed with symptoms varying based on severity. After a time of rest, symptoms usually remit. Given the presentation originates from degradation of acetylcholine receptors, thereby diminishing the levels of the neurotransmitter within the system, medicinal treatment with cholinesterase inhibitors in combination with immunosuppressants is the most common intervention. In some instances, surgical intervention is employed. With treatment, patients live fairly normal lives.

NEUROPATHOLOGY/PATHOPHYSIOLOGY

MG occurs secondary to a degradation of acetylcholinesterase receptors in the neuromuscular junction by buildup of immunoglobulin G antibodies. Idiopathic in nature, no pathogenic cause has been noted.

However, increased risk of MG has been linked with other presentations including diabetes mellitus Type I, rheumatoid arthritis, and lupus. In addition, a high portion of patients present with abnormalities of the thymus, particularly thymomas. This significant correlation is related to the thymus' role in producing T cells that bind to the acetylcholinesterase receptors. These T cells convert B cells into plasma cells, and it is from these plasma cells that the antibodies that block the acetylcholinesterase receptors originate (Richman & Agius, 1994). This reduces the amount of sodium ions that are essential to depolarizing muscle cells and opening sodium channels eventually leading to a release of calcium. The strength of the muscular contraction is dependent upon the amount of calcium present within the muscle cells. Consequently, the hallmark histological features of MG includes decreased numbers of acetylcholine receptors, simplification of the postsynaptic cleft, and widening of the synaptic space in the presence of a normal presynaptic nerve terminal (Drachman, 1994).

NEUROPSYCHOLOGICAL/CLINICAL PRESENTATION

The classic clinical feature of MG is pronounced muscle weakness and increased fatigability. Facial muscles are commonly, but not always, involved. Limb, axial, and respiratory muscles may also be involved. Variability is seen across cases in terms of muscles involved and severity of symptoms (Conti-Fine, Milani, & Kaminski, 2006; Vincent et al., 2001). In some instances, it can be just localized to the eye muscles or simply present as ptosis of either one eye or both. Dysarthria and dysphagia can occur. The severity of symptoms may be classified across five levels. At the mildest level (Class I), only eye weakness is observed. As you move through Classes 2–4, eye muscle weakness may be seen of any severity, but the involvement and severity of other muscle symptoms increases, usually being divided into subclasses based on whether limb and axial muscles are involved or bulbar or respiratory muscles are involved. In Class 5, the weaknesses are of such severity that intubation is needed to maintain integrity of the airway.

Although the presentation is most commonly noted in adults, variations are seen in childhood and adolescence. Neonatal MG occurs when an affected mother passes the problematic antibodies to her unborn child via the placenta. It represents a transient disorder with symptom onset a few days after birth and resolving a few weeks later. Juvenile MG has a similar physiological basis as the adult form but presents unusually early. These variations are distinguished from congenital myasthenia in that the latter is not caused by an autoimmune process. (For more details see the article on Congenital and Childhood Myasthenias.)

DIAGNOSIS

Diagnostic consideration of MG starts with the symptom onset. Given the high prevalence of thymomas MRIs are commonly performed to determine the presence of such tumors. Repeated nerve stimulation tests can be utilized to determine the relative fatigability of muscles. In addition, performance-based assessments may be carried out including tasks such as climbing stairs, doing squats, sustained diverted gaze, and so forth. Single fiber electromyography is frequently used to determine the relative voltage of muscle impulse transmission (Rostedt, Padua, & Stalberg, 2005). A common differential diagnosis is Lambert–Eaton syndrome in which a chest X-ray is often employed to rule out. Stool samples should be evaluated to determine if there is presence of botulinum toxin which may suggest Botulism as the cause of the symptoms (Bartt & Topel, 2007).

TREATMENT

The treatment of MG is largely based on the underlying cause. Given the presentation arises from a relative deficiency of acetylcholine, due to receptor blockade or destruction cholinesterase inhibitors are used with success. This is done in combination with immunosuppressant treatment to prevent the production of the abnormal antibodies. Intravenous immunoglobulins (IVIGs) have been used to target and bind to circulating antibodies (Diaz-Manera, Rojas-García, & Illa, 2009; Gold & Schneider-Gold, 2008; Manfredi, Fasulo, Fulgaro, & Sabbatani, 2008). In those patients who present with an abnormal thymus gland, such as in the case of thymomas, surgical removal of the gland (i.e., thymectomy) may relieve symptoms (Gronseth & Barhon, 2000; Mantegazza, Baggi, Bernasconi, et al., 2003). In severe cases, plasmapheresis may be considered as a means of removing the abnormal antibodies from the blood.

Chad A. Noggle
Amy R. Steiner

Bartt, R. E., & Topel, J. L. (2007). Autoimmune and inflammatory disorders. In C. G. Goetz (Ed.) *Textbook of clinical neurology* (3rd ed., pp. 1155–1184). Philadelphia, PA: Saunders Elsevier.

M

Conti-Fine, B. M., Milani, M., & Kaminski, H. J. (2006). Myasthenia gravis: Past, present, and future. *Journal of Clinical Investigation, 116*, 2843–2854.

Diaz-Manera, J., Rojas-García, R., & Illa, I. (2009). Treatment strategies for myasthenia gravis. *Expert Opinion on Pharmacotherapy, 10*(8), 1329–1342.

Drachman, D. B. (1994). Myasthenia gravis. *New England Journal of Medicine, 330*, 1797–1810.

Gold, R., & Schneider-Gold, C. (2008). Current and future standards in treatment of myasthenia gravis. *Neurotherapeutics, 5*(4), 535–541.

Gronseth, G. S., & Barhon, R. J. (2000). Practice parameter: Thymectomy for autoimmune myasthenia gravis (an evidence-based review): Report of the quality standards subcommittee of the American Academy of Neurology. *Neurology, 55*, 7–15.

Manfredi, R., Fasulo, G., Fulgaro, C., & Sabbatani, S. (2008). Associated thyreoiditis, myasthenia gravis, thymectomy, Chron's disease, and erythema nodosum: Pathogenetic and clinical correlations, immune system involvement, and systemic infectious complications. *Rheumatology International, 28*(11), 1173–1175.

Mantegazza, R., Baggi, F., Antozzi, C., Confalonieri, P., Morandi, L., Bernasconi, P., et al. (2003a). Myasthenia gravis (MG): Epidemiological data and prognostic factors. *Annals of the New York Academy of Sciences, 998*, 413–423.

Mantegazza, R., Baggi, F., Bernasconi, P., Antozzi, C., Confalonieri, P., Novellino, L., et al. (2003b). Video-assisted thoracoscopic extended thymectomy and extended transsternal thymectomy (T-3b) in nonthymomatous myasthenia gravis patients: Remission after 6 years of follow-up. *Journal of the Neurological Sciences, 212*, 31–36.

Richman, D. P., & Agius, M. A. (1994). Myasthenia gravis: Pathogenesis and treatment. *Seminars in Neurology, 14*, 106–110.

Rostedt, A., Padua, L., & Stalberg, E. V. (2005). Correlation between a patient-derived functional questionnaire and abnormal neuromuscular transmission in myasthenia gravis patients. *Clinical Neurophysiology, 116*, 2058–2064.

Vincent, A., Palace, J., & Hilton-Jones, D. (2001). Myasthenia gravis. *Lancet, 357*, 2122–2128.

MYOCLONUS

DESCRIPTION

Myoclonus is defined as a sudden, rapid, involuntary jerking of a muscle or a group of muscles (Factor & Weiner, 2004) and is observed as a presenting symptom of a variety of disorders, often termed hyperkinetic movement disorders or dyskinesias, which may be described as positive or negative suggesting their underlying cause. Specifically, positive myoclonus is caused by muscular contraction whereas negative myoclonus is caused by muscular inhibitions. These jerks or twitches are unable to be controlled by the patient and can be the result of voluntary movement or a simple response to an external event. Due to the sporadic and unpredictable nature of myoclonic jerks, it is often difficult to determine true triggers for their occurrence.

Myoclonus is a symptom that is often classified in a variety of ways. However, due to the great number of situations in which myoclonus presents, it is often difficult to classify in simple terms. The most clear-cut definition of myoclonus is a brief muscle twitch, followed by relaxation. Some common forms of myoclonus are present in patients with multiple sclerosis, Parkinson's disease, Alzheimer's disease, Creutzfeldt–Jakob's disease, epilepsy, and certain sleep disorders (National Institute of Neurological Disorders and Stroke [NINDS], 2000).

NEUROPATHOLOGY/PATHOPHYSIOLOGY

According to research done by the NINDS, there are specific locations in the brain, particularly in the brainstem, that create myoclonic responses. For example, rhythmical myoclonus has been most commonly associated with segmental lesions of the brainstem and spinal cord. These may be the direct result of an injury or they may be genetically influenced. In the case of injury to the brain, one case study reported patients had functional impairment (difficulty holding a cup, tremors in the hands) after the injury, following otherwise normal cognitive and physical development (Balci, Utku, & Cobanoglu, 2007). Similarly, some types of peripheral myoclonus may be related to localized injury to those nerves causing transient inhibition or activation of those corresponding muscles. In most other cases, it is believed that generalized impairment of the central nervous system is the cause of myoclonus. Beyond the brainstem, high-amplitude somatosensory evoked potentials with cortical spikes have been linked with cortical reflexive myoclonus (Fahn, 2007). On a more general level, myoclonus is related to hyperexcitability of neurons causing either sudden muscular contraction or inhibition.

Although it is evident that there is a link between the brain and myoclonus, there also appears to be recent research of types of myoclonus linking to specific genes, especially in regard to myoclonic epilepsy (Striano et al., 2004). Research done in Europe and Japan on autosomal-dominant myoclonus and epilepsy have also corroborated this familial link

(Guerrini, Bonanni, & Patrignani, 2001; Laubage et al., 2002; Uyama, Fu, & Ptacek, 2005, Van Rootselaar et al., 2005)

NEUROPSYCHOLOGICAL/CLINICAL PRESENTATION

As mentioned, there are many disorders in which myoclonus is observed and many ways in which it may present clinically. Simple, nonpathological forms of myoclonus, such as a hiccup or a sudden jerk immediately upon falling asleep, occur in many individuals and are not problematic. However, more severe forms of myoclonus may involve repetitive twitches, several times a minute, that may start in one area of the body and either remain isolated or spread to other muscles (NINDS, 2000). This form of myoclonus may significantly inhibit the patient's gross and fine motor skills, including the ability to walk, eat, write, or talk.

In clinical assessments, the individual may have difficulty completing pencil and paper tasks, have abnormal gait, or slurred speech due to these myoclonic jerks. Patients may report these symptoms to occur very frequently (several times a minute), or infrequently (several times a day). Triggers to the myoclonic jerks may be undetectable to the patient or may be in direct response to certain stimuli, such as bright light, certain sounds, or touch (NINDS, 2000). Often, if triggers are undetectable to the patient, they may be identified with an electroencephalogram (EEG), as they could be the result of low oxygen to the brain (postanoxic myoclonus). They may also report distinguishing patterns or circular movements, or sporadic, isolated events, which are all common presentations of myoclonus.

As is evident, the majority of presenting problems with myoclonus are related to sensorimotor challenges. Striano et al. (2004) looked at cognitive abilities with relation to myoclonic epilepsy and found no significance. They also examined the developmental processes of their small sample and found no link to developmental difficulties with late-onset symptomology. Depending on the severity and time of onset of symptomology, emotional or psychological factors may manifest as a result of difficulties in social and interpersonal situations due to myoclonus.

DIAGNOSIS

Diagnosis of myoclonus can be very difficult due to the great number of similar presenting behaviors. It often requires the use of more sophisticated neuroimaging techniques to differentiate with other disorders. Terminology to describe the outward signs of myoclonus such as tremors, twitches, jerks, tics, and/or seizures are all used by clinicians, further complicating the diagnostic process (Gilbert, 2006). In fact, at times, clinicians may mistake myoclonus for simple seizures, making specific diagnostic criteria a necessity. It appears the simplest way to diagnose myoclonus is to better understand the various classifications, which may then lead to better understanding of etiology and treatment. The following is a brief description of several ways to classify myoclonus.

Location

Cortical reflex myoclonus originates in the cerebral cortex and usually manifests in one part of the body and may be worsened when voluntary movements are attempted. *Spinal* or *segmental myoclonus*, also *reticular reflex myoclonus*, originates around the spinal cord and brainstem, often causing more severe jerks, affecting the entire body. *Palatal myclonus* is a form of segmental myoclonus identified as a twitching or contraction of the soft palate, which may also include other muscles in the face, throat, or mouth, causing repetitive sounds in the ear, often eliciting minor complaints from the individual.

Parts of the Body Involved

Focal myoclonus involves only one part of the body, and *multifocal myoclonus* involves many parts of the body simultaneously. If only one segment of the body is affected, it is considered *segmental myoclonus*, and if the entire body is involved it is considered *generalized myoclonus*.

Muscle Response

Myoclonus can be classified as either a muscle contraction, *positive myoclonus*, or by the muscle relaxation, *negative myoclonus*. These are often observed and identified by neuroimaging techniques, such as EEG.

Related Cause

Some common types of myoclonus, as mentioned, are *physiological* in nature and are experienced by almost everyone, including the startle response, initial sleep jerks, and hiccups. Others may be classified as *primary myoclonus*, as they are not the direct effect of some other medical cause. These forms of myoclonus can be inherited, such as essential myoclonus and generally remain stable over time. *Secondary myoclonus* is the most common form, as this is the case when it is the symptom of a disorder, brain injury, or a reaction to a medication or intervention.

TREATMENT

The best possible treatment for myoclonus is inherent in identification of the cause of the symptom. Treatment is usually an attempt to decrease or eliminate the twitches and typically involves medication such as clonazepam, or similar types of tranquilizers. When epilepsy is identified as the cause, treatment may involve medications specific to the epileptic symptoms, such as certain barbiturates. If peripheral myoclonus is identified, surgical techniques may be used to decompress the injured area. Due to the varying etiology of myclonus, it may require multiple trials of medications, or multiple medications for symptoms to subside.

Beth Trammell
Raymond S. Dean

Balci, K., Utku, U., & Cobanoglu, S. (2007). Two patients with tremor caused by cortical lesions. *European Neurology, 57,* 36–38.

Factor, S. A., & Weiner, W. J. (2004). Hyperkinetic movement disorders. In W. J. Weiner & C. Goetz (Eds.), *Neurology for the non-neurologist* (5th ed., pp. 155–204). Philadelphia, PA: Lippincott, Williams, & Wilkins.

Fahn, S. (2007). Hypokinesia and hyperkinesias. In C. Goetz (Ed.), *Textbook of clinical neurology* (3rd ed., pp. 289–306). Philadelphia, PA: Saunders Elsevier.

Gilbert, D. (2006). Treatment of children and adolescents with tics and Tourette syndrome. *Journal of Child Neurology, 21,* 690–700.

Guerrini, R., Bonanni, P., & Patrignani, A. (2001). Autosomal dominant cortical myoclonus and epilepsy (ADCME) with complex partial seizures and generalized seizures: A newly recognized epilepsy syndrome with linkage to chromosome. *Brain, 124,* 2459–2475.

Laubage, P., Amer, L. O., Simonetta-Moreau, M., Attane, F., Tannier, C., Clanet, M., et al. (2002). Absence of linkage to 8q24 in a European family with familial adult myoclonic epilepsy (FAME). *Neurology, 58,* 941–944.

Martens, P., & Dyken, R. (2007). Storage diseases: Neuronal ceroid-lipofuscinoses, lipidoses, glycogenoses, and leukodystrophies. In C. Goetz (Ed.), *Textbook of clinical neurology* (pp. 612–639). Philadelphia, PA: Saunders Elsevier.

National Institute of Neurological Disorders and Stroke. (2000). *NINDS myoclonus information page.* Retrieved March 8, 2009, from http://www.ninds.nih.gov/disorders/myoclonus/myoclonus.htm

Striano, P., Chifari, R., Striano, S., de Fusco, M., Elia, M., Guerrini, R., et al. (2004). A new benign adult familial myoclonic epilepsy (BAFME) pedigree suggesting linkage to chromosome. *Epilepsia, 45,* 190–192.

Uyama, M. D., Fu, Y. H., & Ptacek, L. (2005). Familial adult myoclonic epilepsy (FAME). In A. V. Delgado-Escueta, R. Guerrini, M. T. Medina, P. Genton, & M. Bureau (Eds.), *Advances in neurology. Myoclonic epilepsies* (Vol. 95, Chap. 22, pp. 281–288). Philadelphia, PA: Lippincott Williams & Wilkins.

Van Rootselaar, A. F., van Schaik, I. N., van den Maagdenberg, A. M., Koelman, J. H., Callenbach, P., & Tijssen, M. (2005). Familial cortical myoclonic tremor with epilepsy: A single syndromic classification for a group of pedigrees bearing common features. *Movement Disorders, 20,* 665–673.

MYOPATHY

DESCRIPTION

The term "myopathy" can be used to define any disease or syndrome in which the patient's symptoms and/or physical signs can be attributed to pathological, biochemical, or electrophysiological changes that are occurring in the muscle fibers (or muscular interstitial tissues) for which there is no evidence that the symptoms are entirely secondary to the disordered function of the central or peripheral nervous system. This group of diseases includes many disorders that are genetically determined, as well as others of metabolic origin, and still others in which the disease process is inflammatory.

Common disorders classified under myopathy would include certain muscular dystrophies, such as Duchenne's dystrophy, congenital myopathies, and mitochondrial myopathies. In general, muscular myopathies are characterized by patterns of proximal shoulder and hip girdle weakness with preservation of distal strength, reduction of reflexes proportionate to reduced strength, and lack of sensory abnormalities (Hammerstaad, 2007).

NEUROPATHOLOGY/PATHOPHYSIOLOGY

It would be impossible to offer a concise discussion of the underlying pathophysiology of the myopathies as it encompasses such a wide variety of disorders. In all cases, the pathological basis corresponds with a disruption of the integrity of muscle fibers. For specifics regarding the individual presentations that fall under this umbrella, readers are recommended to see the respective articles within this text, including Congenital Myopathy, Mitochondrial Myopathies, Mitochondrial Cardiomyopathy, Muscular Dystrophy.

NEUROPSYCHOLOGICAL/CLINICAL PRESENTATION

Patients with some form of myopathy often present with an uncommon syndrome of benign exertional muscle pain for which no cause has been identified (Ropper & Brown, 2005, chapter 51). Atrophy may occur but develops slowly over the years in relation to reduced usage. As previously noted, in general, the myopathies are characterized by patterns of proximal shoulder and hip girdle weakness with preservation of distal strength, reduction of reflexes proportionate to reduced strength, and lack of sensory abnormalities (Eisenchenk, Triggs, Pearl, & Rojiani, 2001; Hammerstaad, 2007; Hund et al., 1997). Ptosis, open mouth expression, and reduced facial mobility are seen at higher rates across the myopathies (Hammerstaad, 2007).

DIAGNOSIS

Clinical data, an electromyogram (EMG), and a muscle biopsy are used in conjunction when a diagnosis of muscle disease is made. None of the three approaches is entirely adequate by itself, but their combined use yields the correct diagnosis in a very high proportion of cases (Eisenchenk et al., 2001; Spuler et al., 2008). Within the clinical data, the genetic history, history of the illness, symptoms of muscle diseases, and the clinical examination are important considerations.

The patient's genetic history is relevant to diagnosis as well as knowledge regarding the muscular dystrophies, congenital myopathies, and inherited metabolic myopathies (Kataeva, Krasik, & Komandenko, 1992). A negative family history, however, does not exclude autosomal recessive inheritance or a new mutation. In autosomal dominant disorders, a negative family history needs to be validated by examination of both parents. The clinical examination of biochemical tests may help in detecting a heterozygote in autosomal recessive or X-linked recessive diseases.

Upon examination of the history of the illness, one should pay particular attention to age of onset, duration, and rate of progression of symptoms. Most benign congenital myopathies, congenital muscular dystrophies, and inherited metabolic myopathies present in infancy. Duchenne's dystrophy usually presents in early childhood. Most inherited myopathies present in childhood or early adult life. Muscle weakness that evolves over a few hours suggests an exogenous intoxication (i.e., poisoning), whereas an abrupt onset of symptoms indicates defects with neuromuscular transmission.

Relatively few symptoms are associated with diverse muscle diseases; these include weakness, decrease of muscle bulk, increased fatigability, muscle pain, cramps, stiffness, and discoloration of urine caused by myoglobinuria. Vague complaints, such as constant fatigue and exhaustion, as well as weakness of the cranial, cervical, torso, and limb muscles present stereotypically. In evaluating abnormal fatigability, it is important to define the duration and intensity of the exercise that provokes fatigue. In patients with defects of neuromuscular transmission, even mild exercise can induce fatigue.

The clinical examination should include inspection and manual muscle testing. Inspection can reveal muscle atrophy, hypertrophy, contractures, fasciculations, and winging of scapulas (Eisencchnk et al., 2001; Hund et al., 1997; Spuler et al., 2008). Inspection provides information on the distribution of weakness, which is confirmed by detailed manual muscle testing. The manual muscle testing part of the examination requires knowledge of the origin, insertion, action, and innervation of the muscles tested, a consistent technique, and a generally accepted rating scale (Ropper & Brown, 2005). This evaluation helps determine the distribution of the weakness and aids in diagnosis because increasing weakness in proximal versus distal muscles suggests a myopathy rather than a neuropathy.

EMG is a test that consists of the analysis of spontaneous, evoked, and voluntarily generated potentials from nerve and muscle. This procedure is useful in distinguishing between broad categories of disease, such as myopathy versus neuropathy. The final approach, the muscle biopsy, makes use of biopsy specimens for light microscopic, ultrastructural, and biochemical studies. Typically, muscles showing mild to moderate weakness are biopsied.

TREATMENT

Because of the nature and diversity of the causes of muscular weakness and wasting, no single suggested medical treatment is viable. Depending upon the specific characteristics and features of the myopathy, numerous treatments may be employed. Unfortunately, no drug has any influence upon the course of the disease, though complications such as respiratory and urinary infections may demand antibiotics. Physical exercise appears to delay the continued

M

weakness and onset of contractures; a regular exercise program of activities may be started under the supervision of a skilled physiotherapist and subsequently continued at home. Such exercise would include regular passive stretching of those tendons that show a tendency to shorten.

In certain cases, operative procedures for the control of scoliosis may be justified, whereas in select cases, surgical lengthening of shortened tendons is advised. However, immobilization or prolonged bed rest resulting from surgery must be avoided as these inevitably cause rapid deterioration. The additional burden of obesity or excess weight should be avoided and caloric requirements are likely to be less than normal.

Physicians working with patients diagnosed with muscle diseases are familiar with harsh complaints of diffuse muscular pain that is induced by minimal effort and greatly restricts activity but for which no physical or biochemical cause has presently been determined. Some individuals are of obsessional and introspective temperament; it is likely that some of their symptoms may have an emotional origin. Treatment with tranquillizing drugs is rarely helpful. Treatment with analgesic and relaxant drugs is often of little if any benefit, and symptoms may prove to be both persistent and disabling. Occasionally, a reflex contraction indicative of myopathies will be accentuated or evoked by anxiety in the patient.

Genetic counseling has been suggested as a treatment option such that the heredity nature of many myopathies can be recognized. Genetic counseling should be no different from counseling by a physician for any other illness. The facts should be clearly presented to all concerned family members so a rational decision about further pregnancies can be made. Information should be presented simply as patients often misunderstand and misinterpret genetic information during counseling sessions. Follow-up visits and written communications are usually helpful.

Psychological management demands considerable patience and understanding on the part of parents and/or family members, doctors, nurses, and social workers. Support, optimism, and encouragement are of great importance in the face of continuing deterioration. Patients and families can be referred for genetic counseling and support counseling by physicians and health care personnel. Patients and families should be made aware of early diagnosis, carrier detection, and prevention.

Matthew Holcombe
Raymond S. Dean
Chad A. Noggle

Eisenchenk, S., Triggs, W. J., Pearl, G. S., & Rojiani, A. M. (2001). Proximal myotonic myopathy: Clinical, neuropathologic, and molecular genetic features, *Annals of Clinical & Laboratory Science, 31*(2), 140–146.

Hammerstaad, J. P. (2007). In C. Goetz (Ed.) *Textbook of clinical neurology* (3rd ed., pp. 243–288). Philadelphia: Saunders Elsevier.

Hund, E., Jansen, O., Kock, M. C., Ricker, K., Fogel, W., Neidermaier, N., et al. (1997). Proximal myotonic myopathy with MRI white matter abnormalities of the brain. *Neurology, 48,* 33–37.

Kataeva, N., Krasik, E., & Komandenko, N. (1992). Neuropsychic syndromes in hereditary neuromuscular pathology. *Zhurnal Nevropatologii i Psikhiatrii imeni S.S. Korsakova, 92*(4), 31–35.

Ropper, A. H. & Brown, R. H. (2005). *Adams and Victor's principles of neurology* (8th ed., Ch. 51, pp. 1230–1243). New York: McGraw-Hill.

Spuler, S., Carl, M., Zabojszcza, J., Straub, V., Bushby, K., Moore, S., et al. (2008). Dysferlin-deficient muscular dystrophy features amyloidosis. *Annals of Neurology, 63*(3), 323–328.

MYOTONIA

DESCRIPTION

Myotonia is an intrinsic disorder of muscle caused by defects in either ion channel or muscle membrane function. Clinically, myotonia in the individual muscle fibers summates to produce a prolonged time for relaxation after voluntary muscle contraction and external mechanical stimulation (Hudson, Ebers, & Bulman, 1995). Patients with myotonia may report painless muscle stiffness immediately upon initiating muscle activity after a period of rest, for example, trouble climbing stairs after a period of sitting. Myotonia may be demonstrated by asking the patient to make tight fists and then to quickly open the hands or inability to release hand grip after a strong handshake. The patient may have a lag in opening the eyes after initial tight eyelid closure. It may be induced by striking the thenar eminence with a percussion hammer, and it may be detected by watching the involuntary drawing of the thumb across the palm. Myotonia may also be demonstrated in the tongue by pressing the edge of the wooden tongue blade against its dorsal surface and by observing the deep furrow that disappears slowly. Myotonia improves with muscle exercise or repeated efforts, the so-called "warm-up phenomenon." Another phenomenon known as paramyotonia, is also a painless muscle stiffness that is associated with exercise rather than improving with exercise, that is, there is no warming-up phenomenon. It is usually not difficult to distinguish them from muscle cramps that present with a sudden and painful focal muscle contracture.

Myotonic disorders are classified into dystrophic myotonias (DM) and nondystrophic myotonias (Figure 1).

NEUROPATHOLOGY/PATHOPHYSIOLOGY

Both myotonia and paramyotonia are associated with myotonic discharge on electromyogram (EMG). The classical myotonic EMG shows spontaneous runs of motor unit potentials with a characteristic waxing and waning of both amplitude and frequency, producing a sound often reminiscent of a World War II dive

bomber or a motor cycle engine when audio-amplified. By definition, myotonic discharges last 500 ms or longer and should be identified in at least three areas of an individual muscle outside of an endplate region (Streib, 1987). Although most patients with myotonia have myotonic dystrophy, myotonia is not specific for this disease and occurs in several rarer conditions. The differential diagnosis may be divided on the basis of presence of electrical myotonia and the clinical picture (myotonia/paramyotonia/both absent) (Miller, 2008). The myotonia is seen in myotonic dystrophies and myotonia congenita. The paramyotonia is seen in paramyotonia congenita (Miller, 2008). Only electrical myotonia without clinical myotonia is seen in acid maltase deficiency (Miller, 2008). Schwartz–Jampel's syndrome (chondrodystrophia myotonia), McArdle's disease (glycogenosis Type 5), Hoffman's disease (myotonia in hypothyroidism), Brody's disease (sarcoplasmic reticulum—Ca2+ATPase deficiency), neuromyotonia, neuroleptic malignant syndromes, and tetanus may mimic clinical myotonia, but they

M

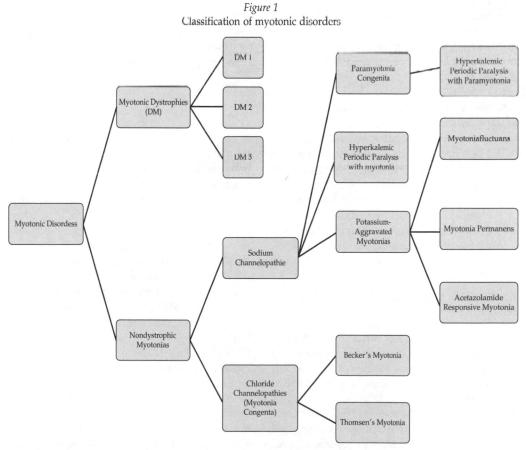

Figure 1
Classification of myotonic disorders

Source: Adapted from (Heatwole & Moxley, 2007).

lack characteristic electrodiagnostic features (pseudo-myotonia) (Heatwole & Moxley, 2007; Trip, Drost, van Engelen, & Faber, 2006).

DM is inherited as an autosomal-dominant trait. It often exhibits a pattern of *anticipation* in which each successive generation has a tendency to be more severely involved (Kliegman, Stanton, Geme, Schor, & Behrman, 2007). DM Types 1 and 2 have RNA-mediated disease mechanism. DM Type 1 is caused by cytosine-thymine-guanosine (CTG) trinucleotide repeat expansion on chromosome 19q13.3 in the 3' untranslated region in the dystrophia myotonica protein kinase (DMPK) gene (Brook et al., 1992). DM Type 2 is caused by cytosine-cytosine-thymine-guanosine repeat expansion in the first intron in zinc finger protein 9 gene on chromosome 3q21 (Liquori et al., 2001). The expanded repeat is transcribed in RNA and forms discrete inclusions in the nucleus. Mutant RNA sequesters MBNL1, a splice regulator protein and depletes MBNL1 from the nucleoplasm. The loss of MBNL1 results in altered splicing of CIC-1 mRNA. Altered splice products do not encode functional CIC-1 protein. This defect causes loss of chloride conductance in the muscle membranes leading to myotonia.

The nondystrophic myotonias are pure skeletal muscle diseases without the involvement of other organ systems. They are ion channel disorders caused by mutations/deletions in the genes encoding chloride (CIC-1) or sodium (SCN4A) channels expressed exclusively in skeletal muscles (Koch et al., 1992; McClatchey et al., 1992; Ptacek et al., 1992, 1994). There are two forms of chloride channel disorders: autosomal recessive myotonia congenita (Becker's disease) and autosomal-dominant myotonia congenita (Thomsen's disease). They are discussed in detail in another article entitled Myotonia Congenita. Sodium channel disorders are all autosomal-dominantly inherited or sporadic. The exact prevalence of sodium channel diseases is not known although the prevalence of paramyotonia congenita has been estimated at 1 per 356,000 (Trip et al., 2006).

NEUROPSYCHOLOGICAL/CLINICAL PRESENTATION

DM 1 commonly presents between 20 and 40 years of age, whereas DM 2 commonly presents between 30 and 40 years of age. Severe congenital form is seen in a minority of cases and to date have had the DM 1 form only (Kliegman et al., 2007). Clinical diagnosis can be easily made by the combination of myotonia and the characteristic pattern of muscle wasting and weakness that include weakness of superficial facial muscle, levator palpebrae superioris, temporalis,

masseter and palate with resultant ptosis, dysarthria and hatchet face. DM 1 has a prominent distal distribution of myopathy while DM 2 has predominant proximal distribution involving limb girdles, the so-called proximal myotonic myopathy. DM causes dysfunction in multiple organ systems. Not only is the striated muscle severely affected but smooth muscle of the alimentary tract and uterus are also involved; cardiac function is altered; and patients have multiple variable endocrinopathies, immunologic deficiencies, cataracts (characteristic Christmas tree–like appearance), dysmorphic facies, frontal balding, and other neurologic abnormalities (Kliegman et al., 2007). About half of the patients with DM are intellectually impaired, but severe mental retardation is unusual. Cognitive impairment may be due to accumulation of mutant DMPK mRNA and aberrant alternative splicing in the neurons (Kliegman et al., 2007).

As noted, the nondystrophic myotonias are pure musculoskeletal diseases without the involvement of other organ systems. The myotonic disorder without progressive weakness, wasting, and dystrophic histopathology fall into this category. Figure 1 shows the classification of nondystrophic myotonias. Nondystrophic myotonia can be dramatic and sometimes disabling. Emotional surprises, cold exposure, potassium ingestion, or exercise are potential triggers of nondystrophic myotonia.

DIAGNOSIS

The primary diagnostic test of DM is a DNA analysis of blood to demonstrate the abnormal expansion of the CTG repeat. The muscle biopsy specimen may be useful in older children, which revels prominent pyknotic nuclear clumps, increased internal nuclei, variable muscle fiber size, muscle fiber atrophy involving Type 1 fiber in DM 1 and Type 2 fiber in DM 2. There is an absence of fibrosis, necrosis, and regeneration. Muscle biopsy is not usually required for diagnosis, which in typical cases can be based on the clinical manifestation.

Diagnosis of nondystrophic myotonia is mostly based on clinical presentation, which includes history and physical examination. Ancillary tests such as EMG and nerve conduction studies may be helpful. Clinical response to cold exposure or exercise testing can help in classification, and it is useful to inquire about these responses before undertaking electrodiagnostic testing. Cold frequently worsens myotonia in paramyotonia congenita and acetazolamide-responsive myotonia (Russell & Hirsch, 1994). Gene tests are usually not required to make the diagnosis, and there is an absence of significant histopathology in the muscle biopsy. Clinically, the nondystrophic myotonias can usually be differentiated based on their inheritance pattern, response to stimuli/triggers, electrodiagnostic features, muscle histology, genetic mutations, and myotonia characteristic (Hudson et al., 1995).

TREATMENT

Myotonia is rarely disabling in DM. Patients often do not require specific medical therapy for myotonia. Sodium channel blockers (procainamide, phenytoin, and mexiletine), tricyclic antidepressive drugs, benzodiazepines, calcium-antagonists, taurine, and prednisone may be of use in reducing myotonia (Trip et al., 2006). To date, we do not have any medication to open chloride channels of the skeletal muscles. Due to insufficient good quality data and lack of randomized studies, it is impossible to determine whether drug treatment is safe and effective in the treatment of myotonia. Small single studies give an indication that clomipramine and imipramine have a short-term beneficial effect and that taurine has a long-term beneficial effect on myotonia (Trip et al., 2006). Management of DM remains at best supportive comprehensive care including patient education, genetic counseling, regular monitoring of cardiac rhythm, early detection of respiratory and swallowing problems, avoidance of anesthesia-related complications, cataract surgery, and provision of physical therapy, occupational therapy, speech and swallowing therapy, and community outreach social welfare programs (Mankodi, 2008).

Myotonia and other symptoms are easily manageable by activity modifications, avoiding certain triggers, and pharmacological therapies (as discussed above). Prognosis is generally excellent.

Gaurav Jain
Sarita Singhal
Chad A. Noggle

Brook, J. D., McCurrach, M. E., Harley, H. G., Buckler, A. J., Church, D., Aburatani, H., et al. (1992). Molecular basis of myotonic dystrophy: Expansion of trinucleotide repeat at the 3′ end of the transcript encoding at protein kinase family member. *Cell, 68,* 799–808.

Heatwole, C. R., & Moxley, R. T., III. (2007). The nondystrophic myotonias. *Neurotherapeutics, IV,* 238–251.

Hudson, A. J., Ebers, G. C., & Bulman, D. E. (1995). The skeletal muscle sodium and chloride channel diseases. *Brain, 118,* 547–563.

Kliegman, R. M., Stanton, B. M. D., Geme, J. S., Schor, N., & Behrman, R. E. (Eds.). (2007). *Nelson textbook of pediatrics* (18th ed., pp. 2544–2546). Philadelphia: Saunders Elsevier.

Koch, M. C., Steinmeyer, K., Lorenz, C., Ricker, K., Wolf, F., Otto, M., et al. (1992). The skeletal muscle chloride channel in dominant and recessive human myotonia. *Science, 257,* 797–800.

Liquori, C. L., Ricker, K., Moseley, M. L., Jacobsen, J. F., Kress, W., Naylor, S. L., et al. (2001). Myotonic dystrophy type 2 caused by a CCTG expansion in intron 1 of ZNF9. *Science, 293,* 864–867.

Mankodi, A. (2008). Myotonic disorders. *Neurology India, 56*(3), 298–304.

McClatchey, A. I., Van den Bergh, P., Pericak-Vance, M. A., Raskind, W., Verellen, C., McKenna-Yasek, D., et al. (1992). Temperature-sensitive mutations in the III-IV cytoplasmic loop region of the skeletal muscle sodium channel gene in paramyotonia congenita. *Cell, 68,* 769–774.

Miller, T. M. (2008). Differential diagnosis of myotonic disorders. *Muscle and Nerve, 37,* 293–299.

Ptacek, L. J., George, A. L. Jr., Barchi, R. L., Griggs, R. C., Riggs, J. E., Robertson, M., et al. (1992). Mutations in an S4 segment of the adult skeletal muscle sodium channel cause paramyotonia congenita. *Neuron, 8,* 891–897.

Ptacek, L. J., Tawil, R., Griggs, R. C., Meola, G., McManis, P., Barohn, R. J., et al. (1994). Sodium channel mutations in acetazolamide-responsive myotonia congenita, paramyotonia congenita, and hyperkalemic periodic paralysis. *Neurology, 44,* 1500–1503.

Russell, S. H., & Hirsch, N. P. (1994). Anaesthesia and myotonia. *British Journal of anaesthesia, 72,* 210–216.

Streib, E. W. (1987). Differential diagnosis of mytonic syndromes. *Muscle Nerve, 10,* 603–615.

Trip, J., Drost, G., van Engelen, B. G., & Faber, C. G. (2006). Drug treatment for myotonia. *Cochrane Database of Systematic Reviews,* (1), CD004762.

MYOTONIA CONGENITA

DESCRIPTION

Myotonia congenita was first described by Thomsen in 1876, whose family, including Thomsen himself, suffered with the disease (Lossin & George, 2008). It is a nondystrophic type of myotonia (see Figure 1 on p. 511) that includes Thomsen's myotonia congenita and Becker's myotonia congenita. The two additional variants of Thomsen's disease are myotonia levior and fluctuating myotonia congenita (Hudson, Ebers, & Bulman, 1995).

All forms of myotonia congenita are caused by mutations that result in impaired functioning of the skeletal muscle chloride channel (ClC-1) that leads to an increase in sarcolemmal excitability that clinically presents as delayed muscular relaxation (myotonia) (Cannon, 2006). The disorder may be transmitted as either an autosomal-dominant or recessive trait with close to 130 currently known mutations (Lossin & George, 2008). They are pure skeletal muscle diseases without multisystem involvement. The estimated worldwide prevalence of myotonia congenita is approximately 1:100,000 (Emery, 1991).

NEUROPATHOLOGY/PATHOPHYSIOLOGY

All forms of myotonia congenita have dysfunction of chloride conductance and have mutations affecting the skeletal muscle voltage-gated chloride channel gene (*CLCN1*) at its chromosome 7q locus (Shapiro & Ruff, 2002). The responsible mutations of *CLCN1* alter the skeletal muscle chloride channel protein, ClC-1 (Lehmann-Horn & Rudel, 1995). A reduction in chloride conductance occurs and leads to membrane hyperexcitability. Myotonia results due to reduced chloride conductance across the transverse tubular system (Shapiro & Ruff, 2002). In normal muscle, a high chloride conductance allows for fast repolarization of the t-tubules, largely eliminating recurrent depolarization. In myotonia congenita, depolarization results in repetitive firing of the muscle fiber and subsequent myotonia.

NEUROPSYCHOLOGICAL/CLINICAL PRESENTATION

The affected individuals describe muscular stiffness upon initiating movements. The stiffness remits with several repetitions of the same movements, giving rise to so called warm-up phenomenon. (Refer to the article on mytonia for further details about myotonia.)

Thomsen's disease is dominantly inherited and is usually evident during early infancy. The first symptom may be delayed relaxation of the eyelids after forceful closure following sneezing or crying (von Graefe's sign or lid lag) (Wakeman, Babu, Tarleton, & Macdonald, 2008). The predominant features of Thomsen's disease are a painless, transient, muscle stiffness with a predilection for both the upper extremity and the facial muscles (Davies & Hanna, 1999). It can vary in severity from mild to moderate. There are no central nervous system manifestations. Social and cognitive regression does not occur, nor does significant occupational limitation (Gutmann & Phillips, 1991). However, a psychiatric burden can be evident, especially in young males where muscular hypertrophy is obvious, mockery and misunderstanding by peers on account of poor physical performance and "clumsiness" can be

problematic (Lossin & George, 2008). Life expectancy is normal, and the affected individual can lead a satisfying and successful life.

Becker's disease, or recessive generalized myotonia, is an autosomal recessive form of myotonia congenita (Lossin & George, 2008). Compared with Thomsen's disease, Becker's disease is more common, more insidious, and has later onset (Heatwole & Moxley, 2007). It is characterized by moderate to severe myotonia with associated transient weakness (typically lasting seconds to minutes), slowly progressive weakness (more common in lower extremities), and eventual wasting in some patients or more pronounced lower extremity hypertrophy in others. Overall, the prognosis is good in Becker's disease, with no reduction in life expectancy (Gutmann & Phillips, 1991). Cognitive regression does not occur. However, some may develop a crippling disability from their lack of strength (Gutmann & Phillips, 1991; Shapiro & Ruff, 2002).

Two additional forms of myotonia congenita have been described: myotonia levior and fluctuating myotonia congenita (Heatwole & Moxley, 2007). Whether these two entities are truly distinct disorders is under debate, and some propose that they are variants of Thomsen's disease (Hudson, Ebers, & Bulman, 1995).

The clinical and diagnostic features of the chloride channel nondystrophic myotonias are summarized in Table 1 (Heatwole & Moxley, 2007; Lossin & George, 2008; Mankodi, 2008).

DIAGNOSIS

The diagnosis of myotonia congenita is mostly based on clinical presentation including a careful history and physical examination (Mankodi, 2008). A family history of myotonia is helpful for distinguishing subtypes in some, but not all, cases, owing to variable expressivity (Lossin & George, 2008). Ancillary tests such as electromyography (EMG) and nerve conduction studies may be helpful. The EMG reveals typically myotonic discharges in many muscles. Motor unit potentials are normal in morphology. Sensory and motor conduction studies are normal. Repetitive nerve stimulation and short exercise test may show decline in compound muscle action potential (larger decline in Becker's subtype). Long exercise tests may reveal a small decrement in Becker's disease but is not a feature of Thomsen's disease (Heatwole & Moxley, 2007). Laboratory tests show a trend toward more pronounced elevation in serum creative phosphokinase in Becker's subtype than in Thomsen's disease (Lossin & George, 2008). Genetic testing usually

Table 1
CLINICAL SUBTYPES OF MYOTONIA CONGENITA

| | Thomsen's Disease | Thomsen's Disease Variants | | |
		Fluctuating Myotonia Congenita	Myotonia Levior	Becker's Disease
Inheritance chromosome	Dominant 7q	Dominant 7q	Dominant 7q	Recessive 7q
Age of onset	Early first decade	Late first decade	First decade to early second decade	Late first decade
Muscles involved	Upper extremity and face > lower extremity	Lower extremity, ocular and masticatory muscles	Predominantly grip	Lower extremity > upper extremity
Severity	Moderate	Mild to moderate (fluctuating)	Mild to moderate	Moderate to severe
Muscle hypertrophy	Yes	No	No	Yes (mostly at lower extremity)
Pain	No	Yes	No	Rare
Provocative stimuli	Movement after prolonged rest, cold, pregnancy, emotional surprise	Movement after rest, cold, pregnancy, fasting state, emotional stress	Movement after rest or maintenance of posture	Movement after rest or maintenance of posture, cold
Nerve conduction studies	Normal; repetitive stimulation may see moderate decremental response	Normal	Normal	Decremental response to repetitive stimulation
Treatment	Mexiletine, quinine, procainamide, acetazolamide	Mexiletine, quinine, procainamide, acetazolamide	Mexiletine, quinine, procainamide, acetazolamide	Mexiletine

confirms the diagnosis. Genetic analysis of *CLCN1* is now commercially available.

TREATMENT

Many individuals with myotonia congenita do not require any pharmacological intervention. Mostly symptoms are easily manageable by activity modifications, relaxation techniques, and avoiding certain triggers. When these maneuvers are insufficient, drugs that reduce the excitability of the sarcolemma can be used. Historically, quinidine and quinine were used as antimyotonic agents (Lossin & George, 2008). They are usually well tolerated in low doses and for short intervals. However, long-term use is not recommended because of side effects that include cinchonism, gastrointestinal upsets, visual and auditory problems. Other drugs that have been used in treating myotonia with varying levels of success include procaine, tocainide, mexiletine, carbamazepine, lithium, and phenytoin (Lossin & George, 2008). All of these

drugs act by use-dependent block of voltage-gated sodium channels. The other approach for ameliorating myotonia due to chloride channel defects is to pharmacologically increase the chloride conductance of skeletal muscle. Taurine and the R (+) isomer of clofibric acid produce modest increase in resting chloride conductance but not sufficient to prevent myotonia (Conte-Camerino et al., 1989; Conte-Camerino, Tortorella, Ferranini, & Bryant, 1984).

Anesthesia should be administered cautiously to patients of myotonia congenita as there is an increased risk for a malignant hyperthermia syndrome.

Gene therapy is currently under research for treatment of myotonia congenita. A major challenge to successful gene therapy remains the great difficulty in systemically targeting skeletal muscle with a gene delivery vector (Lossin & George, 2008).

Gaurav Jain
Sarita Singhal
Chad A. Noggle

Cannon, S. C. (2006). Pathomechanisms in channelopathies of skeletal muscle and brain. *Annual Review Neuroscience, 29,* 387–415.

Conte-Camerino, D., De Luca, A., Mambrini, M., Ferrannini, E., Farconi, F., Giotti, A., et al. (1989). The effects of taurine on pharmacologically induced myotonia. *Muscle Nerve, 12,* 898–904.

Conte-Camerino, D., Tortorella, V., Ferranini, E., & Bryant, S. H. (1984). The toxic effects of clofibrate and its metabolite on mammalian skeletal muscle: An electrophysiological study. *Archives of Toxicology* (Suppl. 7), 482–484.

Davies, N. P., & Hanna, M. G. (1999). Neurological channelopathies: Diagnosis and therapy in the new millennium. *Annals of Medicine, 31,* 406–420.

Emery, A. E. (1991). Population frequencies of inherited neuromuscular diseases—a world survey. *Neuromuscular Disorders, 1,* 19–29.

Gutmann, L., & Phillips, L. H., II. (1991). Myotonia congenita. *Seminars in Neurology, 11,* 244–248.

Heatwole, C. R., & Moxley, R. T., III. (2007). The nondystrophic myotonias. *Neurotherapeutics, 4*(2), 238–251.

Hudson, A. J., Ebers, G. C., & Bulman, D. E. (1995). The skeletal muscle sodium and chloride channel diseases. *Brain, 118,* 547–563.

Lehmann-Horn, F., & Rudel, R. (1995). Hereditary nondystrophic myotonias and periodic paralysis. *Current Opinion in Neurology, 8,* 402–410.

Lossin, C., & George, A. L. (2008). Myotonia congenita. *Advances in Genetics, 63,* 25–55.

Mankodi, A. (2008). Myotonic disorders. *Neurology India, 56*(3), 298–304.

Shapiro, B., & Ruff, R. (2002). Disorders of skeletal muscle membrane excitability: Myotonia congenita, paramyotonia congenita, periodic paralysis, and related disorders. In B. Katirji, H. J. Kaminski, D. C. Preston, R. L. Ruff, & B. E. Shapiro (Eds.), *Neuromuscular disorders in clinical practice* (pp. 987–1020). Boston: Butterworth-Heinemann.

Wakeman, B., Babu, D., Tarleton, J., & Macdonald, I. M. (2008). Extraocular muscle hypertrophy in myotonia congenita. *Journal of the American Academy of Pediatric Ophthalmology, 12,* 294–296.

N

NARCOLEPSY

DESCRIPTION

In 1880, French neurologist Jean-Baptiste Gelineau first coined the term "narcolepsie" to describe a disease (Williams, Karacan, & Moore, 1988). This disorder is now more commonly known as "narcolepsy," but is also referred to as Gelineau's syndrome. Narcolepsy is a chronic neurological disorder caused by the brain's inability to regulate sleep–wake cycles normally (National Institute of Neurological Disorders and Stroke [NINDS], 2008). Narcolepsy is a chronic and potentially disabling disorder that affects approximately 1 in 2,000 individuals (Long-streth, Koepsell, Ton, Hendrickson, & van Belle, 2007). The main symptoms of narcolepsy include uncontrollable, excessive sleep, regardless of the time of day or whether the person had enough sleep the previous night (Swanson, 1999). The *International Classification of Sleep Disorders* (*ICSD-2*) has recognized three forms of narcolepsy: narcolepsy with cataplexy, narcolepsy without cataplexy, and narcolepsy due to a medical condition (American Academy of Sleep Medicine [AASM], 2005).

Narcolepsy with cataplexy includes a sudden episode of loss of muscle function, ranging from slight weakness (such as limpness at the neck or knees, to sagging facial muscles, or inability to speak clearly) to complete body collapse (Swanson, 1999). Narcolepsy without cataplexy is characterized by excessive daytime sleepiness (EDS), naps that are typically refreshing, normal or moderately disturbed nocturnal sleep, and an abnormal tendency for inappropriate transition into rapid eye movement (REM) sleep (AASM, 2005). Narcolepsy without cataplexy is thought to represent between 10% and 50% of all narcolepsy cases, but the precise prevalence is unknown (Billiard, 2008). Narcolepsy due to a medical condition is also known as a secondary or symptomatic narcolepsy, and is diagnosed when the direct cause of the symptoms is a medical condition or neurological disorder (AASM, 2005).

NEUROPATHOLOGY/PATHOPHYSIOLOGY

According to the NINDS (2008), narcolepsy may be secondary to a disease effecting brain mechanisms that regulate REM sleep. For normal sleepers, a typical sleep cycle is about 100–110 min long, beginning with non-REM sleep and transitioning to REM sleep after 80–100 min. People with narcolepsy frequently enter REM sleep within a few minutes of falling asleep (NINDS, 2008).

The pathophysiology of narcolepsy is not confined to REM sleep, but also involves wakefulness and non-REM sleep. During wakefulness, sleep attacks occur often at intervals of 90–120 min similar to the nocturnal non-REM/REM cycle and to the ultraradian sleep–wake cycle of normal newborns (Culebras, 2000). In both wakefulness and sleep, features of the different states of being (wakefulness and REM and non-REM sleep) can intermingle and give rise to such clinical phenomena as sleepwalking, REM sleep-behavior disorder, sleep paralysis, cataplexy, and hallucinations. Narcolepsy therefore appears to represent a disorder of state boundary control (Broughton et al., 1986). Whether or not narcoleptic symptoms represent an exaggeration of normal sleep mechanisms related to insufficient maturation of arousal or to non-REM-sleep mechanisms remains controversial (Culebras, 2000).

A number of variant forms (alleles) of genes located in a region of chromosome 6, known as the HLA complex, have proved to be strongly, although not invariably, associated with narcolepsy (NINDS, 2008). The majority of people diagnosed with narcolepsy are known to have specific variants in certain *HLA* genes (NINDS, 2008). Current evidence strongly supports the pathogenic role of selective loss of hypocretin-containing neurons in the hypothalamus of individuals with narcolepsy with cataplexy (Scammell, 2003). Scientists have found that brains from humans with narcolepsy often contain greatly reduced numbers of hypocretin-producing neurons (NINDS, 2008).

NEUROPSYCHOLOGICAL/CLINICAL PRESENTATION

In most cases, symptoms first appear in individuals between the ages of 10 and 25, but narcolepsy can become clinically apparent at virtually any age (NINDS, 2008). According to Reite, Ruddy, and Nagel (1997), the presenting complaints of narcolepsy include EDS, episodes of irresistible sleepiness, paroxysmal muscle weakness that is often elicited by emotion or surprise (cataplexy), temporary inability to initiate motor movement before sleep on awakening (sleep paralysis), hypnagogic hallucinations, automatic behavior, and disturbed nocturnal sleep. If left undiagnosed and untreated, narcolepsy can pose special problems for children and adolescents, interfering with their psychological, social, and cognitive development, and undermining the ability to succeed at school (NINDS, 2008). Experts have begun to recognize that narcolepsy sometimes contributes to certain childhood behavioral problems, such as ADHD, and must be addressed before the behavioral problem can be resolved (NINDS, 2008).

DIAGNOSIS

The diagnostic criteria for narcolepsy according to the *Diagnostic and Statistical Manual of Mental Disorders* (American Psychiatric Association [APA], 2000) includes: (1) irresistible attacks of refreshing sleep that occur daily over at least 3 months; (2) the presence of one or both of the following: (i) cataplexy, (ii) recurrent intrusions of elements of REM sleep into the transition between sleep and wakefulness, as manifested by either hypnopompic or hypnagogic hallucinations or sleep paralysis at the beginning or end of sleep episodes; and (3) the disturbance is not due to physiological effects of a substance (e.g., drug of abuse and medication) or other general medical condition.

A clinical examination and exhaustive medical history are essential for diagnosis and treatment (NINDS, 2008). A battery of specialized tests, which can be performed in a sleep disorders clinic, is usually required before a diagnosis can be established (NINDS, 2008). Two tests in particular are considered essential in confirming a diagnosis of narcolepsy: the polysomnogram (PSG) and the multiple sleep latency test (MSLT; NINDS, 2008). A PSG is an overnight test that takes continuous measurements while a patient is asleep and can help reveal whether REM sleep occurs at abnormal times in the sleep cycle (NINDS, 2008).

MSLT measures the amount of time it takes a person to fall asleep. Ten minutes or longer is considered a normal amount of time for a person to fall asleep. A latency period of 5 min or less is considered suggestive of narcolepsy (NINDS, 2008).

Rare cases of narcolepsy are known to result from traumatic injuries to parts of the brain involved in REM sleep or from tumor growth and other disease processes in the same regions. Infections, exposure to toxins, dietary factors, stress, hormonal changes (such as those occurring during puberty or menopause), and alterations in a person's sleep schedule are just a few of the many factors that may exert direct or indirect effects on the brain, thereby possibly contributing to disease symptoms (NINDS, 2008).

TREATMENT

Treatment approaches for narcolepsy include behavioral and pharmacological interventions. Behavioral approaches include maximal sleep hygiene, scheduled naps, and education for patient, family, teachers, and employers (Reite et al., 1997). Several recent studies provide evidence that modafinil and sodium oxybate are effective for treatment of hypersomnia due to narcolepsy (Wise, Arand, Auger, Brooks, & Watson, 2007). Despite significant advances in understanding the pathophysiology of narcolepsy, there is still not an identified ideal treatment to restore full and sustained alertness (Wise et al., 2007). New approaches currently being developed include: symptomatic neurotransmitters and endocrine therapy, hypocretin-based therapies, immune-based therapies, and skin warming or cooling (Billiard, 2008). Within the Federal government, NINDS, a component of the National Institutes of Health (NIH), has primary responsibility for sponsoring research on neurological disorders. As part of its mission, the NINDS supports research on narcolepsy and other sleep disorders with a neurological basis through grants to major medical institutions across the country (NINDS, 2008).

Justin Boseck
Raymond S. Dean

American Academy of Sleep Medicine. (2005). *The international classification of sleep disorders: Diagnostic & coding manual* (2nd ed.). Westchester, IL: Author.

American Psychiatric Association. (2000). *Diagnostic and statistical manual of mental disorders* (4th ed., text revision). Arlington, VA: Author.

Billiard, M. (2008). Narcolepsy: Current treatment options and future approaches. *Neuropsychiatric Disease and Treatment*, 4(3), 557–566.

Broughton, R., Valley, V., Aguirre, M., Roberts, J., Suwalski, W., & Dunham, W. (1986). Excessive daytime sleepiness and the pathophysiology of narcolepsy-cataplexy: A laboratory perspective. *Sleep, 9,* 205–215.

Culebras, A. (Ed.). (2000). *Sleep disorders and neurological disease.* New York: Marcel Decker.

Longstreth, W. T., Koepsell, T. D., Jr., Ton, T. G., Hendrickson, A. F., & van Belle, G. (2007). The epidemiology of narcolepsy. *Sleep, 30,* 13–26.

National Institute of Neurological Disorders and Stroke. (2008, September). *Narcolepsy fact sheet.* Retrieved January 19, 2011, from National Institutes of Neurological Disorders and Stroke via: http://www.ninds.nih.gov/disorders/narcolepsy/narcolepsy.htm

Reite, M., Ruddy, J., & Nagel, K. (1997). *Evaluation and management of sleep disorders* (2nd ed.). Washington, DC: American Psychiatric Press.

Scammel, T. E. (2003). The neurobiology, diagnosis, and treatment of narcolepsy. *Annals of Neurology, 53,* 154–166.

Swanson, J. (Ed.). (1999). *Sleep disorders sourcebook.* Detroit, MI: Omnigraphics.

Williams, R. L., Karacan, I., & Moore, C. A. (1988). *Sleep disorders: Diagnosis and treatment.* New York: Wiley-Interscience Publications.

Wise, M. S., Arand, D. L., Auger, R. R., Brooks, S. N., & Watson, N. F. (2007). Treatment of narcolepsy and other hypersomnias of central origin. *Sleep, 30*(12), 1712–1727.

NEUROCANTHOCYTOSIS

DESCRIPTION

Neuroacanthocytosis (NA) is a homogeneous, neurodegenerative disease that refers to a group of conditions first discovered in the 1960s (Bruneau, Lesperance, Chouinard, 2003). The disease presents with acanthocytosis (spiny red blood cells) and neurological features without any lipid abnormalities (Dobson-Stone et al., 2002; Nicholl et al., 2004). The core conditions included in NA are chorea-acanthocytosis (ChAc), McLeod syndrome (MLS), Huntington disease-like 2 (HDL2), and pantothenate kinase-associated neurodegeneration (PKAN) (Danek & Walker, 2005). Symptoms associated with NA include chorea, neuroanatomical atrophy, muscle atrophy and weakness, and cognitive impairments. NA may be more prevalent among men (Balhara, Varghese, & Kayal, 2006). The average life expectancy for a patient with the disease is 5–10 years (Robinson, Smith, & Reddy, 2004). Treatment can only assess the psychological and physiological symptoms; NA is fatal.

NEUROPATHOLOGY/PATHOPHYSIOLOGY

NA is an autosomal recessive disease (Bruneau et al., 2003). The cause of NA appears to be mutations of the *CHAC* gene on chromosome 9q21 (Chowdhury, Saward, & Erber, 2005). In the disease, the red blood cell membrane (erythrocyte membrane) is dysfunctional, which causes the appearance of coarse and irregularly shaped red blood cells, called acanthocytosis (Raina, Salazar, & Micheli, 2007). NA conditions can be divided into two groups based on the occurrence of acanthocytosis. Whereas acanthocytosis is common in ChAc and MLS, it is less prevalent in HDL2 and PKAN. Acanthocytosis occurs only in 10% of patients with PKAN (Schneider, Walker, & Bhatia, 2007). The cause for the erythrocyte membrane dysfunction is relatively unknown.

Neurological dysfunction has to be present to diagnose NA; movement disorders are characteristics of NA. ChAc, MLS, HDL2, and late-onset PKAN present with chorea, parkinsonism, or dystonia. Dysarthia, dystonia, and rigidity are more common in early onset PKAN (Danek & Walker, 2005; Schneider et al., 2007). Neuroimaging has shown general cerebral atrophy in patients with NA (Nicholls et al., 2004). However, the basal ganglia (caudate, putamen, and globus pallidus) is especially affected by atrophy (Robinson et al., 2004). Hypometabolism has been observed in the striatum, but not in the general cerebral cortex (Schneider et al., 2007). A previous study found a reduced glucose metabolism of 60–70% in patients with NA (Hallett, Levey, & Di Chiro, 1989).

Neurochemical changes are present in NA. Decreased levels of dopamine have been found in greater parts of the brain; decreased levels of serotonin have been reported in the caudate nucleus and substantia nigra, while increased levels of norephedrine have been found in globus pallidus and putamen (Balhara et al., 2006). Clinical features include peripheral neuropathy, muscle weakness, reduced motor speed, general seizures, involuntary facial movements, and the eye condition retinitis pigmentosa (Rowland & Merritt, 2005; Dotti, Supple, Danek, & Lawden, 2004). The involuntary facial movements, orofacial dyskinesia, are a key feature of NA and can lead to difficulty swallowing and self-mutilation of the tongue, inside of cheeks, and lips. Orofacial dyskinesia often occurs with lingual dystonia, painful muscle contractions of the tongue (Dykstra, Adams, & Jog, 2007). The neurogeneaology involved in NA differs for the separate conditions. The *VPS13A* gene that encodes the protein chorein has been implemented in ChAc. ChAc patients have reduced amounts of chorein in their tissue (Danek & Walker, 2005).

The function of chorein is unknown. In MLS, absence of Kx red blood cell antigens and the production of weak Kell antigens due to a mutation on the XK gene create a carrier susceptible to the MLS NA condition (Danek & Walker, 2005; Danek, & Frey, 2007). The *junctophilin 3* gene, involved in the formation of junction membrane structures and located on chromosome 16q24.3, has been associated with HDL2. Forty, or more, CAG/CTG repeat expansions at the *junctophilin 3* gene locus cause HDL2 (Holmes et al., 2001). Mutations of the *PKAN2* gene give rise to PKAN. The *PKAN2* gene is located on chromosome 20p13 (Freeman et al., 2007).

NEUROPSYCHOLOGICAL/CLINICAL PRESENTATION

Due to the nonspecific nature of NA, it is important to consider all neuropsychological symptoms that the patient displays when diagnosing the disease. Neuropsychological symptoms tend to be the first symptoms to appear in patients with NA. Behavioral problems due to executive dysfunction such as impulsivity, compulsivity, progressive apathy, irritability, loss of initiative, and impulsiveness are common. Personality changes are often reported by the person's family. Behavioral observations may include adapted behavior due to peripheral neuropathology (burning sensations, numbness, paralysis, or sensitivity to touch) or due to muscle weakness (stiffness and spasms) (National Institute of Neurological Disorders and Stroke [NINDS], 2008).

Constant biting on the lips or tongue, muscle twitches in the face, and loud grunting indicate orofacial dyskinesia, which is irreversible (Kobayashi, 1976). Psychiatric manifestations include anxiety, depression, loss of insight, apathy, and psychosis (Balhara et al., 2006; Kartsounis & Hardie, 1996). Psychotic behavior may also manifest in the form of paranoid delusions in NA (Kartsounis & Hardie 1996). A decline of general intelligence can be expected in patients with NA and speech production impairments are common symptoms. The pattern of cognitive decline and memory disturbances that are present from the beginning of the disease's onset are consistent with cognitive symptoms in subcortical dementias. However, visuoperceptual and some language abilities generally remain preserved (Kartsounis & Hardie, 1996).

DIAGNOSIS

A blood smear has to be performed on peripheral blood in order to diagnose NA and findings of greater than 3% acanthocytosis indicate presence of the disease. Lipoprotein profiles should present as normal, whereas serum creatine kinase-levels should be increased. Electro/echocardiography, muscle biopsy, neuroimagery, and neuropsychological testing should be included in diagnosing NA (Bruneau et al., 2003). Genetic testing should be done to distinguish MLS, PKAN, and HDL2, but genetic testing can be less helpful in diagnosing ChAc since there are several different types of mutations present in this condition (Danek & Walter, 2005). Another finding that can assist in the process of diagnostic narrowing is to measure the creatine-kinase levels, which are elevated in MLS and ChAc. Liver enzymes are also elevated in MLS and ChAc, although when testing, Wilson's disease has to be excluded. By using specific antibodies, the phenotype of the Kell erythrocyte antigens can be identified providing for a diagnosis of MLS (Danek & Walker, 2005). Iron accumulation in the medial globus pallidus lead to a diagnosis of PKAN. It is through the "eye of the tiger" sign on an MRI that the iron accumulation is found (Danek, 2004).

Behavioral observations may include choreiform movements, tics, mood changes, paralysis, stiffness, seizures, and abnormal gait. Slow speech rate and decreased speech intelligibility could be signs of lingual dystonia; presence of lingual dystonia is indicative of NA. (Dykstra et al., 2007). Self-neglect is common among patients with NA; therefore, the patient may arrive at the appointment appearing inappropriately dressed or groomed. Weight loss may be due to impairment ability to swallow, which is indicative of NA and can differentiate the disease from Huntington's disease (Kartsounis & Hardie, 1996). In contrast from Huntington's disease, there are also few pathological findings in the cerebral cortex and the locus coeruleus. Age of onset is another factor that is important to consider. The different NA conditions have different ages of onset: MLS: 40–60 years; ChAc: 20–30 years; PKAN: childhood; HDL2: 30–40 years (Schneider et al., 2007). It is important to consider the lack of research that has been conducted for investigating psychosis in NA. It is therefore difficult to differentiate between psychosis and tardive dyskinesia in schizophrenia, and psychosis with a primary movement disorder such as in NA.

TREATMENT

Treatment of NA is limited to treating the symptoms. Psychopharmacology, such as selective serotonin reuptake-inhibitors in addition to mood stabilizers, can relieve depression, anxiety, or psychosis (Danek & Walker, 2005). Atypical antipsychotics may impact movement disorders and psychosis (Danek & Walker, 2005; Kobayashi, 1976). PKAN has been treated successfully by surgically attaching tiny electrodes to the globus pallidus (pallidotomy) and/or by delivering muscle relaxants directly into the spinal fluid (intrathecal baclofen) (Danek & Walker, 2005). Baclofen can also diminish symptoms of dystonia in NA (Burton, 2000). It is important to bank autologous blood when considering operations on a patient with MLS because blood transfusion reactions can occur. A change in heart rate or weakness of the cardiac muscle can occur; it is therefore important to monitor the person closely. This can potentially be a concern in ChAc (Walker, Saiki, Irvine, Danek, & Hallett, 2008).

Therapy can educate the patient about the symptoms and teach the patient how to deal with them. It is important that the patient understand the prognosis and potential developments in the disease. Maintaining proper nutrition is important for a patient with NA, but as the difficulty swallowing progresses, a feeding tube may be needed (Robinson et al., 2004). Motor speed impairments may affect the person's speech, or even make them lose the ability to speak. Speech therapy, or in extreme cases, a computer-assisted speech system may be necessary (Danek & Walker, 2005). Furthermore, dementia, motor neuron disease, and parkinsonism can also evolve from NA which may addressed by symptom-targeted intervention. Potential causes of death include emaciation due to progressive weakness, dysphagia, and tracheobronchial aspiration (Robinson et al., 2004). Beyond those steps previously noted, therapy may also serve to educate the patient's family about the disease, allowing them to assume a supportive role.

Lena M. F. Prinzi
Charles Golden

Balhara, Y. P. S., Varghese, S. T., & Kayal, M. (2006). Neurocanthocytosis: Presenting with depression. *Journal of Neuropsychiatry and Clinical Neurosciences, 18,* 426.

Bruneau, M.-A., Lesperance, P., & Chouinard, S. (2003). Schizophrenia-like presentation of neurocanthocytosis. *The Journal of Neuropsychiatry and Clinical Neurosciences, 15,* 378–380.

Burton, L. S. (2000). Evaluation and treatment of dystonia. *Southern Medical Journal, 93,* 746–751.

Chowdhury, F., Saward, R., & Erber, W. (2005). Neurocanthocytosis. *British Journal of Haematology, 131,* 285.

Danek, A. (Ed.). (2004). *Neuroacanthocytosis syndromes.* New York: Springer. Reviewed January 2, 2009.

Danek, A., & Walker, R. (2005). Neurocanthocytosis. *Current Opinion in Neurology, 18,* 386–392.

Dobson-Stone, C., Danek, A., Rampoldi, L., Hardie, R. J., Chalmers, R. M., Wood, N. W., et al. (2002). Mutational spectrum of the CHAC gene in patients with chorea-acanthocytosis. *European Journal of Human genetics, 10,* 773–780.

Dykstra, A. D., Adams, S. G., & Jog, M. (2007). The effect of botulinum toxin type A on speech intelligibility in lingual dystonia. *Journal of Medical Speech-Language Pathology, 15,* 173–186.

Freeman, K., Gregory, A., Turner, A., Blasco, P., Hogarth, P., & Hayflick, S. (2007). Intellectual and adaptive behaviour functioning in pantothenate kinase-associated neurodegeneration. *Journal of Intellectual Disability Research, 51,* 417–426.

Holmes, S. E., O'Hearn, E., Rosenblatt, A., Callahan, C., Hwang, H. S., Ingersoll-Ashworth, R. G., (2001). A repeat expansion in the gene encoding of junctophilin-3 is associated with Huntington's disease-like 2. *Natures Genetics, 29,* 377–378.

Kartsounis, L. D., & Hardie, R. J. (1996). The pattern of cognitive impairment in neurocanthocytosis: A subcortical dementia. *Archives of Neurology, 53,* 77–80.

Kobayashi, R. M. (1976). Orofacial dyskinesia. *The Western Journal of Medicine, 125,* 277–288.

National Institute of Neurological Disorders and Stroke. (2008). *Peripheral neuropathy fact sheet.* National Institute of Health Publication No. 04-4853. Reviewed January 2, 2009, from http://www.ninds.nih.gov/disorders/peripheralneuropathy/detail_peripheralneuropathy.htm

Nicholl, D., Sutton, I., Dotti, M., Supple, S., Danek, A., & Lawden, M. (2004). White matter abnormalities on MRI in neurocanthocytosis. *Journal of Neurology, Neurosurgery, and Psychiatry, 75,* 1200–1207.

Robinson, D., Smith, M., & Reddy, R. (2004). Neurocanthocytosis. *American Journal of Psychiatry, 161,* 1716.

Rowland, L. P., & Merritt, H. H. (2005). *Merritt's neurology: Integrating the physical exam and echocardiography.* Philadelphia: Lippincott Williams & Wilkins.

Schneider, S. A., Walker, R. H., & Bhatia, K. P. (2007). The Huntington's disease-like syndromes: What to consider in patients with a negative Huntington's disease gene test. *Nature Clinical Practice: Neurology, 3,* 517–525.

Walker, R. H., Saiki, S., Irvine, G., Danek, A., & Hallett, M. (2008). *Neuroacanthocytosis Syndromes II.* New York: Springer.

NEURODEGENERATION WITH BRAIN IRON ACCUMULATION

DESCRIPTION

Neurodegeneration with brain iron accumulation (NBIA) or pantothenate kinase associate neurodegeneration, previously termed Hallervorden–Spatz disease, is a rare, progressive, and fatal autosomal recessive disease affecting both adults and children. Although sporadic cases have also been cited within the literature, this is extremely rare. NBIA is characterized by excessive iron accumulation and discoloration of the medial globus pallidus and substantia nigra. Clinical features are noted to include extrapyramidal signs (dystonia, rigidity, parkinsonism, dysarthria), corticospinal tract involvement, pyramidal motor symptoms, optic atrophy, retinal pigmentation, psychiatric manifestations, cognitive deficits, dementia later in the course of the disease, and eventually death.

NBIA was first identified in 1922 by Julius Hallervorden and Hugo Spatz. The pair witnessed pigmentation of the basal ganglia in five siblings with progressive dysarthria and dementia. The preferred name, NBIA, evolved from moral concerns raised regarding Hallervorden's involvement in euthanasia during World War II (Hinkelbein, Kalenka, & Alb, 2006).

One hallmark feature of NBIA is the "eye of the tiger" sign observed on T2-weighted MRI due to bilateral low-signal intensities within the globus pallidus and hyperintensity within the central or anteriomedial areas of the pallidum associated with iron accumulation (Hinkelbein et al., 2006). These high-signal intensities have also been attributed to spongiosis and neuronal vacuolization (Bindu, Desai, Shehanaz, Nethravathy, & Pal, 2006; Hinkelbein et al., 2006).

The incidence of NBIA worldwide is estimated to be between one and three per one million population (Freeman et al., 2007; Hinklebein et al., 2006). NBIA appears to affect both genders equally. Although NBIA has been reported in all races, the frequency is unknown because it is quite rare (Hinkelbein et al., 2006).

NEUROPATHOLOGY/PATHOPHYSIOLOGY

Mutations in the pantothenate-kinase 2 gene (*PANK2*) on chromosome 20p13 have been identified as a pathological basis of the presentation (Bindu et al., 2006; Matarin, Singleton, & Houlden, 2006). Deficiency of pantothenate kinase may lead to accumulation of cysteine, which in the presence of iron leads to a cytotoxic event causing free radical production (Mendez & Cummings, 2003; Hinkelbein et al., 2006). Postmortem findings reveal cerebral atrophy, pigmentation, and iron accumulation in the globus pallidus and substantia nigra (Freeman et al., 2007). This accumulation occurs both extracellularly and intracellularly although it is primarily found in astrocytes, microglia, and neurons (Jankovic, 2007). Iron-containing pigment granules, axonal swelling, neuronal loss, gliosis, and demyelination within affected tissues have also been reported (Hinkelbein et al., 2006; Mendez &

Cummings, 2003). Large spheroid bodies are commonly present in the medial globus pallidus, substantia nigra, cortex, and subthalamic nucleus (Pellecchia et al., 2005).

NEUROPSYCHOLOGICAL/CLINICAL PRESENTATION

Heterogeneity in clinical presentation has been well established, particularly within same-age subtypes. However, literature involving neuropsychological and clinical features of the disease has been limited as NBIA is extremely rare and small sample sizes and case studies predominate within the literature. The disease course is usually 10–15 years with onset typically occurring during the first or second decade, though in rare cases may occur up to the seventh decade (Freeman et al., 2006; Mendez & Cummings, 2003). Although variations between classification systems exist, three variants of NBIA have been identified: (1) early-onset childhood type with onset between 1 and 3 years of age (neuroaxonal dystrophy), (2) classic juvenile type with onset between 7 and 12 years of age, and (3) the more rare adult type (Mendez & Cummings, 2003). Among the early-onset childhood type, one study discovered primary motor developmental delays among all participants ($n = 10$) followed by cognitive decline. The juvenile type displayed more variability in presentation, including more behavioral features (e.g., verbal aggression and depression) in addition to extrapyramidal motor signs but without developmental delay (Bindu et al., 2006).

Neuropsychological assessment findings in NBIA has suggested age of onset appears to correlate with disease severity, degree of intellectual impairment, and adaptive functioning, with earlier onset having a poorer prognosis (Bindu et al., 2006; Freeman et al., 2007). Furthermore, diversity in symptom expression has made it difficult to capture a clear picture of neuropsychological presentation in patients with NBIA (Freeman et al., 2007). Slowed processing speed is common with deficits in visuospatial abilities and memory reported; language may be affected later in the course of the disease (Loring, Sethi, Lee, & Meador, 1990). General intellectual functioning often varies between intact to markedly impaired and is often dependent upon disease progression (Freeman et al., 2007). Within the literature, the presence of dysarthria, neuro-ophthalmologic and motor signs almost universally impact formal neuropsychological assessment procedures making nonstandard administration imperative.

Later in the course of the disease, psychiatric manifestations may develop, though one case study of prodromal behavioral symptoms (e.g., anxiety, depression, irritability, mood lability, and verbal aggression) has been identified. These psychiatric manifestations all occurred before the onset of extrapyramidal and pyramidal motor signs, and behavioral symptoms eventually progressed to paranoid delusions that responded well to antipsychotic medications (Panas et al., 2007).

DIAGNOSIS

Prior to advancements in neuroimaging capabilities, confirmation of NBIA was typically given upon autopsy based on the aforementioned iron accumulation and discoloration within the brain in combination with the noted clinical presentation. Neurodiagnostic imaging with T-2 weighted MRI scans may prove useful in the diagnosis of NBIA, although the hallmark "eye of the tiger" sign may be absent in a very small group of NBIA patients. Most recently, identifying the defect on the arm of chromosome 20 has led to positive diagnosis as have pathological results of an affected sibling.

Based on prominent gait disturbance and extrapyramidal signs, differential diagnosis of NBIA includes dementia with Lewy bodies, Parkinson-plus syndromes, progressive supranuclear palsy, Wilson's disease, normal pressure hydrocephalus, and Huntington's disease. In summary, clinical features including progressive course and neuro-ophthalmologic findings, molecular testing, and MRI findings all remain important in the diagnosis of NBIA, with genetic markers being the most recent advancement in differential diagnosis.

TREATMENT

There is no cure for NBIA and no specific treatments exist. Current pharmacological treatments include muscle relaxants, spasticity agents, and dopaminergic medications to control motor symptoms. Within the literature, stereotactic procedures of pallidotomy, thalamotomy, and bilateral pallidothalamotomy have been reported but only in a very small number of patients, and relief appears to be temporary in nature (Hinkelbein et al., 2006; Mendez & Cummings, 2003). Additional treatments are supportive in focus. Physical, occupational, and speech therapies may be utilized to assist in addressing developing deficits that occur with disease progression and to assist in maintaining independent functionality as long as possible. Individualized educational plans can be essential for children with the disease. As the disease progresses, regular modifications are essential. Therapeutic services may be helpful for both patients and their families to aid them in coping with and adjusting to the disease from an emotional and psychosocial standpoint.

Michelle R. Pagoria
Chad A. Noggle

Bindu, P. S., Desai, S., Shehanaz, K. E., Nethravathy, M., & Pal, P. K. (2006). Clinical heterogeneity of Hallervorden-Spatz syndrome: A clinicoradiological study in 13 patients from South India. *Brain and Development, 28,* 343–347.

Freeman, K., Gregory, A., Turner, A., Blasco, P., Hogarth, P., & Hayflick, S. (2007). Intellectual and adaptive behaviour functioning in pantothenate kinase-associated neurodegeneration. *Journal of Intellectual Disability Research, 51,* 417–426.

Hinkelbein, J., Kalenka, A., & Alb, M. (2006). Anesthesia for patients with pantothenate-kinase-associated neurodegeneration (Hallervorden-Spatz disease) — A literature review. *Acta Neuropsychiatrica, 18,* 168–172.

Jankovic, J. (2007). Movement disorders. In C. G. Goetz (Ed.), *Textbook of clinical neurology* (3rd ed.). Philadelphia: Saunders Elsevier.

Loring, D. W., Sethi, K. D., Lee, G. P., & Meador, K. J. (1990). Neuropsychological performance in Hallervorden-Spatz syndrome: A report of two cases. *Neuropsychology, 4,* 191–199.

Matarin, M. M., Singleton, A. B., & Houlden, H. (2006). *PANK2* gene analysis confirms genetic heterogeneity in neurodegeneration with brain iron accumulation (NBIA) but mutations are rare in other types of adult neurodegenerative disease. *Neuroscience Letters, 407,* 162–165.

Mendez, M. F., & Cummings, J. L. (2003). *Dementia: A clinical approach* (3rd ed.). Philadelphia: Butterworth-Heinemann.

Panas, M., Spengos, K., Koutsis, G., Tsivgoulis, G., Sfagos, K., Kalfakis, N., et al. (2007). Psychosis as presenting symptom in adult-onset Hallervorden-Spatz syndrome. *Acta Neuropsychiatrica, 19,* 122–124.

Pellecchia, M. T., Valente, E. M., Cif, L., Salvi, S., Albanese, A., Scarano, V., et al. (2005). The diverse phenotype and genotype of pantothenate kinase associated neurodegeneration. *Neurology, 64,* 1810–1812.

NEUROFIBROMATOSIS

DESCRIPTION

Neurofibromatosis (NF) is an umbrella term encompassing a group of presentations characterized by neurocutaneous lesions. Individual distinction of the different variants is based on the clinicopathological manifestations of each including various types and distributions of lesions. To date, eight different variants are described; however, only NF-1 and NF-2 are definitely recognized by all as falling in this group, as they demonstrate overlapping genetics at a molecular level. Consequently, only these two forms are discussed at this time.

Both NF-1 and NF-2 are autosomal-dominant syndromes characterized by the formation of neural tumors. NF-1 is far more common with a relative prevalence of 1 in 3,000, whereas NF-2 presents in only 1 out of every 40,000–50,000 (MacCollin, 1995). The disorders correspond to abnormalities in the development of neural crest cells producing hypoplasia, neoplasia, and dysplasia of the neuroectodermal elements and their supporting structures (Berg, 2007).

NF-1 presents with multiple café-au-lait spots, multiple peripheral neurofibromas or plexiform, optic gliomas, axillary freckling, and osseous lesions (Riccardi, 1992). Lisch nodules and dysplasias of the skull and spine as well as the extremities are common in adults (Jackson, 1995).

NF-2 is commonly characterized by neoplasms of the central nervous system (CNS) and hallmarked by schwannomas in the region of the eighth cranial nerve bilaterally. Neurofibromas, meningiomas, gliomas, and cerebral calcifications are also quite common (Lantos et al., 2005).

NEUROPATHOLOGY/PATHOPHYSIOLOGY

NF-1 is associated with a number of tumors of the nervous system. These include plexiform neurofibroma, which is the hallmark of NF-1, multiple neurofibromas of other systemic areas including paraspinal neurofibromas, optic gliomas, paraspinal schwannomas, pilocytic astrocytomas of the third ventricle and cerebellum, and astrocytomas of the brain and spinal cord (Russell & Rubenstein, 1989). Hyperintensities of the globus pallidus are often noted on T1-weighted images; basal ganglia, brainstem, and cerebellum hyperintensities are noted on T2 imaging (Truhan et al., 1993).

The NF-1 gene mutations are localized to the 17q11.2 chromosome, which encodes neurofribromin, an amino acid protein that is expressed in most tissues thus explaining the widespread manifestations of the disorder (von Deimling et al., 1995). In the nervous system, neurofribromin is present in oligodendrocytes, Schwann cells, and smooth endoplasmic reticulum of neuronal populations (Nordlund et al., 1993).

NF-2 is most often associated with vestibular schwannomas and the potential of other CNS neoplasms, schwannomas, and meningiomas being the most common. Beyond this, additional neurological features, as seen in NF-1, are not associated with NF-2 (Truhan et al., 1993). Meningioangiomatosis may present in the cortex, meninges, and/or subcortical white matter. It appears as hyperdense lesions with internal calcifications and edema of the adjacent white matter (Aizpuru et al., 1991). Gliomas and microhamartomas may also manifest with the latter more often arising in the basal ganglia, thalamus, cerebellum, and deeper layers of the cerebral cortex and the prior more commonly developing in the spinal cord.

The NF-2 gene mutations are located on chromosome 22q11.1922q13.1. The gene aids in the production of cytoskeletal associated proteins and acts as a tumor suppressor (Louis et al., 1995).

Macrocephaly presents in 10% to 40% of individuals, the middle fossa may be "ballooned," and there may be seen an enlarged or J-shaped sella and dysplastic changes of the sphenoid (Berg, 2007). These features are noted across both types of NF.

NEUROPSYCHOLOGICAL/CLINICAL PRESENTATION

NF-1 presents with cutaneous pigmentation, multiple tumors within both the central and peripheral nervous systems, and lesions of the vascular and other organ systems (Riccardi & Eichner, 1986). As discussed, café-au-lait spots are associated with presentation, arising at birth and becoming more apparent as individuals age. However, café-au-lait spots are not definitive of the presentation as they may arise in other disorders or in isolation. In actuality, for diagnosis of NF-1 more than six spots must be observed. Fibroma molluscum, which are soft or firm papules developing just under the skin, may also occur, as well as Lisch nodules and optic gliomas. Peripheral neurofibromas can present anywhere.

CNS tumors most commonly involve meningiomas and gliomas. Their locality corresponds with neurological symptoms that manifest. Schwannomas may also develop affecting the cranial nerves with the noted dysfunction corresponding with specific cranial nerve affected.

Individuals with NF-2 often become symptomatic in the second or third decade of life. As previously noted, individuals may present with unilateral or bilateral masses of the eighth cranial nerve as well as neurofibromas, meningiomas, gliomas, schwannomas, or posterior subcapsular lenticular opacity (Berg,

2007). Bilateral acoustic neuromas manifest in nearly all patients (>95%). As a result of the latter, tinnitus and hearing loss are common complaints. Café-au-lait spots present in NF-2 as they do in NF-1.

In both forms of NF, mental retardation and seizures can occur. Specifically, approximately 80% of individuals with NF will present with moderate to severe impairments of neurocognition corresponding with the locality of the intracranial tumors (Hyman et al., 2005). These researchers also reported that roughly 50% of individuals demonstrated deficits in reading, spelling, and mathematics, although only 20% meet diagnostic criteria of a specific learning disability.

DIAGNOSIS

Diagnostic practices in NF are multifaceted. CT and MRI are useful evaluations, with preference given to the latter if not contraindicated. They permit evaluation of neurofibromas' locality and infiltration. Imaging should be focused on the peripheral system and internal organs, including the abdomen and chest.

MRI is essential in the evaluation of intracranial masses. As suggested previously, additional neuroanatomical findings may also be observed, particularly in NF-1, including hyperintensities. However, calcifications associated with NF-2 may also be evaluated through these means. In some of these instances, MRI is necessary as CT with contrast has not demonstrated great enough sensitivity to offer full appreciation of some of these lesions (Berg, 2007). Beyond the brain, imaging of the spine is also important in individuals with NF-1. In individuals with NF-2, gadolinium should be used to best evaluate the cerebellopontine region and for acoustic neuromas. Electroencephalogram may be used to document potential seizure activity. Measurement of neurotransmitter metabolites has also been recommended (Berg, 2007). Neuropsychological assessment should be comprehensive as no pure profile of NF exists.

TREATMENT

Treatment of NF is nonspecific. Rather it is symptom-based and supportive. Neurosurgical intervention is utilized to address intracranial and spinal masses. Radiation may also be used. Although most tumors are not malignant, chemotherapy may still be used. Chemotherapy may be employed in cases of optic gliomas that become overly problematic or concerning. However, chemotherapy and/or surgery are only used to treat optic gliomas when absolutely necessary, as demonstrated by documented progression on serial MRIs (Imes & Hoyt, 1986). In fact, for most tumors that present centrally or in the peripheral system, surgery or other means of intervention are only employed when necessary as determined by charted growth rates or locality of presentation. Peripheral neurofibromas rarely require removal unless rapid growth is demonstrated, repeated trauma has been experienced, or for cosmetic reasons. The latter reason is the primary basis for plexiform neuromas to be removed.

Pain medications may be employed to control irritation due to the region of neurofibromas, although often in these instances surgery may be undertaken. Antiepileptic drugs are used to control seizure activity if it remains following surgical removal of the intracranial mass causing the symptoms.

Neuropsychological assessment is an important aspect of treatment, as it permits documentation of the nature and extent of any neurocognitive or learning deficits. Based on findings, appropriate interventions should be enacted. Special education services may be warranted in cases of learning deficits.

Chad A. Noggle

Aizpuru, R. N., Quencer, R. M., Norenberg, M., et al. (1991). Meningioangiomatosis: clinical, radiological, and histopathologic correlation. *Radiology, 179,* 819–821.

Berg, B (2007). Chromosomal Abnormalities and Neurocutaneous Disorders. In Goetz, C., *Textbook of clinical neurology* (pp. 683–697). Philadelphia: Saunders.

Hyman, S. L., Shores, A., North, K. N. (2005). The nature and frequency of cognitive deficits in children with neurofibromatosis type 1. *Neurology, 65,* 1037–1044.

Imes, R. K., Hoyt, W. F. (1986) Childhood chiasmal gliomas: Update on the fate of patients in the 1969 San Francisco study. *British Journal of Ophthalmology, 70,* 179–182.

Jackson, I. T. (1995) Neurofibromatosis of the skull base. *Clinics in Plastic Surgery, 22,* 513–530.

Lantos, P. L., Vandenberg, S. R., & Kleihues, P. (2005). Tumours of the nervous system. In D.I. Graham & P.L. Lantos (Eds.) *Greenfield's neuropathology* (6th ed., vol. 2, pp. 583–879). London: Arnold.

Louis, D. N., Ramesh, V., & Gusella, J. F. (1995). Neuropathology and molecular genetics of neurofibromatosis 2 and related tumors. *Brain Pathology, 5,* 163–172.

MacCollin, M. (1995). CNS Young Investigator Award Lectures: molecular analysis of the neurofibromatosis 2 tumor suppressor. *Brain & Development, 17,* 231–238.

Nordlund, M., Gu, X., Shipley, M. T., Rater, N. (1993). Neurofibromin is enriched in the endoplasmic reticulum of CNS neurons. *Journal of Neuroscience, 13,* 1588–1600.

Riccardi, V. M. (1992). *Neurofibromatosis: Phenotype, natural history, and pathogenesis,* (pp. 1–450). Baltimore: Johns Hopkins University Press.

Riccardi, V. M., & Eichner, J. E. (1986). *Neurofibromatosis-Phenotype, natural history and pathogenesis*. Baltimore: Johns Hopkins University Press.

Russell, D. S., Rubenstein, L. J. (1989). Pathology of tumours of the nervous system (5th ed). London: Edward Arnold.

Truhan, A. P., Filipek, P. A. (1993). Magnetic resonance imaging: Its role in the neuroradiologic evaluation of neurofibromatosis, tuberous sclerosis, and Sturge-Weber syndrome. *Archives of Dermatology*, 129, 219–226.

von Diemling, A., Krone, W., Menon, A. G. (1995). Neurofibromatosis type 1: pathology, clinical features and molecular genetics. *Brain Pathology*, 5: 153–163.

NEUROLEPTIC MALIGNANT SYNDROME

DESCRIPTION

Neuroleptic malignant syndrome (NMS) is a potentially fatal, adverse reaction to antipsychotic medication, typically characterized by muscle rigidity, hyperthermia (pyrexia), alterations in mental status, and autonomic disturbance (Guzofski & Peralta, 2006; Haddad & Dursun, 2008; Susman, 2001). NMS normally occurs 4–11 days after starting an antipsychotic or increasing its dosage (Guzofski & Peralta, 2006). Though less common, NMS cases involving other drugs, including lithium and antidepressants, have been reported (Kohen, 2004). In two-thirds of cases, onset occurs in the first week; however, there are reports of symptoms starting abruptly long after the offending medication was prescribed without changes in dosage. Upon discontinuation of the offending agent, NMS typically resolves in 7–10 days (Guzofski & Peralta, 2006; Kohen, 2004). There is considerable disparity in the literature regarding incidence rates of NMS. Reported rates have varied from 0.007% to 3.23%, with 0.2% being the most widely accepted estimate (Caroff, 2005; Kohen, 2004). The mortality rate of NMS is also unclear, but it is estimated to be around 10% (Caroff, 2005).

NEUROPATHOLOGY/PATHOPHYSIOLOGY

The pathophysiology of NMS is not yet known; however, the most prevalent theory is that it is related to reduced dopaminergic activity subsequent to neuroleptic blockade of dopamine receptors (Caroff, 2005; Kohen, 2004). Hyperthermia is thought to be related to antagonized dopamine receptors of the anterior hypothalamus, an area associated with thermoregulation (Kohen, 2004; Susman, 2001). Dopaminergic blockade of the nigrostriatal pathway is believed to produce muscle rigidity, a contributor to hyperthermia (Guzofski & Peralta, 2006; Kohen, 2004). Changes in state of consciousness may be related to reduced dopaminergic activity in the reticular activating system (Guzofski & Peralta, 2006). NMS symptoms of mutism, akinesia, and decreased arousal could be subsequent to decreased dopamine input to the anterior cingulate-medial orbitofrontal circuit (Kohen, 2004).

NEUROPSYCHOLOGICAL/CLINICAL PRESENTATION

There are a number of symptoms that tend to appear early in the course of NMS. Unexpected changes in mental status often develop such as delirium and obtundation (Caroff, 2005). Early on, such changes in consciousness may take the form of mild confusion and can be difficult to discriminate from existing psychiatric illness and the sedating affects of antipsychotic medication (Kohen, 2004; Pelonero, Levenson, & Pandurangi, 1998). Other common early symptoms include fever, new onset catatonia, tachycardia, diaphoresis, drooling, incontinence, extrapyramidal symptoms refractory to standard treatment, dysphagia, dysarthria, and elevated creatinine phosphokinase (CPK) levels. In a review of the literature, it was found that in 80% of cases ($n = 79$) of NMS, the initial symptoms were changes in mental status and rigidity. Yet, early symptoms are not always helpful in identification, as the course and presentation of NMS are often idiosyncratic, and in rare cases, it can develop abruptly (Caroff, 2005). The clinical picture is further obscured, as symptoms can fluctuate over hours or days and can temporarily remiss completely (Haddad & Dursun, 2008).

DIAGNOSIS

The diagnostic criteria of NMS have proven to be a topic of debate, due to NMS's heterogeneous clinical presentation and variability in severity. The *Diagnostic Statistic Manual IV-TR* outlines criteria for NMS; however, many researchers have proposed their own (Addonizio, Susman, & Roth, 1986; American Psychiatric Association [APA], 2000; Caroff, 2005; Caroff & Mann, 1993; Levenson, 1985; Nierenberg et al., 1991; Pope, Keck, & McElroy, 1986; Sachdev, Mason, & Hadzi-Pavlovic, 1997). No set of criteria has received consensus; thus, much of the diagnostic responsibility relies on a high index of clinician suspicion (Seitz, 2005).

NMS is considered a diagnosis of exclusion, making differential diagnosis essential in the identification of the disorder (Strawn, Keck, & Caroff, 2007; Susman, 2001). Types of ailments most commonly confused with NMS are benign extrapyramidal symptoms, agitated delirium, and infections (Strawn et al., 2007). One condition that can have an identical presentation to NMS is lethal catatonia. In fact, some researchers consider NMS to be a drug-induced iatrogenic form of lethal catatonia (Kohen, 2004; Strawn et al., 2007). The course of lethal catatonia seems to differ from NMS in that it typically begins with psychotic excitement and progresses to exhaustion, as opposed to NMS, which often starts with muscular rigidity (Kohen, 2004; Pelonero et al., 1998).

Another condition that is extremely difficult to discern from NMS is serotonin syndrome. The core features of serotonin syndrome are changes in mental status, autonomic instability, and neuromuscular hyperactivity (Haddad & Durnsun, 2007). It differs from NMS in that it has a rapid onset of about 24 hr, and myoclonus and restlessness is prominent, compared to akinesia and rigidity found in NMS. Also, gastrointestinal symptoms (i.e., nausea, vomiting, and diarrhea) are common in serotonin syndrome unlike NMS. As its name implies, serotonin syndrome normally is induced by medications that increase serotonergic transmission (Guzofski & Peralta, 2006; Haddad & Durnsun, 2007; Kohen, 2004). Patient medication history, behavioral prodrome, and the chronology of symptom presentation are essentials for distinguishing it from NMS (Guzofski & Peralta, 2006).

Other conditions that can mimic NMS are anticholinergic delirium and heat stroke. Like NMS, pyrexia and confusion are symptoms of anticholinergic delirium. However, an individual with anticholinergic delirium will lack rigidity, and their skin will appear dry, in contrast to the sweating that is often observed in NMS (Haddad & Durnsun, 2007; Kohen, 2004). Heat stroke can also look like NMS in that an individual may present with confusion, hyperthermia, agitation, tachycardia, and tachypnea. It differs from NMS in that the skin of the individual will appear red, hot, and dry and typically muscle flaccidity is present (Haddad & Durnsun, 2007; Kohen, 2004; Strawn et al., 2007). For a comprehensive listing of differential diagnoses for consideration, see Strawn et al. (2007).

TREATMENT

Once NMS is suspected, neuroleptic medications should be immediately discontinued, along with other psychotropic medications such as antidepressants and lithium. Withdrawal of anticholinergics should also be considered. A complete medical and neurologic work-up is necessary and supportive treatments should begin promptly. Pulse, blood pressure, and temperature should be evaluated every 2 hours (Kohen, 2004), and monitoring of pulse-oximetry and electrolyte levels should also be conducted regularly. CPK levels should be quickly established and examined daily for the 1st week and every 2 days after that, until returning to normal (Guzofski & Peralta, 2006; Kohen, 2004; Strawn et al., 2007). Rehydration may be required; laryngeal dystonia, dysphagia, respiratory distress, and delirium can impede oral fluid intake; thus, intravenous administration of fluids may be necessary. Electrolyte abnormalities may also require normalization. If hyperthermia is evident, treatment with a cooling blanket is indicated. Chest wall rigidity can impair respiration and may require intubation and ventilator support (Guzofski & Peralta, 2006; Pelonero et al., 1998).

While pharmacological treatment is recommended for NMS, there are conflicting reports regarding the effectiveness of such interventions. Due to the absence of controlled studies of drug therapy, there are no definitive pharmacological guidelines (Pelonero et al., 1998). Nevertheless, potentially beneficial treatment must not be withheld in cases when severity warrants drug therapy. Benzodiazepines are a first-line treatment for catatonia and are also useful for decreasing agitation, and may treat fever and rigidity as well. A 1–2 mg starting dose is recommended. Consistent with the theorized pathophysiology of NMS, a dopamine agonist of amantadine or bromocriptine is suggested. Amantadine can be initiated at 200–400 mg per day, or bromocriptine at 2.5 mg 2–3 times a day (not to exceed 45 mg per day). Bromocriptine can potentially worsen psychosis and hypotension, and should be used cautiously in patients with risk of aspiration, as it may induce vomiting. In addition, the muscle relaxant dantrolene can be used. To start, dantrolene should be administered intravenously at 1–2.5 mg/kg of body weight. If rapid recession of fever and rigidity are observed, it should be continued at 1 mg/kg every 6 hr and then tapered or switched to its oral version after a few days. Dantrolene may be used with both benzodiazepines and dopamine agonists; however, to prevent risk of cardiovascular collapse it should not be used with calcium channel blockers (Strawn et al., 2007). In cases where NMS symptoms are refractory to supportive and pharmacological therapies after 48 hrs, ECT should be considered. For acute NMS, 6–10 treatments with bilateral electrode placement are standard (Strawn et al., 2007).

N

The nature of NMS dictates that most patients with the syndrome will have a diagnosis of severe mental illness, a diagnosis often exacerbated upon its onset. Withdrawal of antipsychotics mandated by treatment generally causes a worsening of psychotic symptoms. Thus, resumption of psychotropic medication upon NMS conclusion is frequently required (Kohen, 2004). Due to the rarity of NMS, there are few studies that have investigated pharmacological rechallenge. This, along with the idiosyncratic nature of the syndrome, makes it difficult to identify predictors for NMS relapse. Nevertheless, antipsychotics (and other psychotropics) can be safely resumed for most patients, if precautions are taken. Psychoactive medications should not be resumed until at least 2 weeks after the NMS episode has resolved. During that time, the costs and benefits of rechallenge should be evaluated and alternatives treatments considered. Once the necessity of antipsychotic treatment has been established, an antipsychotic with a different pharmacodynamic profile than the offending medication should be used. A low-potency typical or atypical (preferably atypical) antipsychotic is recommended, though it should be started at a low dose and titrated slowly (Guzofski & Peralta, 2006; Kohen, 2004; Pelonero et al., 1998). At this time, the patient must be monitored for signs of re-emerging NMS. Assessment for fever, autonomic instability, changes in mental status, extrapyramidal symptoms, dehydration, and monitor temperature, pulse, and blood pressure are important at this time. CPK measurements and white blood cell counts may also be warranted (Guzofski & Peralta, 2006; Kohen, 2004). If agitation is observed, treat promptly with benzodiazepine, as it is a risk factor of NMS (Guzofski & Peralta, 2006).

For a comprehensive review of the NMS literature, visit the Neuroleptic Malignant Syndrome Information Service at http://www.nmsis.org/ that also provides a toll-free hotline for consultation regarding suspected cases of NMS.

Brian Schmitt
Raymond S. Dean

Addonizio, G., Susman, V. L., & Roth, S. D. (1986). Symptoms of neuroleptic malignant syndrome in 82 consecutive inpatients. *American Journal of Psychiatry, 143,* 1587–1590.

American Psychiatric Association. (2000). *Diagnostic and statistical manual of mental disorders* (4th ed., text revision). Washington, DC: Author.

Caroff, S. N. (2005). *Neuroleptic malignant syndrome: An online presentation* [Flash Program]. Retrieved from http://www.nmsis.org/content.asp?type=education&src=pages/NMS_OnlineProgram.asp&title=NMS+Online+Program+Overview

Caroff, S. N., & Mann, S. C. (1993). Neuroleptic malignant syndrome. *Medical Clinics of North America, 77,* 185–202.

Guzofski, S., & Peralta, R. (2006). Neuroleptic malignant syndrome, with attention to its occurrence with atypical antipsychotic medication: A review. *Jefferson Journal of Psychiatry, 20*(1), 53–61.

Haddad, P. M., & Dursun, S. M. (2008). Neurological complications of psychiatric drugs: Clinical features and management. *Human Psychopharmacology: Clinical and Experimental, 23,* 15–26.

Kohen, D. (2004). Neuroleptic malignant syndrome. In P. Haddad, S. Dursun, & B. Deakin (Eds.), *Adverse syndromes and psychiatric drugs: A clinical guide* (pp. 21–36). USA: Oxford University Press.

Levenson, J. L. (1985). Neuroleptic malignant syndrome. *American Journal of Psychiatry, 142,* 1137–1145.

Nierenberg, D., Disch, M., Manheimer, E., Patterson, J., Ross, J., Sivestri, G., et al. (1991). Facilitating prompt diagnosis and treatment of the neuroleptic malignant syndrome. *Clinical Pharmacology and Therapeutics, 50,* 580–586.

Pelonero, A. L, Levenson, J. L., & Pandurangi, A. K. (1998). Neuroleptic malignant syndrome: A review. *Psychiatric Services, 49,* 1163–1172.

Pope, H. G., Jr., Keck, P. E., & McElroy, S. L., Jr. (1986). Frequency and presentation of neuroleptic malignant syndrome in a large psychiatric hospital. *American Journal of Psychiatry, 143,* 1227–1232.

Sachdev, P., Mason, C., & Hadzi-Pavlovic, D. (1997). Case-control study of neuroleptic malignant syndrome. *American Journal of Psychiatry, 154,* 1156–1158.

Seitz, D. P. (2005). Diagnostic uncertainty in a case of neuroleptic malignant syndrome. *Canadian Journal of Emergency Medicine, 7,* 266–272.

Strawn, J. R., Keck, P. E., Jr., & Caroff, S. N. (2007). Neuroleptic malignant syndrome. *American Journal of Psychiatry, 164,* 870–876.

Susman, V. L. (2001). Clinical management of neuroleptic malignant syndrome. *Psychiatric Quarterly, 72,* 325–336.

NEURONAL CEROID LIPOFUSCINOSES

DESCRIPTION

Neuronal ceroid lipofuscinoses (NCLs) represent a group of autosomal recessive neurodegenerative diseases. Often NCLs and Batten's disease are used interchangeably, which is inaccurate. In reality, Batten's disease represents only one of the NCLs (i.e.,

NCL 3), albeit the classic variant that is the chronic juvenile form. Defects in lysosomal enzymes or transporters cause accumulation of proteins within the lysosome. The incidence of disease is 1:100,000 live births worldwide but increases to 1:12,500 in the United States and Scandinavia (Pierret, Morrison, & Kirk, 2008). NCL diseases can be categorized by the type of genetic mutation or by the clinical course of the disease. There are 10 genetic subtypes of NCLs, designated *CLN1-10*. The five major clinical forms are based on the age of onset: congenital (CNCL), infantile (INCL), late infantile (LINCL), juvenile (JNCL) and adults (Kuf's disease or ANCL). All NCLs share a clinical picture consistent with neurologic degeneration, including blindness, motor disturbances, development regression, seizures, and premature death (Jalanko & Braulke, 2009).

NEUROPATHOLOGY/PATHOPHYSIOLOGY

CLN1 is associated with the clinical picture of INCL. It is caused by a mutation on chromosome 1p32 encoding palmitoyl protein thioesterase-1 (PPT1). Over 45 separate mutations have been described; however, missense mutations are the most common. The exact pathophysiological process is not known. It has been theorized that PPT1 may be involved with endocytosis, vesicular trafficking, synaptic function, lipid metabolism, and apoptotic signaling (Jalanko & Braulke, 2009). The proteins accumulated are two types of sphingolipid activator proteins (saposins) A and D. T2-weighted MRI shows decreased signal intensity from the basal ganglia to the thalami. MRI also shows increased intensity on periventricular white matter (Williams et al., 2006). Screening blood tests can be used for *CLN1* diagnosis, and blood samples may show slight changes in calcium concentration (Williams et al., 2006). Changes in electroencephalogram (EEG) correspond with progressing disease. The first finding is decreased reactivity to eye movements, later sleep spindles are lost, and at 3 years of age EEGs become isoelectric. On electron microscopy (EM) of skeletal muscle fibers there are characteristic granular lipopigments, seen only in *CLN1* and rare cases of adult type NCL. These are referred to as granular osmiophilic deposits or GRODs (Jalanko & Braulke, 2009). GRODs are typically associated with saposin A and D protein accumulations (Haltia, 2006).

CLN2 encodes the serine protease, tripeptidyl peptidase protein 1 (TTP1) (Ramirez, Rothberg, & Pearce, 2006). This cleaves tripeptides from the amino-termini of partially unfolded proteins. The major components of stored material include mitochondrial adenosine triphosphate (ATP) synthase

subunit C and minimal amounts of saposins A and D (Ramirez et al., 2006). Preliminary studies show that *CLN2* mutations cause decreased TPP1 activity and hinder processing of mature size peptidase. This results in protein retention in the endoplasmic reticulum (Steinfeld, Steinke, Isbrandt, Kohlschutter, & Gartner, 2004). On EM of neuronal tissue, intraneuronal GRODs characterized by a pure curvilinear patter of lipopigmentation can be seen. These are pathognomonic for CLN2. MRI demonstrates severe cerebellar atrophy that is typical of *CLN2* (Jalanko & Braulke, 2009).

The CLN3 protein, referred to as battenin, is an intrinsic membrane protein that has been localized to the lysosome. However, its role in the pathophysiology of the disease remains unknown. Diagnosis of this variant is considered if EM tissue samples demonstrate the characteristic fingerprint ultrastructure of lipopigments within lysosomal vacuoles (Haltia et al., 2006).

CLN4 is the adult variant of NCL. The chromosome, gene, and gene product remain unknown. However, the stored protein is believed to be the subunit c of mitochondrial ATP synthase. The ultrastructural appearance of intraneuronal storage bodies demonstrates fingerprint bodies and granules (Haltia, 2006).

CLN5 has been localized to chromosome 13q21-q32. In 94% of cases, a 2bp deletion in exon 4 results in a stop codon at Tyr392. *CLN5* represents a Finnish variant of NCL. The function of the CLN5 protein has not yet been identified. EEGs of subjects demonstrate posterior spikes to low frequency photic stimulation and giant somatosensory-evoked potentials. Decreased signal intensity of the thalami and increased signal intensity of the periventricular white matter and posterior limbs of the internal capsule are seen on T2-weighted MRI. (Williams et al., 2006). EM demonstrates *CLN5* avacuolar fingerprint body lipopigments in rectilinear profiles, curvilinear profiles, and fingerprint bodies (Haltia, 2006).

CLN6 is located on chromosome 15q23. The CLN6 protein encoded by this gene is found in the endoplasmic reticulum (ER) and is involved in ER retention signals. It is still unknown how this affects lysosomal function. Autopsy studies demonstrate neuronal loss in layer V of the cerebral cortex (Jalanko & Braulke, 2009). Like *CLN5*, *CLN6* is also associated with avacuolar fingerprint-containing lipopigments and rectilinear and curvilinear profiles (Williams et al., 2006).

CLN7 is located on chromosome 4q28.1-q28.2. CLN7 protein belongs to the large major facilitator super family of transporter proteins. The specific role of *CLN7* is unknown. *CLN7* is also associated with avacuolar fingerprint-containing lipopigments (Williams et al., 2006).

CLN8 is on chromosome 8p23. CLN8 protein is localized in the ER but may travel between the ER and Golgi intermediate complex. It is hypothesized that it may be involved in biosynthesis, metabolism, transport, and detection of lipids (Jalanko & Braulke, 2009).

The *CLN9* gene remains unknown. However, fibroblasts from *CLN9* patients do show rapid growth, sensitivity to apoptosis, a specific cell adhesion defect, and reduced levels of ceramide, dihydro-ceramide, and sphingomyelin (Haltia, 2006).

CLN10 is localized to chromosome 11p15.5 and encodes for major lysosomal aspartic protease cathepsin D(CTSD). CTSD is involved in selective, rather than bulk proteolysis and cleaves prosaposin into saposins A, B, C, and D. CTSD is thought to be involved in cell proliferation, antigen processing, apoptosis, and regulation of plasma HDL cholesterol.

Overall, MRI shows decreased signal intensity from the thalami to the basal ganglia on T2-weighted images and generalized cerebral atrophy (Williams et al., 2006).

NEUROPSYCHOLOGICAL/CLINICAL PRESENTATION

Though all NCLs share a common presentation of progressive neurological deterioration, each clinical profile is unique and disease specific.

CLN1, Santavuori's disease, most commonly causes INCL. However, there are rare cases in which *CLN1* resulted in other phenotypes. INCL is characterized by early and severe onset. The age at first presentation is usually 6–12 months. At birth, children appear normal and prior to 6 months will meet normal developmental milestones. At 6 months of age, deceleration of head growth and muscular hypotonia are detectable. In progressing to the 2nd year of life, children display ataxia, sleep disturbance, visual difficulties, and irritability. Hyperkinesias are common. By 2–3 years of age, patients are usually blind and have lost all social interest. They display with increasing frequency spasticity, seizures, and myoclonic activity. The average age of death is 13 years old (Williams et al., 2006).

CLN2, Bielschowsky's disease, mutations result in late infantile NCL. At birth and during the first 3 years of life, patients appear healthy. However, after 3 years of age, psychomotor delay is common, as is sudden onset epilepsy. Usually, seizures are of a severe myo-clonic type and can be resistant to drug treatment. Retinal degeneration is also characteristic. With appropriate supportive care, children may live up to 10 years (Williams et al., 2006).

CLN3, Batten's disease, mutations cause JNCL. There is a wide variety of clinical presentations asso-ciated with this specific type of mutation. However, the first signs of illness are vision failure from retinal degeneration, which typically occur around 5–10 years of age (Jalanko & Brakle, 2009). Epileptic sei-zures usually begin at approximately 10 years of age. In addition, mental retardation develops slowly over the course of the illness. JNCL patients may also display aggressive behavior, depression, and sleep disorders. Death usually occurs around 20–30 years old (Jalanko & Braulke, 2009).

CLN4, also known as Kuf's disease, represents the adult form of NCL. Symptom onset usually occurs prior to age 40 and is marked by progressive demen-tia. This endmark is preceded by one of two clinical presentations. In one group of individuals, dementia is preceded by late onset myoclonic epilepsy whereas motor functioning is spared (Berkovic, Carpenter, Andermann, Andermann, & Wolfe, 1988). Another group does not commonly manifest seizures, at least in the initial stages. Rather, their presentation is char-acterized by predominant motor dysfunction most commonly involving cerebellar ataxia or progressive rigidity and parkinsonism (Burneo et al., 2003).

CLN5 is the Finnish variant of LINCL. The first symptoms of disease begin with motor clumsiness, progressive visual failure, myoclonia, and seizures around 4–9 years of age. Death occurs between the second and fourth decades of life (Jalanko & Braulke, 2009).

CLN6, Lake's disease, is another variant of LINCL and is most commonly found in people of Eastern European, Pakistani, or Portuguese heritage. In 65% of patients, seizures begin before reaching 5 years old. The age of onset is between 18 months and 8 years. Deterioration is rapid after diagnosis, and most chil-dren die between 5 and 12 years old.

CLN7 is the Turkish variant of LINCL. The age of onset ranges from 2 to 7 years old. The most common presenting symptom is severe epilepsy.

CLN8 is another variant of LINCL and has been reported in Finnish, Turkish, Italian, and Israeli patients. Epileptic symptoms begin at ages 5–10. All patients have generalized tonic-clonic seizures. Progressive mental deterioration and motor problems, as well as more frequent seizure episodes occur during puberty. Patients may survive to between 50 and 60 years of age.

Historically, only four patients in total have been diagnosed with *CLN9*. Symptoms reported are iden-tical to *CLN3* patients (Jalanko & Braulke, 2009).

Only 10 cases of *CLN10*, also called congenital NCL, have been described. These result in infants that present with congenital microcephaly, respiratory distress, and status epilepticus. Death occurs within the first few weeks of life (Williams et al., 2006).

DIAGNOSIS

There is a screening test for *CLN1* and *CLN2* in which TPP1 or PPT1 levels can be measured using a fluorescent substrate enzymatic assay. Samples can be taken as fresh blood, dried blood spots, saliva, or cultured fibroblasts from a skin biopsy. The level of activity of PPT1 or TPP1 is measured. *CLN3* can be suspected in the cases of clinical NCL disease and unremarkable PPT1 and TPP1 assays. Presence of vacuolated lymphocytes in the peripheral smear suggests a *CLN3* diagnosis as well. Final confirmation of this diagnosis can be performed using *CLN3* genetic mutation analysis (Williams et al., 2006).

More extensive genetic screening may be merited if the patient has a clinical picture of an NCL disorder, with normal levels of TTP1 or PPT1 and without vacuolated lymphocytes in the peripheral smear. In this case, *CLN5-CLN10*, mutation analysis can be performed. The patient's ethnicity and clinical picture can provide a basis for which *CLN5-CLN10* testing is necessary. However, not all genetic mutations have been identified, and, as a result, genetic analysis does not detect all NCL disorders (Williams et al., 2006).

Prenatal diagnosis is available and performed using a combination of mutation analysis and enzymatic assays. If necessary, this diagnosis can be confirmed using chorionic biopsies (Williams et al., 2006).

TREATMENT

There are no treatment options available for reversing, slowing, or preventing the neurodegeneration that occurs in NCL disorders. Supportive measures are the mainstay of treatment. This includes effective treatment with anticonvulsants, if necessary. Valproate has been successful in this. It has been suggested that treatment with antioxidants and vitamin D may delay loss of motor function and help to reduce seizure frequency and severity as well. Behavior modification techniques may be useful as well (Maertens & Dyken, 2007).

There are a number of treatment methods being researched at present. One option being considered is enzyme replacement therapy (ERT), which has shown encouraging results in other lysosomal storage disease. However, these exogenous enzymes do not pass through the blood–brain barrier, making ERT less successful in resolving the central nervous system (CNS) pathology of lysosomal storage diseases. Gene therapy is another treatment option being explored. Virus-associated delivery of human PPT1 has shown promising results in mouse models. Clinical trials of human neuronal stem cell injection into children with *CLN3* began in 2006. In terms of pharmacologic treatment, cysteamine and *N*-acetylcystiene combination therapies are in phase II trials (Pierret et al., 2008).

Rebecca Durkin
Chad A. Noggle

Berkovic, S. F., Carpenter, S., Andermann, F., Andermann, E., & Wolfe, L. S. (1988). Kufs' disease: A critical reappraisal. *Brain, 111*, 27–62.

Burneo, J. G., Arnold, T., Palmer, C. A., Kuzniecky, R. I., Oh, S. J., & Faught, E. (2003). Adult-onset neuronal ceroid lipofuscinosis with autosomal dominant inheritance in Alabama. *Epilepsia, 44*, 841–846.

Haltia, M. (2006). The neuronal ceroid-lipofuscinoses: From past to present. *Molecular Basis of Disease, 1762*(10), 850–856.

Jalanko, A., & Braulke, T. (2009). Neuronal ceroid-lipofuscinoses. *Biochimica et Biophysica Acta, 1793*, 697–709.

Martens, P., & Dyken, R. (2007) Lipoidoses. In C. Goetz (Ed.), *Textbook of Clinical Neurology* (pp. 616–625). Philadelphia, PA: Saunders.

Pierret, C., Morrison, J. A., & Kirk, M. D. (2008). Treatment of lysosomal storage disorders: Focus on the neuronal ceroid-lipofuscinoses. *Acta Neurobiologiae Experimentalis, 68*, 429–442.

Ramirez, M., Rothberg, P. G., & Pearce, D. A. (2006). Another disorder finds its gene. *Brain, 129*, 1351–1356.

Steinfeld, R., Steinke, H. B., Isbrandt, D., Kohlschutter, A., & Gartner, J. (2004). Mutations in classical late infantile neuronal ceroid lipofuscinosis disrupt transport of tripeptidyl-peptidase I to lysosomes. *Human Molecular Genetics, 13*, 2483–2491.

Williams, R. E., Aberg, L., Autti, T., Goebel, H. H., Kohlschutter, A., & Lonnqvist, T. (2006). Diagnosis of neuronal ceroid lipofuscinoses: An update. *Biochimica et Biophysica Acta, 1762*, 865–872.

NEUROPATHY

DESCRIPTION

Neuropathy is a neurodegenerative disorder characterized by damage to one or more peripheral nerves.

The peripheral nervous system (PNS) transmits information from the CNS to limbs and organs. Central neuropathy refers to damage sustained by the brain or the spinal cord, both of which are encompassed by the CNS. Though neuropathies may originate in the CNS, the majority originate in the PNS (Uzun, Uluduz, Mikla, & Aydin, 2006). Damage to peripheral nerves causes distortion of information transmitted to and from the body and extremities (i.e., anything beyond the brain and spinal cord), resulting in symptoms ranging from temporary numbness to paralysis and organ or gland dysfunction.

There are several types of neuropathies, each distinguishable by the extent and location of the nerve damage (Andreoli, 2007). When disturbance in function occurs in one nerve, the neuropathy is classified as a mononeuropathy simplex. Mononeuropathy multiplex indicates involvement of several nonadjacent peripheral nerves. Polyneuropathies are more common, concurrently affecting the function of numerous peripheral nerves. The subclassifications of polyneuropathies include axonal neuropathies, principally affecting the axons, demyelinating neuropathies, involving the myelin sheath surrounding the axons, and neuronopathies, involving neurons of the PNS.

NEUROPATHOLOGY/PATHOPHYSIOLOGY

Neuropathy may be acquired or inherited. Idiopathic inflammatory neuropathies are a classification of acquired neuropathies. They are caused by inflammation from activities of the immune system and include acute idiopathic polyneuropathy (Guillain–Barré syndrome) and chronic inflammatory demelinating polyneuropathy (see the entries on Guillain-Barré syndrome and Chronic Inflammatory Demyelinating Polyneuropathy for further review).

Metabolic and nutritional neuropathies can be caused by diabetes, uremia, liver disease, vitamin B12 deficiency, and other endocrinopathies including hypothyroidism and acromegaly. Vitamin B12 is an essential element of healthy nerve function, with a deficiency leading to widespread nerve tissue damage. Peripheral neuropathy is the most common complication of diabetes. Mild neuropathies accompanied by sensory abnormalities are found in up to 70% of diabetic patients, whereas symptomatic neuropathies affect an additional 5–10% (Andreoli, 2007). The clinical form of neuropathy most diabetic patients present with is symmetric polyneuropathy associated with rapid physiologic dysfunction and hyperglycemia.

Infective and granulomatous neuropathies have a variety of causes including AIDS, diphtheria, leprosy, sarcoidosis, sepsis, and multiorgan failure. Though diphtheria and leprosy are rare, Lyme disease is more common and can cause a rapidly developing polyneuropathy.

Mixed connective tissue disease, polyarteritis nodosa, rheumatoid arthritis, and systemic lupus erythematosus are known causes of vasculitic neuropathies. Certain connective tissue disorders, including polyarteritis nodosa and rheumatoid arthritis, may cause mononeuropathy multiplex or even polyneuropathy.

Neoplastic and paraproteinemic neuropathies are caused by compression and infiltration resulting from a tumor, paraneoplastic syndromes, paraproteinemias, and amyloidosis. Neurofibromatoses, genetic diseases involving tumors growing directly on nerve tissue, are often associated with polyneuropathies.

Drug-induced and toxic neuropathies are caused by alcohol, organic compounds such as hexacarbons, and organophosphates, heavy metals such as arsenic, gold, lead, platinum, thallium, and tryptophan. Thiamine deficiency is a common problem associated with alcoholism and can cause neuropathy of the extremities. Excessive alcohol consumption alone may directly cause damage to the peripheral nerves. Peripheral nerve damage is also a side effect of long-term use of anticancer drugs, anticonvulsants, and antibiotics.

Finally, hereditary neuropathies of an idiopathic nature may be caused by Friedreich ataxia and familial amyloidosis, whereas hereditary neuropathies of a metabolic nature may be caused by porphyria, metachromatic leukodystrophy, Krabbe's disease, abetalipoproteinemia, Tangier's disease, Refsum's disease, and Fabry's disease. Hereditary neuropathies result from genetic code errors or new genetic mutations and may begin in infancy in severe cases or in early adulthood for milder forms (Dyck & Thomas, 2005).

NEUROPSYCHOLOGICAL/CLINICAL PRESENTATION

Proper operation of the axon and its myelin sheath is vital for the normal functioning of myelinated nerve fibers. When the axon begins to degenerate as a result of a variety of metabolic, toxic, and heritable causes, the myelin also begins to break down. Axonal degeneration of long nerve fibers is usually the underlying cause of polyneuropathies. When demyelination occurs in peripheral nerves as a result of demyelinating neuropathies, functional deficits identical to those resulting from axonal degeneration are produced. Demyelinating neuropathies are largely caused by inherited disorders of myelin, autoimmune attacks on myelin, and mechanical, toxic, and physical injuries to the nerve (Dyck & Thomas, 2005).

Clinical presentation of the neuropathies depends upon the associated pathophysiologic mechanisms and the anatomical location of the nerve damage. Peripheral nerves have highly specialized functions, leading to a wide array of symptoms when the nerves are damaged. The most common symptom of damage to peripheral motor nerves is muscle weakness, whereas other symptoms may include cramps, muscle loss, bone degeneration, and fasciculations (Andreoli, 2007). Sensory nerve damage generally results in impaired and abnormal sensations and numbness. When involvement of peripheral nerve fibers of a certain size is selective, dissociated sensory loss may occur. In such cases, certain sensory modalities are impaired while others are preserved. Additional sensory and reflex changes associated with the motor neuron deficits suggest peripheral nerve damage.

When small fibers within nerves are affected by the neuropathy, pain is a prominent symptom. Pain is an established symptom of neuropathies related to alcohol use, and diabetes may also be a feature of entrapment neuropathies. Patients with diabetic polyneuropathies generally present with autonomic dysfunction, spontaneous sensations of neuropathic pain including dysesthesias, and reduced pain sensibility. Diabetic neuropathy occurs most often in patients with insulin-requiring long-standing diabetes, and a diagnosis can be confirmed with electrodiagnostic studies. In a study conducted by Turcot, Allet, and Golay (2009), participants with diabetic neuropathy also presented with greater postural instability than control participants. L-periaxin is a protein involved in the stabilization of mature myelin in peripheral nerves. Lawlor, Richards, and De Vries (2002) report the presence of anti-L-periaxin antibodies in patients with diabetes-associated peripheral neuropathy, resulting in morphologic abnormalities of the sensory nerves.

When the neural pathways that mediate reflexes are interrupted, tendon reflexes may be impaired or lost. Patients with polyneuropathies generally experience loss of ankle reflexes first, followed by additional tendon reflex loss.

Symptoms associated with Guillain–Barré syndrome and diabetic neuropathies or those caused by amyloidosis include coldness of extremities, bladder and bowel function disturbances, impotence, and postural hypotension. Along with being an additional symptom of amyloidosis, enlarged peripheral nerves may be an indication of hereditary motor and sensory neuropathies and neuropathies associated with leprosy, Refsum's disease, and acromegaly. Again,

the interested reader is recommended to review these entries within this text.

DIAGNOSIS

Due to high symptom variability, diagnosis of neuropathy can be challenging. Symptoms of a sensory nature are often the first clue of peripheral nerve involvement. Acute development of symptoms usually relates to an inflammatory polyneuropathy, whereas gradual evolution of symptoms is an indication of hereditary or metabolic polyneuropathies. Mononeuropathies with acute symptom presentation generally result from traumatic causes. Symptoms caused by minor traumatic injuries and entrapment of nerves are more likely indications of mononeuropathies of gradual onset. Along with drug and alcohol history, occupational history should also be considered during patient evaluation as certain industrial substances may lead to peripheral neuropathy.

When a diagnosis of neuropathy is suspected, EMG may be used to determine location of denervation. Nerve conduction velocity tests are used to determine whether nerve damage is the result of myelin sheath or axon degeneration. Demyelinating and axonal neuropathies may be differentiated using electrodiagnostic or histopathologic studies. Nerve biopsies may also be conducted to determine the degree of nerve damage. When a diagnosis of peripheral neuropathy is confirmed electrodiagnostically, additional laboratory studies including blood glucose levels, serum vitamin B12, and liver and thyroid function blood tests should be conducted. MRI can detect nerve damage caused by compression and can provide data on muscle size and quality. Abnormal antibodies associated with neuropathies can be identified during examination of CSF, and simple tests to evaluation ability to register sensations may reveal the size of sensory nerve fibers affected.

TREATMENT

Though treatments of inherited forms of neuropathy are limited, depending on classification, acquired neuropathies may be treated in several ways. Generally, the underlying cause of the neuropathy is treated first to limit progression of the symptoms or even reverse the neuropathy itself before symptomatic treatment is initiated.

Adopting a healthy lifestyle, avoiding exposure to toxins, limiting alcohol consumption, correcting vitamin deficiencies, and eating a balanced diet are all helpful strategies to reduce the physical symptoms of many neuropathies. Regular exercise may help in reducing cramps associated with certain neuropathies and improve muscle strength, a vital component of avoiding muscle wasting associated with limb paralysis.

Plasmapheresis shortens recovery time associated with Guillain–Barré syndrome, whereas intravenous immunoglobulin in high doses is an equally effective treatment. Careful monitoring of respiratory function in patients with Guillain–Barré syndrome, diphtheritic neuropathy, and other idiopathic inflammatory neuropathies is essential to effective treatment.

Correction of blood glucose levels is important for preventing and reducing neuropathic symptoms associated with diabetic neuropathy. Anticonvulsants and tricyclic antidepressants have also been found to reduce the painful symptoms of diabetic neuropathy.

J. T. Hutton
Rachel Rock
O. J. Vidal
Antonio E. Puente

Andreoli, T. E. (2007). *Cecil essentials of medicine* (7th ed.). Philadelphia: Saunders Elsevier.

Dyck, P. J., & Thomas, P. K. (2005). *Peripheral neuropathy* (4th ed.). Philadelphia: Saunders Elsevier.

Lawlor, M. W., Richards, M. P., & De Vries, G. H. (2002). Antibodies to L-periaxin in sera of patients with peripheral neuropathy produce experimental sensory nerve conduction deficits. *Journal of Neurochemistry, 83*, 592–600.

Turcot, K., Allet, L., & Golay, A. (2009). Investigation of standing balance in diabetic patients with and without peripheral neuropathy using accelerometers. *Clinical Biomechanics, 24*(9), 716–721.

Uzun, N., Uluduz, D., Mikla, S., & Aydin, A. (2006). Evaluation of asymptomatic central neuropathy in type I diabetes mellitus. *Electromyography and Clinical Neurophysiology, 46*(3), 131–137.

Neurosarcoidosis

DESCRIPTION

Sarcoidosis is a multisystem immune system disorder of unknown etiology characterized by granulomas typically presenting in the lymphatic system and lungs. In rare cases, the central nervous system (CNS) is involved and this is referred to as neurosarcoidosis. Signs of neurologic involvement are usually seen in patients known to have active disease in other systems of the body, occurring in 5% of these patients.

Isolated neurosarcoidosis, without systemic disease, is particularly rare, occurring in only 1% or less of all cases (Burns, 2003; Joseph & Scolding, 2007). The exact cause of sarcoidosis is not known. The disease is associated with an abnormal immune response, but what triggers this response is uncertain. The mechanism of spreading from one system of the body to another is also unclear. Review articles highlight the protean effects of sarcoidosis on the CNS including potential involvement of the meninges, brain parenchyma, cranial nerves, and peripheral nerves (Burns, 2003; Joseph & Scolding, 2007; Nowak & Wideka, 2001). Because of its typical location near the base of the brain, symptoms are variable but can include seizures, endocrine abnormalities, gait and balance disturbance, vision deficits, amnestic syndromes, cranial nerve abnormalities, and neuropathies.

The prevalence of sarcoidosis varies widely according to various demographic groups, but the general incidence rate is 20 per 100,000 persons. Less than 10% of the cases with systemic sarcoid will have neurological involvement, typically occurring later in the disease course, resulting in an incidence rate of less than 2 per 100,000. This prevalence drops significantly for cases of isolated neurosarcoidosis with no other systemic disease occurring in less than 1% of all cases with an incidence rate of less than 0.2 per 100,000 (Nowak & Widenka, 2001). The disease is more common in young adults (20–40 years of age) with predominance in African Americans and slightly greater frequency in women (Joseph & Scolding, 2007; Nowak & Widenka, 2001). Neurosarcoidosis is uncommon in children, particularly those under the age of 9.

NEUROPATHOLOGY/PATHOPHYSIOLOGY

Histologically, neurosarcoidosis is characterized by the formation of granulomas in the CNS. The lesion consists of lymphocytes and mononuclear phagocytes surrounding a noncaseating epithelioid cell granuloma. These granulomas represent an autoimmune response to CNS tissues (Joseph & Scolding, 2007). As described earlier, the presentation of neurosarcoidosis is quite variable with several areas showing vulnerability.

Colover (1948), in his clinical case review, found that the optic nerves and retina; the facial, glossopharyngeal, and vagus nerves; the pars intermedia of the pituitary gland and pituitary stalk; and the peripheral nerves are particularly likely to be affected by neurosarcoisosis. This review also found that the CNS may develop meningoencephalitis or meningomyelitis, may exhibit localized infiltration by sarcoid tissue, or may be affected by tumor-like masses in the dura mater. As outlined in more recent review papers, later studies also confirmed these findings (Burns, 2003; Joseph & Scolding, 2007; Nowak & Widenka, 2001). These reviews highlight the frequent involvement of the cranial nerves, particularly the optic nerve. Additionally, manifestations of tubular-like sarcoid granulomas and intracranial masses in a variety of neurologic areas including intraparenchymal, extra-axial, and diffuse leptomeningeal lesions are also described. The involvement of spinal cord, peripheral nerves and roots, and muscle are less frequent.

NEUROPSYCHOLOGICAL/CLINICAL PRESENTATION

Like most space-occupying focal lesions, the clinical symptoms of neurosarcoidosis are dependent on the location of the lesion. Signs and symptoms may mimic those seen in meningitis, brain neoplasm, subarachnoid hemorrhage, cerebrovascular ischemia, cranial nerve palsy, hydrocephalus, or other focal neurologic conditions. According to the review of Nowak and Widenka (2001), the most common general clinical signs and symptoms of neurosarcoidosis include cranial nerve palsies (50%), headache (30%), seizures (10%), pituitary dysfunction (10%), sensory and motor deficits (10%), neuropsychological deficits (10%), cerebellar symptoms (10%), hydrocephalus (5%), and signs and symptoms of meningitis (5%). As outlined by Joseph and Scolding (2007), specific clinical symptoms are associated with the location of the lesion. Some of the more common specific symptoms include reduced facial motor and sensory functioning due to facial nerve involvement, and reduced visual perception due to optic nerve involvement. Besides, other vision problems are also caused due to obstruction of the normal cerebrospinal fluid (CSF) flow by granulomas. Granulomas in the pituitary gland result in endocrine disturbance including amenorrhoea, diabetes insipidus, hypothyroidism, or hypocortisolism. Meningeal presentations result in headache, nuchal rigidity, and other symptoms of meningitis. If the granulomas are large and tumor-like, a mass effect may occur causing headache, increased risk of seizures, and obstruction of the flow of CSF, which results in increased risk of raised intracranial pressure and hydrocephalus. Focal parenchymal lesions result in abnormalities in the function associated with their presenting location. The involvement of the spinal cord is rare, but when present leads to abnormal sensation or weakness in one or more limbs or cauda equina syndrome.

Neuropsychological deficits are variable and consistent with the site of the lesion. As a result, there is no defined neuropsychological profile for neurosarcoidosis. However, general attention and concentration deficits are common in acute presentations as expected in any acute inflammatory process. Psychiatric problems occur in approximately 20% of the cases. These include various psychiatric signs and symptoms including depression and, in rare cases, acute psychosis in cases with temporal lobe infiltration (Joseph & Scolding, 2007).

DIAGNOSIS

Because of its nonspecific clinical presentation and neuroradiological imaging characteristics, intracranial neurosarcoidosis remains a very difficult diagnosis, particularly in the absence of extracranial signs of the disease (Nowak & Widenka, 2001). Due to the wide spectrum of neuroradiological findings, intracranial sarcoid granulomas can be mistaken for primary brain tumors such as glioma, meningioma, and other masses, as well as an infectious state of the CNS (Nowak & Widenka, 2001). MRI with administration of Gd-Gd-DTPA has been shown to be sensitive in detecting intracranial abnormalities due to neurosarcoidosis, particularly when pathological enhancement of the brain parenchyma and leptomeninges and evidence of periventricular and white matter disease are noted (Zajicek et al., 1999). MRI helps narrow the diagnostic possibilities, but is not conclusive in identifying neurosarcoidosis. Research regarding the usefulness of CSF and other laboratory analysis in the differential diagnosis of neurosarcoidosis has not been promising (Nowak & Widenka, 2001).

A definitive diagnosis for neurosarcoidosis can only be made by biopsy (Burns, 2003; Joseph & Scolding, 2007; Nowak & Wideka, 2001). This would demonstrate granulomas rich in epithelioid cells and surrounded by other immune system cells. According to a classification system developed by Zajicek and colleagues (1999), definite neurosarcoidosis is diagnosed by plausible symptoms, a positive biopsy, and no other possible causes for the symptoms. Probable neurosarcoidosis is diagnosed if the symptoms are suggestive, there is evidence of CNS inflammation, and other diagnoses have been excluded. A diagnosis of systemic sarcoidosis is not essential. Possible neurosarcoidosis may be diagnosed if there are symptoms not due to other conditions, but other criteria are not fulfilled.

TREATMENT

There have been no controlled prospective studies to identify useful therapeutic options for neurosarcoidosis

(Nowak & Widenka, 2001). Corticosteroids are the treatment of choice as they usually suppress inflammation and may relieve acute symptoms. CNS mass lesions may be especially responsive to corticosteroid therapy (Nowak & Widenka, 2001; Zajicek et al., 1999). Whether corticosteroids change the natural course of neurosarcoidosis is unclear. When corticosteroids provide limited benefit, immunosuppressive agents are the next option, although limited research is available regarding the efficacy of these interventions (Nowak & Widenka, 2001). In addition to these treatments, symptom-specific therapies are commonly used to minimize the impact of the disease. In patients unresponsive to medical treatment, radiotherapy may be required. Additionally, if the granulomatous tissue causes obstruction or mass effect, neurosurgical intervention is sometimes necessary to minimize the effects of hydrocephalus and increased intracranial pressure (Joseph & Scolding, 2007).

Mark T. Barisa

Burns, T. M. (2003). Neurosarcoidosis. *Archives of Neurology, 60,* 1166–1168.

Colover, J. (1948). Sarcoidosis with involvement of the nervous system. *Brain, 71,* 451–475.

Joseph, F. G., & Scolding, N. J. (2007). Sarcoidosis of the nervous system. *Practical Neurology, 7,* 234–244.

Nowak, D. A., & Widenka, D. C. (2001). Neurosarcoidosis: A review of its intracranial manifestation. *Journal of Neurology, 248,* 363–372.

Zajicek, J. P., Scolding, N. J., Foster, O., Rovaris, M., Evanson, J., Moseley, I. F., et al. (1999). Central nervous system sarcoidosis — Diagnosis and management. *Quarterly Journal of Medicine, 92,* 103–117.

NEUROSYPHILIS

DESCRIPTION

Neurosyphilis refers to the syphilitic infection of the CNS caused by *Treponema pallidum* (Conde-Sendin, Hernandez-Fleta, Cardenes-Santana, & Amela-Peris, 2002). It is a medically important and frequently encountered sexually transmitted disease (Vieira Santos, Matias, Saraiva, & Goulano, 2005). Much of what we know about neurosyphilis is based on case reports, small series reports, and retrospective reviews (Marra, 2009). Timely intervention is important to help prevent the progression of the disease (Lee,

Lin, Lu, & Liu, 2009). If left untreated, 4–9% of patients go on to develop symptomatic neurosyphilis (Verma & Solbrig, 2006). Neurosyphilis can occur in the secondary stage of the disease process, sometimes called "early neurosyphilis" (O'Donnell & Emery, 2005). Early neurosyphilis can impact the CSF, meninges, and cerebral vasculature (Marra, 2009; O'Donnell & Emery, 2005). Approximately one-third of patients develop tertiary stage or "late neurosyphilis." Late neurosyphilis is a slowly progressive inflammatory disease, which can impact the brain or spinal cord parenchyma (Marra, 2009; O'Donnell & Emery, 2005).

NEUROPATHOLOGY/PATHOPHYSIOLOGY

Identifying the radiological appearance of neurosyphilis is important so that clinical testing and treatment may be initiated (Santos et al., 2005). Russouw, Roberts, Emsley, and Truter (1997) performed MRI on 20 newly diagnosed patients with neurosyphilis, 13 of whom showed radiological abnormalities including generalized atrophy and foci of increased signal intensity on T2-weighted images. They found that frontal lesions were significantly associated with the degree of psychiatric morbidity, suggesting that the location for the burden of lesions may help to determine psychiatric symptoms that frequently accompany the disease process (Russouw et al., 1997). Santos and colleagues (2005) emphasized that imaging findings in neurosyphilis can be similar to those in other conditions that impact the limbic system, such as herpes encephalitis. Pavlović and Milović (1999) found that CT and MRI findings evidenced cortical and subcortical atrophy in the brain parenchyma in four (57%) patients, and multi-ischemic changes in two (29%) patients (seven patients were studied retrospectively). At least 16 patients with medial temporal lobe involvement on neuroimaging findings have been documented in the literature (Lee, Wilck, & Venna, 2005). EEG findings can show generalized periodic epileptiform discharges similar to what is seen in Creutzfeldt–Jacob disease (Anghinah, Camargo, Braga, Waksman, & Nitrini, 2006).

NEUROPSYCHOLOGICAL/CLINICAL PRESENTATION

Neurosyphilis can have a wide array of clinical symptoms, which often mimics better-known neurological conditions (Conde-Sendin, Hernandez-Flet, Cardenes-Santan, & Amela-Peris, 2002). To start, individuals can be asymptomatic or symptomatic. In regard to the former, it is marked by abnormal CSF evaluation with mild lymphocytic or mononuclear pleocytosis, and elevated protein concentration, and a reactive CSF-venereal disease research laboratory (CSF-VDRL) test (CDC, 2007). When individuals are acutely symptomatic, the most common features are that of headache, nausea, stiff neck, and occasional papilledema. Cranial nerves II, III, VI, and VII are most affected, as observed in studies conducted during the pre-antibiotic area (Merritt, Adams, & Solomon, 1946).

Beyond the acute phases, neurosyphilis often resembles psychiatric disorders (Russouw et al., 1997). Personality changes, irritability, depression, and psychosis can occur (O'Donnell & Emery, 2005). The course of the disease can be long and result in a progressive impairment in mental abilities. Very specific deficits can occur due to focal lesions related to the disease (Lezak, 2004); memory loss and concentration difficulties are not uncommon (O'Donnell & Emery, 2005). General paresis is the encephalitic form of neurosyphilis and can result in progressive dementia 15–20 years after the initial infection (range, 5–50 years) (Verma & Solbring, 2004). The clinical manifestation may include dysarthria, delusions, apathy, intention tremor, seizures, myclonus, hyperreflexia, and Argyll Robertson pupils (Verma & Solbring, 2004). Dementia can be a manifestation of late syphilis with associated cognitive and behavioral symptoms (Vargas, Carod-Arfal, Del Negro, & Rodriguez, 2000). Neurosyphilis can also be the cause of epileptic seizures (Anghinah et al., 2006). The clinical findings consistent with neurosyphilis are not clearly defined by the Centers for Disease Control and Prevention (CDC) (Marra, 2009) but in a survey of 49 cases, clinical findings included auditory disease, acute meningitis, stroke, ocular disease, headache, altered mental status, and cranial nerve dysfunction (Wharton, Chorba, Vogt, Morse, & Buehler, 1990). Pavlovic and Milovic (1999) found gait disturbance in five (71%) of seven patients.

DIAGNOSIS

Neurosyphilis can be difficult to diagnose, and it is often further complicated by the co-occurrence of HIV infection (O'Donnell & Emery, 1995). The CDC outlines criteria for "confirmed" and "presumptive" neurosyphilis (Wharton et.al., 1990). Confirmed neurosyphilis is (1) any syphilis stage and (2) a reactive CSF-VDRL. Presumptive neurosyphilis is (1) any syphilis stage, (2) a nonreactive CSF-VDRL, (3) elevated CSF protein or white blood cell count without any other known causes for these abnormalities, and (4) clinical signs or symptoms consistent with neurosyphilis without other known causes for

these abnormalities. Although serologic tests are important in diagnosing syphilis, they can be difficult to interpret. For example, Lyme neuroborreliosis or *Borrelia burgdorferi* is a well-established confound on serologic tests (Scheid, 2006).

TREATMENT

Penicillin is the drug of choice for the treatment of syphilis during all stages, but ceftriaxone is considered a reasonable alternative for those who are allergic to penicillin (Marra, 2009). Efficacious treatment is considered as normalized CSF (which may take longer when HIV is present) and resolution of clinical abnormalities, although these abnormalities may persist, especially if there is tissue damage (Marra, 2009).

Amy R. Steiner
Chad A. Noggle
Amanda R. W. Steiner

Centers for Disease Control and Prevention (CDC). (2007). Symptomatic early neurosyphilis among HIV-positive men who have sex with men—four cities, United States, January 2002–June 2004. *MMWR. Morbidity and Mortality Weekly Report, 56*, 625–628.

Conde-Sendín, M. A., Hernández Fleta, J. L., Cárdenes-Santana, M. A., & Amela-Peris, R. (2002). Neurosyphilis: Forms of presentation and clinical management. *Revista de Neurologia, 35*(4), 380–386.

Lee, C. H., Lin, W. C., Lu, C. H., & Liu, J.W. (2009). Initially unrecognized dementia in a young man with neurosyphilis. *Neurologist, 15*(2), 95–97.

Lee, J. W., Wilck, M., & Venna, N. (2005). Dementia due to neurosyphilis with persistently negative CSF VDRL. *Neurology, 65*, 1838.

Marra, C. (2009). Update on neurosyphilis. *Current Infectious Disease Reports, 11*, 127–134.

Merritt, H. H., Adams, R. D., & Solomon, H.C. (1946). *Neurosyphilis*. New York: Oxford University Press.

O'Donnell, J. A., & Emery, C. L. (2005). Neurosyphilis: A current review. *Current Infectious Disease Reports, 7*, 277–284.

Pavlović, D. M., & Milović, A. M. (1999). Clinical characteristics and therapy of neurosyphilis in patients who are negative for human immunodeficiency virus. *Srpski Arhiv za Celokupno Lekarstvo, 127*(7–8), 236–240.

Russouw, H. G., Roberts, M. C., Emsley, R. A., & Truter, R. (1997). Psychiatric manifestations and magnetic resonance imaging in HIV-negative neurosyphilis. *Biological Psychiatry, 41*(4), 467–473.

Scheid, R. (2006). Differential diagnosis of mesiotemporal lesions: Case report of neurosyphilis. *Neuroradiology, 48*, 506.

Verma, A., & Solbrig, M. V. (2006). Infections of the nervous system. In W. G. Bradley, R. B. Daroff, G. M. Fenichel, & J. Jankovic (Eds.), *Neurology in clinical practice: Principles of diagnosis and management* (Vol. 2, 4th ed., pp. 1496–1498). Philadelphia: Elsevier.

Vieira Santos, A., Matias, S., Saraiva, P., & Goulão, A. (2005). Differential diagnosis of mesiotemporal lesions: Case report of neurosyphilis. *Neuroradiology, 47,* 664–667.

Wharton, M., Chorba, T. L., Vogt., R. L., Morse, D. L., & Buehler, J. W. (1990). Case definitions for public health surveillance. *MMWE. Recommendations and Reports, 39,* 1–43.

NEUROTOXICITY

DESCRIPTION

Neurotoxicant exposure has been associated with an array of deleterious effects on cerebral structures and functions. The range of substances that has been described as "neurotoxic" is considerable, and includes substances that naturally develop and are esoteric such as mold, solvents, metals and pesticides, chemicals prescribed for therapeutic purposes (e.g., chemotherapy), and alcohol and illicit drug use. The nature and extent of empirical support for direct CNS effects of these "toxins" vary considerably. The presentation of behavioral and cognitive dysfunction depends on numerous factors, including the substance ingested, route of exposure (i.e., inhalation, ingestion, dermal, and injection), tissue absorption levels, time frames of absorption (i.e., exposure duration), personality traits, and litigation status. The need to discern both acute and long-term "subclinical" toxin-related neuropsychological dysfunctions and to distinguish such dysfunction from non-CNS etiologies is a critical issue for neuropsychologists.

NEUROPATHOLOGY/PATHOPHYSIOLOGY

Some potentially toxic agents may provoke edema, atrophy, demyelination, infarctions, calcifications, hemorrhages, or changes of perfusion, metabolism, or receptor density (Lang, 2000). The specific pathophysiology seems to depend to some extent on the specific toxin. Solvents, for example, target lipid-rich locations, such as white matter tracts, resulting in demyelination and axonal loss (Rutchik, 2006). With solvent exposure, neuroimaging results are often normal, but have been found to reveal atrophy, particularly volume loss involving the white matter more than gray matter, as well as occasional focal involvement of the temporal lobes, frontal lobes, basal ganglia, thalamus, and cerebellum (Rutchik, 2006).

NEUROPSYCHOLOGICAL/CLINICAL PRESENTATION

Presenting clinical concerns suggestive of CNS dysfunction tend to be changes in personality, memory disturbance, and attentional difficulties (Morrow, Kamis, & Hodgson, 1993; Morrow, Robin, Hodgson, & Kamis, 1992). For most substances, the effects of acute exposure can be distinguished from the more enduring influences of chronic exposure (Morrow, 2006). For example, acute exposure to solvent neurotoxicants tends to produce a constellation of symptoms including headaches and dizziness, easy fatigability, skin rash, nausea, and mental confusion or feeling intoxicated (Morrow, RoBards, Saxton, & Methany, 2008). In contrast, more chronic exposure to these substances, which include chemicals used in cleaning fluids and paints, can appear neuropsychologically as involving deficits in attention and memory, and slowing of responses (Anger, 1992), as well as reduced information-processing capacity (Morrow et al., 1992). Although the threshold values have been established for certain individual solvents and toxins (e.g., lead), it is difficult to precisely determine the dose that causes impairment in any particular person due to many factors such as chemical half-life and individual physiological differences including rates of absorption and clearance (Proctor, Hughes, & Fischman, 1988).

Following exposure, neuropsychological dysfunction tends to be diffusely present, with alterations described on tests of memory and learning, attention, visuospatial and motor functioning and executive capacity (Morrow et al., 2008). Research on causally related cognitive deficits has also produced inconsistent results with methodological problems, perhaps contributing most to the ambiguous interpretations concerning the relationship between toxic exposure and cognitive dysfunction (Lees-Haley & Williams, 1997; Wood & Liossi, 2005). While certain neurotoxic substances have been studied and are known to have adverse neuropsychological effects (e.g., lead, CO, and mercury), opinions concerning the causation of dysfunction stemming from other substances (e.g., mycotoxins) are speculative and are not grounded in the scientific literature (Lees-Haley, 2003).

DIAGNOSIS

Blood and urine assay can provide an objective source for appreciating body burden (e.g., body exposure index), but these data are rarely available, which leaves the clinical interview as the primary means by which information concerning exposure can be gathered. Although neurotoxins exert their impact on a molecular level, their cumulative effect of some toxins on the CNS can be sufficient for detection through neuroimaging at various stages of disease progression (Arora et al., 2008). However, functional and structural imaging techniques have not revealed a consistent pattern of findings that can be applied with diagnostic confidence (Rutchik, 2006). Similarly, EMG and NCS studies have produced mixed and inconsistent results.

The neuropsychological diagnosis of persons reporting problems associated with exposure to a toxic substance typically relies heavily on (1) examinee's self-report of exposure to a substance that in the right amount or for a prolonged period of time can result in compromised CNS functioning; (2) examinee's self-report of symptoms; and (3) deficits on neuropsychological tests. Challenges arise because exposure intensity and duration may not be objectively established, neuropsychological symptoms are nonspecific, deficits on neuropsychological instruments can result from many factors other than neurological damage, and known patterns of neuropsychological performance associated with exposure to various toxins may lack adequate scientific support. The possibility of psychogenic disturbance or dissimulation should be included in the differential diagnosis, with the presence of clear biological markers of high toxicity helping to support a neurological cause or contribution (Greve et al., 2006).

TREATMENT

If symptoms do not subside after the person is no longer exposed to the offending agent, therapeutic efforts should target neurocognitive deficits and both acute and long-standing psychological problems. Approaches to the treatment of persons with toxicant-related neuropsychological changes utilize cognitive rehabilitation techniques, psychotherapy, and psychopharmacologic interventions to reduce symptoms and promote resumption of roles and routines within home, work, and community settings (Rutchik, 2006).

Shane S. Bush
Mark A. Sandberg

Anger, W. K. (1992). Assessment of neurotoxicity in humans. In H. Tilson & C. Mitchell (Eds.), *Neurotoxicology* (pp. 363–386). New York NY: Raven Press.

Arora, A., Neema, M., Stankiewicz, J., Guss, Z. D., Prockop, L., & Bakshi, R. (2008). Neuroimaging of toxic and metabolic disorders. *Seminars in Neurology, 28*, 495–510

Greve, K. W., Bianchini, K. J., Black, F. W., Heinly, M. T., Love, J. M., Swift, D. A., & Ciota, M. (2006). The prevalence of cognitive malingering in persons reporting exposure to occupational and environmental substances. *Neurotoxicology, 27*, 940–950.

Lang, C. J. (2000). The use of neuroimaging techniques for clinical detection of neurotoxicity: A review. *Neurotoxicology, 21*, 847–855.

Lees-Haley, P. R. (2003). Toxic mold and mycotoxins in neurotoxicity cases: Stachybotrys, fusarium, trichoderma, aspergillus, penicillium, cladosporium, alternaria, trichothecenes. *Psychological Reports, 93*, 561–584.

Lees-Haley, P. R., & Williams, C. W. (1997). The implications of limitations in hydrocarbon research for neuropsychological assessment. *Archives of Clinical Neuropsychology, 12*, 207–222.

Morrow, L. A. (2006). Neurotoxicology. In P. J. Snyder & P. D. Nussbaum (Eds.), *Clinical neuropsychology: A pocket handbook for assessment* (2nd ed.). Washington, DC: American Psychological Association.

Morrow, L. A., Kamis, H., & Hodgson, M. J. (1993). Psychiatric symptomatology in persons with organic solvent exposure. *Journal of Consulting and Clinical Psychology, 61*, 171–174.

Morrow, L. A., RoBards, M., Saxton, J. A., & Methany, K. (2008). Toxins in the CNS: Alcohol, illicit drugs, heavy metals, solvents and related exposure. In J. E. Morgan & J. H. Ricker (Eds.), *Textbook of clinical neuropsychology* (pp. 588–598). New York NY: Taylor & Francis.

Morrow, L. A., Robin, N., Hodgson, M. J., & Kamis, H. (1992). Assessment of attention and memory efficiency in persons with solvent neurotoxicity. *Neuropsychologia, 30*, 911–922.

Proctor, N. H., Hughes, J. P., & Fischman, M. L. (1988). *Chemical hazards of the workplace* (2nd ed.). Philadelphia PA: Lippincott.

Rutchik, J. S. (2006). *Organic solvents*. Retrieved October 10, 2009 from http://emedicine.medscape.com/article/1174981-overview

Wood, R. L., & Liossi, C. (2005). Long-term neuropsychological impact of brief occupational exposure to organic solvents. *Archives of Clinical Neuropsychology, 20*, 655–665.

NIEMANN–PICK DISEASE

DESCRIPTION

Niemann–Pick disease (NPD) refers to a group of disorders that impair the body's ability to metabolize sphingolipids, resulting in fatal levels of these lipids within various organs of the body. These sphingolipidoses are part of a larger classification of disorders referred to as lysomal storage diseases. Although as many as six types of NPDs have been described based on presentation and affected organs (Fotoulaki et al., 2007), the following three types of NPDs are most widely referenced in current practice:

■ NPD Type A is a severe neurodegenerative form of NPD that presents in infancy and typically results in death by the age of 3 years (Takahashi, Suchi, Desnick, Takada, & Schuchman, 1992).
■ NPD Type B is characterized by the pathological involvement of the lungs and visceral organs, absent or minimal neurological impairment, and survival into adulthood (McGovern et al., 2008).
■ NPD Type C includes both visceral and neurological involvement with varying life expectancy that is related to the age of onset (Sevin et al., 2007).

NEUROPATHOLOGY/PATHOPHYSIOLOGY

The NPD types can be further conceptualized as belonging to one of two categories based on etiology. NPD Types A and B are sometimes referred to as Type I NPD because they both result from an inherited deficiency of the enzyme acid sphingomyelinase (ASM). This deficiency prevents the effective metabolization of sphingomyelin, subsequently accumulating in the major body organs. Although the prevalence of NPD Types A and B have been estimated to be 0.5–1 per 100,000 live births, this number is thought to be under-representative of the true incidence within the general population (Schuchman, 2007). NPD Type A has demonstrated a higher rate of prevalence amongst the Ashkenazi Jewish population.

NPD Type C, or Type II NPD, results from defective trafficking of lysosomal cholesterol at the intracellular level (Griffin, Gong, Verot, & Mellon, 2004) and is not secondary to an ASM deficiency. These trafficking errors result in excessive accumulation of lysosomal cholesterol and other lipids within the body organs. The prevalence of NPD Type C is estimated to be 1 in 150,000 in Western Europe, although certain populations (i.e., the French Acadians of Nova Scotia and the Spanish-Americans of southern Colorado and New Mexico) demonstrate a much higher incidence (Sun et al., 2001). A fourth type of NPD (NPD Type D) has been used to describe individuals with NPD Type C who are of Nova Scotian descent. However, current research suggests that the etiology and progression of the two types of NPD are the same, making this distinction unnecessary.

NEUROPSYCHOLOGICAL/CLINICAL PRESENTATION

1. NPD Type A presents during infancy and is characterized by a general failure to thrive, psychomotor retardation, hepatosplenomegaly, and neurological deterioration leading to death by 3 years of age (Takahashi et al., 1992).
2. NPD Type B is typically diagnosed during childhood and is characterized by hepatosplenomegaly, respiratory involvement, and absent or minimal neurological involvement. Although progression and severity of NPD Type B is variable, affected individuals typically survive into adulthood and may live into middle age (Levran, Desnick, & Schuchman, 1991).
3. NPD Type C has a highly variable presentation and includes an acute infantile form that rapidly leads to death, a progressive adolescent form resulting in death in the 2nd or 3rd decade, and a rare adult form with a generally slow progression (Battisti et al., 2003). Physical manifestations are equally diverse and include hepatosplenomegaly, pulmonary distress, neurological deterioration, or psychiatric features. Almost all patients with NPD Type C will eventually develop neurological or psychiatric symptoms, which may include dementia, supranuclear gaze palsy, ataxia, dysarthria, dysphagia, and dystonia (Patterson, Porter, Vaurio, & Brown, 2009; Sevin et al., 2007).

DIAGNOSIS

Diagnosis of NPD is based on the observation of the clinical features associated with each type, with hepatosplenomegaly often being the first visible indicator. Diagnosis of NPD Types A and B is confirmed via fluid and tissue cultures that reveal deficient ASM activity (Takahashi et al., 1992). Similarly, the presence of NPD Type C is confirmed by studying cultured fibroblasts and their ability to transport and store lysosomal cholesterol. Advances in DNA analysis also allow for observation of the characteristic mutations in the genes associated with the different types of NPD (Griffin et al., 2004; Schuchman, 2007).

TREATMENT

At the present time, no therapies have been shown to be effective in the treatment of any of the three types of NPDs (Griffin et al., 2004; McGovern, Aron, Brodie, Desnick, & Wasserstein, 2006). Experimental treatments have included the use of enzyme replacement therapies and stem cell transplantation. Treatment is therefore largely supportive and it may help to manage the psychiatric features and loss of cognitive functions that may be present. Counseling may prove beneficial for patients and family members coping with the stress associated with a terminal illness.

Jacob T. Lutz
Raymond S. Dean

Battisti, C., Tarugi, P., Dotti, M. T., De Stefano, N., Vattimo, A., Chierichetti, F., et al. (2003). Adult-Onset Niemann-Pick type C disease: A clinical, neuroimaging, and molecular genetic study. *Movement Disorders, 18*(11), 1405–1409.

Fotoulaki, M., Schuchman, E. H., Simonaro, C. M., Augoustides-Savvopoulou, P., Michelakakis, H., Panagopoulou, P., et al. (2007). Acid sphingomyelinase-deficient Niemann-Pick disease: Novel findings in a Greek child. *Journal of Inherited Metabolic Disease, 30,* 986. doi: 10.1007/s10545-007-0557-3

Griffin, L. D., Gong, W., Verot, L., & Mellon, S. H. (2004). Niemann-Pick disease type C involves disrupted neurosteroidogenesis and responds to allopregnanolone. *Nature Medicine, 10*(7). doi: 10.1038/nm1073

Levran, O., Desnick, R. J., & Schuchman, E. H. (1991). Niemann-Pick type B disease [Electronic edition]. *The Journal of Clinical Investigation, 88,* 806–810.

McGovern, M. M., Aron, A., Brodie, S. E., Desnick, R. J., & Wasserstein, M. P. (2006). Natural history of type A Niemann-Pick disease. *Neurology, 66,* 228–232.

McGovern, M. M., Wasserstein, M. P., Giugliani, R., Bembi, B., Vanier, M. T., Mengel, E., et al. (2008). A prospective, cross-sectional survey study of the natural history of Niemann-Pick disease type B. *Pediatrics, 122*(2). doi: 10.1542/peds.2007-3016

Patterson, M., Porter, F., Vaurio, R., & Brown, T. (2009). Longitudinal study of cognition in subjects with Niemann-Pick disease, type C. *Molecular Genetics and Metabolism, 96*(2), S34. doi: 10.1016/j.ymgme.2008.11.102

Schuchman, E. H. (2007). The pathogenesis and treatment of acid sphingomyelinase-deficient Niemann-Pick disease. *Journal of Inherited Metabolic Disease, 30,* 654–663. doi: 10.1007/s10545-007-0632-9

Sevin, M., Lesca, G., Baumann, N., Millat, G., Lyon-Caen, O., Vanier, M. T., et al. (2007). The adult form of Niemann-Pick disease type C. *Brain, 130,* 120–133. doi: 10.1093/brain/awl260

Sun, X., Marks, D. L., Park, W. D., Wheatley, C. L., Vishwajeet, P., O'Brien, J. F., et al. (2001). Niemann-Pick C variant detection by altered sphingolipid trafficking and correlations with mutations within a specific domain of NPC1 [Electronic version]. *The American Journal of Human Genetics, 68*(6), 1361–1372.

Takahashi, T., Suchi, M., Desnick, R. J., Takada, G., & Schuchman, E. H. (1992). Identification and expression of five mutations in the human acid sphingomyelinase gene causing types A and B Niemann-Pick disease [Electronic version]. *The Journal of Biological Chemistry, 267*(18), 12552–12558.

NONVERBAL LEARNING DISABILITY

DESCRIPTION

Nonverbal learning disability (NLD) is a syndrome characterized by neuropsychological deficits in visuospatial-organizational, tactile-perceptual, complex psychomotor, and nonverbal problem-solving skills that coexist with relative strengths in rote verbal learning, phoneme-grapheme matching, verbal output, and verbal classification (Rourke, 1989, 1995b). Neuropsychological deficits may appear at birth or shortly thereafter or may be caused by significant craniocerebral trauma, such as brain diseases, disorders, and injuries following a period of normal development (Rourke, 1989). NLD syndrome is usually perceived as a subtype of a learning disorder, but does not appear in the *Diagnostic and Statistical Manual of Mental Disorders, fourth edition* (Daley, 2004). Contrary to learning disorders that are more language/phonological based, some language functioning in children with NLD (e.g., word recognition and verbal output) is often well developed, whereas other important language functions (e.g., pragmatics and prosody) are often severely impaired.

The capacity to process information delivered through the auditory modality is the principal neuropsychological strength of children who exhibit the NLD syndrome. Within school settings, the neuropsychological strengths of children with NLD often lead to academic strengths in word decoding, spelling, and verbatim memory, while the neuropsychological deficits usually lead to academic deficits in reading comprehension, mechanical arithmetic, mathematics, and science.

Children with NLD often exhibit difficulty participating in social situations and reading signs of affective and nonverbal communication (Pelletier, Ahmad, & Rourke, 2001). They desire social connection but often lack the ability to self-reflect, make attribution, or monitor their behavior (Forrest, 2004). They are prone to psychosocial dysfunction as they mature (Pelletier et al., 2001) and often develop affective disorders, such as anxiety and depression (Ingalls & Goldstein, 1999). In addition, children with learning

N

disabilities who had well-developed rote verbal skills are very successful using rote repetition to memorize discrete information like vocabulary words or geographic places (Harnadek & Rourke, 1994), which often lead to appearance as a "human encyclopedia." As a result, they often experienced social rejection (Forrest, 2004) and were more likely to exhibit psychopathology than children without NLD (Tsatsanis, Fuerst, & Rourke, 1997).

NEUROPATHOLOGY/PATHOPHYSIOLOGY

The right hemisphere is believed to have a higher concentration of white matter than the left and a greater capacity to integrate complex information and process several models of representation within a single cognitive task (Goldberg-Costa, 1981; Filley, 2001). Based on this theory, Rourke (1989) suggested that NLD represents a manifestation of white matter dysfunction, which compromises the functioning of right hemisphere systems more so than the left hemisphere systems. Extending from this concept, Rourke (1989,1995a) hypothesized that the presentation of the deficits in children with NLD is dependent upon the severity of white-matter involvement and the age at which the damage is sustained. Severe or widespread white-matter disturbance occurring very early in life would be expected to result in deficiencies in virtually all skills and abilities, while mild degrees and extents of dysfunction occurring later in life would be expected to result in a milder impact on a child's neuropsychological abilities. Functions that have been reasonably developed will be less likely affected by white-matter disturbance.

In addition, neuropsychological strengths and deficits of children with NLD change over the course of development (Casey et al., 1991). Progressive deterioration in skills is expected and will become more apparent and more debilitating as individuals approach adulthood (Rourke, 1989; Rourke, van der Vlugt, & Rourke, 2002).

Although NLD syndrome is thought mostly to be congenital, it is also seen in individuals with acquired neurological diseases and disorders, including general deterioration or significant destruction of neuronal white matter (long myelinated fibers) within the right cerebral hemisphere, destruction of access to neuronal intercommunication (e.g., callosal agenesis), head injuries, and some types of hydrocephalus.

Filley (2001) suggested that demyelination of white matter or other abnormalities in white matter volume have been associated with manifestations of emotional dysfunction, often resulting in the development of depression, mania, and psychosis. This association between dysfunctional white matter and affective disorders provides an explanation for the increased risk of emotional and social dysfunction of children with NLD.

NEUROPSYCHOLOGICAL/CLINICAL PRESENTATION

Deriving from his extensive research on NLDs, Rourke outlined the principal clinical manifestations of the NLD syndrome as follows:

1. Well-developed rote verbal capacities, with very well-developed rote verbal-memory skills.
2. Bilateral tactile-perceptual deficits, most noticeably on the left side of the body.
3. Bilateral psychomotor coordination deficiencies, most noticeably on the left side of the body.
4. Considerable deficiencies in visuospatial-organizational abilities.
5. Severe deficits in nonverbal problem solving, concept formation, hypothesis testing, and the ability to benefit from positive and negative informational feedback in various situations.
6. Serious difficulties with cause–effect relationships and deficiencies in the appreciation of incongruities.
7. Significant difficulty adapting to novel and complex situations with overreliance on prosaic, rote behaviors.
8. Deficiencies in mechanical arithmetic despite proficiencies in word decoding/recognition and spelling.
9. Phonetically accurate misspellings.
10. Excessive use of words in a repetitive, rote nature, with poor psycholinguistic pragmatics and little, if any, speech prosody.
11. Reliance on language for social relations, information collection, and anxiety relief.
12. Severe deficits in social perception, judgment, and interaction skills.

DIAGNOSIS

Compared to children without disabilities and children with a phonological-processing subtype of disabilities (e.g., reading and spelling), children with NLD tend to perform more poorly on neuropsychological measures involving visual-perceptual-organizational skills, psychomotor coordination, complex tactile-perceptual skills, and conceptual and problem-solving skills. Clinicians considering making a diagnosis of possible NLD and developing treatment programs should devote attention to children's performance within these realms.

Pelletier et al. (2001) established the following rules for classification of children (ages 9–15) as NLD with the percentage of children classified as having NLD who exhibit each feature (in parentheses):

1. Less than two errors on simple tactile perception and suppression versus finger agnosia, finger dysgraphesthesia, and astereognosis composite greater than 1 SD below the mean (90.9%)
2. WRAT standard score for reading is at least eight points greater than arithmetic (85.7%)
3. Two of WISC/WISC-R vocabulary, similarities, and information are the highest of the verbal scales (77.9%)
4. Two of the WISC/WISC-R block design, object assembly, and coding subtests are the lowest of the performance scales (76.6%)
5. Target test at least 1 SD below the mean (63.6%)
6. Grip strength within 1 SD of the mean or above versus grooved pegboard test greater than 1 SD below the mean (63.6%)
7. Tactual performance test right, left, and both hand times become progressively worse vis-à-vis the norms (59.7%)
8. WISC/WISC-R VIQ exceeds PIQ by at least 10 points (27.3%)

Pelletier et al. (2001) suggested that the 10-point difference between VIQ and PIQ rule may be eliminated from the list without compromising diagnostic accuracy given that it was present only in 27% of the individuals with NLD used to validate these criteria. In addition, it should be noted that many of the tests used to validate the criteria have been revised and are in need of refinement.

Applying the above criteria to younger children (ages 7–8), Drummond, Ahmad, and Rourke (2005) delineated the following rules to identify younger children with NLD. The percentage of children classified as having NLD who exhibit each feature is indicated in parentheses:

1. Target test at least 1 SD below the mean (90.0%)
2. Two of the WISC block design, object assembly, and coding subtests are the lowest of the performance scales (90.0%)
3. Two of WISC vocabulary, similarities, and information are the highest of the verbal scales (80.0%)
4. Tactual performance test right, left, and both hand times become progressively worse vis-à-vis the norms (77.8%)
5. Grip strength within 1 SD of the mean or above versus grooved pegboard test greater than 1 SD below the mean (70.0%)
6. WISC VIQ exceeds PIQ by at least 10 points (70.0%)

7. WRAT standard score for reading is at least eight points greater than arithmetic (60.0%)
8. Less than two errors on simple tactile perception and suppression versus finger agnosia, finger dysgraphesthesia, and astereognosis composite greater than 1 SD below the mean (10.0%)

Drummond et al. (2005) noted that strict application of rules 1 through 3 should result in very few false-positive identification of young children with NLD, and that eliminating rule 8 as a criterion should not affect the accuracy of classification.

TREATMENT

The prognosis of individuals with NLD is limited by the neuropsychological deficits that become progressively more apparent and more debilitating as adulthood approaches (Rourke et al., 2002). Academic difficulties often lead to difficulty in securing and/or sustaining employment in adulthood, and deficits in social information processing and emotional understanding are likely to interfere with opportunities to establish intimate, long-term relationships, both of which tend to increase susceptibility to depression and anxiety. However, early diagnosis with NLD is as critical as it is with other subtypes of learning disorders. An accurate early diagnosis along with an appropriate remedial program can improve the outcome for individuals suffering from the neuropsychological deficits of NLD (Marti, 2004).

Following an accurate and reliable diagnosis, an appropriate remediation treatment plan should be established in the problem areas that may include deficits in social skills, prosody, spatial orientation, problem solving, recognition of nonverbal cues, complex motor skills, attention, initiation, organization, planning, and difficulty with mathematical concepts. A treatment plan should be individually tailored as patterns of specific strengths and weaknesses may not be identical for every individual with NLD. In addition, a treatment plan should be reevaluated and modified as needed to adapt to the problems with NLD that shift across the life span (Marti, 2004).

Parents of children with NLD should teach their child coping, organizational, and problem-solving skills, as well as how to set up routines to deal with daily tasks and responsibilities and how to perform everyday tasks in an efficient manner. Taking the time to make sure that children with NLD master all of the daily living skills necessary to function independently can facilitate a sense of confidence and self-efficacy and may reduce susceptibility to psychiatric problems (e.g., depression and anxiety). Additionally, within the school environment, academic interventions should be provided in the areas of study skills, organizational skills, and how to find main points in reading, make reference, and apply learned skills and knowledge. Physical therapy, occupational therapy, and social skills training should also be beneficial for those with motor difficulties and problems with recognition and interpretation of verbal and nonverbal cues (Marti, 2004).

Psychotherapy is useful when it focuses on helping the individual with NLD understand his/her areas of strengths and weaknesses and develop appropriate ways to manage them. Primary goals for therapy should emphasize coping skills, helping children and their families understand how NLD affects thinking, behavior, and perceptions, and learning how to work with deficits that may be pervasive (Marti, 2004).

Moreover, medication is common in treating the emotional aspect of NLD symptoms because of their resemblance to those seen in a number of psychiatric disorders, such as mood disorders and anxiety disorders, including obsessive-compulsive disorder, social phobia, and panic disorder. Medication also can be prescribed for attention deficits. However, prescribing practitioners should be aware that those with NLD may have trouble processing the complex and multiple factors in the use of medicine; therefore, they should help patients understand the short- and long-term side effects of each prescribed medication. Finally, the combination of medication with behavioral interventions and training has shown to be a more effective long-term strategy in managing neurologically based disorders, including NLD (Marti, 2004).

Mei Chang
Andrew S. Davis

Casey, J. E., Rourke, B. P., & Picard, E. M. (1991). Syndrome of nonverbal learning disabilities: Age differences in neuropsychological, academic, and socioemotional functioning. *Development and Psychology, 3*(3), 329–345.

Daley, S. (2004). *Nonverbal learning disabilities (NLD): Introduction (a disorder of cerebral white matter)*. Retrieved June 23, 2009, from http://gseacademic.harvard.edu/~daleysa/index.htm

Drummond, C. R., Ahmad, S. A., & Rourke, B. P. (2005). Rules for the classification of younger children with nonverbal learning disabilities and basic phonological processing disabilities. *Archives of Clinical Neuropsychology, 20*(2), 171–182.

Filley, C. M. (2001). *The behavioral neurology of white matter*. New York: Oxford University Press.

Forrest, B. J. (2004). The utility of math difficulties, internalized psychopathology, and visual-spatial deficits to identify children with the nonverbal learning disability syndrome: Evidence for a visualspatial disability. *Child Neuropsychology, 10*(2), 129–146.

Goldberg, E., & Costa, L. D. (1981). Hemispheric differences in the acquisition and use of descriptive systems. *Brain and Language, 14*, 144–173.

Harnadek, M., & Rourke, B. P. (1994). Principal identifying features of the syndrome of nonverbal learning disabilities in children. *Journal of Learning Disabilities, 27*(3), 144–154.

Ingalls, S., & Goldstein, S. (1999). Learning disabilities. In S. Goldstein & C. R. Reynolds (Eds.), *Handbook of neurodevelopmental and genetic disorders in children* (pp. 101–153). New York: The Guilford Press.

Marti, L. (2004). Helping children with nonverbal learning disability: What I have learned from living with nonverbal learning disability. *Journal of Child Neurology, 19*(10), 830–836.

Pelletier, P. M., Ahmad, S. A., & Rourke, B. P. (2001). Classification rules for basic phonological processing disabilities and nonverbal learning disabilities: Formulation and external validity. *Child Neuropsychology, 7*(2), 84–98.

Rourke, B. P. (1989). *Nonverbal learning disabilities: The syndrome and the model*. New York: Guilford Press.

Rourke, B. P. (1995a). The NLD syndrome and the white matter model. In B. P. Rourke (Ed.), *Syndrome of nonverbal learning disabilities* (pp. 1–26). New York: Guilford Press.

Rourke, B. P. (1995b). *Syndrome of nonverbal learning disabilities: Neurodevelopmental manifestations*. New York: Guilford Press.

Rourke, B. P., Ahmad, S. A., Collins, D. W., Hayman-Abello, B. A., Hayman-Alello, S. E., & Warriner, E. M. (2002). Child clinical/pediatric neuropsychology: Some recent advances. *Annual Review of Psychology, 53*(1), 309–339.

Rourke, B. P., van der Vlugt, H., & Rourke, S. B. (2002). *Practice of child-clinical neuropsychology: An introduction*. Lisse, The Netherlands: Swets & Zeitlinger.

Tsatsanis, K. D., Fuerst, D. R., & Rourke, B. P. (1997). Psychological dimensions of learning disabilities: External validation and relationship with age and academic functioning. *Journal of Learning Disabilities, 30*, 490–502.

NORMAL PRESSURE HYDROCEPHALUS

DESCRIPTION

Normal pressure hydrocephalus (NPH) is a central nervous system disorder involving interruption in cerebrospinal fluid (CSF) dynamics. Known as the only reversible dementia, NPH is estimated to represent approximately 6% of all dementias, and prevalence is broadly estimated between 0.5% and 1% (Clarfield, 2003, Trenkwalder et al., 1995; Vanneste, Augustiin, Dirven, Tan, & Goedhart, 1992). Clinical presentation typically occurs between the ages of 60 and 80 and is recognized by a classic triad of symptoms including gait ataxia, dementia, and urinary incontinence/urgency. In the presence of the classic triad, neuroradiologic evidence of ventriculomegaly has become a cardinal feature. Current nomenclature describes NPH according to etiology (idiopathic vs. secondary), intracranial pressure (high vs. low), and flow of CSF (communicating vs. obstructive).

NEUROPATHOLOGY/PATHOPHYSIOLOGY

CSF is the protective, nourishing fluid surrounding the brain in the subarachnoid space and circulating through the cerebral ventricles and aqueducts. Healthy CSF dynamics entail the production, distribution, and reabsorption of CSF. By processes of diffusion and pinocytosis, CSF is produced primarily in the choroid plexus at a rate of 0. 2–0.7 mL/min, resulting in an average daily production of 500 mL. Through pulsation of the choroid plexus, CSF is transferred into the ventricular system and circulated via cilia motion of ependymal cells to the arachnoid villi where it is reabsorbed.

NPH is a consequence of disruption in the natural flow and/or absorption of CSF. Instances of NPH resulting from known etiology, such as hemorrhage, infection, and/or head trauma, are branded "secondary NPH." Conversely, many cases of NPH are of unknown etiology, and have been termed "idiopathic NPH" (iNPH). Disruption in CSF dynamics is typically classified according to locus of pathology. Disturbance due to the obstruction in the ventricular system is termed "noncommunicating" hydrocephalus. Alternatively, disruptions occurring in the subarachnoid space or in venous uptake result in "communicating" hydrocephalus. High and low intracranial pressure has been observed in NPH, suggesting that the name "normal pressure" hydrocephalus is a misnomer.

Distinctions regarding the pathophysiology of secondary NPH are more easily made due to the presence of an identifiable precipitant, whereas the pathophysiology of idiopathic NPH remains poorly understood. Early hypotheses of iNPH, proposed a disparity between CSF production and absorption, with expansion of the cerebral ventricles in accommodation of elevated intracranial pressure. Expansion of the cerebral ventricles was considered a normalizing response to elevated intracranial pressure and thought to explain the common finding of "normal pressure" in the CNS. Current mechanistic conceptualizations extend beyond purely hydrodynamic disruption to include hemodynamic pathologies, neurochemical alterations, or multifactorial combinations (Shprecher, Schwalb, & Kurlan, 2008).

Secondary and idiopathic NPH share the neuroradiological finding of ventriculomegaly. Other common neuroradiological findings include bowing of the corpus callosum, flattened gyri, and periventricular hyperintensities (Gallia, Rigamonti, & Williams, 2005). The neuroanatomical changes observed in NPH, principally ventricular dilation, are theorized to produce the symptomatic triad by affecting neuroanatomical areas related to gait ataxia, dementia, and urge/incontinence.

Gait disturbance in NPH has been described as ataxic, magnetic, slow, wide-based, shuffling, and parkinsonian. Disrupted gait is generally cited as the first symptom of the triad to present clinically, and the symptom most amenable to treatment. Originally, gait ataxia was attributed to effects on the primary pyramidal tract; however, current literature implicates extrapyramidal origins involving subcortical/frontal motor pathways. Specifically, the interference in projections from the substantia nigra and basal ganglia to the frontal lobes has been implicated.

The hallmark cognitive disturbance in NPH is described as a subcortical dementia and involves slowed processing, impaired attention, apathy, and poor recall. The cognitive symptoms of NPH are heterogeneous, spanning a broad array of neurocognitive domains, and ranging in severity from mild to profound. The exact pathophysiology of NPH dementia is poorly understood, though the neuropathology appears similar to that of gait disturbance, in that the effects of enlarged ventricles on proximal subcortical projections, parenchyma, and vasculature are thought to underlie the cognitive disturbance.

Urinary symptoms in NPH are "neurogenic" in nature and initiate as increased urgency/frequency, and worsen to incontinence as NPH progresses. While incontinence is considered a classic symptom of NPH, it is not clinically present in all cases and its absence does not rule out a diagnosis of NPH. Urinary urgency is the most common urologic symptom followed by infrequency, frequency, and frank incontinence. Urodynamic investigations cite increased activity of the bladder's detrusor muscle as the cause of urinary symptoms. Detrusor hyperactivity is associated with supraspinal disruption, resulting from the effects of ventriculomegaly on surrounding parenchyma. Incontinence can also result from

N

functional inability secondary to gait disturbance and/or dementia.

Symptoms of the classic triad of NPH are generally attributable to the anatomic, neurochemical, and metabolic effects of ventriculomegaly. However, each of the cardinal symptoms is common among the elderly making diagnosis difficult. Moreover, the presence of each symptom in the triad is not required to consider a diagnosis of NPH. Thus, examination of each of the symptoms on a case-by-case basis is critical and the presence of alternative explanations serves as an important factor in diagnosing NPH.

NEUROPSYCHOLOGICAL/CLINICAL PRESENTATION

The neurocognitive changes associated with NPH are characteristic of subcortical dementias. Clinical descriptions often include apathy, forgetfulness, and bradykinesia/phrenia. Neuropsychological assessment commonly exposes performance impairments across a variety of tasks (Devito et al., 2005). The elemental neurocognitive disturbance of NPH is impaired psychomotor speed; however, dysfunction in attention, memory, executive operations, and visuospatial tasks are also common. Poor attention and concentration often present on tasks such as digit span, letter number sequencing, and arithmetic. Visuospatial deficits are observed on tasks of spatial recognition, design copy, and block design. Impairment in both immediate and delayed verbal recall, with relatively sparred recognition, is an ordinary observation on memory measures. Broad deficits in executive functioning are not unusual; however, impairment on tasks involving initiation, cognitive flexibility, and/or verbal fluency is most typical. Because the features of NPH are a result of disruption in subcortical and frontostriatal systems, cortical functions such as naming are often unaffected.

In addition, depression, mania, aggression, obsessive-compulsive behavior, disinhibition, and psychosis have also been reported. Notably, depression can be neurogenic in nature or a reaction to functional deficits.

DIAGNOSIS

In the elderly population, suspicion of NPH is raised in the presence of the symptomatic triad; however, the entire triad need not be present to consider the diagnosis. Because of the heterogeneity of NPH symptoms and their common occurrence in the elderly,

differential diagnosis and rule out of other possible causes are required before offering a diagnosis of NPH. Diagnosis of secondary NPH differs from iNPH in that symptoms follow a known precipitant warrants investigation of NPH. Clinical guidelines for diagnosing iNPH incorporate historical, neuroradiological, clinical, and physiological information in categorizing the likelihood of NPH as "probable, possible and unlikely" (Relkin, Marmarou, Klinge, Bergsneider, & Black, 2005). Diagnosing NPH requires a minimum of gait disturbance plus one other symptom of the triad, neuroradiologic evidence of ventriculomegaly, and rule out of other etiologies. Ventriculomegaly is typically confirmed by an Evans' Index greater than 0.3 (maximal width of frontal horn divided by transverse diameter of the skull). In the presence of the aforementioned criteria, NPH is typically confirmed through high volume lumbar puncture or external lumbar drain and subsequent observation of symptom reduction. Assessment of symptoms through neuropsychological testing, urodynamic analysis, gait assessment, functional neuroimaging, and other methods, have become common to assist in diagnosis, rule out of other causes, and prognosis.

TREATMENT

Neurosurgical placement of a shunt is the only recognized intervention for NPH. Ventriculoperitoneal or ventriculoatrial shunting are the mainstays of intervention for NPH and involve the diversion of CSF from the ventricular system to a distal site where it can be reabsorbed.

J. Forrest Sanders
Jeffrey T. Barth

Clarfield, A. M. (2003). The decreasing prevalence of reversible dementias: An updated meta-analysis. *Archives of Internal Medicine, 163*(18), 2219–2229.

Devito, E. E., Pickard, J. D., Salmond, C. H., Iddon, J. L., Loveday, C., & Sahakian, B. J. (2005). The neuropsychology of normal pressure hydrocephalus (NPH). *British Journal of Neurosurgery, 19*(3), 217–224.

Gallia, G. L., Rigamonti, D., & Williams, M. A. (2005). The diagnosis and treatment of idiopathic normal pressure hydrocephalus. *Nature Clinical Practice Neurology, 2,* 375–381.

Relkin, N., Marmarou, A., Klinge, P., Bergsneider, M., & Black, P. M. (2005). Diagnosing idiopathic normal-pressure hydrocephalus. *Neurosurgery, 57,* S4–S16

Shprecher, D., Schwalb, J., & Kurlan, R. (2008). Normal pressure hydrocephalus: Diagnosis and treatment. *Current Neurology and Neuroscience Reports, 8,* 371–376.

Trenkwalder, C., Schwarz, J., Gebhard, J., Ruland, D., Trenkwalder, P., Hense, H. W., et al. (1995). Starnberg trial on epidemiology of Parkinsonism and hypertension in the elderly. Prevalence of Parkinson's disease and related disorders assessed by a door-to-door survey of inhabitants older than 65 years. *Archives of Neurology, 52*(10), 1017–1022.

Vanneste, J., Augustijn, P., Dirven, C., Tan, W. F., & Goedhart, Z. D. (1992). Shunting normal-pressure hydrocephalus: Do the benefits outweigh the risks? A multicenter study and literature review. *Neurology, 42*(1), 54–59.

N

OCCIPITAL NEURALGIA

DESCRIPTION

Occipital neuralgia is a form of headache that involves irritation of one or both of the occipital nerves emerging from between the bones of the spine in the upper neck and moving up into the scalp. The occipital nerves are two pairs of nerves that originate in the C2 and C3 vertebrae in the neck. These nerves supply the skin along the base of the skull, and although the nerves are not intertwined with the skull themselves, they are intertwined with other nerves outside of the skull and can affect any area through which any fibers or main nerves pass, forming a neural network. Occipital neuralgia may be either primary or secondary. Primary headaches do not have a clear cause (e.g., migraine and cluster headaches). Within this context, occipital neuralgia is often confused with migraine or cluster headaches. Secondary headaches are due to an underlying disease process, including trauma, tumor, infections, or hemorrhage.

NEUROPATHOLOGY/PATHOPHYSIOLOGY

Patients with occipital neuralgia can be divided into two groups: individuals with structural causes and individuals with idiopathic (unknown) causes. Structural causes may include trauma to the occipital nerves, compression to the occipital nerves or nerve roots (C2&C3), a cervical disc disease, or tumors on the nerve roots, infection, and diabetes. The greater occipital nerve is comprised of fibers from the C2 and C3 nerve roots. The third occipital nerve stems from the posterior area of the C3 nerve and may be involved in occipital neuralgia due to cervical spine changes. Compression of the C2 and C3 nerve roots may also lead to occipital neuralgia. Whiplash or hyperextension injuries are two ways in which this compression may occur. Localized infections, inflammation, diabetes, or gout may also be possible causes of occipital neuralgias. However, most patients fall into the area of "idiopathic" or unknown causes for the disorder.

NEUROPSYCHOLOGICAL/CLINICAL PRESENTATION

Patients present clinically with symptoms including burning, throbbing, and aching pain on one side of the head with intermittent shooting pain. The pain usually originates in the area below the occipital lobe of the brain and radiates to the back of the head or up to the scalp. Patients sometimes complain of pain behind the eyes, in the neck as well as over the temple, and regions of the frontal lobe. Pressure can amplify the pain. Doctors can sometimes find a positive tinel's sign over the occipital nerve. A sensation of "pins and needles" may be apparent if the occipital nerve is tapped lightly. As previously suggested, patients may experience symptoms similar to migraine headaches or cluster headaches. Symptoms further associated with occipital neuralgia include dizziness, sensitivity to light, and burning or tingling in the back of the scalp.

Chronic pain can result in a variety of psychological symptoms that include personality changes, irritability, attention problems, motivational issues, fatigue, and problems with complex, sustained higher cognitive tasks. There is often a debate on idiopathic cases as to whether the disorder has a true neurological cause or is a psychological disorder. Psychological symptoms often can be found with both forms of the disorder whether or not there is a clear physical etiology; hence, the presence of psychological symptoms alone does not rule out a physical cause.

DIAGNOSIS

Complete physical and neurologic exams are necessary in the diagnosis of occipital neuralgia. In this disorder, a diagnosis is typically based on the area of the pain. Finding extra sensitive areas to the pain also helps in determining a diagnosis. Clarification of whether the disorder is structural or idiopathic in nature is important to diagnosis. Structural causes are usually found with abnormal responses to a neurologic exam, in which case a CT scan or MRI may be prescribed for further information with focus placed on the cervical spine and head. If there is a history of

OP

arthritis or trauma, a full spine work-up is recommended.

As previously noted, occipital neuralgia is a constant, burning, aching, shooting pain in occipital and posterior areas of the scalp, either unilaterally or bilaterally, and is usually worse with extension and rotation. Nevertheless, occipital neuralgia is often mistaken for migraine or other types of headaches. A migraine headache is unilateral and hemicranial with throbbing or pulsating pain, sensitivity to light and sound, as well as nausea. Migraines are neurovascular headaches associated with perivascular inflammation through the trigeminal nerve. In comparison, tension headaches are usually bilateral, with a dull, squeezing like pain. Sensitivity to light and sound may also occur. These typically affect frontal and fronto occipital areas. Cluster headaches involve excruciating, painful, drilling pain that is usually incredibly severe. Spain usually is accompanied by one autonomic sign such as lacrimation, nasal congestion, or miosis. Cervicogenic headaches have a similar presentation to occipital neuralgia, cluster, tension, and migraine headaches. Usually, these headaches are unilateral and are constant or intermittent. These headaches are rarely throbbing and are usually caused by neck or head movement.

TREATMENT

If there is structural evidence to the cause of the occipital neuralgia, surgery may be necessary based on the source. However, most patients do not have clear structural causes, and therefore treatment becomes symptomatic. Occipital neuralgia may be difficult to manage due to it often being misconceived as other types of headaches. Nerve blocks, medications, implantation of stimulators, decompression, and/or lesioning are all types of treatment options for occipital neuralgias. Course of treatment usually starts with conservative methods including physical therapy acupuncture, massages, and application of heat. If response is not of a desirable level, conventional therapy involving medicinal interventions may be employed including nonsteroidal anti-inflammatory drugs, neuropathic medication, and sometimes opioids.

Medications most often used include gabapentin (neurontin), carbamazepine (Tegretol), phenytoin (dilantin), valproic acid (Depakote), and baclofen (lioresal). Nerve blocks containing steroids and local anesthetics may also be used. An occipital nerve block is used for both diagnosis and treatment of occipital neuralgias. For the treatment of occipital neuralgia, 3–5 mL of anesthetic is combined with steroids and injected. Anesthesia will typically occur in 10–20 min. Botulism toxin type A (Botox) has been an accepted treatment method for migraine headaches and thus may have a positive effect on occipital neuralgia. The clinical trials in migraines indicate that Botox decreases the duration, length, and severity of headaches and is generally well tolerated.

Surgical options include electrical stimulation, neurolysis, and rhizotomies. Treatment through surgery has been found to be most successful in patients with microvascular nerve decompression. Another widely used treatment measure is radiofrequency thermocoagulation, which has resulted in significant pain relief in patients with occipital neuralgia. The final method of treatment for this disorder is an occipital nerve stimulator implantation. This method includes surgical implantation of an electrode under the skin on the C1–C3 nerve level and has been shown to significantly reduce pain in patients where other treatment methods have failed.

Erin L. Tireman
Charles Golden

Anthony, M. (1992). Headache and the greater occipital nerve. *Clinical Neurology and Neurosurgery, 94*(4), 297–301.

Kuhn, W. F., Kuhn, S. C., & Gilberstadt, H. (1997). Occipital neuralgias: Clinical recognition of a complicated headache. A case series and literature review. *Journal of Orofacial Pain, 11*(2), 158–165.

Loder, E., & Biondi, D. (2002). Use of botulinum toxins for chronic headaches: A focused review. *Clinical Journal of Pain, 18*(6), S169–S176.

Martelletti, P., & Suijlekom, H. V. (2004). Cervicogenic headache: Practical approaches to therapy. *CNS Drugs, 11*(18), 793–805.

Stojanovic, M. (2001). Stimulation methods for neuropathic pain control. *Current Pain and Headache Reports, 5,* 130–137.

Ohtahara's Syndrome

DESCRIPTION

Ohtahara's syndrome was first identified and described by Ohtahara and colleagues in 1976 (Pellock, Dodson, Bourgeois, Sankor, & Nordli, 2008). The disorder is also referred to as early infantile epileptic encephalopathy with suppression-bursts and is an age-dependent epileptic encephalopathy (Pellock et al., 2008). It is one of the earliest and most severe forms of epilepsy (Kato et al., 2007). Around 100 cases have been reported since the disorder was first identified (Jallon, 2003). It is the rarest of the age-dependent epileptic encephalopathies (Yamatogi & Ohtahara, 2002). There is no evidence of gender differences among those with the syndrome and no familial cases have been reported (Wyllie, Gupta, & Lachhwani 2004).

The symptoms begin to appear within the first 10 days of life but could first appear as late as 3 months after birth (Cloherty, Eichenwald, & Stark, 2008). The prevalence of the disorder is very low, and 50% of infants with this disorder will not make it past 1 month of age (Niedermeyer & Lopes da Silva, 2004). The main type of seizure present in Ohtahara's syndrome is a tonic spasm, an involuntary and abnormal contraction of muscles. Partial and generalized seizures can occur as well (Pellock et al., 2008). An infant may experience around 100–300 individual tonic spasms per day. The spasms may also happen in clusters (Binnie et al., 2003). Infants with this syndrome will show a suppression-burst EEG pattern (Pellock et al., 2008). Ohtahara's syndrome often progresses into West's syndrome (Pellock et al., 2008) and from West's syndrome to Lennox–Gastaut's syndrome (LSG) (Yamatogi & Ohtahara, 2002).

NEUROPATHOLOGY/PATHOPHYSIOLOGY

The causes of the syndrome are heterogenous, though structural abnormalities in the form of brain malformations and/or lesions are commonly seen and lead to damage similar to that of cerebral palsy (Cloherty et al., 2008). CT and MRI tend to show irregular lesions and progressive brain atrophy. Other potential causes of Ohtahara's syndrome are cerebral dysgenesis and anoxia (Pellock et al., 2008). Electroencephalogram (EEG) findings show a pattern of variant suppression-burst that occur for every 3–5 seconds and are characterized by increased voltage bursts that alternate with flat patterns (Pellock et al., 2008). These bursts are considered crucial to diagnosing the syndrome (Pellock et al., 2008). There is no sleep–wake cycling with the suppression-burst pattern. The tonic spasms associated with the syndrome occur during a period of suppression as opposed to bursts (Cloherty et al., 2008).

NEUROPSYCHOLOGICAL/CLINICAL PRESENTATION

Ohtahara's syndrome is an epileptic encephalopathy with the presence of a serious underlying disorder with frequent seizures, abnormal EEG patterns, and mental deterioration with the persistence of the seizures. There is a high mortality rate with the incidence of death occurring primarily in infancy but can occur up to adolescence (Pellock et al., 2008). Those who survive Ohtahara's syndrome may suffer from severe mental retardation, may be quadriplegic and/or bedridden, and tend to have frequent infantile spasms (Cloherty et al., 2008; Pellock et al., 2008). Survivors also commonly experience psychomotor retardation (Shorvon, Fish, Pericca & Dodson, 2004). In about half of the cases reported, the seizures subside by school age, but the prognosis is still very poor (Jallon, 2003).

DIAGNOSIS

Detailed neuroimaging is always necessary when Ohtahara's syndrome is suspected (Wyllie et al., 2004). The syndrome is distinguished by tonic spasms, with or without clustering, that appear within the 1st months of life and a suppression-burst pattern in EEG (Yamatogi & Ohtahara, 2002). The suppression burst pattern shown through the EEG is vital to the diagnosis of the syndrome (Pellock et al., 2008).

TREATMENT

With Ohtahara's syndrome, the developmental prognosis is poor with profound physical and mental impairment being present. For survivors, the syndrome evolves into West's syndrome and then to LSG (Pellock et al., 2008; Yamatogi & Ohtahara, 2002). Although the seizures are typically resistant to therapy, some with Ohtahara's syndrome have been treated with adrenocorticotropic hormone (ACTH) therapy. ACTH therapy has been partially effective in some cases (Pellock et al., 2008). Other medications and vitamin therapies have been tried with little success (Pellock et al., 2008). Due to the difficulty of operating on young infants, very little research has examined the usefulness of surgical interventions for Ohtahara's syndrome. Of the surgical cases presented, some evidence of seizure relief after surgery has been shown (Hmaimess et al., 2005). The seizures associated with the syndrome, for most cases, are resistant to therapy (Shorvon et al., 2004).

Jessi H. Robbins
Charles Golden

Binnie, C., Cooper, R., Mauguiere, F., Osselton, J., Prior, P., & Tedman, B. (2003). *Clinical neurophysiology: EEG, paediatric neurophysiology, special techniques and applications.* Boston: Elsevier.

Cloherty, J. P., Eichenwald, E. C., & Stark, A. R. (2008). *Manual of neonatal care*. Philadelphia: Lippincott Williams & Wilkins.

Hmaimess, G., Raftopoulos, C., Kadhim, H., Nassogne, M., Ghariani, S., Tourtchaninoff, M., et al. (2005). Impact of early hemispherotomy in a case of Ohtahara syndrome with left parieto-occipital megalencephaly, *Seizure, 14,* 439–442.

Jallon, P. (2003). *Prognosis of epilepsies*. Montreal: John Libbey Eurotext.

Kato, M., Saitoh, S. Kamei, A., Shiraishi, H., Ueda, Y., Aka-saka, M., et al. (2007). A longer polyalanine expansion mutation in the ARX gene causes early infantile epileptic encephalopathy with suppression burst pattern (Ohtahara syndrome), *The American Journal of Human Genetics, 81,* 361–366.

Niedermeyer, E., & Lopes da Silva, F. (2004). *Electroencephalography*. Philadelphia: Lippincott Williams & Wilkins.

Pellock, J., Dodson, W., Bourgeois, B., Sankar, B., & Nordli, D. (2008). *Pediatric epilepsy*. New York: Demos Medical Publishing.

Shorvon, S., Fish, D., Perucca, E., & Dodson, W. (2004). *The treatment of epilepsy*. Malden, MA: Blackwell Publishing.

Wyllie, E., Gupta, A., & Lachhwani, D. (2004). *The treatment of epilepsy: Principles and practice*. Philadelphia: Lippincott Williams & Wilkins.

Yamatogi, Y., & Ohtahara, S. (2002). Early-infantile epileptic encephalopathy with suppression-bursts, Ohtahara syndrome; its overview referring to our 16 cases, *Brain and Development, 24,* 13–23.

OLIVOPONTOCEREBELLAR ATROPHY

DESCRIPTION

Dejerine and Thomas coined the term olivopontocerebellar atrophy (OPCA) to describe the pathology of a patient who presented with adult-onset progressive cerebellar ataxia. The use of the term OPCA was intended to describe the neuronal degeneration in the cerebellum, pontine nuclei, and inferior olivary nucleus. The patient described by Dejerine and Thomas was over 50 years of age and presented ataxia of gait, dysarthria, impassive face, hypertonia, hyperreflexia, and urinary incontinence. An autopsy revealed an advanced degeneration of the basis pontis, inferior olives, middle cerebellar peduncles, and inferior cerebellar peduncles. Severe atrophy of the Purkinje cells was also noted, with greater atrophy in the cerebellar hemispheres than in the vermis (see Berciano, Bosech, Perez-Ramos, & Wenning, 2006).

The disorder has no definitive treatment, and because motor disruption is a primary feature of OPCA, many of these patients eventually become confined to a bed or wheelchair (Caplan, 1984). The clinical presentation may include a number of different signs and symptoms, including dysphagia (Berciano, 1982; Testa, Tiranti, & Girotti, 2002), respiratory stridor from vocal cord paralysis (Comabella, Montalban, Serena, Lozano, & Codina, 1996; Kneisley & Rederich, 1990; Sundar, Sharma, Arekar, Vimal, & Yeolekar, 2003), dementia, especially later in the disease process (Berciano, 1982; Feher, Inbody, Nolan, & Pirozzolo, 1988), urinary incontinence (Berciano, 1982; Caplan, 1984), and sleep disturbances (Comabella et al., 1996; Kneisley & Rederich, 1990; Tachibana et al., 1995). The predominant signs include progressive gait and limb cerebellar ataxia and dysarthria (Berciano, 1982; Choi, Lee, Kim, & Choi, 1988; Manto, Godaux, Hildebrand, van Naemen, & Jacquy, 1997), with the extrapyramidal and cerebellar signs usually beginning in the lower extremities and subsequently progressing to the upper extremities (Adams & Victor, 1993). Pyramidal signs such as bilateral extensor plantar response, hyperactive deep tendon reflex, and spasticity due to pyramidal tract dysfunction are present early in the course of the disease (Berciano, 1982). Furthermore, position sense (Gatev, Thomas, Lou, Lim, & Hallett, 1996) and vibratory function (Uzunov, Kutchoukov, & Kolchev, 1991) are also reduced, likely secondary to neuropathy.

Greenfield (1954) divided the pathology of ataxias into six different categories, which were aggregated into two different forms, including sporadic (Dejerine–Thomas type) and familial (Menzel type). The sporadic type is more common of the two forms and typically has a later age of onset (Adams & Victor, 1993). Also, the sporadic form does not typically present with nystagmus, optic atrophy, retinal degeneration, ophthalmoplegia, or urinary incontinence (Adams & Victor, 1993), although there are exceptions (Berciano, 1982). A number of other different nosologies have been proposed to subtype and differentiate the various forms of OPCA, each associated with advantages and disadvantages. Following a review of several nosological classifications, Berciano (1982) likened OPCA to a variable progressive cerebellar-plus syndrome, concluding that OPCA is a pathological label that is associated with lesions at all levels of the CNS.

NEUROPATHOLOGY/PATHOPHYSIOLOGY

The term OPCA includes the common sporadic forms as well as the more uncommon genetic forms. Associations between the genetic forms and all three major inheritance patterns have been described in the literature, including autosomal dominant (Choi et al., 1988; Konigsmark & Weiner, 1970), autosomal recessive (Konigsmark & Weiner, 1970), and X-linked (Lutz, Bodensteiner, Schaefer, & Gay, 1989). The sporadic type of OPCA is considered by many to be a subgroup of multiple system atrophy (MSA; Gilman & Quinn, 1996; Penney, 1995; Rinne et al., 1995). Generally, the OPCAs are progressive neurodegenerative conditions. The typical age of onset for the familial form is 28 years and for the sporadic form, the age of onset is 49 years. The duration of OPCA is approximately 15 years for the familial form and 6 years for the sporadic form (Berciano, 1982). The etiology of OPCA is not well-known, but the sporadic forms have been shown to involve abnormalities of alpha-synuclein (Jellinger, 2003; Yoshida, 2007). Also, specific genes have been identified in the familial form, but the precise manner in which these genes exert their influence is not well-known (Burk et al., 1996; Koeppen, 1998). As with other forms of MSA, the five histological features include glial cytoplasmic inclusions, neuronal cytoplasmic inclusions, neuronal nuclear inclusions, glial nuclear inclusions, and neuropil threads (Lowe, Lennox, & Leigh, 1997). Of these, glial cytoplasmic inclusions are the most relevant.

Atrophy predominates in the cerebellum, middle cerebellar peduncles, and the pons. On autopsy, a gray-green discoloration of the putamen can be often seen along with general atrophy of this structure. Also seen is a loss of pigmentation in the substantia nigra and locus coeruleus (Lowe, Lennox, & Leigh, 1997).

NEUROPSYCHOLOGICAL/CLINICAL PRESENTATION

OPCA is primarily a motor-based dysfunction, characterized by cerebellar ataxia; research has also supported changes in memory, cognitive, and emotional functioning. However, the research regarding neuropsychological functioning in OPCA is far from equivocal. Some investigators have reported not only deficits in tasks with motor components but also mild deficits in cognitive functioning (Berent et al., 2002). Brandt, Leroi, O'Hearn, Rosenblatt, and Margolis (2004) reported that patients with cerebellar degeneration were impaired on tests of executive functioning. Similarly, Arroyo-Anllo and Botez-Marquard (1998) found that OPCA patients evidenced lower scores than normal controls on several tests purported to be sensitive to frontal lobe functioning, including hand sequencing, verbal reasoning, and proverb interpretation. Additional deficits were noted with visuoconstructional abilities and visuospatial immediate memory. Other investigators have also reported deficits with

memory and frontal lobe functioning in patients with OPCA (Kish et al., 1988). Botez-Marquard and Botez (1997) reported a pattern of neuropsychological deficits in patients with OPCA that resembles a "subcortical" pattern. Specifically, OPCA patients exhibited impaired executive functioning, slower speed of information processing, and difficulties with memory retrieval. Additional findings included deficits with visuospatial organization and working memory and difficulty with abstract thinking.

Conversely, Moretti et al. (2002) found that OPCA patients, as compared with healthy controls, did not exhibit reduced abstraction, problem-solving abilities, or performance on memory tasks. Rather, they reported that OPCA patients evidenced impaired reading and writing execution. The reason for this discrepancy in research findings regarding the memory and cognitive functioning in OPCA patients is not entirely known. One possibility includes the emotional changes that may accompany this disease. Berent et al. (1990) found that OPCA patients experienced greater depression, anxiety, and subjective emotional distress than normal controls. When education and motor dysfunction were statistically controlled in the analyses, no differences were found between the OPCA patients and normal controls on measures of cognitive and intellectual functioning. Thus, these investigators concluded that OPCA patients may appear to have deficits with memory and cognitive functioning but that these deficits may be due to their motor and emotional functioning. However, it seems worth noting that depression also follows a classic "subcortical" pattern of findings on neuropsychological assessment. Further research will need to be conducted to determine whether the neuropsychological deficits seen in patients with OPCA are due to the neuropathological process of the disease or to emotional changes. This might be accomplished by using scores on measures of depression and anxiety as covariates in statistical analyses or by matching OPCA patients with healthy controls on these variables.

DIAGNOSIS

A number of investigations have examined structural brain changes associated with OPCA. CT scans and MRI have emerged as important tools in identifying the brainstem and cerebellar atrophy that is characteristic of OPCA (Klockgether, Faiss, Poremba, & Dichgans, 1990; Ramos, Quintana, Diez, Leno, & Berciano, 1987; Savoiardo et al., 1990). Not surprisingly, typical findings from CT scans include atrophy of the cerebellum and pons (García de la Rocha,

Moreno Martínez, Garrido Carrión, Fernández, & Martín, 1988; Savoiardo et al., 1983). CT scans conducted in the first year following the onset of cerebellar symptoms may be read as normal, as serial scans are then required to detect infratentorial atrophy (Ormerod et al., 1994). Also, mild cerebellar and pontine atrophy may be necessary but not sufficient for a diagnosis of OPCA. However, the diagnosis becomes more definitive when combined with signal abnormalities in structures that are known to degenerate in OPCA (Savoiardo et al., 1997). Middle cerebellar peduncle diameter seems to be the most sensitive indicator to differentiate OPCA from cortical cerebellar atrophy (Okamoto et al., 2003; Wüllner, Klockgether, Petersen, Naegele, & Dichgans, 1993) and striatonigral degeneration (Naka et al., 2002). Typical findings from MRI investigations have included pancerebellar and brainstem atrophy, flattening of the pons, an enlarged fourth ventricle and cerebellopontine angle, and demyelination of the transverse pontine fibers (Berciano et al., 2006; Giuliani, Chiaramoni, Foschi, & Terziani, 1992; Huang, Tuason, Wu, & Plaitakis, 1993; Savoiardo et al., 1990; Sun, Tanaka, Kondo, Hirai, & Ishihara, 1994). A characteristic "hot cross bun" sign is also seen, resulting from the demyelination of the transverse pontine fibers (Berciano et al., 2006).

Functional imaging may also assist in diagnostic determination. The PET scans of patients with OPCA evidence reduced glucose metabolism rate within the vermis, cerebellar hemispheres, and brainstem (Gilman et al., 1988), including the pons (Sun et al., 1994). Gilman et al. (1995) reported significantly reduced local cerebral blood flow in the cerebellum as well as decreased local cerebral glucose metabolism rate in the cerebellum, brainstem, cerebral cortex, basal ganglia, and thalamus. Other investigators have reported reduced cerebellar hemispheric blood flow and oxygen metabolism in patients with OPCA as compared with normal controls (Yamaguchi et al., 1994).

TREATMENT

The treatment of OPCA largely comprises pharmacological intervention, although one investigation has reported successful treatment with electrostimulation of the spinal cord (Dooley, Sharkey, Keller, & Kasprak, 1978). A number of different medications have been used to treat OPCA. Botez et al. (1999) reported immediate and long-term benefits in motor functioning with amantadine hydrochloride. Subcutaneous lisuride infusion has also been reported to improve motor functioning in patients with OPCA (Heinz, Wöhrle, Schöls, Klotz, Kuhn, & Przuntek, 1992). Carbidopa-levodopa was reported to provide

relief in a patient with OPCA who had developed respiratory distress and inspiratory stridor (Schiffman & Golbe, 1992). A recent review of the literature by Trujillo-Martín, Serrano-Aguilar, Monton-Alvarez, and Carrillo-Fumero (2009) supported the efficacy of 5-hydroxytryptophan in treating patients with OPCA. However, they also found a paucity of research regarding the effectiveness of physical rehabilitation and psychological interventions. However, Landers, Adams, Acosta, and Fox (2009) reported the case of a patient with OPCA who benefited from undergoing 12 weeks of gait and balance training. Certainly, given that these patients have been found to experience changes in mood and anxiety further research will need to be conducted to examine effective treatments for these behavioral symptoms. Furthermore, research regarding the effective treatment of mood and anxiety in OPCA patients will assist in determining whether the neuropsychological effects of OPCA are due more to the underlying neuropathological processes or to changes in mood and anxiety.

Paul S. Foster
Valeria Drago

Adams, R. D., & Victor, M. (1993). *Principles of neurology* (5th ed.). New York: McGraw Hill.

Arroyo-Anllo, E. M., & Botez-Marquard, T. (1998). Neurobehavioral dimensions of olivopontocerebellar atrophy. *Journal of Clinical and Experimental Neuropsychology, 20*, 52–59.

Berciano, J. (1982). Olivopontocerebellar atrophy: A review of 117 cases. *Journal of the Neurological Sciences, 53*, 253–272.

Berciano, J., Boesch, S., Perez-Ramos, J. M., & Wenning, G. K. (2006). Olivopontocerebellar atrophy: Toward a better nosological definition. *Movement Disorders, 21*, 1607–1613.

Berent, S., Giordani, B., Gilman, S., Junck, L., Lehtinen, S., Markel, D. S., et al. (1990). Neuropsychological changes in olivopontocerebellar atrophy. *Archives of Neurology, 47*, 997–1001.

Berent, S., Giordani, B., Gilman, S., Trask, C. L., Little, R. J., Johanns, J. R., et al. (2002). Patterns of neuropsychological performance in multiple system atrophy compared to sporadic and hereditary olivopontocerebellar atrophy. *Brain and Cognition, 50*, 194–206.

Botez, M. I., Botez-Marquard, T., Elie, R., Le Marec, N., Pedraza, O. L., & Lalonde, R. (1999). Amantadine hydrochloride treatment in olivopontocerebellar atrophy: A long-term follow-up study. *European Neurology, 41*, 212–215.

Botez-Marquard, T., & Botez, M. I. (1997). Olivopontocerebellar atrophy and Friedreich's ataxia: Neuropsychological consequences of bilateral versus unilateral cerebellar lesions. *International Review of Neurobiology, 41*, 387–410.

Brandt, J., Leroi, I., O'Hearn, E., Rosenblatt, A., & Margolis, R. L. (2004). Cognitive impairments in cerebellar degeneration: A comparison with Huntington's disease. *Journal of Neuropsychiatry and Clinical Neurosciences, 16,* 176–184.

Burk, K., Abele, M., Fetter, M., Dichgans, J., Skalej, M., Laccone, F., et al. (1996). Autosomal dominant cerebellar ataxia type I clinical features and MRI in families with SCA1, SCA2, and SCA3. *Brain, 119,* 1497–1505.

Caplan, L. R. (1984). Clinical features of sporadic (Dejerine-Thomas) olivopontocerebellar atrophy. *Advances in Neurology, 41,* 21–224.

Choi, I. S., Lee, M. S., Kim, W. T., & Choi, K. K. (1988). Olivopontocerebellar atrophy. *Yonsei Medical Journal, 29,* 233–238.

Comabella, M., Montalban, X., Serena, J., Lozano, M., & Codina, A. (1996). Early vocal cord paralysis in olivopontocerebellar atrophy. *Journal of Neurology, 243,* 670–671.

Dooley, D. M., Sharkey, J., Keller, W., & Kasprak, M. (1978). Treatment of demyelinating and degenerative diseases by electro stimulation of the spinal cord. *Medical Progress Through Technology, 13,* 1–14.

Feher, E. P., Inbody, S. B., Nolan, B., & Pirozzolo, F. J. (1988). Other neurologic diseases with dementia as a sequela. *Clinics in Geriatric Medicine, 4,* 799–814.

García de la Rocha, M. L., Moreno Martínez, J. M., Garrido Carrión, A., Fernández, P. M., & Martín Araguz, A. (1988). Present criteria for the diagnosis of in vivo of olivopontocerebellar atrophy. *Acta Neurologica Scandinavica, 77,* 234–238.

Gatev, P., Thomas, S., Lou, J. S., Lim, M., & Hallett, M. (1996). Effects of diminished and conflicting sensory information on balance in patients with cerebellar deficits. *Movement Disorders, 11,* 654–664.

Gilman, S., Markel, D. S., Koeppe, R. A., Junck, L., Kluin, K. J., Gebarski, S. S., et al. (1988). Cerebellar and brainstem hypometabolism in olivopontocerebellar atrophy detected with positron emission tomography. *Annals of Neurology, 23,* 223–230.

Gilman, S., & Quinn, N. P. (1996). The relationship of multiple system atrophy to sporadic olivopontocerebellar atrophy and other forms of idiopathic late-onset cerebellar atrophy. *Neurology, 46,* 1197–1199.

Gilman, S., St Laurent, R. T., Koeppe, R. A., Junck, L., Kluin, K. J., & Lohman, M. (1995). A comparison of cerebral blood flow and glucose metabolism in olivopontocerebellar atrophy using PET. *Neurology, 45,* 1345–1352.

Giuliani, G., Chiaramoni, L., Foschi, N., & Terziani, S. (1992). The role of MRI in the diagnosis of olivopontocerebellar atrophy. *Italian Journal of Neurological Sciences, 13,* 151–156.

Greenfield, J. G. (1954). *The spinocerebellar degenerations.* Oxford: Blackwell.

Heinz, A., Wöhrle, J., Schöls, L., Klotz, P., Kuhn, W., & Przuntek, H. (1992). Continuous subcutaneous lisuride infusion in OPCA. *Journal of Neural Transmission General Section, 90,* 145–150.

Huang, Y. P., Tuason, M. Y., Wu, T., & Plaitakis, A. (1993). MRI and CT features of cerebellar degeneration. *Journal of the Formosan Medical Association, 92,* 494–508.

Jellinger, K. A. (2003). Neuropathological spectrum of synucleinopathies. *Movement Disorders, 18,* S2–S12.

Kish, S. J., el-Awar, M., Schut, L., Leach, L., Oscar-Berman, M., & Freedman, M. (1988). Cognitive deficits in olivopontocerebellar atrophy: Implications for the cholinergic hypothesis of Alzheimer's dementia. *Annals of Neurology, 24,* 200–206.

Klockgether, T., Faiss, J., Poremba, M., & Dichgans, J. (1990). The development of infratentorial atrophy in patients with idiopathic cerebellar ataxia of late onset: A CT study. *Journal of Neurology, 237,* 420–423.

Kneisley, L. W., & Rederich, G. J. (1990). Nocturnal stridor in olivopontocerebellar atrophy. *Sleep, 13,* 362–368.

Koeppen, A. H. (1998). The hereditary ataxias. *Journal of Neuropathology and Experimental Neurology, 57,* 531–543.

Konigsmark, B. W., & Weiner, L. P. (1970). The olivopontocerebellar atrophies: A review. *Medicine (Baltimore), 49,* 227–241.

Landers, M., Adams, M., Acosta, K., & Fox, A. (2009). Challenge-oriented gait and balance training in sporadic olivopontocerebellar atrophy: A case study. *Journal of Neurologic Physical Therapy, 33,* 160–168.

Lowe, J., Lennox, G., & Leigh, P. N. (1997). Disorders of movement and system degenerations. In D. I. Graham & P. L. Lantos (Eds.), *Greenfield's neuropsychology* (6th ed.). New York: Oxford University Press.

Lutz, R., Bodensteiner, J., Schaefer, B., & Gay, C. (1989). X-linked olivopontocerebellar atrophy. *Clinical Genetics, 35,* 417–422.

Manto, M., Godaux, E., Hildebrand, J., van Naemen, J., & Jacquy, J. (1997). Analysis of single-joint rapid movements in patients with sporadic olivopontocerebellar atrophy. *Journal of the Neurological Sciences, 151,* 169–176.

Moretti, R., Torre, P., Antonello, R. M., Carraro, N., Zambito-Marsala, S., Ukmar, M. J., et al. (2002). Peculiar aspects of reading and writing performances in patients with olivopontocerebellar atrophy. *Perceptual and Motor Skills, 94,* 67–694.

Naka, H., Ohshita, T., Murata, Y., Imon, Y., Mimori, Y., & Nakamura, S. (2002). Characteristic MRI findings in multiple system atrophy: Comparison of the three subtypes. *Neuroradiology, 44,* 204–209.

Okamoto, K., Tokiguchi, S., Furusawa, T., Ishikawa, K., Quardery, A. F., Shinbo, S., et al. (2003). MR features of diseases involving bilateral middle cerebellar peduncles. *American Journal of Neuroradiology, 24,* 1946–1954.

OP

Ormerod, I. E., Harding, A. E., Miller, D. H., Johnson, G., MacManus, D., du Boulay, E. P., et al. (1994). Magnetic resonance imaging in degenerative ataxic disorders. *Journal of Neurology, Neurosurgery, and Psychiatry, 57,* 51–57.

Penney, J. B. (1995). Multiple system atrophy and nonfamilial olivopontocerebellar atrophy are the same disease. *Annals of Neurology, 37,* 553–554.

Ramos, A., Quintana, F., Diez, C., Leno, C., & Berciano, J. (1987). CT findings in pinocerebellar degeneration. *American Journal of Neuroradiology, 8,* 635–640.

Rinne, J. O., Burn, D. J., Mathias, C. J., Quinn, N. P., Marsden, C. D., & Brooks, D. J. (1995). Positron emission tomography studies on the dopaminergic system and striatal opioid binding in the olivopontocerebellar atrophy variant of multiple system atrophy. *Annals of Neurology, 37,* 568–573.

Savoiardo, M., Bracchi, M., Passerini, A., Visciani, A., Di Donato, S., & Cocchini, F. (1983). Computed tomography of olivopontocerebellar degeneration. *American Journal of Neuroradiology, 4,* 509–512.

Savoiardo, M., Grisoli, M., Girotti, F., Testa, D., & Caraceni, T. (1997). MRI in sporadic olivopontocerebellar atrophy and striatonigral degeneration. *Neurology, 48,* 790–791.

Savoiardo, M., Strada, L., Girotti, F., Zimmerman, R. A., Grisoli, M., Testa, D., & Petrillo, R. (1990). Olivopontocerebellar atrophy: MR diagnosis and relationship to multisystem atrophy. *Radiology, 174,* 693–696.

Schiffman, P. L., & Golbe, L. I. (1992). Upper airway dysfunction in olivopontocerebellar atrophy. *Chest, 102,* 1291–1292.

Sun, X., Tanaka, M., Kondo, S., Hirai, S., & Ishihara, T. (1994). Reduced cerebellar blood flow and oxygen metabolism in spinocerebellar degeneration: A combined PET and MRI study. *Journal of Neurology, 241,* 295–300.

Sundar, U., Sharma, A., Arekar, M. A., Vimal, P., & Yeolekar, M. E. (2003). Olivopontocerebellar atrophy presenting with stridor. *Journal of the Association of Physicians of India, 51,* 813–815.

Tachibana, N., Kimura, K., Kitajima, K., Nagamine, T., Kimura, J., & Shibasaki, H. (1995). REM sleep without atonia at early stage of sporadic olivopontocerebellar atrophy. *Journal of the Neurological Sciences, 132,* 28–34.

Testa, D., Tiranti, V., & Girotti, F. (2002). Unusual association of sporadic olivopontocerebellar atrophy and motor neuron disease. *Neurological Sciences, 23,* 243–245.

Trujillo-Martín, M. M., Serrano-Aguilar, P., Monton-Alvarez, F., & Carrillo-Fumero, R. (2009). Effectiveness and safety of treatments for degenerative ataxias: A systematic review. *Movement Disorders, 24,* 1111–1124.

Uzunov, N., Kutchoukov, M., & Kolchev, C. (1991). CT scan and threshold vibrometry in the diagnosis of spinocerebellar degenerations. *Italian Journal of the Neurological Sciences, 12,* 175–179.

Wüllner, U., Klockgether, T., Petersen, D., Naegele, T., & Dichgans, J. (1993). Magnetic resonance imaging in hereditary and idiopathic ataxia. *Neurology, 43,* 318–325.

Yamaguchi, S., Fukuyama, H., Ogawa, M., Yamauchi, H., Harada, K., Nakamura, S., et al. (1994). Olivopontocerebellar atrophy studied by positron emission tomography and magnetic resonance imaging. *Journal of the Neurological Sciences, 125,* 56–61.

Yoshida, M. (2007). Multiple system atrophy: Alpha-synuclein and neuronal degeneration. *Neuropathology, 27,* 484–493.

OPSOCLONUS–MYOCLONUS SYNDROME

DESCRIPTION

Opsoclonus–myoclonus syndrome (OMS) is a rare paraneoplastic syndrome most commonly observed in relation to viral infection affecting the brainstem. It has been noted across the life span, though it is most commonly discussed in pediatric populations with highest rates reported prior to age 2 (Rudnick et al., 2001). Although viral infection of the brainstem is the most common etiology for OMS, it has also been observed in relation to neuroblastomas. In fact, 50% of all children presenting with OMS have a neuroblastoma (Kramer & Pranzatelli, 2005; Rudnik et al., 2001) even though only 2% of children with neuroblastomas develop OMS. In adults, opsoclonus–myoclonus has been associated with breast and small cell lung carcinoma (Posner, 1991).

OMS is associated with an acute onset of myoclonus (i.e., small, frequent, and multifocal jerks of the muscles), opsoclonus (rapid conjugate eye movements that are irregular and involuntary), and ataxia. In children, a rapid loss of motor control and speech, and regression from developmental milestones are commonly noted. Retrospective investigations have suggested that an increased irritability and severe disturbances of sleep precede the hallmark feature of myoclonus and opsoclonus.

OMS has also been referred to as opsoclonus–myoclonus–ataxia, paraneoplastic opsoclonus–myoclonus–ataxia, myoclonic encephalopathy of infants, dancing eyes–dancing feet syndrome, and dancing eyes syndrome.

NEUROPATHOLOGY/PATHOPHYSIOLOGY

Neuropathological correlates of OMS vary. As previously suggested, the primary basis of the presentation is believed to be associated with an immune-mediated antitumor host response, which affects neural cells, with primary susceptibility of those in the cerebellum (Kramer & Pranzatelli, 2005). Some patients are relatively free of identifiable abnormalities, likely due to mild viral infection of the brainstem that is not yet causing anatomical or cellular changes (Ridley, Kennard, & Scholtz 1987). When alterations are seen, they are primarily noted in the cerebellum and brainstem. Loss of Purkinje cells, neuronal loss in the olivary neurons of the brainstem, astrogliosis, and inflammatory infiltration of the brainstem may all be observed (Posner, 1991; Ridley et al., 1987).

An anti-Ri antibody with reactivity to proteins expressed in neuronal nuclei and primary tumor cells may be observed in the serum and CSF (Luque, Furneaux, & Ferzinger, 1991). Similarly, anti-Hu antibodies may also be observed in this same manner, but far less frequently. Anti-Ri antibodies are more commonly noted when the syndrome arises from breast carcinoma, although it has also been seen in gynecological neoplasms (Posner, 1991). Anti-Hu antibodies are often associated with small cell lung cancer. CSF B-cell expansion is a biomarker of disease activity and has been correlated with the presentations clinical severity (Pranzatelli et al., 2006). Still, others have failed to identify associated autoantibodies (Antunes et al., 2000; Blaes et al., 2005; Korfei et al., 2005; Pranzatelli et al., 2004).

NEUROPSYCHOLOGICAL/CLINICAL PRESENTATION

The classic constellation of OMS comprises the subacute onset of jerky eye movements with involuntary, chaotic saccades, and arrhythmic-action myoclonus (Caviness, Forsyth, Layton, & McPhee, 1995). The opsoclonus presents as deficits in ocular motility characterized by spontaneous, arrhythmic, large-amplitude conjugate saccades occurring in all directions of gaze without saccadic interval (Pistoia, Conson, & Sara, 2010). The myoclonus presents as small, frequent, and multifocal jerks of the muscles. However, beyond these features, additional symptoms are known to present. Dysarthria, ataxia, and cortical dysfunction may develop (Pranzatelli, 1992). Other common symptoms include difficulties in ambulation, frequent falls, vertigo, nausea, vomiting, dizziness, blurry vision, and dysphasia (Pistoia et al., 2010).

Over the long term, symptoms may persist, whether associated with neuroblastoma or a paraneoplastic origin (Hayward et al., 2001; Mitchell et al., 2005; Plantaz et al., 2000; Tate, Allison, Pranzatelli, & Verhulst, 2005). These studies as a collective group suggest that ataxia, speech and language

abnormalities, behavioral problems (e.g., irritability and explosiveness), sleep disturbances, inattention, and learning disabilities may remain over the long term without correlation to treatment response. Executive dysfunction, particularly planning, verbal fluency, and working memory, visuospatial organization, visuospatial memory, and personality changes may be seen (Levisohn, Cronin-Golomb, & Schmahmann, 2000; Riva & Giorgi, 2000; Schmahmann & Sherman, 1998). In all, roughly 60% have persisting cognitive deficits.

Variability is seen across outcomes in terms of the percentage of children who demonstrate these residual deficits. What is consistently noted is that multiple relapses are associated with poorer clinical outcomes (Mitchell et al., 2005). In reality, only 12% to 38% of children experience complete recovery (Plantaz et al., 2000).

DIAGNOSIS

Diagnosis is clinically based and corresponds with the symptom profiles exhibited by individuals. Review of medical history is also important given the relationship between the presentation and history of small-cell lung cancer, and, to a lesser extent, gynecological cancers.

MRI of the brain is essential to evaluate for the presence of a neuroblastoma. PET-CT and bone scans may be employed to evaluate for potential metastatic disease related to a history of the small-cell lung cancer or gynecological cancer.

CSF analysis may be undertaken to evaluate for the presence of anti-Ri and anti-Hu antibodies in the serum of the CSF (Luque, Furneaux, & Ferzinger, 1991; Posner, 1991). As previously noted, CSF B-cell expansion is a biomarker of disease activity; thus, its evaluation can be useful for diagnosis. Failure to find such autoantibodies does not rule out the presentation.

TREATMENT

There are no standard protocols or guidelines for the treatment of OMS. In children with neuroblastoma, opsoclonus–myoclonus is approached with treatment of the tumor with chemotherapy and with prednisone, corticotropin, intravenous immunoglobulin (IVIg), and/or rituximab. However, these treatments themselves are associated with high toxicity and adverse event risks.

In adults, paraneoplastic opsoclonus–myoclonus may be treated with IVIg and immunosuppression. Cyclophosphamide, methylprednisolone, and plasmapheresis have also demonstrated utility in this

OP

group as have some of the agents used in children (e.g., prednisone, corticotropin, and rituximab). Gabapentin has also shown some efficacy (Pistoia & Sara, 2009). Better neurological outcomes are seen with prompt tumor treatment. Patient with sleep disturbances may respond to trazodone. Children with OMS associated with neuroblastoma tend to have a better prognosis in terms of symptom resolution as the clinical features dissipate with treatment of the tumor (Telander, Smithson, & Groover, 1989).

Chad A. Noggle

Antunes, N. L., Khakoo, Y., Matthay, K. K., Seeger, R. C., Stram, D. O., Gerstner, E., et al. (2000). Antineuronal antibodies in patients with neuroblastoma and paraneoplastic opsoclonus-myoclonus. *Journal of Pediatric Hematology/Oncology, 22,* 315–320.

Blaes, F., Fuhlhuber, V., Korfei, M., Tschernatsch, M., Behnisch, W., Rostasy, K., et al. (2005). Surface-binding autoantibodies to cerebellar neurons in opsoclonus syndrome. *Annals of Neurology, 58,* 313–317.

Caviness, J. N., Forsyth, P. A., Layton, D. D., & McPhee, T. J. (1995). The movement disorder of adult opsoclonus. *Movement Disorders, 10,* 22–27.

Hayward, K., Jeremy, R. J., Jenkins, S., Barkovich, A. J., Gultekin, S. H., Kramer, J., et al. (2001). Long-term neurobehavioral outcomes in children with neuroblastoma and opsoclonus-myoclonus-ataxia syndrome: Relationship to MRI findings and anti-neuronal antibodies. *Journal of Pediatrics, 139,* 552–559.

Korfei, M., Fuhlhuber, V., Schmidt-Woll, T., Kaps, M., Preissner, K. T., & Blaes, F. (2005). Functional characterisation of autoantibodies from patients with pediatric opsoclonus-myoclonus-syndrome. *Journal of Neuroimmunology, 170,* 150–157.

Kramer, K., & Pranzatelli, M. R. (2005). Management of neurologic complications. In N. K. V. Cheung & S. L. Cohn (Eds.), *Neuroblastoma* (pp. 213–222). Berlin: Springer-Verlag.

Levisohn, L., Cronin-Golomb, A., & Schmahmann, J. D. (2000). Neuropsychological consequences of cerebellar tumour resection in children: Cerebellar cognitive affective syndrome in a paediatric population. *Brain, 123,* 1041–1050.

Luque, F. A., Furneaux, H. M., Ferzinger, R. (1991). Anti-Ri: An antibody associated with paraneoplastic opsoclonus in breast cancer. *Annals of Neurology, 29,* 241–251.

Mitchell, W. G., Brumm, V. L., Azen, C. G., Patterson, K. E., Aller, S. K., & Rodriguez, J. (2005). Longitudinal neurodevelopmental evaluation of children with opsoclonus-ataxia. *Pediatrics, 116,* 901–907.

Pistoia, F., Conson, M., Sara, M. (2010). Opsoclonus-myoclonus syndrome in patients with locked-in syndrome: a therapeutic porthole with gabapentin. *Mayo Clinic Proceedings, 85*(6), 527–531.

Pistoia, K., & Sara, M. (2009). Gabapentin therapy for ocular opsoclonus-myoclonus restores eye movement communication in a patient with a locked-in syndrome. *Neurorehabilitation and Neural Repair, 24,* 493–494.

Plantaz, D., Michon, J., Valteau-Couanet, D., Coze, C., Chastagner, P., Bergeron, C., et al. (2000). Opsoclonus-myoclonus syndrome associated with non-metastatic neuroblastoma. Long-term survival. Study of the French Society of Pediatric Oncologists. *Archives of Pediatrics, 7,* 621–628.

Posner, J. B. (1991). Paraneoplastic syndromes. *Neurology Clinics, 9,* 919–936

Pranzatelli, M. R. (1992). The neurobiology of the opsoclonus-myoclonus syndrome. *Clinical Neuropharmacology, 15,* 186–228.

Pranzatelli, M. R., Tate, E. D., Travelstead, A. L., Barbosa, J., Bergamini, R. A., Civitello, L., et al. (2006). Rituximab (anti-CD 20) adjunctive therapy for opsoclonus-myoclonus syndrome. *Journal of Pediatric Hematology Oncology, 28,* 585–593.

Pranzatelli, M. R., Travelstead, A. L., Tate, E. D., Allison, T. J., Moticka, E. J., Franz, D. N., et al. (2004). B- and T-cell markers in opsoclonus-myoclonus syndrome: Immunophenotyping of CSF lymphocytes. *Neurology, 62,* 1526–1532.

Ridley, A., Kennard, C., Scholtz, C. L. (1987). Omnipause neurons in two cases of opsoclonus associated with oat cell carcinoma of the lung. *Brain, 110,* 1699–1709.

Riva, D., & Giorgi, C. (2000). The cerebellum contributes to higher functions during development: Evidence from a series of children surgically treated for posterior fossa tumours. *Brain, 123,* 1051–1061.

Rudnick, E., Khakoo, Y., Antunes, N. L., Seeger, R. C., Brodeur, G. M., Shimada, H., et al. (2001). Opsoclonus-myoclonus-ataxia syndrome in neuroblastoma: Clinical outcome and antineuronal antibodies—a report from the Children's Cancer Group Study. *Medical and Pediatric Oncology, 36,* 612–622

Schmahmann, J. D., & Sherman, J. C. (1998). The cerebellar cognitive affective syndrome. *Brain, 121,* 561–579.

Tate, E. D., Allison, T. J., Pranzatelli, M. R., & Verhulst, S. J. (2005). Neuroepidemiologic trends in 105 US cases of pediatric opsoclonus-myoclonus syndrome. *Journal of Pediatric Oncology Nursing, 22,* 8–19.

Telander, R. L., Smithson, W. A., Groover, R. V. (1989). Clinical outcome in children with cerebellar encephalopathy and neuroblastoma. *Journal of Pediatric Surgery, 24,* 11–14.

PARANEOPLASTIC SYNDROMES

DESCRIPTION

Paraneoplastic syndromes represent a group of disorders that are varied in their functional impact and clinical presentation. They may affect all levels of the central and peripheral nervous systems. Paraneoplastic syndromes manifest as a result of the immune system's detection and response to a tumor antigen that cross-reacts with similar antigens expressed by the nervous system (Baehering, Quant, & Hochberg, 2007).

It is estimated that paraneoplastic syndromes affect up to 8% of patients with cancer (Baijens & Manni, 2006). Variability is seen based on the location of the onconeural antigen and thus the impact on the system. Based on the clinical features that arise, paraneoplastic syndromes can be divided into four categories: paraneoplastic endocrine syndromes, paraneoplastic hematologic syndromes, paraneoplastic dermatologic and rheumatologic syndromes, and paraneoplastic neurologic syndromes.

NEUROPATHOLOGY/PATHOPHYSIOLOGY

Again, paraneoplastic syndromes arise from an immune response to detected tumor antigens that cross-react with antigens within the nervous system. Individual discrepancies in physiology exist among the subtypes. As tumor cells invade the lymphatic system, this elicits the noted immune detection. Baehring et al. (2007) note that onconeural antigens are classified by their location, either on the cell surface or intracellular, in addition to their subcellular expression pattern. The underlying mechanism across presentations appears to be a serological immune response targeting intracellular antigens that activates cytotoxic T cells directed at peptide sequences arising from the intracellular antigen (Yu et al., 2001).

Pathologically, paraneoplastic syndromes can correspond with neuronal loss that is fairly extensive and irreversible in combination with reactive gliosis, perivascular cuffing by lymphocytes, and meningeal infiltrates affecting the limbic system, brainstem, and spinal cord (Baehring et al., 2007). Again, variability is seen based on the syndrome type and its origin. Pelosof and Gerber (2010), in their review, offered a detailed synthesis of the literature in terms of the types of paraneoplastic syndromes that present, their features, pathology, diagnostic findings, and treatment options that have been adopted in Table 1.

NEUROPSYCHOLOGICAL/CLINICAL PRESENTATION

There is no prototype of paraneoplastic syndromes. Various sites and systems can be affected throughout the system, and the manner in which they are affected corresponds with the clinical features that emerge. Table 1 gives for the main clinical/neuropsychological characteristics observed in conjunction with the various paraneoplastic syndromes.

DIAGNOSIS

Diagnosis of paraneoplastic syndromes can be difficult and requires a synthesis of multiple sources of information including MRI and serological studies in addition to clinical evaluation. In many ways, diagnosis is dualistic in that identification of the paraneoplastic syndrome is important as is the identification of the underlying presentation (e.g., small cell lung cancer). The latter are outlined in Table 1 in terms of their link with specific paraneoplastic syndromes.

MRI can aid in identifying anatomical alterations, including neuronal loss or regional enlargements. PET/CT scans can reveal areas of uptake throughout the body that may suggest cancerous origin/presence. EEG should be utilized in cases where seizures develop (e.g., syndrome of inappropriate secretion of antidiuretic hormone [SIADH]). Spinal tap with CSF analysis is often abnormal in a majority of patients; however, it does not differentiate among paraneoplastic syndromes. Serological studies can be coupled with CSF to narrow diagnostic focus. Specifically, the antibodies revealed on analysis can help direct diagnosis. For example, anti-CRMP-5, anti-Ma, anti-Ma2, and anti-Tr have each demonstrated capabilities in identifying specific cancerous presentations of various types (Bernal et al., 2003; Dalmau et al., 1999; Voltz et al., 1999; Yu et al., 2001). Diagnostic findings and studies based on the type of paraneoplastic syndrome are included in Table 1.

TREATMENT

Treatment and management of paraneoplastic syndrome is often dualistic, requiring simultaneous treatment of the paraneoplastic syndrome itself while attempting to identify and/or treat the cancerous presentation. Plasmapheresis or intravenous immunoglobulin infusion can offer treatment of the paraneoplastic syndrome (Baehring et al., 2007). Immunosuppression with corticosteroids or cyclophosphamide can also be useful, but as noted by Baehring et al. (2007), this can be contraindicated in

OP

Table 1
PARANEOPLASTIC SYNDROME TYPES AND FEATURES

Syndrome	Pathological Correlates	Clinical Features	Diagnostic Findings	Treatment
Paraneoplastic Hematologic Syndromes				
SIADH	Small cell lung cancer, mesothelioma, bladder, ureteral, endometrial, prostate, oropharyngeal, thymoma, lymphoma, Ewing's sarcoma, brain, GI, breast, adrenal	Gait disturbance and falls, seizures, headache, nausea, fatigue, muscle cramps, anorexia, confusion, lethargy, respiratory depression, coma	Hyponatremia: mild, sodium 130–134 mEq/L; moderate, sodium, 125–129 mEq/L; severe, sodium <125 mEq/L Increased urine osmolality (>100 mOsm/k in the context of euvolemic hyponatremia)	Restrict fluids (usually <1,000 mL/d) and encourage adequate salt and protein intake Demeclocycline, 300–600 mg PO twice daily Conivaptan, 20–40 mg/d IV Tolvaptan, ~10–60 mg/d PO Hypertonic (3%) saline at <1–2 mL/kg/h
Hypercalcemia	Breast, multiple myeloma, renal cell, squamous cell cancers (especially lung), lymphoma (including HTLV-associated lymphoma), ovarian, endometrial	Altered mental status, weakness, ataxia, lethargy, hypertonia, renal failure, nausea/vomiting, hypertension, bradycardia	Hypercalcemia: mild, calcium 10.5–11.9 mg/dL; moderate, calcium 12.0–13.9 mg/dL; severe, calcium, <14.0 mg/dL Low to normal (<20 pg/mL) PTH level Elevated PTHrP level	Normal saline, 200–500 mL/h Furosemide, 20–40 mg IV (use with caution and only after adequate fluid resuscitation) Pamidronate, 60–90 mg IV Zoledronate, 4 mg IV Prednisone, 40–100 mg/d PO (for lymphoma, myeloma) Calcitonin, 4–8 IU/kg SC or IM every 12 h Mithramycin, 25 μg/kg IV (often requires multiple doses) Gallium nitrate, 100–200 mg/m²/d IV continuous infusion for 5 days Hemodialysis
Cushing's syndrome	Small cell lung cancer, bronchial carcinoid (neuroendocrine lung tumors account for 50–60% of cases of paraneoplastic Cushing's syndrome), thymoma, medullary thyroid cancer, GI, pancreatic, adrenal, ovarian	Muscle weakness, peripheral edema, hypertension, weight gain, centripetal fat distribution	Hypokalemia (usually <3.0 mmol/L), elevated baseline serum cortisol (>29.0 μg/dL), normal to elevated midnight serum ACTH (>100 ng/L) not suppressed with dexamethasone	Ketoconazole, 600–1,200 mg/d PO Octreotide, 600–1,500 mg/d SC or octreotide LAR, 20–30 mg IM monthly Aminoglutethimide, 0.5–2 g/d PO Metyrapone, ~1.0 g/d PO Mitotane, 0.5–8 g/d PO Etomidate, 0.3 mg/kg/h IV Mifepristone, 10–20 mg/kg/d PO Adrenalectomy

Hypoglycemia	Mesothelioma, sarcomas, lung, GI	Sweating, anxiety, tremors, palpitations, hunger, weakness, seizures, confusion, coma	For non-islet cell tumor hypoglycemia: low glucose, low insulin (often <1.44–3.60 μIU/mL), low C-peptide (often <0.3 ng/mL), elevated IGF-2; IGF-1 ratio (often >10:l) For insulinomas: low glucose, elevated insulin, elevated C-peptide, normal IGF-2:IGF-1 ratio	Glucose (PO and/or parenteral) Dexamethasone, 4 mg 2 or 3 times daily Prednisone, 10–15 mg/d Diazoxide, 3–8 mg/kg/d PO divided into 2 or 3 doses Glucagon infusion, 0.06–0.3 mg/h IV Octreotide, ~50–1,500 μg/d SC or octreotide LAR, 20–30 mg IM monthly (often with corticosteroids) Human growth hormone, 2 U/d SC (often with corticosteroids)

Paraneoplastic Hematologic Syndromes

Eosinophilia	Hodgkin's lymphoma, non-Hodgkin's lymphoma (B and T cell), chronic myeloid leukemia, acute lymphocytic leukemia, lung, thyroid, GI (pancreatic, colon, gastric, liver), renal, breast, gynecologic	Dyspnea, wheezing	Hypereosinophilia (>0.5 × 10⁹/L); elevated serum IL-5, IL-3, IL-2, and GM-CSF	Inhaled corticosteroids Prednisone, 1 mg/kg/d PO
Granulocytosis	GI, lung, breast, gynecologic, GU, brain, Hodgkin's lymphoma, sarcomas	Asymptomatic (no symptoms or signs of such as neurologic deficits or dyspnea)	Granulocyte (neutrophil) count >8 × 10⁹/L, typically without a shift to immature neutrophil forms; elevated LAP; elevated serum G-CSF	Specific treatment not indicated
Pure red cell aplasia	Thymoma, leukemia/lymphoma, myelodysplastic syndrome	Dyspnea, pallor, fatigue, syncope	Anemia (hematocrit, <20 not uncommon), low/absent reticulocytes, bone marrow with nearly absent erythroid precursors, platelet and white blood cell counts in normal ranges	Blood transfusions Prednisone, 1 mg/kg/d PO Antithymocyte globulin, 500 mg daily IV (with corticosteroids and/or cyclophosphamide) Cyclosporine A, 100 mg PO twice daily Cyclophosphamide, 1–3 mg/kg/d PO

(Cont.)

OP

OP

Table 1
PARANEOPLASTIC SYNDROME TYPES AND FEATURES (Continued)

Syndrome	Pathological Correlates	Clinical Features	Diagnostic Findings	Treatment
Pure red cell aplasia (cont.)				Rituximab, 375 mg/m² IV per dose Alemtuzumab, 30 mg IV per dose Plasma exchange Splenectomy
Thrombocytosis	GI, lung, breast, gynecologic, lymphoma, renal cell, prostate, mesothelioma, glioblastoma, head and neck	Asymptomatic (no bleeding or clotting abnormalities)	Elevated platelet count, greater than ~400 × 10⁹/L; elevated serum IL-6	Specific treatment not indicated
Paraneoplastic Dermatologic and Rheumatologic Syndromes				
Acanthosis nigricans	Adenocarcinoma of abdominal organs, especially gastric adenocarcinoma (90% of malignancies in patients with acanthosis nigricans are abdominal); gynecologic	Velvety, hyperpigmented skin (usually on flexural regions); papillomatous changes involving mucous membranes and mucocutaneous junctions; rugose changes on palms and dorsal surface of large joints (e.g., tripe palms)	Skin biopsy: histology shows hyperkeratosis and papillomatosis	Topical corticosteroids
Dermatomyositis	Ovarian, breast, prostate, lung, colorectal, non-Hodgkin's lymphoma, nasopharyngeal	Heliotrope rash (violaceous edematous rash on upper eyelids); Gottron papules (scaly papules on bony surfaces); erythematous rash on face, neck, chest, back, or shoulders (the last of which is known as *shawl sign*); rash may be photosensitive; proximal muscle weakness; swallowing difficulty; respiratory difficulty; muscle pain	Laboratory findings: elevated serum CK, AST, ALT, LDH, and aldolase EMG: increased spontaneous activity with fibrillations, complex repetitive discharges, and positive sharp waves Muscle biopsy: perivascular or interfascicular septal inflammation and perifascicular atrophy	Prednisone, 80–100 mg/d PO Methylprednisolone, up to 1 g/d IV Azathioprine, up to 2.5 mg/kg/d PO Methotrexate, up to 25 mg/wk PO Cyclosporine A, 100–150 mg PO twice daily Mycophenolate mofetil, 2 g/d PO Cyclophosphamide, 0.5–1.0 g/m² IV IVIG, 400–1,000 mg/d to total 2–3 g
Erythroderma	Chronic lymphocytic leukemia, cutaneous T-cell lymphoma (including mycosis fungoides), GI (colorectal, gastric, esophageal, gallbladder), adult T-cell leukemia/lymphoma, myeloproliferative, disorders	Erythematous, exfoliating, diffuse rash (often pruritic)	Skin biopsy: histology shows dense perivascular lymphocytic infiltrate	Topical corticosteroids Narrow-band UVB phototherapy

Hypertrophic osteoarthropathy	Intrathoracic tumors, metastases to lung, metastases to bone, nasopharyngeal carcinoma, rhabdomyosarcoma	Subperiosteal new bone formation on phalangeal shafts ("clubbing"), synovial effusions (mainly large joints), pain, swelling along affected bones and joints	Plain radiography: periosteal reaction along long bones Nuclear bone scan: intense and symmetric uptake in long bones	NSAIDs Opiate analgesics Pamidronate, 90 mg IV Zoledronate, 4 mg IV Localized radiation therapy
Leukocytoclastic vasculitis	Leukemia/lymphoma, myelodysplastic syndromes, colon, lung, urologic, multiple myeloma, rhabdomyosarcoma	Ulceration, cyanosis, and pain, over affected regions (especially digits); palpable purpura, often over lower extremities; renal impairment; peripheral neuropathy	Skin biopsy: histology shows fibrinoid necrosis, endothelial swelling, leukocytoclasis, and RBC extravasation	Methylprednisolone, up to 1 g/d IV Prednisone, 1.0–1.5 mg/kg/d PO Dapsone, ~25–50 mg/d PO Colchicine, ~0.5 mg PO 2 or 3 times daily Methotrexate, 5–20 mg/wk PO Azathioprine, 0.5–2.5 mg/kg/d PO IVIG, 400–1,000 mg/d to total 2–3 g
Paraneoplastic pemphigus	Non-Hodgkin's lymphoma, chronic lymphocytic leukemia, thymoma, Castleman's disease, follicular dendritic cell sarcoma	Severe cutaneous blisters and erosions (predominantly on trunk, soles, palms); severe mucosal erosions, including stomatitis	Serum antibodies to epithelia (against plakin proteins and desmogleins) Skin biopsy: histology shows keratinocyte necrosis, epidermal acantholysis, and IgG and complement deposition in epidermal and basement membrane zones	Prednisone, ~60–120 mg PO daily Azathioprine, ~1.5 mg/kg/d PO Cyclophosphamide, 100–150 mg/d PO Cyclosporine A (target plasma levels 100–150 ng/L) IVIG, 400–1,000 mg/d to total 2–3 g Mycophenolate mofetil, 1–2 g/d PO Plasma exchange Rituximab, 375 mg/m^2 IV per dose
Polymyalgia rheumatic	Leukemia/lymphoma; myelodysplastic syndromes; colon; lung; renal; prostate; breast	Limb girdle pain and stiffness	Laboratory findings: elevated serum ESR (often not as high as in nonparaneoplastic PMR) and CRP	Prednisone, ~15 mg/d PO Methotrexate, ~10 mg/wk PO
Sweet syndrome	Leukemia (especially AML), non-Hodgkin's lymphoma, myelodysplastic syndromes, genitourinary, breast, GI, multiple myeloma,	Acute onset of tender, erythematous nodules, papules, plaques, or pustules on extremities, face, or upper trunk; neutrophilia; fever; malaise	Skin biopsy: histology shows a polymorphonuclear cell dermal infiltrate	Clobetasol propionate, 0.05% topical Triamcinolone acetonide, 3–10 mg/mL intralesional injection(s)

(Cont.)

OP

OP

Table 1
PARANEOPLASTIC SYNDROME TYPES AND FEATURES (Continued)

Syndrome	Pathological Correlates	Clinical Features	Diagnostic Findings	Treatment
Sweet syndrome (cont.)	gynecologic, testicular, melanoma			Methylprednisolone, up to 1 g/d IV; Prednisone, 30–60 mg/d PO; Potassium iodide, 300 mg PO 3 times daily (tablets) or 1,050–1,500 mg/d PO of saturated solution (Lugol solution); Colchicine, ~0.5 mg PO 3 times daily
Paraneoplastic Neurologic Syndromes				
Limbic encephalitis	SCLC (~40–50% of LE patients), testicular germ-cell (~20% of LE patients), breast (~8% of LE patients), thymoma, teratoma, Hodgkin's lymphoma **Associated antibodies:** Anti-Hu (typically with small cell lung cancer) Anti-Ma2 (typically testicular cancer) Anti-CRMP5 (anti-CV2) Anti-amphiphysin	Mood changes, hallucinations, memory loss, seizures, and less commonly hypothalamic symptoms (hyperthermia, somnolence, endocrine dysfunction); onset over days to months	EEG: epileptic foci in temporal lobe(s); focal or generalized slow activity; FDG-PET: increased metabolism in temporal lobe(s); MRI: hyperintensity in medial temporal lobe(s); CSF analysis:pleocytosis, elevated protein, elevated IgG, oligoclonal bands	IVIG, 400–1,000 mg/d to total 2–3 g; Methylprednisolone, up to 1 g/d IV; Prednisone, 1 mg/kg per day PO; Plasma exchange; Cyclophosphamide, ~2 mg/kg/d PO; Rituximab, 375 mg/m² IV per dose
Paraneoplastic cerebellar degeneration	SCLC, gynecologic, Hodgkin's lymphoma, breast **Associated antibodies:** Anti-Yo Anti-Hu Anti-CRMP5 (anti-CV2) Anti-Ma Anti-Tr Anti-Ri Anti-VGCC Anti-mGluRl	Ataxia, diplopia. dysphagia, dysarthria; prodrome of dizziness, nausea, vomiting	FDG-PET: increased metabolism (early stage) and then decreased metabolism (late stage) in cerebellum; MRI: cerebellar atrophy (late stage)	IVIG, 400–1,000 mg/d to total 2–3 g; Methylprednisolone, up to 1 g/d IV; Plasma exchange; Cyclophosphamide, ~2 mg/kg/d PO; Rituximab, 375 mg/m² IV per dose

OP

Lambert–Eaton syndrome	SCLC (~3% of patients have LEMS), prostate, cervical, lymphomas, adenocarcinomas **Associated antibodies:** Anti-VGCC (P/Q type)	Lower extremity proximal muscle weakness, fatigue, diaphragmatic weakness, bulbar symptoms (usually milder than in MG); later in course, autonomic symptoms (ptosis, impotence, dry mouth) in most patients	EMG: low compound muscle action potential amplitude; decremental response with low-rate stimulation but incremental response with high-rate stimulation	3,4-DAP, maximum of 80 mg/d PO Guanidine, ~575 mg/d PO (with pyridostigmine) Pyridostigmine, ~240–360 mg/d PO (with guanidine) Prednisolone, 60–100 mg PO every other day Azathioprine, up to 2.5 mg/kg/d PO IVIG, 400–1,000 mg/d to total 2–3 g Plasma exchange
Myasthenia gravis	Thymoma (in ~15% of MG patients) **Associated antibodies:** Anti-AchR	Fatigable weakness of voluntary muscles (ocular-bulbar and limbs), diaphragmatic weakness	EMG: decremental response to repetitive nerve stimulation	Thymectomy Pyridostigmine, ~600 mg/d PO in divided doses Prednisone, ~1 mg/kg/d PO Azathioprine, up to 2.5 mg/kg/d PO (with corticosteroids) Cyclosporine A, ~3 mg/kg/d PO Tacrolimus, 3–4 mg/d PO Mycophenolate mofetil, 1–3 g/d PO Rituximab, 375 mg/m^2 IV per dose Cyclophosphamide, 50 mg/kg/d IV for 4 d Plasma exchange IVIG, 400–1,000 mg/d to total 2–3 g
Autonomic neuropathy	SCLC, thymoma **Associated antibodies:** Anti-Hu Anti-CRMP5 (anti-CV2) Anti-nAchR Anti-amphiphysin	Panautonomic neuropathy, often subacute onset (weeks), involving sympathetic, parasympathetic, and enteric systems; orthostatic hypotension; GI dysfunction; dry eyes/mouth; bowel/bladder dysfunction; altered pupillary light reflexes; loss of sinus arrhythmia CGP: constipation, nausea/vomiting, dysphagia, weight loss, abdominal distension	Abdominal radiography/barium studies/CT: GI dilatation but no mechanical obstruction (for CGP) Esophageal manometry: achalasia or spasms (for CGP)	For orthostatic hypotension: Water, salt intake Fludrocortisone, 0.1–1.0 mg/d PO Midodrine, 2.5–10 mg PO 3 times daily Caffeine, ~200 mg/d PO For pseduo-obstruction: Neostigmine, 2 mg IV

(Cont.)

OP

Table 1

PARANEOPLASTIC SYNDROME TYPES AND FEATURES (Continued)

Syndrome	Pathological Correlates	Clinical Features	Diagnostic Findings	Treatment
Subacute sensory neuropathy	Lung (~70%–80%), usually SCLC; breast. ovarian; sarcomas; Hodgkin's lymphoma **Associated antibodies:** Anti-Hu Anti-CRMP5 (anti-CV2) Anti-amphiphysin	Parasthesias/pain (typically upper extremities before lower), followed by ataxia; multifocal/asymmetric distribution; all sensory modalities decreased but especially deep sensation/pseudoathetosis of hands; deep tendon reflexes decreased/absent; onset over weeks to months	NCS: reduced/absent sensory nerve action potentials CSF analysis: pleocytosis, high IgG, oligoclonal bands	Methylprednisolone, up to 1 g/d IV Cyciophosphamide, ~3 mg/kg/d PO IVIG, 400–1,000 mg/d to total 2–3 g Plasma exchange

From "Paraneoplastic Syndromes: An Approach to Diagnosis and Treatment" by L. C. Pelosof and D. E. Gerber, 2010, *Mayo Clinic Proceedings*, 85(9), pp. 838–854. Reproduced with permission.

Abbreviations: ACTH, adrenocorticotropic hormone; AML, acute myeloid leukemia; ALT, alanine transaminase; AST, aspartate transaminase; CGP, chronic GI pseudo-obstruction; CK, creatine kinase; CRP, C-reactive protein; EEG, electroencephalogram; EMG, electromyography; GI, gastrointestinal; FDG-PET, fluorodeoxyglucose–positron emission tomography; G-CSF, granulocyte-colony-stimulating factors; HTLV, human T-lymphotropic virus type; IGF, insulin growth factor; IGH, insulin growth factor; IVIG, IV immunoglobin; LAP, leukocyte alkaline phosphatase; LDH, lactate dehydrogenase; NCS, nerve conduction cancer; PMR, polymyalgia rheumatica; PTH, parathyroid hormone; PTHrp, parathyroid hormone–related peptide; SCLC, small cell lung cancer.

those instances where individuals are receiving concurrent chemotherapy, which itself depletes the immune system. Beyond these strategies, symptom-based treatment is recommended. For example, anti-epileptics can be used to control seizures. Treatment specific to each paraneoplastic syndrome is included in Table 1. These would be in addition to those interventions that specifically address the cancerous presentation

Chad A. Noggle

Baehering, J.M., Quant, E., & Hochberg, F.H. (2007). Metastatic neoplasms and paraneoplastic syndromes. In C. Goetz (Ed.) *Textbook of Clinical Neurology* (3rd ed., pp. 1081–1102). Saunders Elsevier: Philadelphia, PA.

Baijens, L. W., & Manni, J. J. (2006). Paraneoplastic syndromes in patients with primary malignancies of the head and neck: Four cases and a review of the literature. *European Archives of Oto-Rhino-Laryngological Societies, 263*, 32–36.

Bernal, F., Shams'ili, S., Rojas, I., et al. (2003). Anti-Tr antibodies as markers of paraneoplastic cerebellar degeneration and Hodgkin's disease. *Neurology, 60(2)*, 230–234.

Dalmau, J., Gultekin, S.H., Voltz, R., et al. (1999). Mal, a novel neuron- and testis-specific protein, is recognized by the serum of patients with paraneoplastic neurological disorders. *Brain, 122* (Pt 1), 27–39.

Pelosof, L. C., & Gerber, D. E. (2010, September). Paraneoplastic syndromes: An approach to diagnosis and treatment. *Mayo Clinic Proceedings, 85(9)*, 838–854.

Voltz, R., Gultekin, S.H., Rosenfeld, M.R., et al. (1999). A serologic marker of paraneoplastic limbic and brainstem encephalitis in patients with testicular cancer. *New England Journal of Medicine, 340(23)*, 1788–1795.

Yu, Z., Kryzer, T.J., Griesmann, G.E., et al. (2001). CRMP-5 neuronal autoantibody: Marker of lung cancer and thymoma-related autoimmunity. *Annals Neurology, 49(2)*, 146–154.

Paresthesias

DESCRIPTION

Paresthesia is a transient condition (Mogyros, Bostock, & Burke, 2000) that refers to a feeling of tingling or numbness on the skin, similar to a feeling of "pins and needles" that commonly results from manifestations of central and peripheral pathological processes involving cutaneous afferent fibers. Cutaneous afferents are more excitable than motor axons due to different biophysical properties. Paresthesias may be produced deliberately by mechanical or electrical stimulation of afferent fibers, or by cutting off circulation to a limb and then releasing and restoring the circulation (Merrington & Nathan, 1949). Sustained pressure placed on an afferent fiber may cause temporary paresthesia, but the feeling of pins and needles quickly goes away once pressure on the afferent fiber is released (National Institute of Neurological Disorders and Stroke [NINDS], 2009).

Paresthesias can occur in many parts of the body. Such sensations commonly occur in the hands, arms, legs, or feet initially, often without warning (NINDS, 2009). The sensations occur spontaneously from ectopic impulse activity in afferent axons, as well as spontaneous activity of afferent fibers that discharge or fire at different times in high-frequency bursts (Merrington & Nathan, 1949; Mogyros et al., 2000).

NEUROPATHOLOGY/PATHOPHYSIOLOGY

Paresthesias may result from disturbances in the function of afferent fibers in the sensory pathway of the central nervous system or the peripheral nervous system. Sensations of touch or pain travel to the brain via afferent fiber pathways; thus, peripheral disturbances are the most common cause of paresthesias. Tactile paresthesias arise from ectopic electrical discharges of A-β- and A-σ-type myelinated primary afferents whereas thermal paresthesias originate from cutaneous receptors arising from C-type unmyelinated primary afferents (Suarez-Roca, Pinerua-Shuhaibar, Morales, & Maxiner, 2003).

Biophysical mechanisms that trigger activity of normal cutaneous afferent fibers have been examined, providing consistent evidence of the neuropathology of paresthesias. Other causes involving peripheral afferent nerves include disturbances associated with diabetes, hypothyroidism, alcoholism, and vitamin B12 deficiency. Differential diagnoses may involve trauma, problems related to connective tissue such as arthritis, Sjögren's syndrome, and symptoms related to carpal tunnel syndrome. Some paresthesias result from hereditary diseases such as porphyria and Charcot–Marie–Tooth disease (Merrigton & Nathan, 1949; NINDS, 2009).

NEUROPSYCHOLOGICAL/CLINICAL PRESENTATION

Although all forms of paresthesias are alike with respect to afferent involvement, individual components influence the manifestation of the sensation.

Tactile paresthesias generally present as tingling and pricking sensations, whereas thermal paresthesias present as warmth/cold sensations (Suarez-Roca et al., 2003). Transient paresthesia is caused by compression of afferent fibers but disappears once pressure is relieved whereas ischemic paresthesia typically results from the arrest of the circulation in a limb. With ischemic paresthesia, the associated sensations are soft, diffuse tingling that is transient, lasting only a few minutes that may disappear with massaging the skin in the affected area, thus restoring circulation. Postischemic paresthesias follow release of the circulation and may consist of thermal paresthesia, buzzing or tingling, pricking or pseudocramp, or feeling of tension. Except for thermal paresthesia, all other sensations are felt peripherally.

Though there are many ways to characterize paresthesias, there are common features with which most patients present. The feeling of having the foot, leg, or arm "fall asleep" is the most common. Continually, a report of some combination of numbness, tingling, pricking, warmth, and cold may occur in any region of the body. Pseudocramps or tension is usually felt in the hand, wrist, and forearm, which may be followed by involuntary muscular contraction (NINDS, 2009).

DIAGNOSIS

Diagnostic evaluation of paresthesias is based on determining the underlying conditions associated with the various sensations. A patient's medical history, physical examination, and laboratory test results are critical for an accurate diagnosis. Often, mental health evaluations may be utilized to obtain further information to help determine the suspected cause (NINDS, 2009). A thorough diagnostic interview should include an assessment of the medical history that includes the onset, duration, and location of symptoms, as well as any other concurrent medical problems, or past exposure to drugs, toxins, infections, or trauma. Furthermore, a family medical history should be obtained to rule out genetically related disorders. Speaking with the patient about daily home and work routines may reveal repetitive motion, chronic vibration, or chemical exposure.

Along with a thorough clinical interview, further examination may be required if a clear diagnosis cannot be made. Neurological examination for symptoms and alterations in reflexes, sensation, or strength may be necessary, or blood tests, a urinalysis, and/or brain imaging studies of the affected area may also be undertaken. More advanced testing such as nerve conduction velocity tests, a nerve biopsy, and an EMG may be utilized as a final resort to ensure a correct diagnosis of paresthesia (NINDS, 2009).

TREATMENT

Treatment of paresthesias is dependent upon the etiology of the presenting conditions. The underlying cause can only be determined by clarifying and categorizing the symptoms that were manifested at the time of onset. Treatment typically involves altering the body's perception of pain; specifically, A-β, A-σ, and C-fibers that are relevant to pain transmission. Simply massaging an affected limb can cause symptoms such as numbness and tingling to resolve and is often a very common recommendation to decrease symptoms. Continually, wearing loose fitting shoes and clothing can release pressure on the nerves and is also a simple intervention. Pharmacological approaches may use pain-reducing medications such as codeine or other opium derivatives or employ anti-inflammatory drugs such as aspirin or ibuprofen. Antidepressant drugs, such as amitriptyline, may also be prescribed. For paresthesias due to nerve damage, human nerve growth factor may be effective in regenerating damaged nerves (Merrington & Nathan, 1949). Nutrition therapy with B complex vitamins and vitamin B12, avoiding alcohol, acupuncture, and massage therapy are alternative forms of treatment.

Angela Dortch
Raymond S. Dean

Icon Health Publications. (2004). *Paresthesia: A medical dictionary, bibliography, and annotated research guide to internet references.* US: Icon Group International.

Merrington, W. R., & Nathan, P. W. (1949). A study of postischemic paresthesias. *Journal of Neurology, Neurosurgery, and Psychiatry, 12,* 1–18.

Mogyoros, I., Bostock, H., & Burke, D. (2000). Mechanisms of paresthesias arising from healthy axons. *Muscle and Nerve, 3,* 310–320.

National Institute of Neurological Disorders and Stroke. (2009). National Institutes of Health. *Paresthesias information page.* Retrieved April 4, 2009, from http://www.ninds.nih.gov/disorders/paresthesia/paresthesia.htm

Suarez-Roca, H., Pinerua-Shuhaibar, L., Morales, M. E., & Maxiner, W. (2003). Increased perception of postischemic paresthesias in depressed subjects. *Journal of Psychosomatic Research, 55,* 253–257.

PARKINSON'S DISEASE

DESCRIPTION

Parkinson's disease (PD) is a neurodegenerative disease caused by a premature deterioration of nerve cells primarily located in the substantia nigra. PD affects approximately 500,000 people in the United States with numbers growing in past years (National Institute of Neurological Disorders and Stroke [NINDS], 2004). As with all neurodegenerative diseases, there is a loss of functioning as a result of the localization of the deterioration. PD is classified as a movement disorder and the loss of cells results primarily in tremors, rigidity, speech deficits, and poor stability in gait and posture. In regards to epidemiology, more men than women are diagnosed and the average age of onset is 60 years, with prevalence increasing with age.

NEUROPATHOLOGY/PATHOPHYSIOLOGY

The most distinguishing feature in the brains of individuals with PD is the lack of a black pigment in the substantia nigra that is caused by the destruction of the cells in this area. In PD, the substantia nigra is also the main site of Lewy bodies, defined as abnormal inclusions inside a cell forming a round or oval structure. Although Lewy bodies can be found in other areas of the brain and in other disorders (i.e., Alzheimer's disease), there is a specific trend of Lewy body formation found in PD, which is often helpful in diagnosis. Cells in the substantia nigra project into the putamen, which is responsible for a large portion of the neurotransmitter dopamine. Therefore, when these cells are destroyed, the dopamine connections between the substantia nigra and the putamen are also destroyed, diminishing the amount of dopamine produced. The loss of dopamine is thought to cause some of the primary symptoms associated with PD. The cell loss in the substantia nigra is caused by a process called apoptosis. Apoptosis is a normal process used in fetal growth to rid the body of unused cells and to remove excess cells to prevent certain autoimmune diseases. However, in PD this process is performed in excess, killing cells needed for normal functioning. The cause of accelerated apoptosis in PD patients is not clear; however, some competing theories include abnormal protein breakdown, genetic influence, toxins in the environment, excitotoxicity, and infection (Rosenbaum, 2006).

Much that is known about the neurological basis of PD has been discovered through the use of functional imaging techniques. F-dopa PET scans or SPECT scans use chemical injections to identify the activity of dopamine neurons during movement compared to activity of neurons at rest. Results from these scans indicate that patients with PD show deficient activation in motor areas, which serve as a valuable tool for the detection of PD (Galvez-Jimenez, 2005). Commonly used CT and MRI scans do not show the degeneration of the substantia nigra and are, therefore, not useful in early-stage diagnosis.

NEUROPSYCHOLOGICAL/CLINICAL PRESENTATION

There are a few symptoms such as constipation, sleepiness, REM behavior disorder, and an inhibited sense of smell, which may serve as preindicators for PD years before motor deficits occur. The motor difficulties are usually asymmetric and are often first experienced in the upper extremities in the form of resting tremors, commonly in a pill-rolling presentation. Typically, these tremors are initially intermittent and increase in regularity over time. Other symptoms include a decrease in dexterity and a feeling of aching or tightness in the muscles that contributes to a bradykinetic presentation. Oftentimes, individuals with PD are observed to have a shorter and unsteady gait, along with unsynchronized swinging of the arms and feet. Later stages of PD may cause difficulties in swallowing, resulting in excess saliva, drooling, and autonomic dysfunction. An inability to voluntarily move and maintain balance is seen in the final stages of the disease (Hauser, Pahwa, Lyons, & Mclain, 2009). Assessments utilized to measure PD include the Unified Parkinson's Disease Rating Scale, the Frontal Assessment Battery, the Dyskinesia Scale, and several other measures of specific symptoms.

Apart from the major symptoms of movement deficits, other cognitive and emotional difficulties can also occur. Symptoms of depression and anxiety are often present when patients are adjusting to and coping with the disease. In addition, a reduction in memory and the ability to retain new knowledge diminishes throughout PD, and dementia is often apparent in the final stages of the disease (Hauser et al., 2009). Therapy is often suggested for patients with PD to help cope with the difficulties associated with life-threatening diseases and chronic illness. The symptoms associated with PD can have a large impact on the individual's functioning, including loss of independence and an inability for social interactions. All these issues can be addressed in a therapeutic setting.

OP

OP

DIAGNOSIS

There are three main signs of PD, of which two must be present to make a clinical diagnosis. The first is the presence of a tremor that is the most extreme when the limb is not being utilized or stressed. The tremor is initially seen in the hand or arm and may be observed as a pill-rolling motion. The second feature is rigidity or increased resistance to the movement of a joint. Rigidity can be tested by flexing and extending a joint to find involuntary resistance to the movement. The third feature is bradykinesia, or slowness and diminished amount of movement that may be manifested as hypomimia, slowed blink rate, and hypophonia. The term "parkinsonian facies" refers to the poverty of automatic facial movements and expression. Other diagnostic features used to identify the progressing severity of the disease include postural instability, an appearance of freezing when initiating walking and turning, and dementia (Hauser et al., 2009).

In the assessment of PD, several differential diagnoses should be considered. Alzheimer's disease is often considered along with PD due to symptoms similar to dementia and impaired cognitive functioning in later stages. In addition, many Parkinson-plus syndromes including multiple system atrophy, diffuse Lewy body disease, and progressive supranuclear palsy have similar symptoms, with quicker progression and more widely spread brain area affected. Other diagnoses that should be considered based on their symptomatic similarities with PD include corticobasalganglionic degeneration, stroke, lacunar syndromes, multiple system atrophy, and striatonigral degeneration (Hauser et al., 2009).

TREATMENT

Currently, there is no cure for PD; thus, the goal of treatment is to diminish the symptoms while also creating the least side effects from medication as possible. The most common treatment for PD is levodopa (L-dopa) coupled with a peripheral decarboxylase inhibitor. L-dopa has several side effects and drawbacks including the wearing-off effect, leading to symptomatic relief becoming shorter as administration becomes more long term. In some instances, catechol-O-methyl transferase (COMT) is administered along with L-dopa to decrease this wearing-off effect. Dyskinesias (involuntary movements) are also a long-term side effect and can be represented through a tic or other repetitive movement. Further side effects include sweating, dizziness, tachycardia, dyspnea, pain, restless legs, anxiety, panic attacks, depression, confusion, and reduced alertness. Other medications used in the early stages of PD include dopamine agonists such as bromocriptine, pergolide, ropinirole, pramipexole, and apomorphine. These are used less frequently than L-dopa because of either decreased effectiveness or a difficult regimen and complex dosing schedules (Galvez-Jimenez, 2005).

Surgical procedures are also used in the treatment of PD. One of these procedures is a pallidotomy. This minimally invasive procedure uses a small electrical probe to destroy a small area of brain cells. Pallidotomy is most commonly done in the internal segment of the globus pallidus and may help decrease dyskinesias caused by L-dopa, though it is rarely in practice today, as less invasive techniques are preferred. A more popular treatment is deep brain stimulation (DBS), often used to target the reduction of tremors. DBS utilizes an implanted pulse generated to send electrical pulses to stimulate neural activity in certain areas of the brain. Each patient must be assessed individually to find exact areas of the brain to be targeted with DBS and certain qualifications (i.e., L-dopa responsive, younger than 65, medically fit) must be met for the procedure to be completed. Research is currently being done on preventive and neurorestorative therapies; however, this research has many challenges and is not expected to be available in the near future (Galvez-Jimenez, 2005).

Mindy Scheithauer
Raymond S. Dean

Galvez-Jimenez, N. (2005). *Scientific basis for the treatment of Parkinson's disease* (2nd ed.). London and New York: Taylor and Francis.

Hauser, R. A., Pahwa, R., Lyons, K. E., & Mclain, T. (2009). *Parkinson disease*. Retrieved March 25, 2009, from http://emedicine.medscape.com/article/1151267-overview

National Institute of Neurological Disorders and Stroke. (2004). *Parkinson's disease: Challenges, progress, and promise*. Retrieved March 25, 2009, from http://www.ninds.nih.gov/disorders/parkinsons_disease/parkinsons_research.htm

Rosenbaum, R. B. (2006). *Understanding Parkinson's disease*. Westport, CT: Praeger Publishers.

PAROXYSMAL CHOREOATHETOSIS

DESCRIPTION

Paroxysmal choreoathetosis (PC) is a movement disorder characterized by sudden brief episodes of unilateral or bilateral involuntary movements, including dystonic posturing, chorea, athetosis, and ballismus. Two different forms present: kinesigenic and nonkinesigenic. In the former, the aforementioned features are induced by voluntary movements and not accompanied by unconsciousness (Demirkiran & Jankovic, 1995; Kato, Sadamatsu, Kikuchi, Niikawa, & Fukuyama, 2006), whereas the latter is not precipitated by movement per se, rather level of arousal in many trigger events. Fatigue, alcohol, or other downers may trigger symptoms as may caffeine, excitement, or emotional stress. The episodes range in duration from seconds to minutes and occur multiple times throughout the day.

Although some consider PC a form of reflexive epilepsy, others have indicted the basal ganglion regions in the presentation given the core features that are similar to other movement disorders. Neuroimaging is often unremarkable (Nagamitsu et al., 1999; Sadamatsu et al., 1999). Cases arise either sporadically or through a familial pattern of inheritance.

NEUROPATHOLOGY/PATHOPHYSIOLOGY

The exact pathophysiology of PC remains unclear. Although some define it as a nonepileptic movement disorder, others have classified it as a reflexive epileptogenic presentation arising in the basal ganglia (Lombroso, 1995) in contrast to the cortex which is where seizures commonly originate. Suggested mechanisms include γ-aminobutyric acid dysregulation, abnormal metabolism of dopamine in the basal ganglia, and dysfunction of the substantia nigra (Demirkiran & Jankovic, 1995). SPECT and PET studies have further supported the role of the basal ganglia in PC as well as the thalamus (Iwasaki, Nakamura, & Hamada, 2004; Ko, Kong, Ngai, & Ma, 2001; Shirane, Sasaki, Kogure, Matsuda, & Hashimoto, 2001; Volonte et al., 2001). Some have further specified localization to the striatum (Vital, Bouillot, Burbaud, Ferrer, & Vital, 2002). Increased perfusion has been specifically noted in the basal ganglia contralateral to the movement symptoms (Ko et al., 2001). Beyond the basal ganglia, paroxysmal kinesigenic choreoathetosis (PKC) has also been associated with lesions of the rostral brainstem (Demirkiran & Jankovic, 1995).

In familial transmission, PC has been associated with autosomal-dominant inheritance with incomplete penetrance (Tomita et al., 1999; Valente et al., 2000). This has been localized within a 12.4-cM region between D16S3093 and D16S416 at 16p11.2-q12.1 (Cuenca-Leon, Cormand, Thomson, & Macaya, 2002; Tomita et al., 1999; Valente et al., 2000).

NEUROPSYCHOLOGICAL/CLINICAL PRESENTATION

OP

PKC is one of the recognized paroxysmal dyskinesias that represent a group of movement disorders characterized by brief yet recurrent attacks of choreoathetosis, dystonia, ballismus, or a combination of these movements (Demirkiran & Jankovic, 1995). As described above, PKC presents with sudden, brief attacks of involuntary movements that are triggered by sudden voluntary movement or mediated by fatigue, alcohol, caffeine, stress, or excitement. Prior to the event(s), individuals will often complain of sensory auras characterized by tension/tightness, cramping, numbness, or tingling.

Dystonic posturing, chorea, athetosis, and ballismus may all present (Kato et al., 2006). Most commonly, this presents unilaterally, although bilateral presentations have been reported. As noted by Kikuchi et al. (2007), attacks can range from seconds to minutes and occur up to 100 times daily. The presentation most commonly arises in childhood and diminishes with maturation. As described by Kinast, Erenberg, and Rothner (1980), "commonly the arm abducts, the wrist dorsiflexes, and the fingers flex. The knee and ankle extend and the foot inverts. These movements may be followed by alternate flexion and extension of the limb in a bizarre writhing manner, facial grimacing, and grotesque posturing."

DIAGNOSIS

Diagnosis of PC has long relied on clinical evaluation and symptom report. These remain the most important aspects of diagnosis to date. Conventional MRI and CT and EEG most often fail to demonstrate neuroanatomical changes definitive of diagnosis, except for a few exceptions (Fahn, 1994). Their use is still highly recommended, yet the absence of findings is not suggestive of an absence of the presentation. Recent research has suggested that diffusion tensor imaging may offer increased sensitivity in defining underlying lesions not shown on conventional MRI. In their study, Zhou, Chen, Gong, Tang, and Zhou (2010) found that diffusion tensor imaging can show changes in the thalamus of patients with idiopathic PKC not otherwise evident on conventional MRI. Specifically, increased fractional anisotropy and decreased mean diffusivity were noted in the thalamus but should not be relied on as definitive diagnosis. Interictal monitoring can also be essential as Joo et al. (2005) found reduced cerebral blood flow in posterior parts of the bilateral caudate nuclei. Invasive measurement has also shown utility in which ictal discharge arose from the supplementary sensorimotor cortex and ipsilateral caudate nucleus (Lombroso, 1995). SPECT has demonstrated utility in identifying lesions that went unrecognized by conventional MRI (Shirane et al., 2001). As suggested earlier, ictal SPECT studies have demonstrated increased perfusion in the contralateral basal ganglia (Ko et al., 2001), whereas ictal–interictal SPECT subtraction studies have shown ictal hyperperfusion in the contralateral thalamus. Similarly, fluorodeoxyglucose-PET studies have shown some uptake during interictal measurement, particularly of the ventral striatum (Volonte et al., 2001).

When considering differential diagnoses, psychiatric disorders, particularly somatoform or conversion disorders, basal ganglion disorders such as Wilson's disease and Huntington's disease, and forms of epilepsy may all be considered. In many instances, the approach to differential diagnosis in these cases is ruling out these competing diagnoses.

TREATMENT

Medicinal intervention remains the most common method of treatment. Both forms of PC respond well to antiepileptic agents such as carbamazepine or phenytoin (Jan, Freeman, & Good, 1995; Wein et al., 1996). Oxcarbazepine has also shown effectiveness in case studies but would likely be considered only after the aforementioned agents. In many instances, symptoms become milder as individuals age. Beyond these previously noted agents, successful treatment has also been reported in conjunction with phenobarbital, primidone, valproic acid, acetazolamide, clonazepam, lamotrigine, levodopa, trihexyphenidyl, flunarizine, and tetrabenazine (Lotze & Jankovic, 2003).

Individuals can attempt to control symptoms by avoiding triggers. Particularly, if alcohol or caffeine elicits symptoms, individuals should avoid them. Adoption of healthy sleep habits and appropriate exercise routines can reduce fatigue, which is also a trigger. In terms of exercise plans, individuals should avoid over-exertion as that too can trigger symptoms. Relaxation techniques and meditation can aid in regulating stress levels, which are also potential triggers.

Chad A. Noggle
Michelle R. Pagoria

Cuenca-Leon, E., Cormand, B., Thomson, T., & Macaya, A. (2002). Paroxysmal kinesigenic dyskinesia and generalized seizures: Clinical and genetic analysis in a Spanish pedigree. Neuropediatrics, 33(6), 288–293.

Demirkiran, M., & Jankovic, J. (1995). Paroxysmal dyskinesias: Clinical features and classification. Annals of Neurology, 38, 571–579.

Fahn, S. (1994). Psychogenic movement disorders. In C. D. Marsden & S. Fahn (Eds.), Movement disorders 3 (pp. 310–345). Oxford, UK: Butterworth-Heinemann.

Iwasaki, Y., Nakamura, T., & Hamada, K. (2004). Late-onset of idiopathic paroxysmal kinesigenic choreoathetosis: A case report. Rinsho Shinkeigaku, 44, 365–368.

Jan, J. E., Freeman, R. D., & Good, W. V. (1995). Familial paroxysmal kinesigenic choreoathetosis in a child with visual hallucinations and obsessive-compulsive disorder. Developmental Medicine & Child Neurology, 37, 366–369.

Joo, E. Y., Hong, S. B., Tae, W. S., Kim, J. H., Han, S. J., & Seo, D. W. (2005). Perfusion abnormality of the caudate nucleus in patients with paroxysmal kinesigenic choreoathetosis. European Journal of Nuclear Medicine and Molecular Imaging, 32(10), 1205–1209.

Kato, N., Sadamatsu, M., Kikuchi, T., Niikawa, N., & Fukuyama, Y. (2006). Paroxysmal kinesigenic choreoathetosis: From first discovery in 1892 to genetic linkage with benign familial infantile convulsions. Epilepsy Research, 70(Suppl. 1), 174–184.

Kikuchi, T., Nomura, M., Tomita, H., Harada, N., Kanai, K., Konishi, T., et al. (2007). Paroxysmal kinesigenic choreoathetosis (PKC): Confirmation of linkage to 16p11-q21, but unsuccessful detection of mutations among 157 genes at the PKC-critical region in seven PKC families. Journal of Human Genetics, 52, 334–341.

Kinast, M., Erenberg, G., & Rothner, A. D. (1980). Paroxysmal choreoathetosis: Report of five cases and review of the literature. Pediatrics, 65(1), 74–77.

Ko, C. H., Kong, C. K., Ngai, W. T., Ma, K. M. (2001). Ictal 99mTc ECD SPECT in paroxysmal kinesigenic choreoathetosis. Pediatric Neurology, 24, 225–227.

Lombroso, C. T. (1995). Paroxysmal choreoathetosis: An epileptic or nonepileptic disorder? Italian Journal of Neurological Sciences, 16, 271–277.

Lotze, T., & Jankovic, J. (2003). Paroxysmal kinesigenic choreoathetosis. Acta Neurologica Scandinavica, 10, 68–79.

Nagamitsu, S., Matsuishi, T., Hashimoto, K., Yamashita, Y., Aihara, M., Shimizu, K., et al. (1999). Multicenter study of paroxysmal dyskinesias in Japan—Clinical and pedigree analysis. Movement Disorders, 14(4), 658–663.

Sadamatsu, M., Masui, A., Sakai, T., Kunugi, H., Nanko, S., & Kato, N. (1999). Familial paroxysmal kinesigenic choreoathetosis: An electrophysiologic and genotypic analysis. Epilepsia, 40(7), 942–949.

Shirane, S., Sasaki, M., Kogure, D., Matsuda, H., & Hashimoto, T. (2001). Increased ictal perfusion of the thalamus in paroxysmal kinesigenic dyskinesia. Journal of Neurology, Neurosurgery & Psychiatry, 71, 408–410.

Vital, A., Bouillot, S., Burbaud, P., Ferrer, X., & Vital, C. (2002). Chorea-acanthocytosis: Neuropathology of brain and peripheral nerve. Clinical Neuropathology, 21, 77–81.

Tomita, H., Nagamitsu, S., Wakui, K., Fukushima, Y., Yamada, K., Sadamitsu, M., et al. (1999). Paroxysmal kinesigenic choreoathetosis locus maps to chromosome 16p11.2-q12.1. *The American Journal of Human Genetics, 65*(6), 1688–1697.

Valente, E. M., Spacey, S. D., Wali, G. M., Bhatia, K. P., Dixon, P. H., Wood, N. W., et al. (2000). A second paroxysmal kinesigenic choreoathetosis locus (EKD2) mapping on 16q13-q22.1 indicates a family of genes which give rise to paroxysmal disorders on human chromosome 16. *Brain, 123*(10), 2040.

Volonte, M. A., Perani, D., Lanzi, R., Poggi, A., Anchisi, D., Balini, A., et al. (2001). Regression of ventral striatum hypometabolism after calcium/calcitriol therapy in paroxysmal kinesigenic choreoathetosis due to idiopathic primary hypoparathyroidism. *Journal of Neurology, Neurosurgery & Psychiatry, 71,* 691–695.

Wein, T., Andermann, F., Silver, K., Dubeau, F., Andermann, E., Rourke-Frew, F., et al. (1996). Exquisite sensitivity of paroxysmal kinesigenic choreoathetosis to carbamazepine. *Neurology, 47,* 1104–1106.

Zhou, B., Chen, Q., Gong, Q., Tang, H., & Zhou, D. (2010). The thalamic ultrastructural abnormalities in paroxysmal kinesigenic choreoathetosis: A diffusion tensor imaging study. *Neurology, 257,* 405–409.

PAROXYSMAL HEMICRANIA

DESCRIPTION

Paroxysmal hemicrania (PH) is a member of the trigeminal autonomic cephalalgias (TACs), a group of primary headache disorders marked by unilateral head pain occurring in conjunction with ipsilateral cranial autonomic features (Cohen, Matharu, & Goadsby, 2007). The TACs are grouped into section 3 of the revised International Classification of Headache Disorders, which includes PH, cluster headache (CH), hemicrania continua (HC), and short-lasting unilateral neuralgiform headache attacks with conjunctival injection and tearing (SUNCT). The TACs are distinguished by attack duration and frequency, as well as differential response to selected therapies. PH is a rare syndrome first described by Sjaastad and Dale in 1974 and is now found worldwide (Rozen, 2009). The hallmarks of PH are the brief attacks and the absolute response to indomethacin therapy (Cittadini, Matharu, & Goadsby, 2008). Prevalence is estimated to be 1 in 50,000; it is diagnosed twice as often in women, and the mean age of onset is 34 years (Paviour & Ellis, 2008).

The clinical phenotype of PH includes severe, relatively brief (paroxysmal), unilateral attacks of pain with cranial autonomic features recurring several times per day (Cohen et al., 2007). The headache is one-sided and often reported in the ophthalmic trigeminal distribution, the orbital and temporal regions, and above or behind the ear (Rozen, 2009). The pain has been described as boring, throbbing, claw-like, or pulsating, and may radiate to the neck or ipsilateral shoulder. Headaches usually persist for 2–30 minutes with abrupt onset and cessation. Although most episodes are spontaneous, some attacks may be provoked by bending or rotating the head as well as applying pressure to the transverse process of C4–C5 or the C2 nerve root on the symptomatic side. Interictal pain or discomfort is noted in 60% of patients and restlessness or agitation in 85% (Cohen et al., 2007).

Cranial autonomic phenomena include lacrimation (62%), nasal congestion (42%), conjunctival injection and rhinorrhea (36%), and ptosis (33%) (Rozen, 2009). Other cranial features may include facial flushing, eyelid edema, forehead sweating, miosis, mydriasis, and swelling of the cheek (Cittadini et al., 2008). PH is classified as episodic or chronic depending upon the presence of a remission period. Approximately 20% of patients are diagnosed with episodic paroxysmal hemicrania (EPH), which is characterized by recurrent bouts of at least 1-week duration separated by remission periods of at least 1 month (Cohen et al., 2007; Paviour & Ellis, 2008). The remaining 80% are diagnosed with chronic paroxysmal hemicrania (CPH, also known as Sjaastad's syndrome) as they do not remit or have remissions lasting less than 1 month.

NEUROPATHOLOGY/PATHOPHYSIOLOGY

Although the mechanisms underlying PH remain unknown, it has been suggested that the pathophysiology of the syndrome centers on the trigeminal-autonomic reflex, the brainstem connection between the trigeminal system and the parasympathetic autonomic nervous system (Cohen et al., 2007; Rozen, 2009). More specifically, the cranial autonomic symptoms of the disorder may be attributable to a central disinhibition of the trigeminal-autonomic reflex by the hypothalamus (Matharu, Cohen, Frackowiak, & Goadsby, 2006). The suggested role of the hypothalamus is plausible given the known hypothalamic-trigeminal connections and its modulatory functions within the nociceptive and autonomic pathways. Lending support to this hypothesis is recent evidence from functional neuroimaging studies (fMRI) implicating posterior hypothalamus and ventral midbrain activation in PH (Cittadini et al., 2008). There is also evidence supporting the involvement of vasoactive neuropeptides such as calcitonin gene-related peptide (CGRP) and vasoactive intestinal polypeptide (VIP) in

OP

OP

PH (Cittadini et al., 2008). Studies have found that both CGRP and VIP levels are elevated during acute attacks (Goadsby & Edvinson, 1996; Paviour & Ellis, 2008;). In addition, indomethacin therapy, which affectively alleviates PH symptoms reduces CGRP, VIP, and intracranial blood flow following administration. In addition, trigeminal sensory C-fibers contain CGRP and neurokinin A, which when released result in meningeal vasodilation, plasma extravasation, platelet activation, and other effects characteristic of neurogenic inflammation (Paviour & Ellis, 2008). Accordingly, trigeminal and parasympathetic neuropeptide release may result in activation of the ipsilateral trigeminovascular system accounting for the abrupt onset of headache and autonomic abnormalities such as miosis, lacrimation, rhinorrhea, as well as increased corneal temperature and intraocular pressure. Autonomic sympathetic involvement is also likely given the presence of symptoms such as sweating and decreased salivation during attacks (Cortelli & Pierangeli, 2003).

NEUROPSYCHOLOGICAL/CLINICAL PRESENTATION

Given the paucity of research regarding the neuropsychological profiles of PH patients and the extracerebrate nature of the pathophysiology within the trigeminal-autonomic reflex, no direct neuropsychological correlates of PH have been established. Nonetheless, the neuropsychological functioning of related chronic pain conditions points to neurocognitive deficits that may be evident in PH. A review of the neuropsychological literature on chronic pain conditions with and without central nervous system dysfunction suggests that mild impairment in attentional capacity, processing speed, and psychomotor speed are typical in chronic pain conditions (Hart, Martelli, & Zasler, 2000). Tests that do not appear sensitive to the effects of pain include the Trail Making Test, WAIS similarities and Block Design Subtests, Number Correction Test, Visual Memory indices, and List-Learning tasks. Observed neuropsychological impairments are known to vary with pain severity and trait anxiety, but not depression or sleep quality. To complicate the study of neurocognitive changes, personality and emotional functioning measures often show signs of somatization, depression, and anxiety.

DIAGNOSIS

Differential diagnosis of the TACs lies in the duration and frequency of attacks, as well as their response to medications. PH is characterized by intermediate duration unilateral headaches (2–30 minutes) of intermediate frequency (1–40/day). CH has the longest attack duration (15–180 minutes) and relative low frequency (1/alternate day–8/day) while SUNCT has the shortest attack duration (5–240 seconds) and highest frequency (3–200/day) (Bigal & Lipton, 2007; Cohen et al., 2007). Unlike CH attacks, which are predominantly nocturnal, PH attacks occur on a regular basis throughout the day. Further, the chronic form of PH (CPH) dominates the clinical presentation in contrast to the more prominent episodic form in CH. In addition, in contrast to the brief episodic nature of PH, patients with HC experience a continuous daily headache present all day, every day of the week (Rozen, 2009). Another difference includes the ability to elicit SUNCT attacks by cutaneous stimulation, which is not typical of other TACs including PH (Cohen et al., 2007).

Perhaps the most distinguishing feature of PH is its absolute response to indomethacin therapy, which is not effective in the treatment of other TACs (Bigal & Lipton, 2007). In addition, CH responds well to oxygen and sumatriptan, and SUNCT to intravenous lidocaine, both of which are largely ineffective in treating HP. Although CT scan or MRI of the brain may help rule out structural pathology, neuroimaging studies are typically normal in PH patients. As noted above, fMRI have reported posterior hypothalamus activation in PH. Such activation is also found in CH and SUNCT; however, HC is characterized by activation in the ventrolateral midbrain (Cittadini et al., 2008).

TREATMENT

Treatment of PH is prophylactic as the brevity and intensity of attacks prevent the effective use of acute oral treatments (Cohen et al., 2007). As noted above, the treatment of choice for PH is indomethacin (Indocin), a nonsteroidal anti-inflammatory drug. Most patients respond to a dosage of 150 mg/day with a dramatic and rapid alleviation of headache symptoms (Rozen, 2009). Individuals normally require continuous dosing as symptoms may recur as soon as 12 hours following cessation of treatment. Following indomethacin, verapamil is the most successful preventive medication. Additional medications that may provide relief include aspirin, naproxen, prednisone, celecoxib, piroxicam, acetazolamide, and ergotamine. PH does not respond to nerve blockade, surgical intervention, oxygen, lithium, carbamazepine, and other anticonvulsant therapies. Although no studies have directly investigated the efficacy of behavioral interventions specific to PH, relaxation and pain management strategies including progressive muscle relaxation and guided imagery may be useful (Kuekkeboom & Gretarsdottir, 2006). In addition, as PH and other pain syndromes are associated with increased anxiety and depression, psychotherapeutic interventions may be considered for mood symptoms.

Kyle Noll
Mark T. Barisa

Bigal, M. E., & Lipton, R. B. (2007). The differential diagnosis of chronic daily headaches: An algorithm-based approach. *Journal of Headache and Pain, 8*, 263–272.

Cittadini, E., Matharu, M. S., & Goadsby, P. J. (2008). Paroxysmal hemicrania: A prospective clinical study of 31 cases. *Brain, 131*, 1142–1155.

Cohen, A. S., Matharu, M. S., & Goadsby, P. J. (2007). *Headache, 47*, 969–980.

Cortelli, P., & Pierangeli, G. (2003). Chronic pain-autonomic interactions. *Neurological Sciences, 24*, 568–570.

Goadsby, P. J., & Edvinson, L. (1996). Neuropeptide changes in a case of chronic paroxysmal hemicrania — evidence for trigemino-parasympathetic activation. *Cephalalgia, 16*, 448–450.

Hart, R. P., Martelli, M. F., & Zasler, N. D. (2000). Chronic pain and neuropsychological functioning. *Neuropsychology Review, 10*, 131–149.

Kuekkeboom, K. L., & Gretarsdottir, E. (2006). Systematic review of relaxation interventions for pain. *Journal of Nursing Scholarship, 38*, 269–277.

Matharu, M. S., Cohen, A. S., Frackowiak, R. S., & Goadsby, P. J. (2006). Posterior hypothalamic activation in paroxysmal hemicrania. *Annals of Neurology, 59*, 535–545.

Paviour, D. C., & Ellis, C. M. (2008). Paroxysmal hemicrania and poems syndrome: Further evidence that neuropeptides are implicated in primary headache?*Cephalalgia, 28*, 1204–1206.

Rozen, T. D. (2009). Trigeminal autonomic cephalalgias. *Neurologic Clinics, 27*, 537–556.

PARRY–ROMBERG'S SYNDROME

DESCRIPTION

Parry–Romberg's syndrome, also known as progressive facial hemiatrophy (PFH) of Romberg, was first described by Caleb Parry in 1825, systematized in 1846 by Moritz Romberg, and named in 1871 by Eulenberg (Dervis & Dervis, 2005; Orozco-Covarrubias et al., 2002; Pearce, 2005). It is a self-limiting, slowly progressive disorder characterized by the loss of fat in the dermal and subcutaneous tissues of the face, occasionally extending to the bone, with hyperpigmentation ("coup de sabre") and alopecia of areas overlying the atrophied tissue (Bilen et al.,

1999; Cory, Clayman, Faillace, McKee, & Gama, 1997; Ropper & Brown, 2005). Age of onset is typically during the first two decades of life (Cory et al., 1997; Hulzebos, Vries, Armbrust, Sauer, & Kerstjens-Frederikse, 2004), but has been documented in individuals as young as 14 months (Chang et al., 1999), and as old as 43 years (Mendonca, Viana, Freitas, & Lima, 2005). Although prevalence of this disorder is unknown it is estimated to be approximately 1:700,000 and affects females more than males at a ratio of approximately 3:1 (Stone, 2006).

The symptomatic expression of the disorder is somewhat heterogeneous. The face is, by definition, affected in all patients, with 10% exhibiting hemiatrophy extending to the trunk, arm, or lower limbs (Aoki, Tashiro, Fujita, & Kajiwara, 2006). This suggests that the neuropathological basis may extend beyond that of the fifth and seventh cranial nerves, which are implicated. In an Internet survey of 205 patients with the syndrome, symptoms reported in addition to the facial hemiatrophy were epilepsy (11%), facial pain (46%), eye problems (46%), migraine (52%), problems with the jaw (35%), depression or anxiety (46%), and sundry autoimmune diseases (Stone, 2003). These are similar to symptoms reported elsewhere in the literature. Epilepsy, frequently experienced by individuals with this disorder, may be of the partial (contralateral to the atrophied side) or Jacksonian variety (Aktekin, Oguz, Aydin, & Senol, 2005). In a review of 54 individual cases, 73% had experienced focal seizures. Other neurologic signs associated with Parry–Romberg's syndrome include movement disorders secondary to brain lesions, masticatory spasms, behavioral changes, intellectual/cognitive decline secondary to cerebral hemiatrophy, and brainstem involvement (Kister, Inglese, Laxer, & Herbert, 2008; Paprocka, Jamroz, Adamek, & Marszal, 2006). The etiology of this disorder is unknown (Larner & Bennison, 1993; Ropper & Brown, 2005).

NEUROPATHOLOGY/PATHOPHYSIOLOGY

The etiology of Parry–Romberg's syndrome remains unknown and contested (Bilen, 1999; Larner & Bennison, 1993; Ropper & Brown, 2005). Numerous postulations persist, including the conceptualization of Parry–Romberg's syndrome as an autoimmune disorder, a malformative disease (maldevelopment of the neural crest), a genetic predisposition disturbing facial development, a disturbance of central or peripheral facial autonomic development, and/or an inflammatory disease (Aoki et al., 2006; Korkmaz, Adapinar, & Uysal, 2005; Larner & Bennison, 1993).

The co-occurrence of PRS with other autoimmune disorders such as uveitis and systemic lupus

OP

erythematosus lends credence to the notion of this syndrome as an autoimmune disorder (Leao & Da Silva, 1994). Conceptualization of PRN as a genetic, autosomal dominant disorder has been largely dismissed as DNA confirmed monozygotic twins have not been found to share the disorder in the only two documented cases (Hulzebos et al., 2004; Larner & Bennison, 1993), and only a small percentage of probands pass the disorder on to their children. Head and facial trauma have been suggested as possible causes as well, but have also been essentially ruled out due to the number of victims of trauma that do not develop PFH, as well as the number of individuals with PFH that have experienced no trauma of any kind (Hulzebos et al., 2004).

Several studies and case reports have incorporated radiological assessment as a means of investigation and clarification of both diagnosis and underlying neurologic pathology. Associated MRI and CT scans have been ambiguous. Nevertheless, cerebral hemiatrophy of the affected side, calcification, enophthalmos, increased signal in the white matter, intracranial calcification, and central cerebral atrophy have also been noted (Cory et al., 1997). In many cases, however, radiological findings reveal no central nervous system anomalies or abnormalities (Bilen, 1999).

It has been postulated that the seventh (facial) and fifth (trigeminal) cranial nerves are involved, as the areas of the face typically affected by PFH are those dermatomes enervated by the trigeminal nerve (Cory et al., 1997; Ropper & Brown, 2005; Sommer et al., 2006), although this is not always the case (Larner & Bennison, 1993). It appears, however, through case reports that the symptom most commonly associated with the cranial nerves may be trigeminal neuralgia.

NEUROPSYCHOLOGICAL/CLINICAL PRESENTATION

There is very little discussion in the literature regarding the neuropsychological characteristics of this disorder (i.e., direct measurements of cognitive impairment, and secondary effects such as poor or diminished academic achievement). Patients in studies have been noted as having learning disorders (Orozco-Covarrubias et al., 2002), progressive cognitive decline (Paprocka et al., 2006), and major depressive disorder (MDD) (Sommer et al., 2006), but these were included only as demographic descriptors, and were not directly assessed. One case study involved an anterior left temporal craniotomy for the treatment of intractable seizures, and included pre- and postoperative neuropsychological testing. An increase in full scale IQ of 10 points was found in the postoperative testing, with a commensurate

increase in verbal memory (DeFelipe et al., 2001); however, this was a single case study, and thus limited the generalizability of the findings.

In some cases, ipsilateral cerebral hemiatrophy or other central nervous system (CNS) involvement has been reported (Bilen et al., 1999; Cory et al., 1997). These findings, especially those involving atrophy of the cortex, are correlated with contralateral hemiparesis, which may involve the trunk, and upper and/or lower limbs; however, this appears as a finding in only a small percentage of cases. In these patients, motor functioning is clearly impaired, but there is no treatment and the slowly progressive disorder runs its course until self-termination (Chang et al., 1999). Such a self-limiting nature threatens the assessment of treatment efficacy of almost any kind.

Other sensory and motor impairments involve the eye and eyelid of the affected side. This expression varies by individual, and may range from a mild, ptosis-like impairment to complete closure of the eyelid (Cory et al., 1997; Sommer et al., 2006). Individuals may also experience enophthalmos, wherein the eye is partially recessed into the orbit secondary to the loss of orbital fat (Aoki et al., 2006; Hulzebos et al., 2004; Kee & Hwang, 2008; Mendonca et al., 2005; Sommer et al., 2006). As in all other symptoms, these reports involve only the affected side of the face, leaving motor and sensory functioning of the contralateral eye intact.

It has been noted in some reports of the psychological difficulty experienced by individuals suffering from this condition due to distress over the disfigurement of the face. Long-term care has been suggested to include psychological intervention for support and prevention of further symptom development (Baskan et al., 2006; Hulzebos et al., 2004; Stone, 2006).

DIAGNOSIS

The presenting symptoms of Parry–Romberg's syndrome are somewhat heterogeneous, and closely associated with localized scleroderma. While all individual cases reported in the literature have wasting of the fat of the affected side of the face, not all involve precisely the same symptom presentation. It is for this reason that the idea has been put forth that Parry–Romberg's syndrome may in fact be a collection of conditions with the underlying commonality of progressive hemiatrophy of one side of the face (Chang et al., 1999). Other distinguishing features that may contribute to diagnosis are the presence of antihistone antibodies and histopathological findings of fibrosis and adnexal atrophy (with accompanying mononuclear cell infiltrates) (Baskan et al., 2006). Autoantibodies were found in 50–75% of patients with linear scleroderma (Kister et al., 2008), again lending support to the hypothesis that PRS is an autoimmune disorder with inflammatory qualities. Serum tests for autoantibodies are recommended when PRS is suspected.

Parry–Romberg's syndrome must be differentially diagnosed from localized scleroderma (localized scleroderma en coup de sabre; LSCS), although it has been noted that the two, distinct disorders are comorbid in 20–37% of the same individuals (Kister et al., 2008). This differential is most effectively accomplished by histological examination of elastic tissue, which is preserved (nonsclerotic) in Parry–Romberg's syndrome (Cory et al., 1997; Jablonska & Blaszczyk, 2005; Orozco-Covarrubias et al., 2002). Several authors note that making the differential between linear scleroderma/SCS is indeed difficult; some go as far as to state that the differential is sometimes not possible, and that the two may indeed be the same pathogenic process, or at the ends of a continuum (Dervis & Dervis, 2005; Jablonska & Blaszczyk, 2005; Kister et al., 2008). Some authors contend that the conditions are essentially considered to overlap, as linear scleroderma tends to progress toward PFH (Baskan et al., 2006; Kister et al., 2008; Stone, 2003).

While several studies have used CT and MRI scans to assess neurologic abnormalities and clarify differential criteria, findings tend to be negative or idiopathic (Cory et al., 1997; Dervis & Dervis, 2005; Mendonca et al., 2005). When abnormalities are detected, they are heterogeneous (Aktekin et al., 2005), thereby limiting the generalizability of the findings. Some of the most frequent findings of MRI and CT scans in the literature revealed individuals with subcortical hyperintensities, calcification, and blurring of white and gray matter (Sommer et al., 2006). This was especially true in those with overt neurologic signs.

TREATMENT

Due to the unknown pathogenesis of PFH, no single, specific treatment intervention is utilized (Kee & Hwang, 2008; Korkmaz et al., 2005). Several methods have been employed as primary interventions to either limit or repair the physical damage of PFH. Surgical intervention, which includes fat and skin grafts to the affected areas of the face, has been reported as a successful treatment. This method of treatment has also been noted to improve the emotional state of sufferers (Guerrerosantos, Guerrerosantos, & Orozco, 2007). Another primary intervention that has been used is oral calcitrol, which was reported as successful in reducing lesions of the face and hyperpigmentation at a 6-month follow-up. Other treatments involve topical agents, immunosuppression, physiotherapy, and phototherapy (Dervis & Dervis, 2005). A more recent treatment for PRS included phototherapy for the reduction of sclerodermic lesioning in individuals with SCS and PRS with some benefit. While the patients in those studies benefited from a reduction in the cutaneous lesioning, atrophy of fat in the face was not halted or slowed (Baskan et al., 2006).

Some cases of PRS have corresponding CNS involvement. It has been noted in the literature that patients with PRS and cerebral lesioning have benefited from the use of immunosuppression, which also speaks to the possibility of an autoimmune etiology of the disorder. Findings have revealed that lesioning regressed over time in these individuals. In contrast, patients with CNS lesions who received no immunosuppressive drugs were reported to have showed no slowing or regression of their lesions (Korkmaz et al., 2005). Unfortunately, none of the patients treated were administered any type of objective assessment of cognitive functioning (that was reported); therefore, the presence and severity of cognitive impairment secondary to the lesions, and the associated changes with treatment were not measured.

To date, the literature is bereft on cognitive and/or behavioral treatments for PFH. It has been noted that the disorder may cause some issues with low self-esteem and possible rejection of facial expression in sufferers of PFH, particularly since the onset is typically during adolescence (Hulzebos et al., 2004). While the literature on the secondary, residual emotional effects of PFH and their treatment is nonexistent, it is possible that the individuals may become preoccupied with their appearance. Given that possibility, the anxiety and depression that might result could lead to MDD, or mimic the course of body dysmorphic disorder (BDD). Compounding that, the onset of BDD is typically during adolescence, which is also the approximate and usual time of onset of PFH. Treatment for such disorders is accomplished via cognitive behavioral therapy (CBT) and/or serotonin-reuptake inhibitors (Phillips, Didie, Feusner, & Wilhelm, 2008; Phillips & Hollander, 2008). While BDD and depression or anxiety secondary to acquired disfigurement cannot be considered as one and the same, it is conceivable that similar treatments may be effective.

W. Howard Buddin Jr.
Charles Golden

Aktekin, B., Oguz, Y., Aydin, H., & Senol, U. (2005). Cortical silent period in a patient with focal epilepsy and Parry-Romberg syndrome. *Epilepsy & Behavior, 6*(2), 270–273.

OP

Aoki, T., Tashiro, Y., Fujita, K., & Kajiwara, M. (2006). Parry-Romberg syndrome with a giant internal carotid artery aneurysm. *Surgical Neurology, 65*(2), 170–173.

Baskan, E. B., Kaçar, S. D., Turan, A., Saricaoglu, H., Tunali, S., & Adim, S. B. (2006). Parry-Romberg syndrome associated with borreliosis: Could photochemotherapy halt the progression of the disease? *Photodermatology, Photoimmunology & Photomedicine, 22*(5), 259–261.

Bilen, N., Efendi, H., Apaydin, R., Bayramgurler, D., Harova, G., & Komsuoglu, S. (1999). Progressive facial hemiatrophy (Parry-Romberg syndrome). *Australasian Journal of Dermatology, 40*(4), 223–225.

Chang, S. E., Huh, J., Choi, J. H., Sung, K. J., Moon, K. C., & Koh, J. K. (1999). Parry-Romberg syndrome with ipsilateral cerebral atrophy of neonatal onset. *Pediatric Dermatology, 16*(6), 487–488.

Cory, R. C., Clayman, D. A., Faillace, W. J., McKee, S. W., & Gama, C. H. (1997). Clinical and radiologic findings in progressive facial hemiatrophy (Parry-Romberg syndrome). *AJNR American Journal of Neuroradiology, 18*(4), 751–757.

DeFelipe, J., Segura, T., Arellano, J. I., Merchán, A., DeFelipe-Oroquieta, J., Martín, P., et al. (2001). Neuropathological findings in a patient with epilepsy and the Parry-Romberg syndrome. *Epilepsia, 42*(9), 1198–1203.

Dervis, E., & Dervis, E. (2005). Progressive hemifacial atrophy with linear scleroderma. *Pediatric Dermatology, 22*(5), 436–439.

Guerrerosantos, J., Guerrerosantos, F., & Orozco, J. (2007). Classification and treatment of facial tissue atrophy in Parry–Romberg disease. *Aesthetic Plastic Surgery, 31*(5), 424–434.

Hulzebos, C., de Vries, T., Armbrust, W., Sauer, P., & Kerstjens-Frederikse, W. (2004). Progressive facial hemiatrophy: A complex disorder not only affecting the face. A report in a monozygotic male twin pair. *Acta Paediatrica, 93*(12), 1665–1669.

Jablonska, S., & Blaszczyk, M. (2005). Long-lasting follow-up favours a close relationship between progressive facial hemiatrophy and scleroderma en coup de sabre. *Journal of the European Academy of Dermatology and Venerology, 19*(4), 403–404.

Kee, C., & Hwang, J. M. (2008). Parry-Romberg syndrome presenting with recurrent exotropia and torticollis. *Journal of Pediatric Ophthalmology and Strabismus, 45*(6), 368–370.

Kister, I., Inglese, M., Laxer, R. M., & Herbert, J. (2008). Neurologic manifestations of localized scleroderma: A case report and literature review. *Neurology, 71*(19), 1538–1545.

Korkmaz, C., Adapinar, B., & Uysal, S. (2005). Beneficial effect of immunosuppressive drugs on Parry-Romberg syndrome: A case report and review of the literature. *Southern Medical Journal, 98*(9), 940–942.

Larner, A. J., & Bennison, D. P. (1993). Some observations on the aetiology of progressive hemifacial atrophy ("Parry-Romberg syndrome"). *Journal of Neurology, 56*, 1035–1039.

Leao, M., & Da Silva, M. (1994). Progressive hemifacial atrophy with agenesis of the head of the caudate nucleus. *Journal of Medical Genetics, 31*(12), 969–971.

Mendonca, J., Viana, S. L., Freitas, F., & Lima, G. (2005). Late-onset progressive facial hemiatrophy (Parry-Romberg syndrome). *Journal of Postgraduate Medicine, 51*(2), 135–136.

Orozco-Covarrubias, L., Guzmán-Meza, A., Ridaura-Sanz, C., Carrasco Daza, D., Sosa-de-Martinez, C., & Ruiz-Maldonado, R. (2002). Scleroderma 'en coup de sabre' and progressive facial hemiatrophy. Is it possible to differentiate them? *Journal of the European Academy of Dermatology and Venerology, 16*(4), 361–366.

Paprocka, J., Jamroz, E., Adamek, D., & Marszal, E. (2006). Difficulties in differentiation of Parry-Romberg syndrome, unilateral facial sclerodermia, and Rasmussen syndrome. *Child's Nervous System, 22*(4), 409–415.

Pearce, J. (2005). Romberg and his sign. *European Neurology, 53*(4), 210–213.

Phillips, K. A., Didie, E. R., Feusner, J., & Wilhelm, S. (2008). Body dysmorphic disorder: Treating an underrecognized disorder. *The American Journal of Psychiatry, 165*(9), 1111–1118.

Phillips, K. A., & Hollander, E. (2008). Treating body dysmorphic disorder with medication: Evidence, misconceptions, and a suggested approach. *Body Image, 5*(1), 13–27.

Ropper, A. H., & Brown, R. H. (2005). *Adams and Victor's principles of neurology* (8th ed.). New York: McGraw-Hill.

Sommer, A., Gambichler, T., Bacharachbuhles, M., Von rothenburg, T., Altmeyer, P., & Kreuter, A. (2006). Clinical and serological characteristics of progressive facial hemiatrophy: A case series of 12 patients. *Journal of the American Academy of Dermatology, 54*(2), 227–233.

Stone, J. (2003). A global survey of 205 patients using the Internet. *Neurology, (61)*, 674–676.

Stone, J. (2006). Parry-Romberg syndrome. *Practical Neurology, 6*(3), 185–188.

PELIZAEUS–MERZBACHER'S DISEASE

DESCRIPTION

Pelizaeus–Merzbacher's disease (PMD) was named after Friedrich Pelizaeus who described the clinical features in 1885 and Ludwig Merzbacher who presented additional observations in 1910, including a postmortem examination (Koeppen & Robitaille, 2002). It is a rare, progressive, degenerative central nervous system (CNS) disorder in which coordination, motor abilities, and intellectual function deteriorate (National Institutes of Health [NIH], 2008). PMD comprises 6.5% of a group of hereditary metabolic disorders occurring in children, known as the leukodystrophies, which affect growth of myelin sheath in varying degrees (Hesselink, 2006; Koeppen & Robitaille, 2002).

NEUROPATHOLOGY/PATHOPHYSIOLOGY

PMD is caused by a mutation in the gene that controls production of proteolipid protein-1 (PLP1), a myelin protein, and is inherited as an X-linked recessive trait, and affected individuals include males and their mothers as carriers of the PLP1 mutation. Depending on the type of PLP1 mutation, severity and onset ranges widely from the neonatal period through the first 5 years of life (Garbern, Krajewsi, & Hobson, 2006). PMD is one of a spectrum of diseases associated with PLP1, which also includes spastic paraplegia type 2 (SPG2). PLP1-related disorders span a continuum of neurologic symptoms ranging from severe central nervous system involvement (PMD) to progressive weakness and stiffness of the legs (SPG2). Noticeable changes in myelination can be detected by MRI analyses of the brain. Phenotypic spectrum ranges from severe infantile-onset disease with lack of any developmental progress and death during the first decade to childhood-onset forms of SPG (Henneke et al., 2008).

NEUROPSYCHOLOGICAL/CLINICAL PRESENTATION

Generally, clinical presentation of PMD may include slow growth, tremor, and failure to develop normal control of head movement, as well as deteriorating speech and mental function. Within the PMD disease spectrum, there are four general classifications ranging in severity, which include connatal PMD, classic PMD, complicated SPG2, and pure (uncomplicated) SPG2. Connatal PMD is the most severe type and involves delayed mental and physical development or deterioration and severe neurological symptoms (i.e., pendular nystagmus, spasticity, and/or convulsions) in the neonatal period (Garbern et al., 2006; NIH, 2008). Often, chorea or athetosis develops and psychomotor development is arrested by the third month, followed by regression (Fenichel, 1988). Limb movements become ataxic and tone spastic, beginning with the legs and then followed by the arms. Optic atrophy and seizures occur later and death occurs by 5–7 years of age. The second type is classic PMD, in which the early symptoms include nystagmus and impaired motor development within the first month of life followed by ataxia, dystonia, dysarthria, and progressive spasticity (Henneke et al., 2008). The course of classic PMD is longer than the neonatal form and survival to adult life is common (Fenichel, 1988; Henneke et al., 2008). The third form, complicated SPG2, features motor development issues and brain involvement (Garbern et al., 2006; NIH, 2008). Symptom presentation is similar, but also includes autonomic dysfunction (spastic urinary bladder) with little to no cognitive impairment. Survival into adulthood is common. The last type, pure (uncomplicated) SPG2 includes cases of PMD that do not have extensive neurologic complications. While autonomic disturbance and spastic gait are present; nystagmus, ataxia, neuropathy, cognitive impairments, and other neurologic signs and symptoms are typically absent.

DIAGNOSIS

In the absence of a family history or a male-inherited neurological illness, it is difficult to diagnose PMD by clinical examination and imaging (Koeppen & Robitaille, 2002). MRI can be helpful in establishing the diagnosis in those who have CNS involvement (Garbern, Krajewsi, & Hobson, 2006), but without family history specific diagnosis can be elusive. For a definitive diagnosis, postmortem examination is required (Fenichel, 1988). As previously mentioned, PMD is one of a group of gene-linked disorders known as the leukodystrophies in which neuroimaging reveals a symmetrical, diffuse, and confluent pattern of white matter involvement. In terms of differential diagnoses, the classic leukodystrophies should be considered as they all affect the growth of myelin sheath (Cecil & Kos, 2006; Henneke et al., 2008). They include adrenoleukodystrophy, Krabbe globoid cell, Alexander's disease, Canavan's disease, Cockayne syndrome, metachromatic leukodystrophy, and PMD (Hesselink, 2006). Other differentials to consider include: ataxia with identified genetic and biochemical defects, cerebral palsy, chorea in adults, chorea in children, complex partial seizures, cortical basal ganglionic degeneration, dopamine-responsive dystonia, Hallervorden–Spatz's disease, inherited metabolic disorders, lysosomal storage disease, multiple sclerosis, Parkinson's disease, Parkinson's disease in young adults, Parkinson-plus syndromes, peroxisomal disorders, progressive supranuclear palsy, striatonigral degeneration, temporal lobe epilepsy, tonic-clonic seizures, and Wilson's disease.

OP

TREATMENT

To date, there is no cure or standard course of treatment for PMD. Treatment typically includes some combination of treating symptoms and supportive therapy, and may include medication for movement disorders (NIH, 2008). Medical care may include supportive care, such as physical therapy, orthotics, and antispasticity agents, including intrathecal baclofen. Physical medicine or orthopedic evaluations, physical therapy, and careful attention to posture and seating help to minimize the development of joint contractures, dislocations, and kyphoscoliosis. Severely affected individuals, such as those who have connatal PMD, may need special attention directed to airway protection and may need anticonvulsant therapy.

In general, developmental assessment is important to maximize cognitive achievement and to assist in appropriate educational program assignment. A specialist in pediatric development should be consulted to optimize the child's educational program and to maximize functional and learning capabilities. Last, genetics counseling is helpful for parents of an affected child in order to educate them about the disorder and any risks to future offspring.

Ana Arenivas
Mark T. Barisa

Cecil, K. M., & Kos, R. S. (2006). Magnetic resonance spectroscopy and metabolic imaging in white matter diseases and pediatric disorders. *Topics in Magnetic Resonance Imaging, 17*(4), 275–293.

Fenichel, G. M. (1988). *Pelizaeus-Merzbacher disease. Clinical pediatric neurology*. Philadelphia, PA: W. B. Saunders Company.

Garbern, J. Y., Krajewsi, K., & Hobson, G. (2006, September). *PLP1-related disorders. Published online through Gene reviews*. Retrieved August 5, 2009, from http://www.ncbi.nlm.nih.gov/bookshelf/picrender.fcgi?book=gene&&partid=1182&blobtype=pdf

Henneke, M., Combes, P., Diekmann, S., Bertini, E., Brockmann, E., Burlina, A. P., et al. (2008). GJA12 mutations are a rare cause of Pelizaeus-Merzbacher-like disease. *Neurology, 7*, 748–754.

Hesselink, J. R. (2006). Differential diagnostic approach to MR imaging of white matter diseases. *Topics in Magnetic Resonance Imaging, 17*(4), 243–263.

Koeppen, A. H., & Robitaille, Y. (2002). Pelizaeus-Merzbacher disease. *Journal of Neuropathology and Experimental Neurology, 61*(9), 747–759.

National Institutes of Health (National Institute of Neurological Disorders and Stroke). (2008).

NINDS Pelizaeus-Merzbacher disease information page. Retrieved August 5, 2009, from http://www.ninds.nih.gov/disorders/pelizaeus_merzbacher/pelizaeus_merzbacher.htm

PERIPHERAL NEUROPATHY

DESCRIPTION

Peripheral neuropathy is a neurodegenerative disorder characterized by damage to one or more peripheral nerves. The peripheral nervous system (PNS) transmits information from the central nervous system (CNS) to limbs and organs. Central neuropathy refers to damage sustained by the brain or the spinal cord, both of which are encompassed by the CNS. Though neuropathies may originate in the CNS, the majority originate in the PNS (Uzun et al., 2006). Damage to peripheral nerves causes distortion of information transmitted to and from the body and extremities (i.e., anything beyond the brain and spinal cord), resulting in symptoms ranging from temporary numbness to paralysis and organ or gland dysfunction.

There are several types of neuropathies, each distinguishable by the extent and location of the nerve damage (Andreoli, 2007). When disturbance in function occurs in one nerve, the neuropathy is classified as a mononeuropathy simplex. Mononeuropathy multiplex indicates involvement of several nonadjacent peripheral nerves. Polyneuropathies are more common, concurrently affecting the function of numerous peripheral nerves. The subclassifications of polyneuropathies include axonal neuropathies, principally affecting the axons, demyelinating neuropathies, involving the myelin sheath surrounding the axons, and neuronopathies, involving neurons of the PNS.

NEUROPATHOLOGY/PATHOPHYSIOLOGY

While there are numerous ways to classify and specify the disorder for diagnosing, the definitive symptoms appear to be caused by the cell body's response to the damage. This occurs most often in either the axon or the myelin sheath of the affected nerve fibers (Cros & Siao, 2001). Often, the neurophysiological features of axonal neuropathy are caused by traumatic injury and are symmetrical sensory and/or motor symptoms. In contrast, demyelinating neuropathies are often a result of nerve compression, creating interruptions in the transmission of nerve impulses (Cros & Siao, 2001).

Peripheral neuropathy is considered to be either an acquired disorder or a hereditary disorder. Idiopathic inflammatory neuropathies are a classification of acquired neuropathies. They are caused by inflammation from activities of the immune system and include acute idiopathic polyneuropathy (Guillain–Barré syndrome) and chronic inflammatory demyelinating polyneuropathy (see these entries within this book for further review).

Metabolic and nutritional neuropathies can be caused by diabetes, uremia, liver disease, vitamin B12 deficiency, and other endocrinopathies including hypothyroidism and acromegaly. Vitamin B12 is an essential element of healthy nerve function, with a deficiency leading to widespread nerve tissue damage. Peripheral neuropathy is the most common complication of diabetes. Mild neuropathies accompanied by sensory abnormalities are found in up to 70% of diabetic patients while symptomatic neuropathies affect an additional 5–10% (Andreoli, 2007). The clinical form of neuropathy most diabetic patients present with is symmetric polyneuropathy associated with rapid physiologic dysfunction and hyperglycemia.

Infective and granulomatous neuropathies have a variety of causes including AIDS, diphtheria, leprosy, sarcoidosis, sepsis and multiorgan failure. Though diphtheria and leprosy are rare, Lyme disease is more common and can cause a rapidly developing polyneuropathy.

Mixed connective tissue disease, polyarteritis nodosa, rheumatoid arthritis, and systemic lupus erythematosus are known causes of vasculitic neuropathies. Certain connective tissue disorders, including polyarteritis nodosa and rheumatoid arthritis, may cause mononeuropathy multiplex or even polyneuropathy.

Neoplastic and paraproteinemic neuropathies are caused by compression and infiltration resulting from a tumor, paraneoplastic syndromes, paraproteinemias, and amyloidosis. Neurofibromatoses, genetic diseases involving tumors growing directly on nerve tissue, are often associated with polyneuropathies.

Drug-induced and toxic neuropathies are caused by alcohol, organic compounds such as hexacarbons and organophosphates, heavy metals such as arsenic, gold, lead, platinum, and thallium, and tryptophan. Thiamine deficiency is a common problem associated with alcoholism and can cause neuropathy of the extremities. Excessive alcohol consumption alone may directly cause damage to the peripheral nerves. Peripheral nerve damage is also a side effect of long-term use of anticancer drugs, anticonvulsants, and antibiotics.

Finally, hereditary neuropathies of an idiopathic nature may be caused by Friedreich's ataxia and familial amyloidosis, while hereditary neuropathies of a metabolic nature may be caused by porphyria, metachromatic leikodystrophy, Krabbe's disease, abetalipoproteinemia, Tangier's disease, Refsum's disease, and Fabry's disease. Hereditary neuropathies result from genetic code errors or new genetic mutations and may begin in infancy in severe cases or in early adulthood for milder forms (Dyck & Thomas, 2005).

NEUROPSYCHOLOGICAL/CLINICAL PRESENTATION

Proper operation of the axon and its myelin sheath is vital for the normal functioning of myelinated nerve fibers. When the axon begins to degenerate as a result of a variety of metabolic, toxic, and heritable causes, the myelin also begins to break down. Axonal degeneration of long nerve fibers is usually the underlying cause of polyneuropathies. When demyelination occurs in peripheral nerves as a result of demyelinating neuropathies, functional deficits identical to those resulting from axonal degeneration are produced. Demyelinating neuropathies are largely caused by inherited disorders of myelin, autoimmune attacks on myelin, and mechanical, toxic, and physical injuries to the nerve (Dyck & Thomas, 2005).

Clinical presentation of the neuropathies depends on the associated pathophysiologic mechanisms and the anatomical location of the nerve damage. Peripheral nerves have highly specialized functions, leading to a wide array of symptoms when the nerves are damaged. The most common symptom of damage to peripheral motor nerves is muscle weakness, while other symptoms may include cramps, muscle loss, bone degeneration, and fasciculations (Andreoli, 2007). Sensory nerve damage generally results in impaired and abnormal sensations and numbness. When involvement of peripheral nerve fibers of a certain size is selective, dissociated sensory loss may occur. In such cases, certain sensory modalities are impaired while others are preserved. Additional sensory and reflex changes associated with the motor neuron deficits suggest peripheral nerve damage.

When small fibers within nerves are affected by the neuropathy, pain is a prominent symptom. Pain is an established symptom of neuropathies related to alcohol use and diabetes and may also be a feature of entrapment neuropathies. Patients with diabetic polyneuropathies generally present with autonomic dysfunction, spontaneous sensations of neuropathic pain including dysesthesias, and reduced pain sensibility. Diabetic neuropathy occurs most often in patients with insulin-requiring long-standing diabetes, and a diagnosis can be confirmed with electrodiagnositic studies. In a study conducted by Turcot et al. (2009), participants with diabetic neuropathy also presented with greater postural instability than control participants. L-Periaxin is a protein involved in the stabilization of mature myelin in peripheral nerves. Lawlor et al. (2002) report the presence of anti-L-periaxin antibodies in patients with diabetes-associated peripheral neuropathy, resulting in morphologic abnormalities of the sensory nerves.

OP

When the neural pathways that mediate reflexes are interrupted, tendon reflexes may be impaired or lost. Patients with polyneuropathies generally experience loss of ankle reflexes first, followed by additional tendon reflex loss.

Symptoms associated with Guillain–Barré syndrome and diabetic neuropathies or those caused by amyloidosis include coldness of extremities, bladder and bowel function disturbances, impotence, and postural hypotension. Along with being an additional symptom of amyloidosis, enlarged peripheral nerves may be an indication of hereditary motor and sensory neuropathies and neuropathies associated with leprosy, Refsum's disease, and acromegaly. Again, the interested reader is referred to these entries within this text.

DIAGNOSIS

Due to high symptom variability, diagnosis of neuropathy can be challenging. Symptoms of a sensory nature are often the first clue of peripheral nerve involvement. Acute development of symptoms usually relates to an inflammatory polyneuropathy, while gradual evolution of symptoms is an indication of hereditary or metabolic polyneuropathies. Mononeuropathies with acute symptom presentation generally result from traumatic causes. Symptoms caused by minor traumatic injuries and entrapment of nerves are more likely indications of mononeuropathies of gradual onset. Along with drug and alcohol history, occupational history should also be considered during patient evaluation as certain industrial substances may lead to peripheral neuropathy.

When a diagnosis of neuropathy is suspected, electromyography may be used to determine location of denervation. Nerve conduction velocity tests are used to determine whether nerve damage is the result of myelin sheath or axon degeneration. Demyelinating and axonal neuropathies may be differentiated using electrodiagnositc or histopathologic studies. Nerve biopsies may also be conducted to determine degree of nerve damage. When a diagnosis of pheripheral neuropathy is confirmed electrodiagnostically, additional laboratory studies including blood glucose levels, serum vitamin B12, and liver and thyroid function blood tests should be conducted. Magnetic resonance imaging can detect nerve damage caused by compression and can provide data on muscle size and quality. Abnormal antibodies associated with neuropathies can be identified during examination of cerebrospinal fluid, and simple tests to evaluation ability to register sensations may reveal the size of sensory nerve fibers affected.

Sabin (2001) notes, however, that if one can establish type of onset, family history, general medical state, and previous exposure to medications or toxins, one can easily diagnose the individual accurately. Burns et al. (2006) also reported a simple way to clarify the varying classifications is by asking "What?," "Where?," "When?," and "What setting?," and by following a type of decision tree based on the responses to those questions.

TREATMENT

Treatment approaches are driven by the accurate diagnosis, as they are either symptomatic or etiological in nature (Vanotti et al., 2007). Though treatments of inherited forms of neuropathy are limited, depending on classification, acquired neuropathies may be treated in several ways. Generally the underlying cause of the neuropathy is treated first to limit progression of the symptoms or even reverse the neuropathy itself before symptomatic treatment is initiated.

Adopting a healthy lifestyle, avoiding exposure to toxins, limiting alcohol consumption, correcting vitamin deficiencies, and eating a balanced diet are all helpful strategies to reduce the physical symptoms of many neuropathies. Regular exercise may help in reducing cramps associated with certain neuropathies and improve muscle strength, a vital component of avoiding muscle wasting associated with limb paralysis.

Plasmapheresis shortens recovery time associated with Guillain–Barré syndrome, while intravenous immunoglobulin in high doses is an equally effective treatment. Careful monitoring of respiratory function in patients with Guillain–Barré syndrome, diphtheritic neuropathy, and other idiopathic inflammatory neuropathies is essential to effective treatment.

Correction of blood glucose levels is important for prevention and reducing neuropathic symptoms associated with diabetic neuropathy. Anticonvulsants and tricyclic antidepressants have also been found to reduce the painful symptoms of diabetic neuropathy

J. T. Hutton
Rachel Rock
O. J. Vidal
Antonio E. Puente

Andreoli, T. E. (2007). *Cecil essentials of medicine* (7th ed.). Philadelphia, PA: Saunders Elsevier.

Burns, J. M., Mauermann, M. L., & Burns, T. M. (2006). An easy approach to evaluating peripheral neuropathy. *The Journal of Family Practice, 55,* 853–861.

Cros, D., & Siao, P. (2001). Electromyography and other neurophysiologic approaches in peripheral neuropathy. In

D. Cros (Ed.), *Peripheral neuropathy: A practical approach to diagnosis and management* (pp. 3–19). Philadelphia, PA: Lippincott, Williams, & Wilkins.

Dyck, P. J., & Thomas, P. K. (2005). *Peripheral neuropathy (4th ed.).* Philadelphia, PA: Saunders Elsevier.

Lawlor, M. W., Richards, M. P., & De Vries, G. H. (2002). Antibodies to l-periaxin in sera of patients with peripheral neuropathy produce experimental sensory nerve conduction deficits. *Journal of Neurochemistry, 83,* 592–600.

Sabin, T. D. (2001). Generalized peripheral neuropathy: Symptoms, signs, and syndromes. In D. Cros (Ed.), *Peripheral neuropathy: A practical approach to diagnosis and management* (pp. 3–19). Philadelphia, PA: Lippincott, Williams, & Wilkins.

Simon, R. P., Greenberg, D. A., & Aminoff, M. J. (2009). *Clinical neurology* (7th ed.). New York, NY: McGraw-Hill Companies, Inc.

Turcot, K., Allet, L., & Golay, A. (2009). Investigation of standing balance in diabetic patients with and without peripheral neuropathy using accelerometers. *Clinical Biomechanics,* 24(9), 716–721.

Uzun, N., Uluduz, D., Mikla, S., & Aydin, A. (2006). Evaluation of asymptomatic central neuropathy in type I diabetes mellitus. *Electromyography and Clinical Neurophysiology,* 46(3), 131–137.

Vanotti, A., Osio, M., Mailland, E., Nascimbene, C., Capiluppi, E., & Mariani, C. (2007). Overview on pathophysiology and newer approaches to treatment of peripheral neuropathies. *CNS Drugs, 21,* 3–12.

Perinventricular Leukomalacia

DESCRIPTION

Periventricular leukomalacia (PVL) refers to necrosis of the white matter adjacent to the lateral ventricles (Volpe, 2008). Although it most commonly occurs in premature infants, PVL has been noted in full-term infants as well, often being those with primary cardiac and pulmonary disease. Premature infants are particularly vulnerable to PVL between 24 and 30 weeks gestation and is often associated with intraventricular hemorrhage (Larroque et al., 2003).

As suggested, the necrotic lesions present in the white matter lateral and posterolateral to the lateral ventricles (Ropper & Brown, 2005). Sensorimotor impairments predominate (e.g., cerebral hemiplegia or diplegia) in combination with a varying degree of neurocognitive impairment with the prior usually exceeding the latter in regard to severity.

NEUROPATHOLOGY/PATHOPHYSIOLOGY

PVL corresponds with necrotic lesions in the white matter usually developing in the perinatal period and presenting as echodensities on ultrasonographic examination. More specifically, the lesions present in the deep watershed territories corresponding with the locality of the cortical and central arteries, lateral and posterolateral to the lateral ventricles (Ropper & Brown, 2005). The most common lesion sites include the area anterior to the frontal horn, angles of the lateral ventricles at the level of the foramen of Monro, and lateral regions of the trigone and occipital horn, including the optic radiation (Kinney & Armstrong, 1997). To a lesser extent, necrotic foci occur in the corpus callosum and internal capsule (Kinney & Armstrong, 1997). Widespread neuronal necrosis is also commonly seen (Kinney & Armstrong, 1997). Theories abound in terms of the physiological basis of the presentation with it most commonly being linked to hypoxic–ischemic burden within arterial border zones (Rorker, 1992). The timeframe of the insult is seen as a result of developing oligodendrocytes' vulnerability to hypoxic event that can promote influxes in glutamate levels, which is toxic to these immature cells (Oka et al., 1993). When infants are born between 24 and 30 weeks gestation the cerebrovascular system remains immature. In particular, border zones such as those around the ventricles, and the developing oligodendrocytes that inhabit these regions, are vulnerable to hypotensive-based ischemic crises in the face of other systemic issues such as infection (Rourke, 1992). As ischemia develops, this causes a cascade of inflammatory responses that include activation of microglia and a release of free radicals that act on cellular production of essential proteins in such a way that it leads to cellular death in the aforementioned regions (Haynes et al., 2003). Clinical presentations that coincide with increased risk of hypoxic–ischemic burden may be risk factors for PVL. This includes, but is not limited to, respiratory disease, maternal infection, maternal chorioamnionitis, and antepartum and peripartum hemorrhage.

NEUROPSYCHOLOGICAL/CLINICAL PRESENTATION

The neuropsychological and functional profile of PVL is variable with no unitary profile emerging. Nevertheless, certain clinical sequelae are seen in greater frequency than others. Epilepsy presents in roughly 25–30% of children with PVL with greater risk associated with greater anatomical compromise (Humphreys et al., 2007; Kohelet et al., 2006). Motor deficits are also

OP

common and are often classified as cerebral palsy. Spastic diplegia affecting the lower limbs more than the upper is the most common form (Ancel et al., 2006; Volpe, 2008). General discoordination and delays in motor development may be seen. From a sensory standpoint, visual deficits are the most common features within this domain. Hyperopia, myopia, astigmatism, deficits of pursuit and saccades, visual field restrictions, strabismus, and nystagmus all present at greater frequency than in the normal population (Edmond & Foroozan, 2006; Jacobsen et al., 1996).

Neurocognitive dysfunction is common in PVL, including general, nonspecific delays in cognitive development and intellectual impairment although some have suggested that a profile emerges similar to a nonverbal learning disability (Iwata et al., 2007; Pisani et al., 2006; Woodward et al., 2006). To some extent, the severity is directly linked to gestational age with greater impairment being associated with greater prematurity. To this sum, greater anatomical disruption is associated with greater intellectual impairment.

DIAGNOSIS

PVL is traditionally identified by way of cranial ultrasound in the neonatal period presenting with echodensities in the periventricular white matter. However, MRI is being used with increasing frequency in these infants and has proven more effective in identifying white matter lesions (Volpe, 2008). EEG should be sought to determine the presence of seizures.

Given the relative prevalence of motor, visual, and cognitive deficits in PVL, thorough assessment of these domains is essential. Evaluation by a physical therapist/occupational therapist can aid in identifying motor delays. Optometry examination is also crucial and may be supplemented by consultation with a neuro-ophthalmologist. Neuropsychological examination should be used to document the nature and extent of any neurocognitive deficits.

TREATMENT

There is no cure for PVL. Treatment is symptombased. Anticonvulsant agents can be effective in controlling seizure activity. Physical and occupational therapy can assist in improving motor functioning, coordination, and ambulation as such deficits present. Special education services are often required.

Chad A. Noggle
Michelle R. Pagoria

Ancel, P. Y., Livinec, F., Larroque, B., Marret, S., Arnaud, C., Pierrat, V., et al. (2006). Cerebral palsy among very preterm children in relation to gestational age and neonatal ultrasound abnormalities: The epipage cohort study. *Pediatrics, 117* (3), 828–835.

DeReuck, J., Chattha, A. S., & Richardson, E. P. J. (1972). Pathogenesis and evolution of periventricular leukomalacia in infancy. *Archives of Neurology, 27,* 229–236.

Edmond, J. C., & Foroozan, R. (2006). Cortical visual impairment in children. *Current opinion in Ophthalmology, 17*(6), 509–512.

Graham, D. I., & Lantos, P. L. (Eds). (1997). *Greenfield's neuropathology* (6th ed.). New York, NY: Oxford University Press, Inc.

Haynes, R., Folkerth, R., Keefe, R., & Sung. I. (2003). Nitrosative and oxidative injury to premyelinating oligodendrocytes is accompanied by microglial activation in periventricular leukomalacia in the human premature infant. *Journal of Neuropathology and Experimental Neurology, 62,* 441–450.

Humphreys, O., Deonandan, R., Whiting, S., Barrowman, N., Matzinger, M. A., Briggs, V., et al. (2007). Factors associated with epilepsy in children with periventricular leukomalacia. *Journal of Child Neurology, 22*(5), 598–605.

Iwata, S., Iwata, O., Bainbridge, A., Nakamura, T., Kihara, H., Hizmune, E., et al. (2007). Abnormal white matter appearance in term FLAIR predicts neuro-developmental outcome at 6 years old following preterm birth. *International Journal of Developmental Neuroscience, 25*(8), 523–530.

Jacobson, L., EK, U., Fernell, E., Flodmark, O., & Broberger, U. (1996). Visual impairments in preterm children with periventricular leukomalacia-Visual, cognitive and neuropaediatric characteristics related to cerebral imaging. *Developmental Medicine and Child Neurology, 38,* 724–735.

Larroque, B., Marret, S., Ancel, P. Y., Arnaud., C., Marpeau, L., Supernant, K., et al. (2003). White matter damage and intraventricular hemorrhage in very preterm infants. The epipage study. *Journal of Pediatrics, 143*(4), 477–483.

Oka, A., Belliveau, M. J., Rosenberg, P. A., & Volpe, J. J. (1993). Vulnerability of oligodendroglia to glutamate: pharmacology, mechanism and prevention. *The Journal of Neurorscience, 13,* 1441–1453.

Pisani, F., Leali, L., Moretti, S., Turco, E., Volante, E., & Bevilsacqua, G. (2006). Transient periventricular echodesnsities in preterms and neurodevelopmental outcome. *Journal of Child Neurology, 21*(3), 230–235.

Ropper, A. H., & Brown, R. H. (2005). Adams and Victor's principles of neurology (8th ed.). McGraw-Hill.

Rorke, L. B. (1992). Anatomic features of the developing brain implicated in pathogenesis of hypoxicischemic injury. *Brain Pathology, 2,* 211–221.

Takashima, S., & Tanaka, K. (1978). Development of cerebrovascular architecture and its relationship to periventricular leukomalacia. *Archives of Neurology*, 35, 11–16.

Volpe, J. J. (2008) *Neurology of the newborn* (5th ed.). Philadelphia, PA: Saunders Elsevier.

Woodward, L. J., Anderson, P. J., Austin, N., Howard, K., & Inder, T. E. (2006). Neonatal MRI to predict neurodevelopmental outcomes in preterm infants. *New England Journal of Medicine*, 355(7), 685–694.

PERSONALITY DISORDERS

DESCRIPTION

A personality disorder is defined as a pattern of pervasive, inflexible thoughts and behaviors that causes interpersonal stress due to social and cultural inappropriateness. As diagnosed by the *Diagnostic and Statistical Manual of Mental Disorders—fourth edition*, Text Revision (*DSM IV-TR*), there are 10 disorders that consist of specific behaviors and treatment implications (American Psychiatric Association [APA], 2000). These 10 disorders are further divided into three clusters based on the similarity of presenting symptoms: Cluster A (Paranoid Personality Disorder, Schizoid Personality Disorder, Schizotypal Personality Disorder), Cluster B (Antisocial Personality Disorder, Borderline Personality Disorder (BPD), Histrionic Personality Disorder, Narcissistic Personality Disorder), and Cluster C (Avoidant Personality Disorder, Dependent Personality Disorder, Obsessive-Compulsive Personality Disorder). Personality Disorder not otherwise specified can also be diagnosed if a subthreshold presentation of symptoms is present and are causing significant functional impairment. The prevalence of personality disorders in the population is estimated at 9.1% (Lenzenweger, Lane, Loranger, & Kessler, 2007; Samuels et al., 2002) although true prevalence is difficult to establish due to comorbidity with other psychiatric disorders, as well as the reluctance of patients to seek treatment. Onset is during adolescence or early adulthood.

NEUROPATHOLOGY/PATHOPHYSIOLOGY

Personality traits are psychological features that are consistent across various environmental contexts and stable over time (APA, 2000), and make each individual unique from others. Although personality traits are not maladaptive by definition, in the case of personality disorders, these traits are often maladaptive or extreme, which in turn creates significant problems, warranting the diagnosis. It is a common belief that biological predispositions of personality are then molded by environmental experiences to create the manifestation of personality traits (Eskedal & Demetri, 2006).

There appears to be a more direct argument for the genetic component to the development of personality disorders, as suggested by results of twin and family studies (Siever, 2009). However, genetic heritability is mostly related to specific components or personality traits that are central to each disorder, such as impulsivity and emotional irregularity, rather than the presence of the disorder itself. Gender differences also appear to be present, with males being more representative in antisocial personality disorder and females in avoidant, dependent, and paranoid personality disorders (Grant et al., 2004). It is also noted in the *DSM-IV-TR* that BPD and histrionic personality disorder are more commonly diagnosed in females (APA, 2000).

While the true etiology of personality disorders is continuing to be explored, there are some findings that link their development to childhood temperament, environmental experiences and trauma. Clark (2005) noted that childhood temperament may play an important role in the development of personality disorders, mostly based on three broad domains of temperament including negative affectivity, positive affectivity, and disinhibition. Environmental experiences and trauma, such as a history of sexual abuse, are often observed in personality disorders, particularly with regard to BPD (APA, 2000). New approaches such as brain imaging techniques are now being implemented to further clarify the relationship between biological aspects of the brain and maladaptive personality traits. A review of the literature by Lis, Greenfield, Henry, and Guile (2007) noted interesting research, specifically within the realm of BPD, which may be promising for future research with other personality disorders.

NEUROPSYCHOLOGICAL/CLINICAL PRESENTATION

Clinical presentation of personality disorders vary according to the type of disorder, though the underlying pervasiveness of the symptoms should be present with each disorder. Therefore, the patient must report the symptoms to be occurring over many months or years, causing interpersonal or occupational difficulties during that time. Cluster A

OP

disorders often share symptoms related to social deficits, cognitive impairment, and perceptual distortions that may be similar to hallucinations. Generally, individuals with these disorders may be considered odd or eccentric. Cluster B disorders often present as impulsive, aggressive, unstable affect regulation, and poor emotional processing. They may be described as erratic or dramatic upon presentation or by peers. Finally, Cluster C disorders may be observed as anxious, fearful, and compulsive, with poor behavioral inhibition.

DIAGNOSIS

The stability of the symptoms is an important factor in diagnosis, particularly with regard to differential diagnosis. Changes in personality that may manifest as a result of a head injury are common (Golden & Golden, 2003), and must be ruled out before the diagnosis of personality disorder is made. Similarly, personality traits directly related to a general medical condition or that are substance-induced are exclusionary criteria for the disorders. Diagnoses of personality disorders are made based on the diagnostic criteria in the *DSM-IV-TR* and a longstanding report of stable personality traits that are maladaptive. Each disorder has signifying characteristics that are important to assess and differentiate before a final diagnosis is made. In addition, the comorbidity of other psychiatric disorders add to the confusion in diagnosis.

TREATMENT

Treatment for patients with personality disorders is often long term and can be quite frustrating for the clinician. Often, individuals with personality disorders do not believe that they have a mental illness and perceive others to be at fault for many of their interpersonal problems. Furthermore, family and friends of a person with a personality disorder often have more distress than the identified patient simply because of the egosyntonic nature of the behavior.

It is well known that patients with personality disorders are some of the most frequent and most expensive to treat in community and hospital settings. Typically, psychotherapy is recommended for treatment, though pharmacological interventions are often implemented to augment therapy. Research often focuses on the entire cluster of disorders, rather than on individual disorders to explore the most effective way to treat the symptoms, each of the disorders within each cluster, respectively. Generally, each personality disorder cluster should be approached in a different therapeutic fashion and with specific treatment interventions. Treatment approaches have included cognitive behavioral therapy, group therapy, family therapy, and psychodynamic therapy, with a focus on developing a more adaptive lifestyle and better interpersonal relationships.

Beth Trammell
Raymond S. Dean

American Psychiatric Association. (2000). *Diagnostic and statistical manual of mental disorders IV-R*. Arlington, VA: American Psychiatric Publishing.

Clark, L. A. (2005). Temperament as a unifying basis for personality and psychopathology. *Journal of Abnormal Psychology, 114*, 505–521.

Eskedal, G. A., & Demetri, J. M. (2006). Etiology and treatment of Cluster C personality disorders. *Journal of Mental Health Counseling, 28*, 1–17.

Golden, Z., & Golden, C. J. (2003). Impact of brain injury severity on personality dysfunction. *International Journal of Neuroscience, 113*, 733–745.

Grant, B. F., Hasin, D. S., Stinson, F. S., Dawson, D. A., Chou, S. P., Ruan, W. J., et al. (2004). Prevalence, correlates, and disability of personality disorders in the United States: Results from the national epidemiologic survey on alcohol and related conditions. *Journal of Clinical Psychiatry, 65*, 948–958.

Lenzenweger, M. F., Lane, M. C., Loranger, A. W., & Kessler, R. C. (2007). DSM-IV personality disorders in the National Comorbidity Survey Replication. *Biological Psychiatry, 62*, 553–564

Lis, E., Greenfield, B., Henry, M., & Guile, J. M. (2007). Neuroimaging and genetics of borderline personality disorder: A review. *Journal of Psychiatry & Neuroscience, 32*, 162–173.

Samuels, J., Eaton, W. W., Bienvenu, O. J., Brown, C. H., Costa, P. T., & Nestadt, G. (2002). Prevalence and correlates of personality disorders in a community sample. *British Journal of Psychiatry, 180*, 536–542.

Siever, L. J. (2009). The neurobiology of personality disorders: Implications for psychoanalysis. *Journal of the American Psychoanalytical Association, 57*, 361–398.

PHENYLKETONURIA

DESCRIPTION

Phenylketonuria (PKU) is an inborn error of metabolism in which phenylalanine, an essential amino acid, builds up due to a deficiency of phenylalanine hydroxylase. The presentation is largely neurological in its impact, although it arises from elevations of liver enzymes. The degree of neurological impact is related to how early and consistent treatment is offered, which mainly involves dietary restrictions. If untreated, the neuropathological effects can be quite severe (Huttenlocher, 2000). However, evidence suggests that even with rigid treatment, neurocognitive residuals and behavioral impairments may be seen (Brumm et al., 2004; Channon, German, Cassina, & Lee, 2004). Given the need and importance of early intervention, routine blood panels drawn in the first 48 hours following birth today include screening for PKU.

NEUROPATHOLOGY/PATHOPHYSIOLOGY

PKU arises from a defect in the phenylalanine hydroxylase activity, which converts phenylalanine to tyrosine (Scriver, Kaufman, Eisensmith, & Woo, 1995). Neurologically, this process is crucial for the biosynthesis of various neurotransmitters and to prevent buildup of phenylalanine, which has a neurotoxic effect when presenting in excess in the system (Pietz, 1998). Consequently, the degree of buildup is directly related to the amount of neurological compromise evidenced on MRI (Thompson et al., 1993). In this instance, MRI findings were also related to the time since dietary treatment had been withdrawn.

In untreated infants, microcephaly commonly develops. With advances in neonatal screening, this has become rare. Still, white matter alterations are often noted presenting as spongiosis, gliosis, and delays in myelination (Thompson et al., 1993). This is due to oligodendrocytes being particularly sensitive to the neurotoxic effects of elevated phenylalanine (Dyer, 1999). Cortical neurons may be smaller than normal and in fewer numbers with fewer Nissl granules, and there are often depleted numbers of dendritic spines (Cordero et al., 1983). Cerebral lipid and proteolipid levels may be low (Lew et al., 1989).

Although early treatment reduces the neurological impact of PKU, it does not offset the effects entirely. White matter abnormalities, with greatest prominence in posterior periventricular regions, are still commonly reported in individuals who received early intervention (Pietz, Kreis et al., 1996). The degree of white matter lesions has been consistently linked with phenylalanine levels throughout life (Pietz, Kreis et al., 1996).

Dopamine, norepinephrine, and serotonin depletions have been consistently reported in relation to PKU, even when early treatment was offered (Burlina et al., 2000; Paans et al., 1996). This has been associated with an interference of elevated phenylalanine levels in the transportation of tyrosine and tryptophan at the blood–brain barrier (Momma, Aoyagi, Rapoport, & Smith, 1987).

NEUROPSYCHOLOGICAL/CLINICAL PRESENTATION

As suggested, PKU is largely neurological in its impact. In regard to the clinical manifestations of PKU, a latency effect is often noted, with developmental delays sometimes not becoming evident until after the first year of life. However, myoclonic seizures in untreated individuals may emerge as early as 4 months of age (Gascon, Ozand, & Cohen, 2007). Furthermore, some delays, such as when an infant sits up on its own, crawls, walks, and says first words, may also be noted sooner. Again, these above features are most noted in untreated individuals. Pitt and Danks (1991) in their review of a cohort of individuals never treated, found that 25% had seizures, 50% were profoundly mentally retarded, and the other half were severely to moderately mentally retarded.

In regard to neuropsychological functioning, executive deficits are potentially the most common features of PKU. Deficits in attention, both selective and sustained (Huijbregts, de Sonneville, Licht, van Spronsen et al., 2002) as well as shifting attention (Weglage et al., 1999) and dividing attention (Huijbregts, de Sonneville, Licht, Sergeant & van Spronsen, 2002) have been reported. In addition, planning and conceptual reasoning (Leuzzi et al., 2004), inhibition (Huijbregts, de Sonneville, Licht, Sergeant et al., 2002), and working memory (White, Nortz, Mandernach, Huntington, & Steiner, 2002) have all been reported although not consistently found across research (e.g., Feldmann, Denecke, Pietsch, Grenzebach, & Weglage, 2002). Processing speed and reaction times are also commonly impacted (Huijbregts, de Sonneville, Licht, van Spronsen et al., 2002). Similarly, retrieval-based memory deficits have been reported (Brumm et al., 2004) as have deficits in immediate memory (Smith, Klim, & Hanley, 2000; White, Nortz, Mandernach, Huntington, & Steiner, 2001). To a lesser extent, language deficits have been reported (Brumm et al., 2004), but these findings have been inconsistently described in the literature.

Learning difficulties are common (Anderson et al., 2004) and may increase in identification as children age, as executive functions are relied on more in their academics. Disabilities in reading and mathematics are reported at far greater rates than seen in the normal population. In comparison, reading deficits are reported more frequently than deficits in mathematics. For example, Azen et al. (1991) found correlations

OP

between phenylalanine levels and performance in intelligence, reading, and spelling performance but not mathematics. In their study, behavior deficits were also linked with phenylalanine. In fact, individuals with PKU demonstrate greater risks for behavioral and psychiatric manifestations (Pietz 1998) including attention deficit hyperactivity disorder and oppositional defiant disorder among others.

DIAGNOSIS

PKU is diagnosed through blood tests nowadays completed within 48 hours of birth. Elevation is indicated by levels greater than 1 μM (i.e., >120 μM) and a blood phenylalanine/tyrosine ratio higher than 2 (Gascon et al., 2007). Beyond urinalysis, MRI and CT of the brain are useful in evaluating neurological correlates, with particular attention placed on white matter tracts. EEG may be useful in cases that go undiagnosed for some time as seizures rates are high. This would be unusual in industrialized countries that check for PKU following birth but may be relevant in those coming from other countries that do not have such neonatal practices. Finally, neuropsychological testing should be used in all cases to determine the nature and extent of neurocognitive deficits given cognitive dysfunction has been found even in well-controlled and early interventions. Particular attention may be placed on executive functions and reaction speed, although comprehensive evaluation is recommended as variable impact of other domains can be observed.

TREATMENT

The primary treatment for PKU following diagnosis is implementation of a controlled diet to reduce phenylalanine intake. This will involve a very low protein diet and use of a phenylalanine-free supplement containing amino acids, minerals, vitamins, and trace elements (Pietz, 1998). For example, aspartame, an artificial sweetener, should be avoided as intestinal hydrolysis liberates phenylalanine (Gascon et al., 2007). The dietary restrictions can be adjusted based on age and severity of the metabolic defect, which is determined through the aforementioned laboratory tests. There are suggestions that as children age, restrictions can be lessened (Azen et al., 1991; Smith, 1994) although this is debated.

When neurological deficits arise, interventions and treatment are consistent with those commonly implemented to counteract such features. Special education services may be required for learning difficulties. Cognitive training may be implemented to teach individuals to better compensate for deficits and to improve functionality.

Chad A. Noggle
Amy R. Steiner

Anderson, P., Wood, S., Francis, D., Coleman, L., Warwick, L., Casanelia, S., et al. (2004). Neuropsychological functioning in children with early-treated phenylketonuria: Impact of white matter abnormalities. *Developmental Medicine & Child Neurology, 46*, 230–238.

Azen, C. R., Koch, R., Friedman, E. G., Berlow, S., Coldwell, J., Krause, W., et al. (1991). Intellectual development in 12 year-old children treated for phenylketonuria. *American Journal of Diseases of Children, 145*, 35–39.

Brumm, V., Azen, C., Moats, R., Stern, A., Broomand, C., Nelson, M., et al. (2004). Neuropsychological outcome of subjects participating in the PKU Adult Collaborative Study: A preliminary review. *Journal of Inherited Metabolic Disease, 27*, 549–566.

Burlina, A., Bonafé, L., Ferrari, V., Suppiej, A., Zacchello, F., Burlina, A., et al. (2000). Measurement of neurotransmitter metabolites in the cerebrospinal fluid of phenylketonuric patients under dietary treatment. *Journal of Inherited Metabolic Disease, 23*, 313–316.

Channon, S., German, C., Cassina, C., & Lee, P. (2004). Executive functioning, memory, and learning in phenylketonuria. *Neuropsychology, 18*, 613–620.

Cordero, M. E., Trejo, M., Colombo, M., & Aranda, V. (1983). Histological maturation of the neocortex in phenylketonuric rats. *Early Human Development, 8*, 157.

Dyer, C. A. (1999). Pathophysiology of phenylketonuria. *Mental Retardation & Developmental Disabilities Research Reviews, 5*, 104–112.

Feldmann, R., Denecke, J., Pietsch, M., Grenzebach, M., & Weglage, J. (2002). Phenylketonuria: No specific frontal lobe-dependent neuropsychological deficits of early-treated patients in comparison with diabetics. *Pediatric Research, 51*, 761–765.

Gascon, G., Ozand, P., & Cohen, B. (2007). Aminoacidopathies and organic acidopathies, mitochondrial enzyme defects, and other metabolic errors. In C. Goetz (Ed). *Textbook of clinical neurology* (pp. 641–681). Philadelphia, PA: Saunders Elsevier.

Huijbregts, S., de Sonneville, L., Licht, R., Sergeant, J., & van Spronsen, F. (2002). Inhibition of prepotent responding and attentional flexibility in treated phenylketonuria. *Developmental Neuropsychology, 22*, 481–499.

Huijbregts, S., de Sonneville, L., Licht, R., van Spronsen, F., Verkerk, P., & Sergeant, J. (2002). Sustained attention and inhibition of cognitive interference in treated phenylketonuria: Associations with concurrent and lifetime phenylalanine concentrations. *Neuropsychologia, 40*, 7–15.

OP

Huttenlocher, P. R. (2000). The neuropathology of phenylk-etonuria: Human and animal studies. *European Journal of Pediatrics, 159*(Suppl. 2), S102–S106.

Leuzzi, V., Pansini, M., Sechi, E., Chiarotti, F., Carducci, C., Levi, G., et al. (2004). Executive function impairment in early-treated PKU subjects with normal mental development. *Journal of Inherited Metabolic Disease, 27,* 115–125.

Lew, E. O., Rozdilsky, B., Munoz, D. G., Perry, G. (1989). A new type of neuronal cytoplasmic inclusion: histologi-cal, ultrastructural, and immunocyctochemical studies. *Acta Neuropathologica (Berl), 77,* 599–604.

Momma, S., Aoyagi, M., Rapoport, S., & Smith, Q. (1987). Phenylalanine transport across the blood-brain barrier as studied with the in situ brain perfusion technique. *Journal of Neurochemistry, 48,* 1291–1300.

Paans, A. M., Pruim, J., Smit, G. P., Visser, G., Willemsen, A. T., & Ullrich, K. (1996). Neurotransmitter positron emission tomographic-studies in adults with phenylk-etonuria, a pilot study. *European Journal of Pediatrics, 155,* S78–S81.

Pietz, J. (1998). Neurological aspects of adult phenylketo-nuria. *Current Opinion in Neurology, 11,* 679–688.

Pietz, J., Kreis, R., Schmidt, H., Meyding-Lamade, U. K., Rupp, A., & Boesch, C. (1996). Phenylketonuria: find-ings at MR imaging and localized in vivo H-1 MR spec-troscopy of the brain in patients with early treatment. *Radiology, 201,* 413–420.

Pitt, D. B., Danks, D. M. (1991). The natural history of untreated phenylketonuria. *Journal of Pediatrics, 27,* 189–190.

Scriver, C., Kaufman, S., Eisensmith, R., & Woo, S. (1995). The hyperphenylalaninemias. In C. Scriver, A. Beaudet, S. Sly, & D. Valle (Eds.), *The metabolic and molecular bases of inherited disease* (pp. 1025–1075). New York NY: McGraw-Hill.

Smith, I. (1994). Treatment of phenylalanine hydroxylase deficiency. *Acta Paediatrica Supplement, 407,* 60–65.

Smith, M., Klim, P., & Hanley, W. (2000). Executive function in school-aged children with phenylketonuria. *Journal of Developmental & Physical Disabilities, 12,* 317–332.

Thompson, A. J., Tillotson, S., Smith, O., Kendall, B., Moore, S. G., Brenton, D. P., et al. (1993). Brain MRI changes in phenylketonuria. *Associations with dietary status. Brain, 116,* 811–821.

Weglage, J., Pietsch, M., Denecke, J., Sprinz, A., Feldmann, R., Grenzebach, M., et al. (1999). Regression of neuro-psychological deficits in early-treated phenylketonurics during adolescence. *Journal of Inherited Metabolic Disease, 22,* 693–705.

White, D., Nortz, M., Mandernach, T., Huntington, K., & Steiner, R. (2001). Deficits in memory strategy use related to prefrontal dysfunction during early develop-ment: Evidence from children with phenylketonuria. *Neuropsychology, 15,* 221–229.

White, D., Nortz, M., Mandernach, T., Huntington, K., & Steiner, R. (2002). Age-related working memory impair-ments in children with prefrontal dysfunction associ-ated with phenylketonuria. *Journal of the International Neuropsychological Society, 8,* 1–11.

PICK'S DISEASE

DESCRIPTION

Arnold Pick first described this disease in 1892 stemming from his observations of a 71-year-old dementing patient with a 3-year history of progressive language problems. At autopsy, the patient was found to have left temporal lobe atrophy and argentophilic intranuclear inclusions, now known as Pick's bodies. For years, all the early onset frontotemporal dementias were subsumed informally under the heading of Pick's disease (as opposed to the later, or senile, onset Alzhei-mer's dementia). Now Pick's disease is considered one of the frontotemporal dementias. The clinical course begins, usually, with changes in personality, including impulsiveness and inappropriate behaviors. There is a distinct decline in social conduct with little tact, poor manners, and inappropriate overt sexual behavior and comments. These patients lack empathy and emotional warmth and appear indifferent, especially to the con-sequences of their behaviors. Even early in the course of the disease, they have little or no insight or concern about their disease or the resultant behaviors. Memory problems, apraxias, and similar more "posterior" neu-ropsychological deficits occur later in the disease, although working memory can become compromised relatively early in the course. They also have difficulty with executive functioning, that is, problems in plan-ning, organizing, and taking into account all the avail-able information before acting. Language becomes nonfluent. The disease begins most often in the 50s, although it has been known to begin in the 20s. It has a life expectancy of 6–7 years after diagnosis, though a fifth of the patients will live more than 10 years. Only 20% of the cases of Pick's disease are familial. Behav-ioral changes may include compulsivity, inappropriate-ness, inability to function, or interact in social or personal situations, problems with personal hygiene, repetitive behavior, withdrawal from social interaction, and the inability to function occupationally and socially. Personal hygiene deteriorates substantially, often with a refusal to wash or bathe and to dress appro-priately. The Kluver–Bucy's syndrome may develop over the course of the disease. Emotional changes can

OP

include abrupt mood changes; decreased interest in daily living activities; failure to recognize changes in behavior; failure to show emotional warmth, concern, empathy, and sympathy; inappropriate mood; and a lack of interest in the environment. Patients often demonstrate amimia, a marked lack of facial expression. They can show a loss of fear and affective responses. Language changes include a decreased ability to read or write, word-finding difficulties, nonfluent aphasia, echolalia, speech sounds that are weak or uncoordinated, and even mutism. Verbal perseveration is common as is stereotyped language.

NEUROPATHOLOGY/PATHOPHYSIOLOGY

There is no definitive premortum test for Pick's disease, as the diagnosis can only be made based on histological evidence. Mendez and Cummings (2003) provided a good description of the neuropathologic changes found in Pick's dementia. These include severe frontotemporal atrophy with knife-like gyri. Histologically, there are Pick's cells (ballooned neurons) and tau positive, ubiquitin-positive Pick's bodies. (The other pathological variants of frontotemporal dementia include motor neuron disease and frontotemporal dementia lacking distinctive histology.) Both the dopaminergic and serotoninergic systems are decreased but not the cholinergic ones. The substantia nigra is small but the concentration of neurons is normal; parkinsonism does not emerge until late in the course of the disease. There is a substantial loss of synapses in the three outer layers of the cortex. Astrocytes surround the cell bodies, and there is demyelination. However, there are no neurofibrillary tangles or senile plaques as seen in Alzheimer's disease.

NEUROPSYCHOLOGY/CLINICAL PRESENTATION

In the past, it has been claimed that it is difficult to differentiate Pick's disease in particular and frontotemporal dementia in general from Alzheimer's disease. In the early stages of the disease, however, this is not true for a skilled neuropsychologist or neurologist. Differentiation is not possible in every case, especially in the later stages, but the initial symptoms usually are quite distinct. Early in Pick's disease, there is a relative sparing of cognitive functions in the face of substantial behavioral changes. Memory and praxic abilities are relatively preserved, and there is no topographic agnosia. Language is also better preserved in the patient with Pick's disease than one with Alzheimer's disease, even if it is less fluent. During the later stages, there is general cognitive decline in Pick's disease, and over the course of time, the two dementias become more and

more similar. The clinical course of Pick's disease consists of three stages (Cummings & Benson, 1983). In the first stage, there are distinct personality and emotional changes. They show poor judgment and usually little insight. Social behavior deteriorates and becomes very inappropriate. Language abnormalities, especially expressive ones, are among the earliest intellectual alterations to occur. Often early in the course Kluver–Bucy's syndrome develops. This is composed of emotional blunting, lack of fear and affective responses, hypermetamorphosis, oral exploratory behavior, sensory agnosia, and hypersexuality. Also often seen after trauma to the temporal lobe, these symptoms can cause substantial embarrassment to the family of the patient. With an insidious onset, the disease often progresses to the point of clear impairment before help is sought and the diagnosis given. In the second stage, the mental status deteriorates further, the aphasia is clear, executive and general cognitive functions are impaired. However, memory (except working memory), visuospatial abilities, and mathematical skills remain relatively intact. In the third stage, intellectual deterioration affects all areas of intellectual function, and the person becomes mute and incontinent. In addition, usually an extrapyramidal syndrome appears. Finally, death occurs, most often from pulmonary, urinary, or decubitus ulcer infection.

DIAGNOSIS

The diagnosis of Pick's disease is usually confirmed at autopsy by the presence of Pick's bodies and cells. Structural imaging studies will show atrophy of the frontal and temporal areas, especially late in the course, and functional imaging studies will show hypometabolism of these areas. Behaviorally the first step in the diagnosis of this dementia is the exclusion of other disorders (e.g., schizophrenia, depression), especially those with frontal involvement (e.g., Huntington's disease, Lewy body dementia, vascular dementia, lesions or tumors of the frontotemporal areas). Clinically, these patients show poor personal regulation and social interactions, emotional blunting, impaired insight, and impaired executive functioning (Neary et al., 1998).

TREATMENT

There is no proven effective treatment for Pick's disease. The goal of treatment is primarily to control symptoms, monitor the patient, assist with self-care and daily living, and maximize the quality of life. Behavior modification (rewarding appropriate or positive behaviors and, as possible, ignoring inappropriate behaviors) may be helpful in controlling some disturbing and unwanted behavior. Formal psychotherapy treatment is not commonly successful because it causes further confusion and disorientation. Medication can be beneficial in addressing dangerous behaviors such as aggression or increased agitation. Antidepressants may help manage mood swings. Given the serotonin and dopamine decrease, the patient may respond well to selective serotonin reuptake inhibitors and similar medications. Major tranquilizers may help those who show aggression or verbal or behavioral outbursts. Disorders that may contribute to confusion should be treated symptomatically. These include anemia, hypoxia, heart failure, infections, nutritional disorders, and psychiatric conditions such as depression. Treating medical and psychiatric disorders will often help to improve the mental functioning of the Pick's patient. Good nursing care and a skilled and empathic caregiver are helpful. Occupational activities and support groups for the patient are also suggested. It is important that the families of Pick's disease patients obtain support and help to assist them in coping. In fact, some say that treatment of the caregiver is as important as treatment for the patient. Even early in the course of the disease, the patient may need assistance with personal hygiene and self-care. Eventually, there may be a need for 24-hour care and monitoring. Sadly, individuals will need legal advice early in the course of the disorder. Advance directives, power of attorney, and other legal actions make it easier to make ethical decisions and enact sensible legal actions regarding the care and other aspects of the life of the person with Pick's disease.

Henry V. Soper
Susan Spicer
Jennifer N. Fiebig

Cummings, J. L., & Benson, D. F. (1983). *Dementia: A clinical approach.* Boston: Butterworth.

Mendez, M. F., & Cummings, J. L. (2003) *Dementia: A clinical approach* (3rd ed.). Boston: Butterworth.

Neary, D., Snowden, J. S., Gustafson, L., Passant, U., Stuss, D., Black, S., et al. (1998). Frontotemporal lobar degeneration: A consensus on clinical diagnostic criteria. *Neurology, 51,* 1546–1554.

PIRIFORMIS SYNDROME

DESCRIPTION

Piriformis syndrome is characterized by hip and buttock pain in individuals with an inflammation of the piriformis muscle. This muscle is located very close to the sciatic nerve at the greater sciatic arch, and the pain is caused by unusual pressure created by inflammation of the muscle. The importance of understanding this disorder can be seen by the estimate that 16% of all work disability evaluations and examinations are performed to rate patients' partial or total disability associated with chronic low back pain, and that the estimation of those patients suffering from low back pain is approximately 6% (Boyajian-O'Neill, McClain, Coleman, & Thomas, 2008). Underdiagnosis can lead to further pain and eventual changes in the surrounding tissue because of the movement pattern the client is forced into because of pain caused by this debilitating problem.

NEUROPATHOLOGY/PATHOPHYSIOLOGY

The piriformis muscle is anatomically located at the sacrum and passes through the sciatic notch where it terminates in the trochanter of the femur. This location allows for a very close proximity with the sciatic nerve. Injuries can vary from minor lifting or lower back injury that inflames it, but in some cases it also arises from severe trauma. There are indications that this injury can occur as a result of sexual assault because of the muscle's location (Scaer, 2007). Piriformis syndrome is thought to occur more commonly among women though it can occur among the male population. Some estimates indicate that among the entire population of lower back pain sufferers, piriformis syndrome might account for 5–36% of these individuals (Boyajian-O'Neill et al., 2008).

The piriformis muscle is crucial to movement. It is thought that it acts as an external rotator, weak abductor, and weak flexor of the hip, which is used both during standing and sitting (Boyajian-O'Neill et al., 2008). The pain that occurs from the inflammation of this muscle can be prevalent through most everyday activities. Many sufferers of piriformis are so debilitated that they can no longer work and in many cases are told that further work could potentially enhance their injury. The nerve pathway associated with the piriformis muscle runs through the sacroiliac joint. The anatomical structure of the sciatic nerve is normally through the inferior surface of the piriformis muscle. However, in some cases it has been known to penetrate the muscle, which may predispose an individual to piriformis syndrome (Boyajian-O'Neill et al., 2008).

Piriformis syndrome is subdivided into two types of piriformis syndrome, primary and secondary. Primary piriformis syndrome can be seen in individuals where the muscle fibers have been split in order for the nerve to pass through. This type is rarer than the secondary type. Secondary piriformis syndrome is caused by the swelling of the muscle, normally as a result of trauma, pinning the muscle against the various surrounding anatomy. This microtrauma can happen from all types of activities of everyday life, such as jogging, light lifting, or a minor sports injury.

NEUROPSYCHOLOGICAL/CLINICAL PRESENTATION

The neuropsychological effects on testing and other psychologically related literature is minimal in regard to the effect of piriformis syndrome. There may be psychological effects on the person related to the etiology of the disorder. As mentioned, there may be a correlation between the symptoms of piriformis syndrome and sexual assault. This conclusion came from investigation into a patient who became nauseous every time the doctor put her into a specific position and eventually led to the patient no longer showing up for sessions (Scaer, 2007).

Pain itself is always something to take into account when conducting neuropsychological or psychological testing. Many of these clients are more comfortable when moving around rather than sitting still, which is part of the criteria for the disorder. This can lead to hurried test performance if forced to sit or signs of inattention if allowed to move around. If the patient can only sit still for a short period of time, testing procedures must adapt in order to accommodate the client, and a clear understanding that the testing period may need to occur over a far longer time than normal protocol must also be taken into account. In addition, chronic pain that is improperly diagnosed and treated can lead to personality change, irritability, sleep loss, fatigue, depression, anxiety, and poor interpersonal relationships.

Paresthesia may also arise from piriformis syndrome. The irritation and compression of the nerve can lead to foot drops and additional gait problems. This can be misinterpreted as a disorder of the central nervous system in some cases. The disorder may also lead to some sexual organ side effects such as dyspareunia in women and impotence in men, all of which can lead to serious psychological consequences.

DIAGNOSIS

The clinical symptoms of this disorder include (1) pain with sitting, standing, or lying longer than 15–20 minutes; (2) pain and/or paresthesias radiating from the sacrum through the gluteus area and down posterior aspects of the thigh, usually discontinuing before the knee; (3) pain improves with ambulation and worsens with no movement; (4) pain when rising from seated or squatting position; (5) pain does not abate completely with change of position; (6) contralateral sacroiliac pain; (7) difficulty walking, antalgic gait, foot drop, numbness in foot, and/or weakness on same side lower extremity; (8) headache, neck pain, abdominal pain, pelvic pain, and inguinal pain; (9) dyspareunia in women; and (10) pain with bowel movements (Boyajian-O'Neill et al., 2008).

Magnetic resonance neurography (MRN) has been used to pinpoint problems associated with the sciatic notch and its comparison to the piriformis muscle. Lewis, Layzer, Engstrom, Barbaro, and Chin (2006) found that MRN was able to visualize the impingement in comparison to normal individuals. These researchers injected a dye into the patient that allowed them to see the piriformis muscle in comparison with the surrounding tissue. Though this is in the research phase, it could become a useful tool in understanding where and why this type of pain occurs in individuals with otherwise normal magnetic resonance imaging results.

TREATMENT

Many different forms of therapy are offered for the treatment of piriformis syndrome. All treatments stress the concept of early treatment. The variations range from stretching, ischemic compression, massage, ultrasound therapy, and injections to surgical release (Travell & Simons, 1992). Stretch therapy requires a certain level of relaxation prior to and after treatment, which is taught to the patient before stretching.

Stretching can be accompanied by massage in order to lengthen the muscle and relieve some of the pressure. Depending upon the area that is problematic and the type of piriformis contraction occurring, the techniques vary. Ischemic compression involves pushing on the outside of the skin over the tenderness of the muscle, which is similar to massage but more forceful in an attempt to loosen the contraction. This technique should be done carefully and by a professional because of the risk of damage to the sciatic nerve resulting in a worse outcome.

Injections, called trigger point injections, involve injecting lidocaine or procaine and sometimes a corticosteroid into the area. The purpose of these injections is to allow the muscle to relax enough and relieve a constant state of spasm. The site of the injections vary depending upon where the piriformis muscle spasms are occurring. At one time, surgical intervention was a viable option but has recently fallen into disfavor because most clinicians now believe that surgery is not an appropriate measure for the reduction of symptoms in association with piriformis syndrome (Travell & Simons, 1992). Others have suggested the use of acupuncture (Spiller, 2007).

In most of the literature, the pressure relief techniques mentioned above provide the most reduction in pain and are the best first defense option. Results are better when the client gets early evaluation and treatment. Though this disorder is currently rarely diagnosed, it is possible that the prevalence rate could be significantly higher than currently recognized.

David M. Scarisbrick
Charles Golden

Boyajian-O'Neill, L. A., McClain, R. L., Coleman, M. K., & Thomas, P. P. (2008). Diagnosis and management of piriformis syndrome: An osteopathic approach. *The Journal of the American Osteopathic Association, 108*(11), 657–664

Lewis, A. M., Layzer, R., Engstrom, J. W., Barbaro, N. M., & Chin, C. T. (2006). Magnetic resonance neurography in extraspinal sciatica. *Archives of Neurology, 63*(10), 1469–1472.

Scaer, R. C. (2007). *The body bears the burden: Trauma, dissociation, and disease.* Haworth Press.

Spiller, J. (2007). Acupuncture, ketamine and piriformis syndrome - a case report from palliative care: A case report. *Acupuncture Medicine, 25,* 109-112.

Travell, J. G., & Simons, D. G., (1992). *Myofascial pain and dysfunction: The trigger point manual.* Lippincott Williams & Wilkins.

POLYARTERITIS NODOSA

DESCRIPTION

Polyarteritis nodosa (PAN) represents a rare complication of hepatitis B infection that develops in roughly l–5% of patients with the virus (McMahon et al., 1989). However, in the reverse, roughly 30% of all cases of PAN are secondary to hepatitis B (Guillevin et al., 1995). PAN presents as a necrotizing vasculitis that demonstrates a preferential targeting of small and medium arteries and veins. The widespread nature of the presentation commonly manifests as peripheral neuropathy, hypertension, weight loss, myalgias, gastrointestinal tract problems, and arthritis (Guillevin et al., 1995). When neurological symptoms are seen

they are primarily motoric based. Overall, prognosis is relatively poor if left untreated.

NEUROPATHOLOGY/PATHOPHYSIOLOGY

PAN manifests as widespread necrotic vasculitis most commonly occurring secondary to hepatitis B infection. The pathophysiological underpinnings of HBV-associated PAN remain unclear. However, immune complexes are often found in patients' sera and endothelia although antineutrophil cytoplasmic antibodies are rarely detected (Guillevin et al., 1993). Neurological involvement is rare, occurring in only 5% of patients, but it is commonly associated with brainstem infiltration. Spinal cord lesions may also present.

The lungs are usually spared, which is key as this can serve as the key differential between PAN and the allergic granulomatous angiitis of Churg–Strauss syndrome (Ropper & Brown, 2005).

NEUROPSYCHOLOGICAL/CLINICAL PRESENTATION

The clinical features of PAN can vary. Arterial and renal hypertension as well as intestinal wall necrosis may be seen. The most common features include peripheral neuropathy, hypertension, unexplained weight loss, myalgias, and arthritis (Guillevin et al., 1995). When the CNS is involved, albeit rare, headache, plegia, and brainstem signs predominate (Ropper & Brown, 2005). As suggested previously, the lungs are spared. When cerebral vessels are involved, patients may present with diffuse encephalopathy, seizure, or stroke (Reichart, Bogousslavsky, & Janzer, 2000). The latter is particularly rare with less than 20 cases being documented prior to 2000 (Reichart et al., 2000). Intracranial aneurysms are also particularly rare (Oomura, Yamawaki, Naritomi, Terai, & Shigeno, 2006; Takahashi et al., 2002).

Neuropsychological deficits are only associated with PAN when the CNS is involved. Focal neurological deficits may present in relation to stroke, which is quite rare. When diffuse encephalopathy manifests, patients commonly present with decreased selective and sustained attention. Psychomotor retardation, processing speed, memory, and executive function deficits may occur.

DIAGNOSIS

Diagnosis is difficult and requires a multifaceted approach. Angiography remains the most essential tool, with more definitive diagnosis being possible if numerous microaneurysms are seen in visceral arteries and potentially in the cerebral circulation (Sharma, Kumar, Mishra, & Gaikwad, 2010).

Specific diagnostic guidelines are also available, including the American College of Rheumatology (ACR) criteria (Lightfoot et al., 1990) and the Chapel Hill Consensus Conference (CHCC) criteria (Segelmark & Selga, 2007), although they have been criticized. Specifically, the ACR criteria is such that many patients end up grouped into more than one disease category, whereas the CHCC guidelines are such that most patients do not meet criteria (Sharma et al., 2010). Surrogate and serologic markers have been included in algorithms as a means of refining these diagnostic flaws (Segelmark & Selga, 2007; Watts et al., 2007; Watts & Scott, 2009). Biopsy of the affected tissue is ideal for diagnosis, permitting confirmation of PAN (Miller, 2000). CT is useful from a diagnostic standpoint in the evaluation of kidneys, whereas MRI of the brain is helpful in the evaluation of intracranial features.

TREATMENT

The treatment of PAN associated with hepatitis B virus remains difficult. Steroids have shown some variable benefit as have therapies with α-interferon, plasma exchange, cyclophosphamide, methotrexate, vidarabine and nucleoside analogs (Bartt & Topel, 2007). Although these therapies have shown some mixed benefit when used singularly, a combination of α-interferon and plasma exchange has been reported previously to contribute to a 50% elimination rate of hepatitis B and a near complete remission of PAN symptoms (Guillevin et al., 1994). As noted, untreated PAN has a poor prognosis with a mean 5-year survival of around 10–20% (Bartt & Topel, 2007). Cutaneous PAN lesions have shown responsiveness to hyperbaric oxygen treatment (Mazokopakis, 2005).

Jacob M. Goings
Chad A. Noggle

Bartt, R. E. & Topel, J. L. (2007). Autoimmune and Inflammatory Disorders. In C.G. Goetz (Ed.) *Textbook of clinical neurology* (3rd ed., pp. 1156–1184). Philadelphia, PA: Saunders Elsevier.

Guillevin, L., Lhote, F., Cohen, P., Sauvaget, F., Jarrousse, B., Lortholary, O., et al. (1995). Polyarteritis nodosa related to hepatitis B virus: a prospective study with long term observation of 41 patients. *Medicine, 74,* 238–253.

Guillevin, L., Lhote, F., Sauvaget, F., Deblois, P., Rossi, F., Levallois, D., *et al.* (1994). Treatment of polyarteritis nodosa related to hepatitis B virus with interferon-alpha and plasma exchanges. *Annals of the Rheumatic Diseases, 53*(5), 334–337.

Guillevin, L., Visser, H., Noel, L. H., Pourrat, J., Vernier, I., Gayraud, M., et al. (1993). Antineutrophil cytoplasm antibodies in systemic polyarteritis nodosa with and without hepatitis B virus infection and Churg-Strauss syndrome-patients. *The Journal of Rheumatology, 20,* 1345–1349.

Lightfoot, R. W. Jr., Michel, B. A., Bloch, D. A., Hunder, G. G., Zvaifler, N. J., McShane, D. J., et al. (1990). The American College of Rheumatology 1990 criteria for the classification of polyarteritis nodosa. *Arthritis & Rheumatism, 33,* 1088–1093.

Mazokopakis, E. (2005). The prophet Jonah as patron saint of divers, and patron saint of diving and hyperbaric medicine, in the Orthodox Church. *European Journal of Underwater Hyperbaric Medicine, 6,* 45–48.

McMahon, B. J., Heyward, W. L., Templin, D. W., Clement, D., Lanier, A. P. (1989). Hepatitis B-associated polyarteritis nodosa in Alaskan Eskimos: clinical and epidemiologic features and long-term follow-up. *Hepatology, 9*(1), 97–101.

Miller, D. L. (2000). Angiography in polyarteritis nodosa. *American Journal of Roentgenology, 175,* 1747–1748.

Oomura, M., Yamawaki, T., Naritomi, H., Terai, T., & Shigeno, K. (2006). Polyarteritis nodosa in association with subarachnoid hemorrhage. *Internal Medicine, 45,* 655–658.

Reichart, M. D., Bogousslavsky, J., & Janzer, R. C. (2000). Early lacunar strokes complicating polyarteritis nodosa Thrombotic microangiopathy. *Neurology, 54,* 883–889.

Ropper, A. H., & Brown, R. H. (2005). Adam's and Victor's Principles of neurology (8th ed.). New York, NY: McGraw-Hill.

Segelmark, M., & Selga, D. (2007). The challenge of managing patients with polyarteritis nodosa. *Current Opinion in Rheumatology, 19,* 33–38.

Sharma, S., Kumar, S., Mishra, N. K., & Gaikwad, S. B. (2010). Cerebral miliary microaneurysms in polyarteritis nodosa: Report of two cases. *Neurology India, 58*(3), 457–459.

Takahashi, J. C., Sakai, N., Iihara, K., Sakai, H., Higashi, T., Kogure, S., et al. (2002). Subarachnoid hemorrhage from a ruptured anterior cerebral artery aneurysm caused by polyarteritis nodosa. Case report. *Journal of Neurosurgery, 96,* 132–134.

Watts, R., Lane, S., Hanslik, T., Hauser, T., Hellmich, B., Koldingsnes, W., et al. (2007). Development and validation of a consensus methodology for the classification of the ANCA-associated vasculitides and polyarteritis nodosa for epidemiological studies. *Annals of the Rheumatic Diseases, 66,* 222–227.

OP

Watts, R. A., & Scott, D. G. (2009). Recent developments in the classification and assessment of vasculitis. *Best Practice & Research Clinical Rheumatology, 23*, 429–443.

POLYMYOSITIS

DESCRIPTION

Polymyositis (PM) is an autoimmune collagen disease, often associated with malignancy that manifests as weakness of the lungs and cardiac system as well as proximal muscles, without skin anomalies. However, some have proposed a more refined definition of PM suggesting it should be restricted to non-dermatomyositis myositis with endomysial infiltrates of T cells often infiltrating nonnecrotic muscle fibers, suggesting a T-cell mediated attack directed against muscle fibers (Briani et al., 2006). The muscle weakness develops subacutely in a diffuse nature, albeit proximal in origin, affecting the upper extremities more so than the lower.

Classified as one of the idiopathic immune-mediated myopathies, PM is relatively rare. In fact, in comparison to the other immune-mediated myopathies, PM is the least common. PM is associated with heightened risk of morbidity and mortality if not properly treated, due to involvement of cardiac and pulmonary systems (Murthy, 2010).

NEUROPATHOLOGY/PATHOPHYSIOLOGY

To date, the pathological basis of PM remains unclear. Research has suggested a combination of CD8$^+$ cells, CD4$^+$ cells, denditric cells, macrophages, and plasma cells contribute to an endomysial-based infiltrating, inflammatory process (Murthy, 2010). Cytotoxic necrosis of muscle fibers is induced by CD8$^+$ lymphocytes, which release perforins and granzymes (Bartt & Topel, 2007). In comparison with dermatomyositis, CD8$^+$ autoinvasive cytotoxic cells recognize antigenic peptides bound to HLA class I molecules on muscle fiber surfaces (Engel et al., 1994). It has been associated with various cancerous presentations, including lymphoma, breast cancer, lung cancer, ovarian cancer, and colon cancer. Links with systemic lupus erythematosus, scleroderma, and rheumatoid arthritis have also been described.

Several autoantibodies are also associated with PM, including antisynthetase antibodies (Jo1, Pl7, PL12), anti-Mi2 antibody, anti-SRP antibody, anti-Ku antibody, anti-Ro, anti-U1-RNP antibodies and, notably, anti-PM-Scl antibody (Weller et al., 1997). Microvasculopathy is seen as a major action in the pathology of PM and is most commonly noted in the form of mononuclear cell infiltrates at perimysial sites around small blood vessels (Weller et al., 1997). These actions target the muscles leading to the aforementioned weakness that occurs in response to the disorder.

The inflammatory infiltrate is mainly perivascular and in the perimysium and endomysium (Weller et al., 1997).

NEUROPSYCHOLOGICAL/CLINICAL PRESENTATION

Muscle weakness is the most common symptom of PM. As suggested, the muscle weakness develops subacutely, and is diffuse in nature, albeit proximal in origin, affecting the upper extremities more so than the lower. In other words, the weakness presents in an inside-to-outside and up-to-down pattern with onset being either gradual or relatively rapid. Furthermore, its chronicity is marked by "flare-ups" in which there are periods of symptom exacerbation throughout the course of the presentation. The end result is general deficits in muscle power and tone, resulting in atrophy in the later stages. Dysphagia may also present related to gastrointestinal involvement. In fact, dysphagia presents in one-third of all cases and is due to involvement of the oropharyngeal muscles and/or upper esophagus striated muscular fibers (De Merieux, Verity, Clements, & Paulus, 1983; Kagen, Hochman, & Strog, 1985).

Pain can be reported in some cases. If the skin becomes involved, in what is termed dermatomyositis, rash may develop from the waist up in most instances, and hard lumps may develop just under the dermis, although this is usually seen in childhood forms.

Cardiac and pulmonary weakness can be commonly seen. Pulmonary symptoms are due to weakness of the thoracic muscles or interstitial lung disease. Although cardiac symptoms are oftentimes subclinical, conduction defects and arrhythmias are reported in as many as 50% of individuals on electrocardiogram (Stern, Goodbold, Chess, & Kagen, 1984). As previously noted, PM is associated with heightened risk of morbidity and mortality if not properly treated, due to involvement of cardiac and pulmonary systems.

Neuropsychological examinations have not been reported. However, assumptions may be made from a clinical standpoint. As cardiac weakness persists, disturbance of cerebrovascular integrity may be seen and raises chances for subcortical issues such as

OP

OP

retrieval-based memory issues and processing speed deficits. Risk of cerebrovascular events is unknown.

DIAGNOSIS

The diagnosis of PM is based on morphological and clinical signs (Dalakas, 1995). Although clinical features, as described above, suggest diagnosis, confirmation is achieved throughout a multifactorial approach, including a number of variables. Muscle biopsy reveals both CD4$^+$ helper T lymphocytes and CD8$^+$ cytotoxic T lymphocytes in the muscle in inflammatory infiltrates or distributed diffusely and remains the gold standard in diagnosis (Lindvall, Dahlbom, Henriksson, Srinivas, & Ernerudh, 2003). Additional laboratory tests for serum muscle enzyme concentrations and presence of autoantibodies are run. Electromyogram is essential to defining the nature and extent of the muscle weakness. In recent years, MRI of the muscles and ultrasound has been introduced in the diagnostic workup (Briani et al., 2006).

TREATMENT

Treatment of PM can be highly successful with very positive outcomes for patients. Corticosteroids are considered to be the preferred drugs of choice in the initial stages of treatment (Amato & Barohn, 2009). This aids in muscle strength recovery after which time the dosage is reduced to low, sustainable dosage. Prednisolone is the most common corticosteroid used. Sometimes azathioprine, an immune suppressor, is used in combination for reduction of relapse risk (Mastaglia, Phillips, Zilko, & Garlepp, 1999; Miro', Laguno, & Grau, 1999). Methotrexate is relatively comparable to azathioprine and may also be used (Cagnoli, Marchesoni, & Tosi, 1991; Joffe et al., 1993; Miller, Sisson, Tucker, deNardo, & Schaller, 1992). When symptoms are particularly severe, or involve more prominent respiratory symptoms, intravenous methylprednisolone may be used in combination with prednisolone (Mastaglia, 2008). For those patients who do not respond effectively to corticosteroids, intravenous immunoglobulin has demonstrated relative efficacy in symptom reduction as has cyclophosphamide (Cherin et al., 1991; Mastaglia, Philips, & Zilko, 1998). Medications including infliximab, etanercept, eculizumab, and alemtuzumab as well as autologous hematopoietic stem cell transplantation have all demonstrated utility in treatment, but remain investigational at this point in time (Joffe et al., 1993).

With proper treatment, individuals with PM can live relatively normal, symptom-free lives. As long as symptoms are controlled, life expectancy remains unaffected in mild cases. As individuals experience more respiratory distress related to PM, life expectancy and quality of life are affected.

Chad A. Noggle
Michelle R. Pagoria

Amato, A. A., & Barohn, R. J. (2009). Evaluation and treatment of inflammatory myopathies. *Journal of Neurology, Neurosurgery & Psychiatry, 80*, 1060–1068.

Bartt, R. E., & Topel, J. L. (2007). Autoimmune and inflammatory disorders. In C. G. Goetz (Ed.), *Textbook of clinical neurology* (3rd ed., pp. 1156–1184). Philadelphia, PA: Saunders Elsevier.

Briani, C., Doria, A., Sarzi-Puttini, P., & Dalakas, M. C. (2006). Update on idiopathic inflammatory myopathies. *Autoimmunity, 39*(3), 161–170.

Cagnoli, M., Marchesoni, A., & Tosi, S. (1991). Combined steroids, methotrexate and chlorambucil therapy for steroid resistant dermatomyositis. *Clinical and Experimental Rheumatology, 9*, 658–659.

Cherin, P., Herson, S., Wechsler, B., Piette, J. C., Bletry, O., Coutellier, A., et al. (1991). Efficacy of intravenous immunoglobulin therapy in chronic refractory polymyositis and dermatomyositis: An open study with 20 adult patients. *American Journal of Medicine, 91*, 162–168.

Dalakas, M. C. (1995). Immunopathogenesis of inflammatory myopathies. *Annals of Neurology, 37*, S74–S86.

De Merieux, P., Verity, M. A., Clements, R. J., & Paulus, H. E. (1983). Esophageal abnormalities and dysphagia in polymyositis and dermatomyositis. *Arthritis Rheumatism, 26*, 961–968.

Engel, A. G., Hohlfeld, R., & Banker, B. Q. (1994). The polymyositis and dermatomyositis syndromes. In A. G. Engel, & C. Franzini-Armstrong (Eds.), *Myology* (pp. 1335–1383). New York: McGraw-Hill.

Joffe, M. M., Love, L. A., Leff, R. L., Fraser, D. D., Targoff, I. N., Hicks, J. E., et al. (1993). Drug therapy of idiopathic inflammatory myopathies: Predictors of response to prednisone, azathioprine, and methotrexate and a comparison of their efficacy. *American Journal of Medicine, 94*, 379–387.

Kagen, L. J., Hochman, R. B., & Strog, E. W. (1985). Cricopharyngeal obstruction in inflammatory myopathy (polymyositis/dermatopolymyositis). *Arthritis Rheumatism, 28*, 630–636.

Lindvall, B., Dahlbom, K., Henriksson, K. G., Srinivas, U., & Ernerudh, J. (2003). The expression of adhesion molecules in muscle biopsies: The LFA-1/VLA-4 ratio in polymyositis. *Acta Neurologica Scandinavica, 107*, 134–141.

Mastaglia, F. L. (2008). Inflammatory muscle diseases. *Neurology India, 56*, 263–270.

Mastaglia, F. L., Philips, B. A., & Zilko, P. J. (1998). Immunoglobulin therapy in inflammatory myopathies. *Journal of Neurology, Neurosurgery & Psychiatry, 65*, 107–110.

Mastaglia, F. L., Phillips, B. A., Zilko, P. J., & Garlepp, M. J. (1999). Relapses in idiopathic inflammatory myopathies. *Muscle Nerve, 22*, 1160–1161.

Miller, L. C., Sisson, B. A., Tucker, L. B., deNardo, B. A., & Schaller, J. G. (1992). Methotrexate treatment of recalcitrant childhood dermatomyositis. *Arthritis Rheumatism, 35*, 1143–1149.

Miro', O., Laguno, M., & Grau, J. M. (1999). Relapses in idiopathic inflammatory myopathies. *Muscle Nerve, 22*, 1159–1160.

Murthy, J. M. K. (2010). Drug treatment of polymyositis and dermatomyositis. *Neurology India, 58*(1), 1–5.

Stern, R., Goodbold, J. H., Chess, Q., & Kagen, L. J. (1984). ECG abnormalities in polymyositis. *Archives of Internal of Medicine, 44*, 2185–2189.

POMPE'S DISEASE

DESCRIPTION

Pompe's disease, also known as type-II glycogenosis, generalized glycogenosis, and/or acid maltase deficiency, is one of the lysosomal enzyme deficiencies. It was first described in 1932 by J. C. Pompe, a pathologist (Pompe, 1932). It presents in infantile, juvenile, and adult forms with the infantile form being more severe and life threatening. Occurring in 1 out of every 40,000 births worldwide, Pompe's disease is often fatal in the end as cardiovascular weaknesses among other issues increase in severity to the point the individual can no longer sustain life (Ausems et al., 1999; Martiniuk et al., 1998).

Pompe's disease specifically arises from a deficiency or absence of a lysosomal enzyme called acid alpha-glucosidase (GAA), also known as acid maltase, which is essential to the breakdown of glycogen into glucose and its removal from the system. As a result, glycogen accumulates skeletal and myocardial cells in the system, thus causing particular susceptibility of skeletal, cardiovascular, and respiratory muscles (Van der Ploeg & Reuser, 2008). The presentation has been divided into two separate variants that are distinguished by the timing of symptom onset, which itself corresponds with the degree of GAA deficiency. Although complete absence usually leads to death within the first year(s) of life due to cardiac or respiratory failure, only partial deficiency of GAA leads to a later onset of symptoms that even then are also milder in presentation (Arad et al., 2005; Haremans, Winkel, Van Doorn et al., 2005; Winkel et al., 2005).

In the early-onset subtype, or infantile Pompe's disease, symptoms present in the first few months, characterized by feeding difficulties and thus poor weight gain or an apparent failure to thrive. Infants may seem lethargic or overly fatigued. Muscle weakness results in floppiness. Again, most die within the first year(s) of life.

In the late-onset subtype, or juvenile/adult Pompe's disease, symptom development has a wide variability in terms of onset. Some may manifest symptoms prior to age 10, whereas others may not manifest features until their 40s or 50s. Similar to the infantile form, muscle weakness and what seems like fatigue are prominently seen. Cardiovascular and respiratory difficulties emerge in relation to increasing weaknesses. Eventually, the disease progresses over the course of several years, marked by increasing cardiorespiratory complications and eventually leading to death, secondary to these issues.

NEUROPATHOLOGY/PATHOPHYSIOLOGY

The genetic mutations associated with Pompe's disease have been localized to chromosome 17q23 (Hermans et al., 1991, 1993). Although over 70 mutations have been reported (e.g., Hermans et al., 2004; Kanazawa et al., 2003; Tsujino et al., 2000), the c.-32-13T>G splice-site mutation has been reported in more than half of adult patients (Becker et al., 1998; Huie et al., 1994). As previously discussed, the presentation arises from deficiencies or absence of GAA with the severity of the disease and the age of onset directly related to the degree of this enzyme deficiency.

Vacuolar myopathy is associated with all forms, owing to the common musculoskeletal weaknesses seen. It tends to be most severe in the infant form, moderate in the juvenile form, and only mild in the adult form (Trende et al., 1985). These vacuoles are filled with glycogen and demonstrate strong acid phosphatase activity. Consequently, capillary endothelial cells and smooth muscle cells demonstrate excessive glycogen and phosphatase activity. Excessive glycogen is also noted in the lysosomes of Kupffer cells in the liver and hepatocytes. Peripheral blood lymphocytes also demonstrate glycogen accumulation in cytoplasmic vacuoles. Severe left ventricular hypertrophy is among the most common features that arise.

Within the central nervous system, glycogen uptake is observed in the neurons of the anterior horn cells of the spinal cord, the motor cranial nerve nuclei, astrocytes of the cerebral cortex, the basal ganglia, and the brainstem. This is observed in both infantile and juvenile forms but often not in adult forms (van der Walt, Swash, Leake, & Cox 1987). Gliosis may be noted in the white matter, but there is no evidence of demyelination.

NEUROPSYCHOLOGICAL/CLINICAL PRESENTATION

Affected infants are symptomatic at birth. They may present with hypotonia, poor motor development and profound muscle weakness, failure to thrive, feeding difficulties, cardiomegaly, macroglossia, hepatomegaly, and respiratory problems often complicated by pneumonia (Raben, Barden, Wong, & Plotz, 2011). Crying becomes increasingly weak. Severe LV hypertrophy is characteristic, often serving as a primary component to the cardiorespiratory issues that lead to death (Arad et al., 2005; van den Hout et al., 2003) but may regress with enzyme replacement therapy (Barker et al., 2010). Death often occurs prior to the first birthday, with a median age of 6–7 months (Kishnani et al., 2006), due to respiratory dysfunction related to cardiac problems or general weakness of the respiratory muscles. Some with an early-onset variant survive to 2–3 years of age, usually because of slightly greater acid GAA levels contributing to a slower progression and less-severe cardiomyopathy (Slonim et al., 2000).

The juvenile form is primarily muscular-based in its dysfunction, mimicking features of muscular dystrophy (MD), which represents a key differential for this group (Maertens & Dyken, 2007; Raben et al., 2011). As with the infantile form, respiratory weakness is commonly noted and becomes progressively worse as does cardiovascular issues. Generalized weakness of the limbs and trunk is a hallmark feature due to limb-girdle myopathy contributing to dyscoordination, reduced strength, difficulties in ambulation, and rising from sitting or lying down (Hagemans, Winkel, Hop, et al., 2005; Winkel et al., 2005).

The adult variant is associated with symptom manifestation in the third decade of life. Again, respiratory weakness is common, and may actually represent the first symptom (Raben et al., 2011). Generalized weakness of the musculoskeletal system follows, becoming progressively worse. Death commonly follows a progressive course of cardiac and respiratory deterioration occurring over the course of a few years.

Few studies have evaluated the neuropsychological correlates of the presentation. In reality, only in the juvenile/onset type would this be relevant. Given the aforementioned features, general decreases of cognitive efficiency may be expected in relation to fatigue and progressive stress related to cardiac and respiratory deterioration. One may anticipate reduced processing speed, psychomotor retardation due to motor weakness, potential weaknesses in sustained attention, retrieval-based memory deficits, and possible variability in executive functioning.

DIAGNOSIS

Diagnosis of Pompe's disease is initially suggested based on clinical presentation, which leads to further diagnostic workup. When considered, measurement of acid GAA enzyme activity (Winchester et al., 2007) can permit exact diagnosis, particularly when used in combination with genetic testing. At that time, it may also be useful for family members of the patient to also undergo genetic testing. Muscle biopsy has also been used as a diagnostic tool, with measurement of glycogen deposits, however, as noted by Lewandowska et al. (2008), diagnosis may be missed when relying on muscle biopsy alone, thus further emphasizing the need to measure acid maltase (GAA) activity for definitive diagnosis.

From a differential diagnosis standpoint, Pompe's disease may be misdiagnosed as MD when presenting as the juvenile variant due to overlap of clinical symptomology. In these instances, the aforementioned laboratory tests can offer differential clarity. Furthermore, MD has its own diagnostic resources that the interested reader is encouraged to review in this text. In adults, polymyositis and mutliple sclerosis may both be considered as potential differentials in which, again, the aforementioned analyses may aid in confirming Pompe's disease. Readers are also encouraged to review these other entries.

Beyond diagnostic clarification, serial MRIs, particularly cardiac MRI, and regular pulmonary work-up may aid in tracking cardiac and respiratory status as they represent the greatest risk factors in terms of mortality. While cardiac MRI has shown particular utility in following the left ventricular mass, because of respiratory issues sedation is risky. However, Barker et al. (2010) as well as others have reported success in this population with minimal or no sedation.

TREATMENT

Treatment is multidimensional and is recommended to involve a combination of cardiology, neurology, and pulmonology as well as physical/occupational therapy, respiratory therapy, genetic counseling, and likely psychology. The combination of these specialties is to offer support and symptom-based treatment.

ERT has been developed with recombinant human GAA (Kishnani et al., 2006; Klinge et al., 2005; Van den Hout et al., 2004), which has shown utility in decreasing heart size, maintaining normal heart function, improving muscle function, tone, and strength, and reducing glycogen accumulation. Myozyme is FDA approved for the treatment of infants and children with Pompe's disease; Lumizyme has been approved for late-onset (noninfantile) Pompe's disease. Although they do not stop the disease from progressing, they have demonstrated capacity to slow progression. For example, clinical trials with Myozyme demonstrate that most infants who were treated with this drug survived significantly longer than those not treated (Kishnani et al., 2007; Nicolino et al., 2009; Van der Ploeg et al., 2008). Furthermore, when infants were identified prior to becoming symptomatic (i.e., identified on genetic testing), time until symptoms emerged and longevity of life were both improved (Nicolino et al., 2009). High-protein diets have also been reported by some as beneficial, but results vary. Similarly, there have been encouraging results in the use of exercise programs to try and offset progressive muscle weakness.

When an individual is diagnosed with Pompe's disease, close relatives should be recommended for genetic counseling so they may be made aware as to their risk of developing the presentation, particularly with emerging evidence that starting previously noted agents may delay onset and lengthen course.

Chad A. Noggle

Arad, M., Maron, B. J., Gorham, J. M., Johnson, W. H. Jr., Saul, J. P., Perez-Atayde, A. R., et al. (2005). Glycogen storage diseases presenting as hypertrophic cardiomyopathy. *The New England Journal of Medicine, 352*, 362–372.

Ausems, M. G., Verbiest, J., Hermans, M. P., Kroos, M. A., Beemer, F. A., Wokke, J. H., et al. (1999). Frequency of glycogen storage disease type II in The Netherlands: Implications for diagnosis and genetic counselling. *European Journal of Human Genetics, 7*, 713–716.

Barker, P., Campbell, M. J., Stephen, D., Li, J., Kim, R., Pasquali, S., et al. (2010). MRI assessment of left ventricular structure and function in children with infantile Pompe disease. *Journal of Cardiovascular Magnetic Resonance, 12*(Suppl. 1), P309.

Becker, J. A., Vlach, J., Raben, N., Nagaraju, K., Adams, E. M., Hermans, M. M., et al. (1998). The African origin of the common mutation in African American patients with glycogenstorage disease type II. *American Journal of Human Genetics, 62*, 991–994.

Hagemans, M. L., Winkel, L. P., Hop, W. C., Reuser, A. J., Van Doorn, P. A., Van der Ploeg, A. T. (2005). Disease severity in children and adults with Pompe disease related to age and disease duration. *Neurology, 64*, 2139–2141.

Hagemans, M. L., Winkel, L. P., Van Doorn, P. A., Hop, W. J., Loonen, M. C., Reuser, A. J., et al. (2005). Clinical manifestation and natural course of late-onset Pompe's disease in 54 Dutch patients. *Brain, 128*, 671–677.

Hermans, M. M., de Graaff, E., Kroos, M. A., Mohkamsing, S., Eussen, B. J., Joosse, M., et al. (1994). The effect of a single base pair deletion (delta T525) and a C1634T missense mutation (pro545leu) on the expression of lysosomal alphaglucosidase in patients with glycogen storage disease type II. *Human Molecular Genetics, 3*, 2213–2218.

Hermans, M. M., de Graff, E., Kross, M. A., Wisselaar, H. A., Oostra, B. A., & Reuser, A. J. (1991). Identification of a point mutation in the human lysosomal alpha — glucosidase gene causing infantile glycogenosis type II. *Biochemical and Biophysical Research Communications, 179*, 919–926.

Hermans, M. M., Kroos, M. A., de Graaff, E., Oostra, B. A., & Reuser, A. J. (1993). Two mutations affecting the transport and maturation of lysosomal alpha-glucosidase in an adult case of glycogen storage disease type II. *Human Mutation, 2*, 268–273.

Hermans, M. M., van Leenen, D., Kroos, M. A., Beesley, C. E., Van der Ploeg, A. T., Sakuraba, H., et al. (2004). Twenty-two novel mutations in the lysosomal alpha-glucosidase gene (GAA) underscore the genotype-phenotype correlation in glycogen storage disease type II. *Human Mutation, 23*, 47–56.

Huie, M. L., Chen, A. S., Tsujino, S., Shanske, S., DiMauro, S., Enge, A. G., et al. (1994). Aberrant splicing in adult-onset glycogen storage disease type II (GSDII): Molecular identification of an IVS1 (–13T®G) mutation in a majority of patients and a novel IVS10 (+1GT®CT) mutation. *Human Molecular Genetics, 3*, 2231–2236.

Kanazawa, N., Miyamoto, T., Ihara, K., Miyoshi, Y., Sakai, N., Inui, K., et al. (2003). Novel mutation and a frequent mutation in Japanese juvenile patients with acid maltase deficiency. *Journal of Inherited Metabolic Disease, 26*(Suppl. 2), 310.

Kishnani, P. S., Corzo, D., Nicolino, M., Byrne, B., Mandel, H., Hwu, W. L., et al. (2007). Recombinant human acid [alpha]-glucosidase: Major clinical benefits in infantile onset Pompe disease. *Neurology, 68*, 99–109.

Kishnani, P. S., Hwu, W. L., Mandel, H., Nicolino, M., Yong, F., Corzo, D., et al. (2006). A retrospective, multinational, multicenter study on the natural history of infantile-onset Pompe disease. *The Journal of Pediatrics, 148*, 671–676.

Kishnani, P. S., Nicolino, M., Voit, T., Rogers, R. C., Tsai, A. C., Waterson, J., et al. (2006). Chinese hamster ovary cell derived recombinant human acid alpha-glucosidase in infantile-onset Pompe disease. *Journal of Pediatrics, 149*, 89–97.

Klinge, L., Straub, V., Neudorf, U., Schaper, J., Bosbach, T., Gorlinger, K., et al. (2005). Safety and efficacy of recombinant acid alpha-glucosidase (rhGAA) in patients with classical infantile Pompe disease: Results of a phase II clinical trial. *Neuromuscular Disorders, 15,* 24–31.

Lewandowska, E., Wierzba-Bobrowicz, T., Rola, R., Modzelewska, J., Stepień, T., Lugowska, A., et al. (2008). Pathology of skeletal muscle cells in adult-onset glycogenosis type II (Pompe disease): Ultrastructural study. *Folia Neuropathologica, 46*(2), 123–133.

Maertens, P., & Dyken, R. (2007). Storage diseases: Neuronal ceroid-lipofuscinoses, lipidoses, glycogenoses, and leukodystrophies. In C. Goetz (Ed.), *Textbook of clinical neurology* (pp. 613–639). Philadelphia, PA: Saunders Elsevier.

Martiniuk, F., Chen, A., Mack, A., Arvanitopoulos, E., Chen, Y., Rom, W. N., et al. (1998). Carrier frequency for glycogen storage disease type II in New York and estimates of affected individuals born with the disease. *American Journal of Medical Genetics, 79,* 69–72.

Nicolino, M., Byrne, B., Wraith, J. E., Leslie, N., Mandel, H., Freyer, D. R., et al. (2009). Clinical outcomes after long-term treatment with alglucosidase alfa in infants and children with advanced Pompe disease. *Genetics in Medicine, 11,* 210–219.

Pompe, J. C. (1932). Over idiopatische hypertrophie van het hart. *Nederlands Tijdschrift Geneeskunde, 76,* 304–311.

Raben, N., Barden, M., Wong, A., & Plotz, P. H. (2011). Pompe disease and the contribution of autophagy to its pathogenesis. *Lysosomal Storage Diseases, 9*(1), 1–8.

Slonim, A. E., Bulone, L., Ritz, S., Goldberg, T., Chen, A., Martiniuk, F., et al. (2000). Identification of two subtypes of infantile acid maltase deficiency. *The Journal of Pediatrics, 137,* 283–285.

Trend, P. S., Wiles, C. M., Spencer, G. T. Morgan-Hughes, J. A., Lake, B. D., & Patrick, A. D. (1985). Acid maltase deficiency in adults. Diagnosis and management in five cases. *Brain, 108,* 845–860.

Tsujino, S., Huie, M., Kanazawa, N., Sugie, H., Goto, Y., Kawai, M., et al. (2000). Frequent mutations in Japanese patients with acid maltase deficiency. *Neuromuscular Disorders, 10,* 599–603.

Van den Hout, H. M., Hop, W., van Diggelen, O. P., Smeitink, J. A., Smit, G. P., Poll-The, B. T., et al. (2003). The natural course of infantile Pompe's disease: 20 original cases compared with 133 cases from the literature. *Pediatrics, 112,* 332–340.

Van den Hout, J. M., Kamphoven, J. H., Winkel, L. P., Arts, W. F., De Klerk, J. B., Loonen, M. C., et al. (2004). Long-term intravenous treatment of Pompe disease with recombinant human alphaglucosidase from milk. *Pediatrics, 113,* e448–e457.

Van der Ploeg, A. T. & Reuser, A. J. (2008). Pompe's disease. *Lancet, 372,* 1342–1353.

van der Walt, J. D., Swash, M., Leake, J., & Cox, E. L. (1987). The pattern of involvement of adult-onset acid maltase deficiency in autopsy. *Muscle & Nerve, 10,* 272–281.

Winchester, B., Bali, D., Bodamer, O. A., Caillaud, C., Christensen, E., Cooper, A., et al. (2007). Methods for a prompt and reliable laboratory diagnosis of Pompe disease: Report from an international consensus meeting. *Molecular Genetics and Metabolism,* 1–7.

Winkel, L. P., Hagemans, M. L., Van Doorn, P. A., Loonen, M. C., Hop, W. J., Reuser, A. J., et al. (2005). The natural course of non-classic Pompe's disease: A review of 225 published cases. *Journal of Neurology, 252,* 875–884.

PORENCEPHALY

DESCRIPTION

Porencephaly is a rare congenital brain defect in which a cyst or cavity develops within the brain and is filled with CSF. The nature in which the lesions initially arise are classified as either genetic or encephalophaloplastic (Ho et al., 1998; Stevenson & Hall, 2006; Tonni, Ferrari, Defelice, & Gentini, 2005). In the former, porencephaly develops secondary to disturbances of early neuronal migration to the area of cystic development. In encephalophaloplastic porencephaly, the CSF-filled cyst or cavity is seen as a consequence of later prenatal or perinatal vascular lesioning resulting from hypoxic, ischemic, or thrombotic trauma. Regardless of the etiology, the cysts may present in either hemisphere and any lobe or lobes (Tonni et al., 2005). When the hemispheres are nearly completely replaced with CSF-filled sacs, it is commonly referred to as hydranencephaly.

Although clinical presentation may vary based on the locality of the cysts, congenital hemiparesis and intractable epilepsy are common (Harding & Copp, 1997; Kolawole, Patel, & Mahdi, 1987). In addition, severe mental retardation, blindness, and tetraplegia or decerebrate rigidity can be seen. Many individuals can survive into adulthood, but life span, as with other such congenital disorders, is shortened.

NEUROPATHOLOGY/PATHOPHYSIOLOGY

The genetic form of porencephaly is not as well understood. In these instances, no pathological basis has been well described beyond a general suggestion of neuronal migration disruption. In comparison,

encephalophaloplastic porencephaly is best conceptualized as a hypoxic–ischemic injury that may arise
from a number of factors including hypoxia, systemic
vascular occlusion, placental bleeding, maternal
toxemia, cystic periventricular leukomalacia, intracranial hemorrhage, necrotizing enterocolitis, prenatal
viruses, endotoxins, trauma and drug abuse (Stanava
et al., 2002; Vohr et al., 2000). In all cases, they result in
brain necrosis that is replaced by the porencephalic
cyst that fills with CSF roughly 2–6 weeks later
(Bejar, Vaucher, Benirschke, & Berry, 1992; Low,
1993).

Porencephalic cysts are usually seen bilaterally,
centering most commonly around the sylvian fissure,
but may be observed unilaterally. The cysts are
smooth, and surrounded by cortical ribboning that
on microscopic examination demonstrate disorganization in the form of clusters of gray matter or polymicrogyria. Polymicrogyria may in fact be noted in
areas throughout the brain. There is a deficiency or
complete absence of the septum pellucidum, and the
thalamus is often undersized (Harding & Copp, 1997).
Although these abnormalities are noted, the basal
ganglia, brainstem, and cerebellum remain largely
unaffected. The cyst often terminates just above the
ventricle with only a thin layer separating the cyst
from the ventricular space. Nodular gray heterotopias
are often present just beneath the ventricular wall
(Harding & Copp, 1997).

NEUROPSYCHOLOGICAL/CLINICAL PRESENTATION

Although clinical presentation may vary based on the
locality of the cysts, congenital hemiparesis and intractable epilepsy are common (Harding & Copp, 1997;
Kolawole et al., 1987). In addition, severe mental retardation, blindness, and tetraplegia or decerebrate rigidity can be seen (Harding & Copp, 1997). Nevertheless,
neurocognitive functioning in some instances can
approach or even reach normal levels depending
upon the location of the porous cyst, although this
profile of milder cognitive dysfunction is rare.

DIAGNOSIS

Diagnosis is most attainable with MRI. Prenatal ultrasound is also capable of identifying the porous cysts
associated with the presentation prior to birth. Electroencephalogram should be used to determine the
presence and nature of seizures. Neuropsychological
assessment and physical therapy evaluations should
be undertaken to identify cognitive, academic, and
motoric deficits.

TREATMENT

Oftentimes treatment is purely focused on seizure
control. This is most commonly done through anticonvulsant medications in lieu of surgical intervention,
as localization of seizures foci is difficult in porencephaly (Ho et al., 1997). When surgery is utilized, the
nature of the individual's symptoms determines the
nature and extent of the approach. Hemispherectomy
is indicated in individuals with intractable seizures,
moderate to severe hemiparesis, and hemianopsia
(Andermann, 1997; Schramm, Behrens, & Entzian,
1995; Villemure & Peacock, 1997). When hemiparesis
is simply mild, partial hemispherectomy or lobec-
tomies may be considered (Cendes et al., 1995;
Raymond et al., 1995). Special education services,
physical therapy, and speech therapy may all be useful depending on the nature of the functional deficits.

Chad A. Noggle
Javan Horwitz

Andermann, F. (1997). Functional hemispherectomy: Clinical indications and outcome. In E. Wylie (Ed.), *The
treatment of epilepsy: Principles and practice* (pp. 1074–
1080). Baltimore: Williams & Wilkins.

Banh, P. G. (1984). Prenatal classic encephalopathies. *Clinical
Neurology, 6*, 65–75.

Bejar, R. F., Vaucher, Y. E., Benirschke, K., & Berry, C. C.
(1992). Postnatal white matter necrosis in preterm
infants. *Journal of Perinatology, 12*, 3–8.

Cendes, F., Cook, M. J., Watson, C., Andermann, F., Fish,
D. R., Shorvon, S. D., et al. (1995). Frequency and characteristics of dual pathology in patients with lesional
epilepsy. *Neurology, 45*, 2058–2064.

Harding, B., Copp, A. J. (1997). Malforniaiioris. In D. I.
Graham & P. L. Lantos (Eds.), *Greenfield's neuropathology* (pp. 455–459). London: Arnold.

Ho, S. S., Kuzniecky, R. I., Gilliam, F., Faught, E., Bebin, M., &
Morawetz, R. (1997). Congenital porencephaly and
hippocampal sclerosis. Clinical features and epileptic
spectrum. *Neurology, 49*, 1382–1388.

Ho, S. S., Kuzniesky, R. I., Gilliam, F., Faught, E., Bebin, M., &
Morawetz, R. (1998). Congenital porencephaly: MR
features and relationship to hippocampal sclerosis.
American Journal Neuroradiology, 19(1), 135–141.

Hunter, A. (2006). Porencephaly. In R. E. Stevenson & J. G.
Hall (Eds.), *Human malformations and related anomalies*
(2nd ed., pp. 645–654). Oxford, UK: Oxford University
Press.

OP

Kolawole, T. M., Patel, P. J., & Mahdi, A. H. (1987). Poren-cephaly: Computed tomography (CT) scan findings. *Computerized Radiology, 11,* 53–58.

Lorenzo, N. Y., Parisi, J. E., Cascino, G. D., Jack, C. R., Jr., Marsh, W. R., & Hirschorn, K. A. (1995). Intractable frontal lobe epilepsy: Pathological and MRI features. *Epilepsy Research, 20*(2), 171–178.

Low, J. A. (1993). Relationship of fetal asphyxia to neuropa-thology and deficits in children. *Clinical and Investigative Medicine, 16,* 133–140.

Oisuho, H., Ochi, A., Elliott, I., Chuang, S. H., Rutka, J. T., Jay, V., et al. (2001). MEG predicts epileptic zone in lesional extrahippocampal epilepsy: 12 pediatric sur-gery cases. *Epilepsia, 42,* 1523–1530.

Raymond, A. A., Fish, R. D., Sisodiya, S. M., Alsanjari, N., Stevens, J. M., & Shorvon, S. D. (1995). Abnormalities of gyration, heterotopias, tuberous sclerosis, focal cortical dysplasia, microdysgenesis, dysembryoplastic neuroe-pithelial tumour and dysgenesis of the archicortex in epilepsy. Clinical, EEG and neuroimaging features in 100 adult patients. *Brain, 18,* 629–660.

Salamnii, V., Andemiann, F., Rasinusscn, T., Olivier, A., & Quesney, L. F. (1995). Parietal lobe epilepsy. Clinical manifestations and outcome in 82 patients treated surgically between 1929 and 1988. *Brain, 118*(Pt. 3), 607–627.

Salanova, V., Andermann, F., Olivier, A., Rasmussen, T., & Quesney, L. F. (1992). Occipital lobe epilepsy: Electro-clinical manifestations, electrocorticography, cortical stimulation and outcome in 42 patients treated between 1930 and 1991. Surgery of occipital lobe epilepsy. *Brain, 115*(Pt. 6), 1655–1680.

Schramm, J., Behrens, E., & Entzian, W. (1995). Hemisphe-rical deafferentation: An alternative to functional hemi-spherectomy. *Neurosurgery, 36,* 509–516.

Stanava, K. N., Hartmann, S., Uhlemann, M., Diete, H., Reschke, E., Koepe, E., et al. (2002). Neonatal ultrasono-graphic cerebral findings: Association with risk factor for cerebral palsy. *Zeitschrift für Geburtshilfe und Neona-tologie, 206,* 142–150.

Tonni, G., Ferrari, B., Defelice, C., & Gentini, G. (2005). Neo-natal porencephaly in very low birth weight infants: Ultrasound timing of asphyxial injury and neurodeve-lopmental outcome at two years of age. *The Journal of Maternal-Fetal and Neonatal Medicine, 18*(6), 361–365.

Villemure, J. G., & Peacock, W. (1997). Multilobar resections and hemispherectomy. In J. Engel Jr. & T. A. Pedley (Eds.), *Epilepsy: A comprehensive textbook.* Philadelphia: Lippincott-Raven. 1829–1839.

Vohr, B. R., Wright, L. L., Dusick, A. M., Mele, L., Verter, J., Steichen, J. J., et al. (2000). Neurodevelopmental and functional outcomes of extremely low birth weight infants in the Neonatal Institute of Child Health and Human Development Neonatal Research Network, 1993–1994. *Pediatrics, 105,* 1216–1226.

POSTCONCUSSION DISORDER/SYNDROME

DESCRIPTION

Postconcussion disorder (PCD) or postconcussion syn-drome (PCS) is a complex presentation of mixed symp-tomology that arises following a head injury. Patients who sustain a head injury of any severity will often initially develop symptoms associated with postcon-cussional syndrome. Complaints of somatic, affective, and cognitive symptoms are common, often resolving 3–12 months following the injury (Carroll et al., 2004; van der Naalt, van Zomeren, Sluiter, & Minderhoud, 1999). Additional symptoms may include headaches, dizziness (usually precipitated by assuming an upright position), nervousness, inability to concentrate, irrita-bility, fatigue, and anxiety.

Research varies on the etiology, prognosis, and pro-gression of PCS. Some have argued for a neurological basis while others suggest the persistence of symptoms, beyond the time of normal resolution, is due to psycho-genic factors (Ferrari, Constantoyannis, & Papadakis, 2001; Mittenberg & Strauman, 2000; Ruff, 2005).

With the possibility of a variety of presentations of symptomology, typical cases of PCS can have remarkably different progressions. Some have argued for a fairly short time span for experiencing PCD with symptoms lasting from 2 to 6 months. Other research, however, has argued for a slower progression of 6 months to 1 year with the possibility of no recovery from a PCS experience.

NEUROPATHOLOGY/PATHOPHYSIOLOGY

The neuropathology of PCS is not well understood. There is little agreement over which symptoms repre-sent organic factors associated with the pathology and which are psychogenic in nature. Some researchers have argued that early onset symptoms associated with PCS are to be associated with the pathology of the syndrome while late onset symptoms should be attributed to psychological factors.

There is some research using brain-imaging tech-niques such as fMRI and SPECT scans, which suggest that PCS can be linked to a reduction of glucose in the brain, which concomitantly lowers the cerebral blood flow. This research, as does other research related to the syndrome, has its detractors in that many clients with PCS show no abnormal changes in brain func-tioning. Cortical contusions arising from coup and countercoup trauma and diffuse axonal injury repre-sent the initial biomechanical effects of head injury, but this is also believed to set into motion a cascade of neurochemical changes. Release of excitatory neurotransmitters including acetylcholine, glutamate, and aspartate have been proposed as neurochemical substrates of PCS (Evans, Wilberger, & Bhatia, 2007) What is important to know is that a negative CT or MRI does not rule out PCD/PCS. In fact, structural imaging techniques are often negative, with potential neuropathological features being more diffuse (Brazarian, Blyth, & Cimpello, 2006).

NEUROPSYCHOLOGICAL/CLINICAL PRESENTATION

Personality changes, irritability, anxiety, and depression present in more than half of patients within the first 3 months following a head injury (Evans et al., 2007). As patients become irritable and frustrated when experiencing the symptoms, they are usually met with a lack of understanding from friends and family. This exacerbates the disorder and creates a cycle of disability. Some of these features have led authors to suggest that certain patients experiencing postconcussional syndrome have an underlying neurotic personality disorder, or were under stress at the time of the accident that the accident subsequently exacerbated, thus explaining the persistence of symptoms. Anxiety and depression present at higher rates following head injury (McCauley, Boake, Levin, Contant, & Song, 2001), which some have associated with premorbid personality features. Still, there is substantial evidence that associates these behavioral features with anatomical susceptibility, particularly of the frontal and temporal regions, to head injury due to the combination of biomechanical forces and these regions proximity to the cranial fossas.

Cognitively, individuals present with "fogginess" of mentation. Speed of processing and reaction time are often down. Inattention and poor concentration are usually noted, and likely represent the most frequent cognitive complaints. These factors contribute to memory deficits in regard to the acquisition of new information.

Migraine headaches are commonly reported as is fatigue and dizziness. Cranial nerve signs can be observed but tend to be mild. Similarly, patients may have reports of blurred vision, hearing loss, and even loss of smell, but these are relatively uncommon, each being noted in less than 15% of patients (Evans et al., 2007).

DIAGNOSIS

Diagnosis is made by noting the multiplicity of symptoms and the exclusion of a significant structural lesion. CT and MRI scans can exclude lesions such as hematomas or intracranial bleeds. Patients should be followed up every few days in the initial week to ensure no prominent changes in behavior arise, in terms of decline. Patients with mild head injury who report postconcussional symptoms exhibit measurable deficits on neuropsychological instruments, and these can be extremely useful in identifying deficits. Both the *International Classification of Diseases–10th edition* (*ICD-10*; World Health Organization, 1993) and the *Diagnostic and Statistical Manual of Mental Disorders–4th edition* (*DSM-IV*; American Psychiatric Association, 1994) have established criteria for diagnosis. The initial difference between these two sources is that the presentation is referred to as postconcussion disorder in the *DSM-IV* and postconcussion syndrome in the *ICD-10*.

Criteria are not consistent across the two sources. In comparing the two, Boake et al. (2005) actually found that PCS was diagnosed six times as much using the *ICD-10* criteria compared with the *DSM-IV* in individuals 3 months post-injury. Still, even the *DSM-IV* criteria lacked specificity.

TREATMENT

Rest is usually prescribed following injury. In addition, tranquilizers, antidepressants, and benzodiazepines may be prescribed. Headaches can be treated with common nonprescribed agents. Patients and families should understand that there is a possibility that the patient may experience personality changes, concentration problems, and so forth, that may need to be compensated for by modifications in the environment, at least over the short term (Mittenberg, Canyock, Condit, & Patton, 2001). The patient should be made aware that returning to work may be difficult at first and may only be possible at a reduced workload. Informing the patient and family of possible future implications of the head injury can help to avoid the emotional impact of the disorder that can be more debilitating than the physical trauma.

Matt Holcombe
Chad A. Noggle

American Psychiatric Association. (1994). *Diagnostic and statistical manual of mental disorders* (4th ed.). Washington, DC: Author.

Boake, C., McCauley, S. R., Levin, H. S., Pedroza, C., Contant, C. F., Song, J. X., et al. (2005). Diagnostic criteria for postconcussional syndrome after mild to moderate traumatic brain injury. *Journal of Neuropsychiatry and Clinical Neurosciences, 17*, 350–356.

Brazarian, J. J., Blyth, B., & Cimpello, L. (2006). Bench to bedside: Evidence for brain injury after concussion—looking beyond the computed tomography scan. *Academic Emergency Medicine, 13*, 199–214.

Carroll, L. J., Cassidy, J. D., Peloso, P. M., Borg, J., von Holst, H., Holm, L., et al. (2004). Prognosis for mild traumatic brain injury: Results of the WHO Collaborating Centre Task Force on Mild Traumatic Brain Injury. *Journal of Rehabilitation Medicine, 36*(Suppl. 43), 84–105.

Evans, R. W., Wilberger, J. E., & Bhatia, S. (2007). Traumatic disorders. In C. Goetz (Ed.), *Textbook of clinical neurology* (3rd ed., pp. 1185–1211). Philadelphia, PA: Saunders Elsevier.

Ferrari, R., Constantoyannis, C., & Papadakis, N. (2001). Cross-sectional study of symptom expectation following minor head injury in Canada and Greece. *Clinical Neurology & Neurosurgery, 103*, 254–259.

McCauley, S. R., Boake, C., Levin, H. S., Contant, C. F., & Song, J. X. (2001). Postconcussional disorder following mild to moderate traumatic brain injury: Anxiety, depression, and social support as risk factors and comorbidities. *Journal of Clinical and Experimental Neuropsychology, 23*, 792–808.

Mittenberg, W., Canyock, E. M., Condit, D., & Patton, C. (2001). Treatment of post-concussion syndrome following mild head injury. *Journal of Clinical and Experimental Neuropsychology, 23*, 829–836.

Mittenberg, W., & Strauman, S. (2000). Diagnosis of mild head injury and the postconcussion syndrome. *Journal of Head Trauma Rehabilitation, 15*, 783–791.

Ruff, R. (2005). Two decades of advances in understanding of mild traumatic brain injury. *Journal of Head Trauma Rehabilitation, 20*, 5–18.

van der Naalt, J., van Zomeren, A. H., Sluiter, W. J., & Minderhoud, J. M. (1999). One year outcome in mild to moderate head injury: The predictive value of acute injury characteristics related to complaints and return to work. *Journal of Neurology, Neurosurgery, and Psychiatry, 66*, 207–213.

World Health Organization. (1993). *The ICD-10 classification of mental and behavioural disorders: Diagnostic criteria for research*. Geneva, Switzerland: World Health Organization.

POSTURAL ORTHOSTATIC TACHYCARDIA SYNDROME

DESCRIPTION

Postural orthostatic tachycardia syndrome (POTS) mainly affects women between the ages of 20 and 50 (Mathias, 2002). Its main feature, orthostatic intolerance, is brought about by standing and resolved by reclining. Orthostatic intolerance occurs when standing because of physical stressors that require immediate vascular and neurologic compensation to maintain blood pressure, cerebral blood flow, and consciousness. People who suffer from orthostatic intolerance do so because they lack the mechanisms for such compensation. POTS is separated from other forms of orthostatic intolerance by the occurrence of tachycardia (rapid beating of the heart) when the person stands. During this change of position, the heart rate of a patient may increase by 30 beats per minute or more (Mathias, 2002).

NEUROPATHOLOGY/PATHOPHYSIOLOGY

This syndrome is characterized by a type of orthostatic tachycardia which, unlike traditional orthostatic hypotension, does not involve a fall in pressure or loss of consciousness on standing. It can be characterized by increased heart rate and other signs that mimic symptoms of insufficient blood flow to the brain (Raj, 2006). Because many pathophysiological illnesses include symptoms of tachycardia and weakness when coming up to a standing position, many believe POTS is better viewed as a syndrome rather than a disease. Different forms of this syndrome have been found and must be taken into account during diagnosis and treatment.

NEUROPSYCHOLOGICAL/CLINICAL PRESENTATION

Patients complaining of this syndrome may report symptoms such as tunnel or blurred vision, nausea, "mental clouding," and feelings of fainting although most do not lose consciousness (Raj, 2006). They may also exhibit a bluish color in their extremities upon standing (caused by blood pooling in those areas during the change of position). Many patients report that their symptoms began after acute stressors such as surgery or pregnancy. Comorbid disorders may include autoimmune diseases, chronic fatigue, and irritable bowel syndrome (Raj, 2006). Symptoms are transient and can be relieved by sitting or lying down.

Psychologically, those afflicted with POTS may have been diagnosed with an anxiety disorder at some point in their lives. Their scores on the Beck Anxiety Inventory, an assessment used to measure the severity of anxiety symptoms, were significantly raised compared with the normal population (Raj, 2006). However, the Beck Inventory includes physical symptoms of anxiety which overlap with

OP

the actual symptoms of the disorder, which may result in overdiagnosis. When a more cognitive rather than physical measure was used, patients with POTS displayed less anxiety than the general population rather than more. Evidence has been found to indicate that patients with POTS have reduced attention and concentration than the normal population, based on results from the Connors Adult ADHD Rating Scale (Raj, 2006). However, this is a self-report measure that does not distinguish between the temporary lapses in attention that are clearly characteristic of the disorder and more chronic symptoms that might exist in between episodes.

DIAGNOSIS

In order to diagnose patients with postural tachycardia, they must exhibit complaints of "orthostatic intolerance" for at least 6 months in conjunction with an unusual increase in heart rate of at least 30 beats per minute occurring within 5–30 minutes of standing up or getting in an upright position (Raj, 2006). The patient should show no evidence of orthostatic hypotension (drop in blood pressure), nor should they be taking medications that are known to disrupt regulation of the autonomic nervous system, be on extended bed rest, or have other chronic conditions that may cause tachycardia such as hyperthyroidism. Thus, though the presence of orthostatic tachycardia is required for a diagnosis, its presence is not by itself enough to fulfill the diagnostic requirements. In its more severe forms, POTS can be quite disabling and may interfere with a person's everyday activities such as bathing or exercising.

Features of the autonomic nervous system such as the levels of norepinephrine, epinephrine, and dopamine may be measured during both the standing and sitting positions for patients thought to have hyperadrenergic POTS (Grubb, 2008, p. 2815). This form of POTS is less frequent and is often described as having a slower onset. Those afflicted with this subtype of the disorder seem to have a poor reuptake mechanism for norepinephrine, the excess of which produces the hyperadrenergic state. Patients will present with both orthostatic hypertension and orthostatic tachycardia (Grubb, 2008).

Postural orthostatic tachycardia should be differentiated from pheochromocytoma. People suffering from that disorder will have higher levels of norepinephrine than those with POTS, and they may experience symptoms while lying down (Raj, 2008). The hyperadrenergic form of POTS should be differentiated from inappropriate sinus tachycardia (IST) (Grubb, 2008). Much like POTS, IST is prevalent in women and even has many of the same symptoms as the hyperadrenergic form. However, POTS patients exhibit a higher heart rate than patients with IST during changes in posture and do not have the same degree of change in levels of norepinephrine as those with hyperadrenergic POTS (Grubb, 2008).

TREATMENT

Treatment should begin by finding any causes that are deemed reversible such as medications the person may be using, chronic disease, inadequate hydration, extended bed rest, and so forth (Raj, 2006, p. 93). The type of treatment depends on which form of POTS is present. POTS patients are encouraged to undergo "physical reconditioning" where they will work toward such achievements as improving their ability to perform an aerobic activity for an extended amount of time. Patients are asked to hydrate more by drinking at least 2 L of fluids every day and to consume 3–5 g of salt a day as well (except for those with the hyperadrenergic form).

If it is believed that a patient's POTS is too severe for such treatments, then medication must be considered. In general, medication will be the main form of treatment until they are stable enough to pursue the nonmedication treatments discussed above. Currently, there is no medication approved for treatment of POTS; therefore, any treatment is "off-label" and differs from client to client. Many patients are given serotonin reuptake inhibitors (SSRIs) or norepinephrine reuptake inhibitors to alleviate symptoms of POTS with mixed serotonin and norepinephrine abnormalities. For patients so severely affected by POTS where no other therapy is effective, Grubb (2008) has suggested erythropoietin, a medication used to treat orthostatic disorders as well as anemia. The hyperadrenergic form of POTS can be treated by medication that will block the neurotransmitter norepinephrine and its effects such as clonidine HCl (Grubb, 2008).

Josie Bolanos
Charles Golden

Grubb, B. P. (2008). Postural tachycardia syndrome. *Circulation: Journal of the American Heart Association. 117,* 2814–2817.

Mathias, C. J. (2002). Postural tachycardia syndrome (PoTS). In A. K. Asbury, G. M. McKhann, W. I. McDonald, P. J. Goadsby, & J. C. McArthur (Eds.), *Diseases of the nervous system: Clinical neuroscience and therapeutic principles*

(3rd ed., pp. 789–793). Cambridge, UK: Cambridge University Press.

Raj, S. R. (2006). The postural tachycardia syndrome (POTS): Pathophysiology, diagnosis & management. *Indian Pacing and Electrophysiology Journal, 6*(2), 84–99.

PRADER–WILLI SYNDROME

DESCRIPTION

Prader–Willi syndrome (PWS) is a genetic disorder influencing multiple body systems whose primary phenotypic expressions include (a) hypotonia with poor suck and poor weight gain in infancy (i.e., failure to thrive), (b) cognitive dysfunction often summarized as mild mental retardation, (c) hypogonadism, (d) growth hormone insufficiency with concomitant delayed or absent puberty, (e) early childhood-onset hyperphagia and obesity, and (f) neurobehavioral disturbance. PWS is described as a genetic condition involving chromosome 15, more specifically the q11.2-q13 region, which involves an absent expression of paternally inherited genes (Cassidy & Driscoll, 2009). It has two modes of inheritance (paternally derived deletion, DEL; maternal uniparental disomy, mUPD), only one of which (UPD) is associated with an increased risk of autistic symptomology (Halit, Grice, Bolton, & Johnson, 2008). According to the Prader–Willi Association and consistent with other estimates, the incidence of PWS reported is 1 in 10,000–15,000 live births.

NEUROPATHOLOGY/PATHOPHYSIOLOGY

Genetic testing is paramount to accurate diagnosis. The defining characteristics of PWS are variable, in large part dependent upon the phenotypic expression of the specific variant. For example, psychotic symptomatology is strongly associated with the mUPD genetic variant of PWS, whereas persons with the DEL subtype are more likely to experience affective features without accompanying psychosis (Soni et al., 2008). Infants with PWS have been shown to experience delays in their neural maturity as reflected in EEG development of defined sleep stages (Heussler et al., 2008). Woodcock, Oliver, and Humphreys (2008) examined the deficit in attentional switching among persons diagnosed with PWS using among other measures, MRI technology. They found abnormalities in specific frontal regions in individuals with PWS, and functional images revealed significant differences in switch-related activation in individuals

with PWS compared with controls. Miller et al. (2007) studied the clinical feature of appetite dysregulation by comparing functional MRI blood oxygen level dependent (BOLD) responses while viewing pictures of food after ingestion of an oral glucose load. They found that individuals with PWS had an increased BOLD response in the ventromedial prefrontal cortex compared with normal weight controls when viewing pictures of food after an oral glucose load. Butler et al. (2002), utilizing neuroanatomical autopsy studies, suggested that the paraventricular nucleus (a region involved in the control of appetite and sexual behavior) may be reduced in size, with fewer oxytocin expressing neurons.

NEUROPSYCHOLOGICAL/CLINICAL PRESENTATION

Persons with PWS have an average IQ of 70, with a range from severely deficient to average (Butler et al., 2006). One-third are described as functioning within the borderline to average range (IQs 70–100), 61% in the mild-to-moderate ranges of mental retardation (IQs 50–70), and 6% in the severe-profound range (Whitman & Thompson, 2006). Syndromal variants (DEL & mUPD) are also seen concerning behavioral and cognitive dimensions. Roof et al. (2000) examined neurocognitive skills by genetic subtype (DEL vs. mUPD) and found that persons with mUPD have significantly higher verbal scores and those with DEL have significantly higher visualperceptual-spatial scores. The work of Key and Dykens (2008) focused on how persons with PWS perceive visual food stimuli. They studied neural responses to food stimuli using the visual event-related potentials (ERP). They found that the mUPD group functioned more like controls, focusing on the suitability of food for consumption, with differences noted even in the first milliseconds of stimuli exposure. Distinguishing phenotypic features were also supported by the work of Halit et al. (2008) in regard to face and gaze processing. Using electrophysiological (ERP) technology and behavioral assessments, they found that although behavioral measures did not distinguish the two groups, ERP's did provide differential information regarding the processing of facial images.

DIAGNOSIS

Essential diagnostic features include chromosomal microdeletion of 15q11-q13 ascertained through genetic testing, with a range of cognitive, physical, and behavioral characteristics that are phenotypically prototypical of PWS. Newborn presentation tends to coincide with subtle dysmorphism and nonspecific findings such as hypotonia, somnolence, and weak sucking reflex, which can delay diagnostic identification. The trajectory of development, which includes a delay in the acquisition of milestones and conversion to hyperphagia, promotes detection and recommendation for genetic assessment. PWS is observed in all races and ethnic groups, but is reported most often in Caucasians (Butler et al., 2006).

TREATMENT

PWS has no cure; therapeutic methods, however, can be employed at various developmental junctures to address relevant clinical issues. During infancy, early intervention services promoting muscle tone and nutritional adequacy are important strategies to implement. As the child enters a more hyperphagic stage, behavioral methods utilizing applied behavioral analysis techniques will need to be implemented. Behavioral methods targeting other maladaptive behaviors will also be necessary. Self-injurious skin-picking is a distinctive PWS feature among other repetitious, compulsion-like behaviors that are thought to be reflective of damage to the orbitofrontal cortices and anterior temporal lobes or to circuits involving them (Ogura, Shinohara, Ohno, & Mori, 2008). Pharmacological intervention supplementing behavioral intervention and family support is a commonly used method of intervention. Persons with PWS are also at risk for sleep disorders including excessive daytime sleepiness and insomnia involving disordered breathing. Persons with PWS should be referred for sleep study with appropriate intervention initiated as required. Academically, children with PWS present a variety of needs in school settings (Kundert, 2008), and they tend to benefit from a highly structured learning environment, supplemental support, and intervention to promote adaptive social development. Later, transition planning to include vocational planning and training is indicated, with multidisciplinary efforts likely required across the life span.

Shane S. Bush
Mark A. Sandberg

Butler, J. V., Whittington, J. E., Holland, A. J., Boer, H., Clarke, D., & Webb, T. (2002). Prevalence of, and risk factors for, physical ill-health in people with Prader-Willi syndrome: A population-based study. *Developmental Medicine & Child Neurology, 44,* 248–255.

Cassidy, S. B., & Driscoll, D. J. (2009). Prader-Willi syndrome. *European Journal of Human Genetics, 17*(1), 3–13.

Halit, H., Grice, S. J., Bolton, R., & Johnson, M. H. (2008). Face and gaze processing in Prader-Willi syndrome. *Journal of Neuropsychology, 2,* 65–77.

Heussler, H., Suresh, S., Harris, M., Cooper, D., Dakin, C., Williams, G., et al. (2008). Developmental aspects of sleep in Prader-Willi Syndrome. *Journal of Intellectual Disability Research, 52,* 815.

Key, A. P., & Dykens, E. M. (2008). "Hungry Eyes": Visual processing of food images in adults with Prader-Willi syndrome. *Journal of Intellectual Disability Research, 52,* 536–546.

Kundert, D. K. (2008). Prader-Willi syndrome. *School Psychology Quarterly, 23,* 246–257.

Miller, J. L., James, G. A., Goldstone, A. P., Couch, J. A., He, G., Driscoll, D. J., et al. (2007). Enhanced activation of reward mediating prefrontal regions in response to food stimuli in Prader–Willi syndrome. *Journal of Neurology, Neurosurgery, and Psychiatry, 78,* 615–619.

Ogura, K., Shinohara, M., Ohno, K., & Mori, E. (2008). Frontal behavioral syndromes in Prader-Willi syndrome. *Brain & Development, 30,* 469–476.

Roof, E., Stone, W., MacLean, W., Feurer, I. D., Thompson, T., & Butler, M. G. (2000). Intellectual characteristics of Prader-Willi syndrome: Comparison of genetic subtypes. *Journal of Intellectual Disability Research, 44,* 25–30.

Soni, S., Whittington, J., Holland, A. J., Webb, T., Maina, E. N., Boer, H., & Clarke, D. (2008). The phenomenology and diagnosis of psychiatric illness in people with Prader-Willi syndrome. *Psychological Medicine, 38,* 1505–1514.

Whitman, B. Y., & Thompson, T. (2006). Neurodevelopmental and neuropsychological aspects of Prader-Willi syndrome. In M. G. Butler, P. D. K. Lee, & B. Y. Whitman (Eds.), *Management of Prader-Willi syndrome* (3rd ed., pp. 245–271). New York: Springer.

Woodcock, K., Oliver, C., & Humphreys, G. (2008). Associations between repetitive questioning, resistance to change, temper outbursts and anxiety in Prader-Willi and Fragile-X syndromes. *Journal of Intellectual Disability Research, 53,* 265–278.

PRIMARY LATERAL SCLEROSIS

DESCRIPTION

Primary lateral sclerosis (PLS) has been described as a syndrome of progressive upper motor neuron dysfunction when no other cause can be attributed to the condition (Singer, Statland, Wolfe, & Barohn, 2007). Although motor symptoms predominate, cognitive deficits are also seen, with the functional constellation presenting similarly to frontotemporal dementias. Consequently, emotional and behavioral alterations can also be seen, but are not considered a specific characteristic of the presentation until later in the disease progression and early on may be more reactionary to functional changes as opposed to neurological disruption. Eventually, patients become dependent on a caregiver or family and the social economy is affected.

NEUROPATHOLOGY/PATHOPHYSIOLOGY

The most common functional changes associated with PLS involve leg weakness and spasticity, as well as spastic bulbar weakness. However, sensory symptoms should be carefully considered in case of alternative diagnosis such as amyotrophic lateral sclerosis (ALS). Thus, it still remains unclear if exclusively limb or bulbar cases are present or if the disease would progress become spinobulbar spasticity with time (Singer et al., 2007). Furthermore, initial symptoms associated with PLS have included dysarthria, dysphagia, inappropriate laughing or crying, and hyperactive muscle-stretch reflexes (Beal & Richardson, 1981). In addition, Beal and Richardson reported some pathological changes in a case report that include atrophy of the precentral gyri, a depletion of Betz cells, and loss of myelinated fibers through the pyramidal system, although there were no signs of loss of cranial nerve neurons or spinal cord anterior horn cells. Laminar gliosis in the external and internal pyramidal cell cortical layers have also been noted (Pringle et al., 1992). In contrast, the substantia nigra is not affected, and lower motor neuron abnormalities are not typically found in hypoglossal or spinal gray nuclei (Pringle et al., 1992).

Similarly, Gastaut, Michel, Figarella-Branger, and Somma-Mauvais (1988) reported five PLS cases using clinical and laboratory data. As a result, the following pathological changes were consistently indicated: (a) dysarthria, (b) difficulty chewing, (c) salivary stasis, (d) speech difficulty, (e) moderate disability in all four limbs, (f) rigid movement, (g) fixed facial expressions, (h) inability of closing mouth due to excess of saliva, (i) cheek and jaw movement were limited, (j) stiffness in walking, and (h) inability to talk due to dysphagia.

NEUROPSYCHOLOGICAL/CLINICAL PRESENTATION

The onset of PLS starts at middle age, ranging from 45 to 55 years. It is predominantly seen in males. The first symptoms that appear in the clinical picture are spastic bulbar weakness as manifested in dysarthria,

followed by dysphagia that progresses to anarthria. Progressive spasticity and weakness of limbs have also been noted as early symptoms. The course of the disease has a slow and insidious progression with several studies reporting periods of stability or improvement lasting months or even years (Floeter & Mills, 2009). Survival after the onset ranges from 1 to 15 years but the causes of deaths have not been attributed directly to this disease (Le Forestier et al., 2001; Singer et al. 2007).

The work of Singer et al. (2007) described the clinical manifestations that are typically reported by patients. They indicate stiffness, clumsiness, and poor coordination as the initial limb movement loss. Generally, the most common clinical symptoms are spasticity, hyperreflexia, and mild weakness. Electromyography (EMG), muscle biopsy, and motor evoked potentials are recommended to confirm diagnosis as well as other laboratory studies such as the normal serum chemistries, vitamin B_{12} levels, cerebrospinal fluid examination, and magnetic resonance imaging (MRI) (Le Forestier et al., 2001).

In more advanced stages of the disease, affective symptoms such as emotional instability, inappropriate laughing and crying emerge. Neurocognitive functioning is also compromised during the course of the illness with memory and executive functioning deficits presenting similar to that seen in the frontotemporal dementias. As a result, sensitive neurocognitive tests are needed to detect these deficits, thus brief and standard psychological test such as WAIS do not identify the impairment (Piquard et al., 2006).

In a study regarding neuropsychological functioning, Caselli, Smith, and Osborn (1995) studied the nine patients with PLS. The individuals underwent a neuropsychological assessment between 3 and 20 years after the onset of the spasticity symptom. They found mild cognitive deficits in executive functioning and memory that were noticed only by using sensitive neuropsychological tools such as the Controlled Oral Word Association Test, Wisconsin Card Sorting Test, Booklet Category Test, Stroop, and Trail Making Test. Other studies confirm the presence of more severe neurocognitive symptoms that are associated to frontotemporal atrophy and it suggests a form of dementia syndrome (Murphy et al., 2008; Tan et al., 2003).

DIAGNOSIS

Previously, Pringle et al. (1992) proposed the following diagnostic criteria for PLS: (a) insidious onset of spastic paresis in upper and more commonly lower extremities; (b) an adult onset, commonly by the age of 50 or later; (c) lack of family history; (d) progressive course is gradual instead of sudden; (e) duration is at least

3 years or more; (f) clinical findings are mainly associated with corticospinal dysfunction; and (g) the individual develops severe spastic spinobulbar paresis with symmetrical distribution.

Despite the diagnostic criteria, the concept of PLS remains controversial and the condition is attributed to other central nervous diseases. According to Gastaut et al. (1988), PLS is still considered a rare condition although it was first described by Charcot over a century ago. As a result of the controversy, numerous studies have been conducted with the objective of distinguish PLS diagnosis. For instance, Caselli et al. (1995) reviewed the results of cognitive and neuropsychological testing in nine patients (seven males and two females) with no signs of dementia and who were clinically diagnosed with PLS to determine if functions of the frontal lobe were normal using the criteria set by Pringle et al. (1992), although not all the patients had every test that Pringle et al. listed in their diagnosis criteria. Findings from Caselli et al. supported the following: (a) PLS is accompanied by mild cognitive deficits, (b) neuropsychological testing is useful in the diagnosis and management of patients with PLS, (c) many other causes of progressive spasticity can be differentiated from PLS by using modern techniques such as MRI or EMG.

In recent years, the number of studies comparing PLS and ALS has increased with the objective of differentiating the diseases. In order to distinguish between PLS and ALS, Le Forestier et al. (2001) investigated evidence of involvement of lower motor neurons using electrophysiological examinations and muscle biopsy in 20 patients who were diagnosed with PLS according to the diagnostic criteria from Pringle et al. findings. Le Forestier et al. revealed that PLS is part of the continuum of motor neuron disease instead of a separate condition.

Overall, the diagnostic criteria of PLS are still controversial because the distinction among other conditions is unclear. For instance, although Beal and Richardson (1981) presented a case report of a 66-year-old female who met the criteria of PLS, the absence of modern technologies for pathologic confirmation might question the PLS diagnosis. Furthermore, the application of MRI, EMG, and modern neurodiagnostic techniques is recommended in order to establish a clear distinction among PLS and other conditions such as ALS, multiple sclerosis, structural cerebral lesions, as well as spinal cord lesions (Caselli et al., 1995).

TREATMENT

Although there is no cure for PLS, treatment can improve both the quality and length of life. Because PLS is a complex disease, caring of PLS patients is best provided at multi-compound treatment (Veldink, Van den Berg, & Wokke, 2004). It requires a multidisciplinary approach with specialists in each branch of pneumology, nutrition, palliative care, psychology, neuropsychology, neurology, neuropsychology, psychiatry, speech therapist, social workers, and nurses (Rodríguez, Grande, & García-Caballero, 2007); each one is responsible for treating physical, behavioral, cognitive, spiritual, and emotional symptomatology of the patient, their caregiver and family. Professionals also serve to inform, guide, treat, rehabilitate, and follow-up in each of the different stages of the disease.

The treatment of spasticity is the main aspect of medical care. The spastic paresis of origins has been treated with gamma-aminobutyric acid agonists, in particular, baclofen (Marquiardt & Seifert, 2000). Riluzole, an anti-glutamate drug, has proven to be effective in slowing the disease, which restrains the release of glutamate, decreasing its citotoxic effect (Veldink et al., 2004). Drugs such as tricyclics, inhibitors of the reuptake of serotonin, psychotropics, muscle relaxants or corticoids, and so forth are used to alleviate other symptoms such as muscle stiffness, the cramps, the problems of salivation, swallowing, weakness, respiratory problems, and psychiatric symptoms, such as depression (Gil, 2007).

Nevertheless, more studies are needed to expand the evidence-based approaches in supportive treatments, including radiotherapy and the effect on sialorrhoea, the effect of medications on symptoms, the effects of noninvasive ventilation, and the comparison of percutaneous endoscopic gastrostomy with radiologically inserted gastrostomy and a hybrid gastrostomy technique (per-oral imagine-guided gastrostomy) (Veldink et al., 2004).

In conclusion, the combination of different imaging modalities such as volumetric MRI with perfusion MRI or functional MRI, or volumetric MRI with SPECT/PET will not only add to the understanding of the disease processes but also help to improve interpretation of treatment effects. Finally, magnetic resonance measures might also be helpful to identify patients at risk of developing adverse effects during the treatments (Gil, 2007).

Carlos Ojeda
Mónica Muzquiz
Javier Gontier
Antonio E. Puente

Beal, M., & Richardson, E. (1981). Primary lateral sclerosis. A case report. *Archives of Neurology, 38,* 630–633.

Caselli, R., Smith, B., & Osborn, D. (1995). Primary lateral sclerosis: A neuropsychological study. *Neurology, 45,* 2005–2009.

OP

Floeter, M., & Mills, R. (2009). Progression in primary lateral sclerosis: A prospective analysis. *Amyotrophic Lateral Sclerosis, 10*(5–6), 339–346.

Gastaut, J., Michel, B., Figarella-Branger, D., & Somma-Mauvais, H. (1988). Chronic progressive spinobulbar spasticity. A rare form of primary lateral sclerosis. *Archives of Neurology, 45,* 509–513.

Gil, R. (2007). *Neuropsicología.* Ed. Elsevier Masson.

Le Forestier, N., Maisonobe, T., Piquard, A., Rivaud, S., Crevier-Bushman, L., Salachas, F., et al. (2001). Does primary lateral sclerosis exist? A study of 20 patients and a review of the literature. *Brain, 124,* 1989–1999.

Marquiardt, G. & Seifert, V. (2000). Use of intrathecal baclofen for treatment of spasticity in amyotrophic lateral sclerosis. *Journal of Neurology, Neurosurgery and Psychiatry, 72,* 275–276.

Murphy, M., Grace, G., Tartaglia, M., Orange, J., Chen, X., Rowe, A., et al. (2008). Cerebral haemodynamic changes accompanying cognitive impairment in primary lateral sclerosis. *Amyotrophic Lateral Sclerosis, 9*(6), 359–368.

Piquard, A., Le Forestier, N., Baudoin-Madec, V., Delgadillo, D., Salachas, F., Pradat, P., et al. (2006). Neuropsychological changes in patients with primary lateral sclerosis. *Amyotrophic Lateral Sclerosis, 7*(3), 150–160.

Pringle, C., Hudson, A., Munoz, D., Kierman, J., Brown, W., & Ebers, G. (1992). Primary lateral sclerosis. Clinical features, neuropathology and diagnostic criteria. *Brain, 115,* 495–520.

Rodríguez, F. J., Grande, M., & García-Caballero, J. (2007). Desarrollo de una vía clínica para la atención a pacientes con esclerosis lateral amiotrófica en un ámbito regional. Red de Atención de ELA-Comunidad de Madrid. *Neurología, 22*(6), 354–361.

Singer, M., Statland, J., Wolfe, G., & Barohn, R. (2007). Primary lateral sclerosis. *Muscle & Nerve, 35,* 291–302.

Tan, C., Kakita, A., Piao, Y., Kikugawa, K., Endo, K., Tanaka, M., et al. (2003). Primary lateral sclerosis: A rare upper-motor-predominant form of amytrophic lateral sclerosis often accompanied by frontotemporal lobar degeneration with ubiquitinated neuronal inclusions? *Acta Neuropathologica, 105,* 615–620.

Veldink, J., Van den Berg, L., & Wokke, J. (2004). The future of motor neuron disease. The challenge is in the genes ALS. *Journal of Neurology, 251,* 491–500.

PRIMARY PROGRESSIVE APHASIA

DESCRIPTION

Primary progressive aphasia (PPA) is a neurodegenerative disease of insidious onset, marked by increasing deficits in word finding, object naming, syntax, or comprehension in the absence of generalized dementia within the initial 2 years of the presentation. Considered part of the frontal lobe or frontotemporal dementias (FTDs), PPA presents in three different forms including progressive nonfluent aphasia (PNFA), semantic dementia (SD, i.e., fluent PPA), and logopenic progressive aphasia (LPA). These subtypes are so described as they differ based on their clinical presentation as discussed below. Although variability is seen in the clinical presentation, PPA as a general disorder is linked with neuroanatomical abnormalities, predominately of the language areas of the brain, not attributed to stroke or infarction.

Onset is usually between 50 and 75 years of age (Westbury & Bub, 1997). As with other dementing diseases, there is no known cure. Treatment is focused on slowing disease progression while providing accommodations to prolong individuals' capacity for independence and a quality life.

NEUROPATHOLOGY/PATHOPHYSIOLOGY

The neuropathological basis of PPA is variable. In some respects, the differential anatomical origin corresponds with the clinical presentation and resulting subtypes. Although bilateral decay is common, involvement of the left hemisphere greater than the right is typical (Westbury & Bub, 1997). The left perisylvian region has been linked with all subtypes of PPA on neuroimaging studies (Galton, Patterson, Xuereb, & Hodges, 2000; Neary et al., 1998). When comparing the three subtypes, different anatomical profiles emerge. Semantic dementia is linked with more prominent atrophy in medial and anterior temporal; PNFA more commonly corresponds with left frontal hypometabolism and atrophy in the motor and premotor cortex; LPA is associated with atrophy of the left inferior and medial parietal lobe regions, the posterior third of the middle temporal gyrus, the superior temporal sulcus, and the left hippocampus (Rogalski & Mesulam, 2009).

In most cases of PPA, the presentation is sporadic. In those instances were a familial or genetic predisposition has been proposed, point mutations on chromosome 17q21 and 17q22 in the genes that encode either tau or progranulin have been noted (Basun et al., 1997; Lendon et al., 1998; Mesulam et al., 2007).

NEUROPSYCHOLOGICAL/CLINICAL PRESENTATION

The clinical presentation of PPA has been well described in the literature (e.g., Mesulam, 2001; Neary et al., 1998).

PPA is characterized by an insidious and progressive course of impairment in word finding, naming, syntax, or word comprehension during conversation or through assessment that remain isolated for 2 or more years while activities of daily living and other cognitive functions remain relatively intact. However, ideomotor apraxia and acalculia may still present. After the first 2 years, additional cognitive domains are commonly affected, but language remains the most impaired.

As noted, PPA has been divided into three subtypes that differ in their underlying neuropathology that corresponds with differences in their clinical presentation. In SD, what some refer to as fluent-PPA, individuals present with a prominent loss in the meaning of words and objects in the presence of grammatically correct speech and preserved syntactic comprehension. Spontaneous speech is fluent despite the aforementioned loss of object and word meaning (Hodges, Patterson, Oxbury, & Funnell, 1992) making output empty. Articulation, syntax, and repetition remain intact in the early stages (Hodges et al., 1992).

Nonfluent PPA in comparison is characterized by poor and difficult articulation, disrupted fluency and prosody, paraphasias (most commonly phonemic), agrammatism, and variable anomia in the presence of preserved comprehension (Gorno-Tempini et al., 2004). High-order sentence comprehension may be impeded as well (Hodges & Patterson, 1996; Neary et al., 1998; Turner, Kenyon, Trojanowski, Gonatas, & Grossman, 1996). Apraxia of speech and anarthria have both been associated with this variant (Broussolle et al., 1996; Fukui, Sugita, Kawamura, Shiota, & Nakano, 1996; Gorno-Tempini et al., 2004).

Finally, logopenic PPA manifests as slowed speech and frequent word finding pauses that are noted in the presence of relatively normal articulation (Gorno-Tempini et al., 2004). This is viewed as related to short-term phonological memory deficits owing to the fact that in conversation these word finding pauses are observed, yet on multiple-choice examination, individuals identify the correct words (Gorno-Tempini et al., 2004). Phonemic paraphasias are common (Kertesz, Davidson, McCabe, Takagi, & Munoz, 2003). Syntax and comprehension are impaired aside from the simplest incidences.

Beyond language, the PPAs are commonly associated with secondary behavioral and motor disturbances. The nonfluent PPA subtype may demonstrate behavioral manifestations similar to FTD aside from the fact that they do not become overly disrespectful or mean. Depression, disinhibition, impulsivity, and emotional blunting have all been associated with fluent PPA, that is, semantic dementia (Caselli, Beach, Sue, Connor, & Sabbagh, 2002; Rosen et al.,

2006; Thompson, Patterson, & Hodges, 2003). Fewer behavioral disturbances have been associated with the logopenic subtype. Limb apraxia may present in any of the three PPA variants and is consequently, as previously noted, one of only two features including acalculia that may present even in the earliest stages of disease progression (Joshi, Roy, Black, & Barbour, 2003). Motoric retardation, subtle rigidity, and diminished control are sometimes noted in conjunction with nonfluent aphasia, usually affecting the right more than the left owing to the pathological origin in the left hemisphere. Semantic dementia and logopenic variants are not associated with additional motor deficits beyond the aforementioned potential of apraxia.

DIAGNOSIS

Diagnosis of PPA is largely based on clinical history and presentation, including both positive and negative findings on neuropsychological assessment and neuroimaging. Just as there are inclusionary criteria, there are exclusionary criteria. The former can be generalized as increasing deficits in word finding, object naming, syntax, or comprehension in the absence of generalized dementia within the initial 2 years of the presentation. In terms of exclusionary criteria, the onset may not be abrupt, the presentation is not related to a focal lesion that is suggestive of a traumatic event such as cerebrovascular accident, and the features may not be accompanied in the initial 2 years with more widespread dementia and neurological features aside from possibly apraxia and/or acalculia (Rogalski & Mesulam, 2009).

Neuropsychological assessment can be essential to diagnosis, although testing can be difficult to interpret if clinicians are not experienced with the presentation. Limitations may occur as performance-based test results may be skewed depending on the nature of the verbal deficits. Nonverbal tests may be incorporated into the assessment to offer further comparison between verbal and nonverbal domains.

MRI and CT scans may be utilized with particular attention placed on the left hemisphere, particularly the perisylvian region to evaluate for atrophy. PET or SPECT may be used to evaluate metabolism in this same region, and EEG can evaluate electrical activity, with positive findings consisting of hypometabolism on the former and slowing in frontal and/or temporal regions on the latter.

TREATMENT

Similar to cortical dementias such as Alzheimer's disease, there is no specific treatment or cure for PPAs. In comparison, acetylcholinesterase inhibitors such as Aricept, Namenda, and/or Exelon, which are usually useful in slowing the progression of presentations such as Alzheimer's disease, are ineffective in PPAs. Alternative communication strategies may be employed under guidance of a speech therapist (Rogalski & Mesulam, 2009). Patient and family support and education is strongly recommended. If behavioral symptoms arise, depending upon their presentation, medicinal strategies may prove useful. Depression may respond to traditional selective serotonin reuptake inhibitors, whereas antiepileptic drugs may serve as a means of controlling disinhibition or impulsivity, although, as noted previously, individuals often remain polite.

Chad A. Noggle
Michelle R. Pagoria

Basun, H., Almkvist, O., Axelman, K., Brun, A., Campbell, T. A., Collinge, J., et al. (1997). Clinical characteristics of a chromosome 17-linked rapidly progressive familial frontotemporal dementia. *Archives of Neurology, 54*(5), 539–544.

Broussolle, E., Bakchine, S., Tommasi, M., Laurent, B., Bazin, B., Cinotti, L., et al. (1996). Slowly progressive anarthria with late anterior opercular syndrome: A variant form of frontal cortical atrophy syndromes. *Journal of Neurological Sciences, 144*(1–2), 44–58.

Caselli, R. J., Beach, T. G., Sue, L. I., Connor, D. J., & Sabbagh, M. N. (2002). Progressive aphasia with Lewy bodies. *Dementia and Geriatric Cognitive Disorders, 14*(2), 55–58.

Fukui, T., Sugita, K., Kawamura, M., Shiota, J., & Nakano, I. (1996). Primary progressive apraxia in Pick's disease: A clinicopathologic study. *Neurology, 47*(2), 467–473.

Galton, C. J., Patterson, K., Xuereb, J. H., & Hodges, J. R. (2000). Atypical and typical presentations of Alzheimer's disease: A clinical, neuropsychological, neuroimaging and pathological study of 13 cases. *Brain, 123*(3), 484–498.

Gorno-Tempini, M. L., Dronkers, N. F., Rankin, K. P., Ogar, J. M., Phengrasamy, L., Rosen, H. J., et al. (2004). Cognition and anatomy in three variants of primary progressive aphasia. *Annals of Neurology, 55*(3), 335–346.

Hodges, J. R., & Patterson, K. (1996). Nonfluent progressive aphasia and semantic dementia: A comparative neuropsychological study. *Journal of the International Neuropsychological Society, 2*(6), 511–524.

Hodges, J. R., Patterson, K., Oxbury, S., & Funnell, E. (1992). Semantic dementia. Progressive fluent aphasia with temporal lobe atrophy. *Brain, 115*(6), 1783–1806.

Joshi, A., Roy, E. A., Black, S. E., & Barbour, K. (2003). Patterns of limb apraxia in primary progressive aphasia. *Brain Cognition, 53*(2), 403–407.

Kertesz, A., Davidson, W., McCabe, P., Takagi, K., & Munoz, D. (2003). Primary progressive aphasia: Diagnosis, varieties, evolution. *Journal of the International Neuropsychological Society, 9*(5), 710–719.

Lendon, C. L., Lynch, T., Norton, J., McKeel, D. W., Jr., Busfield, F., Craddock, N., et al. (1998). Hereditary dysphasic disinhibition dementia: A frontotemporal dementia linked to 17q21-22. *Neurology, 50*(6), 1546–1555.

Mesulam, M. M. (2001). Primary progressive aphasia. *Annals of Neurology, 49*(4), 425–432.

Mesulam, M. M., Johnson, N., Krefft, T. A., Gass, J. M., Cannon, A. D., Adamson, J. L., et al. (2007). Progranulin mutations in primary progressive aphasia: The PPA1 and PPA3 families. *Archives of Neurology, 64*(1), 43–47.

Neary, D., Snowden, J. S., Gustafson, L., Passant, U., Stuss, D., Black, S., et al. (1998). Frontotemporal lobar degeneration: A consensus on clinical diagnostic criteria. *Neurology, 51*(6), 1546–1554.

Rogalski, E. J., & Mesulam, M. M. (2009). Clinical trajectories and biological features of primary progressive aphasia (PPA). *Current Alzheimer Research, 6*, 331–336.

Rosen, H. J., Allison, S. C., Ogar, J. M., Amici, S., Rose, K., Dronkers, N., et al. (2006). Behavioral features in semantic dementia vs other forms of progressive aphasias. *Neurology, 67*(10), 1752–1756.

Thompson, S. A., Patterson, K., & Hodges, J. R. (2003). Left/right asymmetry of atrophy in semantic dementia: Behavioral cognitive implications. *Neurology, 61*(9), 1196–1203.

Turner, R. S., Kenyon, L. C., Trojanowski, J. Q., Gonatas, N., & Grossman, M. (1996). Clinical, neuroimaging, and pathologic features of progressive nonfluent aphasia. *Annals of Neurology, 39*(2), 166–173.

Westbury, C., & Bub, D. (1997). Primary progressive aphasia: A review of 112 cases. *Brain Language, 3*, 381–406.

PROGRESSIVE MULTIFOCAL LEUKOENCEPHALOPATHY

DESCRIPTION

Progressive multifocal leukoencephalopathy (PML), also referred to as progressive multifocal leukoencephalitis, is a rare and highly fatal demyelinating disease affecting the central nervous system (CNS). PML is an opportunistic infection caused by the common polyomavirus JC (JC virus) that is generally latent in healthy individuals. The JC virus may be reactivated in patients with severely compromised immune systems, and is most often seen in patients with HIV, but also occurs in patients with certain types of cancer and those undergoing immunosuppressive therapy (e.g., organ transplant patients). The reactivated JC virus causes a lysis of oligodendrocytes leading to a breakdown of myelin, which produces expanding lesions within the brain (McCalmont & Bennett, 2007). Although rare, the incidence of PML is increasing as the number of individuals living with persistently compromised immune systems also increases.

NEUROPATHOLOGY/PATHOPHYSIOLOGY

Current research suggests that the seroprevalence of the JC virus varies depending on age, with older individuals demonstrating the highest seropositive rate (Chang et al., 2002). The JC virus may be carried by as many as 85% of adults (Weber et al., 1997) but is asymptomatic in individuals with normally functioning immune systems. PML is caused by the reactivation of the JC virus in individuals experiencing severe immunosuppression. The reactivated JC virus targets and subsequently destroys oligodendrocytes, resulting in the rapid deterioration of white matter within the CNS (Paul et al., 2007). The lysis of oligodendrocytes in PML results in more rapidly coalescing lesions than is typically seen with diseases such as multiple sclerosis where the myelin (rather than the glial cells which produce it) is attacked. This rapid deterioration results in multifocal lesions throughout the CNS and has been found to involve areas such as the cerebral hemispheres, cerebellum, brainstem, and cervical spinal cord (von Einsiedel et al., 1993). If untreated, individuals with a dual diagnosis of HIV and PML typically experience only a 10% survival rate beyond 1 year (Koralnik, 2004).

NEUROPSYCHOLOGICAL/CLINICAL PRESENTATION

Presentation of PML varies and is dependent upon the location of lesions within the CNS. Symptoms observed with PML may include gait abnormalities, loss of higher order cognitive functioning, poor memory, seizures, emotional lability, hemiparesis, speech dysarthria, and visual changes (Roberts, 2005; Salvan, Confort-Gouny, Cozzone, & Vion-Dury, 1999). PML occurs most often in individuals with AIDS, which is estimated to be the underlying disease in approximately 55-85% of individuals with PML (Berger, Pall, Lanske, & Whiteman, 1998). This complicates diagnosis as the initial symptoms of PML may be misdiagnosed as HIV-related cerebral lesions (Engsig et al., 2009).

DIAGNOSIS

Diagnosis of PML is typically made on the basis of clinical symptomatology combined with MRI results showing the characteristic focal lesions associated with the loss of white matter. CT scans are often also employed but demonstrate less sensitivity than MRIs in detecting PML (Leswick, Robinson, & Harder, 2006). Cerebrospinal fluid analysis may be conducted but tends to produce many false negatives (von Einsiedel et al., 1993). Brain biopsy allows for histological confirmation of PML but is not preferred due to its invasive nature.

TREATMENT

There is currently no treatment for the JC virus that causes PML in immunosuppressed individuals. However, in individuals with dual HIV/PML diagnosis, highly active antiretroviral therapy (HAART) has been shown to significantly improve survival rates (De Luca et al., 2000). HAART works indirectly against PML by preventing replication of HIV and allowing for recovery of the immune system (Koralnik, 2004). Additional treatment considerations include aiding in the management of physical symptoms such as difficulty walking or speaking, and addressing the social/emotional difficulties that may result from a diminished quality of life.

Jacob T. Lutz
Raymond S. Dean

Berger, J. R., Pall, L., Lanska, D., & Whiteman, M. (1998). Progressive multifocal leukoencephalopathy in patients with HIV infection [Electronic version]. *Journal of Neurovirology, 4,* 59–68.

Chang, H., Wang, M., Tsai, R. T., Lin, H. S., Huan, J. S., Wang, W. C., et al. (2002). High incidence of JC viruria in JC-seropositive older individuals. *Journal of Neurovirology, 8,* 447–451. doi: 10.1080/13550280290100824

De Luca, A., Giancola, M. L., Ammassari, A., Grisetti, S., Paglia, M. G., Gentile, M., et al. (2000). The effect of potent antiretroviral therapy and JC virus load in cerebrospinal fluid on clinical outcome of patients with AIDS-associated progressive multifocal leukoencephalopathy. *The Journal of Infectious Diseases, 182,* 1077–1083. doi: 0022-1899/2000/18204-009

Engsig, F. N., Hansen, A. B., Omland, L. H., Kronborg, G., Gerstoft, J., Laursen, A. L., et al. (2009). Incidence, clinical presentation, and outcome of progressive multifocal leukoencephalopathy in HIV-infected patients during the highly active antiretroviral therapy era:

A nationwide cohort study. *The Journal of Infectious Diseases, 199*, 77–83. doi: 10.1086/595299

Koralnik, I. J. (2004). New insights into progressive multifocal leukoencephalopathy. *Current Opinion in Neurology, 17*, 365–370. doi: 10.1097/01.wco.0000130306.82387.60

Leswick, D. A., Robinson, C. A., & Harder, S. L. (2006). Answer to case of the month #112 progressive multifocal leukoencephalopathy with characteristic magnetic resonance imaging and magnetic resonance spectroscopy findings [Electronic version]. *Canadian Association of Radiologists Journal, 57*(4), 249–253.

McCalmont, V., & Bennett, K. (2007). Progressive multifocal leukoencephalopathy: A case study [Electronic version]. *Progress in Transplantation, 17*(2), 157–160.

Paul, R. H., Laidlaw, D. H., Tate, D. F., Lee, S., Hoth, K. F., Gunstad, J., et al. (2007). Neuropsychological and neuroimaging outcome of HIV-associated progressive multifocal leukoencephalopathy in the era of antiretroviral therapy [Electronic version]. *Journal of Integrative Neuroscience, 6*(1), 191–203.

Roberts, M. T. M. (2005). AIDS-associated progressive multifocal leukoencephalopathy: Current management strategies. *CNS Drugs, 19*(8), 671–682. doi: 1172-7047/05/0008-0671

Salvan, A. M., Confort-Gouny, S., Cozzone, P. J., & Vion-Dury, J. (1999). Atlas of brain proton magnetic resonance spectra: Part III viral infections [Electronic version]. *Journal of Neuroradiology, 26*, 154–161.

von Einsiedel, R. W., Fife, T. D., Aksamit, A. J., Cornford, M. E., Secor, D. L., Tomiyasu, U., et al. (1993). Progressive multifocal leukoencephalopathy in AIDS: A clinicopathologic study and review of the literature [Electronic version]. *Journal of Neurology, 240*, 391–406.

Weber, T., Trebst, C., Frye, S., Cinque, P., Vago, L., Sindic, C. J., et al. (1997). Analysis of the systemic and intrathecal humoral immune response in progressive multifocal leukoencephalopathy. *The Journal of Infectious Diseases, 176*, 250–254. doi: 0022–1899/97/7601–0033

PROGRESSIVE SUPRANUCLEAR PALSY

DESCRIPTION

Progressive supranuclear palsy (PSP) is one of the most common parkinsonism-plus syndromes. Acknowledging the seminal contributions of the three physicians who first described the condition (Steele, Richardson, & Olszweski, 1964), PSP is also referred to as Steele–Richardson–Olszweski syndrome. PSP is a rapidly progressive degenerative disease. The characteristic syndrome consists of supranuclear ophthalmoplegia, pseudobulbar palsy, and axial dystonia, although it may take over a year for these features to develop fully (Ropper & Brown, 2005). Early prominent features include postural instability, falls, executive dysfunction, and slowed information processing. The hallmark symptom is a vertical gaze palsy that is often downward but can sometimes occur only upward. Typical age of onset is in the 60s (range 45–75 years) with a median survival time of approximately 6 years from the initial onset of symptoms (Litvan, Agid, et al., 1996; Litvan, Mangone, et al., 1996). There are conflicting reports whether males or females are more likely to develop PSP (Bower, Maraganore, McDonnell, & Roca, 1997; Golbe, 1996). Overall prevalence is estimated between 1.4 and 6.4 per 100,000 (Golbe, Davis, Schoenberg, & Duvoisin, 1988; Schrag, Ben-Shlomo, & Quinn, 1999).

NEUROPATHOLOGY/PATHOPHYSIOLOGY

The pathophysiology of PSP involves severe neuronal degeneration of subcortical structures and minimal cortical lesions. Lesion sites are somewhat variable and typically occur between the upper brainstem and basal ganglia. Broadly, there is evidence of neuronal loss in the striatum and substantia nigra, and degeneration of structures in the basal ganglia, upper brainstem, and cerebellum (Agid, Ruberg, DuBois, & Pillon, 1987). Lesions may compromise the nigrostriatal pathway, basal forebrain, pedunculopontine nucleus, subnucleus compactus, mesencephalopontine tegmental nuclei, and locus ceruleus (Grafman, Litvan, & Stark, 1995). Dopamine levels drop drastically during the course of the illness leading to parkinsonian-type symptoms.

Degeneration impacts ascending pathways from subcortical structures to the prefrontal cortex. Grafman et al. (1995) hypothesized that pathology in the dorsolateral frontal, lateral-orbitofrontal, and anterior cingulate circuits contributes to specific cognitive dysfunctions (executive functioning, social-cognitive, and attention).

Although frontal lobe pathology is not prominent, multiple positron emission tomography (PET) studies have revealed frontal hypometabolism (Bhatt, Snow, Martin, Peppard, & Calne, 1991; Blin et al., 1990; Blin et al., 1992), and some imaging studies have reported significant frontal cortical atrophy (Cordato, Halliday, Harding, Hely, & Morris, 2000; Cordato et al., 2002; Gröschel et al., 2004). MRI studies have found atrophy of midbrain structures most pronounced in the superior colliculi and pons (Masucci, Borts, Smirniotopoulos, Kurtzke, & Schellinger, 1985; Schonfeld, Globe, Sage, Safer, & Duvoisin, 1987).

NEUROPSYCHOLOGICAL/CLINICAL PRESENTATION

Consistent with subcortical dysfunction, common manifestations of PSP reflect executive dysfunction, including cognitive slowing, impaired set-shifting, and decreased verbal fluency (Grafman et al., 1995; Jacobs, Levy, & Marder, 2003). It is generally believed that these deficits are related to frontal deafferentation secondary to subclinical lesions, although some researchers have hypothesized a more direct relationship between frontal lobe pathology and behavioral deficits (Cordato et al., 2002). Immediate and delayed recall of information can vary from normal to impaired, whereas recognition memory is improved or intact (Jacobs et al., 2003). Primary language abilities are typically preserved, though word-finding problems may develop years following formal diagnosis (Lezak, Howieson, & Loring, 2004). Not surprisingly given ocular involvement, visuospatial skills are often impaired. Visual attention impairment is typically related to duration of PSP (Kertzman, Robinson, & Litvan, 1990).

The course of physical symptoms consists of postural instability and falls several years prior to formal diagnosis. The hallmark physical symptom of PSP is a vertical gaze palsy that typically occurs relatively late in the disease process. Compensation for visual limitations can frequently lead to falls. Bradykinesia, rigidity, impaired control of mouth/ neck are also relatively common later in the course. It is notable that the development of core symptoms may present late, or never develop, during the course of the disease (Litvan et al., 2003). For example, histological confirmed cases of PSP have been reported without ophthalmoplegia (Santacruz, Uttl, Litvan, & Grafman, 1998). Respiratory arrest may occur due to a degenerative process involving the brainstem respiratory centers, or be secondary to pneumonia. Unlike Parkinson's disease, patients with PSP tend to have more of an erect rather than a stooped posture and lack tremor (Ropper & Brown, 2005).

Consistent with executive dysfunction, two of the most common behavioral manifestations of PSP are apathy and disinhibition. One study administered the Neuropsychiatric Inventory to 22 patients with PSP and found apathy to be the most prevalent neuropsychiatric feature, present in 91% of patients (Litvan, Mega, Cummings, & Fairbanks, 1996). Disinhibition was exhibited by one-third of patients, followed by dysphoria (18%) and anxiety (18%). Impaired metacognitive awareness has also been observed and is attributed to the disruption of frontostriatal feedback loops (O'Keeffe et al., 2007). Obsessive behaviors, euphoria, and depressive symptoms are also possible (Destee et al., 1990). Sleep abnormalities are prevalent as well and are most often characterized by shortened total sleep time, frequent awakenings, and decreased REM sleep (Cummings, 2003).

DIAGNOSIS

Although multiple diagnostic criteria have been proposed (e.g., Collins, Ahlskog, Parisi, & Maraganore, 1995; Tolosa, Valldeoriola, & Marti, 1994), those set forth by Litvan et al. (1996) are the most frequently cited in the literature and form the basis for the National Institute of Neurological Disorders and Stroke and Society for Progressive Supranuclear Palsy (NINDS-SPSP; Litvan et al., 2003) clinical criteria. Diagnosis of "possible PSP" requires either vertical supranuclear palsy *or* both slowing of vertical saccades and postural instability with falls during the 1st year of disease onset. "Probable" diagnosis of PSP requires vertical supranuclear palsy *and* prominent postural instability with falls within the 1st year of disease onset. Diagnosis of possible or probable PSP requires symptom onset at or after age 40, and it is necessary that there be a gradual progression of symptoms. "Definite" diagnosis of possible or probable PSP requires histopathologic confirmation at autopsy.

NINDS-SPSP clinical criteria provide a number of supportive criteria to assist in differential diagnosis. Supportive motor features include symmetric akinesia or rigidity (proximal greater than distal) and neck dystonia. An early onset of two or more of the following cognitive symptoms is also supportive of PSP diagnosis: impaired abstraction, decreased verbal fluency, "utilization or imitation behavior," "frontal release" signs, and apathy. In addition, PSP may be considered if motor symptoms do not respond, or minimally respond, to levodopa therapy and if there are early symptoms of dysphagia or dysarthria.

PSP is often misdiagnosed early in the course of the disease as Parkinson's disease or confused with other parkinsonian disorders. Severity and pattern of executive deficits characterized by slowed information processing, impaired accuracy in carrying out plans, and difficulty in set shifting tends to differentiate PSP patients from others with basal ganglia lesions (Robbins et al., 1994). The combination of postural instability leading to falls early in the course of the disease and vertical gaze palsy are also key symptoms in differentiating PSP from other disorders with parkinsonism and dementia.

OP

Neuroimaging techniques can be useful in differential diagnosis. Diffusion-weighted imaging has shown promise in differentiating PSP from Parkinson's disease early in disease onset based on increased regional apparent diffusion coefficients in the putamen, globus pallidus, and caudate nucleus (Seppi et al., 2003). An additional reliable manner to differentiate PSP from Parkinson's disease is significantly lower anteroposterior diameter of the midbrain on axial T2-weighted magnetic resonance images (Warmuth-Metz, Naumann, Csoti, & Solymosi, 2001).

Differential diagnosis between PSP and corticobasal degenerative syndrome (CBDS) is challenging. These conditions have numerous factors in common including similar neuropsychological profiles (Pillon et al., 1995), pathological features (Feany, Mattiace, & Dickson, 1996), and the finding that both conditions are considered to be predominantly 4-repeat tauopathies (Kertesz & Munoz, 2004). Further complicating the differential diagnosis, individuals with CBDS may exhibit vertical gaze palsy, falls, and symmetrical extrapyramidal syndrome (Litvan, Goetz, & Lang, 2000). One possible distinguishing feature between these syndromes is greater atrophy of the midbrain, pons, thalamus, and striatum in PSP relative to CBDS (Boxer et al., 2006).

TREATMENT

Unfortunately, PSP is a treatment-resistant and degenerative condition. Although dopaminergic agents can improve the parkinsonian features, they can also induce adverse side effects, such as orthostatic hypotension, hallucinations/delusions, and gastrointestinal complaints (Kompoliti, Goetz, Litvan, Jellinger, & Verny, 1998). It is recommended that anticholinergic agents be avoided (Cummings, 2003). There is no significant improvement with levodopa therapy.

Anita H. Sim
James B. Hoelzle

Agid, Y., Ruberg, M., DuBois, B., & Pillon, B. (1987). Anatomoclinical and biochemical concepts of subcortical dementia. In S. M. Stahl, S. D. Iversen, & E. C. Goodman (Eds.), *Cognitive neurochemistry*. Oxford: Oxford University Press.

Bhatt, M. H., Snow, B. J., Martin, W. R., Peppard, R., & Calne, D. B. (1991). Positron emission tomography in progressive supranuclear palsy. *Archives of Neurology, 48*, 389–391.

Blin, J., Baron, J. C., Dubois, B., Pillon, B., Cambon, H., Cambier, J., et al. (1990). Positron emission tomog-

raphy study in progressive supranuclear palsy. Brain hypometabolic pattern and clinicometabolic correlates. *Archives of Neurology, 47*, 747–752.

Blin, J., Vidailhet, M. J., Pillon, B., Dubois, B., Feve, J. R., & Agid, Y. (1992) Corticobasal degeneration and asymmetrical glucose consumption as studied with PET. *Movement Disorders, 7*, 348–354.

Bower, J. H., Maraganore, D. M., McDonnell, S. K., & Roca, W. A. (1997) Incidence of progressive supranuclear palsy and multiple systems atrophy in Olmsted County, Minnesota, from 1976 to 1990. *Neurology, 49*, 1284–1288.

Boxer, A. L., Geschwind, M. D., Belfor, N., Gorno-Tempini, M. L., Schauer, G. F., Miller, B. L., et al. (2006). Patterns of brain atrophy that differentiate corticobasal degeneration syndrome from progressive supranuclear palsy. *Archives of Neurology, 63*, 81–86.

Collins, S. J., Ahlskog, J. E., Parisi, J. E., & Maraganore, D. M. (1995). Progressive supranuclear palsy: Neuropathologically based diagnostic clinical criteria. *Journal of Neurology, Neurosurgery, and Psychiatry, 58*, 167–173.

Cordato, N. J., Halliday, G. M., Harding, A. J., Hely, M. A., & Morris, J. G. (2000). Regional brain atrophy in progressive supranuclear palsy and Lewy body disease. *Annals of Neurology, 47*, 718–728.

Cordato, N. J., Pantelis, C., Halliday, G. M., Velakoulis, D., Wood, S. J., Stuart, G. W., et al. (2002). Frontal atrophy correlates with behavioural changes in progressive supranuclear palsy. *Brain, 125*, 789–800.

Cummings, J. L. (2003). *The neuropsychiatry of Alzheimer's disease and related dementias*. New York: Taylor & Francis Group.

Destee, A., Gray, F., Parent, M., Neuville, V., Muller, J. P., Verier, A., et al. (1990). Comportement compulsif d'allure obsessionnelle et paralysie supranucleaire progressive [Obsessive-compulsive behavior and supranuclear palsy]. *Revue Neurologique, 146*, 12–18.

Feany, M. B., Mattiace, L. A., & Dickson, D. W. (1996). Neuropathologic overlap of progressive supranuclear palsy, Pick's disease and corticobasal degeneration. *Journal of Neuropathology and Experimental Neurology, 55*, 53–67.

Golbe, L. I. (1996). The epidemiology of progressive supranuclear palsy. *Advances in Neurology, 69*, 25–31.

Golbe, L. I., Davis, P. H., Schoenberg, B. S., & Duvoisin, R. C. (1988). Prevalence and natural history of progressive supranuclear palsy. *Neurology, 38*, 1031–1034.

Grafman, J., Litvan, I., & Stark, M. (1995). Neuropsychological features of progressive supranuclear palsy. *Brain and Cognition, 28*, 311–320.

Gröschel, K., Hauser, T. K., Luft, A., Patronas, N., Dichgans, J., Litvan, I., et al. (2004). Magnetic resonance imaging-based volumetry differentiates progressive supranuclear palsy from corticobasal degeneration. *Nueroimage, 21*, 714–724.

Jacobs, D. M., Levy, G., & Marder, K. (2003). Dementia in Parkinson's disease, Huntington's disease and related disorders. In T. E. Feinberg & M. J. Farah (Eds.), *Behavioral neurology and neuropsychology* (2nd ed.). New York: McGraw-Hill.

Kertesz, A., & Munoz, D. (2004). Relationship between frontotemporal dementia and corticobasal degeneration/ progressive supranuclear palsy. *Dementia and Geriatric Cognitive Disorders, 17,* 282–286.

Kertzman, C., Robinson, D. L., & Litvan, I. (1990). Effects of physostigmine on spatial attention in patients with progressive supranuclear palsy. *Archives of Neurology, 47,* 1346–1350.

Kompoliti, K., Goetz, C. G., Litvan, I., Jellinger, K., & Verny, M. (1998). Pharmacological therapy in progressive supranuclear palsy. *Archives of Neurology, 55,* 1099–1102.

Lezak, M. D., Howieson, D. B., & Loring, D. W. (2004). *Neuropsychological Assessment* (4th ed.). New York: Oxford University Press.

Litvan, I., Agid, Y., Jankovic, J., Goetz, C., Brandel, J. P., Lai, E. C., et al. (1996). Accuracy of clinical criteria for the diagnosis of progressive supranuclear palsy (Steele-Richardson-Olszewski syndrome). *Neurology, 46,* 922–930.

Litvan, I., Bhatia, K. P., Burn, D. J., Goetz, C. G., Lang, A. E., McKeith, I., et al. (2003). Movement Disorders Society Scientific Issues Committee report: SIC Task Force appraisal of clinical diagnostic criteria for Parkinsonian disorders. *Movement Disorders, 18,* 467–486.

Litvan, I., Goetz, C., & Lang, A. (2000). *Advances in neurology: Corticobasal degeneration and related disorders.* Lippincott, Williams, & Wilkins.

Litvan, I., Mangone, C. A., McKee, A., Verny, M., Parsa, A., Jellinger, K., et al. (1996). Natural history of progressive supranuclear palsy (Steele-Richardson-Olszewski syndrome) and clinical predictors of survival: A clinicopathological study. *Journal of Neurology, Neurosurgery, and Psychiatry, 60,* 615–620.

Litvan, I., Mega, M. S., Cummings, J. L., & Fairbanks, L. (1996). Neuropsychiatric aspects of progressive supranuclear palsy. *Neurology, 47,* 1184–1189.

Masucci, E. F., Borts, F. T., Smirniotopoulos, J. G., Kurtzke, J. F., & Schellinger, D. (1985). Thin section CT of midbrain abnormalities in progressive supranuclear palsy. *AJNR American Journal of Neuroradiology, 6,* 767–772.

O'Keeffe, F. M., Murray, B., Coen, R. F., Dockree, P. M., Bellgrove, M. A., Garavan, H., et al. (2007). Loss of insight in frontotemporal dementia, corticobasal degeneration, and progressive supranuclear palsy. *Brain, 130,* 753–764.

Pillon, B., Blin, J., Vidailhet, M., Deweer, B., Sirigu, A., DuBois, B., et al. (1995). The neuropsychological pattern of corticobasal degeneration: Comparison with progressive supranuclear palsy and Alzheimer's disease. *Neurology, 45,* 1477–1483.

Robbins, T. W., James, M., Owen, A. M., Lange, K. W., Lees, A. J., Leigh, P. N., et al. (1994). Cognitive deficits in progressive supranuclear palsy, Parkinson's disease, and multiple system atrophy in tests sensitive to frontal lobe dysfunction. *The Journal of Neurology, Neurosurgery, and Psychiatry, 57,* 79–88.

Ropper, A. H., & Brown, R. H. (2005). *Adams and Victor's principles of neurology* (8th ed.). New York: McGraw-Hill.

Santacruz, P., Uttl, B., Litvan, I., & Grafman, J. (1998). Progressive supranuclear palsy: A survey of the disease course. *Neurology, 50,* 1637–1647.

Schonfeld, S. M., Globe, L. I., Sage, J. I., Safer, J. N., & Duvoisin, R. C. (1987). Computed tomographic findings in progressive supranuclear palsy: Correlation with clinical grade. *Movement Disorders, 2,* 263–278.

Schrag, A., Ben-Shlomo, Y., & Quinn, N. P. (1999). Prevalence of progressive supranuclear palsy and multiple system atrophy: A cross-sectional study. *Lancet, 354,* 1771–1775.

Seppi, K., Schocke, M. F., Esterhammer, R., Kremser, C., Brenneis, C., Mueller, J., et al. (2003). Diffusion-weighted imaging discriminates progressive supranuclear palsy from PD, but not from parkinson variant of multiple system atrophy. *Neurology, 60,* 922–927.

Steele, J. C., Richardson, J. C., & Olszweski, J. (1964). Progressive supranuclear palsy: A heterogenous degeneration involving the brainstem, basal ganglia, and cerebellum, with vertical gaze and pseudobulbar palsy, nuchal dystonia, and dementia. *Archives of Neurology, 10,* 333–359.

Tolosa, E., Valldeoriola, F., & Marti, M. J. (1994). Clinical diagnosis and diagnostic criteria of progressive supranuclear palsy (Steele-Richardson-Olszewski syndrome). *Journal of Neural Transmission: Supplementum, 42,* 15–31.

Warmuth-Metz, M., Naumann, M., Csoti, I., & Solymosi, L. (2001). Measurement of the midbrain diameter on routine magnetic resonance imaging. *Archives of Neurology, 58,* 1076–1079.

PSEUDOTUMOR CEREBRI

DESCRIPTION

Pseudotumor cerebri represents a syndrome that is characterized by persisting headache and papilledema (unilateral or bilateral) in the absence of focal neurologic signs, abnormal CSF composition, and enlarged ventricles or an intracranial mass. The presentation is associated with increased intracranial hypertension, most commonly idiopathic in nature.

Pseudotumor cerebri is most frequently observed in overweight young women with a relative prevalence of 19–21 out of 100,000, although the condition has also been found to occur in children and adolescents, with no sex predominance, and in men (Digre & Corbett, 1988). In the general population, prevalence is reported at a rate of 1–2 per 100,000 (Radhakrishan, Ahlskog, Garrity, & Kurland, 1994).

NEUROPATHOLOGY/PATHOPHYSIOLOGY

Idiopathic, the underlying pathology of pseudotumor cerebri is relatively unknown. The most prevalent theories suggest a disruption of the outflow on the venous sinuses with cerebral venous pressure being consistently noted in prior studies (e.g., Karahalios, Rekate, Khayata, & Apostolides, 1996). In their sample, half their patients presented with venous outflow obstruction, which Karahalios and colleagues proposed, increases the resistance of CSF absorption leading to the heightened pressure and the resulting presentation. This proposal may be explained by findings of Mann, Johnson, Butler, and Bass (1979) who suggested dysfunction is in the absorption function of the arachnoid villi. Although the basis of this absorption dysfunction itself is under dispute, King, Mitchell, Thomson, and Tress (2002) have suggested that increased venous pressure is actually a secondary feature of venous stenosis, although this does not apply in all cases. The increased intracranial pressure is said to develop over a period of weeks or months.

Beyond this, the presentation has a number of other pathogenic associations including cerebral venous hypertension (e.g., occlusion of superior sagittal or lateral venous sinus, increased blood volume due to high-flow arteriovenous malformation, dural fistulas, and other vascular anomalies), meningeal disease (e.g., carcinomatous and lymphamatous meningitis, chronic infectious and granulomatous meningitis), gliomatosis cerebri, toxins (hypervitaminosis, lead, tetracycline), metabolic disturbances (e.g., administration or withdrawal of corticosteroids, hyper- and hypoadrenalism, mysedema, hypoparathyroidism), and associated with greatly elevated protein concentration in the CSF (e.g., Guillain–Barré syndrome, spinal oligodendroglioma, systemic lupus erythematosus) (Ropper & Brown, 2005).

NEUROPSYCHOLOGICAL/CLINICAL PRESENTATION

Pseudotumor cerebri is characterized by a constellation of persistent and unremitting headache and papilledema. Less frequently seen complaints may include blurred vision, a vague dizziness, minimal horizontal diplopia, transient visual obscurations that often coincide with the peak intensity of the headache, a trifling numbness of the face on one side, and/or nasal CSF leak (Clarke, Bullock, Hui, & Firth, 1994).

Neurological examination is generally unremarkable aside from occasional unilateral or bilateral abducens palsy, fine uninterpretable nystagmus, or far lateral gaze, or a minor sensory change (Ropper & Brown, 2005). Neurocognitive functioning is unaffected. In rare cases, more so in children than adolescents and adults, Bell's palsy may be observed (Chutorian, Gold, & Braun, 1977).

Visual loss is often seen and characterized by peripheral constriction and blind spot enlargement. In fact, visual loss represents the most probable long-term defect. Deficits may be severe, presenting as blindness. Still, the most typical presentation demonstrates preservation of visual acuity and color in the presence of optic nerve-related visual field defects. This presents in more than 90% of patients and includes enlarged blind spots, generalized peripheral constriction, and inferior nasal field loss (Osborne, Liu, & Newman, 2007). If intracranial hypertension and papilledema are left untreated, permanent visual loss is possible.

DIAGNOSIS

Diagnosis is made by meeting the following criteria: (1) signs and symptoms due to elevated intracranial pressure, (2) a normal result on neurological examination except for an abducens palsy, (3) modern neuroimaging excluding a mass lesion or other cause of elevated intracranial pressure, and (4) normal CSF parameters except an elevated opening pressure (>250 mm H_2O) (Osborne et al., 2007). As suggested, when symptoms of persisting headaches and papilledema arise with a normal neurological examination, neuroimaging is recommended to evaluate for an intracranial mass. If MRI and/or CT are negative for an intracranial mass, one must consider occlusion of the dural venous sinuses, gliomatosis cerebri, and occult arteriovenous malformation (Ropper & Brown, 2005). Lumbar puncture should be utilized to rule presentations such as meningitis and to determine CSF pressure. In pseudotumor cerebri, the CSF opening pressure should exceed 250 mm H_2O, which is the upper limit of normal for most obese and nonobese people (Corbett & Mehta, 1983). In order to determine potential visual loss, quantitative perimetry can be helpful in better determining the integrity of the visual fields. Additionally, fundus photographs are useful in assessing papilledema course.

TREATMENT

Treatment is focused on relieving headache, reducing risk of permanent visual loss, and eliminating potential for future complications. As noted, quantitative perimetry can be helpful in better determining visual field loss. Additionally, fundus photographs are useful in assessing papilledema course. Given obesity has been associated with heightened risk of the presentation, weight management is commonly employed. Although this may not serve as treatment for acute symptoms, it is seen as an essential long-term treatment component. This may include dietary management, exercise programs, and in severe cases, surgical intervention such as gastric bypasss.

Medicinal intervention is commonly employed and may include singular or combined application of corticosteroids, oral hyperosmotic agents, and/or carbonic anhydrase inhibitors as a means of reducing CSF levels. In more severe cases, lumbar-peritoneal shunting may be employed to offer more immediate and continuous reduction of CSF pressure. This is rarely employed due to the risks associated.

Chad A. Noggle
Amy R. Steiner

Chutorian, A. M., Gold, A. P., & Braun, C. W. (1977). Benign intracranial hypertension and Bell's palsy. *New England Journal of Medicine, 296,* 1214.

Clarke, D., Bullock, P., Hui, T., & Firth, J. (1994). Benign intracranial hypertension: A cause of CSF rhinorrhea. *Journal of Neurology, Neurosurgery, and Psychiatry, 57,* 847.

Corbett, J. J., & Mehta, M. P. (1983). Cerebrospinal fluid pressure in normal obese subjects and patients with pseudotumor cerebri. *Neurology, 33,* 1386–1388.

Digre, K. B., & Corbett, J. J. (1988). Pseudotumor cerebri in men. *Archives of Neurology, 45,* 866.

Karahalios, D. G., Rekate, H. L., Khayata, M. H., & Apostolides, P. J. (1996). Elevated intracranial venous pressure as a universal mechanism in pseudotumor cerebri of varying etiologies. *Neurology, 46,* 198.

King, J. O., Mitchell, P. J., Thomson, K. R., & Tress, B. M. (2002). Manometry combined with cervical puncture in idiopathic intracranial hypertension. *Neurology, 58,* 26.

Mann, J. D., Johnson, R. N., Butler, A. B., & Bass, N. H. (1979). Impairment of cerebrospinal fluid circulatory dynamics in pseudotumor cerebri and response in steroid treatment. *Neurology, 29,* 550.

Osborne, B. J., Liu, G. T., & Newman, N. J. (2007). Cranial nerves II and afferent visual Pathways. In C. G. Goetz (Ed.), *Textbook of clinical neurology* (3rd ed.). Philadelphia PA: Saunders Elsevier

Radhakrishnan, K., Ahlskog, J. E., Garrity, J. A., & Kurland, L. T. (1994). Idiopathic intracranial hypertension. *Mayo Clinic Procedures, 69,* 169.

Ropper, A. H., & Brown, R. H. (2005). Adams and Victor's principles of neurology (8th ed., pp. 529–545). New York NY: McGraw-Hill.

PSYCHOTIC DISORDERS

DESCRIPTION

Psychotic disorders constitute a group of psychiatric disorders that significantly affect the mind and impede normal functioning and, at times, distort reality in the context of particular symptoms. Psychotic disorders are now recognized as neurologically based in many respects. This coincides with consistency in literature demonstrating patterns of neuroanatomical alterations and cognitive dysfunction.

They are seen as chronic entities, with lifelong treatment being required once initiated. Oftentimes symptom onset is not until late adolescence or early adulthood, but cases of childhood onset have been reported and are considered particularly severe and predictive of poorer prognosis.

NEUROPATHOLOGY/PATHOPHYSIOLOGY

A multitude of studies has been undertaken to delineate the pathological basis of schizophrenia and psychoses. As a result, emerging literature has suggested a number of factors that have demonstrated some relationship to the manifestation of clinical features. In terms of schizophrenia, disconnection of areas that modulate positive and negative symptoms have been reported, owning to the constellation of symptoms commonly seen (Bartzokis, 2002; Bullmore, Frangou, & Murray, 1997). Reductions in the power and synchrony of evoked gamma osculations have been included in the support of this notion (Kwon et al., 1999; Spencer et al., 2004).

Anatomical abnormalities have been reported in relation to the frontal-striatal-thalamic-cerebellar axis and temporolimbic regions (Keshavan, Kennedy, & Murray, 2004) although abnormalities have been discussed throughout the brain (Harrison, 1999). For example, in early-onset cases, reduced parenchymal volume and ventricular enlargement have been reported (Mehler & Warnke, 2002). Focally, the temporal lobes and frontal lobes have received a fair amount of the attention. Reductions in temporal lobe volume and neuron proliferation, density and size have all been reported (Zaidel, Esiri, & Harrison, 1997). Neuronal arrangement has been reported to be in disarray with ectopic expression of neurons regionally (Akbarian et al., 1993). Similarly, decreased cell and neuronal density, size, and number in frontal regions have been reported (Rajkowska, Selemon, Goldman-Rakic, 1998; Selemon, Rajkowska, & Goldman-Rakic,, 1995) as has hypoactivity in this region on functional imaging (Weinberger, 1993; Weinberger & Lipska, 1995).

On a chemical level, the dopaminergic system has long been associated with schizophrenia and psychosis as has the glutaminergic system. Schizophrenia and primary psychotic disorders appear to demonstrate a strong genetic predisposition with elevated rates of the disorders with relative risk ranging from 3% to 15% (Gottesman & Shields, 1982; Kendler, Gruenberg, & Tsuang, 1985). Biological sex of the proband has been identified as a mediator in this regard. Specifically, women with schizophrenia have higher rates of schizophrenia and related psychotic spectrum disorders among their first-degree relatives than men, whereas men with schizophrenia have significantly higher rates of schizotypal personality disorder and flat affect in their first-degree relatives (Goldstein, Faraone, Chen, & Tsuang, 1995).

When considering schizoaffective disorder, less evidence is seen in terms of evaluating the neuropathological basis of the presentation. Arguments can be found about schizophrenia and schizoaffective disorder representing the same disease and that the latter is termed when individuals demonstrate more prominent affective disturbance. Consequently, overlapping of pathology has been suggested, with some mainly suggesting potential greater involvement of serotonin and/or norepinephrine systems in schizoaffective disorder, owning to their increased affective disturbance. This has been merely proposed from a theoretical standpoint however.

NEUROPSYCHOLOGICAL/CLINICAL PRESENTATION

The clinical presentation of the psychotic disorders is commonly conceptualized by their positive psychotic

features such as hallucinations; however, the past 20 years has demonstrated the full spectrum of characteristics associated with these presentations. Among them, neuropsychological deficits have been well documented. In his review of the literature, Heinrichs (2005) suggested that cognitive dysfunction was actually one of the most consistent features of schizophrenia. The pattern of dysfunction suggests fairly diffuse cognitive compromise. Impairments has been noted in attention (both selective and sustained), working memory, executive functioning, memory, and learning (Marcopulos et al., 2008; Seaton, Goldstein, & Allen, 2001).

These features are in addition to those psychiatric features that define the presentations. In the case of schizophrenia, it is marked by a chronic (>6 months) pattern of two or more of the following: delusions, hallucinations, disorganized speech, grossly disorganized or catatonic behavior, or negative symptoms (American Psychiatric Association, 2001). In regard to schizophreniform, the potential features are largely consistent with that of schizophrenia except for the fact that active phase symptoms occur concurrently with episodes of mood disturbance. Furthermore, there must be a 2-week period in which psychotic features are seen outside the confines of mood disturbance.

DIAGNOSIS

Diagnosis of the psychotic disorders remains dependent upon description of clinical features and their adherence to *DSM-IV* criteria. However, a neurological/physiological source should be ruled-out first. Particularly in those cases where symptom onset is reported as more rapid, neurological correlates must be evaluated. Some suggest an easy way of differentiating psychiatric from neurological in terms of hallucinations lies in whether there are auditory hallucinations present. Purely visual hallucinations have been reported in neurological presentations such as Lewy body dementia, peduncular hallucinosis, some seizure disorders, and so forth. In comparison, it is far more rare for auditory hallucinations to occur in association with anything but psychotic disorders. In presentations like temporal lobe epilepsy where Heschl's gyrus is involved, some individuals will experience preictal auditory aura. Thus, clinical history should be very detailed outlining any or all symptoms and their features including experiences prior to and after their occurrence if such observations have been made. MRI and CT can be used to rule out specific structural

OP

abnormalities. EEG may be sought in instances where seizures/epilepsy is considered as part of the differential. Lumbar puncture with CSF analysis can aid in ruling-out an infectious or similar process. Many of these latter technologies are used for completeness sake.

TREATMENT

Treatment of psychotic disorders remains largely medicinally based. Although historically other methods such as psychosurgery were used, the prominent negative effects of these interventions, in combination with the advancement and effectiveness of modern day medicinal control, have limited such practices. Both typical and atypical antipsychotics are used today, although the prior is used on a very limited basis. Their mechanisms of action are slightly different, but in general, the term *antipsychotic* suggests an antagonistic effect on brain dopamine receptors (Ivanov & Charney, 2008). In the case of typical antipsychotic, they block dopamine D2 receptors (Surja, Tamas, & El-Mallakh, 2006). Although they are quite effective in controlling positive symptoms, they carry a significant adverse risk profile that includes akathisia, acute dystonias and dyskinesias, and gradually evolving parkinsonian bradykinesia as well as tardive dyskinesia and chronic dystonias (Gardner, Baldessarini, & Waraich, 2005). In comparison, atypical antipsychotics demonstrated equal, if not greater effectiveness in comparison to typical antipsychotics yet do not carry the same negative consequences. They differ from typical antipsychotics in that they demonstrate a mixed dopamine and serotonin blockade (Surja et al., 2006).

Beyond medicinal treatment, there is a significant role of cognitive-behavioral interventions through a therapeutic modality. Neuropsychological assessment can identify strengths and from that define strategies for individual to compensate for cognitive weaknesses. The combination of these strategies can be essential to helping individuals maintain independence and success socially, educationally, and occupationally.

Chad A. Noggle

Akbarian, S., Vinuela, A., Kim, J. J., Potkin, S. G., Bunney, W. E. Jr., & Jones, E. G. (1993). Distorted distribution of nicotinamide-adenine dinucleotide phosphate-diaphorase neurons in temporal lobe of schizophrenics implies anomalous cortical development. *Archives of General Psychiatry, 50,* 178–187.

American Psychiatric Association. (2001). *Diagnostic and Statistical Manual of Mental Disorders (Fourth Edition-Text Revision)*. Washington, D.C.: Author.

Bartzokis, G. (2002). Schizophrenia: breakdown in the well-regulated lifelong process of brain development and maturation. *Neuropsychopharmacology, 27,* 672–683.

Bullmore, E. T., Frangou, S., & Murray, R. M. (1997). The dysplastic net hypothesis: an integration of developmental and dysconnectivity theories of schizophrenia. *Schizophrenia Research, 28,* 143–156.

Gardner, D. M., Baldessarini, R. J., & Waraich, P. (2005). Modern antipsychotic drugs: A critical overview. *Canadian Medical Association Journal, 172* (13), 1703–1711.

Goldstein, J. M., Faraone, S., Chen, W., & Tsuang, M. (1995). Genetic heterogeneity may in part explain sex differences in the familial risk for schizophrenia. *Biological Psychiatry, 38,* 808–813.

Gottesman, I. I., & Shields, J. (1982). *The epigenetic puzzle.* Cambridge, MA: Cambridge University Press.

Harrison, P. J. (1999). The neuropathology of schizophrenia. A critical review of the data and their interpretation. *Brain, 122,* 593 624.

Heinrichs, R. W. (2005). The primacy of cognition in schizophrenia. *American Psychologist, 60,* 229–242.

Ivanov, I., & Charney, A. (2008). Treating pediatric patients with antipsychotic drugs: Balancing benefits and safety. *Mount Sinai Journal of Medicine, 75,* 276–286.

Kendler, K. S., Gruenberg, A. M. & Tsuang, M. T. (1985). Psychiatric illness in first-degree relatives of schizophrenia and surgical control patients. *Archives of General Psychiatry, 42,* 770–779.

Keshavan, M. S., Kennedy, J. L., & Murray, R. M. (2004). *Neurodevelopment and schizophrenia.* New York NY: Cambridge University Press.

Kwon, J. S., O'Donnell, B. F., Wallenstein, G. V., Greene, R. W., Hirayasu, Y., Nestor, P. G., et al. (1999). Gamma frequency range abnormalities to auditory stimulation in schizophrenia. *Archives of General Psychiatry, 56,* 1001–1005.

Marcopulos, B. A., Fuji, D., O'Grady, J., Shaver, G., Manley, J., & Aucone, E. (2008). Providing neuropsychological services for person with schizophrenia: A review of the literature and prescription for practice. In J. E. Morgan & J. H. Ricker (Eds.), *Textbook of clinical neuropsychology* (pp. 743–761). New York NY: Taylor & Francis.

Mehler, C. & Warnke, A. (2002). Structural brain abnormalities specific to childhood-onset schizophrenia identified by neuroimaging techniques. *Journal of Neural Transmission, 109,* 219–234.

Rajkowska, G., Selemon, L. D., & Goldman-Rakic, P. S. (1998). Neuronal and glial somal size in the prefrontal cortex: A postmortem morphometric study of schizophrenia and

Japanese Society of Neuropathology Huntington disease. *Archives of General Psychiatry, 55,* 215–224.

Seaton, B. E., Goldstein, G., & Allen, D. N. (2001). Sources of heterogeneity in schizophrenia: The role of neuropsychological functioning. *Neuropsychology Review, 11,* 45–67.

Selemon, L. D., Rajkowska, G., & Goldman-Rakic, P. S. (1995). Abnormally high neuronal density in the schizophrenic cortex. A morphometric analysis of prefrontal area 9 and occipital area 17. *Archives of General Psychiatry, 52,* 805–818.

Spencer, K. M., Nestor, P. G., Perlmutter, R., Niznikiewicz, M. A., Klump, M. C., Frumin, M., et al. (2004). Neural synchrony indexes disordered perception and cognition in schizophrenia. *Proceedings of the National Academic of Sciences of the United States of America, 101,* 17288–17293.

Subuh Surja, A. A., Tamas, R. T., & El-Mallah, R. S. (2006). Antipsychotic medications in the treatment of bipolar disorder. *Current Drug Targets, 7,* 1217–1224

Weinberger, D. R. (1993). A connectionist approach to the prefrontal cortex. *The Journal of Neuropsychiatry and Clinical Neurosciences, 5,* 241–253.

Weinberger, D. R., Lipska, B. K. (1995). Cortical maldevelopment, anti-psychotic drugs, and schizophrenia: A search for common ground. *Schizophrenia Research, 16,* 87–110.

Zaidel, D. W., Esiri, M. M., & Harrison, P. J. (1997). Size, shape, and orientation of neurons in the left and right hippocampus: Investigation of normal asymmetries and alterations in schizophrenia. *The American Journal of Psychiatry, 154,* 812–818.

Rasmussen's Encephalitis

DESCRIPTION

Rasmussen's encephalitis is a rare brain disorder that involves severe epileptic seizures, hemispheric atrophy, hemianopsia, hemiparesis, and aphasia if the left hemisphere is affected (Granata, 2003). The epileptic seizures in Rasmussen's encephalitis are most commonly simple partial motor seizures, although tonic-clonic, complex partial, postural, and somatosensory seizures may be present as well (Bien et al., 2005). Very often, seizure activity progresses to epilepsia partialis continua (EPC) in children, which is defined as a persistent seizure involving consistent motor activity. EPC is often one of the first symptoms that inform clinicians of the presence of Rasmussen's encephalitis.

Rasmussen's encephalitis has long been thought to be a disorder that solely affects children. However, recent advancements in the ability to diagnose and distinguish the presence of Rasmussen's encephalitis has revealed that this disorder does primarily affect children, but can take an adult onset also (Bien et al., 2005). In children, Rasmussen's encephalitis typically takes a predictable course, involving three proposed phases. The first phase of the disorder involves infrequent seizure activity and mild hemiparesis characterized as a weakness in one side of the body. This initial phase of the disorder typically lasts for about 8 months (Bien et al., 2005). The second phase is typified by much more frequent seizure activity, usually simple partial motor seizures, severe hemiparesis, and/or hemianopsia (i.e., blindness in one-half of the visual field of either one or both eyes). After an average of 8 months, the third chronic phase begins, which causes considerable cognitive deficits, as well as epileptic seizure activity (Bien et al., 2005). In contrast, adult onset Rasmussen's encephalitis manifests itself in exactly the same way, though it exhibits milder seizure activity, usually occipital lobe seizures, and less cognitive deficits (Hart et al., 1997).

NEUROPATHOLOGY/PATHOPHYSIOLOGY

There are several competing theories as to the etiology of this unusual condition, though there is currently no validated explanation. Debate persists as to the basis for Rasmussen's encephalitis. Specifically, though some suggest Rasmussen's encephalitis is caused by a viral infection that then leads to a localized immune response, there is also suggestion that the disorder is caused by an autoimmune deficiency that is unrelated to viral infection (Tran, Day, Eskin, Carney, & Maria, 2000). Most researchers agree that viral infection must be involved in the etiology due to many histopathological symptoms such as microglial nodules, and neuronophagia (neuronal death due to phagocytes), which are both common in central nervous system infection (Tran et al., 2000).

Neuropathological findings indicate hemispheric atrophy occurs in Rasmussen's encephalitis, and, more specifically, degeneration of the caudate nucleus is commonly seen. Further observation of the brain in Rasmussen's encephalitis has revealed that often microglial nodules are present, which are nodules of necrotic tissue (Bien et al., 2005). In addition, significant brain inflammation has been found to be present, along with glial scarring, gyral necrosis, the presence of perivascular round cells, and neuronal death (Roger, Bureau, Genton, Tassinari, & Wolf, 2001). This significant brain inflammation is mainly caused by the infiltration of T cells and microglial cells.

According to MRI studies, Rasmussen's encephalitis begins by affecting the temporal or anterior parietal lobes, which leads to partial motor seizures (Deb et al., 2005). Robitaille and colleagues have suggested conceptualizing Rasmussen's encephalitis pathology in four stages or steps. The most severe proposed stage of this chronic encephalitis is the "active disease" stage, which is defined as a stage of the disease causing glial scarring, the presence of perivascular cells, and nodules of necrotic brain tissue (Deb et al., 2005). The second stage, known as the "active and remote" stage is comprised of less microglial nodules than the former stage, round cell infiltration, and gyral necrosis (Deb et al., 2005). The third, known as the "remote stage" presents with still less glial scarring, some neuronal atrophy, and brain inflammation. Lastly, the "nonspecific change" stage is the most benign form of Rasmussen's encephalitis with mild glial scarring, and mild neuronal damage (Deb et al., 2005).

NEUROPSYCHOLOGICAL/CLINICAL PRESENTATION

Previous research has indicated that 90% of children with Rasmussen's encephalitis maintain an average intelligence quotient before the onset of epileptic activity (Tran et al., 2000). The presence of focal seizures severely damages neuropsychological functioning and intellectually impairs 85% of individuals with the chronic encephalitis (Tran et al., 2000). Paralleling the rapid cognitive decline in Rasmussen's encephalitis, are overt sensory and motor deficiencies such as hemianopsia. Due to the excessive neuronal damage among Rasmussen's encephalitis patients, significant neuropsychological deficits are inevitable. Among children with this disorder, performance intelligence is commonly higher than verbal intelligence (Hennessy et al., 2001). This disparity between verbal and performance intelligence may be due to the temporal lobe focus of this disorder. As discussed previously, Rasmussen's encephalitis often affects the temporal lobe specifically. Damage to the left temporal lobe may cause aphasia or dysphasia as delineated by neuropsychological testing (Deb et al., 2005). In addition, verbal comprehension may be impacted by focal temporal neuronal damage (Hennessy et al., 2001). Also, cases of memory loss, specifically short-term memory, and working memory have been reported due to hippocampal and parahippocampal damage (Hennessy et al., 2001).

DIAGNOSIS

Diagnosing Rasmussen's encephalitis is based on the clinical presence of seizures (especially EPC and by electroencephalocardiogram (EEG), MRI, or biopsy evaluation (Bien et al., 2005). Abnormal EEG patterns include an overwhelming amount of delta wave activity, and ictal discharge, which is indicative of seizure activity (Granata, 2003). MRI studies have contributed to the diagnosis of Rasmussen's encephalitis by discovering several important MRI abnormalities in patients. First, the inner and outer cerebrospinal fluid compartment tends to be unilaterally enlarged (Bien et al., 2005). These studies have also provided evidence that cortical swelling occurs possibly due to viral infection. Lastly, in some cases, specific atrophy of the caudate nucleus can be seen in MRI scanning.

Brain biopsy is regarded as the last resort, or measure taken to appropriately diagnose the presence of Rasmussen's encephalitis. Most commonly, frontal or temporal biopsies are performed due to the histopathological localization of affected tissue in these areas. The use of all four of these methods should be enough to derive the diagnosis of Rasmussen's encephalitis. The activity of EPC seizures is probably the most useful indicator when assessing for Rasmussen's encephalitis.

When assessing for differential diagnoses, one must consider the possibility of other unilateral or unihemispheric neurological disorders such as Sturge–Weber's syndrome (Bien et al., 2005). Secondly, other possibilities for the occurrence of EPC should be taken into account. For example, EPC is also seen in diabetes mellitus (Bien et al., 2005). Lastly, alternative diseases that cause brain inflammation such as multiple sclerosis should be considered (Bien et al., 2005).

TREATMENT

Due to the persistent nature of the seizures in Rasmussen's encephalitis, one of the major goals of treatment is to alleviate or eradicate seizure activity. One extreme way that this is done is by performing a functional hemispherectomy. This involves the removal of the temporal lobe of the affected hemisphere and surgically disabling the connection of one hemisphere to the other (Bien et al., 2005). This operation almost invariably ceases seizure activity, though causes many secondary symptoms such as significant cognitive decline, lack of interhemispheric tasks, and hemiparesis or hemiplegia. Current research offers disparate ideas about the implementation of the hemispherectomy, due to the significant cognitive impact that it can cause. The most common view is that a hemispherectomy should be avoided when dealing with individuals who have maintained average intelligence and cognitive functioning due to the degree of expected residuals that may themselves impede functioning and quality of life. In cases where cognition has already been detrimentally influenced, a hemispherectomy is generally recommended simply because of its ability to reduce seizure activity.

Recently, the use of corticosteroids has increased in cases of Rasmussen's encephalitis. These corticosteroids are thought to positively alter the course of the disorder by reducing epileptic activity and reducing brain inflammation (Tran et al., 2000). The use of steroids may be the first line of defense in treatment, because anticonvulsants alter the course of the disorder (Bien et al., 2005).

Lastly, interferon therapy has been shown to alleviate Rasmussen's encephalitis symptoms. Interferon therapy is applied intraventricularly and may reduce symptoms for several weeks. Previous research has provided evidence that interferon therapy reduces the frequency and severity of seizure activity (Bien et al., 2005). A major disadvantage of this treatment is the perpetual requirement of receiving this therapy every 3 weeks or so. This weakness in the treatment is what makes a functional hemispherectomy such a viable choice for many patients.

Ryan Boddy
Charles Golden

Bien, C. G., Granata, T., Antozzi, C., Cross, J. H., Dulac, O., Kurthen, M., et al. (2005). Pathogenesis, diagnosis and treatment of Rasmussen encephalitis: A European consensus statement. *Brain, 128,* 3, 454–471.

Deb, P., Sharma, M. C., Gaikwad, S. M., Tripathi, P., Chandra, S., Jain, S., et al. (2005). Neuropathological spectrum of Rasmussen encephalitis. *Neurology India, 53*(2), 156–161.

Granata, T. (2003). Rasmussen's syndrome. *Neurological Sciences, 1*(24), 239–243.

Hart, Y. M., Andermann, F., Fish, D. R., Dubeau, F., Robitaille, Y., Rasmussen, T., et al. (1997). Chronic encephalitis in adults and adolescents: A variant of Rasmussen's syndrome? *Neurology, 48,* 418–424.

Hennessy, M. J., Koutroumanidis, M., Dean, A. F., Jarosz, J., Elwes, R., Binnie, C. D., et al. (2001). Chronic encephalitis and temporal lobe epilepsy: A variant of Rasmussen's syndrome? *Neurology, 56,* 678–681.

Rasmussen, T., Olszwewski, J., & Lloyd-Smith, D. (1958). Focal seizures due to chronic localized encephalitis. *Neurology, 8*(6), 435–445.

Roger, J., Bureau, M., Dravet, C., Genton, P., Tassinari, C., &Wolf, P. (2001). *Epileptic syndromes in infancy, childhood and adolescence* (3rd ed.). Montrouge, France: Eurotext.

Tran, T., Day, J., Eskin, T., Carney, P. R., & Maria, B. L. (2000). Rasmussen's syndrome: Aetiology, clinical features and treatment options.*CNS Drugs, 14*(5), 343–354.

READING DISORDERS

DESCRIPTION

According to the American Psychiatric Association's (APA) *Diagnostic and Statistical Manual of Mental Disorders*, fourth edition, text revision (APA, 2000), to meet criteria for Reading Disorder an individual's reading achievement (reading accuracy or comprehension) must be substantially below the expected level given the person's age, age-appropriate education, and measured intelligence. Reading achievement must be measured via individually administered standardized tests, and the disturbance must significantly interfere with academic achievement or daily activities that require reading skills. An estimated 4% of school children meet criteria for Reading Disorder, and among those diagnosed, between 60% and 80% are male (APA, 2000). Though reading difficulties may be present as early as kindergarten (e.g., poor letter identification skills or poor association of letters with phonemes), formal reading instruction usually begins in the middle of first grade and, thus, Reading Disorder is rarely diagnosed prior to this point. When an individual with high IQ experiences Reading Disorder, symptoms may go undetected until the fourth grade or later. Early identification and intervention typically proves successful in a significant number of cases (APA, 2000).

In 2001, the National Center for Education Statistics revealed that 37% of fourth-grade students are below the reading level necessary to work effectively at their grade level (Torgesen, 2002). Given that low reading achievement hinders vocabulary growth (Cunningham & Stanovich, 1998), negatively affects children's motivation to read (Oka & Paris, 1986), and leads to diminished opportunities for developing comprehension strategies (Brown, Palincsar, & Purcell, 1986), early identification and early intervention is essential.

NEUROPATHOLOGY/PATHOPHYSIOLOGY

Neuroradiological findings have shown that specific types of brain activity are correlated with reading skills. Turkeltaub, Gareau, Flowers, Zeffiro, and Eden (2003) found that phonological awareness correlated with activity in the left posterior superior temporal cortex (grapheme-phoneme translation and phonology) and the inferior frontal gyrus (articulation). Further, activity in this network increased as a child's phonological skill level increased. Cohen and Dehaene (2004) also found that the "visual word form area" becomes increasingly active as reading expertise develops.

Simos et al. (2002) noted that children with developmental dyslexia demonstrate underactivation of phonological brain areas and that phonics-based interventions improve activation in these areas. They examined dyslexic children who had shown significant improvement following 80 hours of intensive phonological intervention. Prior to intervention, the children exhibited expected hypoactivation in the

QR

left temporoparietal regions (Goswami, 2008). Following intervention, a dramatic increase of activation in this area occurred, particularly in the left posterior superior temporal gyrus (which supports grapheme-phoneme coding in normally developing readers; Turkeltaub et al., 2003).

Regarding the time course of neuronal activation and the development of reading skill (Goswami, 2008), Simos et al. (2005) found that individuals at high risk for reading difficulties were significantly slower in exhibiting neural activity in the occipitotemporal region when presented with both nonwords and letters in kindergarten. Further, the high-risk individuals demonstrated atypical activation in the left inferior frontal gyrus, as the onset of activity significantly increased from kindergarten to 1st grade. Typically, developing readers showed no such increase.

Pennington, McGrath, and Smith (in press) note that researchers have identified candidate genes for dyslexia as these risk alleles have been linked to the development of poor neuronal connections. Functional neuroimaging studies reveal that reading involves the integration of several brain areas, including the anterior and posterior portions of the fusiform word area and language cortex. Given that integration is dependent upon connections between and within brain areas, malformations in neuronal connectivity produced by these risk alleles may cause interference with the integration of brain areas required for reading (Pennington, 2009).

NEUROPSYCHOLOGICAL/CLINICAL PRESENTATION

Torgesen (2002) notes that in order to comprehend the meaning of text, an individual must have both of the following skills: general language comprehension and accurate and fluent identification of words in print. Fluent and accurate reading is preceded by an ability to implement accurate phonemic decoding skills, which then aid the child in acquiring specific memories for words, which is crucial in automatic recognition (Ehri, 1998). Weaknesses in phonemic awareness are found both in children of average intelligence and children of low intelligence. Children with low general oral language skills, such as those of lower socioeconomic status, present with an additional deficit as they are deficient in the critical language knowledge required for good reading comprehension (Gough, 1996; Whitehurst & Lonigan, 1998).

Reading Disorder is highly comorbid with Attention Deficit Hyperactivity Disorder (Donfrancesco, Mugnaini, & Dell'Uomo, 2005). In addition to behavioral impulsivity, children with Reading Disorder

have demonstrated higher levels of cognitive impulsivity versus controls. Consequently, impulsivity assessments are useful when assessing children with Reading Disorder as such work enables one to devise a more specific rehabilitation program (Donfrancesco et al., 2005).

Parents and teachers often view problematic behavior in the classroom as a factor that exacerbates academic struggle. What often goes unrecognized is that a mismatch between academic needs and instructional program can result in problematic behavior from the child. Such circumstances as excessive failure, frustration, and negative feedback from the teacher can exacerbate clinical concerns in the child. As such, it is imperative to properly assess a child's academic performance in order to adequately assess a behavioral deficit (Noell, 2003).

DIAGNOSIS

Children at risk for reading deficits can be identified in kindergarten through screeners that assess letter-sound knowledge, phonemic awareness, and vocabulary. In order to reduce false negatives, Torgesen (2002) recommends screenings in kindergarten through third grade, three times per year. Minimal time can be used through implementation of measures such as the *Test of Word Reading Efficiency* (Torgesen, Wagner, & Rashotte, 1999), which requires 45 seconds to assess phonemic decoding efficiency and 45 seconds to measure sight word vocabulary growth.

Another efficient assessment tool is called Dynamic Indicators of Basic Early Literacy Skill (DIBELS). DIBELS involves short (1 minute) standardized fluency measures that assess student alphabetic understanding, phonological awareness, and fluency. DIBELS is comprised of three subtests: Letter Naming Fluency, Initial Sound Fluency, and Phonemic Segmentation Fluency. These subtests have demonstrated reliability and have proven to be useful tools in identifying children with low reading achievement. Given its high levels of sensitivity, DIBELS is recommended as an initial screening tool. Subsequently, tests of higher specificity should be used with those positively identified in order to screen false positives (Hintze, Ryan, & Stoner, 2003).

Though teacher referral (TR) is commonly used for identification of low-achieving children in the classroom, universal screening methods such as Problem Validation Screening (PVS) are currently available. VanDerHeyden and Witt (2005) compared TR with PVS and found that PVS maximizes the discovery of true positives. Further, though TR yields higher predictive power estimates in low-achieving classrooms, PVS outperformed TR as an identification tool in both high- and low-performing classrooms.

TREATMENT

In 2004, the Individuals with Disabilities Education Act was reauthorized to allow schools to use response to intervention (RTI) to determine eligibility for learning disabled classification (Daly, Martens, Barnett, Witt, & Olson, 2007). RTI involves the continuous evaluation of a student's response to evidence-based interventions. RTI models involve a three-tier, fixed sequence of delivery of type and strength of intervention (Daly et al., 2007). The first tier involves universal intervention that is delivered school and class-wide, ruling out inadequate instruction as a source of low performance and also serving as a universal screen (Gresham, 2004). In the second tier, children not adequately responding to the first tier are administered selected interventions. A third level provides more intensive intervention to children not responding the first two tiers.

It is imperative that school-based intervention teams correctly adapt instruction to the student. The Instructional Hierarchy (IH) conceptualizes proficiency as progression through three steps: acquisition, fluency, and generalization (Daly, Lentz, & Boyer, 1996). The IH guides choice of intervention, and correct responses from the student are elicited through modeling, prompting, error correction, and feedback. Fluency is strengthened through repeated practice and reinforcement for meeting fluency goals. Gradually, assistance is withdrawn until the skill is performed not just accurately but also independently (Daly et al., 2007). Martens and Eckert (2007) note that the strongest effects are found when a combination of methods is utilized, such as combining modeling, contingent error correction, and repeated practice. In order to monitor the success of fluency-based interventions, curriculum-based measurement probes are reliable and valid tools that measure progress (e.g., Chard, Vaughn, & Tyler, 2002). Such measures have been used to identify effective interventions for various subtypes of low-performing readers (e.g., low fluency–high accuracy versus low fluency–low accuracy; Chafouleas, Martens, Dobson, Weinstein, & Gardner, 2004).

Audrey L. Baumeister
William Drew Gouvier

American Psychiatric Association. (2000). *Diagnostic and statistical manual of mental disorders (DSM-IV-TR)*. Washington, DC: Author.

Brown, A. L., Palincsar, A. S., & Purcell, L. (1986). Poor readers: Teach, don't label. In U. Neisser (Ed.), *The school achievement of minority children: New perspectives* (pp. 105–143). Hillsdale, NJ: Erlbaum.

Chafouleas, S. M., Martens, B. K., Dobson, R. J., Weinstein, K. S., & Gardner, K. B. (2004). Fluent reading as the improvement of stimulus control: Additive effects of performance-based interventions to repeated reading on students' reading and error rates. *Journal of Behavioral Education, 13,* 67–81.

Chard, D. J., Vaughn, S., & Tyler, B. J. (2002). A synthesis of research on effective interventions for building reading fluency with elementary students with learning disabilities. *Journal of Learning Disabilities, 35,* 386–406.

Cohen, L., & Dehaene, S. (2004). Specialization within the ventral stream: The case for the visual word form area. *NeuroImage, 22,* 466–476.

Cunningham, A. E., & Stanovich, K. E. (1998). What reading does for the mind. *American Educator, 22*(Spring/Summer), 8–15.

Daly, E. J., III, Lentz, F. E., & Boyer, J. (1996). The instructional hierarchy: A conceptual model for understanding the effective components of reading interventions. *School Psychology Quarterly, 11,* 369–386.

Daly, E. J., Martens, B. K., Barnett, D., Witt, J. C., & Olson, S. C. (2007). Varying intervention delivery in response to intervention: Confronting and resolving challenges with measurement, instruction, and intensity. *School Psychology Review, 36*(4), 562–581.

Donfrancesco, R., Mugnaini, D., & Dell'Uomo, A. (2005). Cognitive impulsivity in specific learning disabilities. *European Child and Adolescent Psychiatry, 14,* 270–275.

Ehri, L. C. (1998). Grapheme-phoneme knowledge is essential for learning to read words in English. In J. Metsala & L. Ehri (Eds.), *Word recognition in beginning reading* (pp. 3–40). Hillsdale, NJ: Erlbaum.

Goswami, U. (2008). Reading, dyslexia and the brain. *Educational Research, 50,* 135–148.

Gough, P. B. (1996). How children learn to read and why they fail. *Annals of Dyslexia, 46,* 3–20.

Gresham, F. M. (2004). Current status and future directions of school-based behavioral interventions. *School Psychology Review, 33,* 326–343.

Hintze, J. M., Ryan, A. L., & Stoner, G. (2003). Concurrent validity and diagnostic accuracy of the dynamic indicators of basic early literacy skills and the comprehensive test of phonological processing. *School Psychology Review, 32*(4), 541–556.

Martens, B. K., & Eckert, T. L. (2007). The instructional hierarchy as a model of stimulus control over student and teacher behavior: We're close but are we close enough? *Journal of Behavioral Education, 16,* 82–90.

Noell, G. H. (2003). Direct assessment of clients' instructional needs: Improving academic, social, and emotional

QR

outcomes. In M. L. Kelley, D. Reitman, & G. H. Noell (Eds.), *Practitioner's guide to empirically based measures of school behavior* (pp. 63–82). New York: Kluwer Academic/Plenum Publishers.

Oka, E., & Paris, S. (1986). Patterns of motivation and reading skills in underachieving children. In S. Ceci (Ed.), *Handbook of cognitive, social, and neuropsychological aspects of learning disabilities* (Vol. 2). Hillsdale, NJ: Erlbaum.

Pennington, B. F. (2009). How neuropsychology informs our understanding of developmental disorders.*The Journal of Child Psychology and Psychiatry, 50,* 72–78.

Pennington, B. F., McGrath, L. M., & Smith, S. D. (2009). Genetics of dyslexia: Cognitive analysis, candidate genes, comorbidities, and etiologic interactions. In T. Goldberg & D. R. Weinberger (Eds.), *Genetics of cognitive neuroscience* (pp. 177–194). Boston: MIT Press.

Simos, P. G., Fletcher, J. M., Bergman, E., Breier, J. I., Foorman, B. R., Castillo, E. M., et al. (2002). Dyslexia-specific brain activation profile becomes normal following successful remedial training. *Neurology, 58,* 1203–1213.

Simos, P. G., Fletcher, J. M., Sarkari, S., Billingsley, R. L., Castillo, E. M., Pataraia, E., et al. (2005). Early development of neurophysiological processes involved in normal reading and reading disability: A magnetic source imaging study. *Neuropsychology, 19*(6), 787–798.

Torgesen, J. K. (2002). The prevention of reading difficulties. *Journal of School Psychology, 40*(1), 7–26.

Torgesen, J. K., Wagner, R. K., & Rashotte, C. A. (1999). *Test of word reading efficiency.* Austin, TX: PRO-ED.

Turkeltaub, P. E., Gareau, L., Flowers, D. L., Zeffiro, T. A., & Eden, G. F. (2003). Development of neural mechanisms for reading. *Nature Neuroscience, 6*(6), 767–773.

VanDerHeyden, A. M., & Witt, J. C. (2005). Quantifying context in assessment: Capturing the effect of base rates on teacher referral and a problem-solving model of identification. *School Psychology Review, 34*(2), 161–183.

Whitehurst, G. J., & Lonigan, C. J. (1998). Child development and emergent literacy. *Child Development, 69,* 335–357.

REDUPLICATIVE PARAMNESIA

DESCRIPTION

Reduplicative paramnesia (RP) is the delusional belief that a place or location has been duplicated, existing in two or more places simultaneously, or that it has been "relocated" to another site. It is one of the delusional misidentification syndromes along with Capgras syndrome where an individual believes that a person, most often a loved one, has been replaced by an identical looking imposter. RP differs from Capgras syndrome in that though the person believes that a place or person has been duplicated, there is no sense of replacement and therefore the imposter belief is not present. First described by Pick in 1903, RP is not a rare syndrome, as was once thought, with prevalence estimates of up to 8% in neurological patients (Hakim, Verma, & Greiffenstein, 1988; Murai, Toichi, Sengoku, Miyoshi, & Morimune, 1997). It is most commonly associated with traumatic brain injury (TBI) and stroke, particularly when there is simultaneous damage to the right cerebral hemisphere and to both frontal lobes. It is usually a transient phenomenon occurring in the acute to subacute stages of acquired brain injury. Although typically seen in acute TBI and stroke, this syndrome has been described in a variety of other neurologic conditions including intracerebral hemorrhages, tumors, dementias, encephalopathies, and various psychiatric conditions (Forstl, Almeida, Owen, Burns, & Howard, 1991).

NEUROPATHOLOGY/PATHOPHYSIOLOGY

Pick initially used the term RP to describe reduplicative beliefs in a patient presumed to have diffusely cortical neurodegenerative disease (Pick, 1903). Weinstein and Kahn (1955) described cases with nonspecific focal brain lesions and described a reduplicative phenomenon as a form of denial of illness expressed in metaphorical language. More recent research reflects a consensus that acute right hemisphere and bilateral frontal pathology are necessary and sufficient for RP to occur (Alexander, Stuss, & Benson, 1979; Benson, Gardner, & Meadows, 1976; Hakim et al., 1988; Makiko, Murai, & Ohigashi, 2003; Moser, Cohen, Malloy, Stone, & Rogg, 1998; Murai et al., 1997; Ruff & Volpe, 1981). Although many theories have been advanced to explain how these lesions could produce this syndrome, the specific pathophysiology is unknown. From a clinical point of view, RP is generally a transient phenomenon and should not be confused with more persistent neurobehavioral problems. Recovery of RP is noted in conjunction with postinjury recovery and resolution of acute and subacute neuropsychological and other deficits (Kapur, Turner, & King, 1988; Ruff & Volpe, 1981).

NEUROPSYCHOLOGICAL/CLINICAL PRESENTATION

No single neuropsychological deficit, such as amnesia, can fully explain the development and resolution of RP. Benson et al. (1976) outline how the right hemispheric dysfunction alters spatial coding of the environment and severe frontal dysfunction prevents recognition of this alteration. In addition, anosognosic tendencies or monitoring deficits in self-produced errors are likely to be a prerequisite of the syndrome, and contingencies in life history might determine the content of delusion. Further research including neuropsychological analysis highlights the frontal and right hemispheric involvement of RP. Patterson and Mack (1985) found that RP represents a combination of perceptual and memory deficits as well as impaired ability to integrate information. Consistent with this finding, Kapur et al. (1988) identified three sets of cognitive impairments noted in a case of RP including memory disturbance, visuospatial deficits with a significant degree of left-sided inattention, and impaired reasoning ability. Hakim et al. (1988) found that patients with RP showed selective deficits in spatial reasoning with relative sparing of verbal reasoning. Moser et al. (1998) found learning, memory and frontal-executive functions were deteriorated with or without RP, but these impairments were more severe after the onset of RP. Some select studies have provided neuropsychological data before and after recovery from RP, suggesting that resolution of RP coincided with at least partial recovery of the underlying neuropsychological impairments (Hakim et al., 1988; Kapur et al., 1988).

DIAGNOSIS

It is important to note that RP is a sign or symptom of underlying neurologic disturbance, but it is not specific to any single diagnostic group. Identification of RP is based on observation and patient and collateral report of the reduplicative phenomenon. Follow-up interview and observation are valuable to document the persistence and eventual resolution of this misidentification syndrome in conjunction with objective neurocognitive measures.

TREATMENT

RP is typically a transient syndrome found in the acute to subacute stages of an acquired brain injury. Resolution of the reduplicative phenomena typically occurs across the natural course of brain injury recovery. Small doses of neuroleptics might be beneficial when RP is associated with sleep–wake cycle disturbance (Makiko et al., 2003).

Mark T. Barisa

Alexander, M. P., Stuss, D. T., & Benson, D. F. (1979). Capgras syndrome: A reduplicative phenomenon. *Neurology, 29*, 334–339.

Benson, D. F., Gardner, H., & Meadows, J. C. (1976). Reduplicative paramnesia. *Neurology, 26*, 147–151.

Forstl, H., Almeida, O. P., Owen, A. M., Burns, A., & Howard, R. (1991). Psychiatric, neurological, and medical aspects of misidentification syndromes: A review of 260 cases. *Psychiatric Medicine, 21*, 905–910.

Hakim, H., Verma, N. P., & Greiffenstein, M. F. (1988). Pathogenesis of reduplicative paramnesia. *Journal of Neurology, Neurosurgery, and Psychiatry, 51*, 839–841.

Kapur, N., Turner, A., & King, C. (1988). Reduplicative paramnesia: Possible anatomical and neuropsychological mechanisms. *Journal of Neurology, Neurosurgery, and Psychiatry, 51*, 579–581.

Makiko, Y., Murai, T., & Ohigashi, Y. (2003). Postoperative reduplicative paramnesia in a patient with a right frontotemporal lesion. *Psychogeriatrics, 3*, 127–131.

Moser, D. J., Cohen, R. A., Malloy, P. F., Stone, W. M., & Rogg, J. M. (1998). Reduplicative paramnesia: Longitudinal neurobehavioral and neuroimaging analysis. *Journal of Geriatric Psychiatry and Neurology, 11*, 174–180.

Murai, T., Toichi, M., Sengoku, A., Miyoshi, K., & Morimune, S. (1997). Reduplicative paramnesia in patients with focal brain damage. *Neuropsychiatry, Neuropsychology, and Behavioral Neurology, 10*, 190–196.

Patterson, M. B., & Mack, J. L. (1985). Neuropsychological analysis of a case of reduplicative paramnesia. *Journal of Clinical and Experimental Neuropsychology, 7*, 11–21.

Pick, A. 1903. Clinical studies: III. On reduplicative paramnesia. *Brain, 26*, 260–267.

Ruff, R. L., & Volpe, B. T. (1981). Environmental reduplication associated with right frontal and parietal lobe injury. *Journal of Neurology, Neurosurgery, and Psychiatry, 44*, 387–391.

Weinstein, E. A., & Kahn, R. L. (1955). *Denial of illness: Symbolic and physiological aspects*. Springfield, IL: Charles C. Thomas.

REPETITIVE MOVEMENT DISORDERS

DESCRIPTION

As the name suggests, repetitive movement disorders (RMDs), also known as repetitive motion disorders, are impairments in motor functions caused by repetitive activities (National Research Council and Institute of Medicine [NRCIM], 2001). Other terms that have been used to describe this syndrome include repetitive or cumulative trauma disorders, repetitive strain injuries, overuse syndrome, work-related disorders, and regional musculoskeletal disorders (NRCIM, 2001). Symptoms of the disorder tend to be pain in the area, typically a joint or multiple joints, associated with overuse. Occupations that require repetitive actions place workers at higher risk for RMDs.

Prevalence rates of RMDs vary according to the specific type of RMD syndrome, and there is no clear evidence that race or sex differences exist (Hogan & Gross, 2003). The latter differences that are reported in the literature are thought to be largely due to occupation or activity selection rather than endogenous sex differences. Differences in prevalence rates based on age does exist with carpal tunnel syndrome being more common in middle age and trigger finger being more common in the 50s and 60s (Tallia & Cardone, 2003). In 1992, RMDs were responsible for 60% of all occupational illness, with an 880% increase of reported RMDs over the previous decade to approximately 44 cases per 10,000 workers (NRCIM, 2001). RMDs result in approximately $27 million and $45 million per year in the United States (NRCIM, 2001).

NEUROPATHOLOGY/PATHOPHYSIOLOGY

The pathophysiology of RMDs focuses on repetition of movement and may be exacerbated by motion that is unnatural or overextended, poor posture, or muscle fatigue (Beers & Berkow, 2002). Other etiologies include trauma, friction, and systemic degenerative diseases. The development of RMDs is from microscopic tears in the tissue (Hogan & Gross, 2003). Specifically, microtears may occur in the muscle fibers, nerve fibers, tendons, and ligaments, or compression of that tissue, resulting in inflammation and a sensation of pain.

The most frequently noted injuries from repetitive movements are tendinitis and bursitis. Tendinitis is characterized by pain secondary to an inflamed tendon, which may be exacerbated by motion (Hogan & Gross, 2003). Typical tendinitis conditions include tennis elbow, golfer's elbow, and damage to the bicep or rotator cuff region. Bursitis is characterized by pain, tenderness, and decreased range of motion, and the typical areas of impairment include the knee, elbow, and hip (Hogan & Gross, 2003).

NEUROPSYCHOLOGICAL/CLINICAL PRESENTATION

The clinical presentation of RMDs includes pain, paresthesias (abnormal sensations), numbness, dyspraxia or motor weakness, impaired range of motion, popping or clicking in the joints, and swelling or redness in the associated area (Tallia & Cardone, 2003). For some individuals, no presence of injury may be detected; however, performing basic and essential tasks may be difficult.

There is no evidence of cognitive impairments associated with RMDs.

DIAGNOSIS

Diagnosis of RMDs typically occurs from clinical evaluation followed by imaging — which may provide evidence of derangement or compression of the tissue (Beers & Berkow, 2002). Electromyography may be utilized to evaluate nerve conduction, whereas lab tests may be utilized to rule out diabetes, anemia, or a thyroid dysfunction. Psychological evaluation may be warranted to rule out job dissatisfaction or other psychosomatic etiology.

Numerous variants of RMDs include bursitis and tendonitis, as well as presentations such as carpal tunnel syndrome, epicondylitis, ganglion cyst, tenosynovitis, and trigger finger (Tallia & Cardone, 2003). Bursitis and tendonitis may be difficult to differentiate and often coexist (Hogan & Gross, 2003).

TREATMENT

Treatment for RMDs usually includes reducing or stopping the motions that cause the symptoms. This may include resting the affected area and implementing appropriate ergonomics. Appropriate warm-up prior to intense physical exertion may reduce the pain and swelling experienced. Applying ice on the affected area and utilizing anti-inflammatory medications or analgesics may alleviate some pain experienced. Splints may also be utilized to reduce pressure on nerves and muscles. Physical therapy may be prescribed to alleviate symptoms, and corrective surgery may be considered in extreme and intractable cases.

Treatment outcomes for those with RMDs tends to be good with typically complete recovery; however, without treatment the injury may be permanent resulting in complete loss of function (Beers & Berkow, 2002). Changes in the manner in which one performs the movement may also reduce the chance of reinjury.

Javan Horwitz
Natalie Horwitz
Chad A. Noggle

Beers, M., & Berkow, R. (2002). Neurovascular syndromes: Carpal tunnel syndrome. In *The Merck manual of diagnosis and therapy*. Whitehouse Station, NJ: Merck Research Laboratories.

Hogan, K., & Gross, R. (2003). Overuse injuries in pediatric athletes. *Orthopedic Clinics of North America, 34,* 405–415.

National Research Council and Institute of Medicine. (2001). *Musculoskeletal disorders and the workplace: Low back and upper extremities.* Washington, DC: National Academy Press.

Tallia, A., & Cardone, D. (2003). Diagnostic and therapeutic injection of the wrist and hand region. *American Family Physician, 67,* 745–750.

Restless Legs Syndrome

DESCRIPTION

Restless legs syndrome (RLS) is a neurological disorder that primarily affects the sensorimotor functions and involves a powerful urge to move the legs in response to an uncomfortable and unpleasant sensation (Pearson et al., 2008; Silber et al., 2004; Smith & Tolson, 2008; Thomas & Watson, 2008), seemingly related to psychiatric disorders. These uncomfortable symptoms of RLS are usually more intense in the evening or at night, though individuals with the disorder often report fewer or less severe symptoms with increased movement of the legs (Silber et al., 2004; Smith & Tolson, 2008; Thomas & Watson, 2008). The prevalence of RLS in the general population has been reported to be between 5% and 10% and it is generally more prevalent in women than in men (Sajita & Ondo, 2008; Smith & Tolson, 2008; Thomas & Watson, 2008).

NEUROPATHOLOGY/PATHOPHYSIOLOGY

The precise etiology of RLS is still unclear, though there is evidence that central dopaminergic dysfunction is one possibility of the cause of RLS symptoms (Smith & Tolson, 2008; Thomas & Watson, 2008). The pattern of RLS symptoms coincides with the circadian pattern of dopamine levels as evidenced by the symptoms being the worst at night, when dopamine levels are at their lowest. Furthermore, certain agents that block dopaminergic pathways can exacerbate the symptoms of RLS (Smith & Tolson, 2008; Thomas & Watson, 2008). The results of brain imaging studies are often conflicting, but some have shown abnormal dopamine receptor binding or dopamine hyperactivity in individuals with RLS (Smith & Tolson, 2008).

Iron has also been shown to be a factor in the etiology of RLS (Smith & Tolson, 2008; Thomas & Watson, 2008). RLS symptoms can be triggered by the conditions associated with iron deficiency, as studies have suggested that patients with RLS have lower iron levels in their brains compared to their control counterparts (Sajita & Ondo, 2008; Smith & Tolson, 2008). Studies have also supported a genetic component of RLS (Sajita & Ondo, 2008; Silber et al., 2004; Smith & Tolson, 2008; Thomas & Watson, 2008). A positive family history of RLS has been associated with a younger onset of symptoms (Sajita & Ondo, 2008) as well as increased risk for developing the disorder (NINDS, 2009). The concordance rates of RLS among monozygotic twin pairs range from 54% to 83%, further enhancing the argument that genetics is a factor in the etiology (Sajita & Ondo, 2008; Thomas & Watson, 2008). Genome-wide scans have led to the discovery of the first three genes that cause RLS; specifically: *BTBD9, MEIS1,* and *MAP2K5/LBXCOR1.* All these genes have been linked to 70% of genetic RSL cases (Sajita & Ondo, 2008).

NEUROPSYCHOLOGICAL/CLINICAL PRESENTATION

There are two forms of RLS: primary and secondary. The primary form is idiopathic, and the age of onset varies. In the secondary form, the symptoms of RLS are caused by another condition, which may include renal failure, iron deficiency, neuropathy, and normal pregnancy (Pearson et al., 2008; Smith & Tolson, 2008; Thomas & Watson, 2008). The two forms are similar in presentation; however, treatment for each form can be quite different. For instance, resolving the underlying condition of the secondary form of RLS may lead to the resolution of RLS symptoms (Smith & Tolson, 2008). Therefore, it is important to rule out other conditions when diagnosing RLS.

According to a revision by the International RLS Study Group (IRLSSG) in 2003, there are four essential diagnostic criteria for RLS, all of which focus on sensory symptoms. The first criterion is an urge to move the legs, which is usually accompanied or caused by uncomfortable and unpleasant sensations in the legs. The second criterion is that the urge to move or the unpleasant sensations begin, or worsen, during periods of rest or inactivity. The third criterion is relief, either partial or total, from the urge to move or unpleasant sensations for as long as the activity continues. The fourth criterion is that symptoms are worse, or only exclusively experienced, in the evening or night hours (Sajita & Ondo, 2008; Thomas & Watson, 2008). There are additional criteria that are not necessary for diagnosing RLS, but may help with differential diagnosis. Supportive criteria for an RLS diagnosis include periodic limb movements (PLMs), positive family history of RLS, and positive therapeutic response to dopaminergic drugs (Sajita & Ondo, 2008; Smith & Tolson, 2008; Thomas & Watson, 2008).

DIAGNOSIS

The diagnosis of RLS involves examining the patient's history as well as assessing the patient for the afore-mentioned symptoms. There are several procedures that could be utilized to exclude other causes for the symptoms and to identify signs of secondary RLS. Some suggested procedures include neurological examination, routine laboratory tests, and electro-myographic evaluation (Sajita & Ondo, 2008). There are several conditions with symptoms similar to those of RLS and differential diagnoses for RLS include akathisia, peripheral neuropathy, peripheral vascular disease, and nocturnal leg cramps (Sajita & Ondo, 2008; Smith & Tolson, 2008; Thomas & Watson, 2008).

TREATMENT

There are both nonpharmacological and pharmacolo-gical treatments for the symptoms of RLS, but there is currently no cure for the disorder. Nonpharmacological treatments can be utilized as the primary treatment for RLS or in conjunction with medication. These treatments include avoiding caffeine, alcohol, and nicotine; engaging in mentally challenging activities; and taking iron replacement. Continually, regular exer-cise, countersensory measures, and discontinuation of antihistamines have also been shown to be effective nonpharmacological treatments (Sajita & Ondo, 2008; Thomas & Watson, 2008). Dopaminergic drugs tend to be the pharmacological treatment of choice; levodopa (L-dopa) being the first of this type to be used effec-tively to treat RLS (Sajita & Ondo, 2008; Silber et al., 2004). The only U.S. FDA approved treatments for RLS are ropinirole and pramipexole, which are both dopa-mine agonists (Smith & Tolson, 2008). Other drug therapies that may be helpful include low-potency opioids, benzodiazepines, and antiepileptic drugs (Sajita & Ondo, 2008; Silber et al., 2004).

Silber et al. (2004) developed an algorithm for the management of RLS symptoms by dividing patients into three groups: intermittent, daily, and refractory. In intermittent RLS, the symptoms are bothersome enough when present to require treatment, but do not occur frequently enough to necessitate daily therapy. On the contrary, symptoms in daily RLS are frequent and troublesome enough to require daily ther-apy. Refractory RLS is defined as daily RLS that is cur-rently being treated with a dopamine agonist. This agonist results in one or more of the following out-comes: inadequate initial response despite adequate doses, response that has become inadequate with time despite increasing doses, intolerable adverse effects, and/or augmentation that is not controlled with additional earlier doses of the drug.

Amy Zimmerman
Raymond S. Dean

Pearson, V. E., Gamaldo, C. E., Allen, R. P., Lesage, S., Hening, W. A., & Earley, C. J. (2008). Medication use in patients with restless legs syndrome compared with a control population. *European Journal of Neurology, 15,* 12–17.

Satija, P., & Ondo, W. G. (2008). Restless legs syndrome pathophysiology, diagnosis, and treatment. *CNS Drugs, 22*(6), 497–518.

Silber, M. H., Ehrenberg, B. L., Allen, R. P., Buchfuhrer, M. J., Earley, C. J., Hening, W. A., et al. (2004). An algorithm for the management of restless legs syndrome. *Mayo Clinic Proceedings, 79*(7), 916–922.

Smith, J. E., & Tolson, J. M. (2008). Recognition, diagnosis, and treatment of restless legs syndrome. *Journal of American Academy of Nurse Practitioners, 20,* 396–401.

Thomas, K., & Watson, C. B. (2008). Restless legs syndrome in women: A review. *Journal of Women's Health, 17*(5), 859–868.

RETT'S SYNDROME

DESCRIPTION

Rett's syndrome (RS) is a neurodevelopmental disorder of infancy almost exclusively affecting females. RS is characterized by severe regression of cognitive, motor, language, and social abilities between the age of 4 and 18 months, following a see-mingly normal period of development. Hallmark fea-tures include stereotypic hand movements (hand wringing), microencephaly, and autistic-like beha-viors. Prevalence ranges from 1:10,000 to 1:22,000 with diverse representation among the world popula-tion. The syndrome is named after Andreas Rett who, in 1966, first described its clinical features.

NEUROPATHOLOGY/PATHOPHYSIOLOGY

RS is a genetic disorder caused by mutation on the X-linked *MECP2* gene, and subsequent MeCP2 protein deficiency (Amir et al., 1999; Hagberg, 2002). The majority of cases occur sporadically; inherited cases are rare. Genotype–phenotype studies have identi-fied different clinical abnormalities associated with different *MECP2* mutations (Percy, 2008a; Zhang & Minassian, 2008).

Studies to determine the specific neuropathology/neurophysiology of RS have found decelerated head growth starting at 3–6 months leading to microencephaly, decreased size of the dendrites of pyramidal neurons in the frontal and temporal lobes, and abnormalities in the substantia nigra. Neuropathology also involves the precentral gyrus, frontal cortex, superior temporal area, and parietal cortex (Brodmann areas 4, 45, 22 and 40). MRI findings have revealed atrophy in selective regions of gray and white matter in the prefrontal, frontal, and anterior temporal regions (Ibrahim & Khan, 2008; Pizzamiglio et al., 2008). EEG findings are characterized by the appearance of focal, multifocal, and generalized epileptiform abnormalities and the occurrence of theta activity in the frontal-central regions. Frequent seizure activity is reported; however, video EEG monitoring is critical because many apparent seizures are not correlated with EEG activity (Glaze, 2002).

NEUROPSYCHOLOGICAL/CLINICAL PRESENTATION

There are four clinical stages of RS (Hagberg, 2002): (1) *early onset* stage, between the age of 6 and 18 months, which involves subtle hypotonia with decreased sitting or crawling, beginning loss of eye contact, disinterest in toys, subtle hand wringing, and decreased head growth; (2) *rapid destruction* stage, between the age of 1 and 4 years, involving loss of purposeful hand movement; emergence of the characteristic hand wringing, clasping, or clapping; repetitive hand movements to the mouth; loss of communication; autistic-like, repetitive and stereotyped behaviors; irritability; emotional outbursts; and disturbed sleep; gait apraxia; and breathing abnormalities; (3) *plateau* or *pseudo stationary* stage, between the age of 2 and 10 years, involving epileptic seizures, with improvements in awareness, attention, communication skills, and emotional state; and (4) *late motor deterioration* stage, involving loss of ambulation in previous walkers, spasticity, muscle weakness, rigidity and stiffness, dystonia, and scoliosis, with improvements in eye gaze and hand wringing.

Overall cognitive and functional abilities are profoundly impaired. Most persons with RS communicate through eye gaze and hand gestures rather than language. Global cognitive skills are generally developed to an age level equivalent to 9 months. Daily living abilities generally correspond with age of 12–14 months. Psychological and behavioral health features of RS include anxiety and panic, lack of interest in play, and self-injury that is mostly in the form of hand-biting and face-hitting (Pizzamiglio et al., 2008). Survival through 10 years of age is typical, with at least 80% survival to the age of 20 years and 50% survival for those over the age of 50 years (Percy, 2008b). Sudden death has been described in RS. Although the specific cause of death is often unclear, it may well involve autonomic dysfunction or a cardiac conduction system abnormality.

DIAGNOSIS

Specific guidelines are used in the clinical diagnosis of RS (Ben Zeev Ghdoni, 2007; Hagberg, Aicardi, Dias, & Ramos, 1983; Hagberg et al., 1985; Hagberg & Witt-Engerstrom, 1986; Hagberg & Skjeldal, 1994). Essential criteria include normal head circumference at birth and apparently normal development, followed by deceleration of head growth, loss of purposeful hand skills with repetitive hand movements, severely impaired expressive language, gait apraxia, and torso apraxia/ataxia between the age of 1 and 4 years. Supportive evidence is present in some RS cases, but is not necessary for the diagnosis. Such evidence includes seizures, EEG changes, epileptiform discharges, scoliosis, teeth grinding, breathing difficulties, muscle rigidity, spasticity, abnormal sleep patterns, chewing and swallowing difficulties, growth retardation, and poor circulation of the lower extremities with cold feet or hands.

The presence of any one of the following exclusion criteria rules out a diagnosis of classic RS: microcephaly at birth, loss of vision due to retinal disorder or optic atrophy, acquired brain damage after birth, evidence of growth retardation in utero, metabolic disorders or acquired neurological disorder from severe infection or head trauma, or any other degenerative disorder. Differential diagnosis with autism is important (Mount, Charman, Hastings, Reilly, & Cass, 2003). Genetic testing can confirm a clinical diagnosis in 70% to 80% of RS cases.

TREATMENT

Treatment interventions have focused on the alleviation of core medical symptoms through medication management of breathing difficulties, sleep problems, seizure disorder, and motor difficulties. Occupational therapy, physiotherapy, and hydrotherapy are used to assist individuals with self-directed activities and mobility (Ben Zeev Ghidoni, 2008). Music therapy has been shown to interrupt hand movements and sooth individuals, but only while treatment is in progress. Therapeutic horseback riding has promoted balance and created positive emotional states (Pizzamiglio

QR

et al., 2008). Cognitive rehabilitation has focused on improving visual-motor and communication skills.

Shane S. Bush
Donna Rasin-Waters

Amir, R. E., Van den Veyver, I. B., Wan, M., Tran, C. Q., Francke, U., & Zoghbi, H. Y. (1999). Rett syndrome caused by mutations in X-linked MECP2, encoding methyl-CpG-binding protein 2. *Nature Genetics, 23,* 185–188.

Ben Zeev Ghidoni, B. (2007). Rett syndrome. *Child and Adolescent Psychiatric Clinics of North America, 16,* 723–743.

Glaze, D. G. (2002). Neurophysiology of Rett syndrome. *Journal of Child Neurology, 20,* 740–746.

Hagberg, B., & Witt-Engerstrom, I. (1986). Rett syndrome: A suggested staging system for describing impairment profile with increasing age towards adolescence. *American Journal of Medical Genetics, 26,* 47–59.

Hagberg, B., & Sjeldal, O.H. (1994). Rett variants: A suggested model for inclusion criteria. *Pediatric Neurology, 1,* 5-11.

Hagberg, B. (2002). Clinical manifestations and stages of Rett syndrome. *Mental Retardation and Developmental Disabilities, 8,* 61–65.

Hagberg, B., Aicardi, J., Dias, K., & Ramos, O. (1983). A progressive syndrome of autism, dementia, ataxia, and loss of purposeful hand use in girls: Rett's syndrome: Report of 35 cases. *Annals of Neurology, 14,* 471–479.

Ibrahim, S., & Khan, S. G. (2008). Rett syndrome: A classic presentation. *Journal of Pediatric Neurology, 6,* 191–194.

Mount, R. H., Charman, T., Hastings, R. P., Reilly, S., & Cass, H. (2003). Features of autism in RS and severe mental retardation. *Journal of Autism and Developmental Disorders, 33,* 435–442.

Percy, A. K. (2008a). Rett syndrome: Recent research progress. *Journal of Child Neurology, 23,* 543–549.

Percy, A. K. (2008b). *Rett syndrome: From recognition to diagnosis to intervention.* Retrieved April 28, 2009, from www.medscape.com/viewarticle/576129

Pizzamiglio, M. R., Nasti, M., Piccardi, L., Zotti, A., Vitturini, C., Spitoni, G., et al. (2008). Sensory-motor rehabilitation in Rett syndrome: A case report. *Focus on Autism and Other Developmental Disabilities, 23,* 49–62.

Zhang, Y., & Minassian, B. A. (2008). Will my Rett syndrome patient walk, talk, and use her hands? *Annals of Neurology, 70,* 1302–1303.

REYE'S SYNDROME

DESCRIPTION

Reye's syndrome (RS), first identified in 1963, is predominantly a childhood disease characterized by severe, noninflammatory encephalopathy with altered levels of consciousness and transient liver dysfunction. Although specific etiology is unknown, onset of the disorder typically occurs after a prodromal disease (e.g., upper respiratory infection, chickenpox, gastroenteritis) has begun to improve. During the 1970s, RS was second only to encephalitis as the most fatal virus-related illness of the developing nervous system. Salicylate use has been linked to the development of RS; consequently, decreased use of aspirin seems to have resulted in a dramatic decrease in cases during the 1980s (Evans, 1998).

In the United Sates, most cases are seen in the late fall and winter with geographic clustering. Widespread outbreaks have been associated with influenza epidemics. Affected children are predominantly White; the disease is uncommon among Black children. There is no sex difference. Mortality has been estimated at approximately 30%; however, if the child survives the acute stage of the illness with no or low-grade coma, the long-term neurological consequences are limited.

NEUROPATHOLOGY/PATHOPHYSIOLOGY

RS is almost exclusively a disorder of childhood. There is some evidence to suggest that RS is linked to the use of salicylates in children suffering from chickenpox. During the 1980s, research in the United Kingdom linked the occurrence of RS to aspirin exposure (Soumerai et al., 2002). Similar findings have also been found in French studies. Epidemiological research has linked the presentation most commonly with influenza A, influenza B, and varicella-zoster. Little is known or understood with regard to specific neuropathology of the syndrome. Nevertheless, the most salient evidence suggests a multiorgan etiology secondary to diffuse mitochondrial injury—itself of unknown origins (DeVivo, 1978; VanCoster et al., 1991). This has been proposed as histological damage and has been noted in mitochondria in the liver (e.g., hepatocytes) and the pancreas as well as cardiac and skeletal muscle fibers (Gascon, Ozand, & Cohen, 2007). Neurologically, similar damage has been noted in neurons and brain capillary endothelial cells.

NEUROPSYCHOLOGICAL/CLINICAL PRESENTATION

During the prodrome phase of the disease, symptom presentation may correspond with the potential etiological disease (e.g., influenza A, B, or, varicella-zoster). Upper respiratory infection is commonly seen as is vomiting. The latter has been proposed as a potential feature of brainstem involvement as the onset is sudden and often unremitting even in the face of pharmacological intervention that is often useful in halting such features when occurring secondary to systemic illness. In many instances, patients will recover and not progress beyond these features. However, in some instances symptoms worsen with the child soon developing prominent restlessness, disorientation, dysautonomia, tachycardia, sweating, and dilated pupils (Gascon et al., 2007). For those that progress beyond this presumed second stage, coma usually develops and seizures present in over 50% of patients in stage 3, followed by cerebrate posturing and respiratory dysfunction in stage 4, and "deeper" coma in stage 5 with no response to painful stimuli and absence of brainstem reflexes (Gascon et al., 2007). Upon recovery, the liver resumes functioning within normal limits; however, the secondary complications can cause long-term changes in cortical functioning. The majority of children who manifest mild levels of the disease and see remission prior to stage 3 appear to experience no long-term neurological sequelae (Hartlage et al., 1980). However, follow-up with survivors of coma grades III and IV have demonstrated the potential for psychomotor retardation, subtle perceptual difficulties, mental retardation, hyperactive disorder, and seizures (Preston et al., 1982). Emotional disturbance related to the onset of these permanent changes in the child's functioning should be expected.

DIAGNOSIS

RS is suspected in any child exhibiting sudden onset of coma and accompanying liver dysfunction. Clinical diagnosis is made when criteria outlined by the Centers for Disease Control are present. These include a prodromal illness, acute onset of vomiting 3–7 days after the onset of the prodromal illness, extreme changes in blood serum levels of glutamic-oxaloacetic transaminase (SGOT) and glutamic-pyruvic transaminase (SGPT) or serum ammonia concentrations, and microvesicular fatty deposits in the tissues, particularly the liver. Although laboratory findings are not diagnostic, they are essential for systemic care and consideration. Common findings include: (1) alanine aminotransferase and aspartate aminotransferase levels 20–30 times higher than normal once vomiting commences, (2) ammonia levels three times higher than normal at onset of coma, (3) increased lactic and organic acids due to respiratory and metabolic acidosis, (4) diffuse EEG slowing that is common in encephalopathic presentations, and (5) diffuse cerebral edema and ventricular compression on CT or MRI (Gascon et al., 2007).

As noted, lethargy, combativeness, and/or coma are the most obvious physical signs. Depth and rate of progression of coma appear to be related to prognosis. As the prodromal illness abates and vomiting commences, some patients remain at the "mild" stage of RS with lethargy but no loss of consciousness. Other patients experience a more severe stage of RS that involves a deep comatose state. Seizure activity may occur in patients experiencing deeper comas. Encephalopathy may persist from 1 to 4 days with gradual neurological improvement. Few, if any, long-term effects have been reported among survivors who exhibited mild stages of RS (i.e., no coma). Permanent neurological deficits have been linked with deeper comatose states.

TREATMENT

Early recognition of the possibility of RS, before the development of serious neurological signs, is recommended. Indeed, avoiding the use of aspirin with children has dramatically cut the incidence of RS. Children who present with vomiting after a respiratory infection or chickenpox should be considered at high risk for RS. A physical, including measurement of blood serum levels of SGOT or SGPT, should be completed. If serum levels show SGOT or SGPT elevations greater than three times normal, hospitalization is indicated. Although no standard treatment regimen exists, hyperventilation and dehydrating agents (e.g., mannitol) have been used to reduce cerebral edema; intravenous administration of vitamin K and glucose are designed to correct liver dysfunction. If coma is present, a lumbar puncture is indicated to exclude the possibility of infection. A percutaneous liver biopsy will positively diagnose RS.

For those children with no secondary complications from coma, no intervention other than treatment of the disease may be mandated. However, coma survivors and their families may need supportive services to adjust to their altered level of functioning. Counseling may address the anger and frustration felt with perceptual-motor and/or cognitive changes. Modifications of expectations both of the family and the educational system may need to be addressed. Depending upon the type of sequelae present, occupational therapy/physical therapy services and medication may also be required.

Matthew Holcombe
Raymond S. Dean
Chad A. Noggle

DeVivo, D. C. (1978). Reye's syndrome: A metabolic response to an acute mitochondrial insult? *Neurology, 28,* 105–108.

Evans, J. (1998). Reye's syndrome. Health-related disorders in children and adolescents: *A guidebook for understanding and educating* (pp. 558–563). Washington, DC, US: American Psychological Association.

Gascon, G. G., Ozand, P. T., & Cohen, B. H. (2007). Aminoacidopathies and organic acidopathies, mitochondrial enzyme defects, and other metabolic errors. In C. G. Goetz (Ed.), *Textbook of neurology* (3rd ed., pp. 641–682). Philadelphia: Saunders Elsevier.

Hartlage, L., Stovall, K., & Hartlage, P. (1980). Age related neuropsychological sequelae of Reye's Syndrome. *Clinical Neuropsychology, 2*(2), 83–85.

Preston, G., Sarnaik, A., & Nigro, M. (1982). Transient intellectual and psychosocial regression during recovery phase of stage V Reye's syndrome.*Journal of Developmental and Behavioral Pediatrics, 3*(4), 206–208.

Soumerai, S., Ross-Degnan, D., & Kahn, J. (2002). The effects of professional and media warnings about the association between aspirin use in children and Reye's syndrome. In R. C. Hornik (Ed.) *Public health communication: Evidence for behavior change* (pp. 265–288). Mahwah, NJ US: Lawrence Erlbaum Associates Publishers.

Van Coster, R. N., DeVivo, D. C., Blake, D., Lombes, A., Barrett, R., & DiMauro, S., et al. (1991). Adult Reye's syndrome: A review with new evidence for a generalized defect in intramitochondrial enzyme processing. *Neurology, 41*, 1815–1821.

RHEUMATOID ARTHRITIS

DESCRIPTION

Rheumatoid arthritis (RA) is a chronic, autoimmune, inflammatory disease that affects the connective tissues of the body (Akil & Amos, 1995; American College of Rheumatology [ACR], 2002; National Institute of Arthritis and Musculoskeletal and Skin Diseases [NIAMS], 2004). Often confused with osteoarthritis (OA), RA is a systemic disorder with symptoms including pain, swelling, stiffness, fatigue, muscle weakness, weight loss, anemia, occasional fevers, and loss of function in the joints (NIAMS, 2004). Symptoms wax and wane and may last only a few months without long-term damage. Some mild or moderate cases can have periods of severe symptoms, flares, and times when symptoms subside. In other cases, the symptoms remain active, last many years or a lifetime, and cause severe joint damage (NIAMS, 2004).

RA is the most common inflammatory arthritis (Akil & Amos, 1995; Emery et al., 2002). It occurs two to three times more frequently in women than in men, with an overall national prevalence of 2.1 million people, or approximately 1% of the adult population according to NIAMS. The disease usually begins in middle age and occurs more frequently in older populations, though children and young adults are also susceptible (NIAMS, 2004; Rindfleisch & Muller, 2005). Symptoms tend to decrease during pregnancy and flare up after childbirth (Akil & Amos, 1995; NIAMS, 2004).

NEUROPATHOLOGY/PATHOPHYSIOLOGY

Although the etiology of RA is not entirely understood, research often shows an interaction between environment and genetics (Akil & Amos, 1995; Rindfleisch & Muller, 2005). Researchers also believe an infection can be a likely cause, though the exact agent is not yet clear (NIAMS, 2004). Based on symptomatic changes during pregnancy, researchers are also hypothesizing that hormones may be a factor. Specifically, the tumor necrosis factor-alpha (TNF-α) and the immune system molecules interleukin 12 (IL-12) change along with hormone levels, possibly contributing to swelling and tissue damage (NIAMS, 2004).

Joints of the hands and feet are usually the first areas to experience difficulties associated with RA. Symptoms generally occur in a symmetrical pattern; therefore, if one hand is affected, the other is also affected (NIAMS, 2004). Gradually, wrists, knees, and/or shoulders can become affected. Before prominent symptoms develop, the person may experience coolness of hands and feet as well as numbness and tingling, as these are signs of compression of the vasomotor nerve. Symptoms tend to appear over a period of weeks to months and usually begin in a single joint. The most frequently affected joints are those with the highest ratio of synovium to articular cartilage (Rindfleisch & Muller, 2005).

The inflammation of the delicate anatomy of the joints is often the cause of redness, swelling, and pain in patients with RA. Joints are protected and surrounded by capsules and these capsules are lined with tissue called synovium. Synovium produces fluid that lubricates the joints and when the synovium becomes inflamed as a result of RA, the above mentioned symptoms occur (NIAMS, 2004). Prolonged inflammation can cause irreversible damage to the joint capsule and cartilage, and scar-like tissue called pannus may develop. Pannus can cause joints to become fixed in place (ankylosed) and may cause displacement and deformity of the joints. Continually, tissues near the joints, such as skin, bones, cartilage, ligaments, and muscles, can suffer from atrophy from the disuse (NIAMS, 2004). Osteoporosis can occur from generalized bone loss due to damaging consequences of RA (Akil & Amos, 1995; NIAMS, 2004).

NEUROPSYCHOLOGICAL/CLINICAL PRESENTATION

Daily suffering is a likely product of RA, including constant pain. In some instances, RA can negatively affect daily routines and tasks of family life and decrease employment opportunities. Some people experience feelings of helplessness, anxiety, and depression related to the disease (NIAMS, 2004). Research indicates patients with RA in combination with a history of multiple episodes of depression experience more chronic pain and also tend to be more vulnerable to stress-related pain (Zautra et al., 2007). Consequently, both chronic pain and depression have been linked with difficulties in select domains of memory, attention, visuospatial ability, processing speed, and executive functioning on a day-to-day basis but not necessarily secondary to a neurological origin.

DIAGNOSIS

In the early stages, RA is often difficult to diagnose, as the symptoms vary from case to case. Symptoms may be similar to other types of arthritis and joint conditions and thus other conditions need to be ruled out. Physician and rheumatologists use a variety of methods to diagnose RA and rule out other conditions. A patient's medical history and description of the symptoms is imperative for the initial assessment. A physical examination includes examination of the joints, reflexes, and muscle strength. Furthermore, X-rays can be helpful as the disease progresses to determine the severity of joint deterioration (NIAMS, 2004).

Blood tests are often used to help in diagnosing because many people with RA have autoantibodies in their blood called rheumatoid factors (NIAMS, 2004). These autoantibodies indicate that an autoimmune reaction is part of the disease process. An autoimmune reaction attacks the body's own tissues, and an antibody is a protein that usually helps the body fight foreign substances (NIAMS, 2004). The rheumatoid factor is not detected in everyone diagnosed with RA, and it is especially difficult to detect in the early stages of the disease. In addition, some people who test positive for rheumatoid factor will never develop clinical symptoms of the disease (NIAMS, 2004).

Possible causes of positive test results for rheumatoid factor include other connective tissue diseases, viral infections, leprosy, liver disease, and tuberculosis (Akil & Amos, 1995).

Physicians also utilize other laboratory tests when diagnosing, including a white blood count, a test for anemia, and an erythrocyte sedimentation rate test. An erythrocyte sedimentation rate measures inflammation of the body (NIAMS, 2004). An increased erythrocyte sedimentation rate and the presence of acute phase proteins are often found in patients with RA (Akil & Amos, 1995).

RA must be differentiated from several disorders. These include scleroderma, lupus, fibromyalgia, infectious endocarditis, polyarticular gout, polymyalgia rheumatica, reactive arthritis, Still disease, thyroid disease, and psoriatic arthritis (Akil, & Amos, 1995; Rindfleisch & Muller, 2005).

TREATMENT

Deterioration of the joints can occur within a few weeks of the onset of symptoms, thus early treatment is encouraged. Early treatment can decrease the rate of disease progression and improve the outcome and quality of life (ACR, 2002; Emery et al., 2002). Physicians and rheumatologists use a variety of treatments for RA, but the goals of treatment are to slow or stop joint deterioration, alleviate pain, and reduce inflammation, as there is no known cure for the disease (ACR, 2002; NIAMS, 2004).

In treating symptoms of RA, medications can be used for pain relief and inflammation reduction. Taking disease modifying antirheumatic drugs (DMARDs) during the early stages can lessen joint damage (ACR, 2002; Emery et al., 2002). DMARDs are used to slow the course of the disease (NIAMS, 2004) and should be considered for all patients with RA (Rindfleisch & Muller, 2005). Furthermore, combinations of DMARDs can be more effective than single-drug prescriptions. Women of childbearing age should take precautions when taking DMARDs, as they can be harmful to fetuses (Rindfleisch & Muller, 2005).

Other treatments considered include nonpharmacological interventions such as rest and exercise, stress reduction, and healthy diet (ACR, 2002; NIAMS, 2004). Splints and other orthopedic appliances are used to prevent or correct deformity of the joints, and physical therapy helps alleviate pain and swelling (ACR, 2002). Different types of surgeries are available to correct severe joint damage. Joint replacement, tendon reconstruction, and synovectomies are some common procedures. A synovectomy is the removal of inflamed synovial tissue, but is rarely performed since the tissue will eventually grow back by itself (ACR, 2002; NIAMS, 2004).

Andrea Stephen
Raymond S. Dean

Akil, M., & Amos, R. S. (1995). Rheumatoid arthritis—I: Clinical features and diagnosis. *British Medical Journal. (International edition), 310*(6979), 587.

American College of Rheumatology. (2002). Guidelines for the management of rheumatoid arthritis. *Arthritis & Rheumatis, 46*(2), 328–346.

Emery, P., Breedveld, F. C., Dougados, M., Kalden, J. R., Schiff, M. H., & Smolen, J. S. (2002). Early referral recommendation for newly diagnosed rheumatoid arthritis: Evidence based development of a clinical guide. *Annals of the Rheumatic Diseases, 61,* 290–297.

National Institute of Arthritis and Musculoskeletal and Skin Diseases. (2004). *Rheumatoid arthritis.* Retrieved March 13, 2009, from http://purl.access.gpo.gov/GPO/LPS80325

Rindfleisch, J. A., & Muller, D. (2005). Diagnosis and management of rheumatoid arthritis. *American Family Physician, 72*(6), 1037–1047.

Zautra, A. L., Parrish, B. P., Van Puymbroeck, C. M., Tennen, H., Davis, M. C., Reich, J. W., et al. (2007). Depression history, stress, and pain in rheumatoid arthritis patients. *Journal of Behavioral Medicine, 30*(3), 187–197. Retrieved March 14, 2009, from ProQuest Nursing & Allied Health Source database. (Document ID: 1291750991).

SANDHOFF'S DISEASE

DESCRIPTION

Sandhoff's disease is a rare and progressive genetic lysosomal storage dysfunction that leads to delayed myelination or demyelination of the central nervous system (CNS; Alkan et al., 2003; McKusick, 1998; Van der Kaamp & Valk, 1995). The disorder was first described and studied by Sandhoff, Andreae, and Jatzkewitz (1968); however, a series of subsequent studies allowed distinguishing the disorder's specific types and their clinical symptomatology (GM2-gangliosidoses variant 0; hexosaminidases A and B deficiency; hexosaminidases B deficiency; Sandhoff–Jatzkewitz–Pilz disease; total hexosaminidase deficiency; Sandhoff's disease, infantile type; Sandhoff's disease, juvenile type; Sandhoff's disease adult type; McKusick, 1998).

The most common form of Sandhoff's disease manifests in infancy at approximately 3–6 months of age. The first symptoms include slow motoric and cognitive development and muscle weakness. Affected infants may lose voluntary motor skills (i.e., turning over, sitting, and crawling) and develop an exaggerated startle reaction. As the disease progresses, children with Sandhoff's disease develop seizures, vision and hearing loss, intellectual disability, paralysis, and eventual death around age of 3. Other forms of Sandhoff's disease, which tend to be less common, affect individuals in childhood, adolescence, or adulthood and are usually milder than Sandhoff's infantile form (McKusick, 1998; National Institute of Health [NIH], 2009).

NEUROPATHOLOGY/PATHOPHYSIOLOGY

Sandhoff's disease is an inherited disorder of sphingolipid metabolism characterized by an autosomal recessive pattern of inheritance. In Sandhoff's disease, genetic mutations in the hexosaminidase beta-chain gene result in a hexosaminidase A (alpha beta) and B (beta beta) deficiency (Arfi et al., 2006; Caliskan, Ozmen, Beck, & Apak, 1993). The deficiency further leads to the inactivity of hexosaminidase enzymes and the intracellular accumulation of GM2 ganglioside in lysosomes (Alkan et al., 2003; Yuksel, Yalcinkaya, Islak, Gunduz, & Seven, 1999). Eradication of the intracellular accumulation of lysosomal enzyme substrates, ganglioside GM2, and other glycolipids is not possible in Sandhoff's disease (Kroll et al., 1995; Yuksel et al., 1999), and the genetic lysosomal storage impairment leads to delayed myelination or demyelination of the CNS (Alkan et al., 2003) causing a number of coordination, muscle control, and cognitive deficits. In addition to the widespread demyelination, the condition results in neuroaxonal loss, and anaerobic metabolism, affecting both white matter and grey matter (Alkan et al., 2003).

Neuroimaging studies suggest that acute forms of Sandhoff's disease result in homogeneous thalamic hyperdensity, mild cortical atrophy, a thin corpus callosum, and abnormal signal intensities in the caudate nucleus, globus pallidum, putamen, cerebellum, and brainstem (Yuksel et al., 1999). In some cases, signs of heart impairment, such as heart murmur and cardiomegaly, are present before the neurologic deterioration (Krevit et al., 1972).

NEUROPSYCHOLOGICAL/CLINICAL PRESENTATION

Onset of Sandhoff's disease usually occurs no earlier than 6 months of life, and the disease is not limited to any ethnic group. It is characterized by rapid progressive neurodegeneration; however, the symptoms differ depending upon the type of genetic mutation and time of onset.

Sandhoff's disease is generally classified into three main forms: infantile, juvenile, and adult, all referring to the onset of the condition. The infantile form of Sandhoff's disease, the most common and acute form of the disease, is characterized by relatively early onset and appears in the first 6–18 months of life. Main clinical features include motor weakness and progressive motor retardation, exaggerated startle reactions to sound, early blindness, progressive mental deterioration, macrocephaly (an abnormally enlarged head), macular red cherry spots in the eyes, seizures, and myoclonus (shock-like contractions of a muscle).

Other symptoms may include frequent respiratory infections, doll-like facial appearance, and an enlarged liver and spleen (Alkan et al., 2003; Yuksel et al., 1999). Although the life expectancy differs depending upon the severity of the condition, it typically leads to death by 3 years of age (Alkan et al., 2003).

The juvenile form of Sandhoff's disease is considered milder than the infantile form, with onset that occurs after the period of infancy and before adulthood. It is characterized by muscle weakness, hyperflexia of lower extremities, and impaired thermal sensitivity. In addition, impaired sexual functions, urinary incontinence, and postural dizziness are commonly reported (Neote, Brown, Mahuran, & Gravel, 1992). Juvenile Sandhoff's may also be associated with mental retardation (Wakamatsu, Kobayashi, Miyatake, & Tsuji, 1992) and/or spinal muscular atrophy (Banerjee et al., 1991). Individuals affected with this form of the disease tend to survive to late adulthood (McKusick, 1998).

The adult type has a less pronounced presentation as compared to other forms of Sandhoff's disease. It is usually discovered later in life (i.e., in the early 30s), and the symptoms can include slowly progressive weakness of lower extremities and diffuse fasciculations. These symptoms may be further accompanied by moderate reduction in strength, widespread spontaneous fasciculations, and hyperactive deep tendon reflexes. Cognitive functioning tends to be unaffected (Gomez-Lira et al., 1995).

Sandhoff's disease is often confused and has similar presentation to Tay–Sachs's disease. Unlike Tay–Sachs's disease, which is characterized by the deficiency of hexosaminidases A, Sandhoff's disease is known for the lack of hexosaminidases A and B; thus, the differentiation between the diseases is usually conducted through biochemical analysis and the activity measurement of the two hexosaminidase enzymes (McKusick, 1998).

DIAGNOSIS

For a child to suffer from Sandhoff's, both parents must be carriers and both must transmit the genetic mutation to the child. Thus, if both parents have the mutation, there is 25% chance their child will inherit the condition. Frequently, parents are given the opportunity to have a DNA screening if they are at high risk to determine their carrier status before they have children. The diagnosis of Sandhoff's disease can be conducted both prenatally and after birth. Prenatal diagnosis of Sandhoff's disease (infantile onset) is possible at about 16 weeks gestation through the detection and analysis of N-acetylglucosaminyl-

oligosaccharides in amniotic fluid and using high performance liquid chromatography (Warner, Turner, Toone, & Applegarth, 1985).

Before the condition becomes apparent through physical examination, postnatal diagnosis can be conducted through the following procedures: a biopsy removing a sample of tissue from the liver, genetic testing, molecular analysis of cells and tissues (to determine the presence of a genetic metabolic disorder), enzyme essay, and occasionally a urinalysis to determine if the above-noted compounds are abnormally stored within the body.

TREATMENT

There is no definitive or specific treatment for Sandhoff's disease other than supportive therapy (Alkan et al., 2003), including proper nutrition and hydration. In order to prevent breathing problems, it is often recommended to keep the airway open. Anticonvulsants may help to control seizures. Generally, the development of treatment or cure of the Sandhoff's disease, and other lysosomal storage diseases that affect the CNS, is extremely challenging. Due to the limitations imposed by the blood–brain barrier, the enzyme replacement therapy is not a feasible option (Arfi et al., 2006).

In some ongoing clinical studies, a small number of affected children have received an experimental treatment using transplants of stem cells from umbilical cord blood. Other investigated treatment possibilities include gene therapy. Gene therapy, which is based on the ability of genetically modified calls to overexpress a particular enzyme, aims at restoring normal cellular metabolism (Arfi et al., 2005, 2006). Although the trials have not yet produced a treatment or cure, scientists continue to study these and other investigational approaches with a hope for cure or effective treatment (NIH, 2007).

Anya Mazur-Mosiewicz
Raymond S. Dean

Alkan, A., Kutlu, R., Yakinci, C., Sigirci, A., Aslan, M., &, Sarac, K. (2003). Infantile Sandhoff's disease: Multivoxel magnetic resonance spectroscopy findings. *Journal of Child Neurology, 18,* 425–428.

Arfi, A., Bourgoin, C., Basso, L., Emiliani, C., Tancini, B., Chigomo, V., et al. (2005). Bicistronic lentiviral vector corrects β-hexosaminidase deficiency in transduced and cross-corrected human Sandhoff fibroblasts. *Neurobiology of Disease, 20,* 583–593.

Arfi, A., Zisling, R., Richard, E., Batista, L., Poenaru, L., Futerman, A. H., et al. (2006). Reversion of the biochemical defects in murine embryonic Sandhoff neurons using a bicistronic lentiviral vector encoding hexosaminidase alpha and beta. *Journal of Neurochemistry*, 6, 1572–1579.

Caliskan, M., Ozmen, M., Beck, M., & Apak, S. (1993). Thalamic hyperdensity: Is it a diagnostic marker for Sandhoff disease. *Brain and Development*, 15, 387–388.

Gomez-Lira, M., Sangalli, A., Mottes, M., Perusi, C., Pignatti, P. F., Rizzuto, N., et al. (1995). A common beta hexosaminidase gene mutation in adult Sandhoff disease patients. *Human Genetics*, 96, 417–422.

Krivit, W., Desnick, R. J., Lee, J., Moller, J., Wright, F., Sweeley, C. C., et al. (1972). Generalized accumulation of neutral glycosphingolipids with GM2 ganglioside accumulation in the brain. Sandhoff's disease (variant of Tay-Sachs disease). *American Journal of Medicine*, 52, 763–770.

Kroll, R. A., Pagel, M. A., Roman-Goldstein, S., Barkovich, A. J., D'Agostino, A. N., & Neuwelt, E. A. (1995). White matter changes associated with feline GM2 gangliosidosis (Sandhoff disease): Correlation of MR findings with pathologic and ultrastructural abnormalities. *American Journal of Neuroradiology*, 16, 1219–1226.

McKusick, V. A. (1998). *Mandelian inheritance in man: A catalog of human genes and genetic disorders* (12th ed.). Baltimore: The John Hopkins University Press.

National Institutes of Health. (2009). *Sandhoff disease*. Retrieved February 21, 2009, from http://ghr.nlm.nih.gov/condition = sandhoffdisease

Neote, K., Brown C. A., Mahuran, D. J., & Gravel, R. A. (1991). Translation initiation in the HEXB gene encoding the beta-subunit of human beta-hexosaminidase. *Journal of Biological Chemistry*, 265, 20799–20806.

Sandhoff, K., Andreae, U., & Jatzkewitz, H. (1968). Deficient hexozaminidase activity in an exceptional case of Tay-Sachs disease with additional storage of kidney globoside in visceral organs. *Life Sciences*, 7(6), 283–288.

Van der Kaamp, M. S., & Valk, J. (1995). GM, gangliosidosis. In M. S. Van der Kaamp & G. M. Valk (Eds.), *Magnetic resonance of myelin, myelination, and myelin disorders* (Vol. 10, 2nd ed., pp. 81–89). Berlin, Germany: Springer Verlag.

Wakamatsu, N., Kobayashi, H., Miyatake, T., & Tsuji, S. (1992). A novel exon mutation in the human beta-hexosaminidase beta subunit gene affects 3′ splice site selection. *Journal of Biological Chemistry*, 267, 2406–2413.

Warner, T. G., Turner, W., Toone, J., & Applegarth, J. (1985). Prenatal diagnosis of infantile GM 2 gangliosidosis type II (Sandhoff disease) by detection of N-acetylglucosaminyl-oligosaccharides in amniotic fluid with high-performance liquid chromatography. *Prenatal Diagnosis*, 6, 393–400.

Yuksel, A., Yalcinkaya, C., Islak, C., Gunduz, E., & Seven, M. (1999). Neuroimaging findings of four patients with Sandhoff disease. *Pediatric Neurology*, 21, 562–565.

SCHILDER'S DISEASE

DESCRIPTION

Schilder's disease, also known as diffuse myelinoclastic sclerosis, is a rare demyelinating disease most commonly found in children. It is primarily characterized by dementia, poor attention, aphasia, tremors, balance instability, personality changes, incontinence, muscle weakness, headaches, vomiting, speech impairment, cortical blindness, signs of intracranial pressure, and psychiatric disturbances (Afifi, Follett, Greenlee, Scott, & Moore, 2001). Schilder's disease is a progressive disease of the central nervous system, considered to be a variant of multiple sclerosis. Affecting males and females equally, the average age of onset is between 5 and 10 years of age. The onset of the disease is abrupt and commonly followed by a rapid deterioration of overall health. Death often occurs within months to years after onset (Kotil, Kalayci, Koseoglu, & Tugrul, 2002).

Schilder's disease was first termed in 1912 by Paul Schilder. Originally, however, the term was used to describe three separate diseases: adrenoleukodystrophy, subacute sclerosing panencephalitis, and myelinoclastic diffuse sclerosis (Poser, Goutieres, Carpentier, & Aicardi, 1986). Schilder's disease was used to describe several demyelinating disorders of differing etiologies until eventual diagnostic criterion was created in 1985. The development of clinical diagnostic criteria limited the term to solely include instances consistent with subacute or chronic myelinoclastic diffuse sclerosis and the formation of at least one large plaque. Developed criteria made the term Schilder's disease less ambiguous and emphasized clear criteria that distinguished myelinoclastic sclerosis from the original group of diseases that were incorporated under the same name. Diagnosis is difficult and one that is made by exclusion.

NEUROPATHOLOGY/PATHOPHYSIOLOGY

Neuroimaging techniques may reveal variable characteristics of Schilder's disease. Specifically, imaging techniques may reveal large, focal lesions located in the parieto-occipital regions of the brain. Images that are indicative of the disease are those that present with an overall sparing of the brainstem, ring enhancement that is incomplete, both brain hemispheres that are generally involved equally and, lastly, images that are diffusion weighted, have a low signal, and a minimal mass effect (Canellas, Gols, Izquierdo, Subirana,

S

& Gairin, 2007). The CT image will often reveal large bilateral or unilateral lesions of the white matter that are predominately within the centrum semiovale. However, there is not a specific neuroimaging pattern that is characteristic of Schilder's disease (Afifi et al., 2001). The supratentorial lesions in the centrum semiovale that are large and spherical often mimic tumors, but they are able to be recognized and classified as a demyelinating disease due to the absence of mass effect and edema that is displayed through CT images (Garell et al., 1998). Overall, lesions of Schilder's disease are distinctly outlined, large, and play a major role in the destruction of the myelin. Lesions typically involve an entire cerebral hemisphere and are often large enough to extend across the corpus callosum to the opposing hemisphere (Kotil et al., 2002).

Lesions that are consistent with multiple sclerosis are often detected through examination of the spinal cord, brainstem, and optic nerves. The demyelination of white matter, microglial proliferation with fibrillar gliosis, a single focus that is large, and lymphocytic perivascular infiltrate are histological characteristics of multiple sclerosis that often present in Schilder's disease (Kotil et al., 2002). White matter involvement generally becomes widespread and, as a result, various neurological deficits become apparent.

The underlying neuropathology of Schilder's disease is apparent through the neurological deficits that are associated with its presentation. In severe cases, progressive deterioration may present with dementia, bowel and bladder dysfunction, as well as papilledema. Increased cranial pressure is characteristic of the pseudotumoral type; the polysclerotic type will involve a progression that is consistent with multiple sclerosis. Lastly, a psychiatric form of the disease will present itself as mainly psychiatric symptoms, with major deficits in visual loss, including cortical blindness and hemianopia (Afifi et al., 2001).

NEUROPSYCHOLOGICAL/CLINICAL PRESENTATION

Neuropsychological aspects of Schilder's disease include the presence of aphasia, ataxia, hemiplegia, progressive dementia, memory disturbances, confusion, irritability, disorientation, and changes in personality. Increasing symptoms occur with the progression of the disease, and with the deterioration of the myelin. As the disease progresses effects of damage to the brainstem and cerebellum are apparent through the development of vertigo, dysarthria, dysphagia, and often paralysis of eye movement (Afifi et al., 2001). Diagnosis of the disease following the initial clinical presentation involves electoencephalogram (EEG), MRI, lumbar puncture, and

brain biopsy. It is a diagnosis made by exclusion; that is, all other possibilities must be ruled out before Schilder's disease can be diagnosed. Neuropsychological assessment measures are not included in the diagnostic process. However, neuropsychological assessment of cognitive decline may reveal deficits similar to that of multiple sclerosis (NINDS, 2008).

DIAGNOSIS

The common presentation of Schilder's disease often appears similar to that of acute disseminated encephalomyelitis (ADEM), tumor, abscess, amyotrophic leukodystrophy (ALD), and multiple sclerosis. Appropriate diagnosis must include a histological assessment, biopsy, neuroimaging, laboratory tests, and history due to the commonality between diseases. Onset, duration of illness, co-occurring psychiatric disorders, history of previous treatment, family history, history of vaccinations, and viral infections are essential features that should be included in the appropriate assessment and diagnosis of Schilder's disease (Garrell et al., 1998).

Multiple sclerosis will present with abnormal immunoglobulin in the cerebral spinal fluid, which differentiates from Schilder's disease in that there are no abnormalities of immunoglobulin in Schilder's disease. Large areas of demyelination within the centrum semiovale are characteristic of Schilder's disease that is different than the confluent and periventricular plaques that involve infratentorial and supratentorial structures of multiple sclerosis. Outside of the demyelinating lesions of Schilder's disease, the brain will appear normal on an MRI, which is not characteristic of multiple sclerosis (Afifi et al., 2001).

Schilder's disease may also appear similar to a cerebral tumor or neoplasm on radiological images. The use of brain biopsy is then required to determine the correct diagnosis. Schilder's disease must also be differentiated from ADEM. In comparison, ADEM usually is associated with a history of immunizations or viral infections and does not generally present with the generally large and symmetrical plaques in the centrum semiovale of both cerebral hemispheres, and does not typically include the lesions of the brainstem with which Schilder's disease presents (Miyamoto et al., 2006). Of interest, the MRI of Schilder's disease is consistent with that of ALD, with the distinction between the two relying on the fact that ALD lesions are primarily on the occipital lobes and appear more symmetrical. Furthermore, the presence of long chain fatty acids that are abnormal will indicate a diagnosis of ALD, in contrast to the normal chain of fatty acids that are diagnostically indicative of Schilder's disease (Kotil et al., 2002).

All other demyelinating disorders must be eliminated before exclusionary criteria can be met and a diagnosis of Schilder's disease can be made. The diagnostic criterion that was established by Poser et al. (1986) was able to provide a clearer distinction between the demyelinating disorders.

TREATMENT

There is currently no cure for Schilder's disease; therefore, treatment is focused on managing the symptoms that are associated with the rate of progression. The course of Schilder's disease is unpredictable, and the prognosis depends on its course. Progression of the disease has several possibilities including, progressive, monophasic remitting and not remitting, and all types have the additional possibility of fatality. As the disease progresses, the severity and number of deficits increases (NINDS, 2008). Progression of Schilder's disease is similar to that of multiple sclerosis, and therefore treatment methods are similar.

Corticosteroids are the initial choice of treatment for Schilder's disease and have proven to be the most effective. Alternative treatment methods include beta-interferon and immunosuppressive therapy. Cases of Schilder's disease that are of the progressive type tend to be less responsive to treatment of all types, and therefore neurological functioning continues to deteriorate regardless of treatment (Garrell et al., 1998). Further treatment focuses on symptomatic management, in which the primary concern is relief of symptoms in attempt to increase the level of daily functioning. Additional support is mainly in the form of occupational therapy, physiotherapy, and eventually nutritional support (NINDS, 2008). Pharmacological treatment is the initial choice and most effective throughout all levels of Schilder's disease.

Jamie Rice
Charles Golden

Afifi, A. K., Follett, K. A., Scott, W. E., & Moore, S. A. (2001). Optic Neuritis: A novel presentation of Schilder disease. *Journal of Child Neurology, 16*(9), 693–696.

Canellas, A. R., Gols, A. R., Izquierdo, R., Subirana, M. T., & Gairin, X. M. (2007). Idiopathic inflammatory-demyelinating diseases of the central nervous system. *Neuroradiology, 49*, 393–409.

Garell, P. C., Menezes, A. H., Baumbach, G., Moore, S. A., Nelson, G., Mathews, K., et al. (1998). Presentation, management and follow-up of Schilder disease. *Pediatric Neurosurgery, 29*, 86–91.

Kotil, K., Kalayci, M., Koseoglue, T., & Tugrul, A. (2002). Myelinoclastic diffuse sclerosis (Schilder disease):

Report of a case and review of the literature. *British Journal of Neurology, 16*(5), 516–519.

Miyamoto, N., Kagohashi, M., Nishioka, K., Fujishima, K., Kitada, T., Tomita, Y., et al. (2006). An autopsy case of Schilder's variant of multiple sclerosis (Schilder disease). *European Neurology, 55*, 103–107.

Poser, C. M., Goutieres, F., Carpentier, M., & Aicardi, J. (1986). Schilder's myelinoclastic diffuse sclerosis. *Pediatrics, 77*(1), 107–112.

SCHIZENCEPHALY

DESCRIPTION

Schizencephaly is a rare disease that leads to abnormal brain development (clefts) in one or both cerebral hemispheres. There are two types of schizencephaly, closed-lip (Type I) and open-lip (Type II). In both instance, schizencephaly is so rare that recent prevalence estimates are 1.54 per 100,000 people (Curry, Lammer, Nelson, & Shaw, 2005). Although the specific cause is unknown, it is currently classified as a neuronal migration problem and it is believed that this problem occurs during fetal development (1–7 months).

NEUROPATHOLOGY/PATHOPHYSIOLOGY

The defining features of schizencephaly are the cerebral clefts, either closed or open, lined with gray matter that extend from the pial surface of the cerebral cortex to the ependymal surface at the lateral ventricle. The clefts can occur in any region of the brain; however, they most commonly occur in the perisylvian regions (Close & Naul, 2009).

Heterotopias (collection of gray matter in abnormal locations) and polymicrogyria (neurons that are abnormally distributed) line the clefts. Arachnoid cysts can also be associated with the disorder. Microcephaly has also been noted in some patients. Another interesting fact is that in 80% to 90% of such patients the septum pellucidum is not present, suggesting that schizencephaly may coexist with septo-optic-dysplasia (Close & Naul, 2009; Rajderkar, Phatak, & Kolwadkar, 2006).

Two main theories surround the organic basis of schizencephaly: (1) neuronal migration fails at the point of the germinal matrix and (2) vascular trauma occurs postmigration. In comparison, neuronal migration dysfunction is the primary cause of this rare disorder. The neural migration causes clefts that are filled with CSF and the cleft is lined with gray matter (Close & Naul, 2009).

The most prominent theory proposes that schizencephaly occurs because of an early focal destruction of the germinal matrix and surrounding brain tissue before the hemispheres are fully developed (Ross & Walsh, 2001). The origins of schizencephaly are not definitive. Some suspect that the lesions, or more accurately clefts, have multiple origins that can be metabolic, toxic, vascular, and infectious in origin (Curry et al, 2005; Rocella & Testa, 2003; Tietjen et al., 2007). Others focus on the *LHX2* and *EMX2* genes believing that this disease has a more genetic basis (Brunelli et al., 1996; Ho, 2001; Tietjen et al., 2007).

NEUROPSYCHOLOGICAL/CLINICAL PRESENTATION

The defining feature in all cases of schizencephaly is the formation of clefts in the cerebral hemispheres; however, the presentation varies among patients. General features include developmental delay, mental retardation, motor deficits, and epilepsy (Barkovich, 2000; Denis et al., 2000). Patients with unilateral clefts and fused lips may have mild hemiparesis and seizures, but otherwise experience normal development. In closed-lip schizencephaly, a deep furrow exists that is lined with gray matter (Dubey, Gupta, Sharma, & Sharma, 2001; Wolpert & Barnes, 1992). Open cleft patients will most often have mild-to-moderate mental delay and hemiparesis. In the open-lip schizencephaly, the missing cerebral hemisphere creates a cavity that becomes filled with CSF. The severity of the manifestations is related to how much of the cortex is involved in the defect.

DIAGNOSIS

Schizencephaly is most often diagnosed in childhood, although in a few instances it has been diagnosed in adulthood because of seizure onset. An interesting aspect of schizencephaly is the array of anomalies that can exist including ventriculomegaly, microcephaly, polymicogyria, gray matter heterotopias, dysgenesis of corpus callosum, absence of septum pellucidum, and optic nerve hypoplasia (Close & Naul, 2009; Rajderkar et al., 2006).

The primary diagnostic features of closed-lip schizencephaly are defined by a few key features. Only a small area of the cerebral hemisphere is affected, there is no hydrocephalus, and there is a thin seam of gray matter (pial-ependymal cells) close together, explaining the name closed-lip schizencephaly. In closed-lip schizencephaly, the cleft walls that are lined with gray matter on each side block the CSF

space within the cleft. Closed clefts may be unilateral or bilateral (Close & Naul, 2009).

According to Naidich (1988), there are two primary features in diagnosing open-lip schizencephaly: (1) presence of continuous ependymal gray matter and (2) lining of the cleft by a seam comprised of epidermal cells.

From a differential diagnosis standpoint, several other medical conditions can be confused with schizencephaly. Specifically, it is important to rule out the following possible conditions: holoprosencephaly, porencephaly, hydranencephaly, and arachnoid cysts. Holoprosencephaly is characterized by facial anomalies and a thalamic midline mass within the monoventricular cavity. Hydranencephaly is characterized by a mostly absent cerebrum, with the meninges and cranial vault intact. Porencephaly is most similar in appearance to schizencephaly. It presents bilaterally in the vicinity of the Sylvian's fissure. However, MRI or CT scans will show that there is no gray matter present along the clefts in porencephaly. Arachnoid cysts are not symmetrical in shape and do not communicate with the lateral ventricles (Hayashi, Tsutsumi, & Barkovich, 2002).

TREATMENT

Unfortunately there is no cure for schizencephaly. The treatment focuses on the symptoms resulting from the abnormal brain development. A common treatment for all cases of schizencephaly is physical therapy to improve movement, ambulation, and symptoms of paralysis, spasticity, and/or hand movement difficulties. In cases where seizures occur, medication is the frontline treatment choice. If the seizures are not adequately managed with medication, surgery that would remove abnormal tissue surrounding the cleft is recommended (Guerrini & Carrozzo, 2001). In some cases of schizencephaly where hydrocephalus is present a ventricular shunt may be needed. The shunt helps relieve the accumulation of fluid and pressure.

Teri J. McHale
Henry V. Soper

Barkovich, A. (2000). Congenital malformations of the brain and skull. In A. J. Barkovich(Ed.), *Pediatric Neuroimaging* (Vol. 3e, pp. 289–292).

Brunelli, S., Faiella, A., Capra, V., Nigro, V., Simeone, A., Cama, A., et al. (1996). Germline mutations in the homeobox gene EMX2 in patients with severe schizencephaly. *Nature Genetics, 12,* 94–96.

Close, K., & Naul, L. (2009). Schizencephaly. eMedicine Specialties-Radiology. Retrieved from http://emedicine.

medscape.com/article/413051-overview on April 22, 2009.

Curry, C., Lammer, E., Nelson, V., & Shaw, G. (2005). Schizencephaly: Heterogeneous etiologies in a population of 4 million California births. *American Journal of Medical Genetics, 137A,* 181–189.

Denis, D., Maugey-Laulom, B., Carles, D., Pedespan, J. M., Brun, M., & Chateil, J. F. (2001). Prenatal diagnosis of schizencephaly by fetal magnetic resonance imaging. *Fetal Diagnosis and Therapy, 16*(6), 354–359.

Dubey, A., Gupta, R., Sharma, P., & Sharma, R. (2001). Schizencephaly type-1. *Indian Pediatrics, 38,* 949–951.

Guerrini, R., & Carrozzo, R. (2001). Epilepsy and genetic malformations of the cerebral cortex. *American Journal of Medical Genetics, 106,* 160–173.

Hayashi, N., Tsutsumi, Y., & Barkovich, A. (2002). Morphological features and associated anomalies of schizencephaly in the clinical population: detailed analysis of MR images. *Neuroradiology, 44,* 5.

Ho, A. (2001). A genetic basis for schizencephaly: Lhx2 may play a role in schizencephaly, septo-optic dysplasia, and Joubert Syndrome. *The Harvard Brain, 8,* 1–18.

Naidich, T. (1988). The neuro image quiz. *Pediatric Neuroscience, 14,* 54–56.

Oh, K., Kennedy, A., Frias, A., & Byrne, J. (2005). Fetal Schizencephaly: Pre- and postnatal imaging with a review of the clinical manifestations. *RadioGraphics, 25,* 647–657.

Rajderkar, D., Phatak, S., & Kolwadkar, P. (2006). Septo-optic dysplasia with unilateral open lip Schizencephaly: A case report. *Indian Journal of Radiology Imaging, 16*(3), 321–323.

Rocella, M., & Testa, D. (2003). Fetal alcohol syndrome in developmental age. Neuropsychiatric aspects. *Minerva Pediatrics, 55,* 63–69.

Ross, M., & Walsh, C. (2001). Human brain malformations and their lessons from neuronal migration. *Annual Review of Neuroscience, 24,* 1041–1070.

Tietjen, I., Bodell, A., Apse, K., Mendonza, A., Chang, B., Shaw, G., et al. (2007). Comprehensive EMX2 genotyping of a large schizencephaly case series. *American Journal of Medical Genetics Part A, 143A,* 1313–1316.

Wolpert, S., & Barnes, P. (1992). *MRI in pediatric neuroradiology.* St. Louis, MO: Mosby Year Book.

SCLERODERMA

DESCRIPTION

Scleroderma is a chronic group of rare autoimmune rheumatic diseases characterized by hardening and tightening (sclerosis) of the skin and connective tissues (the fibers that provide framework and support to the body). The most visible symptom of the disorder is hardening of the skin. There are two forms of scleroderma, localized and systemic. Localized scleroderma, sometimes known as morphea, affects only the skin. This form is disabling but most often tends not to be fatal. It is characterized by hardening of the skin and sometimes a reduction in joint movement due to the hardening.

Systemic scleroderma, or systemic sclerosis, is the generalized type of the disease. This form of the disease can be fatal as a result of damage to internal organs including the heart, lung, kidney, or intestinal tract. Systemic sclerosis is characterized by varying degrees of tissue scarring, hardening (fibrosis), and chronic inflammation within the internal organs. A large number of patients (85–95%) may experience Raynaud's phenomenon, disorder that affects the blood vessels in the extremities, fingers, toes, ears, and nose. It is characterized by vasospastic spasms that cause the blood vessels to constrict and change color.

It is estimated that about 250 people per million have some form of scleroderma. Scleroderma may run in families, but most often occurs without any known family history of the disease. Mortality can occur and is most often due to pulmonary hypertension and renal crisis. Survival is based on disease subtype and extent of organ involvement and averages about 12 years from diagnosis (Valentini & Black, 2002).

NEUROPATHOLOGY/PATHOPHYSIOLOGY

Sclerosis affects the organ systems; most obvious is the skin, but the disease can also affect the heart, lungs, kidneys, and GI tract. The symptoms are due to inflammation and occlusion due to an excessive production of collagen. The overproduction of collagen may be the result of a dysfunction in the autoimmune system, where the immune system would start to attack its own chromosomes. This chromosomal deterioration can cause genetic malfunction, and T cells would then accumulate that stimulate collagen depositing.

Studies have determined that stimulation of the fibroblast cells is crucial to the disease process. Transforming growth factor (TGFb) begins to be overproduced in this disease process and the fibroblast then overexpresses the receptor. A secondary messenger system that begins transcription of proteins and enzymes responsible for collagen production is developed through an intracellular pathway that consists of SMAD2/SMAD3, SMAD4, and an inhibitor SMAD7. In systemic sclerosis, vascular dysfunction is one of the earliest symptoms. Vascular changes are usually

S

seen in small arteries and arterioles. Severe changes in small blood vessels of the skin and internal organs are always present in systemic sclerosis. These changes may include formation of excess connective tissue (fibrosis) and T cell infiltration. The cause of systemic sclerosis is unclear; however, the following mechanisms are present in all areas: endothelial cell injury, fibroblast activation, and cellular derangement. Environmental factors may be a cause including silica and solvent exposure, and radiation or radiotherapy exposure.

NEUROPSYCHOLOGICAL/CLINICAL PRESENTATION

Localized scleroderma presents with skin appearing tight, reddish, or scaly. Skin pigmentation alternates from hyperpigmentation to hypopigmentation. The blood vessels may be dilated and appear more visible, most obvious is the face. The skin of the hands may appear swollen or "puffy" at first. Skin may appear tight and shiny, and patients may present with loss of hair, decreased sweating, and an inability to fold or bend skin. There is a great variation amongst patients in terms of severity. Diffuse scleroderma can cause complications in numerous other organ systems throughout the body. Problems can occur in the musculoskeletal, pulmonary, gastrointestinal, and renal systems, along with other areas such as eyes and ears. Individuals have greater involvement of internal tissues and organs if they have a larger involvement of skin in the course of the disease. Over 80% of patients have vascular symptoms and reports of Raynaud's phenomenon (Herrick, 2004). Deposits of calcium under the skin are also common in systemic sclerosis.

Scleroderma may cause a decrease in saliva production and a greater prevalence of oropharyngeal and esophageal cancers. Musculoskeletal symptoms often begin with pain in the joints and morning stiffness. The first joint pains are typically nonspecific and can possibly lead to arthritis and cause discomfort in tendons and muscles. Palpable tendon friction rubs may be detected over moving joints. Pulmonary impairment is very common and the leading cause of mortality in the disease. Shortness of breath during physical activity and dry cough are the most common pulmonary symptoms found in scleroderma. Pulmonary hypertension or elevations in arterial pressure may also develop in some patients. Patients with rapidly developing diffuse scleroderma have a much higher risk of developing renal crisis. Renal involvement in scleroderma is considered a poor prognostic factor and is a frequent cause of death. Symptoms of a renal crisis include high blood pressure with organ damage, high renin levels, kidney failure with accumulation of waste products in the blood, and destruction of red blood cells. Excess blood and proteins may also be found in the urine. Gastrointestinal symptoms include esophageal reflux, esophagitis, gastroesophageal reflux disease (GERD), bacterial overgrowth in the intestine, ischemic colitis, malabsorption, and a symptom called watermelon stomach (atypical blood vessels proliferate in a symmetrical pattern around the stomach). Finally, scleroderma may cause some neurological difficulties. In rare occasions, trigeminal neuralgia may occur. Trigeminal neuralgia is a neuropathic disorder that causes great pain in the facial features: eyes, nose, lips, jaw, scalp, and forehead. Other neurologic symptoms include possible carpal tunnel syndrome due to peripheral neuropathies.

DIAGNOSIS

Criteria for classification of scleroderma have been determined by the American College of Rheumatology. Classification requires one major criterion or two minor criteria. The major criterion is proximal scleroderma that is characterized by thickening and tightening of the fingers. These changes may affect the face, neck, trunk, or entire extremity. Minor criteria include thickening, hardening and tightening of the skin, limited only to the fingers (sclerodactyly), scarring of the fingers, loss of substances from the finger pad, or pulmonary hardening at the base of the lungs (bibasilar pulmonary fibrosis) (Klippel, 2008).

Diagnosis of the disease process may also be determined through the presence of autoantibodies, such as anti-centromere and anti-scl 70/anti-topoisomerase antibodies. Biopsies may also be conducted in order to determine diagnosis. Differential diagnoses include eosinophilia, eosinophilia-myalgia syndrome, primary biliary cirrhosis, pulmonary hypertension, reflex sympathetic dystrophy, and mycosis fungoides. Other disorders that need to be considered in differentiating scleroderma include: toxic oil syndrome, digital sclerosis of diabetes mellitus, vibration disease, radiation exposure, intestinal obstruction, infiltrative cardiomyopathy, and amyloidosis. Laboratory workups for diagnosis may include hamogram (to reveal anemia), urinalysis (proteinuria, hematuria), chest X-rays (pulmonary fibrosis), CT scans (alveolitis), and ECHO (pulmonary arterial pressure).

TREATMENT

The US Food and Drug Administration has not approved any therapies for systemic sclerosis (Oliver &

Winkelmann, 1989). Skin thickening can be treated with topical treatments that may improve pain and ulceration but do not alter the disease course. Nonsteroidal anti-inflammatory drugs, such as naproxen, can be used to ease painful symptoms associated with the disease. Prednisone is sometimes used but has been shown to provide limited benefit. Skin thickening can also be treated with D-penicillamine. Raynaud's phenomenon can be treated with calcium channel blockers. Pruritus (itching) can be treated with moisturizers. Acute renal failure and high blood pressure with evidence of organ damage due to scleroderma are often treated with dialysis (Steen & Medsger, 2000). However, angiotensin-converting enzyme (ACE) inhibitors are beneficial and may benefit enough to discontinue renal replacement therapy. Pulmonary problems are often treated with a combination of cyclophosphamide and a small dose of steroids (Tashkin, Elashoff, & Clements, 2006). Pulmonary hypertension is treated with Bosentan and has proved significant in patients with systemic sclerosis related pulmonary hypertension (Steen, 2005). Surgery may be used in patients with severe Raynaud's phenomenon. Amputation may be required in infected hand lesions. Hand surgery is used to correct flexion difficulties. Occasionally, removal or draining of calcium deposits is required.

Erin L. Tireman
Charles Golden

Herrick, A. L. (2005). Pathogenesis of Raynaud's phenomenon. *Rheumatology, 44*(5), 587–596.

Jimenez, S. A., & Derk, C. T. (2004). Following the molecular pathways toward an understanding of the pathogenesis of systemic sclerosis. *Annals of Internal Medicine, 140*(1), 37–50.

Klippel, J. H. (2008). *Primer on the rheumatic diseases* (11th ed.). Atlanta, GA: Arthritis Foundation.

Oliver, G. F., & Winkelmann, R. K. (1989). The current treatment of scleroderma. *Drugs, 37*(1), 87–96.

Steen, V. D. (2005). The lung in systemic sclerosis. *Journal of Clinical Rheumatology, 11*(1), 40–46

Steen, V. D., & Medsger, T. A., Jr. (2000). Long term outcomes of scleroderma renal crisis. *Annals of Internal Medicine, 133*(8), 600–603.

Tashkin, D. P., Elashoff, R., Clements, P. J., Goldin, J., Roth, M. D., Furst, D. E., et al. (2006). Cyclophosphamide versus placebo in scleroderma lung disease. *New England Journal of Medicine, 354*(25), 2655–2666.

Valentini, G., & Black, C. (2002). Systemic sclerosis. *Best practice and research in Clinical rheumatology, 16*(5), 807–816.

SEMANTIC DEMENTIA

DESCRIPTION

Semantic dementia (SD) was first discovered in 1975. It is one of the main variants of frontotemporal dementia (FTD) (Rascovsky, Growdon, Pardo, Grossman, & Miller, 2009). SD involves degradation of conceptual knowledge and difficulties in understanding the meaning of objects and words, as well as naming (Coulthard et al., 2006). Other aspects of cognition, including visuospatial abilities, perceptual reasoning, executive functioning, and episodic memory may remain generally intact (Laisney et al., 2009). Understanding this disorder is important due to the increasing aging population, the often insidious onset, and diverse clinical presentation (Amici, Gorno-Tempini, Ogar, Dronkers, & Miller, 2006). Differential diagnosis can be challenging for the different dementia syndromes but neuropsychological testing as well as radiological findings may be helpful tools.

NEUROPATHOLOGY/PATHOPHYSIOLOGY

SD is a clinical syndrome and therefore there is not always a specific underlying pathology that can be identified (Garrard & Hodges, 2000). Pereira and colleagues (2009) note that although atrophy patterns for variants of FTD are observed, histologic FTD do not evidence clear differences. In general, SD is viewed as having non-Alzheimer's type pathology. At the macroscopic level, abnormalities of the white and gray matter in the left temporal lobe have been observed, particularly the inferolateral portions and the pole (Garrard & Hodges, 2000). At a microscopic level, gliotic degeneration or nonspecific spongiotic changes have been discovered, as well as histological patterns common to Pick's disease (Hodges, Garrard, & Patterson, 1998). Neuropathological findings have also revealed ubiquitin-positive, tau-negative neuronal inclusions (Hodges & Patterson, 2007).

Radiological findings of SD have resulted in a number of observations regarding patterns of atrophy. Cortical atrophy has been found to remain relatively isolated to the inferior and anterior portions of the temporal lobe earlier in the disease process, but later affecting the temporal cortex more extensively (Reilly & Peelle, 2008). MRI findings have revealed left hemisphere atrophy, most prominent around the sylvian fissure of the temporal lobe (Hodges, Patterson, Oxbury, & Funnell, 1992; Hodges,

Patterson, & Tyler, 1994). Cortical thickness analysis from volumetric MRI has found significant cortical thinning in the left temporal lobe, especially in the entorhinal cortex, temporal pole, and fusiform, para-hippocampal and inferior temporal gyri (Rohrer et al., 2009). CT findings have illustrated diffuse ventricular enlargement and widening, most marked in the left anterior temporal region (Cummings & Duchen, 1981). PET studies have also shown atrophy in the temporopolar and perirhinal cortices (Hodges & Patterson, 2007). Pronounced hypoperfusion of the entire left hemisphere has been noted in SPECT (Poeck & Luzzatti, 1988).

NEUROPSYCHOLOGICAL/CLINICAL PRESENTATION

SD is often referred to as "fluent aphasia" as spontaneous speech is often grammatically correct and fluent, despite a loss of semantic knowledge. Semantic paraphasias are quite common, however (Hodges et al., 1992). For example, a person may refer to a pencil as a pen. As the disease progresses, speech may become "empty" with limited use of nouns and reliance on vague fillers, such as "that," "thing," and "this" (Amici et al., 2006). Patients may use clichés, which may be strangely appropriate to the situation (e.g., "I don't understand") (Hodges, Patterson, Graham, & Dawson, 1996). Associated behavioral symptoms in SD can be quite diverse, with the most frequently seen features including depression, repetitive motor behaviors, overeating, or changes in food preference (e.g., increased craving for sweets), emotional blunting, and changes in social interactions (Rosen et al., 2002).

Neuropsychological findings have revealed decreased word retrieval on confrontation naming tasks, with little benefit from even multiple choice cues (Gorno-Tempini et al., 2004). Wilson and colleagues (2009) note impairment in reading low frequency words, with atypical spelling-to-sound translation. Patients may have difficulty with naming fingers, body parts, and shapes and they may be unable to discriminate left and right. Semantic fluency is often severely impaired, and depressed scores are found on phonemic fluency (Amici et al., 2006). Sentence repetition may be intact, as well as executing multi-step commands. Calculations may be normal, as well as digits backward. However, praxis may be impaired due to impaired object recognition (Amici et al., 2006). On bedside examination, patients may be oriented and be able to recall recent events although language deficits may greatly interfere with formal assessment (Garrard & Hodges, 2000).

In a longitudinal study by Libon and colleagues (2009), researchers found that group differences were notable between SD and other variants of frontotemporal lobar degeneration, and these were maintained over the duration of the illness, and suggest that the various disorders do not converge into one subtype over time. Hodges and colleagues (1999) found a distinct clinical profile when differentiating temporal and frontal variants of FTD from early Alzheimer's disease. Those with SD evidenced isolated but profound anomia and surface dyslexia, but they are indistinguishable from the AD group when assessing story recall.

DIAGNOSIS

Diagnosis is based on demonstration of the clinical features of SD that have been defined as: (1) selective impairment in semantic memory, resulting in severe anomia, impaired written and spoken single-word understanding, reduced general fund of knowledge about word-meaning, objects and persons, and diminished category fluency; (2) generally intact functions in other aspects of language comprehension and production; (3) intact working memory, visuospatial, and problem-solving skills; (4) generally intact episodic and autobiographical memory (Hodges et al., 1992).

Other common variants of SD include progressive nonfluent aphasia (PNFA) that is characterized by agrammatism in speech production and/or comprehension, and labored speech, as well as logopenic progressive aphasia, which presents as word-finding difficulties, impaired sentence comprehension, and simple but accurate language output (Amici et al., 2006). The frontal variant of fronto-temporal dementia (fv-FTD) results in prominent changes in personality and social functioning, and common cognitive deficits involve executive dysfunction and working memory (Boxer & Miller, 2005; Coulthard et al., 2006).

TREATMENT

To date, the Food and Drug Administration (FDA) has not established an approved treatment for SD. Boxer and colleagues (2009) investigated the use of Memantine in three subtypes of FTD, including SD. Unfortunately, SD groups declined on most of the cognitive and behavioral outcome measures. Cholinesterase inhibitors have been used in variants of FTD. There was no evidence of cognitive improvements, and in some cases, behavioral symptoms actually worsened

(Amici et al., 2006). Amici and colleagues (2006) found out that serotonin-specific-reuptake inhibitors (SSRIs) can be helpful in addressing behavioral symptoms. Clearly there is a need for pharmacological advancement in the treatment of SD.

Efficacious treatment is limited for those with focal brain damage due to stroke, let alone language-based neurodegenerative conditions (Henry, Beeson, & Rapcsak, 2008). In a review by Henry and colleagues (2008), it is noted that learning is possible in SD patients but greater reliance on autobiographic and perceptual information is important for vocabulary learning. They add that treatment may actually help to slow the rate of decline, particularly in the early stages of the process when aspects of semantic knowledge are accessible and episodic memory is generally intact.

Amy R. Steiner
Chad A. Noggle
Amanda R. W. Steiner

Amici, S., Gorno-Tempini, M., Ogar, J. M., Dronkers, N. F., & Miller, B. L. (2006). An overview on Primary Progressive Aphasia and its variants. *Behavioural Neurology, 17,* 77–87.

Boxer, A. L., Lipton, A. M., Womack, K., Merrilees, J., Neuhaus, J., Pavlic, D., et al. (2009).

An Open-label Study of Memantine Treatment in 3 subtypes of Frontotemporal Lobar Degeneration. *Alzheimer Disease and Associated Disorders,* July-Sep: 23 (3): 211–217.

Boxer, A. L., & Miller, B. L. (2005). Clinical features of frontotemporal dementia. *Alzheimer Disease Association Discord, 19*(Suppl. 1), S3–S6.

Coulthard, E., Firbank, M., English, P., Welch, J., Birchall, D., O'Brien, J., et al. (2006). Proton magnetic resonance spectroscopy in frontotemporal dementia. *Journal of Neurology, 253,* 861–868.

Cummings, J. L., & Duchen, L. W. (1981). Kluver-Bucy syndrome in Pick's disease: Clinical and pathological correlations. *Neurology, 31,* 1415–1422.

Garrard, P., Hodges, J.R. (2000). Semantic dementia: clinical, radiological, and pathological perspectives. *Journal of Neurology,* 247: 409–422.

Gorno-Tempini, M.L., Dronkers, N.F., Rankin, K.P., Ogar, J.M., Phengrasamy, L. et al. (2004). Cognition and anatomy in three variants of primary progressive aphasia. *Annals of Neurology,* 55 (3), 335–346

Henry, M. L., Beeson, P. M., & Rapcsak, S. Z. (2008). Treatment for anomia in semantic dementia. *Seminars in Speech and Language, 29*(1), 60–70.

Hodges, J. R., Garrard, P., & Patterson, K. (1998). Semantic dementia and Pick complex. In A. Kertesz & D. Munoz (Eds.), *Pick's disease and Pick's complex.* New York: Wiley Liss.

Hodges, J. R., & Patterson, K. (2007). Semantic dementia: A unique clinicopathological syndrome. *Lancet Neurology, 6*(11), 1004–1014.

Hodges, J. R., Patterson, K., Graham, N., & Dawson, K. (1996). Naming and knowing in dementia of Alzheimer's type. *Brain Language, 54,* 302–325.

Hodges, J. R, Patterson, K., Oxbury, S., & Funnell, E. (1992). Semantic dementia: Progressive fluent aphasia with temporal lobe atrophy. *Brain, 115,* 1783–1806.

Hodges, J. R., Patterson, K., & Tyler, L. K. (1994). Loss of semantic memory: Implications for the modularity of mind. *Cognitive Neuropsychology, 11,* 505–542.

Hodges, J. R., Patterson, K., Ward, R., Garrard, P., Bak, T., Perry, R., et al. (1999).

The differentiation of semantic dementia and frontal lobe dementia (temporal and frontal variants of frontotemporal dementia) from early Alzheimer's disease: A comparative neuropsychological study. *Neuropsychology, 13*(1), 31–40.

Laisney, M., Matuszewski, V., Mézenge, F., Belliard, S., de la Sayette, V., Eustache, F., et al. (2009). The underlying mechanisms of verbal fluency deficit in frontotemporal dementia and semantic dementia. *Journal of Neurology, 256*(7), 1083–1094.

Libon, D. J., Xie, S. X., Wang, X., Massimo, L., Moore, P., Vesely, L., et al. (2009). Neuropsychological decline in frontotemporal lobar degeneration. A longitudinal analysis. *Neuropsychology, 23*(3), 337–346.

Pereira, J. M., Williams, G. B., Acosta-Cabronero, J., Pengas, G., Spillantini, M. G., Xuereb, J. H., et al. (2009). Atrophy patterns in histologic versus clinical groupings of frontotemporal lobar degeneration. *Neurology, 72*(19), 1653–1660.

Poeck, K., & Luzzatti, C. (1988). Slowly progressive aphasia in three patients: The problem of accompanying neuropsychological deficit. *Brain, 111,* 151–168.

Rascovsky, K., Growdon, M. E., Pardo, I. R., Grossman, S., & Miller, B. L. (2009). The quicksand of forgetfulness': Semantic dementia in one hundred years of solitude. *Brain,* Sep:132 (Pt 9): 2609–2616.

Reilly, J., & Peelle, J. (2008). Effects of semantic impairment on language processing in semantic dementia. *Seminars in Speech and Language, 29*(1), 32–43.

Rohrer, J.D., Warren, J.D., Modat, M., Ridgway, G.R., Douiri, A. (2009). Patterns of cortical thinning in the language variants of frontotemporal lobar degeneration. *Neurology,* May 5; 72 (18): 1562–1569.

Rosen, H. J., Kramer, J. H., Gorno-Tempini, M. L., Schuff, N., Weiner, M., & Miller, B. L. (2002). Patterns of cerebral atrophy in primary progressive aphasia. *American Journal of Geriatric Psychiatry,* 89–97.

Wilson, S. M., Brambati, S. M., Henry, R. G., Handwerker, D. A., Agosta, F., Miller, B. L., et al. (2009). The neural basis of surface dyslexia in semantic dementia. *Brain, 132*(1), 71–86.

S

SHAKEN BABY SYNDROME

DESCRIPTION

Shaken baby syndrome (SBS), or inflicted traumatic brain injury (TBI), is caused by violent and forceful shaking of a child with or without contact of the child's head against a hard surface. The whiplash type motion results in brain trauma including subdural hematoma, retinal hemorrhage, and diffuse axonal injury. The term "nonaccidental head injury" is used synonymously to emphasize that SBS does not refer to an accidental trauma. For example, when an infant sustains brain damage in a car accident, this would not be referred to as SBS, but rather a TBI. In short, SBS results from abusive shaking of an infant or child.

NEUROPATHOLOGY/PATHOPHYSIOLOGY

The original triad for understanding the SBS was characterized by subdural hemorrhage, retinal hemorrhage, and encephalopathy all of which coincide with the shaking. Over time this triad has been questioned as having to occur in a consistent pattern (Squier, 2008). Recent studies have documented that parenchymal lesions are associated with SBS and further brain damage can include edema, bleeding, stroke, white matter contusional tears, and axonal injury (Bonnier et al., 2003). Even if brain damage can be objectified on neuroimaging, it is often challenging to determine if the brain was damaged due to an inadvertent drop versus someone intentionally shaking the baby. Geddes, Hacksaw, Vowles, Nickols, and Whitwell (2001) classified the following five categories for establishing SBS or nonaccidental brain injury: (1) brain injury where there was a confession by the perpetrator; (2) cases where SBS was established in criminal courts; (3) cases with unexplained brain injuries, but no conviction was made; (4) no permanent brain injury was objectified (i.e., neuroimaging), but caretaker(s) were convicted of inflicting physical injuries to the infant's head or neck; and (5) major discrepancy remained unresolved between the caretaker's explanation and a significant injury, such as a skull fracture.

One of the greatest protections against common forms of brain trauma is the ability to keep the head stationary in response to an impact to the head or movements of the body. Consequently, because an infant has a proportionately large head in conjunction with weak neck muscles, there is less protection from severe acceleration–deceleration forces to the brain. Particularly, severe rotational forces can have deleterious effects. The constellation of these factors is such that a baby's brain cannot withstand severe shaking that would unlikely harm an older child or adult.

NEUROPSYCHOLOGICAL/CLINICAL PRESENTATION

A full recovery applies to the patient having no long-term physical, cognitive, and emotional residuals. The detrimental sequelae associated with SBS include cerebral palsy, ongoing seizures, visual problems (secondary to retinal hemorrhages), speech and language problems, and behavioral problems (Karandikar, Coles, Jayawant, & Kemp, 2004). The sequelae associated with SBS is undoubtedly worse if the shaking takes place on more than one occasion.

The signs and symptoms of SBS range on a continuum from a "low-dose" shaking/impact to a "high-dose" shaking/impact. The effects of severe craniocerebral injuries vary and can include decreased responsiveness, poor feeding, irritability, lethargy and hypotonia, seizures, vomiting, tachypnea, hypothermia, bradycardia, coma, fixed dilated pupils, and death (Karandikar et al., 2004). Associated injuries may also be seen outside of the brain itself. Specifically, prominent and multilayered retinal hemorrhages are present in the majority of cases. Acute skull fractures indicate that impact has accompanied the shaking (Talvik et al., 2007). Seizures and apnea were the most common symptoms noted by emergency health care personnel (Starling et al., 2004).

The incidence of SBS varies across studies from 15–40.5 per 100,000 children (Talvik et al., 2007). The morbidity rates across studies ranges between 38–40% and 58–70%. Yet some studies even reported morbidity as high as 80–100%. This variable range is due to zcultural differences (studies were conducted in Scotland, North Carolina, and Estonia), magnitude of sample size, and the sensitivity of the outcome measures. The literature has pointed out that even if some of the infants or children "may look well immediately following the trauma, the child may be left with serious and permanent disabilities" (Talvik et al., 2007, p. 1164). Approximately one-third of the SBS survivors present with severe neurological disorders. Nearly a quarter of the victims die within a few hours to a few days of their brain injury. Fifty to ninety percent of the survivors are left with varying degrees of disabilities ranging from serious learning disabilities and behavioral disorders to paralyses, blindness, and permanent vegetative states (Talvik et al., 2007).

DIAGNOSIS

The diagnosis of a brain trauma is based on loss of consciousness, posttraumatic amnesia, disorientation, and neurological signs (American Congress of Rehabilitation Medicine, 1993). Because infants are unable to respond to questions that are essential to retrospectively assess posttraumatic amnesia and disorientation, the diagnosis for milder brain traumas is far more challenging. Moreover, problems related to SBS are sometimes not detected until the child enters the educational system and behavioral problems and learning difficulties are observed by their teachers. But years later, the link between these learning and behavioral problems and SBS may never be convincingly established. Diagnosis cannot be confirmed unless the perpetrator confesses, reliable witnesses come forth, and/or there is conclusive objective evidence of brain damage consistent with SBS.

A majority of the infants with SBS are under 2 years old (Talvik et al., 2007). Therefore, formal neuropsychological testing is extremely limited in this age group; however, long-term follow-up evaluations have documented that many survivors suffer from severe disabilities including a plethora of cognitive residuals. Predictors of poor outcome include shaking while the infant is under 6 months, apnea, impaired consciousness, and depending upon auxiliary respiratory support at presentation (Jennet & Bond, 1975). When testing a group of school-aged children who were shaken in their infancy, cognitive residuals included weaknesses in intelligence, working memory, attention, reasoning, mental planning and organization, and mental inhibition (Sitpanicic, Nolin, Fortin, & Gobeil, 2008).

Careful investigation by medical professionals, child protective agencies, investigators, and prosecutors is important, since the legal consequences can be severe. Child protective services routinely refer cases suspected of SBS for court-ordered family medical and psychological evaluations. The medical evaluation includes a review of the medical findings in the case and a determination of the nature and cause of the injuries. Psychological evaluations of the adults assess current psychological functioning, parenting competencies, and risk factors for abuse such as substance abuse, personality factors, and the parent's ability to provide predictable, consistent, and emotionally attuned caretaking. Parents are interviewed for medical history and, if forthcoming, a history of how the injuries occurred. Psychological evaluations are not used by the team to solely determine who injured the child. Fault and intentionality of the injury are determined by analyzing the injuries, access to the child, and witness and perpetrator statements.

These findings and recommendations regarding child placement and mental health interventions are conveyed to the parents, the courts, and child protective services for implementation. Collaborative decision making between physicians and psychologists enhance each discipline's conclusions and minimize the likelihood of error. To this end, improved decision making protects children from abusive caretakers and, when appropriate, preserves families if a caretaker has not abused the child and is not at risk to abuse the child. When a parent is the perpetrator, the likely separation or limited contact with this parent can result in attachment issues.

TREATMENT

SBS should be viewed from a family system's perspective. If an innocent parent is accused of SBS, it can be emotionally devastating to the entire family to be questioned about the possibility of intentional abuse. For parents who already blame themselves for an inadvertent fall, this questioning can exacerbate their self-blame. Although this is potentially detrimental to the already stressed family system, it is nonetheless an unavoidable component of intervening in abusive situations. Additionally, if a nonfamily caregiver is determined to be responsible for SBS, then the parents' feelings of guilt, anger, and depression will likely affect the family system. If a partner or spouse has caused SBS, then this severely strains — if not permanently damages — the partnership. Overall, criminal investigations often take several months, if not years, before decisions are finalized, and during this time period, the family is constantly anchored to the tragedy of an innocent infant having been harmed. Having family issues that may have contributed to this trauma being played out in a court room strains the family system exponentially. If the couple separates, then the loss of a parent will alter the family dynamic, not only for the abused child but also for any siblings.

Potential risk factors that trigger SBS should be dealt with by both education and therapeutic care. Risk factors can include, but are not limited to, unwanted pregnancy and/or poor coping mechanisms including uncontrolled anger reactions, substance abuse, and unrealistic expectations about a child's behavior, particularly inappropriate reaction to or misinterpretation of crying as rejection or disobedience. For example, when an infant has colic and is difficult to soothe, and the sleepless nights are the rule rather than an exception, parents' coping mechanisms are often maximally stressed. Thus, risk factors should be identified for expectant parents before and after pregnancy regarding preventive steps they can take. For example, the National Center on Shaken Baby Syndrome has developed the Period of PURPLE Crying program (Barr et al., 2009). This program identifies the triggers associated with crying in order to help caregivers understand and avoid negative responses to crying infants. The letters in PURPLE each stand for a property of crying in healthy infants that frustrates caregivers; that is, P for peak pattern, in which crying increases, peaks during the 2nd month and then declines; U for unexpected timing of prolonged crying bouts; R for resistance to soothing; P for pain-like look on the child's face; L for long crying bouts; and E for late afternoon and evening clustering. The PURPLE materials reinforce that these cycles are normal and suggest ways for caregivers to soothe and cope with a baby's inconsolable crying. First, parents are encouraged to use typical calming responses such as carrying, comforting, walking, and talking. Second, if the crying is too frustrating it is okay to put the baby down in a safe place, walk away, calm yourself, and then return to check on the baby. Third, never shake your baby.

Parents need to be educated as to the possibility of severe postpartum imbalances that can result in severe depression and occasionally even psychotic reactions. Accordingly, they should have access to treatment in the event these symptoms occur. In sum, education and treatment are essential in order to reduce the frequency of SBS, which permanently harms innocent babies and devastates families. Continued research should be aimed at identifying the circumstances and triggers that caused caretakers to shake an infant.

Ronald Ruff
Saralyn Ruff
Christina Weyer Jamora
Ann M. Richardson

American Congress of Rehabilitation Medicine, Mild Traumatic Brain Injury Committee, A. C. R. M., Head Injury Interdisciplinary Special Interest Group. (1993). Definition of mild traumatic brain injury. *Journal of Head Trauma Rehabilitation, 8*, 86–87.

Barr, R. G., Rivara, F. P., Barr, M., Cummings, P., Taylor, J., Lengua, L. J., et al. (2009). Effectiveness of educational materials designated to change knowledge and behaviors regarding crying and shaken-baby-syndrome in mothers of newborns: A randomized controlled trial. *Pediatrics, 123*, 972–980.

Bonnier, C., Nassogne, M. C., Saint-Martin, C., Mesples, C., Kadhim, H., & Sébire, G. (2003). Neuroimaging of intraparenchymal lesions predicts outcome in shaken baby syndrome. *Pediatrics, 112*, 808–814.

Geddes, J. F., Hacksaw, A. K., Vowles, G. H., Nickols, C. D., & Whitwell, H. L. (2001). Neuropathology of inflicted head injury in children. *Brain, 124*, 1290–1298.

Jennet, B., & Bond, M. (1975). Assessment of outcome after severe brain damage. *Lancet, 1*, 480–484.

Karandikar, S., Coles, L., Jayawant, S., & Kemp, A. M. (2004). The neurodevelopmental outcome in infants who have sustained a subdural hemorrhage from non-accidental head injury. *Child Abuse Review, 13*, 178–187.

Sitpanicic, A., Nolin, P., Fortin, G., & Gobeil, M. F. (2008). Comparative study of the cognitive sequelae of school-aged victims of Shaken Baby Syndrome. *Child Abuse and Neglect, 32*, 415–428.

Squier, W. (2008). Shaken Baby Syndrome: The quest for evidence. *Developmental Medicine and Child Neurology, 50*, 10–14.

Starling, S., Patel, S., Burke, B., Sirotnak, A., Stronks, S., & Rosquist, P. (2004). Analysis of perpetrator admissions to inflicted traumatic brain injury in children. *Archives of Pediatrics & Adolescent Medicine, 158*, 454–458.

Talvik, I., Männamaa, M., Jüri, P., Leito, K., Põder, H., Hämarik, M., et al. (2007). Outcome of infants with inflicted traumatic brain injury (shaken baby syndrome) in Estonia. *Acta Paediatrica, 96*, 1164–1168.

SHINGLES

DESCRIPTION

Shingles, or herpes zoster, is a latent reaction to the varicella zoster virus (chickenpox) and is a member of the herpes virus family (Urman & Gottlieb, 2008). In order to develop shingles, the person must have first been infected with chickenpox (Urman & Gottlieb, 2008). People commonly contract chickenpox through inhalation; however, when the disease has returned in the form of shingles, it can no longer be transmitted to others (Urman & Gottlieb, 2008). Shingles is a relatively common disease, with 600,000 to 1 million cases being reported in the United States each year (Urman & Gottlieb, 2008) and a lifetime prevalence rate of 10–20% (Oaklander, 2001). Prevalence rates increase with age and in those with suppressed autoimmune function (Christo, Hobelmann, & Maine, 2007; Oaklander, 2001; Urman & Gottlieb, 2008).

The most notable characteristic of shingles is the unique rash, which has a unilateral, dermatomal distribution and forms in the mid to lower thoracic region (Bajwa & Ho, 2001; Christo et al., 2007; Urman & Gottlieb, 2008). This rash may also be vesicular or bullous in nature (Bajwa & Ho, 2001). In some cases, there may be prodromal symptoms before the rash, such as fever, malaise, headache, and preherpetic neuralgia, or pain (Urman & Gottlieb, 2008). Pain can appear 7–100 days before other symptoms, although this is uncommon (Bajwa & Ho, 2001). Neuralgia can also occur while the rash is present or after it has disappeared, called postherpetic neuralgia (PHN) (Bajwa & Ho, 2001; Urman & Gottlieb, 2008). PHN can begin 30 days after skin lesions have disappeared and can last for over a year (Urman & Gottlieb, 2008). PHN is more common in the elderly, those suffering from immunosuppression diseases, trauma, X-irradiation, and malignancy (Bajwa & Ho, 2001; Kennedy, 2002; Urman & Gottlieb, 2008). Another risk factor is significantly lower levels of immunoglobulin G (Wrensch et al., 2005). Less common symptoms may include a bacterial super infection and ocular and neurological impairment (Urman & Gottlieb, 2008). In extreme cases, encephalitis can occur; however, this is much more likely in individuals with previously compromised immune systems (Kennedy, 2002).

A common complication of shingles, PHN causes deficits in thermal, tactile, pinprick, and vibration sensations in the affected skin areas (Bajwa & Ho, 2001). Common symptoms of PHN are altered sensation, ongoing pain not produced by stimuli, and mechanical allodynic pain, pain to light skin touch but normal sensation to thermal stimulation (Christo et al., 2007; Kennedy, 2002; Oaklander, 2001). PHN may in part stem from the dorsal horn atrophy caused by the reactivation of the herpes zoster virus (Kennedy, 2002). It can cause cutaneous neuritis, can decrease sensitivity in nerve endings, and can decrease innervations (Oaklander et al., 1998). Individuals are more likely to develop PHN if their rash was more severe, or if they had increased neurosensitiviy disturbance, a prodrome to symptom presentation, demyelization with fibrosis, or dorsal horn atrophy (Christo et al., 2007). The number of sensory nerve terminals lost or affected by the herpes zoster virus is strongly correlated to the presence of PHN pain; the more terminals lost, the greater the likelihood the person will experience PHN pain (Oaklander et al., 1998).

NEUROPATHOLOGY/PATHOPHYSIOLOGY

After the initial varicella zoster virus infection begins to subside, the virus lies dormant for years to decades in the dorsal root or trigeminal root ganglia in the cranial and spinal nerves (Bajwa & Ho, 2001; Kennedy, 2002). While it is dormant, the virus's DNA is still integrated into the carrier's DNA, but the viral proteins are not made (Urman & Gottlieb, 2008).

Because the virus contains double-stranded DNA, when it reactivates it is able to cause new and different symptoms from the chickenpox presentation (Christo et al., 2007; DeLengocky & Bui, 2007). During the acute stage, as the herpes zoster virus reactivates it travels along from the dorsal root ganglia to the central nervous system (CNS) then to the peripheral nerves (Bajwa & Ho, 2001). Eventually, the virus is transmitted to the sensory neurons and ultimately the skin (Urman & Gottlieb, 2008). Once the virus reaches the skin, it can travel more directly between skin cells or along the extracellular matrix (Urman & Gottlieb, 2008).

This viral procession causes abnormalities in the CNS, such as an inflammation (Kennedy, 2002). Thoracic nerve areas 4 and 6 are commonly affected by the virus as well as the cranial sensory ganglia (Bajwa & Ho, 2001; DeLengocky & Bui, 2007). In the peripheral nervous system, the disease causes deafferentation, a persistent pain where sensory loss has occurred (Christo et al., 2007), or aberrant activity of peripheral neurons, which can cause sensitivity of these neurons and cell necrosis (Christo et al., 2007; Oaklander, 2001).

Both the spinal and peripheral axons affected by the herpes zoster virus degenerate, replaced by collagen (Oaklander, 2001). This causes the intense burning and shooting pain associated with shingles (Christo et al., 2007). As the disease continues to spread, vesicles form, which eventually hemorrhage and crust over. The eruption of these vesicles is another source of pain for infected individuals (Christo et al., 2007).

NEUROPSYCHOLOGICAL/CLINICAL PRESENTATION

Shingles and PHN can be associated with anxiety, depression, impaired sleep, decrease in appetite, and diminished libido (Bajwa & Ho, 2001). Research has also shown that shingles can decrease a person's quality of life (Katz, Cooper, Walther, Sweeney, & Dworkin, 2004). One study has found that 42% of those with shingles surveyed reported horrible and excruciating pain (Katz et al., 2004). It was found that this pain contributed to not only poorer physical functioning but also poorer social functioning (Katz et al., 2004).

The more pain an individual reported, the higher the person's emotional distress level was found to be (Katz et al., 2004). Overall, participants in higher amounts of pain reported decreased emotional well-being (Katz et al., 2004). Increased education on shingles and its symptoms was found to help

S

decrease pain perception in affected individuals (Katz et al., 2004).

Another neuropsychological symptom found in those with shingles is sensory response changes (Fleetwood-Walker et al., 1999). The sensory abnormalities, which develop as a result of the herpes zoster virus, cause increases in sensitivity to sensory stimuli in the affected extremities (Fleetwood-Walker et al., 1999). Most commonly, an increased sensitivity to thermal sensation has been found (Fleetwood-Walker et al., 1999).

DIAGNOSIS

The most common method for diagnosis of shingles is clinical observation of the distinctive rash (Novatnack & Schweon, 2007). However, shingles is much harder to diagnose before the rash is present, and some individuals never develop a rash, named zoster sine herpete (Roxas, 2006). If shingles is suspected, a sample of fluid will be removed from a vesicle for testing (Novtnack & Schweon, 2007). Two common tests are the fluorescent antibody test or the polymerase chain reaction (PCR) test (Novtnack & Schweon, 2007). A viral culture can also be used but it is not as accurate because the varicella zoster virus is labile (Roxas, 2006).

The PCR test has been found to be the most sensitive in detecting the herpes zoster virus's DNA (Noratnack & Schweon, 2007; Roxas, 2006). This test can also aid in differential diagnosis. Pleurisy, cardiac complications, herniated nucleus pulposus, trigeminal neuralgia, and Bell's palsy are all commonly considered during differential diagnosis (Roxas, 2006). Other differential diagnoses for shingles include herpes simplex or coxsackie virus (Bajwa & Ho, 2001). A Tzanck test can help discriminate between these diseases for accurate diagnosis (Bajwa & Ho, 2001). Common misdiagnoses for shingles include appendicitis, myocardial infarct, renal colic, and choletithiasis (Roxas, 2006).

TREATMENT

Early intervention is essential in order to control and eliminate pain as quickly as possible (Bajwa & Ho, 2001). Due to the vast number of associated disorders, a combination of medications can provide the most thorough relief, such as antivirals, antidepressants, corticosteroids, opioids, and topical crèmes such as lidocaine (Bajwa & Ho, 2001; Christo et al., 2007). For pain management, many of these medications are used along with nerve blockade, in which local anesthetics are injected in peripheral nerves to produce relief (Bajwa & Ho, 2001). However, corticosteroids have not been shown to be effective relief for pain symptoms (Christo et al., 2007). Other treatments include capsaicin (the extract of hot chili peppers), a topical ointment that aids in the release of substance P and other neuropeptides, and ketamine, which aids in relieving pain by acting on calcium channels (Christo et al., 2007). For patients with compromised immune systems who experience pain, antiviral medications, such as acyclovir, valacyclovir HCl, and famciclovir have been found to be most effective in treating pain and healing lesions quickly (Bajwa & Ho, 2001).

Because treatments for shingles can be costly and do not completely prevent PHN (Urman & Gottlieb, 2008), preventing the development of shingles and chickenpox has become essential (Christo et al., 2007). In 1995, a new vaccine Varivax (Merck) was developed and is now routinely administered to children (Christo et al., 2007; Urman & Gottlieb, 2008). In the future, the prevalence rates of both shingles and chickenpox are expected to decline (Christo et al. 2007). Research has also found that vaccinating elderly individuals at higher risk for development of shingles can help reduce the likelihood of developing the disease (Christo et al., 2007). The newer vaccine Zostavax (Merck) has been shown to decrease the incidence rate of shingles and of PHN in 50% of those who received the treatment (Christo et al., 2007). However, vaccines can also be costly and the duration of their effectiveness can vary (Urman & Gottlieb, 2008).

Sarah E. West
Charles Golden

Bajwa, Z. H., & Ho, C. C. (2001). Herpetic neuralgia: Use of combination therapy for pain relief in acute and chronic herpes zoster. *Geriatrics, 56,* 18–24.

Christo, P. J., Hobelmann, G., & Maine, D. N. (2007). Postherpetic neuralgia in older adults: Evidence-based approaches to clinical management. *Drugs and Aging, 24,* 1–19.

DeLengocky, T., & Bui, C. M. (2008). Complete ophthalmoplegia with puillary involvement as an initial clinical presentation of herpes zoster ophthalmicus. *The Journal of the American Osteopathic Association, 108,* 615–621.

Fleetwood-Walker, S. M., Quinn, J. P., Wallace, C., Blackburn-Munro, G., Kelly, B. G., Fiskerstrand, C. E., et al. (1999). Behavioural changes in the rat following infection with varicella-zoster virus. *Journal of General Virology, 80,* 2433–2436.

Katz, J., Cooper, E. M., Walther, R. R., Sweeney, E. W., & Dworkin, R. H. (2004). Acute pain in herpes zoster and its impact on health-related quality of life. *Clinical Infection Diseases, 39,* 342–348.

Kennedy, P. G. (2002). Varicella-zoster virus latency in human ganglia. *Reviews in Medical Virology, 12,* 327–334.

Novatnack, E., & Schweon, S. (2007). Shingles: What you should know. *Registered Nurses, 70,* 27–31.

Oaklander, A. L. (2001). The density of remaining nerve endings in human skin with and without postherpetic neuralgia after shingles. *Pain, 92,* 139–145.

Oaklander, A. L., Romans, K., Horasek, S., Stocks, A., Hauer, P., & Meyer, R. A. (1998). Unilateral postherpetic neuralgia is associated with bilateral sensory neuron damage. *Annals of Neurology, 44,* 789–795.

Roxas, M. (2006). Herpes zoster and postherpetic neuralgia: Diagnosis and therapeutic considerations. *Alternative Medicine Review, 11,* 102–113.

Urman, C. O., & Gottlieb, A. B. (2008). New viral vaccines for dermatologic disease. *Journal of the American Academy of Dermatology, 58,* 361–370.

Wrensch, M., Weinberg, A., Wiencke, J., Miike, R., Sison, J., Wiemels, J., et al. (2005). History of chickenpox and shingles and prevalence of antibodies to varicella-zoster virus and three other herpes viruses among adults with glioma and controls. *American Journal of Epidemiology, 161,* 929–938.

SICKLE CELL DISEASE

DESCRIPTION

Sickle cell disease (SCD) is a group of inherited blood disorders caused by a genetic change in hemoglobin, the oxygen-carrying protein in red blood cells. These disorders are characterized by a loss of red blood cells and the destruction of the cell membrane causing a release of hemoglobin (Beulter, 2002; Bojanowski & Frey, 2002). The most common SCD is sickle cell anemia (Bojanowski & Frey, 2002; Uthman, 1998). Other forms of SCD include, S/beta thalassemia, hemoglobin SC disease, hemoglobin SD disease, and hemoglobin SO disease and are caused by the inheritance of the sickle cell gene and an altered beta-globin gene (Beulter, 2002; Bojanowski & Frey, 2002).

The sickle cell gene is highly prevalent in the United States, but a very small percentage of the population has SCD because the individual must inherit the sickle gene from both parents to have the disease. Those who inherit a single sickle cell gene are said to have the sickle cell trait (SCT) (Uthman, 1998). SCT is a condition that occurs when one sickle hemoglobin (hemoglobin S) gene and one normal hemoglobin gene are inherited. With SCT, the red cells contain about 60% of the normal hemoglobin and 40% of the hemoglobin S (Beulter, 2002).

There appears to be a strong relationship between SCT and malaria. Specifically, the SCT may help protect against malaria as those who had the trait survived malaria more frequently than those who did not in areas where malaria was present and the trait originated (Beulter, 2002; Bloom, 1995; Bojanowski & Frey, 2002; Uthman, 1998). Continually, malaria and the prevalence of SCD tend to be distributed along the same geographic regions (Bloom, 1995). There is evidence to suggest that SCT migrated with people, as about 1 in 12 African Americans are carriers of the mutation (Bojanowski & Frey, 2002), or 7.8–9% of African Americans (Beulter, 2002; Uthman, 1998).

In contrast to those with the disease, individuals with SCT do not have vaso-occlusive (painful) symptoms and tend to have a normal life expectancy (National Institute of Health [NIH], 2002). Extreme physiological stress, including intense exercise can increase problems associated with SCT (NIH, 2002), and in rare cases, traces of blood can appear in the urine (Bojanowski & Frey, 2002).

Globally, it is estimated that 1 in 250,000 infants are born with SCD each year. The diseases mainly affect African, Mediterranean, Middle Eastern, and Asian Indian populations, but it occurs in people from other ethnic backgrounds and is increasing in Latino populations (Bojanowski & Frey, 2002).

NEUROPATHOLOGY/PATHOPHYSIOLOGY

SCD is caused when sickle cell hemoglobin replaces normal hemoglobin (Bloom, 1995). This replacement is initiated by a mutation in the beta-globlin, producing sickle hemoglobin (hemoglobin S) (Beulter, 2002; Bojanowski & Frey, 2002). Sickle hemoglobin polymerizes into rod-like structures and change the shape of normal red blood cells into the resemblance of an agricultural tool, called the sickle, thus the name SCD.

Hemoglobin S tends to have a shorter life span, which can cause chronic anemia because of the reduced levels of hemoglobin and red blood cells. Hemoglobin S can also become trapped in blood vessels, limiting blood flow and decreasing oxygen. The lack of oxygen damages tissues and organs and can result in excruciating pain, which is often one of the chief complaints of individuals with SCD (Bloom, 1995; Bojanowski & Frey, 2002). When this impedes blood flow to the brain, ischemic stroke may occur. In fact, SCD is one of the more common risk factors of stroke in children, particularly African Americans as they are at greatest risk for SCD in general. Vascular obstruction associated with the sickling process contributes to both large and small infarctions when they occur. Although this proposes an ischemic presentation, cerebral venous thrombus and hemorrhage can occur. Individuals with SCD are at risk for frequent infections and tend to have a shorter life span (Bloom, 1995).

NEUROPSYCHOLOGICAL/CLINICAL PRESENTATION

One of the most reported symptoms of SCD is painful episodes, lasting a few days up to a few weeks. The pain can range from annoying to agonizing (Bloom, 1995) and the specific pain associated with SCD can develop as early as infancy (NIH, 2002). Painful episodes are the leading cause of emergency room visits and hospitalizations for individuals with SCD (Bojanowski & Frey, 2002; NIH, 2002). SCD pain can be categorized as acute, chronic, or mixed (NIH, 2002). The majority of the pain is caused when sickle cells block blood vessels, creating oxygen deprivation in some parts of the body. If blood flow is not restored, tissue can become inflamed and damaged. As sickle cells can cause blockage in any small blood vessel, pain and damage can occur in any part of the body. However, the chest, bones, and abdomen are where the painful episodes are most reported (Bloom, 1995).

Individuals with SCD are especially vulnerable to infections. The spleen, which helps fight infections, can be severely damaged in patients with SCD due to oxygen loss (Bloom, 1995; Bojanowski & Frey, 2002), causing surgical removal of the spleen in extreme cases. Damage or removal of the spleen is especially dangerous for children based on its connection to the immune system. The younger the children when damage occurs, the more vulnerable they are to life-threatening infections. Furthermore, once an infection occurs, individuals with SCD are more difficult to treat, and the infection can be more severe than for healthy individuals (Bloom, 1995).

As mentioned, sickle cell anemia is the most prevalent SCD (Bojanowski & Frey, 2002; Uthman, 1998). Once red blood cells become sickle shaped, they are destroyed. This then creates a deficiency in red blood cells and anemia develops (Bloom, 1995). Fatigue, shortness of breath, and a pale complexion are common symptoms of anemia (Bojanowski & Frey, 2002), though the first symptom of sickle cell anemia in an infant is often dactylitis. Dactylitis is caused by limited circulation to small bones in the fingers and toes and results in painful swelling. The consequences of sickle cell anemia are related to limited oxygen reaching organs due to the jamming of sickled red cells known as an infarctive crisis. The loss of tissue resulting from plugged blood vessels is known as an infarction. This can create pain and organ function may suffer, including leg ulcers that can be the result of a loss of circulation. In fact, these infections are the most common cause of death related to sickle cell anemia (Uthman, 1998).

Neurological complications are common in sickle cell anemia due to damage of the brain caused by decreased blood flow. The decreased blood flow can cause cerebral infarction and lead to a stroke for individuals with SCD. Acute hemiplegia is the most common residual, although all focal cerebral presentations can occur (Ropper & Brown, 2005). Common manifestations of stroke caused by SCD include hemiparesis, aphasia, visual difficulties, and seizures (Mankad & Dyken, 1992).

DIAGNOSIS

Neonatal screening, when incorporated with diagnostic testing and appropriate care, has a key impact on the quality of life for individuals with SCD. In the United States, most states automatically provide genetic screenings for newborns, including SCD, and screenings can be requested in the other states. Most screening programs utilize isoelectric focusing to screen for disorders (NIH, 2002), whereas other programs use high-performance liquid chromatography (HPLC) (Bojanowski & Frey, 2002; NIH, 2002). HPLC separates the normal hemoglobin from the sickle hemoglobin and helps determine which types of hemoglobin are present in the blood. A complete blood count may also be useful because it describes many aspects of an individual's blood. SCD will show a lower hemoglobin level and other red blood cell abnormalities. SCD can also be identified through the use of prenatal diagnosis, including chorionic villus sampling and amniocentesis (Bojanowski & Frey, 2002). Preimplantation genetic diagnosis is a technique that involves genetic testing of developing embryos before implantation occurs (Bloom, 1995; Bojanowski & Frey, 2002).

TREATMENT

Several interventions are used to prevent and treat symptoms of SCDs. Antibiotics are used to prevent infections. Penicillin is utilized to prevent pneumococcal infections and is particularly important for children with SCD. Routine vaccinations are also recommended for individuals with SCD, though they may also require additional immunizations to help prevent infections (Bojanowski & Frey, 2002; NIH, 2002). As pain is one of the most common concerns with sickle cell anemia, pain management may be a critical aspect in treatment planning. Often, nonsteroidal anti-inflammatory drugs and opioids are used to manage pain (NIH, 2002).

Blood transfusions are an option for individuals with frequent and severe painful episodes and severe anemia (Bojanowski & Frey, 2002; NIH, 2002). When used correctly, blood transfusions can prevent organ damage because transfusions may raise the oxygen in the blood and decrease the number of sickle cells (NIH, 2002). Furthermore, regular transfusions can reduce symptoms associated with SCD (Bojanowski & Frey, 2002). Cerebral circulatory disorder due to SCD occurring to red blood cell sludging related to the sickling process is most commonly treated with intravenous hydration and transfusion (Ropper & Brown, 2005).

Andrea Stephen
Raymond S. Dean

Beutler, E. (2002). Sickle cell disease. In L. Breslow (Ed.), *Encyclopedia of public health* (Vol. 4, pp. 1099–1100). New York: Macmillan Reference USA. Retreived March 15, 2009, from http://find.galegroup.com/gvrl/infomark.do?&contentSet=EBKS&type=retrieve&tabID=T001&prodId=GVRL&docId=CX3404000780&source=gale&userGroupName=munc80314&version=1.0

Bloom, M. (1995). *Understanding sickle cell disease.* Jackson, MS: University Press of Mississippi.

Bojanowski, J., & Frey, R. J. (2002). Sickle cell disease. In S. L. Blachford (Ed.), *Gale encyclopedia of genetic disorders* (Vol. 2, pp. 1048–1056). Detroit, MI: Gale. Retrieved March 15, 2009, from http://find.galegroup.com/gvrl/infomark.do?&contentSet=EBKS&type=retrieve&tabID=T001&prodId=GVRL&docId=CX3405500351&source=gale&userGroupName=munc80314&version=1.0

Mankad, V. N., & Dyken, P. R. (1992). Neurological complications of sickle cell disease. In V. N. Mankad & R. B. Moore (Eds.), *Sickle cell disease: Pathophysiology, diagnosis, and management* (pp. 300–306). Westport, CT: Praeger.

National Institutes of Health, National Heart, Lung and Blood Institute. (2002). *The management of sickle cell disease.* Retrieved March 21, 2009, from http://purl.access.gpo.gov/GPO/LPS22097

Ropper, A., & Brown, R. H. (2005). *Adams and Victor's principles of neurology* (8th ed., pp. 660–746). New York: McGraw-Hill. [Cerebrovascular Disease]

Uthman, E. (1998). *Understanding anemia* (pp. 95–98). Jackson, MS: University Press of Mississippi.

SJÖGREN'S SYNDROME

DESCRIPTION

Sjögren's syndrome is a chronic autoimmune disorder that has a primary manifestation of dry mouth and dry eyes. The body's immune cells attack and destroy exocrine glands that produce bodily fluids, resulting in poor tear and saliva production. The incidence is 1 in 70 Americans or about 40 million people. Sjögren's syndrome is the second most common autoimmune disorder of the class of rheumatic disorders that affect the musculoskeletal system (Wallace, 2005). Approximately 90% of patients with Sjögren's syndrome are women. The average age of onset is in the late 40s and perimenopausal women are the highest risk group (Wallace, Bromet, & Sjögren's Syndrome Foundation, 2005). Primary Sjögren's syndrome occurs in isolation and secondary occurs with another rheumatic or autoimmune disorder such as lupus or rheumatoid arthritis.

NEUROPATHOLOGY/PATHOPHYSIOLOGY

Sjögren's syndrome is an autoimmune disorder in which the body's white blood cells attack the endocrine system, particularly the lachrymal glands of the eyes and the saliva glands of the mouth. The cell death of these moisture-producing glands limits the fluids the body can produce, creating dryness and inflammation. Due to the high concentration of cases in women, it is hypothesized that hormonal factors play a role in the development of Sjögren's syndrome, such as the decrease in androgen levels that occur during states of elevated estrogen levels like menopause (Sullivan, Dartt, & Meneray, 1998). This research has largely been based upon experimental studies with animals.

Human leukocyte antigen genes have been hypothesized to be a heritable, genetic component of Sjögren's syndrome. The gene *HLA-DR3* is frequently found in persons of European descent with primary Sjögren's syndrome (Dyson, 2005). The antinuclear antibodies SS-A (Ro) and SS-B (La) are found in 60–70% and 40% of patients, respectively (Dyson, 2005). There is no clear evidence that the disorder is heritable, but multiple family members can have conditions within the class of autoimmune rheumatic disorders.

NEUROPSYCHOLOGICAL/CLINICAL PRESENTATION

A number of authors describe the impairments in daily functioning that patients with Sjögren's syndrome face

(Dyson, 2005; Hanger & Schneebaum, 2003; Wallace, 2005). Patients are unable to wear contact lenses and have to apply eye drops regularly. They may be sensitive to light and have blurred vision, with severe cases resulting in corneal ulcers. Patients complain of bad breath due to the lack of saliva to cleanse the teeth and prevent plaque buildup. Dietary habits change due to loss of taste, difficult and painful swallowing, and excessive need to drink fluids. Some patients have gastrointestinal symptoms such as gas, frequent urination, and diarrhea, which are embarrassing and limit their social contact. Female patients may complain of pain during sexual intercourse due to poor lubrication. Skin rashes may develop due to vascular conditions that affect blood flow and content.

The development of arthritis may make it difficult for the patient to perform fine motor tasks without pain. Joint pain and frequent nighttime urination lead to unsatisfying sleep and fatigue that may be misinterpreted as depression when it is combined with reports of muscle pain and poor appetite. Patients may develop a raspy, hoarse voice due to inflammation of the larynx. It is estimated that 50% of patients report social isolation due to their symptoms (Wallace et al., 2005).

Patients with Sjögren's syndrome, as with other chronic medical conditions, report higher incidence of emotional distress such as grieving the loss of identity and physical functioning, denial, anger, depression, suicidal ideations, and anxiety (Fremes & Carteron, 2003).

DIAGNOSIS

In about 50% of cases, Sjögren's syndrome is secondary to or comorbid with rheumatoid arthritis, systemic lupus erythematosus, scleroderma, and other rheumatic disorders (Wallace et al., 2005). Primary Sjögren's syndrome occurs independently of other autoimmune or neurological disorders. However, it is so highly associated with these conditions that patients diagnosed with primary Sjögren's syndrome are frequently evaluated for systematic lupus erythematosus, scleroderma, rheumatoid arthritis, polymyositis, dermatomyositis, thyroid disease, and autoimmune liver disease (Dyson, 2005). The presence of one of these disorders warrants further evaluation over the next several years.

It is estimated that up to 40% of older adults report symptoms of dry eyes and mouth without confirmation of Sjögren's syndrome or any other disorder (Pompei, Murphy, & American Geriatric Society, 2006). The symptoms are subtle and difficult to identify with a mean onset of 6 years before diagnosis

(Wallace, 2005). The most common symptoms are severe dry eyes (keratoconjunctivitis sicca) and mouth (xerostomia). Other symptoms include dry nose or throat, swelling, difficulty swallowing and chewing food, and thrush (yeast infections of the mouth) (Yu & Scherer, 2007).

In addition to the eyes (lachrymal glands) and mouth (salivary glands), the lungs, heart, gastrointestinal tract, pancreas, liver, kidney, and vagina may be affected (Pompei et al., 2006). Poor hydration of these organs and systems causes pain, fatigue, and poor performance of their respective functions (Yu & Scherer, 2007). Unexplained symptoms of bloating, indigestion, and constipation serve as symptoms and show gastrointestinal involvement (Fremes & Carteron, 2003). Irritable bladder syndrome, causing urgency, frequency, pain, and nighttime urination, is a symptom of kidney dysfunction, as are renal stones (Fremes & Carteron, 2003). Dehydrated blood vessels can lead to cutaneous vasculitis, swelling of the blood vessels that lead to skin rash; hyperviscosity, blood that is too thick; or blood conditions such as cryoglobulinemia (Wallace, 2005). Inflammation of the joints leads to arthritis, sometimes chronic, in up to 50% of patients (Fremes & Carteron, 2003). Inflammation of nerve cells can lead to carpal tunnel syndrome or neuropathy (Dyson, 2005). Wallace et al. (2005) reported that 62% of patients have serious dental complications such as excessive caries.

Sjögren's syndrome may be diagnosed with a number of measures (Wallace, 2005). The Schirmer's eye test measures the amount of cornea tearing. The eyes can also be assessed for keratoconjunctivitis sicca, inflammation of the cornea and conjunctiva due to dryness. The Rose Bengal staining test assesses the cornea for scarring, pitting, or other abnormalities such as ulcers. Tests of saliva production as well as clinical observation are utilized. A lip biopsy can also be performed to evaluate for chemical signs of inflammation. This procedure is rarely utilized because it is very painful. Full blood analyses should be conducted regularly to assess for rheumatic markers such as Ro antibodies, La antibodies, or HLA-DR3 markers (Wallace, 2005). Inflammation is evaluated through the erythrocyte sedimentation rate (ESR), which requires a small blood sample (Dyson, 2005).

Some authors distinguish between Sjögren's syndrome and Sjögren's disease. Sjögren's disease indicates the involvement of exocrine glands throughout the body that are connected through the lymph system. Up to 5–10% of Sjögren's patients may develop this lymphoproliferative malignancy, leading to chronic and severe complications. The presence of Ro and La antinuclear antibodies put the patient at increased risk for developing lymphoma. This tendency to result in lymphoma is unique among autoimmune disorders.

A rare subtype of Sjögren's syndrome is Mikulicz's disease, which is readily diagnosed by enlarged parotid or salivary glands. These patients appear to have the mumps, have salivary glands that are tender to the touch, and excessive inflammation of the salivary glands (Wallace, 2005).

TREATMENT

Wallace (2005) describes the treatment of Sjögren's syndrome as primarily symptomatic. He stated that traditional treatments include the use of artificial tears to moisten the eyes as needed. Mouth gels, hard candies, and sipping on water hydrate the mouth and throat and help to prevent dental decay by washing away bacteria and food particles. Humidifiers are used to treat the primary symptoms as well as the dry nose and throat that can result. Patients are encouraged to visit their optometrist and dentist regularly. Medications have shown some success at increasing salivation and soothing dry eyes. These are pilocarpine, cevimeline, and cyclosporine eye drops. Hydroxychloroquine may treat the immune process itself. Nonsteroidal anti inflammatory medications may be utilized to treat musculoskeletal symptoms such as arthritis (Fremes & Carteron, 2003).

It is important to evaluate and treat the emotional and cognitive symptoms associated with Sjögren's syndrome due to its chronic nature (Fremes & Carteron, 2003). Much research has confirmed the fact that treatment compliance is increased when the patient has a sense of control and optimism, which may be provided through education concerning symptoms, medical procedures, and treatment options. Psychotropic medications, therapy, and relaxation techniques should be recommended. Patients may feel isolated and need additional social support, increasing the need for family therapy or support groups.

Jessie L. Morrow
Charles Golden

Dyson, S. (2005). *Positive options for Sjogren's syndrome: Self help and treatment*. Alameda, CA: Hunter House.

Fremes, R., & Carteron, N. (2003). *A body out of balance: Understanding and treating Sjogren's Syndrome*. New York: Avery.

Hanger, N. C., & Schneebaum, A. B. (2003). *The first year — Lupus: An essential guide for the newly diagnosed*. Emeryville, CA: Marlowe and Company.

Pompei, P., Murphy, J. B., & American Geriatric Society. (2006). *Geriatrics review syllabus: A core curriculum in geriatric medicine*. Hoboken, NJ: Blackwell Publishing.

Sullivan, D. D., Dartt, D. A., & Meneray, M. A. (1998). *Lacrimal gland, tear film, and dry eye syndromes 2: Basic science and clinical relevance*. New York: Springer.

Wallace, D. J. (2005). *The lupus book: A guide for patients and their families* (3rd ed.). New York: Oxford University Press.

Wallace, D. J. (Ed.). Bromet, E. J., Sjogren's Syndrome Foundation. (2005). *The new Sjogren's syndrome handbook*. New York: Oxford University Press.

Yu, W., & Scherer, W. (2007). *What to eat for what ails you: How to treat illnesses by changing the food and vitamins in your diet*. Beverly, MA: Fair Winds.

SLEEP APNEA

DESCRIPTION

Sleep apnea is usually a chronic (ongoing) condition that disrupts sleep three or more nights each week. One often moves out of deep sleep and into light sleep when one's breathing pauses or becomes shallow resulting in poor sleep quality and consequently fatigue during the day. In fact, sleep apnea is one of the leading causes of excessive daytime sleepiness. The Greek word "apnea" literally means "without breath." There are three types of apnea: obstructive, central, and mixed; of the three, obstructive is the most common. Despite the difference in the root cause of each type, in all three, people with untreated sleep apnea pause in breathing or take shallow breaths, sometimes hundreds of times during the night, which can last for a few seconds to minutes often occurring 5–30 times or more an hour. Typically normal breathing resumes with a loud snort or choking sound as air tries to squeeze past the blockage (American Sleep Apnea Association, 2008).

NEUROPATHOLOGY/PATHOPHYSIOLOGY

The underlying physiology of sleep apnea varies based on the type of sleep apnea presented. Obstructive sleep apnea occurs when the muscles in the back of the throat relax. These muscles support the soft palate, the triangular piece of tissue hanging from the soft palate (uvula), the tonsils, and the tongue. When the muscles relax, the airway narrows or closes when taking a breath, and breathing momentarily stops. This may lower the level of oxygen in the blood. The brain senses this inability to breathe and

S

briefly rouses the patient from sleep so that the patient can reopen the airway. This awakening is usually so brief that most patients don't remember it. Obstructive sleep apnea is caused by repetitive upper airway obstruction during sleep as a result of narrowing of the respiratory passages. Patients with the disorder are most often overweight, with associated peripharyngeal infiltration of fat and/or increased size of the soft palate and tongue. Some patients have airway obstruction because of a diminutive or receding jaw that results in insufficient room for the tongue. These anatomic abnormalities decrease the cross-sectional area of the upper airway. Decreased airway muscle tone during sleep in combination with the pull of gravity in the supine position further decreases airway size, impeding airflow during respiration. Initially, partial obstruction may occur and lead to snoring. As tissues collapse further or the patient rolls over on his or her back, the airway may become completely obstructed. Whether the obstruction is incomplete (hypopnea) or total (apnea), the patient struggles to breathe and is aroused from sleep. Often, arousals are only partial and are unrecognized by the patient, even if they occur hundreds of times a night. The obstructive episodes are often associated with a reduction in oxyhemoglobin saturation.

With each arousal event, the muscle tone of the tongue and airway tissues increases. This increase in tone alleviates the obstruction and terminates the apneic episode. Soon after the patient falls back to sleep, the tongue and soft tissues again relax, with consequent complete or partial obstruction and loud snoring (Patil, Schneider, Schwartz, & Smith, 2007).

The combinations of the physiological characteristics causing obstructive sleep apnea may vary considerably among patients. Most obstructive apnea patients have an anatomically small upper airway with augmented pharyngeal dilator muscle activation maintaining airway patency awake, but not asleep. However, individual variability in several phenotypic characteristics may ultimately determine who develops apnea and how severe the apnea will be. These include: (1) upper airway anatomy, (2) the ability of upper airway dilator muscles to respond to rising intrapharyngeal negative pressure and increasing CO_2 during sleep, (3) arousal threshold in response to respiratory stimulation, and (4) loop gain (ventilatory control instability). As a result, patients may respond to different therapeutic approaches based on the predominant abnormality leading to the sleep-disordered breathing.

Occasionally, obstructive sleep apnea can be caused by less common medical problems, including hypothyroidism, acromegaly, and renal failure.

Neuromuscular disorders such as postpolio syndrome can result in inadequate neuromuscular control of the upper airway and lead to obstructive sleep apnea. Restrictive lung disease from scoliosis has also been associated with the disorder.

Central sleep apnea, which is far less common, occurs when the brain fails to transmit signals to the breathing muscles. The patient may awaken with shortness of breath or have a difficult time getting or staying asleep. Like obstructive sleep apnea, snoring and daytime sleepiness can occur. Central sleep apnea, in its various forms, is generally the product of an unstable ventilatory control system (high loop gain) with increased controller gain (high hypercapnic responsiveness) generally being the cause. High plant gain can contribute under certain circumstances (hypercapnic patients). The most common cause of central sleep apnea is heart disease, and less commonly, stroke. People with central sleep apnea may be more likely to remember awakening than people with obstructive sleep apnea (White, 2005).

Mixed (complex) apnea, as the name implies, is a combination of the two. With each apnea event, the brain briefly arouses people with sleep apnea in order for them to resume breathing, but consequently sleep is extremely fragmented and of poor quality. People with complex sleep apnea have upper airway obstruction just like those with obstructive sleep apnea, but they also have a problem with the rhythm of breathing and occasional lapses of breathing effort (Mayo Clinic, 1998).

In general, sleep apnea may occur whether the patient is young or old, male or female. Even children can have sleep apnea. But certain factors put individuals at increased risk. In the case of obstructive sleep apnea, risk factors include: excess weight; neck circumference; high blood pressure (hypertension); a narrowed airway; being male; being older (sleep apnea occurs two to three times more often in adults older than 65); family history; use of alcohol, sedatives or tranquilizers; and smoking. In the case of central sleep apnea, risk factors include: being male, heart disorders, and stroke or brain tumor (these conditions can impair the brain's ability to regulate breathing).The same risk factors for obstructive sleep apnea are also risk factors for complex sleep apnea. In addition, complex sleep apnea may be more common in people who have heart disorders (Mayo Clinic, 1998).

NEUROPSYCHOLOGICAL/CLINICAL PRESENTATION

The most common complaints associated with sleep apnea involve loud snoring, disrupted sleep, and excessive daytime sleepiness. Patients with apnea suffer from fragmented sleep and may develop cardiovascular abnormalities because of the repetitive cycles of snoring, airway collapse, and arousal. The snoring and apneic episodes may be worse after the patient drinks alcohol or takes sleeping pills because these sedatives decrease pharyngeal muscle tone and can exacerbate obstructive sleep apnea. Although most patients are overweight and have a short, thick neck, some are of normal weight but have a small, receding jaw. Because many patients are not aware of their heavy snoring and nocturnal arousals, obstructive sleep apnea may remain undiagnosed; therefore, it is helpful to question the bedroom partner of a patient displaying symptoms such as chronic sleepiness and fatigue.

People with sleep apnea may also complain of memory problems, morning headaches, mood swings or feelings of depression, a need to urinate frequently at night (nocturia), and impotence. Gastroesophageal reflux disease (GERD) may be more prevalent in people with sleep apnea. Children with untreated sleep apnea may be hyperactive and may be diagnosed with attention deficit hyperactivity disorder (ADHD).

Daytime fatigue and sleepiness are the most significant complaints of the patient with obstructive sleep apnea with symptoms ranging along a continuum, for example, the patient falls asleep during sedentary activities, such as watching television or sitting in a movie theater. This can progress to falling asleep in embarrassing situations, such as during meals or when sitting in a car stopped at a traffic light. The patient often has to nap during the day, but typically wakes up unrefreshed.

Patients with obstructive sleep apnea show neuropsychological impairments ranging from vigilance decrements, attentional lapses, and memory gaps to decreased motor coordination. In terms of neurobehavioral performance, studies have revealed objective daytime somnolence but little impairment in memory and motor domains (Kelly, Claypoole, & Coppel, 1990). Cerebral data have shown gray matter loss in the frontal and temporo-parieto-occipital cortices, the thalamus, hippocampal region, some basal ganglia and cerebellar regions, mainly in the right hemisphere. A decrease in brain metabolism is generally right-lateralized, but more restricted than gray matter density changes, and involves the precuneus, the middle and posterior cingulate gyrus, and the parieto–occipital cortex, as well as the prefrontal cortex. Even in cases of patients displaying only minor memory and motor impairments, there are still significant cerebral changes in terms of both gray matter density and metabolic levels, indicating that these patients

may benefit from cognitive reserve and compensatory mechanisms. Therefore, it is possible that cerebral changes in obstructive sleep apnea patients may precede the onset of notable neuropsychological consequences (Khalid, 2009).

Neuropsychological evaluations can address the general deficits associated with sleep apnea such as the Beck Depression Inventory to assess depression, the Hopkins Verbal Learning Task to assess memory, and the Stroop Test to assess attention, mental speed, and mental control. Alternatively, a battery of tests such as the Halstead–Reitan or Luria–Nebraska Neuropsychological Battery, assessing a broad range of functional domains may be administered. These evaluations could be repeated after a treatment protocol has been instituted in order to assess pre- and post-functioning. The neuropsychological evaluation may also be tailored according to the specific needs of the patient. For example, if the effects of a treatment were being assessed in terms of a patient's driving ability, specific tests would be used to measure cognitive abilities accessed while driving a car. (1) Vigilance: subjects have to watch a beam on a screen moving up and down. They have to react on rarely occurring higher swings by pressing a button. (2) Alertness: simple reaction on a lamp flashing upwards. (3) Divided attention: patients have to press colored lamps when the corresponding color flashes on a board. In addition, they have to react to acoustic signs by pressing buttons and foot pedals when indicated by signals (Orth et al., 2005).

DIAGNOSIS

A physician may make an evaluation based on the symptoms or may refer the patient to a sleep disorder center to undergo further evaluation that often involves overnight monitoring of breathing and other body functions during sleep. Tests to detect sleep apnea may include nocturnal polysomnograph, where the patient is hooked up to equipment that monitors heart, lung, and brain activity, breathing patterns, arm and leg movements, and blood oxygen levels asleep.

Oximetry is another screening method that involves using a small machine that monitors and records the oxygen level in the blood while the patient is asleep. If the results are abnormal, the doctor may prescribe polysomnography to confirm the diagnosis. Oximetry doesn't detect all cases of sleep apnea, so the doctor may still recommend a polysomnogram even if the oximetry results are normal.

Portable cardiorespiratory testing has also demonstrated utility. Under certain circumstances, the doctor may provide the patient with simplified tests to be used at home to diagnose sleep apnea. These tests usually involve oximetry, measurement of airflow, and measurement of breathing patterns.

A patient with obstructive sleep apnea may be referred by his or her doctor to an ear, nose, and throat doctor (otolaryngologist) to rule out any blockage in the nose or throat. An evaluation by a heart doctor (cardiologist) or a doctor who specializes in the nervous system (neurologist) may be necessary to look for causes of central sleep apnea.

TREATMENT

For milder cases of sleep apnea, the doctor may recommend lifestyle changes such as losing weight, quitting smoking, avoiding alcohol and medications such as tranquilizers and sleeping pills (Veasey et al., 2006). Other recommendations include sleeping on one's side or abdomen rather than on one's back. Nasal passages can be kept open at night by using a saline nasal spray, nasal decongestants, or antihistamines. These medications, however, are generally recommended only for short-term use.

If these measures don't improve signs and symptoms or if apnea is moderate to severe, a number of other treatments are available. Certain devices can help open up a blocked airway. In other cases, surgery may be necessary (Mayo Clinic, 1998). Most alternative medicines for sleep apnea have not been well studied. Acupuncture has shown some benefit but also needs more study and should therefore be used in conjunction with standard treatments rather than as a replacement.

Gershom T Lazarus
Antonio E. Puente

American Sleep Apnea Association. (2008). *Sleep apnea.* Retrieved February 2009, from American Sleep Apnea Association Web site: http://www.sleepapnea.org/

Kelly, D. A., Claypoole, K. H., & Coppel, D. B. (1990). Sleep apnea syndrome: Symptomatology, associated features, and neurocognitive correlates. *Neuropsychology Review, 1*(4), 323–342.

Mayo Clinic. (1998). *Sleep apnea.* Retrieved February 2009, from Mayo Clinic. Web site: http://www.mayoclinic.com/health/sleep-apnea/DS00148

Orth, M., Duchna, H. W., Leidag, M., Widdig, W., Rasche, K., Bauer, T. T., et al. (2005). Driving simulator and neuropsychological testing in OSAS before and under CPAP therapy. *The European Respiratory Journal, 26* 898–903.

Patil, S., Schneider, H., Schwartz, A., & Smith, P. (2007). Adult obstructive sleep apnea pathophysiology and diagnosis. *Chest, 132*(1), 325–337.

Veasey, S. C., Guilleminault, C., Strohl, K. P., Sanders, M. H., Ballard, R. D., & Magalang, U. J. (2006). Medical therapy for obstructive sleep apnea: A review by the medical therapy for obstructive sleep apnea task force of the standards of practice committee of the American Academy of Sleep Medicine. *Sleep: Journal of Sleep and Sleep Disorders Research, 29*(8), 1036–1044.

White, D. (2005). Pathogenesis of obstructive and central sleep apnea. *American Journal of Respiratory and Critical Care Medicine, 172,* 1363–1370.

Yaouhi, K., Bertran, F., Clochon, P., Mézenge, F., Denise, P., Foret, J. et al (2009). A combined neuropsychological and brain imaging study of obstructive sleep apnea. *Journal of Sleep Research, 18*(1), 36–48.

SOMATOFORM AND CONVERSION DISORDERS

DESCRIPTION

Somatoform disorders are characterized by persistent bodily symptoms and concerns that cannot be fully accounted for by a diagnosable medical condition (Janca, Isaac, & Ventouras, 2006). The physical symptoms "suggest a general medical condition," but "are not fully explained by a general medical condition, by the direct effects of a substance, or by another mental disorder" (*Diagnostic and Statistical Manual of Mental Disorders, 4th Edition, Text Revision* [*DSM-IV-TR*]; American Psychiatric Association [APA], 2000, p. 485). The *DSM-IV-TR* lists the following somatoform disorders: somatization, undifferentiated somatoform, conversion, pain, hypochondriasis, body dysmorphic disorder, and somatoform disorder not otherwise specified (APA, 2000, p. 485). These will be described in detail.

The *DSM-IV-TR* (APA, 2000) reports the following lifetime prevalence rates for the somatoform disorders: somatization disorder, 0.2–2% among women and less than 0.2% in men; conversion disorder, 0.01–0.5% in general population samples, up to 3% of outpatient referrals to mental health clinics, and 1–14% in general medical/surgical inpatients; hypochondriasis, 1–5% in the general population and 2–7% among primary care outpatients; and body dysmorphic disorder, 5–40% in clinical mental health settings in individuals with anxiety or depressive disorders; and 6–15% in cosmetic surgery and dermatology settings (APA, 2000, p. 509). The prevalence rates of somatoform disorders reported in the *DSM-IV-TR* are significantly lower than those reported in other research studies.

Somatoform disorders are often comorbid with anxiety (Karvonen et al., 2007; Leiknes, Finset, Moum, & Sandanger, 2007) and depression (Leiknes et al., 2007) at rates approaching 50%. High prevalence rates of somatoform disorders leads to increased usage of medical care. Patients with somatization had approximately twice the outpatient and inpatient medical care utilization and twice the annual medical care costs of patients without such difficulties (Barsky, Orav, & Bates, 2005). When Barsky et al. (2005) extrapolated their findings to the national level, they estimated that $256 billion a year in medical care costs are attributable to the incremental effect of somatization alone in the United States.

Somatization is associated with female gender, lower level of education (Hiller, Rief, & Brahler, 2006; Karvonen et al., 2007), age greater than 45, lower household income, and a rural residence (Hiller et al., 2006). Research by Hiller et al. (2006) found that the most common complaints in patients with somatoform disorders were pain (e.g., back, head, joints, and extremities), food intolerance, sexual indifference, painful menstruation, and erectile/ejaculatory dysfunction.

NEUROPATHOLOGY/PATHOPHYSIOLOGY

Research demonstrates increased levels of physiological arousal and subjective feelings of tension when compared with controls in patients with tendencies toward somatization (Rief, Shaw, & Fichter, 1998). Rief et al. (1998) found that persons demonstrating symptoms of somatization had higher morning salivary cortisol concentrations, higher pulse rates, lower levels of finger pulse volume, and subjective feeling of tension. They also found that during a mental stress task, these persons reported more subjective distress and had higher pulse rates, whereas controls exhibited habituation to the experimental situation. Campayo et al. (2007) found mean P300 latency was significantly higher in persons with somatization disorder compared with controls, demonstrating electrophysiological disturbances in the cognitive processing of information, particularly attention and memory.

Rief et al. (2004) found that reduced amounts of certain amino acids are correlated with medically unexplained symptoms. In this study, persons with medically unexplained symptoms had significantly lower levels of plasma tryptophan (a principal precursor of serotonin), and individuals with diagnosable somatoform disorder exhibited the lowest scores of branched chain amino acids (BCAAs). The researchers hypothesized that because BCAA oxidation supplies energy to the muscle and nitrogen for the glucose alanine cycle, BCAAs may have an important function as a peripheral factor contributing to the development of unexplained physical symptoms.

Neuroimaging studies suggest differences between individuals with somatoform disorders versus controls. Structural neuroimaging (morphometric MRI) in 10 individuals with conversion disorder revealed smaller mean volumes of the left and right basal ganglia and a smaller right thalamus than controls (LaFrance, 2009). Deficits in attention and inhibition have been observed in patients with sensory and motor conversion disorders (LaFrance, 2009). Using with SPECT and functional MRI, LaFrance (2009) identified that the anterior cingulate gyrus and the orbitofrontal cortex potentially mediate the hypothesized attention and inhibition findings observed in patients with sensory and motor conversion disorders. In addition, a PET study by Hakala et al. (2002) demonstrated that the patients diagnosed with somatization disorder or undifferentiated somatoform disorder had lower cerebral metabolism rates of glucose in bilateral caudate nuclei, left putamen, and right precentral gyrus compared with healthy volunteers.

NEUROPSYCHOLOGICAL/CLINICAL PRESENTATION

Research on the neuropsychological performance of persons with somatoform disorders is inconclusive, possibly because of questionable test effort. One study comparing 10 women diagnosed with somatization disorder or undifferentiated somatoform disorder and 10 controls concluded that those with somatic symptoms performed significantly below controls in tests of semantic memory, verbal episodic memory, and visuospatial tasks and were slower to complete attentional tasks (Niemi, Portin, Aalto, Hakala, & Karlsson, 2002). However, Drane et al. (2006) found that many patients with psychogenic nonepileptic seizures (NES) did not put forth maximum effort during neuropsychological assessment based on the Word Memory Test and that when they did put forth valid effort, they demonstrated less objective evidence of neuropathology than did patients with bona fide epileptic seizures (ES).

Research using Minnesota Multiphasic Personality Inventory-2 (MMPI-2) profiles of patients with somatoform disorders found that participants with pain disorder associated with psychological factors had elevated scores on MMPI-2 scales: Hs (Hysteria), D (Depression), and Hy (Hypochondriasis), with Hs and Hy higher than D (Monsen, 2001). Patients with conversion disorder have produced elevated scores on the MMPI-2 Hs Scale (Shiri, Tsenter, Livai, Schwartz, & Vatine, 2003).

The Personality Assessment Inventory (PAI) has demonstrated utility in the diagnosis of NES. Wagner, Wymer, Topping, and Pritchard (2005) created a NES indicator by subtracting the Somatic Health Concerns Scale from the Somatic Conversion Scale (SOM-C), where a score greater than zero suggests NES based on the notion that NES participants present with greater conversion symptoms relative to overall health concerns. The NES indicator produced sensitivity of 84% and specificity of 73% for the diagnosis of NES versus ES (Wagner et al., 2005). However, research by Thompson, Hantke, Phatak, and Chaytor (2010) found the SOM-C scale alone to be just as useful at diagnosing NES.

DIAGNOSIS

In the *DSM-IV-TR* (APA, 2000) common features of somatoform disorders include the presence of medically unexplainable physical symptoms that also cannot be explained by the direct effects of a substance or by another mental disorder (p. 485). As with other *DSM-IV-TR* diagnoses, "The symptoms must cause clinically significant distress or impairment in social, occupational, or other areas of functioning" (p. 485). The *DSM-IV-TR* (to which readers are directed for thorough diagnostic criteria) includes the following seven somatoform disorders (APA, 2000, p. 485):

1. Somatization disorder is a polysymptomatic disorder that begins with onset before age 30 extends over a period of years, and characterized by a combination of four or more pain symptoms: two or more gastrointestinal symptoms, one or more sexual symptom, and one or more pseudo-neurological symptom.
2. Undifferentiated somatoform disorder is characterized by unexplained physical complaints, which last at least 6 months and are below the threshold for a diagnosis of somatization disorder.
3. Conversion disorder involves unexplained symptoms or deficits affecting voluntary motor or sensory function, suggesting a neurological condition or a general medical condition. Psychological factors are judged to be associated with the symptoms or deficits.
4. Pain disorder is characterized by pain as the focus of clinical attention. In addition, psychological factors

are judged to have an important role in pain's onset, severity, exacerbation, or maintenance.
5. Hypochondriasis is the preoccupation with the fear or idea of having a serious disease based on the patient's misperceptions of bodily symptoms or bodily functions.
6. Body dysmorphic disorder is the preoccupation with an imagined or exaggerated defect in physical appearance.
7. Somatoform disorder not otherwise specified is included for coding disorders with somatoform symptoms that do not meet the criteria for any specific somatoform disorders.

The *DSM-5* somatic symptoms disorders work group proposes replacing somatoform disorders with somatic symptom disorders and subsuming psychological factors affecting medical conditions and factitious disorders in this section because they involve presentation of physical symptoms and/or concern about medical illness (May 10, 2010, http://www.dsm5.org/Pages/Default.aspx). The work group also proposes integrating somatization disorder, hypochondriasis, undifferentiated somatoform disorder, and pain disorder as complex somatic symptom disorder as they each share common features of somatic symptoms and cognitive distortions characterized by persistent (at least 6 months) multiple somatic symptoms (or one severe symptom) that are distressing to the patient, in addition to misattributions, excessive concern or preoccupation with symptoms and illness, and that the state of being symptomatic is chronic and persistent.

The *DSM-5* somatic symptoms disorders work group also proposes modifying the diagnostic criteria for conversion disorder, including removing the requirements that the clinician actively establish that the patient is not feigning and that there are associated psychological factors, and include the importance of obtaining positive evidence of the diagnosis from appropriate neurological assessment and testing (http://www.dsm5.org/Pages/Default.aspx). Lastly, body dysmorphic disorder is being given consideration as an anxiety and obsessive-compulsive spectrum disorder. It remains to be seen, however, which if any of these changes will be incorporated in the *DSM-5*.

TREATMENT

Multiple strategies consisting of psychosocial and pharmacological treatments as well as educational interventions have been effective at managing somatoform disorders (Janca et al., 2006). In particular, cognitive behavioral therapy (CBT) has been effective across a spectrum of somatoform disorders including somatization disorder and its lower threshold variants, and also for the broader category of medically unexplained symptoms, reducing physical symptoms, psychological distress, and disability (Kroenke, 2007; LaFrance, 2009; Sumathipala, 2007). Group CBT for the treatment of body dysmorphic disorder and somatization disorder has also been found to be effective (LaFrance, 2009). In addition, Nanke and Rief (2003) found that using biofeedback in conjunction with individual CBT, physical therapy, and medical care in patients with somatization symptoms showed substantial reduction of catastrophizing of somatic sensations and a higher acceptance of psychosocial casual attributions.

In addition to cognitive behavioral intervention, research has also demonstrated psychopharmacological interventions to be effective in the treatment of somatoform disorders. For example, Altamura et al. (2003) found that the use of levosulpiride, a selective antagonist of central dopamine receptors, led to reduced total number of somatoform disorder symptoms when compared with placebo. In addition, patients with somatoform disorders that include an obsessional component (e.g., hypochondriasis, body dysmorphic disorder) tend to respond well to selective serotonin reuptake inhibitors (Fallon, 2004). Luo et al. (2009) found that persistent somatoform pain disorder patients with comorbid depression demonstrated a superior analgesic response than the individuals without depression when taking fluoxetine, which they attributed to the antidepressant effect. Other randomized, controlled trials have also demonstrated efficacy of antidepressant compounds (e.g., St. John's wort, opipramol [a tricyclic compound available in Germany]) in managing the symptoms of somatoform disorders (LaFrance, 2009).

Melissa M. Swanson
Mary E. Haines
Timothy F. Wynkoop

Altamura, A. C., DiRosa, A., Ermentini, A., Guaraldi, G. P., Invernizzi, G., Rudas, N., et al. (2003). Levosulpiride in somatoform disorders: A double-blind, placebo-controlled cross-over study. *International Journal of Psychiatry in Clinical Practice, 7,* 155–159.

American Psychiatric Association. (2000). *Diagnostic and statistical manual* (4th ed., text revision). Washington, DC: Author.

Barsky, A. J., Orav, E. J., & Bates, D. W. (2005). Somatization increases medical utilization and costs independent of psychiatric and medical comorbidity. *Archives of General Psychiatry, 62,* 903–910.

Campayo, J. G., Lopez, A. P., Lafita, C. A., Bara, I. M., Zaera, I. D., & Alvarez-Manzaneda, E. D. (2007). P300 endogen evoked potentials in somatization disorder: A controlled study. *Actas Espanolas de Psiquiatria, 35,* 52–58.

Drane, D. L., Williamson, D. J., Stroup, E. S., Holmes, M. D., Jung, M., Koerner, E., et al. (2006). Cognitive impairment is not equal in patients with epileptic and psychogenic nonepileptic seizures. *Epilepsia, 47,* 1879–1886.

Fallon, B. A. (2004). Pharmacotherapy of somatoform disorders. *Journal of Psychosomatic Research, 56,* 455–460.

Hakala, M., Karlsson, H., Ruotsalainen, U., Koponen, S., Bergman, J., Stenman, H., et al. (2002). Severe somatization in women is associated with altered cerebral glucose metabolism. *Psychological Medicine, 32,* 1379–1385.

Hiller, W., Rief, W., & Brahler, E. (2006). Somatization in the population: From mild bodily misperceptions to disabling symptoms. *Social Psychiatry and Psychiatric Epidemiology, 41,* 704–712.

Janca, A., Isaac, M., & Ventouras, J. (2006). Towards better understanding and management of somatoform disorders. *International Review of Psychiatry, 18,* 5–12.

Karvonen, J. T., Joukamaa, M., Herva, A., Jokelainen, J., Laksy, K., & Veijola, J. (2007). Somatization symptoms in young adult Finnish population: Associations with sex, educational level and mental health. *Nordic Journal of Psychiatry, 61,* 219–224.

Kroenke, K. (2007). Efficacy of treatment for somatoform disorders: A review of randomized controlled trials. *Psychosomatic Medicine, 69,* 881–888.

LaFrance, W. C. (2009). Somatoform disorders. *Seminars in Neurology, 29,* 234–246.

Leiknes, K. A., Finset, A., Moum, T., & Sandanger, I. (2007). Current somatoform disorders in Norway: Prevalence, risk factors, and comorbidity with anxiety, depression, and musculoskeletal disorders. *Social Psychiatry and Psychiatric Epidemiology, 42,* 698–710.

Luo, Y., Zhang, M., Wu, W., Li, C., Lu, Z., & Li, Q. (2009). A randomized double-blind clinical trial on analgesic efficacy of fluoxetine for persistent somatoform pain disorder. *Progress in Neuro-Psychopharmacology & Biological Psychiatry, 33,* 1522–1525.

Monsen, K. (2001). Psychological functioning and bodily conditions in patients with pain disorder associated with psychological factors. *British Journal of Medical Psychology, 74,* 183–195.

Nanke, A., & Reif, W. (2003). Biofeedback-based interventions in somatoform disorders: A randomized control trial. *Acta Neuropsychiatrica, 15,* 249–256.

Niemi, P. M., Portin, R., Aalto, S., Hakala, M., & Karlsson, H. (2002). Cognitive functioning in severe somatization—a pilot study. *Acta Psychiatrica Scandinavica, 106,* 461–463.

Rief, W., Pilger, F., Ihle, D., Verkerk, R., Scharpe, S., & Maes, M. (2004). Psychobiological aspects of somatoform

S

disorders: Contributions of monoaminergic transmitter systems. *Neuropsychobiology, 49,* 24–29.

Rief, W., Shaw, R., & Fichter, M. M. (1998). Elevated levels of psychophysiological arousal and cortisol in patients with somatization syndrome. *Psychosomatic Medicine, 60,* 198–203.

Shiri, S., Tsenter, J., Livai, R., Schwartz, I., & Vatine, J. J. (2003). Similarities between the psychological profiles of complex regional pain syndrome and conversion disorder patients. *Journal of Clinical Psychology in Medical Settings, 10,* 193–199.

Sumathipala, A. (2007). What is the evidence for the efficacy of treatments for somatoform disorder? A critical review of previous intervention studies. *Psychosomatic Medicine, 69,* 889–900.

Thompson, A. W., Hantke, N., Phatak, V., & Chaytor, N. (2010) The Personality Assessment Inventory as a tool for diagnosing psychogenic nonepileptic seizures. *Epilepsia, 51,* 161–164.

Wagner, M. T., Wymer, J. H., Topping, K. B., & Pritchard, P. B. (2005). Use of the Personality Assessment Inventory as an efficacious and cost-effective diagnostic tool for nonepileptic seizures. *Epilepsy & Behavior, 7,* 301–304.

SOTOS' SYNDROME

DESCRIPTION

Sotos' syndrome, also referred to as cerebral gigantism, is an overgrowth syndrome characterized by rapid growth during prenatal and postnatal phases, without an identified endocrine disorder. A person afflicted with the disorder will likely exhibit distinctive facial features, such as a protrusive forehead, greater than average distance between the eyes, and the eyes may have a downward slant. Advanced bone age, developmental delay and mental retardation are also common features of the disorder. Affected children may exhibit behavioral and learning difficulties. This is a nonprogressive neurological and genetic disorder (Brooks, Clayton, Brown, & Savage, 2005; Harris, 1998; National Organization for Rare Disorders [NORD], 2002).

Sotos' syndrome affects males and females equally, occurring in all ethnic groups throughout the world. The syndrome appears sporadically, although familial hereditary cases are not uncommon. In instances where familial inheritance is evident, an autosomal dominance has been suggested. There have been many cases where there is parent-to-child transmission over several generations (NORD, 2002; Rourke, 1995).

NEUROPATHOLOGY/PATHOPHYSIOLOGY

Although Sotos' syndrome is thought to be a hereditary disorder, the mode of transmission has been debated. The exact cause is unknown, and it is not clear whether all patients have the same root defect. Sixty to seventy-five percent of patients have shown a deletion or point mutation of a single gene, *NSD1*, located at chromosome 5q35. This indicates that haplo-insufficiency of *NSD1* is possibly a major cause of Sotos' syndrome. Furthermore, although a number of cases appear sporadic, it is likely that some cases go undiagnosed because of less pronounced dysmorphic facial features. Therefore, some cases that appear to be sporadic may, in fact, have a genetic link that has gone undetected (Brooks et al., 2005; NORD, 2002; Rourke, 1995).

NEUROPSYCHOLOGICAL/CLINICAL PRESENTATION

Sotos' syndrome is detected primarily by physical characteristics. There is rapid growth in the first 4 years of life, as well as prenatal overgrowth. The excessive growth is commonly evident at birth, even though growth hormone levels usually fall within a normal range. Growth rate is excessive in the first few years and then parallels the average height. Hypotonia, or low muscle tone, is usually present during infancy. Sitting, crawling, walking and other developmental milestones are often delayed. The hypotonia may improve as children get older.

Bone age is usually advanced by the 4th year, and puberty will possibly occur early, yet within the normal age range. There is a distinctive craniofacial configuration possibly including a prominent forehead, a receding frontoparietal hairline, a dolichocephalic large head, increased distance between the eyes (hypertelorism), down-slanting of palpebral fissures, high narrow palate and a small, pointed chin. X-rays show a larger-than-average skull size, a high-orbital roof, and an increased interorbital distance. ECGs are commonly abnormal. Most patients will have a premature eruption of teeth. Around 50% of cases will also have a seizure disorder. As adults, those affected will reach a height 50% greater than that of the average adult height, yet the average excessive height will still fall within the upper range for normal height (Brooks et al., 2005; Gillberg, 2003; NORD, 2002).

Behavioral problems and learning difficulties are prominent. Common behavioral problems may include aggressiveness, poor social relationships, destructiveness, compulsivity, and irritability. More than half display a low-frustration tolerance and sleep difficulties. There will likely be a delay in language and motor development, and 80–85% of patients will have a mental deficiency. Language is also deficient with a likelihood of echolalia, slurred speech, and poor articulation. There seems to be a large discrepancy between verbal and performance IQ, with performance IQ being lower than verbal IQ, probably as a result of perceptual problems. Two-thirds of those affected by Sotos' syndrome will have an IQ ranging from 50 to 70, whereas the remaining one-third will have an IQ ranging from 70 to 90. Children will likely have behavioral problems, attention deficits, and cognitive dysfunction (Harris, 1998).

DIAGNOSIS

There are no biochemical markers for Sotos' syndrome. The diagnosis is made based on clinical grounds with the most characteristic manifestations being the excessive growth and the distinctive facial and cranial malformations. Without these physical characteristics, a diagnosis for Sotos' syndrome will not be made. There are diagnostic tests used in differential diagnosis in order to exclude other possibilities including Fragile X syndrome, which can be ruled out or accepted by means of DNA analysis (NORD, 2002).

There is often significant variation in the presentation of the disorder. In some cases, the signs may be so mild that a diagnosis is never made. According to Harris (1998), the classic diagnostic criteria for Sotos' syndrome include rapid growth within the 1st year of life resulting in infants being over the 97th percentile for height. Accelerated growth rate continues for the next 4 years and then levels off to a normal rate of growth (NORD, 2002).

Diagnosis is generally made in younger children based on the excessive growth, facial features, and developmental delay. According to Brooks et al. (2005), diagnosis will not likely be made if at least one of the following criteria are not met: height above the 97th percentile based on age, head circumference larger than the 97th percentile, and/or bone-age greater than the 90th percentile. Any of the symptoms combined with developmental delay will likely lead to a diagnosis of Sotos' syndrome (Brooks et al., 2005; Harris, 1998; NORD, 2002).

TREATMENT

Important interventions include social skills training, behavior management, and management of mental retardation. Individual therapies including speech therapy, occupational therapy, special education support, physical therapy, and behavioral therapy will help with the management of any mental retardation and behavioral problems. Although excessive height is not usually a concern for male children, some feel that it is a problem in female children and suggest high doses of estrogen to lessen linear growth. Psychological counseling is useful for those affected who exhibit behavioral problems and act immaturely for their age (Harris, 1998; NORD, 2002). Family therapy is essential to help parents understand and deal with the children's difficulties.

Kelly R. Pless
Charles Golden

Brooks, C. G. D., Clayton, P. E., Brown, R. S., & Savage, M. O. (2005). *Brook's clinical pediatric endocrinology.* Oxford: Blackwell Publishing.

Gillberg, C. (2003). *Clinical child neuropsychiatry.* New York: Cambridge University Press.

Harris, J. C. (1998). *Developmental neuropsychiatry: Assessment, diagnosis and treatment of developmental disorders* (Vol. II). New York: Oxford University Press.

National Organization for Rare Disorders. (2002). *NORD Guide to rare disorders.* Philadelphia: Lippincott Williams & Wilkins.

Rourke, B. P. (1995). *Syndrome of nonverbal learning disabilities: Neurodevelopmental manifestations* New York: Guilford Press.

SPINA BIFIDA

DESCRIPTION

Spina bifida, which literally means "cleft spine" in Latin, is the most common birth defect related to the central nervous system (CNS). Spina bifida results from a malformation of the osseous (bony) spine (Izenberg, 2000; Wong, 1997), often developing during the first 28 weeks of pregnancy (Wong et al., 1999). Specifically, spina bifida involves the failure to close at the caudal end of the neural tube, which results in malformation of the spinal cord, vertebral column and individual vertebrae (Evans, 1987). Because spina bifida involves the CNS, it can manifest as a range of physical, psychological, and cognitive problems. The condition often affects the development of the brain, spinal cord, and/or their protective coverings (i.e., meninges) (Botto, Moore, Khoury, & Erickson, 1999).

Although the causes of spina bifida are not fully known, it is commonly accepted that the disorder has a multifactorial etiology and may involve a combination of genetic, nutritional, and environmental causes. One of the primary environmental risks is insufficient intake of folic acid in the mother's diet during pregnancy, which corresponds with about 70% of cases of all neural tube defects. The other 30% of cases are related to factors that may include maternal age, maternal fevers, intrauterine viral infections, hormonal effects, vitamin deficiencies, excess of vitamin A, maternal diabetes, maternal alcohol use, and other teratogens (Botto et al., 1999; Riccio & Pizzitola-Jarratt, 2005).

Spina bifida is the most common neural tube defect in the United States and affects about 1,500–2,000 of the more than 4 million babies born in the country each year. There is a significantly higher incidence of spina bifida in Caucasians than in African Americans (Riccio & Pizzitola-Jarratt, 2005; Shin, Besser, & Correa, 2008).

NEUROPATHOLOGY/PATHOPHYSIOLOGY

Although the primary defect in spinal bifida is related to a failure of the neural tube to close during embryonic development, there is evidence that the defect may also be related to splitting of the already closed neural tube. The splitting may be a result of an abnormal increase in cerebrospinal fluid (CSF) pressure during the first trimester of the pregnancy (Wong, 1997; Wong et al., 1999).

The degree of neurological abnormality is positively correlated with the level of anatomic defects. As is the case with most neural tube disorders, spina bifida is related to a wide range of primary and secondary deficits. Infants born with spina bifida often suffer early complications, including problems related to walking and coordination, skeletal malformations, incontinence of urinary and bowel functions, limb numbness, hydrocephalus, and paralysis. (Chiartti et al., 2008; Riccio & Pizzitola-Jarratt, 2005; Shin et al., 2008). Secondary complications may include scoliosis, seizures, shunt complications, urinary tract infections, allergies, skin ulcerations, obesity, decreased growth, learning and cognitive problems, and emotional difficulties (Hoeman, 1997; Klingbeil, Baer, & Wilson, 2004; Simeonsson, McMillen, & Huntington, 2002). In addition, about 80% to 90% of children with spina bifida develop hydrocephalus (Riccio & Pizzitola-Jarratt, 2005; Wong, 1997).

Depending upon whether the neural tissue is exposed to the external environment or covered by the skin, spina bifida has different presentations; thus, it is categorized into two major groups: open and closed (Chiaretti et al., 2008). Spina bifida occulta, or the closed neural tube defect, refers to a defect that is not visible externally. This type of spina bifida is the "mildest" and most common form in which one or more vertebrae are malformed. Often the malformations within the vertebrae do not affect the spinal cord. It is estimated that about 10% to 30% of the general population have this form of spina bifida (Rauen, 1995). Spina bifida occulta rarely causes disability and may not be noticed unless there are associated neuromuscular manifestations, such as pain, muscle weakness, and bowel dysfunctions (Wong et al., 1999).

Spina bifida cystica refers to the visible defects that are manifested by an external sac-like protrusion. On average, 1 out of 1,000 babies in the United States is born with this form of spinal bifida (Izenberg, 2000). Cystica, also referred to as spina bifida manifesta, has two forms: meningocele and myelomeningocele. In meningocele, the meninges protrude from the spinal opening, and the malformation may or may not be covered by a layer of skin. The protrusion is filled with the CSF and forms a balloon through a gap in the vertebrae. Meningocele may be harmless to the nervous system if the sac contains only CSF; however, if the sac traps nerves, the condition may cause difficulties controlling bladder and muscles. Meningocele usually requires surgery during infancy to place the meninges back inside and close the gap in the vertebrae (Izenberg, 2000). Some patients with meningocele may have few or no symptoms, whereas others may experience symptoms similar to closed neural tube defects (Wong, 1997).

Myelomeningocele is the most severe type of spina bifida. As in meningocele, the meninges protrude through the gap in vertebrae forming a sac, but in myelomeningocele the spinal cord bulges as well. The sac can be covered by skin or the nerves with the spinal cord can be exposed. In myelomeningocele, the higher the gap occurs in the spinal column, the more severe the neuromuscular and cognitive disturbances. Usually, the affected individuals suffer paralysis below the abdominal vertebrae, have problems with the control of their bladder or bowel, and develop hydrocephalus (Izenberg, 2000). Myelomeningocele requires surgery within 24–48 hours of birth (Izenberg, 2000; Wong et al., 1999). In addition, individuals with myelomeningocele are at high risk of meningitis, an infection in the meninges. Children with myelomeningocele who also suffer from hydrocephalus may have cognitive difficulties and learning disabilities, including difficulties paying attention, problems with language and reading comprehension, and trouble learning math (Wong et al., 1999).

NEUROPSYCHOLOGICAL/CLINICAL PRESENTATION

Spina bifida is associated with significant clinical complications that often affect the quality of life and survival chances of the affected individuals (Shin et al., 2008). Complications in spina bifida range from minor physical problems to severe physical and mental disabilities. However, most people with spina bifida are of normal intelligence. The clinical manifestation of spina bifida vary depending upon the type and degree of spinal defect, the size and location of the malformation, whether or not skin covers it, whether or not spinal nerves protrude from it, and the type of involved spinal nerves. In general, all nerves located below the malformation are affected, and the higher the malformation occurs on the back, the greater the amount of neurologic damage and neuromuscular abnormality (Wong et al., 1999).

Sensory disturbances, such as impaired pain perception, may accompany motor and muscular dysfunction. Moreover, defective nerve supply to the bladder involves sphincter and detrusor tone, which can cause dribbling of urine. Poor anal sphincter tone and poor anal skin reflex can result in a lack of bowel control and rectal prolapse. The abnormal nervation of the muscles in the lower extremities may produce joint deformities in utero. These usually involve flexion or extension contractures, talipes valgus or varus contractures, kyphosis, lumbosacral scoliosis, and dislocation of the hips (Wong et al., 1999).

DIAGNOSIS

Prenatal Diagnosis

There are several methods of testing for spina bifida prenatally. The most common screening methods are maternal serum alpha fetoprotein (MSAFP) screening, fetal ultrasound, and amniocentesis (Izenberg, 2000). nig.com is not in refs. The MSAFP test is usually performed between 16 and 18 weeks of pregnancy and assesses the level of a protein called alpha fetoprotein (AFP), which is produced by the fetus and placenta. Abnormally high levels of AFP in the mother's bloodstream may indicate a possibility of developmental defect, including spina bifida. If high levels of AFP are detected, an ultrasound or amniocentesis is recommended for confirmation of diagnosis. Although amniocentesis cannot reveal the severity of spina bifida, finding high levels of AFP in the amniotic fluid may indicate the presence of the disorder.

Postnatal Diagnosis

The symptoms of spina bifida vary from person to person; however, the postnatal diagnosis is based on clinical manifestations and examination of the meningeal sac. Closed forms of spina bifida often have no outward signs of the disorder but may be recognized due to an abnormal tuft or clump of hair or a small dimple or birthmark on the skin at the site of the spinal malformation (Wong et al., 1999). The primary methods used in diagnosis are MRI, CT scans, and myelography (not in refs Wong et al., 1999). Mild cases of spina bifida not diagnosed during prenatal testing may be detected postnatally by X-ray during routine examination.

TREATMENT

Currently, there is no cure for spina bifida because the nerve tissue cannot be replaced or repaired. Treatment for spina bifida may include surgery, medication, and physiotherapy and may involve a multidisciplinary approach involving specialties of neurology, neurosurgery, pediatrics, urology, orthopedics, rehabilitation, physical therapy, occupational therapy, and social services. The treatment usually focuses on the three most crucial areas: (1) difficulties associated with primary disorders, which include hydrocephalus, paralysis, orthopedic abnormalities, and genitourinary abnormalities; (2) possible secondary problems such as meningitis, hypoxia, and hemorrhage; and (3) other abnormalities, including cardiac or gastrointestinal malformations (Wong et al., 1999). Many individuals with spina bifida need assistive devices such as braces, crutches, or wheelchairs. Ongoing therapy and medical care are often necessary throughout the affected individual's life. Surgery to close the newborn's spinal opening is performed within 24–48 hours after birth to minimize the risk of infection and maximize the neurological outcome (Izenberg, 2000; Wong et al., 1999)

The main preventive factor for spina bifida is folic acid supplementation. Studies have shown that by adding folic acid to their diets, women of childbearing age can reduce the risk of having a child with spina bifida and other neural tube defects (Wong, 1997; Wong et al., 1999). The current recommendation for women of childbearing age is to consume 400 µg of folic acid daily.

Anya Mazur-Mosiewicz
Raymond S. Dean

Botto, L., Moore, C., Khoury, M., & Erickson, J. (1999). Neural-tube defects. *New England Journal of Medicine, 341,* 1509–1919.

Chiaretti, A., Rendeli, C., Antonelli, A., Barone, G., Focarelli, B., Tobacco, F., et al. (2008). GDNF plasma levels in spina bifida: Correlation with severity of spinal damage and motor function. *Journal of Neurotrauma, 25,* 1477–1481.

Evans, O. B. (1987). *Manual of child neurology.* Edinburgh, UK: Churchill Livingstone.

Hoeman, S. (1997). Primary care of children with spina bifida. *Nurse Practitioner, 22,* 60–62.

Hunter, A. (1993). Brian and spinal cord. In R. E. Stevenson, J. G. Hall, & R. M. Goodman (Eds.), *Human malformation and related abnormalities* (pp. 127–130). New York: Oxford University Press.

Izenberg, N. (2000). *Human diseases and conditions.* New York: Charles Scribner's Sons.

Klingbeil, H., Baer, H., & Wilson, P. (2004). Aging with disability. *Archives of Physical Medicine and Rehabilitation, 85,* 68–73.

Rauen, K. (1995). *Guidelines for spina bifida health care services throughout life.* Washington, DC: Spina Bifida Association of America.

Riccio, C. A., & Pizzitola-Jarratt, K. (2005). Abnormalities of neurological development. In R. C. D'Amato, E. Fletcher-Janzen, & C. R. Reynolds (Eds.), *Handbook of School Psychology.* Hoboken, NJ: Wiley.

Shin, M., Besser, L. M., & Correa, A. (2008). Prevalence of spina bifida among children and adolescents in metropolitan Atlanta. *Birth Defects Research, 82,* 748–754.

Simeonsson, R. J., McMillen, J., & Huntington, G. S. (2002). Secondary conditions in children and youth with disabilities. *Research in Mental Retardation and Developmental Disabilities, 8*(3), 198–205.

Wong, D. (1997). *Pedatric nursing* (5th ed.). Tulsa, OK: Mosby.

Wong, D., Hockenberry-Eaton, M., Wilson, D., Winkelstein, M. L., Ahmann, E., & Divito-Thomas, D. (1999). *Nursing car of infants and children* (6th ed.). Tulsa, OK: Mosby.

SPINAL CORD INJURY

DESCRIPTION

Spinal cord injury (SCI) involves damage to the spinal cord that results in a loss or interruption of normal sensation and/or motor function. Motor vehicle accidents are the most frequent cause of SCI. Other causes include falls, work-, sports-, and violence-related injuries. Males and young adults between the ages of 21 and 30 are at an increased risk of suffering from an SCI. Additional risk factors include alcohol and drug use (Sekhon & Fehlings, 2001). The etiology, level, and grade of injury, as well as the individual's age at the time of the injury, are factors that influence prognosis. SCIs most commonly occur at the cervical level. Injuries affecting the first, second, or third cervical vertebrae are most frequently associated with mortality. More severe neurogenic deficits and injury at a younger age (equal to or less than 15 years of age) are also associated with increased mortality (Shavelle, DeVivo, Paculdo, Vogel, & Strauss, 2007). Effective management of spinal cord injuries, including immobilization and the administration of methylprednisolone, improves survival rates and prognosis.

NEUROPATHOLOGY/PATHOPHYSIOLOGY

The primary mechanism of injury refers to the initial insult to the spinal cord. The initial impact may lead to a contused, compressed, lacerated, disrupted, and/or transected spinal cord. Cell injury and death result, as well as axonal demyelization. Neurons in the central nervous system are very limited in their ability to regenerate. The obstructing presence of oligodendrocytes and astrocytes are thought to play a role in restricting axonal regeneration.

Secondary mechanisms refer to various processes or changes that follow an SCI. These changes or processes, which include vascular changes, electrolyte changes, biochemical changes, loss of energy metabolism, loss of neurotrophic factor support, free radical formation, and glutamate excitotoxity exacerbate the initial injury. Hemorrhage, edema, and ischemia may occur resulting in additional cell death through necrosis or apoptosis. Vascular changes result from the release of cytokines. SCI may initially result in hypertension and an increase in heart rate followed by an extended period of bradycardia and hypotension. Individuals with spinal cord injuries may also experience spinal shock, neurogenic shock, and/or thrombosis. Electrolyte changes that accompany spinal cord injuries include increased intracellular calcium and sodium levels and increased extracellular potassium levels (Agrawal & Fehlings, 1996; Yong & Koreh, 1986). After a SCI, macrophages remove cellular debris and a cavity is formed. Glial scar formation ensues creating an obstacle for neuroregeneration (Ao et al., 2007).

X-rays, CT scans, MRI, and myelograms are radiographic studies used to identify spinal cord injuries (Brant-Zawadzki, Miller, & Federle, 1981; Kulkarni et al., 1987; Virapongse & Kier, 1982). Spinal cord injuries have been associated with intraspinal hemorrhage, cord edema, and contusion. On T2-weighted magnetic resonance images, intraspinal hemorrhage reveals reduced signal intensity, and cord edema and contusion reveal elevated signal intensity (Kulkarni et al., 1987). In instances where obvious cord abnormalities cannot be visualized, CT scans, MRIs, and myelograms may reveal skeletal and/or ligament injuries (Kulkarni et al., 1987).

NEUROPSYCHOLOGICAL/CLINICAL PRESENTATION

Signs and symptoms of spinal cord injuries include edema of the cord, loss of movement, loss of sensation, pain, difficulty breathing, and loss of bowel or bladder control. Urinary infections, pressure ulcers, and pulmonary embolisms are common complications of spinal cord injuries (Harkonen, Lepisto, Paakkala, Patiala, & Rokkanen, 1979).

The degree of motor and sensory impairment resulting from an SCI depends upon the severity and vertebral level of the injury. Individuals with incomplete spinal cord injuries have some intact sensory and/or motor function below the level of the injury, whereas individuals with complete spinal cord injuries have no sensory or motor function below the level of the injury. Complete injuries are associated with more severe impairments, as are injuries at higher levels of the vertebral column. Tetraplegia results from an injury to the cervical level of the spinal column, whereas paraplegia is the consequence of injury to the thoracic, lumbar, or sacral level of the spinal column. The level of sensory loss typically corresponds to the level of motor loss in individuals with complete spinal cord injuries. Respiratory support is often necessary for individuals with tetraplegia from C1-, C2-, or C3-level injuries, particularly if the injury is complete. Also, these individuals require great assistance in activities of daily living. Individuals injured at the C4 level can typically breathe independently; however, they, too, require aid in performing most daily activities. Mobility of the shoulders and upper arms are seen in individuals with injuries below the C5 level, and when aided by assistive devices, these individuals may be able to feed themselves and perform other activities of daily living. Injuries below the C6 level allow individuals use of their hands. Though finger movement is impaired, these individuals can drive with special equipment and may be able to live independently. The prospect of an independent life is even greater if the C7 level is uninjured. Injuries to the upper thoracic region (T1–T6) allow for normal movement of the upper extremities. Individuals with these injuries can use manual wheelchairs and live independently, though they may have difficulties with balance. Individuals with injuries below the T11 level may be able to walk with leg braces and other assistive devices (Trieschmann, 1988). The Functional Independence Measure and the Spinal Cord Independence Measure (SCIM) are two instruments used to evaluate the functional capabilities and progress of individuals with spinal cord injuries. Research suggests the SCIM may be more effective in detecting some functional changes in individuals with tetraplegia, paraplegia, and incomplete spinal cord injuries (Catz, Itzkovich, Agranov, Ring, & Tamir, 2001).

Besides physical deficits, there are also neuropsychological impairments related to spinal cord injuries. Spinal cord injuries have been associated with deficits in processing speed, motor speed, and verbal learning, as assessed by the Symbol Digit Modalities Test-Written, Grooved Pegboard, and Rey Auditory Learning Test, respectively (Hess, Marwitz, & Kreutzer, 2003). Even many years post-injury (M = 17 years), research reveals that individuals with spinal cord injuries demonstrate impairments in processing speed; however, in that same study, no deficits in memory, visuospatial skills, attention, or executive functioning were demonstrated (Dowler et al., 1995). These abnormal neuropsychological findings can be attributed to the frequently occult comorbid occurrence of traumatic brain injury, which occurs in as many as 40% to 50% of persons presenting with SCI (Davidoff, Roth, Morris, Bleiberg, & Meyer, 1986; Richards, Brown, Hagglund, Bua, & Reeder, 1988).

DIAGNOSIS

Initial indications that an individual may have suffered an SCI include dilated pupils, paralysis, signs of shock, edema, and head, neck, or back pain. X-rays, CT scans, MRIs, and/or myelograms are helpful in diagnosing spinal cord injuries, as they allow for the visualization of fractures and/or soft-tissue lesions.

If an SCI is suspected, the individual should be immobilized and evaluated to see if their respiratory and circulatory systems are compromised. This evaluation often includes an assessment of the person's vital signs, blood pressure, skin color, nail bed color, respiration, and responsiveness. A comprehensive neurological exam should also be conducted. The International Standards for Neurological Classification of Spinal Cord Injury, also called the American Spinal Injury Association (ASIA) Standards, can be used to assess the extent and level of sensory and motor impairments (Ditunno, Young, Donovan, & Creasey, 1994). The sensory examination involves a pinprick and light touch to key points corresponding to the 28 dermatomes. These points are tested bilaterally. Absent, impaired, or normal perception of the stimulus is scored as a 0, 1, or 2, respectively. Whether or not the individual is able to perceive sensation at the anal sphincter should also be noted. The motor examination involves the assessment of ten paired muscles, which are examined bilaterally. A 6-point scale, ranging from 0, total paralysis, to 6, normal movement with no limitation in range of motion, is used to rate the strength of the muscle pair. Whether or not the sphincter is able to contract should also be noted. The ASIA impairment scale has five grades, A, B, C, D, and E. Grade A denotes a complete injury. Grades B through D denote incomplete injuries of decreasing severity, and Grade E indicates normal functioning. Besides a neurological examination, an assessment of the autonomic nervous system is also recommended for individuals with spinal cord injuries, as autoregulation may be impaired (Alexander et al., 2009). Areflexia, hypotension, and/or bradycardia may be present as well as bowel, bladder, or sexual dysfunction.

TREATMENT

Pharmacological and conservative treatments are available to individuals with spinal cord injuries. Methylprednisolone given in high doses within 8 hours of an acute SCI has been shown to be an effective pharmacological treatment associated with improved recovery (Bracken, 2001). To reduce the risk of further injury to the spinal cord, individuals with spinal injuries should be immobilized and receive appropriate treatment for orthopedic problems. Tetraplegia may be treated conservatively with skull traction and an orthopedic neck brace (Harkonen et al., 1979). Electronic wheelchairs, computers, leg braces, and other assistive devices as well as physical and occupational therapy may be helpful in improving the mobility and functional capacity of individuals with spinal cord injuries (Hulsebosch, 2002; Kakulas, 2004).

New treatments focusing on regeneration of the spinal cord are presently being investigated. One strategy is the implantation of neuronal stem cells that could differentiate into healthy replacement neurons (Okano et al., 2003). Another approach to neuronal regeneration is the use of olfactory ensheathing cells, which are glial cells capable of promoting axonal growth (Ao et al., 2007). Other research is investigating factors that guide axonal growth during development in hopes that these factors may be able to promote regeneration later in life (Harel & Strittmatter, 2006). Neurotropic factors, including brain-derived neurotropic factor, neurotrophin-3, and neurotropin-4, have been found to stimulate axonal growth (Bregman, McAtee, Dai, & Kuhn, 1997).

Alyse Barker
Mandi Musso
William Drew Gouvier

Agrawal, S. K., & Fehlings, M. G. (1996). Mechanisms of secondary injury to spinal cord axons in vitro: Role of Na+, Na+-K+-ATPase, the N+-H+ exchanger, and the Na+-Ca2+ exchanger. *Journal of Neuroscience, 16*(2), 545–552.

Alexander, M. S., Biering-Sorensen, F., Bodner, D., Brackett, N. L., Cardenas, D., Charlifue, S., et al. (2009). International standards to document remaining autonomic function after spinal cord injury. *Spinal Cord, 47*(1), 36–43.

Ao, Q., Wang, A. J., Chen, G. Q., Wang, S. J., Zuo, H. C., & Zhang, X. F. (2007). Combined transplantation of neural stem cells and olfactory ensheathing cells for the repair of spinal cord injuries. *Medical Hypotheses, 69*(6), 1234–1237.

Bracken, M. B. (2001). Methylprednisolone and acute spinal cord injury — an update of the randomized evidence. *Spine, 26*(24), 47–54.

Brant-Zawadzki, M., Miller, E. M., & Federle, M. P. (1981). CT in the evaluation of spine trauma. *American Journal of Roentgenology, 136*(2), 369–375.

Bregman, B. S., McAtee, M., Dai, H. N., & Kuhn, P. L. (1997). Neurotropic factors increase axonal growth after spinal cord injury and transplantation in the adult rat. *Experimental Neurology, 148*(2), 475–494.

Catz, A., Itzkovich, M., Agranov, E., Ring, H., & Tamir, A. (2001). The spinal cord independence measure (SCIM): Sensitivity to functional changes in subgroups of spinal cord lesion patients. *Spinal Cord, 39*(2), 97–100.

Davidoff, G., Roth, E., Morris, J., Bleiberg, J., & Meyer, P. R. (1986). Assessment of closed head injury in trauma-related spinal cord injury. *Paraplegia, 24*(2), 97–104.

Ditunno, J. F., Young, W., Donovan, W. H., & Creasey, G. (1994). The international standards booklet for neurological and functional classification of spinal cord injury. *Paraplegia, 32*(2), 70–80.

Dowler, R. N., O'Brien, S. A., Haaland, K. Y., Harrington, D. L., Feel, F., & Fiedler, K. (1995). Neuropsychological functioning following a spinal cord injury. *Applied Neuropsychology, 2*(3–4), 124–129.

Harel, N. Y., & Strittmatter, S. M. (2006). Can regenerating axons recapitulate developmental guidance during recovery from spinal cord injury? *Nature Reviews Neuroscience, 7*(8), 603–616.

Harkonen, M., Lepisto, P., Paakkala, T., Patiala, H., & Rokkanen, P. (1979). Spinal-cord injuries associated with vertebral fractures and dislocations: Clinical and radiological results in 30 patients. *Archives of Orthopaedic and Traumatic Surgery, 94*(3), 185–190.

Hess, D. W., Marwitz, J. H., & Kreutzer, J. S. (2003). Neuropsychological impairments after spinal cord injury: A comparative study with mild traumatic brain injury. *Rehabilitation Psychology, 48*(3), 151–156.

Hulsebosch, C. E. (2002). Recent advances in pathophysiology and treatment of spinal cord injury. *Advances in Physiology Education, 26*(4), 238–255.

Kakulas, B. A. (2004). Neuropathology: The foundation for new treatments in spinal cord injury. *Spinal Cord, 42*(10), 549–563.

Kulkarni, M. V., McArdle, C. B., Kopanicky, D., Miner, M., Cotler, H. B., Lee, K. F., et al. (1987). Acute spinal cord injury: MR imaging at 1.5 T[1]. *Radiology, 164*(3), 837–843.

Okano, H., Ogawa, Y., Nakamura, M., Kaneko, S., Iwanami, A., & Toyama, Y. (2003). Transplantation of neural stem cells into the spinal cord after injury. *Seminars in Cell and Developmental Biology, 14*(3), 191–198.

Richards, J. S., Brown, L., Hagglund, K., Bua, B. G., & Reeder, K. (1988). Spinal cord injury and concomitant traumatic brain injury: Results of a longitudinal investigation. *American Journal of Physical Medicine and Rehabilitation, 67*(5), 211–216.

Sekhon, L. H. S., & Fehlings, M. G. (2001). Epidemiology, demographics, and pathophysiology of acute spinal cord injury. *Spine, 26*(245), S2–S12.

Shavelle, R. M., DeVivo, M. J., Paculdo, D. R., Vogel, L. C., & Strauss, D. J. (2007). Long-term survival after childhood spinal cord injury. *Journal of Spinal Cord Medicine, 30*, S48–S54.

Trieschmann, R. B. (1988) *Spinal cord injuries: Psychological, social, vocational rehabilitation* (2nd ed.). New York: Demos Publication.

Virapongse, C., & Kier, E. L. (1982). Mitrizamide myelography in cervical-spine trauma—a modified technique using lateral fluoroscopy. *Radiology, 144*(3), 636–637.

Yong, W., & Koreh, I. (1986). Potassium and calcium changes in injured spinal cords. *Brain Research, 365*(1), 42–53.

SPINAL MUSCULAR ATROPHIES

DESCRIPTION

Spinal muscular atrophies (SMA) are a group of rare neuromuscular diseases that correspond with progressive degeneration of lower motor neurons of the medulla and spinal cord. The presentation arises from a defect in the survival motor neuron gene (*SMN1*), located on chr5q (Sumner, 2007), which causes a deficiency in essential proteins that feed the lower motor neurons (Lefebvre et al., 1995; Lefebvre et al., 1997; Lunn & Wang, 2008;). SMA presents with an annual incidence of 1 in 10,000 births (Wirth, 2000), and is a leading genetic cause of infant death. As the lower motor neurons degenerate in SMA, the affected individual's muscles atrophy, leading to symmetrical, proximal weakness. Global hypotonia, pulmonary insufficiency, and autonomic and bulbar dysfunction may also present (Graham, Athiraman, Laubach, & Sethna, 2009).

Four different variants of SMA have been described. They are differentiated by the age of onset, the severity of symptoms, and the maximal motor function attained (Zerres & Davies, 1999). In SMA-1, symptoms develop in infancy and progress rapidly. Individuals are never able to sit or walk on their own. In severe cases, when the lungs become involved, infants may die due to respiratory distress. SMA-2 arises prior to 18 months of age and while infants may sit up on their own, they never are able to walk unaided. SMA-3 sufferers eventually can walk without assistance, but often exhibit muscular weakness. SMA-4 onset is not until adulthood and is associated with minimal symptoms (Lunn & Wang, 2008; Sumner, 2007).

NEUROPATHOLOGY/PATHOPHYSIOLOGY

SMAs arise from degeneration of the anterior horn cells of the spinal cord and bulbar motor neurons. In rare instances, degeneration of the dorsal root ganglion cells and sensory columns and loss of neurons in the posteroventral nucleus of the thalamus may be seen. Neurogenic muscular atrophy develops characterized by groupings of small round fibers and type-I hypertrophied fibers on biopsy (Crawford & Pardo, 1996).

The genetic basis for the SMAs have been mapped to 5q-11.2-13.3 leading to reduced levels of SMN protein because of mutations in the *SMN1* gene . It is inherited in an autosomal recessive fashion. While *SMN1* mutation is hallmark of the presentation, oweing to deficits in the SMN protein, the latter is not completely absent – one would not be able to live without any SMN protein (Schrank et al., 1997). Small amounts are produced by the *SMN2* gene, which is nearly identical to *SMN1*. In fact, the number of *SMN2* gene copies expressed by an individual in many respects determines the subtype of SMA, as greater numbers of *SMN2* copies leads to higher amounts of SMN protein. which reduces symptom severity; lower numbers of *SMN2* copies corresponds with lower SMN protein levels and greater severity of symptoms (Campbell et al., 1997).

NEUROPSYCHOLOGICAL/CLINICAL PRESENTATION

Degeneration of spinal anterior horn neurons and occasionally brainstem nuclei correspond to a range of clinical characteristics, but the hallmark features include hypotonia, weakness, and cranial nerve palsies. Differentiation among the types is largely linked to age of onset and severity of symptoms, which both correspond with the amount of residual *SMN2*. For example, while type 1 manifests in infancy and leads to death, often before infants are 1 year old, type IV does not demonstrate symptom onset until the fourth decade of life and is not strongly linked to reduced life expectancy.

Across all types, onset and progression is insidious, leading to somewhat generalized weakness, affecting proximal muscles prior to distal and caudal regions prior to rostral. Siddique, Sufit, and Siddique (2007) summarized the differences among groups, which are summarized in Table 1.

Diagnosis

The diagnosis of SMA is most appropriately done through a combination of EMG and muscle biopsy and histochemistry. As noted by Siddique et al. (2007), homozygous deletion of SMN is a sensitive test for confirming diagnosis across all types in comparison to one another and potential differentials. Fibrillation and normal-sized residual motor units present in denervated muscle fibers in type 1, whereas types 2 and 3 manifest large motor units with absence of spontaneous activity (Siddique, et al., 2007). Age of onset, nature of symptoms, and the amount of residual *SMN2* can all aid in differentiating between the subtypes.

TREATMENT

The SMAs are incurable and currently treatment is limited. The primary goal, if it can be achieved, is to increase SMN levels, the depletion of which serves as the basis of the disorder. Different strategies have been proposed including the use of gene therapy vectors to provide a continuous source of exogenous SMN or activating the *SMN2* promoter to modulate the endogenous *SMN2* gene (Grzeschik, Ganta, Prior, Heavlin, & Wang, 2005; Hahnen et al., 2006; Riessland et al., 2006; Avila et al., 2007). However, while these have shown some efficacy in the laboratory, largely through animal models, there has been a lack of clearly positive evidence in translational research within the clinical setting (Oskoui & Kaufmann, 2008). Mildly positive findings have been reported in relationship to sodium butyrate, valproic acid, and potentially riluzole (Siddique et al., 2007).

Given the lack of effective treatment to halt progression, interventions are often directed at symptom resolution. Physical and occupation therapy is often recommended to aid in maintaining ambulation and independence from a motoric standpoint. Braces may be required on the legs and used in combination with forearm crutches as the arms are affected less and may offer some means of compensation in ambulation. Eventually individuals may need to rely on wheelchairs. Oxygen and potentially even ventilation may be required as the disease progresses based on the extent of respiratory weakness. Feeding tubes are often needed in SMA type 1. Genetic counseling is recommended for parents who have a child with SMA or

Table 1
DIFFERENTIATION AMONG SPINAL MUSCULAR ATROPHIES

Type	*Age of Onset*	*Symptoms*	*Prognosis*
SMA type 1	In utero–6 mos	Hypotonia Generalized weakness Poor sucking Poor swallowing Poor breathing Never able to sit up	95% die within first year
SMA type 2	3–15 mos	Proximal leg weakness Fasciculations Fine hand tremor Never able to walk No facial weakness	Often die prior to age 10 Some survive into adolescence and even adulthood Dependent upon respiratory symptoms
SMA type 3	15 mos–teens	Proximal leg weakness delayed obtainment of motor development milestones	Life expectancy shortened, but not specific Dependent upon respiratory symptoms
SMA type 4	20–40 years on average	Proximal weakness	Life expectancy not shortened

Adapted from Siddique et al. (2007).

for SMA patients themselves who may be thinking of having children, most usually are types 3 or 4.

Chad A. Noggle
Michelle R. Pagoria

Avila A. M., Burnett, B. G., Taye, A. A., Gabanella, F., Knight, M. A., Hartenstein, P., . . . Sumner CJ. (2007). Trichostatin A increases SMN expression and survival in a mouse model of spinal muscular atrophy. *The Journal of Clinical Investigation, 117*(3), 659–671.

Campbell, L., Potter, A., Ignatius, J., Dubowitz, V., & Davies, K. (1997). Genomic variation and gene conversion in spinal muscular atrophy: implications for disease process and clinical phenotype. *American Journal of Human Genetics, 61*(1), 40–50.

Crawford, T. O., & Pardo, C. A. (1996). The neurobiology of childhood spinal muscular atrophy. *Neurobiology of Disease, 3,* 97–110.

Graham, R., Athiraman, U., Laubach, A. E., & Sethna, N. F. (2009). Anesthesia and perioperative medical management of children with spinal muscular atrophy. *Pediatric Anesthesia, 19,* 1054–1063

Grzeschik, S. M., Ganta, M., Prior, T. W., Heavlin, W. D., & Wang, C. H. (2005). Hydroxyurea enhances SMN2 gene expression in spinal muscular atrophy cells. *Annals of Neurology, 58*(2), 194–202.

Hahnen, E., Eyüpoglu, I. Y., Brichta, L., Haastert, K., Tränkle, C., Siebzehnrübl, F. A., . . . Blümcke, I. (2006). In vitro and ex vivo evaluation of second-generation histone deacetylase inhibitors for the treatment of spinal muscular atrophy. *Journal of Neurochemistry, 98*(1), 193–202.

Lefebvre, S., Burglen, L., Reboullet, S., Clermont, O., Burlet, P., . . . Zeviani., M. (1995). Identification and characterization of a spinal muscular atrophy-determining gene. *Cell, 80,* 155–165.

Lefebvre, S., Burlet, P., Liu, Q., Bertrandy, S., Clermont, O., . . . Melki, J. (1997). Correlation between severity and SMN protein level in spinal muscular atrophy. *Nature Genetics, 16,* 265–269.

Lefebvre, S., Burlet, P., Liu, Q., Bertrandy, S., Clermont, O., Munnich, A., . . . Melki, J. (1997). Correlation between severity and SMN protein level in spinal muscular atrophy. *Nature Genetics, 16*(3), 265–269.

Lunn, M. R., & Wang, C. H. (2008). Spinal muscular atrophy. *Lancet, 371,* 2120–2133.

Oskoui, M., & Kaufmann, P., (2008). Spinal muscular atrophy. *Neurotherapeutics, 5*(4), 499–506

Riessland, M., Brichta, L., Hahnen, E., & Wirth, B. (2006). The benzamide M344, a novel histone deacetylase inhibitor, significantly increases SMN2 RNA/protein levels in spinal muscular atrophy cells. *Human Genetics, 120*(1), 101–110.

Schrank, B., Gotz, R., Gunnersen, J. M., Ure, J. M., Toyka, K. V., . . . Sendtner, M. (1997). Inactivation of the survival motor neuron gene, a candidate gene for human spinal muscular atrophy, leads to massive cell death in early mouse embryos. *Proceedings of the National Academy of Sciences of the United States of America, 94,* 9920–9925.

Siddique, N., Sufit, R., & Siddique, T. (2007). Degenerative motor, sensory, and autonomic disorders. In C. G. Goetz (Ed.), *Textbook of clinical neurology* (pp. 785–787). Philadelphia, PA: WB Saunders.

Sumner, C. J. (2007). Molecular mechanisms of spinal muscular atrophy. *Journal of Child Neurology, 22,* 979–989.

Wirth, B. (2000). An update of the mutation spectrum of the survival motor neuron gene (SMN1) in autosomal recessive spinal muscular atrophy (SMA). *Human Mutation, 15,* 228–237.

Zerres, K., & Davies, K. E. (1999). 59th ENMC International Workshop: Spinal Muscular Atrophies: Recent progress and revised diagnostic criteria 17–19 April 1998, Soestduinen, The Netherlands. *Neuromuscular Disorders: NMD, 9,* 272–278.

SPINOCEREBELLAR DEGENERATIVE DISORDERS

DESCRIPTION

The spinocerebellar degenerative disorders are a group of diseases that, as their name suggests, involve neurodegeneration of the posterior regions of the brain including the cerebellum and spinal cord. However, degeneration of the brainstem and/or the basal ganglia may also occur similar to that seen in multiple system atrophy (MSA; Gilman & Quinn, 1996). In fact, most sporadic cases of spinocerebellar degeneration are now considered MSA. This grouping includes spinocerebellar ataxia types 1, 2, 3, 6, 7, and 17, as well as dentatorubral-pallidoluysian atrophy (DRPLA), Friedrich's ataxia, and MSA. While variability across presentations is seen in terms of the clinical features, limb and truncal ataxia, dysarthria, dysphagia, dystonia, pyramidal and extrapyramidal signs, and autonomic dysfunction are common. Cognitive deficits may also occur (Schmahmann & Sherman, 1998).

NEUROPATHOLOGY/ PATHOPHYSIOLOGY

The spinocerebellar degenerative disorders are similar in that all presentations demonstrate relatively similar pathological features of deterioration of the cerebellum and/or other posterior brain regions. However, variability is seen across disease types in terms of their specific pathology, owing to their clinical differences.

SCA1 demonstrates a constellation of pathological changes including loss of Purkinje and granule cells in the cerebellum; neuronal loss and gliosis of the dentate gyrus, inferior olives and pontine nuclei; and neuronal loss in the substantia nigra, putamen, pallid, and subthalamic nucleus (Schöls, Amoiridis, Büttner, Przuntek, Epplen, & Riess, 2004). These changes have been associated with diffuse hypoperfusion involving the caudate and putamen of the basal ganglia as well as the cerebellum and brainstem (Gilman, Sima, Junck, Kluin, Koeppen, Lohman, & Little, 1996). These changes have also been noted in the cerebral cortex as well.

SCA2 commonly presents with degeneration of the supratentorial and infratentorial regions (Brenneis, Bösch, Schocke, Wenning, & Poewe, 2003). This includes the cerebellum (including Purkinje and granular cells and cerebellar peduncles), thalamus, pons, mesencephalon, nondominant orbitofrontal and tempromesial cortices, sensorimotor cortex bilaterally, inferior olives, and the cerebral cortex (Schöls et al., 2004; Wüllner et al., 2005).

SCA3 consists of degeneration involving the globus pallidus, substantia nigra, red nucleus, pontine nuclei, subthalamic nucleus, superior cerebellar peduncle, dentate nucleus, oculomotor nucleus, medial longitudinal fasciculus, anterior horn, spinocerebellar tracts, Clark's nuclei, intermediolateral column, and lateral reticular nucleus (Rüb, de Vos, Schultz, Brunt, Paulson, & Braak, 2002).

SCA6, unlike the first three types of spinocerebellar ataxia, is not associated with more widespread degeneration. Rather, this type is characterized by fairly focal degeneration of the cerebellum including loss of Purkinje and granular cells although deterioration of the dentate nucleus is also commonly seen (Takahashi, Ikeuchi, Honma, Hayashi, & Tsuji, 1998). Some studies have also reported reduced metabolism in the cerebral cortex (Soong, Liu, Wu, Lu, & Lee, 2001), while others have not (Honjo et al., 2004).

SCA7, presents with a causative gene mutation of a translated CAG repeat expansion in gene coding for ataxin-7, which is expressed throughout the brain in the cytoplasm of neurons. This type present with primary atrophy of an olivopontocerebellar origin.

SCA17 is associated with neuronal loss and atrophy of the caudate nucleus, putamen, thalamus, and both the frontal and temporal lobes, as well as loss of Purkinje cells in the cerebellum (Bruni et al., 2004; Rolfs et al., 2003). Reduced metabolism in the

basal ganglia and cerebellum are commonly noted (Minerop et al., 2005).

Dentatorubral-pallidoluysian atrophy (DRPLA) presents in conjunction with leukodystrophic changes and calcifications in the regions of the basal ganglia in addition to cerebellar and brainstem atrophy. DNA analysis reveals multiple CAG repeats (Ikeuchi, Onodera, Oyake, Koide, Tanaka, & Tsuji, 1995). Degeneration of the dentatorubral pallidoluysian and fatigio-vestibular systems are hallmark features (Schöls et al., 2004).

Finally, Friedrich's ataxia, is most commonly caused by loss of function mutations in the frataxin gene and corresponds with mutation on chromosome 9q13. Interestingly, cerebellar degeneration is not seen; rather, it affects the spinocerebellar tracts, posterior columns, and corticospinal tracts.

NEUROPSYCHOLOGICAL/CLINICAL PRESENTATION

Across all forms of spinocerebellar degeneration, although variability is seen, neurocognitive residuals very much adhere to a profile indicative of prefrontal dysfunction that is consistent with what is recognized as cerebellar cognitive affective syndrome. Within this model and on functional imaging the cerebellum has demonstrated activation and thus a role in attention (Allen, Buxton, Wong, & Courchesne, 1997), general cognitive and verbal processing (Kim, Ugurbil, & Strick, 1994), semantic fluency and word generation (Klein, Milner, Zatorre, Meyer, & Evans, 1995), motor sequence learning (Jenkins, Brooks, Nixon, Frackowiak, & Passingham, 1994), and verbal and working memory (Desmond, Gabrieli, Wagner, Ginier, & Glover, 1997) among other areas. The cognitive influence of the cerebellum in these areas is not necessarily a one-to-one link with the region and the function; rather, through indirect disruption of broader systems and loops including cerebrocerebellar circuitry, corticostriatal-thalamocortical circuitry and the frontal lobe. Schmahmann and Sherman (1998) have found deficits in executive functioning, language, and higher-order cognition in addition to personality changes as a result of cerebellar lesions. However, they further noted, that the nature of the deficits corresponded with the locality of the lesions, with posterior lesions corresponding with cognitive and behavioral/affective disturbances, and minor deficits in executive and visual-spatial functions corresponding with anterior lesions (Schmahmann & Sherman, 1998). Beyond this general profile of neurocognitive dysfunction, neuropsychological and other functional deficits vary based on the type of spinocerebellar degeneration.

SCA1, as with most of the spinocerebellar degenerations, is associated with both cognitive and noncognitive residuals. General deficits in cognitive functioning and intellect have been reported in association with this type (Kish, el-Awar, Schut, Leach, Oscar-Berman, & Freedman, 1988), although it presents as one of the types with the lowest risk of dementia (Tang, Liu, Shen, Dai, Pan, Jing, Ouyang, & Xia, 2000). Consistent with what would be expected given the findings of Schmahmann and Sherman (1998), executive dysfunctions have been associated with SCA1 (Burk et al., 2001). In addition, these researchers noted verbal memory deficits (Burk et al., 2001). These cognitive deficits are noted in conjunction with additional neurological dysfunctions including ataxia, dysarthria, and bulbar deficits primarily. Spasticity, hyperreflexia, extensor plantar responses, and oculomotor signs may also be seen.

SCA2 has been associated with deficits in immediate recall of non-contextual or non-categorized information such as list learning as well as delayed recall (Burk et al., 1999). Similar to that which is seen in frontal or subcortical patterns of memory dysfunction, improvement is seen when offered cueing and/or recognition. Simultaneously, executive function deficits were also observed. Dementia is seen in 20–40% of patients (Burk et al., 1999). In terms of features beyond cognition, ataxia is the other main neurological feature.

The primary clinical manifestations of SCA3 include ataxia, hyperrefelxia, and spasticity. Dystonia, parkinsonism, ophthalmoplegia, and myotrophy are also commonly seen among other infrequent features. REM sleep disorder has been reported at higher rates in association with SCA3. From a cognitive standpoint, SCA3 has been associated with deficits in verbal and visual memory, verbal fluency, set-shifting, verbal and visual attention, and visuospatial and constructional abilities (Zawacki, Grace, Friedman, & Sudarsky, 2002; Kawai, Takeda, Abe, Washimi, Tanaka, & Sobue, 2004).

SCA6, in comparison to all other types of spinocerebellar degeneration, is the least associated with cognitive dysfunction (Lee et al., 2003). Nevertheless, deficits have been noted, consistent with those features commonly noted in cerebellar dysfunction. Mild executive dysfunction has been reported in conjunction with the SCA6 type (Globas, Bösch, Zühlke, Daum, Dichgans, & Bürk, 2003). In addition, retrieval based memory deficits, immediate memory deficits, and semantic and verbal fluency deficits have all been noted through research (Suenaga et al., 2008). Neurologically, ataxia, dysarthria, extrapyramidal signs and horizontal nystagmus are all seen in relation to SCA6.

SCA7 has an onset at approximately 25 years of age and initially presents with ataxia. However, as progression occurs, gradual loss of vision is seen. This is initially due macular degeneration that then eventually involves the retina and optic nerve. In comparison to other types, dementia is not commonly seen (Enevoldson et al., 1994). Tendon reflexes are commonly absent. Gaze palsy, dysphagia, and generalized muscle weakness often present.

SCA17 is the least research type of spinocerebellar degeneration as it is the newest in terms of being recognized as a separate variation. Consequently, more specific findings regarding the neurocognitive profile associate with SCA17 could not be found. Dementia is commonly seen, and presents as early as 20 years of age (Schöls et al., 2004). Executive dysfunction and deficits in higher-order cognition may be anticipated because of the cerebellar involvement (Schmahmann & Sherman, 1998), but it has not been specifically reported. What have been reported are affective and psychiatric disturbances in association with SCA17. Depression, irritability, aggression, personality changes, delusions, and hallucinations have been suggested in conjunction with the presentation (De Michele et al., 2003). Beyond ataxia, other neurological features have not been fully described.

DRPLA is characterized by ataxia, chorceoathcto sis, myoclonus, and epilepsy (Schöls et al., 2004). Cognitively, patients often present with a profile similar to that seen in conjunction with subcortical dementias in that patients demonstrate diminished executive functioning and retrieval-based memory deficits (Ikeuchi et al., 1995). Bradykinesia and bradyphrenia are often descriptive of the behavioral presentations of patients. DRPLA is strongly linked with psychiatric manifestations as well. Patients may develop visual or auditory hallucinations, but more commonly mood swings, irritability and immaturity, to the extent that individuals who almost act like children can be seen.

Friedrich's ataxia has been associated with a range of cognitive and other functional deficits. Impairments in attention, processing speed, visuoconstructive and visuospatial abilities, planning, and implicit learning have all been noted (Mantovan et al., 2006). Mantovan and colleagues (2006) also noted deficits in verbal fluency that was also noted by de Nobrega, Nieto, Barroso and Monton (2007) in semantic, phonemic, and action fluencies. Executive dysfunction commonly presents. Gait and limb ataxia, dysarthria, and lower extremity weakness are common. Medically, heightened risk of cardiomyopathy and diabetes have been reported (Fogel & Perlman, 2007).

DIAGNOSIS

Clinically, differential diagnosis between the various types of spinocerebellar degeneration is difficult given the significant overlap. Thorough clinical interview and history taking as well as evaluation are essential. Some traits are more hallmark of certain SCAs and thus can aid in diagnosis. Laid out some points of differentiation. For example, pyramidal tract signs, dysphagia, and pale discs are indicative of SCA1. Slow saccades, axonal neuropathy, and severe pontine atrophy on MRI are more suggestive of SCA2. Pure cerebellar involvement is more suggestive of SCA6. Ataxia with progressive visual loss is more consistent with SCA7. Ataxia, chorea, and seizures are usually indicative of DRPLA.

MRI is important in identifying atrophy related to the entire group of SCAs. However, in trying to differentiate the various types, focus must be placed on genetic assessment such as the locality of CAG repeats. Demonstration of CAG repeat expansion at the SCA1 locus is definitive of SCA1; when it is at the SCA2 locus it is indicative of SCA2; at locus SCA3, it suggests SCA3; SCA6 demonstrates the CAG repeat expansion at the *CACNA1A* gene; SCA7 demonstrates CAG repeat expansion at locus SCA7; SCA17 demonstrates CAG/CAA repeat expansion of the *TBP/SCA17* gene; and DRPLA demonstrates CAG repeat at the DRPLA locus.

TREATMENT

There is no cure or specific treatment for any of the spinocerebellar degenerations. They are progressive in nature. Symptoms are addressed in accordance with standard practices. For example, parkinsonian symptoms are addressed medicinally similar to the manner in which they are treated in other presentations. When seizures arise, such as in the case of DRPLA, anticonvulsants are beneficial. Antipsychotic and antidepressant agents may be used to address psychotic and mood disturbances. Literature could not be found regarding the potential utility of psychostimulants in offsetting some of the frontal-appearing cognitive residuals.

Physical therapy is often required to aid in maintaining independence in ambulation. Individuals can often end up bound to a wheelchair. Speech therapy may also be utilized.

Chad A. Noggle
Michelle R. Pagoria

Allen, G., Buxton, R. B., Wong, E. C., & Courchesne, E. (1997). Attentional activation of the cerebellum independent of motor involvement. *Science, 275,* 1940–1943.

Bürk, K., Bösch, S., & Globas, C., et al. (2001). Executive dysfunction in spinocerebellar ataxia type 1. *Eur Neurol, 46,* 43–48.

Bürk, K., Globas, C., Bösch, S., et al. (1999). Cognitive deficits in spinocerebellar ataxia 2. *Brain, 122,* 769–777.

Brenneis, C., Bösch, S. M., Schocke, M., Wenning, G. K., & Poewe, W. (2003). Atrophy pattern in SCA2 determined by voxel-based morphometry. *Neuroreport, 14,* 1799–1802.

Bruni, A. C., Takahashi-Fujigasaki, J., Maltecca, F., Foncin, J. F., Servadio, A., Casari, G., . . . Duyckaerts, C. (2004). Behavioral disorder, dementia, ataxia, and rigidity in a large family with TATA box-binding protein mutation. *Arch Neurol, 61,* 1314–1320.

Desmond, J. E., Gabrieli, J. D., Wagner, A. D., Ginier, B. L., & Glover, G. H. (1997). Lobular patterns of cerebellar activation in verbal workingmemory and finger-tapping tasks as revealed by functional MRI. *J Neurosci, 17,* 9675–9685.

De Michele, G., Maltecca, F., Carella, M., Volpe, G., Orio, M., De Falco, A., . . . Bruni, A. (2003). Dementia, ataxia, extrapyramidal features, and epilepsy: Phenotype spectrum in two Italian families with spinocerebellar ataxia type 17. *Neurol Sci, 24,* 166–167.

de Nobrega, E., Nieto, A., Barroso, J., & Monton, F. (2007). Differential impairment in semantic, phonemic, and action fluency performance in Friedreich's ataxia: Possible evidence of prefrontal dysfunction. *J Int Neuropsychol Soc, 13,* 944–952.

Fogel, B. L., & Perlman, S. (2007). Clinical features and molecular genetics of autosomal recessive cerebellar ataxias. *Lancet Neurol, 6,* 245–257.

Gilman, S., Sima, A. A., Junck, L., Kluin, K. J., Koeppen, R. A., Lohman, M. E., & Little, R. (1996). Spinocerebellar ataxia type 1 with multiple system degeneration and glial cytoplasmic inclusions. *Ann Neurol, 39,* 241–255.

Gilman, S., & Quinn, N. P. (1996). The relationship of multiple system atrophy to sporadic olivopontocerebellar atrophy and other forms of idiopathic late-onset cerebellar atrophy. *Neurology, 46,* 1197–1199.

Globas, C., Bösch, S., Zühlke, Ch., Daum, I., Dichgans, J., & Bürk, K. (2003). The cerebellum and cognition: Intellectual function in spinocerebellar ataxia type 6 (SCA6). *J Neurol, 250,* 1482–1487.

Honjo, K., Ohshita, T., Kawakami, H., Naka, H., Imon, Y., Maruyama, H., . . . Matsumoto, M. (2004). Quantitative assessment of cerebral blood flow in genetically confirmed spinocerebellar ataxia type 6. *Arch Neurol, 61,* 933–937.

Ikeuchi, T., Onodera, O., Oyake, M., Koide, R., Tanaka, H., & Tsuji, S. (1995). Dentatorubral-pallidoluysian atrophy (DRPLA): Close correlation of CAG repeat expansions with the wide spectrum of clinical presentations and prominent anticipation. *Semin Cell Biol, 6,* 37–44.

Jenkins, I. H., Brooks, D. J., Nixon, P. D., Frackowiak, R. S., & Passingham, R. E. (1994). Motor sequence learning: A study with positron emission tomography. *J Neurosci, 14,* 3775–3790.

Kawai, Y., Takeda, A., Abe, Y., Washimi, Y., Tanaka, F., & Sobue, G. (2004). Cognitive impairments in Machado-Joseph disease. *Arch Neurol, 61,* 1757–1760.

Kim, S. G., Ugurbil, K., & Strick, P. L. (1994). Activation of a cerebellar output nucleus during cognitive processing. *Science, 265,* 949–951.

Kish, S. J., el-Awar, M., Schut, L., Leach, L., Oscar-Berman, M., & Freedman, M. (1988). Cognitive deficits in olivopontocerebellar atrophy: Implications for the cholinergic hypothesis of Alzheimer's dementia. *Ann Neurol, 24,* 200–206.

Klein, D., Milner, B., Zatorre, R. J., Meyer, E., & Evans, A. C. (1995). The neural substrates underlying word generation: A bilingual functional imaging study. *Proc Natl Acad Sci USA, 92,* 2899–2903.

Lee, W. Y., Jin, D. K., Oh, M. R., Lee, J. E., Song, S. M., Lee, E. A., . . . Lee, K. H. (2003). Frequency analysis and clinical characterization of spinocerebellar ataxia types 1, 2, 3, 6, and 7 in Korean patients. *Arch Neurol, 60,* 858–863.

Mantovan, M. C., Martinuzzi, A., Squarzanti, F., Bolla, A., Silvestri, I., Liessi, G., . . . Angelini, C. (2006). Exploring mental status in Friedreich's ataxia: A combined neuropsychological, behavioral and neuroimaging study. *Eur J Neurol, 13,* 827–835.

Minnerop, M., Joe, A., Lutz, M., Bauer, P., Urbach, H., Helmstaedter, C., . . . Wüllner, U. (2005). Putamen dopamine transporter and glucose metabolism are reduced in SCA17. *Ann Neurol, 58,* 490–491.

Rolfs, A., Koeppen, A. H., Bauer, I., Bauer, P., Buhlmann, S., Topka, H., . . . Riess, O. (2003). Clinical features and neuropathology of autosomal dominant spinocerebellar ataxia (SCA17). *Ann Neurol, 54,* 367–375.

Rüb, U., de Vos, R. A., Schultz, C., Brunt, E. R., Paulson, H., & Braak, H. (2002). Spinocerebellar ataxia type 3 (Machado-Joseph disease): Severe destruction of the lateral reticular nucleus. *Brain, 125,* 2115–2124.

Schmahmann, J. D., & Sherman, J. C. (1998). The cerebellar cognitive affective syndrome. *Brain, 121,* 561–579.

Schöls, L., Bauer, P., Schmidt, T., Schulte, T., & Riess, O. (2004). Autosomal dominant cerebellar ataxias: Clinical features, genetics, and pathogenesis. *Lancet Neurol, 3,* 291–304.

Soong, B., Liu, R., Wu, L., Lu, Y., & Lee, H. (2001). Metabolic characterization of spinocerebellar ataxia type 6. *Arch Neurol, 58,* 300–304.

Suenaga, M., Kawai, Y., Watanabe, H., Atsuta, N., Ito, M., Tanaka, F., . . . Sobue, G. (2008). Cognitive impairment

in spinocerebellar ataxia type 6. *J Neurol Neurosurg Psychiatry, 79,* 496–499.

Takahashi, H., Ohama, E., Naito, H., Takeda, S., Nakashima, S., Makifuchi, T., & Ikuta, F. (1988). Hereditary dentatorubral-pallidoluysian atrophy: Clinical and pathologic variants in a family. *Neurology, 38,* 1065–1070.

Tang, B., Liu, C., Shen, L., Dai, H., Pan, Q., Jing, L., Ouyang, S., & Xia, J. (2000). Frequency of SCA1, SCA2, SCA3/MJD, SCA6, SCA7, and DRPLA CAG trinucleotide repeat expansion in patients with hereditary spinocerebellar ataxia from Chinese kindreds. *Arch Neurol, 57,* 540–544.

Wüllner, U., Reimold, M., Abele, M., Bürk, K., Minnerop, M., Dohmen, B. M., . . . Klockgether, T. (2005). Dopamine transporter positron emission tomography in spinocerebellar ataxias type 1, 2, 3, and 6. *Arch Neurol, 62,* 1280–1285.

Zawacki, T. M., Grace, J., Friedman, J. H., & Sudarsky, L. (2002). Executive and emotional dysfunction in Machado-Joseph disease. *Mov Disord, 17,* 1004–1010.

Stiff-Person Syndrome

DESCRIPTION

Formerly called stiff-man syndrome, stiff-person syndrome (SPS) was identified by Moersch and Woltman over 50 years ago (Tinsley, Barth, Black, & Williams, 1997). This rare condition is a progressive autoimmune disorder that is characterized by two sets of symptoms: (1) symmetrical muscle rigidity and stiffness of axial and distal muscles, and (2) episodic muscular spasms (Dalakas, 2008). Epidemiological data are limited; one clinic in Germany reviewed their records from a decade (1988–1998), and identified 52 SPS cases in 25,000 cases seen (Meinck, 2001).

NEUROPATHOLOGY/PATHOPHYSIOLOGY

The pathogenesis of this condition is uncertain, but it is hypothesized to be an autoimmune-mediated chronic encephalomyelitis. Glutamic acid decarboxylase (GAD) antibodies have been found in the majority of cases presenting with this syndrome, with a minority of cases also showing other antibodies (Ab), including amphiphysin Ab (Murinson & Guarnaccia, 2008). Antibodies are located in both the central and peripheral nervous systems; within the peripheral nervous system, there is a high concentration of Ab against pancreatic beta cells. The enzyme (i.e., GAD)

S

plays a vital role in the conversion of glutamic acid to GABA, which is an inhibitory neurotransmitter found throughout the CNS (Darnell, Victor, Rubin, Clouston, & Plum, 1993). A link between SPS and type 1 diabetes, and SPS and other autoimmune disorders (e.g., thyroiditis and pernicious anemia) have also been reported. In addition, genetic evidence, for example, specific human leukocyte antigen (HLA) alleles, is noted in the literature supporting the co-occurrence of SPS and diabetes mellitus. Insulin-dependent diabetes is reported in upward of 35% of patients who are diagnosed with SPS.

Both tetanus and SPS share pathophysiological features in that they have been associated with sympathetic hyperactivity secondary to a lack of synaptic inhibition of pregangliotic autonomic neurons (Benarroch, Freeman, & Kaufman, 2007). A primary association has been made between SPS and excessive firing of the motor unit, implicating disinhibition of the descending pathways to the Renshaw cells of the gamma motor system (Thompson, 1994).

NEUROPSYCHOLOGICAL/CLINICAL PRESENTATION

Onset has been noted to be insidious, most commonly during the fourth or fifth decades of life (Meinck, 2001). In addition, SPS has been noted to occur more frequently in women than in men. Initial symptoms include muscle stiffness in one or in both legs; unexplained falls, or difficulty initiating gait, especially when emotionally stressed. With symptom development, stiffness and rigidity occur initially in the axial extremities moving to distal extremities. Therefore, hyperlordosis and ankylosis are common. Spasms are also frequent, and they may occur spontaneously or in association with a range of activities, including exposure to stimuli including noise and touch, experience of emotional upset, and brisk movement. Spasms are generally bilateral, occur axially or in the proximal limbs, have "violent [and] jerky," myoclonic characteristics, and are reduced in sleep. Other commonly associated features include eye movement disturbances, ataxia, exaggerated startle response, positive head retraction reflex, and the Babinski response to the plantar reflex. Fractures are also seen in this population. Paroxysmal autonomic dysfunction is seen in some patients.

Variants of the condition exist, and they are termed stiff limb syndrome (SLS), progressive encaphalomyelitis with rigidity and myoclonus (PERM), and paraneoplastic SPS. According to Meincke (2001), these three syndromes represent variations of

SPS, although he states that there is some controversy within the field regarding this classification. For SLS, the stiffness exists in only one limb, whereas in PERM, the stiffness occurs axially and in the extremities, and sensory loss occurs. In SLS and PERM, there are spasms and autoimmunity against GAD. In paraneoplastic conditions, the anti-GAD antibodies are not always present and are more commonly present against amphiphysin.

Limited information is available on neuropsychological presentations of this condition. One study of 10 patients, using standardized assessments of intelligence, memory, attention, and executive function, reported no substantive neuropsychological features (Ameli, Snow, Rakovcevic, & Dalakas, 2005). However, examinations of psychological status have noted the co-occurrence of phobias, in particular fears of open spaces and agoraphobia (Ameli et al., 2005; Tesch, Severus, & Holdorff, 1998). Some researchers (Ameli et al., 2005) have reported that concerns regarding the environment could be considered realistic, given the functional limitations (e.g., limited ability to engage in behaviors such as crossing streets) that co-occur with SPS.

Other reports, primarily case and small-group studies, have identified depression, anxiety, and alcohol abuse co-occurring with SPS (Black, Barth, Williams, & Tinsley, 1998; Tinsley et al., 1997). For example, Gerschlager, Schrag, & Brown (2002) examined the psychological health of 24 persons diagnosed with SPS. In their study, self-reported quality of life, as measured by the Short Form-36 (SF-36) survey, was significantly reduced when compared with general population mean scores on this scale. In addition, scores on the SF-36 were correlated with the duration of the disease process and with scores on the Beck Depression Inventory.

One case study also reported the presence of post-traumatic stress disorder in a patient who subsequently developed SPS (Dinnerstein, Collins, & Berman, 2007). Another retrospective report of nine patients found historical features in the majority of cases, including a major stressful life change happening within 6 months before permanent SPS symptoms began (in seven of nine cases), the presence of transient motor symptoms occurring years before the onset of SPS (five of nine), and childhood history of loss of home or loss/invalidation of one or both parents (seven of nine) (Henningsen, Clement, Kuchenhoff, Simon, & Meinck, 1996). Interestingly, eight cases were initially diagnosed with a psychiatric condition. Such a finding is consistent with other reports that 60% of patients with SPS have a comorbid psychiatric diagnosis (Kyriakos & Franco, 2002).

DIAGNOSIS

Diagnosis is based on the clinical criteria of symptoms (i.e., rigidity and spasms). Standard neurological diagnostic procedures (e.g., CT, MRI) often produce limited differentiation of persons with this syndrome, with the exception of exclusion of other conditions. For example, few patients show abnormalities on MRI and evoked potential studies. The primary diagnostic procedure is assessment of serum autoantibodies to GAD-65 through immunocyctochemistry, Western blot or radioimmunoassay (Dalakas, 2008), as elevations have been reported in 60–80% of patients seen (Meinck, 2001). Another diagnostic feature is involvement of muscles without the presence of extrapyramidal or pyramidal tract signs but instead low-frequency motor unit firing at rest in agonist and antagonist muscles. SPS must be differentially distinguished from other conditions with similar symptoms (e.g., multiple sclerosis, tetanus, neuromyotonia, spinal cord tumors) and movement disturbances of psychogenic origin.

TREATMENT

The most commonly used treatment is benzodiazepines (e.g., diazepam). Diazepam and other GABA agonists, specifically barbiturates, have been shown to diminish neurological and psychiatric symptoms (Kyriakos & Franco, 2002). The use of substances that enhance GABA transmission (e.g., vigabatrin and baclofen) are also noted to reduce symptoms. Antispasmodic agents (e.g., tizanidine) and steroid medications, for example, methylprednisolone have been shown to decrease muscle stiffness and spasms. Via case reports, intravenous immunoglobulin has been associated with reports of reduced pain, and improved social functioning, general mental health, and vitality (Gerschlager et al., 2002).

Jacqueline Remondet Wall
Jennifer Mariner

Ameli, R., Snow, J., Rakocevic, G., & Dalakas, M. C. (2005). A neuropsychological assessment of phobias in patients with stiff person syndrome. *Neurology, 61*(11), 1961–1963.

Benarroch, E., Freeman, R., & Kaufman, H. (2007). Autonomic Nervous System. In C. G. Goetz (Ed.), *Textbook of clinical neurology* (3rd ed., pp. 383–404). Philadelphia: Saunders Elsevier.

Black, J. L., Barth, E. M., Williams, D. E., & Tinsley, J. A. (1998). Stiff-man syndrome: Results of interviews and psychologic testing. *Psychosomatics, 39*(1), 38–44.

Dalakas, M. C. (2008). Advances in the pathogenesis and treatment of patients with stiff person syndrome. *Current neurology and neuroscience reports, 8*(1), 48–55.

Darnell, R. B., Victor, J., Rubin, M., Clouston, P., & Plum, F. (1993). A novel antineuronal antibody in stiff-man syndrome. *Neurology, 43*, 114–120.

Dinnerstein, E., Collins, D., & Berman, S. A. (2007). A patient with post-traumatic stress disorder developing stiff person syndrome: Is there a correlation? *Cognitive and Behavioral Neurology, 20*(2), 136–137.

Gerschlager, W., Schrag, A., & Brown, P. (2002). Quality of life is stiff-person syndrome. *Movement Disorders, 17*(5), 1064–1067.

Henningsen, P., Clement, U., Küchenhoff, J., Simon, F., & Meinck, H. M. (1996). Psychological factors in the diagnosis and pathogenesis of stiff-man syndrome. *Neurology, 47*(1), 38–42.

Kyriakos, C. R., & Franco, K. N. (2002). Stiff-man syndrome: A case report and review of the literature. *Psychosomatics, 43*(3), 243–244.

Meinck, H. M. (2001). Stiff man syndrome. *CNS Drugs, 15*(7), 515–526.

Murinson, B. B., & Guarnaccia, J. B. (2008). Stiff-person syndrome with amphiphysin antibodies: Distinctive features of a rare disease. *Neurology, 9*(71), 1938–1939.

Tesch, M., Severus, E., & Holdorff, B. (1998). Agoraphobia and "psychogenic"—attributed gait disorder as symptoms of "stiff-man" syndrome. *Psychiatrische Praxis, 25*(6), 310–311. Abstract obtained from *Medline*, PMID No. 9885845.

Thompson, P. D. (1994). Stiff people. In C.D. Marsden & S. Fahn (Eds.), *Movement disorders* (3rd ed., pp. 373–405). Oxford: Butterworth.

Tinsley, J. A., Barth, E. M., Black, J. L., & Williams, D. E. (1997). Psychiatric consultations in stiff-man syndrome. *Journal of Clinical Psychiatry, 58*(10), 444–449.

STRIATONIGRAL DEGENERATION

DESCRIPTION

Striatonigral degeneration is a progressive neurodegenerative disorder (Multiple System Atrophy, 2008). Striatonigral degeneration, Shy–Drager's syndrome, and olivopontocerebellar atrophy comprise a class of disorders called multiple systems atrophy (MSA) (Adams & Jenkins, 2008; Cohen & Freedman, 2005). There is significant overlap between these disorders. Striatonigral degeneration is often referred to as MSA-p (parkinsonian type) as the initial predominant features are similar to those of Parkinson's disease (PD), although autonomic failure and cerebellar dysfunction emerge over time (Adams & Jenkins, 2008; Appenzeller & Oribe, 1997; Multiple System Atrophy, 2008;).

Because striatonigral degeneration presents as similar to PD, many researchers believe individuals with striatonigral degeneration are sometimes mistakenly diagnosed with PD due to the similarities. Common symptoms are those associated with parkinsonism, including poverty of movement (akinesia), slowed movements (bradykinesia), a flexed/stooped posture, and rigidity (Braffman, 1993; Lishman, 1998). A tremor may be present, but it is not a prominent sign as in PD (Shulman, Minagar, & Weiner, 2004). Cerebellar and autonomic difficulties develop over time and are common in the later stages. Cerebellar dysfunction includes a loss of muscle coordination (ataxia) and difficulties with movement and balance (Cohen & Freedman, 2005; Shulman et al., 2004). Gait ataxia and ocular difficulties develop where there are involuntary, jerky movements, making it difficult for the individual to have a steady gaze (Appenzeller & Oribe, 1997).

Autonomic failure symptoms include urinary problems (frequency, urgency, and retention), breathing abnormalities while sleeping, erectile dysfunction, swallowing difficulties (dysphagia), and loss of sphincter control (Adams & Jenkins, 2008; Calabresi, Cupini, Mercuri, & Bernardi, 1993; Lishman, 1998). Orthostatic hypotension causing fainting is common, which can lead to complications from injuries sustained during falls (Adams & Jenkins, 2008; Lishman, 1998). Speech difficulties are also present, consisting of slowed, dysfluent speech with difficulties in articulation due to muscle incoordination. Speech impairment worsens with time as the disorder progresses. About one-third of cases present with inhalatory stridor, which is when a harsh sound is made upon inhalation (Adams & Jenkins, 2008). Onset of striatonigral degeneration is always in adulthood, usually between the ages of 50 and 60 (Adams & Jenkins, 2008; Berman, 2007). To date, there is no sex or racial preference (Shulman et al., 2004). The exact prevalence is unknown although estimates suggest 4 cases per 100,000 individuals (Adams & Jenkins, 2008; Appenzeller & Oribe, 1997). The mean survival rate is less than 10 years (Berman, 2007; Shulman et al., 2004).

NEUROPATHOLOGY/PATHOPHYSIOLOGY

Although the etiology is unknown, diffuse small neuronal loss and degeneration in the substantia nigra, caudate nucleus, putamen, and basal ganglia are commonly noted (Adams & Jenkins, 2008; Berman, 2007; Braffman, 1993; Shulman et al., 2004). Gray matter shows a decrease in neurons and white matter shows a decrease in myelination (Adam & Jenkins, 2008). Autonomic failure is associated with neuronal loss in the spinal cord and brainstem (Blass, 2006; Lishman, 1998). Cerebellar dysfunction is associated with cerebellar and brainstem atrophy and olivopontocerebellar lesions. Cytoplasmic inclusions (glial cells with internal protein tangles) have been reported in the substantia nigra and other basal ganglia structures. Decreased dopamine levels resulting in bradykinesia are present. Research has also suggested abnormalities in the protein of alpha-synuclein (Adams & Jenkins, 2008).

Autopsy reports have found neuron loss in the basal ganglia structures. Damaged areas have shown a proliferation of astrocytes with a corresponding increase in cell density. In striatonigral degeneration, no Lewy bodies (abnormal aggregates of protein inside nerve cells) are present and there is a lack of neurofibrillary tangles—a distinguishing characteristic from PD. Autopsy has confirmed degenerative changes in the putamen and caudate nucleus. The hallmark characteristic found upon autopsy is the presence of glial cytoplasmic inclusion bodies in affected structures involved in movement, balance, autonomic control, and cerebellar function (Berman, 2007; Shulman et al., 2004).

NEUROPSYCHOLOGICAL/CLINICAL PRESENTATION

Clinically, individuals with striatonigral degeneration present with slow, stiff movements similar to those found in individuals with PD (Lishman, 1998). Their posture is stooped, and they tend to walk with a shuffling gait (Shulman et al., 2004). As such, frequent falls are common (Hannay, Howieson, Loring, Fischer, & Lezak, 2004). Limb movement is reduced (e.g., not using arm gestures when speaking, holding arms stiffly near body when walking) (Hannay et al., 2004) and, in general, individuals have difficulty initiating directed movement and performing tasks smoothly and slowly. Handwriting is messy and decreases in size (i.e., micrographia) (Shulman et al., 2004). Poor hygiene may be evident. Speech is halting. Anxiety, fatigue, and stimulants can exacerbate difficulties (Hannay et al., 2004).

Neuropsychological testing has shown some cognitive deterioration over time that is generally dependent upon the level of cerebellar degeneration (Soliveri et al., 2000). As a result, global cognitive disturbance has not been reported (Adams & Jenkins, 2008). Measures requiring motor skills show impairment due to the effects of ataxia. Motor sequencing is particularly difficult (Soliveri et al., 2000). Difficulties with visual and visual-motor tasks have been reported (Berman, 2007; Cohen & Freedman, 2005) as have memory impairments, particularly verbal and figural working memory (Lange et al., 2003). Furthermore, there are executive problems similar to those seen in frontal lobe lesions (Cohen & Freedman, 2005; Shulman et al., 2004); attentional difficulties have been reported on the Stroop Color-Word Test (Meco, Gasparini, & Dorrichi, 1996). Oral reading is slow and verbal fluency is reduced (Meco et al., 1996; Soliveri et al., 2000). There has been inconsistency in reporting mood disturbances (Berman, 2007; Cohen & Freedman, 2005).

DIAGNOSIS

Striatonigral degeneration is similar to PD and is commonly mistaken for it due to the similarity of symptoms (Appenzeller & Oribe, 1997). Several differences in symptoms make differential diagnosis possible, though conclusions are often not definitive. There is a poor response to the use of L-DOPA for treatment (Appenzeller & Oribe, 1997; Cohen & Freedman, 2005; Shulman et al., 2004). Striatonigral degeneration presents with inhalatory stridor, which rarely occurs in patients with PD. There is less of a resting tremor and more symptoms of autonomic system failure (Berman, 2007; Cohen & Freedman, 2005; Shulman et al., 2004). Lewy bodies are not present although they are characteristic of PD (Shulman et al., 2004).

Although there is a lack of specific diagnostic tests for striatonigral degeneration currently, the utility of CT scans, MRIs, positron emission tomography (PET) scans, and electroencephalograms (EEGs) is being explored. Specifically, CT scans can show evidence of cerebellar or brain atrophy (Appenzeller & Oribe, 1997), and MRIs have shown evidence of cerebellar, striatum, and brainstem atrophy. Small neuron loss in the putamen and caudate nucleus has also been found, as has a diminished pars compacta in the substantia nigra (Braffman, 1993). Furthermore, decreased signal atrophy in the putamen has been noted (Shulman et al., 2004). From a functional imaging standpoint, PET scans have found evidence of down-regulation of postsynaptic D2 receptor binding and a lower than normal concentration of D1 and D2 receptors in the striatum (Appenzeller & Oribe, 1997). In addition, there is evidence of decreased glucose utilization in the frontal lobe, as well as decreased glucose utilization in the striatum (Cohen & Freedman, 2005). Finally, minor EEG abnormalities were found in the sleeping state, typically associated with autonomic sleep difficulties.

TREATMENT

There is no cure for striatonigral degeneration; treatments focus on alleviating symptoms. Medication can be used to assist with parkinsonian symptoms, including dopamine agonists such as pramipexole, ropinirole, and amantadine (Shulman et al., 2004). In comparison, L-DOPA has proven to be ineffective in alleviating symptoms; some cases have even reported a worsening of the condition after such treatment. Neuromuscular blocking agents can be used to improve transmission of impulses at the myoneural junction, thereby increasing muscular function. Occupational, physical, and speech therapy are recommended adjuncts to assist with walking/movement difficulty, dysfluent speech, and activities of daily living (Adams & Jenkins, 2008). Individuals often need assistance obtaining health services, and case management is advisable.

Orthostatic hypotension is treated with a combination of pharmacotherapy and behavior management (Shulman et al., 2004). Sympathomimetic agents are used to increase standing blood pressure, and mineralocorticoids are used to enhance the reabsorption of sodium, thereby increasing blood pressure and reducing risk of lightheadedness and fainting. As falls are a common occurrence that can result in injury, safety precautions should be taken, including having access to emergency services, and caution when rising and walking. Individuals are advised to avoid common triggers of low blood pressure, such as dehydration and hot weather. Increased fluid and sodium intake is recommended. Other suggestions include sleeping with the head in an elevated position and wearing pressure stockings if necessary (Shulman et al., 2004).

Christine Corsun-Ascher
Charles Golden

Adams, S. G., & Jenkins, M. E. (2008). Multiple system atrophy and Shy-Drager syndrome. In M. R. McNeil (Ed.), *Clinical management of sensorimotor speech disorders* (pp. 348–349). New York: Thieme.

Aotsuka, A., & Paulson, G. W. (1993). Striatonigral degeneration. In M. B. Stern & W. C. Koller (Eds.), *Parkinsonian syndromes* (pp. 33–40). New York: Informa Health Care.

Appenzeller, O., & Oribe, E. (1997). *The autonomic nervous system*. Philadelphia: Elsevier Health Sciences.

Berman, S. A. (2007). *eMedicine: Striatonigral degeneration*. Retrieved December 5, 2008, from www.emedicine.com/neuro/topic354.htm

Blass, J. P. (2006). *Concise clinical pharmacology: CNS therapeutics*. New York: McGraw-Hill Professional.

Braffman, B. (1993). Neurodegenerative disorders. In J. Kucharczyk, M. E. Moseley, & A. James (Eds.),

Magnetic resonance neuroimaging (p. 229). Boca Raton, FL: CRC Press.

Calabresi, P., Cupini, L. M., Mercuri, N. B., & Bernardi, G. (1993). Age-related disorders of the autonomic nervous system. In F. Amenta (Ed.), *Aging of the autonomic nervous system* (pp. 304–305). Boca Raton, FL: CRC Press.

Cohen, S., & Freedman, M. (2005). Cognitive and behavioral changes in the Parkinson's-plus syndromes. In K. E. Anderson, W. J. Weiner, & A. Lang (Eds.), *Behavioral neurology of movement disorders* (pp. 172–174). Philadelphia: Lippincott Williams & Wilkins.

Hannay, H. J., Howieson, D. B., Loring, D. W., Fischer, J. S., & Lezak, M. D. (2004). Neuropathology for neuropsychologists. In M. D. Lezak, D. B. Howieson, D. W. Loring (with H. J. Hannay, & J. S. Fischer) (Eds.), *Neuropsychological assessment* (4th ed., pp. 225–231). Oxford: Oxford University Press.

Lange, K. W., Tucha, O., Alders, G. L., Preier, M., Csoti, I., Merz, B., et al. (2003). Differentiation of parkinsonian syndromes according to difference in executive functions. *Journal of Neural Transmission, 110*(9), 983–995.

Lishman, W. A. (1998). *Organic psychiatry: The psychological consequences of cerebral disorder*. Hoboken, NJ: Blackwell Publishing.

Meco, G., Gasparini, M., & Doricchi, F. (1996). Attentional functions in multiple system atrophy and Parkinson's disease. *Journal of Neurology, Neurosurgery, and Psychiatry, 60*(4), 393–398.

Pahwa, R., & Koller, W. C. (1995). Defining Parkinson's disease and parkinsonism. In J. H. Ellenberg, W. C. Koller, & J. W. Langston (Eds.), *Etiology of Parkinson's disease* (pp. 17–18). New York: Informa Health Care.

Shulman. L. M., Minagar, A., & Weiner, W. J. (2004). Multiple-system atrophy. In R. L.Watts & W. C. Koller (Eds.), *Movement disorders: Neurologic principles and practice* (pp. 359–360). New York: McGraw-Hill Professional.

Soliveri, P., Monza, D., Paridi, D., Carella, F., Genitrini, S., Testa, D., et al. (2000). Neuropsychological follow up in patients with Parkinson's disease, striatonigral degeneration-type multisystem atrophy, and progressive supranuclear palsy. *Journal of Neurology, Neurosurgery, and Psychiatry, 69*(3), 290–291.

Vinters, H. V. (1998). *Diagnostic neuropathology*. New York: Informa Health Care.

STURGE–WEBER SYNDROME

DESCRIPTION

Sturge–Weber syndrome (SWS) is a progressive congenital disease that is commonly associated with the port wine stain, an auburn colored birthmark, among other neurological and psychological deficits. SWS was first described by Sturge in 1879, as partial epilepsy caused by a lesion in the vasomotor brain center along with a characteristic neurocutaneous nevus. In 1922 and 1929, Weber described another case of SWS, although he named it "encephalotrigeminal angiomatosis." Genetic causes of SWS are unknown, although rare monozygotic twin studies have led scientists to speculate that the syndrome originates from somatic gene mutation during early neonatal trimesters (Maiuri, Gangemi, Jaconetta, & Maiuri, 1989). SWS occurs in all sexes and races sporadically and equally. Treatments for SWS are symptomatically based and include aspirin, anticonvulsants, and dermal laser procedures.

NEUROPATHOLOGY/PATHOPHYSIOLOGY

The most common and apparent symptom associated with SWS is the trigeminal port wine stain, a birthmark most likely caused by agenesis of the cephalic venous plexus during the first neonatal trimester (Kossoff, Hatfield, Ball, & Comi 2004; McIntosh & Morse, 2006). Although the birthmark is seen in most cases of SWS, the majority (more than 50%) of infants born with the port wine stain birthmark do not have the associated neurological deficits found in SWS (Comi, 2003). The birthmark most frequently occurs unilaterally, although it does occur bilaterally, and develops on the face near the eyes. The port wine stain is caused by an overabundance of capillaries under the dermal layers. The birthmark has normal texture and can appear in a variety of colors, from light pink to deep red (Comi, 2003; McIntosh & Morse, 2006). The birthmark itself does not pose any neuropsychological or neurological symptoms.

The most common neurolopathological feature of SWS is angioma, which is the excessive and abnormal growth of blood vessels on the surface of the brain. Research suggests that the angioma found in SWS results from abnormal maturation of the most primitive cephalic venous plexus during the first neonatal trimester (Comi, 2003, pp. 9, 19). Animal models of the angioma seen in SWS have been replicated in horses, although few have been scientifically researched (Comi, 2003). Further studies regarding abnormal brain structures of SWS have shown abnormal vascular structures in the leptomeninges, showing atrophic tissue and brain calcifications (Comi, 2003). Evidence also indicates that the meninges are significantly more thin and narrow in SWS patients (Di Trapani, Di Rocco, & Abbamondi, 1982).

Brain calcifications frequently occur in SWS and are most commonly found in the cortical layers, which include the outermost layers of the brain. Brain calcifications consist of calcium and phosphorus deposits near parenchymal vessels and form within subcortical tissues in the cortex and vary greatly among patients (Comi, 2003). Although the structure of the brain calcifications is known, the origin and neuropsychological effect of brain calcifications in SWS are currently unknown and greatly disputed within scientific literature. According to Comi (2003), research suggests that SWS is caused by the complicated interplay between abnormal extracellular matrix, vascular innervations, and endothelium alongside the leptomeningeal angioma.

Other physical abnormalities associated with SWS include glaucoma, increased vascularity of jaw tissue, and growth hormone deficits. Various oral manifestations are also frequently present in SWS patients. These include increased vascularity of the jaw tissue, swelling of soft oral tissue, enlargement of the jawbone, and arched palate. Secondary symptoms associated with increased vascularity include the premature loss of permanent teeth (Comi, 2003).

Study results attribute abnormal brain structure to noradrenergic innervations in regard to the increased constriction in cortical vessels. It is hypothesized that such abnormalities would put SWS patients at a higher risk for chronic ischemia and seizures and in turn, brain injury (Comi, 2003). Studies have also shown that there is a high prevalence of growth hormone deficiency in SWS patients (61% in the SWS population and 0.03% in the general population) (Miller, Ball, Comi, & Germain-Lee, 2009).

NEUROPSYCHOLOGICAL/CLINICAL PRESENTATION

SWS is associated with several commonly occurring clinical symptoms including seizures, mental retardation (MR), migraines, glaucoma, and stroke-like episodes (Comi, 2003; Kossoff et al., 2004; McIntosh & Morse, 2006). Seizures are a frequent neurological symptom of SWS (occurring in approximately 70–80% of SWS patients), nearly 75% experiencing onset prior to 12 months of age, the mean age of onset being 9 months (Cody & Hynd, 1998; Kossoff, Buck, & Freeman, 2003; Morse & McIntosh, 2006). Seizures are not experienced by all SWS patients; while some SWS patients experience frequent and numerous seizures, others experience infrequent episodes. Seizures associated with SWS are generally focal in onset; however, they tend to generalize to other brain regions over time (McIntosh & Morse,

2006). Seizure type varies between patients. Seizure onset typically occurs within the first 2 years of the child's life, with the majority occurring prior to age 1 (approximately 75%) (Cody & Hynd, 1998; Comi, 2003; McIntosh & Morse, 2006).

Although SWS is not considered a fatal syndrome, seizures frequently give rise to the onset of morbid secondary symptoms, including motor delays, hemiatrophy and hemiplegia (30–50%) and brain lesions (Cody & Hynd, 1998; McIntosh & Morse, 2006). Hemiparesis and hemiplegia often occur as a result of acute seizure episodes and leave the SWS patient with either severe muscle weakness or paralysis of one or both sides of the body. Hemiatrophy and hemiplegia often cause permanent motor delays (Comi, 2003; McIntosh & Morse, 2006). Comi (2003) recently evidenced that SWS patients often experience weakness in the face or body that is contralateral to the port wine stain. In some cases, researchers have examined patients who have suffered acute ischemic brain injury resulting from acute seizure episodes (Comi, 2003). Studies show that the abnormal synaptic plasticity caused by seizures in the cortical tissue may lead to reoccurring epileptic episodes, supporting earlier research that seizures in SWS become more intense over time (Comi, 2003).

In addition, approximately 60–80% of SWS patients have mild to severe MR, with only 8% of patients considered to have average cognitive functioning (Cody & Hynd, 1998; Comi, 2003; McIntosh & Morse, 2006). A strong correlation between age of seizure onset and cognitive functioning has been shown; although there is also scientific speculation that age of seizure onset is not as predictive of cognitive functioning as seizure intensity (Cody & Hynd, 1998; McIntosh & Morse, 2006). Seizures occurring during the child's first year have been shown to significantly increase the risk for MR (Comi, 2003). This research is supported by the fact that MR is rarely seen in SWS patients who do not experience seizures (Aicardi, 1990).

Headaches are another secondary symptom of seizures. Approximately 50% of SWS patients complain of headaches, the majority of which are diagnosed as migraines. Headaches commonly occur directly after the onset of a seizure. In some cases, headaches are symptomatic of the pressure experienced as a result of glaucoma (Cody & Hynd, 1998; Comi, 2003; McIntosh & Morse, 2006). According to Kossoff et al. (2004), the most common symptomology associated with headache in SWS includes unilateral pain, nausea, photophobia, phonophobia, and throbbing sensations. Kossoff et al. (2004) also found that the most common type of headache was the migraine.

Neuropsychological symptoms associated with SWS include an increased risk for academic, intellectual, and behavioral problems. SWS patients are at a significantly high risk for pervasive developmental disorders (PDDs), particularly autism spectrum, MR, learning disabilities, and attention deficit hyperactivity disorder (ADHD) (close to 20% in SWS population and only 5–6% in the general population). PDDs develop at a significantly higher risk in SWS (Cody & Hynd, 1998). The most common PDD is autism, or autism spectrum disorders (Cody & Hynd, 1998). Depression has also been commonly seen in older children and adolescents. In general, early development appears more normal than later developmental stages in children diagnosed with SWS (Cody & Hynd, 1998). SWS patients often exhibit behavioral issues including increased disinhibition (Cody & Hynd, 1998). The majority of these children need to have specialized educational plans created for them. There is currently little research on specific neuropsychological deficits found in SWS.

DIAGNOSIS

SWS is categorized into three types. Type 1 is classified by the presence of the port wine stain along with leptomeningeal angioma, which consists of blood vessel tumors in the membranes covering the brain and spinal cord. In some Type 1 cases glaucoma is present. Type 2 consists of only the facial angioma, and glaucoma is sometimes present. Type 2 is categorized as having only the leptomeningeal angioma. Glaucoma is hardly ever present in Type 3 patients (Cody & Hynd, 1998; Comi, 2003; McIntosh & Morse, 2006). There are currently no known preventive methods for the development of SWS, and infants born with the port wine stain should be screened periodically throughout infancy and into early childhood for diagnostics, since certain neurological symptoms associated with SWS, including brain calcifications and lesions, may not be present or visible in early neuro-imaging scans (Comi, 2003). Diagnostic methods most frequently used in the diagnosis of SWS include positron emission tomography (PET), MRI, and single-photon emission computed tomography (SPECT) (Comi, 2003).

TREATMENT

Laser treatment procedures are used to treat or decrease the visibility of the port wine stain. In certain circumstances, these procedures can be done on infants as early as 1 month old (McIntosh & Morse, 2006). The seizures found in SWS patients frequently intensify in severity and frequency as age increases, often becoming untreatable with anticonvulsants (Cody & Hynd, 1998). A study conducted by Wilfong, Buck, and Ball (2008) shows that the most common form of anticonvulsant prescribed to SWS patients are sodium channel blockers, including levetiracetam, carbamazepine, and oxcarbazepine. In acute cases, vagus nerve stimulation or epilepsy surgery, known as hemispherectomy, can be used to treat seizures. A study by Wilfong et al. (2008) found that 81% of SWS patients who had undergone vagus nerve stimulation or hemispherectomy experience no postoperative seizures, with 53% of these patients no longer having to take anticonvulsants. Surgery is still highly controversial and considered to be a last resort for treating SWS, since studies show that approximately 47% of patients experience postoperative complications (Wilfong et al., 2008). Glaucoma is often treated with eye drops, corrective lenses, as well as surgery. Headaches are generally treated with aspirin.

Ashley L. Ware
Antonio E. Puente

Aicardi, J. (1990). Epilespy in brain-injured children. *Developmental Medicine and Child Neurology, 32*, 191–202.

Cody, H., & Hynd, G. W. (1998). Sturge-Weber syndrome. In L. Phelps (Ed.), *Health-related disorders in children and adolescents: A guidebook for understanding and educating* (pp. 624–628). Washington, DC: American Psychological Association.

Comi, A. M. (2003). Pathophysiology of Sturge-Weber syndrome. *Journal of Child Neurology, 18*(8), 509–516.

Di Trapani, G., Di Rocco, C., & Abbamondi, A. L. (1982). Light microscopy and ultrasound studies of Sturge-Weber disease. *Childs Brain, 9*, 23–36.

Kossoff, E. H., Buck, C., & Freeman, J. M. (2003). *Outcomes of 32 hemispherectomies for Sturge-Weber syndrome worldwide.* Study funded by the Sturge-Weber Foundation. Baltimore: Johns Hopkins.

Kossoff, E. H., Hatfield, L. A., Ball, K. L., & Comi, A. M. (2004). Comorbidity of epilepsy and headache in patients with Sturge-Weber syndrome. *Journal of Child Neurology, 20*, 678–682.

Maiuri, F., Gangemi, M., Jaconetta, G., & Maiuri, L. (1989). Sturge-Weber disease without facial nevus. *Journal Neurosurgery Science, 33*, 215–218.

McIntosh, D. E., & Morse, M. M. (2006). Neurocutaneous syndromes. In L. Phelps (Ed.), *Chronic health-related disorders in children: Collaborative medical and psychoeducational interventions* (pp. 157–173). Washington, DC: American Psychological Association.

Miller, R. S., Ball, K. L., Comi, A. M., & Germain-Lee, E. L. (2009). *Growth hormone deficiency in children with Sturge-Weber syndrome.* Study funded by the Sturge-Weber Foundation. Unpublished manuscript.

Wilfong, A., Buck, C., & Ball, K. (2008). *Sturge-Weber syndrome: Trends in epilepsy therapy.* Study funded by the Sturge-Weber Foundation. Unpublished manuscript.

SUBCORTICAL VASCULAR DEMENTIA

DESCRIPTION

Cerebral atherosclerosis has been known since the late 19th century. The vascular dementias represent the second most common form of dementia in the United States and Europe and are the leading cause of dementia in some sections of Asia. Vascular dementia also commonly co-occurs with Alzheimer's disease. Subcortical vascular dementia is a particular subtype involving the small blood vessels of the brain that can mimic the primary neurodegenerative disorders by causing degradation of the white matter (Martinez-Lage & Hacinski, 1998). Consequently, it is marked by a more frontal-subcortical cognitive dysfunction profile owing to the predominance of white matter within this cerebral region. Furthermore, the presentation occurs most often in the setting of one or more vascular risk factors such as hypertension and/or diabetes mellitus (Caselli & Boeve, 2007). Current treatment focuses on controlling vascular risks and symptomatic treatment.

NEUROPATHOLOGY/PATHOPHYSIOLOGY

The small arteries that feed the deep structures of the brain, the white matter tracts, and subcortical nuclei are vulnerable to lipohyalinosis and venous collagenosis due to vascular disease (Munoz, 2003). The most common causes are hypertension, hypercholesterolemia, diabetes mellitus, obstructive sleep apnea, and smoking. Microvascular disease has been associated with white matter changes on brain imaging (white matter hyperintensities on MRI, hypointensities on CT) and microhemorrhages as evinced by hemosiderin deposits. Small lacunar infarcts can also be seen in subcortical vascular dementia due to the same underlying pathophysiology. Rarely, in patients without common risk factors, other possible vascular etiologies must be explored. The prototype of this is cerebral autosomal-dominant arteriopathy with subcortical infarcts and leukoencephalopathy.

NEUROPSYCHOLOGICAL/CLINICAL PRESENTATION

Patients suffering from subcortical vascular dementia present with a similar onset and progression to that of primary neurodegenerative disorders, with a gradual onset and progressive decline as opposed to the sudden onset and stepwise decline seen in multi-infarct dementia. Symptoms that suggest a subcortical vascular etiology include early gait involvement, urinary incontinence, and emotional/personality changes. Psychomotor slowing, a poor learning curve, impeded delayed recall with general improvement with cueing and/or recognition, and relative sparing of naming and other language skills have also been noted (Graham, Emery, & Hodges, 2004). Patients with vascular risk factors as part of their past medical history should also be suspected. Careful neurological examination may discern focal neurological deficits, though this is more common in multi-infarct dementia. As a result, neuropsychological assessment can be essential in evaluating neurocognitive status and the potential of a subcortical vascular dementia diagnosis. In this regard, the cognitive profile on testing tends toward more frontal-subcortical deficits and executive dysfunction. The degree of white matter disease seen on MRI correlates with the cognitive profile of patients, with more white matter disease accompanying more problems with working memory, especially compared with episodic memory (Libon et al., 2008), and executive and visuoconstructive tests as compared with memory and language tests (Price, Jefferson, Merino, Heilman, & Libon, 2005).

DIAGNOSIS

The diagnosis of subcortical vascular dementia is largely based on a combination of clinical judgment and neuroimaging. Before making a diagnosis of subcortical vascular dementia, the patient should have multiple cognitive deficits that are causing significant functional decline in his or her day-to-day life. This may be best accomplished through a comprehensive neuropsychological assessment that permits the evaluation of a variety of cognitive domains. Reversible causes should be ruled out, predominantly by laboratory studies including a complete metabolic panel, blood count, thyroid function, antinuclear antibody profile, sedimentation rate, B-12 level, and syphilis serology. In addition, the contribution of potential psychogenic factors, such as depression, must also be considered. Neuroimaging serves a capacity of both inclusion and exclusion. Regarding the latter, differentials including normal pressure hydrocephalus, tumors, and other potential causes may be ruled out via imaging. In regard to inclusionary criteria, neuroimaging can reveal whether there is enough subcortical vascular changes to support a diagnosis of subcortical vascular dementia. In comparison of the potential methods of imaging, the presence of white matter disease is more easily discerned on MRI

S

imaging with FLAIR. In general, involvement of 25% or more of the white matter is believed to be enough to cause some cognitive disruption, whereas white matter changes of 50% or more is consistent with outright subcortical vascular dementia. Multiple lacunar infarcts in the white matter and subcortical structures can also be seen.

TREATMENT

There are no proven treatments for subcortical vascular dementia. Conventional practice focuses on control of presumed vascular risk factors leading to the vascular damage. Diet and exercise can improve several common vascular risk factors, and smokers should be counseled on cessation. In models of secondary stroke prevention, statins have proved useful and are certainly of use in patients with hypercholesterolemia. Patients with obstructive sleep apnea should be placed on continuous positive airway pressure (CPAP). Antiplatelet agents can be used to reduce the risk of further vascular insult. Antihypertensives should be used for those with high blood pressure. Antiglycemics should be used for those with diabetes mellitus.

Symptomatic treatment can be attempted. The most commonly used drugs are those currently used to treat Alzheimer's disease, acetylcholinesterase inhibitors, and memantine (Erkinjuntti, Román, & Gauthier, 2004). Another possible treatment is the vasodilator hydergine (Olin, Schneider, Novit, & Luczak, 2001).

Glen Finney

Caselli, R. J., & Boeve, B. F. (2007). The degenerative dementias. In C. G. Goetz (Ed.), *Textbook of clinical neurology* (3rd ed., pp. 699–733). Philadelphia, PA: Saunders Elsevier.

Erkinjuntti, T., Román, G., & Gauthier, S. (2004). Treatment of vascular dementia—evidence from clinical trials with cholinesterase inhibitors. *Journal of the Neurological Sciences, 226*(1–2), 63–66.

Graham, N. L., Emery, T., & Hodges, J. R. (2004). Distinctive cognitive profiles in Alzheimer's disease and subcortical vascular disease. *Journal of Neurology, Neurosurgery, and Psychiatry, 75*, 61–71.

Libon, D. J., Price, C. C., Giovannetti, T., Swenson, R., Bettcher, B. M., Heilman, K. M., et al. (2008). Linking MRI hyperintensities with patterns of neuropsychological impairment: Evidence for a threshold effect. *Stroke, 39*, 806–813.

Martinez-lage, P., & Hacinski, V. (1998). Multi-infarct dementia. In H. J. M. Barnett, J. P. Mohr, B. M. Stein, & F. M. Yatsu (Eds.), *Stroke pathophysiology, diagnosis, and management* (3rd ed., pp. 875–894). Philadelphia, PA: Churchill Livingstone.

Munoz, D. G. (2003). Small vessel disease: Neuropathology. *International Psychogeriatric, 15*(Suppl. 1), 67–69.

Olin, J., Schneider, L., Novit, A., & Luczak, S. (2001). Hydergine for dementia. *Cochrane Database of Systematic Reviews*, (2), CD000359.

Price, C., Jefferson, A. L., Merino, J., Heilman, K., & Libon, D. J. (2005). Towards an operational definition of the "Research Criteria for Subcortical Vascular Dementia": Integrating neuroradiological and neuropsychological data. *Neurology, 65*, 376–382.

Roman, G. C., Tatemichi, T. K., Erkinjuntti, T., Cummings, J. L., Masdeu, J. C., Garcia, J. H., et al. (1993). Vascular dementia: Diagnostic criteria for research studies— Report of the NINDS-AIREN International Workshop. *Neurology, 43*, 250–260.

SUNCT HEADACHE SYNDROME

DESCRIPTION

SUNCT headache syndrome stand for short-lasting unilateral neuralgiform headache attacks with conjunctival injection and tearing. It is a relatively rare chronic headache syndrome (Sjaastad et al., 1989). First described in 1989 by Sjaastad and colleagues, the presentation constitutes a pattern of repeated (20 or more episodes), severe stabbing or throbbing pain in the temporal or orbital regions of the head in a unilateral formation that coincides with ipsilateral conjunctival injection and lacrimation. It is more commonly observed in males versus females, with symptom onset usually occurring in the fifth or sixth decade of life (Matharu, Cohen, Boes, & Goadsby, 2003).

Of all the primary headache disorders, SUNCT headaches are most resistant to treatment (Goadsby & Lipton, 1997). Lidocaine, lamotrigine, gabapentin, topiramate, and oxcarbazepine have shown minimal yet positive results, as have others as discussed in the following (Cohen, 2007).

NEUROPATHOLOGY/PATHOPHYSIOLOGY

The neuropathological basis of SUNCT headaches has been localized to the inferior posterior hypothalamus (Cohen, Matharu, Kalisch, Friston, & Goadsby, 2004; Sprenger et al., 2005). More specifically, the headaches arise on the ipsilateral side of the hypothalamic activation. This has been demonstrated through functional MRI and blood oxygenation level dependent (BOLD) imaging. However, it is worth noting that this is etiology is not definitive of SUNCT, as similar activation has been noted in cluster headaches and paroxysmal hemicrania (Matharu, Cohen, Frackowiak, & Goadsby, 2006; Sprenger et al., 2004). Vascular-based structural lesions have also been documented in the area of the posterior fossa, either extra-axial or intra-axial, mostly vascular disturbances/malformations.

NEUROPSYCHOLOGICAL/CLINICAL PRESENTATION

As previously discussed, SUNCT headaches present as unilateral pain that coincides with conjunctival injection and tearing that are short lasting in duration. Ipsilateral cranial autonomic features accompany the presentation, most commonly lacrimation and conjunctival injection that are essential to diagnosis. The pain is most commonly localized to the temporal or orbital regions, although spread past midline as well as extension posteriorly to the occipital region have been noted (Manzoni et al., 1983). Patients often describe it as stabbing, throbbing, burning, or electrical pain lasting 10 to 60 seconds (Pareja & Sjaastad, 1997). Over the long term, individuals may experience periods of clustering where numerous headaches are experienced, while at other times they may remain asymptomatic. Phonophobia and photophobia commonly occur in conjunction with the headaches (Cohen, Matharu, & Goadsby, 2006). Ptosis may present.

Neuropsychological deficits have not been directly related to the presentation. During symptomatic periods, individuals may present with deficits in attention, concentration, and retrieval-based memory. Visuospatial dysfunction may also be observed in conjunction with visual disturbances secondary to the headaches. During asymptomatic periods neuropsychological dysfunction has not been strongly associated with the presentation.

DIAGNOSIS

Diagnosis of SUNCT headache syndrome is symptom based as are the vast majority of primary headache presentations. Consequently, specific diagnostic criteria for SUNCT headache syndrome have been established (Goadsby & Lipton, 1997). As it stands, the diagnosis of SUNCT headache syndrome require 20 to 30 attacks of unilateral, moderately severe, orbital or temporal, stabbing or throbbing pain, lasting for 15–120 seconds and associated with at least one of the following cranial autonomic features: conjunctival injection, lacrimation, nasal congestion, rhinorrhoea, ptosis, or eyelid edema (Matharu, Cohen, & Goadsby, 2004; May, Bahra, Büchel, Turner, & Goadsby, 1999; Olesen, 2001).

In some ways, the presentations lack of response to medicinal intervention may also be seen as diagnostic in nature (Mondéjar et al., 2006).

Beyond the constellation of symptoms, as with other primary headache syndromes, diagnostic workup should include neuroimaging in the form of CT and/or MRI. This is recommended to rule-out and evaluate for the presence of intracranial lesions including aneurysms, other arteriovenous malformations, tumors/neoplasm, hydrocephalus, as well as other factors that may contribute to increased intracranial pressure.

TREATMENT

Of all primary headache syndromes, SUNCT headache syndrome is recognized as the most highly refractory to treatment. Commonly used agents including sumatriptan, indomethacin, prednisone, aspirin, and carbamazepine (Goadsby & Lipton, 1997). Lamotrigine, gabapentin, topiramate, intravenous lidocaine and intravenous phenytoin have demonstrated the most encouraging results in treating SUNCT headaches (May et al., 2006). Combined treatment of some these agents with prednisone or prednisolone have also yielded positive results in more refractory cases (De Benedittis, 1996; Gardella, Viruega, Rojas, & Nagel, 2001; Graff-Radford, 2000; Morales-Asín et al., 2000; Pareja, Kruszewski, & Sjaastad, 1995). Several case reports have also suggested a potential efficacy of calcium antagonists including nifedipine, verapamil, diltiazem, and flunarizine (Gardella et al., 2001; Graff-Radford, 2000; Pareja et al., 1995; Raimondi & Gardella, 1998). Nonsteroidal, anti-inflammatory drugs such as ibuprofen, piroxicam, and naproxen have not shown benefit (Gardella et al., 2001; Pareja et al., 1995).

Chad A. Noggle
Michelle R. Pagoria

Cohen, A. S. (2007). Short-lasting unilateral neuralgiform headache attacks with conjunctival injection and tearing. *Cephalalgia, 27,* 824–832.

Cohen, A. S., Matharu, M. S., & Goadsby, P. J. (2005). Suggested guidelines for treating SUNCT and SUNA. *Cephalalgia, 25,* 1200.

Cohen, A. S., Matharu, M. S., & Goadsby, P. J. (2006). Short-lasting unilateral neuralgiform headache attacks with conjunctival injection and tearing (SUNCT) or cranial autonomic features (SUNA) — a prospective clinical study of SUNCT and SUNA. *Brain, 129,* 2746–2760.

Cohen, A. S., Matharu, M. S., Kalisch, R., Friston, K., & Goadsby, P. J. (2004). Functional MRI in SUNCT shows differential hypothalamic activation with increasing pain. *Cephalalgia, 24,* 1098–1099.

De Benedittis, G. (1996). SUNCT syndrome associated with cavernous angioma of the brainstem. *Cephalalgia, 16,* 503–506.

Gardella, L., Viruega, A., Rojas, H., & Nagel, J. (2001). A case of a patient with SUNCT syndrome treated with the Janneta procedure. *Cephalalgia, 21,* 996–999.

Goadsby, P. J., & Lipton, R. B. (1997). A review of paroxysmal hemicranias, SUNCT syndrome and other short-lasting headaches with autonomic feature, including new cases. *Brain, 120,* 193–209.

Graff-Radford, S. B. (2000). SUNCT syndrome responsive to gabapentin (Neurontin). *Cephalalgia, 20,* 515–517.

Manzoni, G. C., Terzano, M. G., Bono, G., Micieli, G., Martucci, N., & Nappi, G. (1983). Cluster headache: Clinical findings in 180 patients. *Cephalalgia, 3,* 21–30.

Matharu, M. S., Cohen, A. S., Boes, C. J., & Goadsby, P. J. (2003). SUNCT syndrome: A review. *Current Pain Headache Reports, 7,* 308–318.

Matharu, M. S., Cohen, A. S., Frackowiak, R. S., & Goadsby, P. J. (2006). Posterior hypothalamic activation in paroxysmal hemicrania. *Annals of Neurology, 59,* 535–545.

Matharu, M. S., Cohen, A. S., & Goadsby, P. J. (2004). SUNCT syndrome responsive to intravenous lidocaine. *Cephalalgia, 24,* 985–992.

May, A., Bahra, A., Büchel, C., Turner, R., & Goadsby, P. J. (1999). Functional magnetic resonance imaging in spontaneous attacks of SUNCT: Short-lasting neuralgiform headache with conjunctival injection and tearing. *Annals of Neurology, 46,* 791–794.

May, A., Leone, M., Afra, J., Linde, M., Sandor, P. S., Evers, S., & Goadsby, P. J. (2006). EFNS guidelines on the treatment of cluster headache and other trigeminal-autonomic cephalalgias. EFNS Task Force. *European Journal of Neurology, 13,* 1066–1077.

Mondéjar, B., Cano, E. F., Pérez, I., Navarro, S., Garrido, J. A., Velásquez, J. M., & Alvarez, A. (2006). Secondary SUNCT syndrome to a variant of the vertebrobasilar vascular development. *Cephalalgia, 26,* 620–622.

Morales-Asín, F., Espada, F., López-Obarrio, L. A., Navas, I., Escalza, I., & Iñiguez, C. (2000). A SUNCT case with response to surgical treatment. *Cephalalgia, 20,* 67–68.

Olesen, J. (2001). Revision of the international headache classification. An interim report. *Cephalalgia, 21,* 261.

Pareja, J. A., Kruszewski, P., & Sjaastad, O. (1995). SUNCT syndrome: Trials of drugs and anesthetic blockades. *Headache, 35,* 138–142.

Pareja, J. A., & Sjaastad, O. (1997). SUNCT syndrome: A clinical review. *Headache, 37,* 195–202.

Raimondi, E., & Gardella, L. (1998). SUNCT syndrome: Two cases in Argentina. *Headache, 38,* 369–371.

Sjaastad, O., Saunte, C., Salvesen, R., Fredriksen, T. A., Seim, A., Røe, O. D., . . . Zhao JM. (1989). Shortlasting unilateral neuralgiform headache attacks with conjunctival injection, tearing, sweating, and rhinorrhea. *Cephalalgia, 9,* 147–156.

Sprenger, T., Boecker, H., Tolle, T. R., Bussone, G., May, A., & Leone, M. (2004). Specific hypothalamic activation during a spontaneous cluster headache attack. *Neurology, 62,* 516–517.

Sprenger, T., Valet, M., Platzer, S., Pfaffenrath, V., Steude, U., & Tolle, T. R. (2005). SUNCT: Bilateral hypothalamic activation during headache attacks and resolving of symptoms after trigeminal decompression. *Pain, 113,* 422–426.

SYDENHAM'S CHOREA

DESCRIPTION

Sydenham's chorea (also known as hyponic-hyperkinetic syndrome, rheumatic chorea, chorea minor, and St. Johannis chorea) was first described by Thomas Sydenham's in his book *Schedula Monitoria de Noval Febris Ingressa* published in 1686 (Jummani & Okun, 2001; Weiner & Normandin, 2007). Sydenham's chorea is characterized by the spontaneous, jerking movements that occur and can be caused by medication, cerebral palsy, or most commonly, acute rheumatic fever (ARF) due to group A streptococcal (GAS) throat infection (Golden, Haut, & Moshe, 2006; Weiner & Normandin, 2007).

Sydenham's chorea is one of the most distinguishing features of ARF and prevalence rates of Sydenham's chorea in those with ARF range from 10–30% (Golden et al., 2006; Pavone, Parano, Rizzo, & Trifiletti, 2006; Walker et al., 2007). This disorder occurs most commonly during childhood with the average age of onset ranging between 9 and 11 years of age (Jummani & Okun, 2001; Kiliç et al., 2007; Walker et al., 2007; Weiner & Normandin, 2007). Although cases of Sydenham's chorea are rarer under the age of 5 and over the age of 18, symptoms of the disorder have been reported to manifest anytime between 2 and 21 years of age (Kiliç et al., 2007; Walker et al., 2007). Most cases of Sydenham's chorea (up to two-thirds) are reported in females (Kiliç et al., 2007; Pavone et al., 2006; Walker et al., 2007).

Disorders associated with Sydenham's chorea are carditis and polyarthritis, which commonly occur during ARF as well; however, some research has shown that those who have ARF and chorea may be much less likely to develop carditis or arthritis (Kiliç et al., 2007; Walker et al., 2007). Other more rare associated disorders include mild mitral insufficiency and mitral regurgitation (Kiliç et al., 2007; Walker et al., 2007).

NEUROPATHOLOGY/PATHOPHYSIOLOGY

Although the exact pathogenesis of Sydenham's chorea is unknown, it is suspected to be caused by an antibody response to an infection of the GAS carbohydrate and rheumatic fever (Kirvan, Swedo, Heuser, & Cunningham, 2003; Pavone et al., 2006). Researchers have asserted that this infection causes a cross-reactive immune response that attacks neurons in the brain, especially in the basal ganglia, which may explain the motor symptoms (Kirvan et al., 2003). The antibodies attack brain neurons because of the molecular similarity between streptococcal antigens and the neuronal antigens of the basal ganglia proteins (Kiliç et al., 2007; Pavone et al., 2006). Both clinical and MRI studies have shown that antibodies that attack the streptococcal infection are found in the basal ganglia and the cortex, and the number of antibodies present is associated with the severity and duration of symptoms (Jummani & Okun, 2001; Kirvan et al., 2003).

These antibodies may cause further impairments in the central nervous system (CNS) through neuronal signal transduction and cell signaling (Kirvan et al., 2003). This impairment in signaling may be a result of the antibodies interfering with the gangliosides' ability to bind with the neuronal receptors (Kirvan et al., 2003). The antibodies increase signal transduction causing the release of excitatory neurotransmitters, which may elicit dopamine release and play a role in the obsessive-compulsive symptoms, tics, and attention problems (Kirvan et al., 2003). Although the antibodies drastically interfere with the basal ganglia and the CNS, they do not cause permanent damage (Kirvan et al., 2003). The swelling caused by the infection appears to subside when properly treated, and no evidence of glial scarring or neuronal loss has been found (Pavone et al., 2006).

NEUROPSYCHOLOGICAL/CLINICAL PRESENTATION

Early signs and symptoms include limping or unsteadiness in one leg in which the affected leg is dragged and shaking in the hand(s), which cannot be steadied (Jummani & Okun, 2001). Softer neurological symptoms that occur early in the development of the disease can include "milkmaid's grip," the inability to hold a fist for a prolonged period (Weiner & Normandin, 2007), and "darting tongue" (Pavone et al., 2006). The hallmark symptom is the involuntary, spontaneous, and choreiform movements, which occur in the face and extremities (Golden et al., 2006; Jummani & Okun, 2001; Kiliç et al., 2007; Weiner & Normandin, 2007).

Gait disturbances, hypotonia, muscle weakness, and incoordination are also characteristics of Sydenham's chorea (Jummani & Okun, 2001; Kiliç et al., 2007). Psychological symptoms such as attention problems, emotionally lability, and obsessive-compulsive symptoms are commonly seen as deficits in reading, writing, and speaking (dysarthric speech difficulties) (Jummani & Okun, 2001; Kiliç et al., 2007; Kirvan et al., 2003; Pavone et al., 2006). In severe cases, ballistic movements, the inability to ambulate, and motor and vocal tics may be present (Pavone et al., 2006).

Symptoms are considered to be mild through severe based on the activities that are affected by the disease, for example, the inability to ambulate would be indicative of severe symptoms (Kiliç et al., 2007). Chorea symptoms can be general, involving the whole body, or specific, affecting only part of the body (Kiliç et al., 2007). These symptoms usually subside after approximately 4 months but have been reported to last between 1 week to 2 years (Kiliç et al., 2007; Pavone et al., 2006).

Psychological symptoms such as personality changes, obsessive-compulsive disorder (OCD), anxiety and mood swings as well as attention disorders have been noted in the literature (Kiliç et al., 2007; Walker et al., 2007; Weiner & Normandin, 2007). These symptoms are thought to occur because the antibodies, generated to attack the streptococcal infection, attack basal ganglia, increasing signal transduction causing the release of excitatory neurotransmitters, which may elicit dopamine release (Da Rocha, Correa, & Teixeria, 2008). One of the most common psychological disorders is OCD; behavioral symptoms of OCD may present 2–4 weeks before the symptoms of chorea (Da Rocha et al., 2008; Weiner & Normandin, 2007) and up to 70% of those with Sydenham's chorea will develop the symptoms of OCD (Asbahr et al., 2005). Research has shown that OCD occurring with Sydenham's chorea is very similar to childhood-onset OCD (Asbahr et al., 2005).

The most common obsessions reported in those with Sydenham's chorea are thoughts of aggression, contamination, hoarding, religion, symmetry, and somatization (Asbahr et al., 2005). Common compulsions that have been reported are cleaning, checking, repeating, counting, ordering, and hoarding (Asbahr et al., 2005). Motor and verbal tics have also been reported in those with Sydenham's chorea (Asbahr et al., 2005). Common tic-like symptoms described are touching, blinking, rubbing, and staring (Asbahr et al., 2005). Symptoms of separation anxiety, although much less common, have been reported along with OCD symptoms, and the obsessions in these children are much more likely to be aggressive in nature than those without separation anxiety symptoms (Asbahr et al., 2005).

DIAGNOSIS

Diagnoses of Sydenham's chorea are made by clinical observations (Pavone et al., 2006). At this time, there are no confirmatory tests available; however, increases in levels of antistreptococcal titers have been shown to be present in 80% of those with the disease (Pavone et al., 2006). Because GAS respiratory infections are usually a precursor to the development of Sydenham's chorea, close clinical examination is recommend post infection in order to diagnosis this disease as soon as possible (Pavone et al., 2006). Other factors associated with developing ARF and subsequent Sydenham's chorea, especially in third world countries are poverty, malnutrition, and overcrowding (Walker et al., 2007). However, there have been more recent increases in ARF in the United States, which most likely cannot be attributed to the previously mentioned factors (Walker et al., 2007). In more highly developed countries with first-rate health care systems, interactions of different strains of streptococcus and/or genetic predispositions to ARF may be able to explain these increases (Walker et al., 2007).

TREATMENT

Although the symptoms of Sydenham's chorea usually spontaneously remit with treatment in 1–6 months, long-term treatment is often needed, especially for the accompanying ARF infection (Pavone et al., 2006; Walker et al., 2007). Pharmacological interventions are recommended in cases where symptoms are severe and interfere with daily functioning, or significant weight loss is experienced (Walker et al., 2007). One treatment for moderate to severe symptoms is the medication haloperidol for chorea and penicillin prophylaxis for the associate ARF (Kiliç et al., 2007). One study showed that remission of symptoms occurred within 1–12 months after treatment with haloperidol; however, treatment may

take longer, over a year, if other associated disorders, such as carditis, are present (Kiliç et al., 2007). Other studies have shown the recovery rate to be 50% for those treated with haloperidol (Golden et al., 2006).

Other drugs, such as valproic acid and carbamazepine, and corticosteroids (prednisone), are increasingly being used (Kiliç et al., 2007; Walker et al., 2007). Corticosteroids have been shown to significantly decrease the course of chorea symptoms as well (Walker et al., 2007). Studies have shown that valproic acid and carbamazepine have shown improvement rates of 85% or higher, although relapses have been reported (Golden et al., 2006). Research has also provided evidence that the recovery rate for antiepileptic drugs is 83%, but they have found that valproate may lead to a much more rapid recovery, and, thus, is the recommended medication of choice for treatment of chorea (Golden et al., 2006). Carbamazepine, haloperidol, and sodium valproate may be effective in treating chorea symptoms because they operate on the dopaminergic or γ-aminobutryic acid (GABA) pathways (Walker et al., 2007). However, corticosteroids act on the antibodies or mechanisms of the immune system, which leads to the neuronal dysfunction present in chorea (Walker et al., 2007). Although Sydenham's chorea symptoms usually remit without permanent damage with or without medication, damage to the heart valves due to ARF may persist in 63–94% of patients (Weiner & Normandin, 2007).

Sarah E. West
Charles Golden

Asbahr, F. R., Garvey, M. A., Snider, L. A., Zanetta, D. M., Elkis, H., & Swedo, S. E. (2005). Obsessive-compulsive symptom among patients with Sydenham chorea. *Biological Psychiatry, 57,* 1073–1076.

Da Rocha, F. F., Correa, H., & Teixeira, A. L. (2008). Obsessive-compulsive disorder and immunology: A review. *Progress in Neuro-Psychopharmacology & Biological Psychiatry, 32,* 1139–1146.

Golden, A. S., Haut, S. R., & Moshé, S. L. (2006). Nonepileptic uses of antiepileptic drugs in children and adolescents. *Pediatric Neurology, 34,* 421–432.

Jummani, R. R., & Okun, M. S. (2001). Sydenham chorea. *Archives of Neurology, 58,* 311–313.

Kiliç, A., Unüvar, E., Burak, T, Gökçe, M, Omeroğlu, R. E., Oğuz, F., et al. (2007). Neurologic and cardiac findings in children with Sydenham chorea. *Pediatric Neurology, 36,* 159–164.

Kirvan, C. A., Swedo, S. E., Heuser, J. S., & Cunningham, M. W. (2003). Mimicry and autoantibody-mediated neuronal cell signaling in Sydenham chorea. *Nature Medicine, 9,* 914–920.

Pavone, P., Parano, E., Rizzo, R., & Trifiletti, R. R. (2006). Autoimmune neuropsychiatric disorders associated with streptococcal infection: Sydenham chorea, PANDAS, and PANDAS variants. *Journal of Child Neurology, 21,* 727–736.

Walker, A. R., Tani, L. Y., Thompson, J. A., Firth, S. D., Veasy, L. G., & Bale, J. F. (2007). Rheumatic chorea: Relationship to systemic manifestations and response to corticosteroids. *The Journal of Pediatrics, 151,* 679–683.

Weiner, S. G., & Normandin, P. A. (2007). Sydenham chorea: A case report and review of the literature. *Pediatric Emergency Care, 23,* 20–24.

SYNCOPE

DESCRIPTION

Syncope represents the medical term for fainting, and it is accompanied by a collection of physiological symptoms resulting from decreased or interrupted blood flow to the brain. It is characterized by a brief loss of consciousness and postural tone, most often occurring while standing.

NEUROPATHOLOGY/PATHOPHYSIOLOGY

A defining feature of all syncopal episodes is a rapid and sudden reduction or cessation of blood flow to the brain. In syncope, the blood hypoperfusion to the cerebral hemispheres and/or the brainstem reticular activating system results in a failure to maintain consciousness. Hypoperfusion can occur when there is cerebral vasoconstriction or global hypotension (Brignole et al., 2004; Kenny, 2002).

In general, a series of neurohormonal events take place upon changes in body position, such as standing. The neurohormonal activity assists in maintaining cerebral perfusion in healthy individuals. In optimum situations when there is a decreased venous return, the resulting decreased filling of the left ventricle responds by increasing sympathetic tone and hypercontracting of the left ventricle. However, the hypercontracted left ventricle may, in some people, detect the left ventricular volume overload and inhibit sympathetic stimulation while still engaging the parasympathetic system, which can lead to hypotension, brachycardia, and syncope (Brignole et al., 2004; Kenny, 2002; Linzer et al., 1997b).

NEUROPSYCHOLOGICAL/CLINICAL PRESENTATION

Those with syncope often experience specific physiological symptoms that result in a rapid loss of consciousness followed by a quick recovery. Clinical features of syncope, regardless of cause, are commonly related to posture, time of day, and precipitating factors such as emotions, injury, pain, and heat. Skin pallor and cardiovascular signs are also common (Brignole et al., 2004; Linzer et al., 1997a; Zaqqa & Massumi, 2000). In general, most syncopal events are precipitated by an overall feeling of weakness, lightheadedness, sweating, giddiness, blurry vision, tinnitus, or gastrointestinal symptoms. Regardless of the causes of syncope, all types end with cerebral hypoperfusion. During the syncopal event, most people are motionless after the loss of consciousness, but some may also exhibit myoclonic jerks. The pulse rate will be slow with shallow breathing and excessively low blood pressure.

DIAGNOSIS

The diagnosis of syncope requires the assessment of the underlying causes; however, the most common diagnostic protocol involves a comprehensive history, physical examination, and ECG. This protocol helps identify 56–85% of cases (Kapoor, 2000; Linzer et al., 1997). Brignole et al. (2004) advised that three questions are mandatory in assessment: (1) Is the loss of consciousness related to syncope or not? (2) Does heart disease exist or not? and (3) Do the clinical features obtained in the history relate to the diagnosis? The assessment needs to identify the precursors to the syncopal event, the onset, the attack, and the end of the attack (Miller & Kruse, 2005) as well as any history of heart disease and/or other illnesses.

In addition, it is important to differentiate syncope from other conditions that are nonsyncopal but also result in loss of consciousness. Nonsyncopal events that can lead to unconsciousness include disorders that have behavioral manifestations that are similar to syncope, such as seizures and attacks related to carotid origins (Brignole et al., 2004). Similar, nonsyncopal events that do not result in consciousness include falls and psychogenic pseudo-symptoms.

The most common forms of syncope are reflex mediated, cardiac, orthostatic, and cerebrovascular (Limmer, Mistouich, & Krost, 2009; Miller & Kruse, 2005). According to Farwell and Sulke (2002) and Cadman (2001), 36–62% of syncopal episodes are reflex mediated, 10–30% are cardiac related, 2–24% are orthostatic related, and 1% are cerebrovascular related. The

S

prognosis for most cases of syncope without cardiac disorder is positive. When a cardiac condition is identified, there is a 20–30% mortality rate within 1 year of the original event. There is also a 33% chance for sudden death within 5 years (Soteriades et al., 2002).

Reflex-mediated syncope is often a result of autonomic reflex dysfunction caused by stress secondary to fear and/or pain. This results in an increase of vagal tone instead of increasing sympathetic tone. The three subtypes of reflex-mediated syncope are vasovagal, carotid sinus, and situational. Vasovagal syncope consists of three specific phases: prodrome symptoms, loss of consciousness, and the postsyncopal phase. In vasovagal syncope, an outside event most often precipitates the episode, such as prolonged standing, emotional stress, pain, physical straining, or trauma. Once the outside event triggers an episode, the first prodrome phase can consist of diaphoresis, gastric problems, fatigue, weakness, yawning, nausea, dizziness, and vertigo (Brignole et al., 2004). Loss of consciousness occurs in the next phase. The third phase, postsyncopal, can often last for hours, and rarely days. This phase can include protracted confusion, disorientation, nausea, dizziness, and an overall sense of not feeling well (Kenny, 2002). If the postsyncopal phase lasts more than a few days, it may indicate a more serious condition than vasovagal syncope and extensive evaluation should be given.

Carotid sinus syncope is most often diagnosed if the patient has a history of syncopal events in connection with head movements, wearing tight collars, and even shaving, and mostly occurs in older patients (Miller & Kruse, 2005).

Situational syncope is most often associated with micturition, defecation, coughing, or gastrointestinal problems. Cardiac syncope involves two basic subtypes: dysrhythmia-mediated and structural cardiopulmonary lesions. The common feature associated with both subtypes is the heart being unable to increase cardiac output to meet the associated demand.

Neurologic syncope is the least common form of syncope and often occurs as a result of the reticular activating system of the brainstem becoming ischemic. It could also be a result of subarachnoid hemorrhage or subclavian steal.

Psychiatric syncope occurs at a high rate in psychiatric patients. It is most often related to Axis I disorders, such as anxiety, panic, and major depressive disorders. Orthostatic syncope occurs when a person is in the upright position and their blood flow pools. In healthy individuals, sympathetic tone would be increased upon standing. In others, adequate sympathetic tone is not achieved, resulting in syncope. Possible causes can be related to neurological insult and drugs.

TREATMENT

Due to the fact that most people diagnosed with syncope (children and adults) do not have an underlying heart disease or abnormal heart rhythm (arrhythmia), extensive medical workup is not often needed. Most causes of syncope will be discovered with a thorough physical examination, as mentioned previously.

The treatment for neurally mediated syncope is counterintuitive to our American diet. Consuming increased amounts of salt along with increased fluid intake assists in reducing the chance of dehydration and helps to maintain blood volume. People with syncope should become aware of the presyncope warning signs, such as sweaty palms, dizziness, and nausea. When the presyncope events are experienced, it is best to lie down with legs elevated (Atiga, Rowe, & Calkins, 1999; National Institute of Neurological Disorders and Stroke [NINDS], 2008).

Overall it is best to reduce events that can exacerbate syncope, such as avoiding extreme heat, limiting alcohol intake, and not standing for long periods of time. Di Girolamo, Di Iorio, Leonzio, Sabatini, and Barsotti (1999) and Mahanonda et al. (1995) recommended tilt table training for those who have frequent syncope attacks. Zaqqa and Massumi (2000) indicated that medication treatment should be individualized. They state that considering the age of the patient, co-occurring disorders, and the side effects and safety of each medication is essential. Common first-line medications for adults are beta blockers and for children fludrocortisones (Scott et al., 1995).

Teri J. McHale
Stephen E. Prover
Henry V. Soper

Atiga, W., Rowe, P., & Calking, H. (1999). Management of vasovagal syncope. *Journal of Cardiovascular Electophysiology, 10,* 874–886.

Bloomfield, D., Sheldon, R., Grubb, B., Calkins, H., & Sutton, R. (1999). Putting it together: A new treatment algorithm for vasovagal syncope and related disorders. *American Journal of Cardiology, 84,* 833–839.

Brignole, M., Alboni, P., Benditt, D., Gergfeldt, L., Blanc, J., Bloch et al. (2004). Guidelines on management (diagnosis and treatment) of syncope—Update 2004. *Europace, 6*(6), 467. Retrieved from http://www.guideline.gov/summary/summary.aspz?doc_id=6468

Cadman, C. S. (2001). Medical therapy of neurocardiogenic syncope. *Cardiology Clinics, 19,* 203–213.

Di Girolamo, E., Di Iorio, C., Leonzio, L., Sabatini, P., & Barsotti, A. (1999). Usefulness of a tilt training program for the prevention of refractory neurocardiogenic syncope in adolescents: A controlled study. *Circulation, 100,* 1798–1801.

Farwell, D., & Sulke, N. (2002). How do we diagnose syncope? *Journal of Cardiovascular Electrophysiology*, 13(Suppl. 1), S9–S13.

Kapoor, W. (2000). Syncope. *The New England Journal of Medicine, 343*, 1856–1862.

Kenny, R. (2002). Neurally mediated syncope. *Clinics in Geriatric Medicine, 18*, 191–210, vi.

Limmer, D., Mistovich, J., & Krost, W. (2009). Beyond the basics: Syncope. *EMS Magazine. Cygnus Business Media, 38*(2), 52–55.

Linzer, M., Yang, E., Estes, M., Wang, P., Vorperian, V., & Kapoor, W. (1997a). Clinical guideline: Diagnosing syncope: Part 1: Value of history, physical examination, and electrocardiography. *Annals of Internal Medicine, 126*(12), 989–996.

Linzer, M., Yang, E., Estes, M., Wang, P., Vorperian, V., & Kapoor, W. (1997b). Clinical guideline: Diagnosing syncope: Part 2: Unexplained syncope. *Annals of Internal Medicine, 127*(1), 76–86.

Mahanonda, N., Bhuripanyo, K., Kangkagate, C., Wansanit, K., Kulchot, B., & Nademanee, K. (1995). Randomized double-blind, placebo-controlled trial of oral atenolol in patients with unexplained syncope and positive upright tilt table test results. *American Heart Journal, 130*, 1250–1253.

Miller, T., & Kruse, J. (2005). Evaluation of syncope. *American Family Physician, 1*–12.

National Institute of Neurological Disorders and Stroke. (2008). NINDS Syncope Information page. Retrieved from the world wide web on March 16, 2009 www.ninds.nih.gov/disorders/syncope/cyncope.htm

Scott, W. Pongiglione, G., Bromberg, B., Schaffer, M., Deal, B., Fish, F., et al. (1994). Randomized comparison of atenolol and fludrocortisone acetate in the treatment of pediatric neurally mediated syncope. *American Journal of Cardiology, 76*, 400.

Soteriades, E., Evans, J., Larson, M., Chen, M., Chen, L., Benjamin, E., et al. (2002). Incidence and prognosis of syncope. *New England Journal of Medicine, 347*, 878–885.

Zaqqa, M., & Massumi, A. (2000). Neurally mediated syncope. *Texas Heart Institute Journal, 27*(3), 268–272.

SYRINGOMYELIA

DESCRIPTION

Syringomyelia results from a cyst, also called a syrinx, which develops and grows in the spinal cord leading to damage over time (Greitz, 2006). The disorder, which often occurs between the ages of 25 and 40, commonly develops gradually; however, onset may be rapid following injury (i.e., straining or trauma). Symptoms include progressive—sometimes intermittent—weakness ranging to paralysis in the arms and legs, decline in sensation, bladder or bowel dysfunction, and severe pain (Madsen, Green, & Bowen, 1999).

Syringomyelias may result from a number of conditions, but it is estimated that prevalence is 8.4 per 100,000, and more men than women manifest this disorder (Greitz, 2006). Prognosis following treatment shows modest improvements for most individuals; however, this is dependent upon the etiology, significance of neurologic impairment, and size and location of the syrinx (Attal, Parker, Tadie, Aghakani, & Bouhassira, 2004).

NEUROPATHOLOGY/PATHOPHYSIOLOGY

Although the exact pathophysiology of syringomyelia is unknown, multiple theories of pressure and flow gradients exist (Chang & Nakagawa, 2003). In essence, the spinal cord is surrounded by the cerebrospinal fluid (CSF), which serves to transport nutrients, remove waste, and protect the central nervous system. During the development of the nervous system, CSF fills the central canal. This canal ultimately closes, yet if CSF is obstructed in the spinal cord, the extra fluid will be diverted into the central canal and eventually develops into a syrinx (Madsen et al., 1999). Continued obstruction results in continued growth and ultimately spinal cord damage.

Depending upon the area of impairment involved by the expansion of the syrinx, different regions and fiber tracts may be involved resulting in a variety of symptoms. Syrinx tends to impinge the spinothalamic fibers that moderate appreciation of pain and temperature, whereas medial lemniscus fibers, which moderate appreciation of touch, vibration, and position, remain intact until much later in the disease process (Koyanagi, Iwasaki, Hida, & Houkin, 2005). Damage to the anterior horns of the motor neurons in the spinal cord causes muscle atrophy, typically beginning in the hands and progressing proximally (Koyanagi et al., 2005). Horner syndrome may also be present secondary to damage to the intermediolateral cell column of sympathetic neurons (Koyanagi et al., 2005).

NEUROPSYCHOLOGICAL/CLINICAL PRESENTATION

Depending upon the location and growth of the syrinx, nerve fibers may be affected that can result in a variety of symptoms. In general, pain, weakness, and stiffness may predominate in locations depending on

S

the relative dermatomes involved (i.e., arms, legs, shoulders, and back). Motor functions tend to be compromised by the associated muscle atrophy and as a result, claw hand or spasticity in the lower extremities may be present (Madsen et al., 1999). In addition, reflexes in the arms may be diminished early in the disease process (Madsen et al., 1999).

Sensory disturbance, usually lack of appreciation of temperature may occur, and, in particular, a "cape-like" pattern of loss of temperature and pain sensation along the back and arms may be present (Koyanagi et al., 2005). Typically, syringomyelia does not impact the dorsal column of the spinal cord (medial lemniscus), which moderates pressure, vibration, touch, and proprioception in the upper extremities, until much later in the disease process when astereognosis may be evident upon clinical evaluation (Koyanagi et al., 2005).

Other manifestations of syringomyelia may include headaches, ulcers (particularly on the hands), edema, hyperhidrosis, neurogenic arthropathies, or scoliosis may be present (Madsen et al., 1999). Generally, there is no reported cognitive or academic impairments noted in syringomyelia; however, a variant occurring when the syrinx manifests near the brainstem results in a different condition called syringobulbia, which has reported cognitive impairments (Madsen et al., 1999).

DIAGNOSIS

In the past, diagnosis of syringomyelia may have been difficult due to the fact that many early symptoms of this disorder are apparent in other more frequent disorders. With the advent of MRI, diagnosis of syringomyelia in the early stages of the disease process is much easier and is often the diagnostic tool of choice (Yeom et al., 2007). Other tests include electromyography (EMG) (which measures nerve conduction in the muscle and its weakness), lumbar puncture (to measure CSF pressure), or myelogram (which takes an X-ray within the context of an injection of contrast dye into the subarachnoid space).

Two major variants of syringomyelia exist: communicating and noncommunicating syringomyelia (Oldfield et al., 1994). Communicating syringomyelia, named from the perception of connection between the brain and spinal cord, is characterized by the development of a syrinx in the cervical region of the spinal cord near the Chiari I malformation, which is part of the cerebellum that protrudes through the foramen magnum (Oldfield et al., 1994). Onset tends to be in early adulthood and may be caused by fluctuations of CSF or straining activities. Some individuals with communicating syringomyelia may experience hydrocephalus due to inflammation of the arachnoid membrane surrounding the brain (Oldfield et al., 1994). Noncommunicating syringomyelia occurs following either direct or indirect trauma to the spinal cord from a potential of multiple etiologies (i.e., meningitis, hemorrhage, tumor, arachnoiditis, or direct trauma), where the syrinx begins to grow and onset of symptoms may be immediate or even delayed several years following injury (Madsen et al., 1999).

Differential diagnosis of syringomyelia include, but are not limited to, acute inflammatory demyelinating polyradiculoneuropathy, amyotrophic lateral sclerosis, ankylosing spondylitis, arteriovenous malformations, atlantoaxial instability associated with Down's syndrome, brainstem gliomas, central pontine myelinolysis, cervical spondulosis, chronic inflammatory demyelinating polyradiculoneuropathy, diabetic neuropathy, ependymoma, hydrocephalus, limb-girdle muscular dystrophy, medulloblastoma, meningioma, multiple sclerosis, neural tube defects, spinal cord hemorrhage, spinal cord infarction, trauma, spinal epidural abscess, and spinal muscular atrophy (Greitz, 2006).

TREATMENT

Treatment for syringomyelia, if symptomatic, tends to involve surgery, either singular or multiple, which may focus on enlarging the foramen magnum in the case of communicating syringomyelia, shunting and draining the syrinx fluid to alleviate symptoms, or even resecting a tumor in order to eliminate obstruction (Rhoton & Hamilton, 1999). In the past, surgeons would also shunt trauma-induced syringomyelias, yet this procedure often requires multiple surgeries. Currently, surgeons expand the space around the spinal cord by removing tethers, realigning the vertebrae, and adding "patches" that reinforce the dura surrounding the spine (Rhoton & Hamilton, 1999).

Other forms of treatment, such as medications or radiation, are not therapeutic; however, medication may be prescribed to alleviate pain. Opioids are often combined with other medications utilized for treating neuropathic pain (Rhoton & Hamilton, 1999). In general, prognosis following surgery results in modest improvements for most individuals; however, treatment delays may have irreversible outcome on spinal cord damage (Attal et al., 2004).

Javan Horwitz
Natalie Horwitz
Chad A. Noggle

Attal, N., Parker, F., Tadie, M., Aghakani, N., & Bouhassira, D. (2004). Effects of surgery on the sensory deficits of syringomyelia and predictors of outcome: A long term prospective study. *Journal of Neurology, Neurosurgery, and Psychiatry, 75*(7), 1025–1030.

Chang, H., & Nakagawa, H. (2003). Hypothesis on the pathophysiology of syringomyelia based on simulation of cerebrospinal fluid dynamics. *Journal of Neurology, Neurosurgery, and Psychiatry, 74*(3), 344–347.

Greitz, D. (2006). Unraveling the riddle of syringomyelia. *Neurosurgery Review, 29*(4), 251–264.

Koyanagi, I., Iwasaki, Y., Hida, K., & Houkin, K. (2005). Clinical features and pathomechanisms of syringomyelia associated with spinal arachnoiditis. *Surgical Neurology, 63*(4), 350–356.

Madsen, P., III., Green, B., & Bowen, B. (1999). Syringomyelia. In H. Herkowitz, S. Garfin, & R. Balderston (Eds.), *The spine* (4th ed., pp. 1431–1459). Philadelphia, PA: W.B. Saunders Company.

Oldfield, E., Muraszko, K., Shawker, T. H., & Patronas, N. (1994). Pathophysiology of syringomyelia associated with Chiari I malformation of the cerebellar tonsils: Implications for diagnosis and treatment. *Journal of Neurosurgery, 80*(1), 3–15.

Rhoton, A., & Hamilton, A. (1999). Chiari malformation and syringomyelia. In E. Benzel (Ed.), *Spine surgery: Techniques, complication avoidance, and management* (pp. 793–812). Boston: Churchill-Livingstone.

Yeom, J. S., Lee, C., Park, K. W., Lee, J. H., Lee, D. H., Wang, K. C., et al. (2007). Scoliosis associated with syringomyelia: Analysis of MRI and curve progression. *European Spine Journal, 16*(10), 1629–1635.

SYSTEMIC LUPUS ERYTHEMATOSUS

DESCRIPTION

Systemic lupus erythematosus (SLE) is a chronic and potentially fatal multisystem autoimmune disease with a varied spectrum of neurological, neuropsychiatric, and cognitive presentations. Lesions within the central nervous system (CNS) may produce headache, seizures, psychosis, aseptic meningitis, cerebral vascular accidents (CVAs), transient ischemic attacks (TIAs), microvascular changes, white matter lesions, thrombosis, chorea, demyelinization syndromes, transverse myelitis, and cranial or peripheral neuropathies (Coín-Mejías et al., 2008; Leritz, Brandt, Minor, Reis-Jensen, & Petri, 2002; Loukkola et al., 2003; Schrott & Crnic, 1996). Affective disturbance (e.g., depression and anxiety) is also common (Schrott &

Crnic, 1996) as are skin rashes, joint ailments, and renal failure. The course of SLE is a fluctuating one, and although many may experience periods of remission, a number of individuals experience ongoing and disabling sequelae (Iverson, 1995). Individuals with SLE have a reduced life expectancy, in part, due to the increased risk of infection due to autoimmune suppression (Breitbach et al., 1998).

Worldwide prevalence of SLE ranges between 15 and 50 per 100,000 with more cases cited in the United States than elsewhere and women eight times more likely to be diagnosed with SLE than men (Skeel, Johnstone, Yangco, Walker, & Komatireddy, 2000). Increased incidence has also been found in African Americans (up to three times more likely than White females) with increased mortality rates noted at a younger age in non-White females (Breitbach et al., 1998; Skeel et al., 2000). It remains uncertain whether these differences reflect genetic vulnerability or are a manifestation of other socioeconomic factors (Breitbach et al., 1998). Finally, SLE has an increased incidence in women of childbearing age, suggesting hormonal factors as a causative factor (Schrott & Crnic, 1996).

SLE often presents with and without CNS involvement; neuropsychiatric SLE (NPSLE) is another term used to differentiate between these individuals with neuropsychological impairment included within the umbrella of CNS or neuropsychiatric involvement. Depending upon the criteria used, it is estimated that between 14–75% of SLE cases present with CNS involvement and those with CNS involvement are more likely to exhibit cognitive dysfunction (Coín-Mejías et al., 2008; Leritz et al., 2002).

NEUROPATHOLOGY/PATHOPHYSIOLOGY

The precise etiology of SLE remains uncertain; however, the most accepted proposal is that of it being multifactorial including vascular causes, autoantibodies, and inflammatory mediators (Benedict, Shucard, Zivadinov, & Shucard, 2008). Antiphospholipid antibodies (aPLs), both lupus anticoagulant (LA) and anticardiolipin (aCL), have been identified as a contributor to vascular risk factors in SLE due to immune-mediated hypercoagulability (Leritz et al., 2002). This increases risk of thrombosis, which itself promotes focal symptoms such as CVA, TIA, and seizures. A noninflammatory vasculopathy involving small vessels may permit such antibodies to enter the CNS at which point they react with cell-surface or serum components (Mills, 1994). Cytokines have been proposed as an inflammatory mediator in the disease and have been established in the literature as being related to increased risk of cognitive deficits, both acute and over the long term.

MRI abnormalities include diffuse hyperintensities within the deep white matter and cerebral atrophy with greater disease severity associated with positive aPLs (Benedict, Shucard, Zivadinov, & Shucard, 2008; Loukkola et al., 2003). Neural injury and death may be due to the production of antinuclear antibodies (ANA) and pro-inflammatory cytokines (Benedict et al., 2008; Schrott & Crnic, 1996).

NEUROPSYCHOLOGICAL/CLINICAL PRESENTATION

Cognitive dysfunction in SLE patients has been well documented. Estimates suggest that 81% of individuals with CNS involvement or NPSLE, and 42% of those without CNS involvement demonstrate cognitive dysfunction (Loukkola et al., 2003; Skeel et al., 2000). Common cognitive complaints within the domains of attention, psychomotor speed, executive functioning, verbal fluency, and retrieval-based memory have been well documented (Holliday et al., 2003; Loukkola et al., 2003). Some researchers also note deficits in visuospatial skills and worse visual learning and memory relative to new learning and memory for verbal material (Benedict et al., 2008; Coín-Mejías et al., 2008; Mendez & Cummings, 2003). The presence of aPLs in SLE individuals has also been associated with a worse neuropsychological outcome (Leritz et al., 2002). Poorer neuropsychological performance in African American patients has also been attributed to psychosocial factors (Breitbach et al., 1998). Affective complaints are a common feature of SLE and may further adversely impact cognitive functioning (Breitbach et al., 1998). However, it appears that cognitive manifestations remain even when these factors are controlled for (Leritz et al., 2002) and do not fully explain deficits in processing speed, attention, and memory. The possible adverse affects of corticosteriod treatment (e.g., psychiatric manifestations and cognitive decline) should also be considered. Clinical manifestations are varied and represent a systemic disease process with a relapsing remitting course affecting multiple areas, as discussed earlier.

Beyond cognitive domains, seizures represent another salient issue along neurological lines in patients with SLE, occurring in 25% of patients (Kaell, Shetty, Lee, & Lockshin, 1986).

DIAGNOSIS

The diagnosis of SLE is made via the presence of ANA and double-stranded DNA titers, and elevated aPLs in blood serum. Cerebrospinal fluid (CSF) may also show mild protein and lymphocyte elevations (Mendez & Cummings, 2003). MRI may show structural changes, including cerebral infarction, diffuse white matter changes, and cerebral atrophy. The clinical presentation of SLE is varied and neuropsychological assessment is a most sensitive tool in determining neurocognitive and functional status in these patients (Breitbach et al., 1998).

TREATMENT

Corticosteroids and anti-inflammatory agents are currently the treatments of choice for SLE. Psychiatric manifestations are common among persons with SLE, though it remains uncertain if these are related to primary CNS involvement, psychological factors associated with illness, or both (Iverson, 1995). As such, efforts to manage psychological factors and behaviors are warranted. Finally, the etiology of increased incidence in non-White females remains uncertain but may be attributed to socioeconomic status. Therefore, support, psychoeducation, and promotion of health promoting behaviors (e.g., maintaining proper diet, exercise, maintaining stress, medication adherence) are important in the treatment and maintenance of symptoms in persons with SLE (Iverson, 1995).

Michelle R. Pagoria
Chad A. Noggle

Benedict, R. H. B., Shucard, J. L., Zivadinov, R., & Shucard, D. W. (2008). *Neuropsychology Review, 18,* 149–166.

Breitbach, S. A., Alexander, R. W., Daltroy, L. H., Liang, M. H., Boll, T. J., Karlson, E. W., et al. (1998). Determinants of cognitive performance in systemic lupus erythematosus. *Journal of Clinical and Experimental Neuropsychology, 20,* 157–166.

Coín-Mejías, M. A., Peralta-Ramírez, M. I., Santiago-Ramajo, S., Morente-Soto, G., Ortego-Centeno, N., Callejas Rubio, J. L., et al. (2008). Alterations in episodic memory in patients with systemic lupus erythematosus. *Archives of Clinical Neuropsychology, 23,* 157–164.

Holliday, S. L., Navarrete, M. G., Hermosillo-Romo, D., Valdez, C. R., Saklad, A. R., Escalante, A., et al. (2003). Validating a computerized neuropsychological test battery for mixed ethnic lupus patients. *Lupus, 12,* 697–703.

Iverson, G. L. (1995). The need for psychological services for persons with systemic lupus erythematosus. *Rehabilitation Psychology, 40,* 39–49.

Kaell, A.T., Shetty, M., Lee, B. C., & Lockshin, M. D. (1986). The diversity of neurological events in systemic lupus erythematosus. Prospective clinical and computed tomographic classification of 82 events in 71 patients. *Archives of Neurology, 43,* 273–276.

Leritz, E., Brandt, J., Minor, M., Reis-Jensen, F., & Petri, M. (2002). Neuropsychological functioning and its relationship to antiphospholipid antibodies in patients with systemic lupus erythematosus. *Journal of Clinical and Experimental Neuropsychology, 24,* 527–533.

Loukkola, J., Laine, M., Ainiala, H., Peltola, J., Metänoja, R., Auvinen, A., et al. (2003). Cognitive impairment in systemic lupus erythematosus and neuropsychiatric systemic lupus erythematosus: A population-based neuropsychological study. *Journal of Clinical and Experimental Neuropsychology, 25,* 145–151.

Mendez, M. F., & Cummings, J. L. (2003). *Dementia: A clinical approach* (3rd ed.). Philadelphia: Butterworth-Heinemann.

Mills, J. A. (1994). Systemic lupus erythematosus. *New England Journal of Medicine, 330,* 1871–1879.

Schrott, L. M., & Crnic, L. S. (1996). Increased anxiety behaviors in autoimmune mice. *Behavioral Neuroscience, 110,* 492–502.

Skeel, R. L., Johnstone, B., Yangco, D. T., Walker, S. E., & Komatireddy, G. R. (2000). Neuropsychological deficit profiles in systemic lupus erythematosus. *Applied Neuropsychology, 7,* 96–101.

S

Takayasu's disease

DESCRIPTION

Takayasu's disease, also known as Takaysu's arteritis, is a rare and chronic inflammatory vascular disorder that primarily affects the aorta and its main branches as well as the pulmonary arteries and results in absent limb pulses and retinopathy (Bassa, Desai, & Moodley, 1995). Takayasu's disease predominantly affects Asian females with an overall male-to-female ratio of 1 to 8.5. In the majority of cases, the age of onset is between 10 and 20 years of age; however, there is still a sizeable variety in presenting age (Batchelor & Dean, 1996; Tann, Tulloh, & Hamilton, 2008). The incidence of Takayasu's arteritis is estimated to be 2.6 cases per 1 million persons each year (Hall et al., 1985).

NEUROPATHOLOGY/PATHOPHYSIOLOGY

Takayasu's arteritis emerges in response to aortic burden, in addition to involvement of the aorta's main branches, resulting in systemic vascular and potential immune response. Degradation of these structures has been associated with invasion of the media and adventitia of the vessels by giant cells (Bartl & Topel, 2007). Infectious processes, particularly tuberculosis, have been linked to the pathophysiology of the disease. Takayasu's arteritis can be divided into two stages: acute and chronic. Inflammation of the adventitial vessels of the arterial walls occurs in the acute stage. This initial phase is usually followed by a prolonged chronic phase, in which the elastic tissue is replaced by fibrosis. In addition, thickening exists in all three layers (Tann et al., 2008). At that point, there is typically a progressive and gradual deterioration of function due to vascular occlusion (Batchelor & Dean, 1996).

NEUROPSYCHOLOGICAL/CLINICAL PRESENTATION

There are many signs and symptoms of Takayasu's arteritis, including a diminished pulse, hypertension, vascular bruits, and angina. Patients may present with neurological symptoms, such as transient ischemic attacks, hypertensive encephalopathy, seizures, dizziness, vertigo, and/or headaches (Batchelor & Dean, 1996; Kerr et al., 1994; Tann et al., 2008). Furthermore, patients may complain of fatigue, pain in the extremities, or unexplained weight loss.

DIAGNOSIS

Diagnosis of Takayasu's arteritis can be quite difficult, as the symptoms and signs are nonspecific, and the course of the disease varies from patient to patient (Kerr et al., 1994). In many cases, blood pressure is elevated and abnormal blood movement can be heard with a stethoscope (The Johns Hopkins Vasculitis Center, 2009). Furthermore, blood tests may reveal anemic conditions that are also common in Takayasu's arteritis. Conventional catheterization angiography is a popular procedure for the initial diagnosis for Takayasu's arteritis, though it may be unreliable in the early phase of the disease because it may not detect significant abnormalities. In addition, research on the use of MRI with 3-D contrast-enhanced angiography has shown the method to be exceptionally helpful in the early diagnosis and follow-up of Takayasu's arteritis. These diagnostic procedures reveal morphological changes, as well as subtle pathological changes in the arterial wall (Halefoglu & Yakut, 2005).

TREATMENT

Treatment for Takayasu's arteritis is often focused on inducing remission and/or managing complications of the disease. Medical treatment typically involves high-dose corticosteroids with immunosuppressants. Glucocorticoid therapy alone is usually the first line of treatment for Takayasu's arteritis patients. If this is unsuccessful, other agents can be added, including cyclophosphamide, azathioprine, and methotrexate. Hypertension is exacerbated by glucocorticoid therapy, making treating patients with this condition as well as Takayasu's arteritis difficult. Some patients require surgical and endovascular procedures, which relieve ischemic complications (Batchelor & Dean, 1996; Tann et al., 2008). If left untreated,

Takayasu's arteritis can result in death from cerebral hemorrhage, renal failure, heart failure, myocardial infarction, cerebral thrombosis, or aneurysm rupture (Fields et al., 2006).

Amy Zimmerman
Raymond S. Dean

Bartt, R. E., & Tropel, J. L. (2007). Autoimmune and inflammatory disorders. In C. G. Goetz (Ed.), *Textbook of clinical neurology* (3rd ed., pp. 1155–1184). Philadelphia, PA: Saunders Elsevier.

Bassa, A., Desai, D. K., & Moodley, J. (1995). Takayasu's disease and pregnancy. *South African Medical Journal, 85,* 107–112.

Batchelor, E. S., Jr., & Dean, R. S. (1996). *Pediatric neuropsychology: Interfacing assessment and treatment for rehabilitation.* Needham Heights, MA: Allyn & Bacon.

Fields, C. E., Bower, T. C., Cooper, L. T., Hoskins, T., Noel, A. A., Panneton, J. M., et al. (2006). Takayasu's arteritis: Operative results and influence of disease activity. *Journal of Vascular Surgery, 43*(1), 64–71.

Halefoglu, A. M., & Yakut, S. (2005). Role of magnetic resonance imaging in the early diagnosis of Takayasu arteritis. *Australasian Radiology, 49,* 377–381.

Hall, S., Barr, W., Lie, J. T., Stanson, A. W., Kazmier, F. J., & Hunder, G. G. (1985). Takayasu arteritis: A study of 32 North American patients. *Medicine, 64,* 89–99.

Kerr, G. S., Hallahan, C. W., Giordano, J., Leavitt, R. Y., Fauci, A. S., Rottem, M., & Hoffman, G. S. (1994). Takayasu arteritis. *Annals of Internal Medicine, 120*(11), 919–929.

Tann, O. R., Tulloh, R. M. R., & Hamilton, M. C. K. (2008). Takayasu's disease: A review. *Cardiology in the Young, 18,* 250–259.

The Johns Hopkins Vasculitis Center. (2009). *Takayasu's arteritis.* Retrieved May 5, 2009, from http://vasculitis.med.jhu.edu/typesof/takayasu.html#symptoms

TARDIVE DYSKINESIA

DESCRIPTION

Beginning in the 1950s, neuroleptic medication revolutionized the treatment of schizophrenia; however, it quickly became apparent that one major risk of treatment with neuroleptic medication was the development of tardive dyskinesia (TD). In early descriptions of the disorder, TD was characterized by (1) involuntary, abnormal movements of the body; (2) occurrence either late in the treatment regimen or after the discontinuation of medication, persistence of motor abnormalities for months or years; and (3) poor response to treatment (Crane, 1969). Although some advances have been made in understanding the pathophysiology of TD, researchers still debate underlying mechanisms, and there is no consistently effective treatment for the disorder. The development of atypical antipsychotics and their widespread use as an alternative to phenothiazine-based antipsychotics has greatly reduced the incidence of TD.

Prevalence of TD among patients receiving chronic pharmacotherapy with antipsychotics is approximately 20% after the first 3 years of exposure, with a 5% increase in new cases per year of treatment with neuroleptic medication. Individuals at higher risk for developing TD include the elderly, females, persons with affective disorders, alcohol abuse, sensitivity to acute extrapyramidal symptoms, and mutations of D2 and D3 receptor genes. A longitudinal study examined patients with and without TD over 10 years and found a relatively benign long-term course for most, with some patients entering remission and others maintaining a relatively stable course (Gordos et al., 1994). For others, however, TD symptoms proved intractable and severely disabling.

NEUROPATHOLOGY/PATHOPHYSIOLOGY

TD is associated with degeneration of neurons in the mesencephalon, primarily the basal ganglia and subthalamic nucleus. To date, researchers have yet to reach a consensus on the mechanism(s) underlying TD. Two theories dominate TD literature, the dopamine hypersensitivity hypothesis and a free radical hypothesis.

The most prominent theory is the dopamine hypersensitivity theory that proposes that long-term use of antipsychotic medication results in an upregulation of postsynaptic dopamine receptors in the basal ganglia. One study, using positron emission tomography (PET) scans to assess D2 receptor binding in eight schizophrenics who had never been exposed to antipsychotic medication and nine schizophrenics who had taken antipsychotics for a mean of 16 years, found a 34% increase in D2-binding potential in patients subjected to long-term exposure of antipsychotic medication (Silvestri et al., 2000). In this study, the patient with the highest D2-binding potential developed TD. One researcher found enlarged caudate nuclei in the early stages of treatment of young schizophrenics and proposed that it is possible that the enlargement may be the result of interaction between treatment with neuroleptics and neuronal plasticity of the DA system Chakos and colleagues (1994) proposed that enlargement of the caudate nuclei may be the result of interaction between treatment with neuroleptics and neuronal plasticity. Inconsistencies in the DA supersensitivity hypothesis include the fact that the number of DA receptors increases over a course of days, but symptoms of TD do not typically develop for months or years. Second, in many instances receptor concentrations do return to normal densities, but the symptoms of TD persist.

The free radical hypothesis of TD suggests that neuronal degeneration may result from oxidative damage caused by free radical formation. The free radical hypothesis holds that by blocking dopamine receptors, antipsychotics cause an increase in dopamine production resulting in increased free radical production by monoamine oxidase inhibition in areas of the brain that receive large quantities of oxygen, such as the basal ganglia (Lohr, Kuczenski, & Niculescu, 2003). Lohr et al. (2003) further suggests that certain antipsychotics may cause increases in reactive oxygen via mitochondria.

Other mechanisms proposed for increased risk of TD include decreases in or damage to neurons that release GABA, especially in the striatum, and increased release of glutamate and aspartate as a result of D2 receptor blockage that normally inhibits the release of glutamate. One study examined cerebrospinal fluid from individuals with and without TD and found increased levels of N-acetylaspartate, aspartate, and N-acetylglutamate. Some research has found relationships between loss of striatal cholinergic neurons and TD (Margolese, Chouinard, Kolivakis, Beauclair, & Miller, 2005). Also, recent evidence suggests that reduced levels of brain-derived neurotrophic growth factor (BDNF) are found in schizophrenic patients with TD and that levels of BDNF are inversely correlated with dyskinetic movements (Tan, Zhou, & Zhang, 2005).

NEUROPSYCHOLOGICAL/CLINICAL PRESENTATION

TD is marked by severe motor impairment primarily affecting the tongue, lips, jaw, face, trunk, extremities, and the respiratory system; the onset of symptoms has been documented in patients after a short time of treatment with neuroleptic medication (months), after discontinuing neuroleptic medication, or after reinstatement of neuroleptic medication after a period of time without administration. Spontaneous dyskinesias are rare but have been reported in patients who have never received neuroleptic medication. Involuntary movements are most frequently seen in

the oral region of patients with TD and may escalate in severity to effect speech. Stereotypical features of the oral-facial region include protrusion of the tongue, grimacing, rolling, pursing, sucking motions of the lips, or contractions of the jaw. Other anatomical regions may present with jerky or choreiform movements, atheosis, and uncoordinated movements of the respiratory muscles. Swallowing may become difficult as well as maintaining balance. Many patients present with a peculiar, shuffling gait.

Involuntary movements made by patients with TD may be socially unacceptable and may cause awkwardness in social situations, not only to the patients, but to relatives and friends of the patient as well. Patients vary in the degree to which they are disturbed by the abnormal and involuntary motions, though most patients are at least somewhat bothered.

DIAGNOSIS

The Abnormal Involuntary Movement Scale (AIMS) was published in 1976 and is the most commonly used assessment instrument in the diagnosis of TD. Clinicians rate overall severity of movements as well as the severity of movements in seven anatomical positions (tongue, lips, jaw, face, upper extremities, lower extremities, and trunk) on 5-point rating scales (0 = none, 1 = minimal, 2 = mild, 3 = moderate and 4 = severe). Lane, Glazer, Hansen, Berman, and Kramer (1985) proposed several conventions in order enhance interrater reliability including rating severity based on three dimensions (amplitude, severity, and frequency) as well as criteria for distinguishing abnormal movements in various anatomical parts. A score of 2 "mild" or 1 "moderate" on the AIMS is indicative of TD.

Another widely used TD assessment is the Dyskinesia Identification System, Condensed User Scale (DISCUS: Kalachnik & Sprague, 2006), which has been shown to be of particular value in assessing for TD among persons with intellectual deficiency. The DISCUS examination has more stringent rules for standardized administration and interpretation than the AIMS or other available scales, and, thus, is psychometrically preferable to other assessment scales for TD.

Schooler and Kane (1982) suggest using prerequisites in order to make diagnoses on a progressive scale. They first state that patients must meet three criteria: a history of 3 months of neuroleptic medication, at least moderate abnormal, involuntary motor functions, and the absence of other conditions that may account for the abnormal movements. These criteria in culmination with information pertaining to the persistence of abnormal movements, the dose history of the patient, and the time in which patients have been on medication and exhibited movements may allow diagnoses to be assigned. The progressive diagnoses that they suggest include probable TD, masked probable TD, transient TD, withdrawal TD, persistent TD, and masked persistent TD.

TREATMENT

Some research suggests that medications that reduce free radical formation may be effective in preventing TD. Tacopherol is an antioxidant that counteracts free radicals and shows promise in the treatment and, possibly, the prevention of TD. Researchers have examined possible effects of using vitamin E, a free radical scavenger, as a treatment of TD. Results of such studies have been mixed, and no consistent consensus has been reached on the efficacy of vitamin E treatment for TD. Given the relatively low risks associated with its use, many clinical authors suggest treatment with vitamin E is a safe "add-on" for patients with TD, since it might be of value and is unlikely to be of any detriment to the client.

Paradoxically, medication-induced TD is often treated using low doses of the same medications that purportedly caused the disorder in the first place. Although no drugs have proven to effectively eliminate symptoms of TD, the incidence of TD has been reduced since the development of newer, atypical, antipsychotic medications that have a reduced propensity toward the development of TD. Olanzapine is a newer antipsychotic that has shown promise for the treatment of schizophrenia with reduced incidence in TD as well as less change in brain volume (Lieberman et al., 2005), less damage to striatal neurons (Margolese et al., 2005), and fewer extrapyramidal symptoms (Geddes, Freemantle, Harrison, & Bebbington, 2000). Olanzapine may protect the brain against free radical formation (Tollefson, Beasley, Tamura, Tran, & Potvin, 1997).

Mandi Musso
Alyse Barker
William Drew Gouvier

Chakos, M. H., Lieberman, J. A., Bilder, R. M., Borenstein, M., Lerner, G., Bogerts, B., et al. (1994). Increase in caudate nuclei volumes of first-episode schizophrenic patients taking antipsychotic drugs. *American Journal of Psychiatry, 151*(10), 1430–1436.

Crane, G. E., Ruiz, P., Kernohan, W. J., Wilson, W., & Royalty, N. (1969). Effects of drug withdrawal on tardive dyskinesia. *Activitas Nervosa Superior, 11*(1), 30–35.

Elkashef, A. M., Buchanan, R. W., Gellad, F., Munson, R. C., & Breier, A. (1994). Basal ganglia pathology in schizophrenia and tardive dyskinesia: An MRI quantitative study. *American Journal of Psychiatry, 151*(5), 752–755.

Geddes, J., Freemantle, N., Harrison, P., & Bebbington, P. (2000). Atypical antipsychotics in the treatment of schizophrenia: Systematic overview and meta-regression analysis. *British Medical Journal, 321,* 1371–1376.

Gordos, G., Casey, D. E., Cole, J. O., Perenyi, A., Kocsis, E., Arato, M., et al. (1994). Ten-year outcome of tardive dyskinesia. *American Journal of Psychiatry, 151*(6), 836–841.

Kalachnik, J. E., & Sprague, R. L. (2006). The Dyskinesia Identification System Condensed User Scale: Reliability, validity, and a total cut-off score for mentally ill and mentally retarded populations. *Journal of Clinical Psychology, 49,* 177–189.

Lane, R. D., Glazer, W. M., Hansen, T. E., Berman, W. H., & Kramer, S. I. (1985). Assessment of tardive-dyskinesia using the Abnormal Involuntary Movement Scale. *Journal of Nervous and Mental Disease, 173*(6), 353–357.

Lieberman, J. A., Tollefson, G. D., Charles, C., Zipursky, R., Sharma, T., Kahn, R. S., et al. (2005). Antipsychotic drug effects on brain morphology in first-episode psychosis. *Archives of General Psychiatry, 62,* 361–370.

Lohr, J. B., Kuczenski, R., & Niculescu, A. B. (2003). Oxidative mechanisms and tardive dyskinesia. *CNS Drugs, 17*(1), 47–62.

Margolese, H. C., Chouinard, G., Kolivakis, T., Beauclair, L., & Miller, R. (2005). Tardive dyskinesia in the era of typical and atypical antipsychotics: Part 1: Pathophysiology and mechanisms of induction. *Canadian Journal of Psychiatry, 50*(9), 541–547.

Schooler, N. R., & Kane, J. M. (1982). Research diagnoses for tardive dyskinesia (letter). *Archives of General Psychiatry, 39,* 486–487.

Silvestri, S., Seeman, M. V., Negrete, J. C., Houle, S., Shammi, C. M., Reminton, G. J., et al. (2000). Increased dopamine D2 receptor binding after long-term treatment with antipsychotics in humans: A clinical PET study. *Psychopharmacology, 152,* 174–180.

Tan, Y. L., Zhou, D. F., & Zhang, X. Y. (2005). Decreased plasma brain-derived neurotrophic factor levels in schizophrenic patients with tardive dyskinesia: Association with dyskinetic movements. *Schizophrenia Research, 74*(2–3), 263–270.

Tollefson, G. D., Beasley, C. M., Tamura, R. N., Tran, P. V., & Potvin, J. H. (1997). Blind, controlled, long-term study of the comparative incidence of treatment-emergent tardive dyskinesia with olanzapine or haloperidol. *American Journal of Psychiatry, 154,* 1248–1254.

TARLOV CYSTS

DESCRIPTION

Tarlov cysts, also known as sacral perineural cysts, are a rare cause of localized or radiating back pain and leg pain, caused by the development of cerebrospinal fluid–filled cysts in the sacral area of the spine. They often cause dull, nebulous sciatic pain, which makes both assessing and diagnosing Tarlov cysts difficult (Landers & Seex, 2002). Frequently, they are asymptomatic, meaning that their existence causes no pain, and therefore may need no intervention. The prevalence of Tarlov cysts represents about 4.5% out of all cases of back pain (Prashad, Jain, & Dhammi, 2007). Of all cases of Tarlov cysts, only about 20% of cases are symptomatic and may require treatment (Prashad et al., 2007). It should be noted that the relevant literature uses the terms Tarlov cysts, sacral cysts, and perineural cysts interchangeably; thus, these terms should be treated as synonymous.

Specifically, Tarlov cysts are spinal root lesions, most often seen in the sacral area of the spine at about S-2 or S-3 (Voyadzis, Bhargava, Fraser, & Henderson, 2001). Both injury and congenital etiologies can cause spinal root lesions that fill up with cerebrospinal fluid. In contrast with a diverticula, which is an open fluid-filled lesion, Tarlov cysts are closed, meaning that they fill gradually (Voyadzis et al., 2001). For this reason, the use of radiopaque dye during myelography studies to locate the cyst has been largely unsuccessful.

NEUROPATHOLOGY/PATHOPHYSIOLOGY

Isadore Tarlov, who initially discovered the presence of Tarlov cysts while studying autopsy cases, identified several unique characteristics of Tarlov cysts. First, he found that Tarlov cysts always form between the endoneurium and perineurium, which are both layers of connective tissue enclosing nerve fibers. He also noted that there can be cases of multiple Tarlov cysts that impinge spinal nerves (Voyadzis et al., 2001). Cases of multiple Tarlov cysts can encapsulate a spinal nerve and affect neighboring nerves, which often causes radiculating back, leg, and buttocks pain.

The pathogenesis of Tarlov cysts remains greatly debated. Originally, Tarlov speculated that the perineural cysts were due to inflammation within the nerve root sheath (Acosta, Hinojosa, Schmidt, & Weinstein, 2003). Another possible etiology that Tarlov suggested was hemorrhaging of the subarachnoid space, which can lead to cyst formation.

More recent research has yielded two major hypotheses. First, much research suggests that subarachnoid hemorrhaging and cyst formation can be caused by localized injury or trauma to the lumbar area (Acosta et al., 2003). Another common presumption is that Tarlov cysts are congenital, caused by either a natural propensity to form spinal cysts, or a type of congenital connective tissue disorder (Acosta et al., 2003). Although disparity remains among researchers, the idea of multiple etiologies is commonly espoused. Although sacral cysts are the most common, Tarlov cysts have been found in multiple places along the spinal column (Voyadzis et al., 2001).

NEUROPSYCHOLOGICAL/CLINICAL PRESENTATION

Tarlov cysts can cause a wide range of possible symptoms and pathologies. Most patients with either one or multiple Tarlov cysts report experiencing some sort of radiculopathy or neuropathy, which is to generally say that most patients experience some nerve dysfunction. Specific symptomatology includes either a dull or more intense pain in the back, legs, sacrum, buttocks, or genital area. In addition, Tarlov cysts can cause motor weakness and bladder incontinence (Acosta et al., 2003). Frequently, patients report sensory disturbances such as hypesthesia or paresthesia. Hypesthesia is a reduction in tactile sensitivity, whereas paresthesia is described as a persistent itching or burning condition. Both of these symptoms can be induced by nerve damage caused by the expansion of Tarlov cysts in the sacral area of the anterior spinal column.

Given the multiple locations in which Tarlov cysts can be found, symptomatology is extremely variable in this medical condition. Depending on cyst location, dyspareunia may be a reported symptom, which is the experience of pain during sexual intercourse, usually due to a physical condition. The prevalence of dyspareunia and Tarlov cysts are more common in women than men; generally, 80% of all cases of perineural cysts are women (Acosta et al., 2003). Due to the consistent saturation of cerebrospinal fluid in the sacrum, erosion and sacral fractures can occur, causing a greater amount of lumbar pain (Acosta et al., 2003).

Patients often describe Tarlov cysts as causing a nebulous pain that is exacerbated by standing, sitting, or even coughing. These actions can impose pressure on the subarachnoid space, which stores cerebrospinal fluid. This compression on the subarachnoid space forces cerebrospinal fluid down to the S-2 or S-3 area, where the Tarlov cysts are harbored. As the cerebrospinal fluid begins to fill the spinal root lesion

(Tarlov cyst), swelling occurs, which can impact surrounding nerves (Acosta et al., 2003).

Current research suggests that Tarlov cysts rarely present with neurological symptoms, though it does happen. Common neurological complaints include general or localized motor weakness, hypesthesia, and paresthesia. Due to their sensory symptomatology, Tarlov cysts do not overtly mediate cognitive functioning; however, they may impact neuropsychological testing in indirect ways, such as distractibility due to excessive pain or dysfunctional sensory feedback. Sitting, especially for long durations, can be painful and difficult for patients with Tarlov cysts, making cooperation through a long battery of testing unlikely.

DIAGNOSIS

Diagnosis of Tarlov cysts tends to be incidental in nature, due to their asymptomatic nature. Tarlov cysts are most often identified through the use of CT or MRI scans, which both successfully locate perineural cysts (Voyadzis et al., 2001). Radiopaque dye is also used but tends to be less successful. Because Tarlov cysts are closed lesions, radiopaque dye may take weeks to flow into the cysts, enabling the identification of Tarlov cysts. More recently, water-based dye is being used, which facilitates diagnosis fairly quickly (Acosta et al., 2003). Recently, a classification system was introduced to give further description to sacral cysts and to assist their accurate diagnosis. Type I sacral cysts are known as extradural cysts, which do not contain spinal nerve roots. Type II cysts are extradural cysts with spinal nerve roots, and Type III cysts are intradural (Nabors, Pait, & Byrd, 1988).

The differential diagnoses for Tarlov cysts tend to be more common than symptomatic perineural cysts. One relatively frequent differential diagnosis is that of meningocele. It is a rare form of spina bifida, involving meningeal cysts. These cysts appear quite similar to Tarlov cysts and can present with similar symptoms (Smith & Davis, 1980). Arachnoid cysts, which are cerebrospinal fluid-filled cysts, grow on the arachnoid layer of the spinal cord and should be considered as a differential diagnosis when assessing the presence of spinal cysts. Lastly, neurofibroma is a nerve sheath tumor caused by dysfunctional Schwann cells. The symptomatology of neurofibroma tends to be more severe than Tarlov cysts, causing significant cognitive deficits.

Because Tarlov cysts are usually asymptomatic, they are quite often discovered accidentally through the use of CT or MRI. Previous research argues that though the cysts cause no overt symptoms, they should be consistently monitored for cyst expansion or increased subarachnoid pressure (Landers et al.,

2002). Monitoring asymptomatic perineural cysts are important, due to their potential to expand impinging surrounding bone, tissue, and nerve roots.

TREATMENT

Treatment for Tarlov cysts remains disputed, though several empirically studied options do exist. One non-surgical intervention that is used quite often is draining the accumulated cerebrospinal fluid from the cyst or cysts. This is done through the use of a lumboperitoneal shunt that has been found to be successful as a short-term therapy (Acosta et al., 2003). In order for this treatment to remain efficacious, continuous draining must take place to avoid the inevitable accumulation of cerebrospinal fluid from subarachnoid pressure. Another possible treatment is through the use of corticosteroids or other anti-inflammatory medication. Typically, this would be the first step of treatment taken, though it may not suffice in more malignant cases.

Isadore Tarlov promulgated complete excision of the cyst, the affected nerve root, and the attached ganglion. After Tarlov's discovery of Tarlov cysts, he began to surgically excise the cysts, and found that this method was longitudinally more successful than shunting (Acosta et al., 2003). Presently, cyst excision is practiced, though the surgical risk is disputed. Because Tarlov cysts are fairly benign, many argue that excision is too drastic an intervention. Cyst excision should be an intervention reserved for individuals who experience a great amount of pain due to either multiple or enlarged cysts and have experienced no alleviation from either anti-inflammatory medication or cerebrospinal fluid shunting.

Ryan Boddy
Charles Golden

Acosta, F. L., Hinojosa, A., Schmidt, M. H., & Weinstein, P. R. (2003). Diagnosis and management of sacral Tarlov cysts: Case report and review of the literature. *Journal of Neurosurgery, 15*(2), 1–7.

Landers, J., & Seex, K. (2002). Sacral perineural cysts: Imaging and treatment options. *British Journal of Neurosurgery, 16*(2), 182–185.

Nabors, M. W., Pait, T. G., & Byrd, E. D. (1988). Updated assessment and current classification of spinal meningeal cyst. *Journal of Neurosurgery, 68,* 366–377.

Prashad, B., Jain, A. K., & Dhammi, I. K., (2007). Tarlov cyst: Case report and review of the literature. *Indian Journal of Orthopedics, 41*(4), 401–403.

Smith, H. P., & Davis, C. (1980). Anterior sacral meningocele: Two case reports and discussion of surgical approach. *Neurosurgery, 7*(1), 61–67.

Voyadzis, J. M., Bhargava, P., & Henderson, F. (2001). Tarlov cysts: A study of 10 cases with review of the literature. *Journal of Neurosurgery, 95*(1), 25–32.

TAY–SACHS' DISEASE

DESCRIPTION

Tay–Sachs' disease is a genetic neurodegenerative disorder of lipid storage, corresponding with deficient activity of hexosaminidase A (Hex-A) (Kolodny, 1997). This activity serves to catalyze gangliosides, thus this decreased activity results in a buildup of ganglioside G_{M2} in tissues throughout the body as well as nerve cells in the brain. Although cases have been reported across the globe, Tay–Sachs' disease presents most commonly in Ashkenazi Jews with a carrier prevalence of 3.3% (Petresen, Rotter, & Cantor, 1983).

The classic description of Tay–Sachs' disease has focused on the early-onset variant in which infants develop normally for the first few months of life, but as ganglioside G_{M2} builds up in the brain, mentation, and physical functioning regress. Eventually infants present with blindness, deafness, dysphagia, and decerebrate posturing prior to death. In the rarer, late-onset variant where symptoms manifest when the individual is in their 20s, and sometimes early 30s, progressive neurological deterioration in conjunction with disturbed gait and psychiatric features are observed (Hurowitz, Silver, Brin, Williams, & Johnson, 1993; Rosebush et al., 1995). Emerging evidence also suggests that carriers of Tay–Sachs' disease, who have long been believed to be asymptomatic, actually demonstrate increased prevalence of mild psychiatric and neurological features (Federico et al., 1988). To date, there is no cure or effective treatment for the presentation (Desnick & Kaback, 2001).

NEUROPATHOLOGY/PATHOPHYSIOLOGY

Once considered no different from gangliosidosis, Tay-Sachs' disease is now considered an infantile form of this grouping with distinct enzyme deficiencies and genetic mutations (Lake, 1997). Inherited as an autosomal recessive trait, it is relatively common in Ashkenazi Jews.

G_{M2}-ganglioside levels may be more than 100 times their regular state. Hexosaminidase activity is deficient leading to residual N-acetylgalactosamine on G_{M2}-gangliosidose (Okada & O'Brien, 1969).

Anatomically, infants develop megalencephaly by 2 years of age if they survive that long. Prior to this, the brain may appear microcephalic at birth or even normal in size and swells as the disease progresses. The volumetric growth is due to neuronal swelling and hyperplasia of astrocytes due to the excessive levels of G_{M2}-ganglioside. Meganeurite formation in the cerebral cortex also occurs related to these increased levels (Siegel & Walkley, 1994).

Demyelination occurs disrupting the differentiation between gray and white matter. On MRI with subsequent phosphorus spectroscopy, high signal intensity and severe metabolic changes in the subcortical white matter membrane-bound phosphates and in the basal ganglia have been reported (Mugikura et al., 1996; Schengrund, 1990). Cerebellar atrophy has been reported by some as the most common finding, primarily involving the cerebellar vermis (Streifler, Gornish, Hadar, & Gadoth, 1993). Mutations, which permit residual activity of Hex-A, result in juvenile and adult onset of Tay–Sachs' disease, whereas no activity results in the infantile form (Yacubian et al., 2000).

NEUROPSYCHOLOGICAL/CLINICAL PRESENTATION

Clinically, infants demonstrate normal development for the first few months of life. A heightened startle response may be noted during this asymptomatic period. As the disease progresses, a plateau of psychomotor development is reached followed by retardation. Hypotonia and spasticity eventually develop. Seizures also develop within the first 2 years of life. In the later stages, infants become blind, oftentimes deaf, and exhibit decerebrate posturing prior to death. In comparison, the late-onset subtype is marked by signs of motor neuron and cerebellar involvement as well as dysarthria and psychiatric features (Gravel, Clark, Kaback, Mahuran, & Sandhoff, 1995; Hurowitz et al., 1993; Rosebush et al., 1995).

Emerging findings suggest that even carriers of Tay–Sachs' disease present with neurological and psychiatric residuals. Cognitive impairment, cerebellar ataxia, and psychiatric manifestations have all been said to present at higher rates in Tay–Sachs' disease carriers as opposed to noncarriers (Zelnika, Khazanovb, Sheinkmanc, Karpatid, & Pelegd, 2000).

DIAGNOSIS

Diagnosis is initially suggested based on clinical presentation, demographic, and medical history including family history given more than 80% are of Jewish decent. Amniotic fluid and chorionic villi may be removed early in pregnancy for analysis, in which Tay–Sachs' disease may be determined (Maertens & Dyken, 2007). DNA testing in combination with enzyme analysis can be definitive (Eiris, Chabas, Coll, & Castr- Gato, 1999).

In regard to differential diagnosis, cerebroretinal syndromes, leukodystrophies, and other gangliosidoses variants should be considered, but the combination of the aforementioned DNA testing and enzyme analysis can prove definitive.

TREATMENT

There is no cure or standard treatment for Tay–Sachs' disease. The approach is supportive and symptom based. Anti-epileptic drugs may be used to control seizure activity. Feeding tubes may be needed if dysphagia develops. Gene transfer and cell engraftment of neural stem cells have been tested in animal models as a means of express Hex-A (Guidotti et al., 1999), but it is not being tested in humans yet. Haloperidol, phenothiazines, and other D2 receptor blockers as well as tricyclic antidepressants might promote storage of gangliosides in the neurons (Rosebush, 1995; Renshaw, Stern, Welch, Schouten, & Kolodny, 1992) and thus should be avoided in late-onset Tay–Sachs' disease if considered to treat psychiatric features. For example, Navon and Baram (1987) demonstrated that imipramine caused cellular depletion of Hex-A.

Chad A. Noggle

Desnick, R. J., & Kaback, M. M. (2001). Future perspectives for Tay-Sachs disease. *Advances in Genetics, 44*, 349–356.

Eliris, J., Chabas, A., Coll, M. J., & Castr- Gato, M. (1999). Late infantile and juvenile form of GM2-gangliosidosis variant B1. *Revista de Neurologia, 29*, 435–438.

Federico, A., Palmeri, S., Mangano, L., Mondelli, M., Rossi, A., & Guazzi, G. C. (1988). Clinical and neurophysiological changes in carriers from a family with type O chronic GM2 gangliosidosis with ALS phenotype. In R. Savayre, L. Douste-Blazy, & S. Gatt (Eds.), *Lipid storage disorders. Biological and medical aspects* (pp. 253–258). New York: Plenum Press.

Gravel, R. A., Clark, J. T. R., Kaback, M. M., Mahuran, D. J., & Sandhoff, K. (1995). The GM2 gangliosidoses. In C. R. Scriver, A. L. Beaudet, W. S. Sly, & D. Valle (Eds.), *The metabolic and molecular basis of inherited disease* (pp. 2839–2879). New York: McGraw-Hill.

Guidotti, J. E., Mignon, A., Haase, G., Caillaud, C., McDonell, N., Kahn, A., et al. (1999). Adenoviral gene therapy of the Tay-Sachs disease in hexosaminidase A-deficient knock-out mice. *Human Molecular Genetics, 8*, 831–838.

Hurowitz, G. I., Silver, J. M., Brin, M. F., Williams, D. T., & Johnson, W. G. (1993). Neuropsychiatric aspects of adult onset Tay-Sachs disease: Two case reports with several new findings. *The Journal of Neuropsychiatry and Clinical Neurosciences, 5*, 30–36.

Kolodny, E. H. (1997). The GM2 gangliosidoses. In R. N. Rosenberg, S. B. Pruisner, S. Di Mauro, R. L. Barchi, L. M. Kunkel (Eds.), *The molecular and genetic basis of neurological disease* (pp. 531–540). Boston: Butterworth-Heinemann.

Lake, B. (2007). Lysosomal and peroxisomal disorders. In Goetz, C. (Ed.), *Textbook of clinical neurology* (pp. 657–753). Philadelphia, PA: Saunders Elsevier.

Lichtenberg, P., Navon, R., Wertman, E., & Lerer, B. (1988). Postpartum psychosis in adult GM2 gangliosidosis. A case report. *The British Journal of Psychiatry, 153*, 387–389.

Maertens, P., & Dyken, R. (2007). Storage diseases: Neuronal ceroid-lipofuscinoses, lipidoses, glycogenoses, and leukodystrophies. In Goetz, C. (Ed.), Textbook of clinical neurology (pp. 613–639). Philadelphia, PA: Saunders Elsevier.

Mugikura, S., Takahashi, S., Higano, S., Kurihara, N., Kon, K., & Sakamoto, K. (1996). MR findings in Tay-Sachs disease. *Journal of Computer Assisted Tomography, 20*, 551–555.

Navon, R., & Baram, D. (1987). Depletion of cellular betahexosaminidase by imipramine is prevented by dexamethasone: Implication for treating the psychotic hexosaminidase A deficient patients. *Biochemical and Biophysical Research Communications, 148*, 1098–1103.

Okada, S., & O'Brien, J. S. (1969). Tay-Sachs's disease: generalized absence of a beta-D-N-acetylhexosaminidase component. *Science, 165*, 698–700.

Petresen, G. M., Rotter, J. I., & Cantor, R. M. (1983). The Tay-Sachs gene in North American Jewish population: Geographic variations and origin. *American Journal of Human Genetics, 35*, 1258–1269.

Renshaw, P. F., Stern, T. A., Welch, C., Schouten, R., & Kolodny, E. H. (1992). Electroconvulsive therapy treatment of depression in a patient with adult GM2 gangliosidosis. *Annals of Neurology, 31*, 342–344.

Rosebush, P. I., MacQueen, G. M., Clarke, J. T., Callahan, J. W., Strasbery, P. M., & Mazurek, M. F. (1995). Late onset Tay-Sachs disease presenting as catatonic schizophrenia: Diagnostic and treatment issues. *Journal of Clinical Psychiatry, 56*, 347–353.

Schengrund, C. L. (1990). The role(s) of gangliosides in neural differentiation and repair: A perspective. *Brain Research Bulletin, 24*, 131–141.

Siegel, D. A., & Walkley, S. U. (1994). Growth of ectopic dendrites on cortical pyramidal neurons in neuronal storage diseases correlates with abnormal accumulation of Gm2 ganglioside. *Journal of Nuerochemistry, 62,* 1852–1862.

Streifler, J. Y., Gornish, M., Hadar, H., & Gadoth, N. (1993). Brain imaging in late-onset GM2 gangliosidosis. *Neurology, 43,* 2055–2058.

Yacubian, E., Rosemberg, S., Garrido Neto, T., Suely, K. N., Valério, R., & Jorge, C. (2000). Phosphorus magnetic resonance spectroscopy in late-onset Tay-Sachs disease. *Journal of Child Neurology, 16*(5).

Zelnika, N., Khazanovb, V., Sheinkmanc, A., Karpatid, A. M., & Pelegd, L. (2000). Clinical manifestations of psychiatric patients who are carriers of Tay-Sachs disease possible role of psychotropic drugs. *Neuropsychobiology, 41,* 127–131.

TETHERED SPINAL CORD SYNDROME

DESCRIPTION

Tethered spinal cord syndrome is characterized by extraneous tissue attachments that limit and abnormally stretch the spinal cord, resulting in anomalous lower limb sensorimotor functions, incontinence, and musculoskeletal deformities (Iskandar & Oakes, 2001). The disorder is related to spina bifida myelomeningocele, yet other etiologies exist including dermal sinus tract, diastematomyelia, lipoma, tumor, thickened or tight filum terminale, history of spine trauma, and history of spine surgery (Iskandar & Oakes, 2001).

A tethered spinal cord results from abnormal development of the neural tube, where the lower portion of the spinal cord remains attached to the skin near the posterior lumbar vertebrae and fails to ascend as in normal development (Barson, 1970). Thus, the spinal cord remains connected to the thecal sac, where the spinal nerves' roots exist. As growth occurs, the spinal cord is tethered at that location, leading to stretching and resulting in damage to the spinal cord and blood supply disruption.

Prevalence for tethered spinal cord is approximately 5–25 per 100,000; and prognosis varies based on severity and etiology of the tethering, yet most individuals will live a generally full and fairly normal life (Iskandar & Oakes, 2001).

NEUROPATHOLOGY/PATHOPHYSIOLOGY

The pathophysiology of tethered spinal cord syndrome is characterized by the mechanical stretching of an inelastic spinal cord that is anchored on the caudal end, preventing movement toward the head of the individual. Stretching can occur due to differences in growth rates or flexion and extension of the area.

Neurochemical changes — impairments in oxidative metabolism — are central to this syndrome and relate to depressed electrophysiological activity, leading to changes in ratios of the enzyme, cytochrome oxidase (Fuse, Patrickson, & Yamada, 1989). The effects of these changes result in hypoxemia and brain and spinal cord ischemia (Yamada, Zinke, & Sanders, 1981).

NEUROPSYCHOLOGICAL/CLINICAL PRESENTATION

Clinical presentation of tethered spinal cord syndrome includes abnormalities on the lower back (i.e., hairy patches, tumors, lesions, or dimples), spinal (i.e., scoliosis) and foot deformities, weakness in the lower limbs, and incontinence (French, 1983). While symptoms are typically evident in childhood, sensorimotor problems and incontinence may not develop until adulthood (French, 1983). Etiology may be varied as described previously, and symptoms may include lower limb movement or sensory impairments, pain in the lower extremities or back, muscle weakness, and may include incontinence of bowel and bladder.

With regard to sensorimotor impairments, motor dysfunction in the individual with tethered spinal cord syndrome may manifest as lower extremity muscle atrophy, hyperreflexia, and pathologic plantar response (also known as the Babinski response) which is indicative of compromise to the central nervous system (Schneider, 1996). Sensory dysfunctions typically manifest as abnormal pain, temperature, and proprioception often in a patchy distribution (Schneider, 1996).

Neuropathic bladder, which tends to worsen with age (70% for adults versus 20–30% for children), results in urinary urgency and frequency, incomplete voiding, and incontinence (French, 1983). With dysfunctional bladder, there is frequently associated recurrent and chronic infection that may lead to renal failure. Females with tethered spinal cord may suffer from ineffective labor and postpartum rectal prolapse secondary to an atonic pelvic floor (Schneider, 1996).

With the exception of previously noted impairments, cognitive and academic functions are typically in the normal ranges for tethered spinal cord syndrome.

T

DIAGNOSIS

Tethered spinal cord is often diagnosed through an MRI, which will conclusively reveal a tethered spinal cord on the distal end. This tethering will result in abnormal stretching of the spinal cord, which can lead to previously discussed symptoms. Other diagnostic measures include a myelogram, which is an X-ray following contrast injection of the spinal canal's thecal sac, or ultrasound for the purposes of demonstrating pressure on the nerves of the spinal cord (McCullough, Levy, DiChiro, & Johnson, 1991). Diagnosis is generally considered accurate following imaging; thus, differential diagnosis is often not problematic.

A positive diagnosis of tethered cord syndrome warrants ruling out Chiari malformation and Ehlers–Danlos syndrome due to the correlation of these diagnoses (Schneider, 1996).

TREATMENT

Surgical treatment is considered paramount with tethered spinal cord syndrome due to the often irreversible nature of the neurologic symptoms (Johnson & Levy, 1995). The goal of surgery in children is to prevent further deterioration, while the goal of surgery in adults is to restore function and alleviate symptoms. In general, sensorimotor improvements are noted following surgical detethering (Johnson & Levy, 1995).

Additional treatment tends to be supportive and to alleviate symptoms. NSAIDs, opiates, synthetic opiates, Cox-2 inhibitors, atypical tricyclic antidepressants, and anticonvulsive medications are often prescribed but there is little evidence that these provide consistent and persisting relief (Huttmann, Krauss, Collmann, Sorensen, & Roosen, 2001). Transcutaneous Electrical Nerve Stimulation units may provide some benefit, but this has not been fully validated (Huttmann et al., 2001).

Javan Horwitz
Natalie Horwitz
Chad A. Noggle

Barson, A. (1970). The vertebral level of termination of the spinal cord during normal and abnormal development. *Journal of Anatomy, 106,* 489–497.

French, B. (1983). The embryology of spinal dysraphism. *Clinical Neurosurgery, 30,* 295–340.

Fuse, T., Patrickson, J., & Yamada, S. (1989). Axonal transport of horseradish peroxidase in the experimental tethered spinal cord. *Pediatric Neuroscience, 15,* 296–301.

Huttmann, S., Krauss, J., Collmann, H., Sorensen, N., & Roosen, K. (2001). Surgical management of tethered spinal cord in adults: Report of 54 cases. *Journal of Neurosurgery, 95,* 173–178.

Iskandar, B., & Oakes, W. (2001). Anomalies of the spine and spinal cord. In D. McLone (Ed.), *Pediatric neurosurgery: The surgery of the developing nervous system* (4th ed., pp. 307–324). Philadelphia, PA: W.B. Saunders.

Johnson, D., & Levy, L. (1995). Predicting outcome in the tethered cord syndrome: A study of cord motion. *Pediatric Neurosurgery, 22,* 115–119.

McCullough, D., Levy, L., DiChiro, G., & Johnson, D. (1991). Toward the prediction of neurological injury from tethered cord: Investigation of cord motion with magnetic resonance. *Pediatric Neurosurgery, 16,* 3–7.

Schneider, S. (1996). Tethered cord syndrome: The neurological examination. In S. Yamada (Ed.), *Tethered cord syndrome* (pp. 49–54). Park Ridge, IL: AANS.

Yamada, S., Zinke, D., & Sanders, D. (1981). Pathophysiology of "tethered cord syndrome." *Journal of Neurosurgery, 54,* 494–503.

THORACIC OUTLET SYNDROME

DESCRIPTION

Thoracic outlet syndrome (TOS) occurs when nerves and/or vessels are compressed in the core of the neck resulting in problems with nerve and vascular functions, both locally and distally (Ruckley, 1983). TOS has a number of possible origins including pressure due to a cervical rib, a defect in the clavicle or first rib, an aneurysm, a tumor, problems with the anterior scalene muscle, a contraction of the costoclavicular space, and/or other space-inhabiting lesions (Woods, 1978). Consequently, compression occurs at different areas including the thoracic outlet, the cubital tunnel, the carpal tunnel, and Guyon's canal. In some cases, several points of compression may occur between the cervical spine and hand with less pressure producing symptoms in each area. In fact, multiple crush syndrome exists when a patient has concomitant TOS, carpal tunnel syndrome, and ulnar nerve compression at the elbow (Urchel & Kourlis, 2007).

Women, particularly those who are slim and/or have dropping shoulders, are more likely to have TOS than men (Ruckley, 1983). According to Woods (1978), 71% of the cases he reviewed were women, while 29% were men. In addition, the range of the patients' ages was 10–84, with 37 being the mean (Woods, 1978).

NEUROPATHOLOGY/PATHOPHYSIOLOGY

As suggested, TOS originates from compression of nerves or blood vessels, or both, because of a disruption of the passageway through the area between the base of the neck and the armpit known as the thoracic outlet. The anatomical location of the thoracic outlet is surrounded by muscle (e.g., anterior scalene muscle), bone (e.g., clavicle or ribs), and other tissue. Any defect or alteration of these tissues that infringes upon the thoracic outlet, thereby compressing the nerves (i.e., brachial plexus) and/or vessels (subclavian artery and veins) that pass through the tunnel leads to TOS. Given that this can occur at different sites from different tissues, functional outcomes can vary, therefore TOS may be best classified as an umbrella diagnosis representing an entire group of disorders.

Eighty to 90% of TOS cases are comprised of neurological defects, which occur more in women, whereas vascular compression occur more in men. However, vascular symptoms present more serious health issues, as irreversible hand injury and damage to the entire arm may occur. Neurological symptoms are usually less critical, as an aching pain in the neck, arm, and/or shoulder is most often reported (Ruckley, 1983).

The compression against the first rib causes several vascular and nerve problems including edema, venous distension, Paget–Schroetter's syndrome, loss of a pulse, aneurysm, paresthesias, motor weakness, Raynaud's phenomenon, ischemia, and temperature changes (Urchel & Kourlis, 2007).

In a study by Urchel and Kourlis (2007), no patients died due to TOS. One of the main complications occurred when the remains of a rib were left in the first surgery, which caused TOS to recur. In very few patients, a large amount of bleeding, nerve injuries, and Horner's syndrome occurred. In their study on 5,102 patients with TOS, Urchel and Kourlis (2007) found that the outcome was good in 85%, fair in 12%, and poor in only 3%. In addition, 95% of the patients reported progress shortly after surgery (Urchel & Kourlis, 2007).

Repetitive motions, especially of the hands and shoulders, often cause TOS. Clavicular trauma from pregnancy, polio, and bad posture can also cause TOS. Furthermore, breast surgery, such as radical mastectomies and implants, can contribute to TOS. Two other causes include hypertrophy and extreme opening of the median sternotomy retractor (Urchel & Kourlis, 2007). The most common cause of TOS is a neck injury resulting from an auto accident, which accounted for 61% of the 459 cases Woods (1978) reviewed. More specifically, rear-end collisions,

resulting in a whiplash injury accounted for 44% of the cases. Industrial accidents were responsible for 23% of the TOS cases, and miscellaneous trauma accounted for 8% (Woods, 1978).

NEUROPSYCHOLOGICAL/CLINICAL PRESENTATION

Woods (1978) reviewed 459 patients with TOS, documenting the various symptoms that appeared related to the disorder. There were several symptoms that occurred in the majority of TOS patients, such as arm pain, neck pain/stiffness, numbness and tingling of the hand, weakness of grip, and anterior scalene pressure (Woods, 1978). These represent the hallmark symptoms that correspond with the anatomical abnormalities of TOS impacting the subclavian artery and/or veins and the brachial plexus. In comparison, the clinical presentation in vascular TOS is usually acute, and depends upon whether the compression is arterial or venous (Sessions, Ranavaya, & Brooks, 2002).

Beyond those sensory and motor symptoms noted above, Woods (1978) reported several neuropsychological effects the disorder had on his patients. Forty-eight percent reported postural vertigo, 44% reported blurred vision, 54% reported retro-orbital pain, and 31% reported problems with concentration, focusing, and memory. Moreover, 85% reported occipital headaches, 18% stated their gait had become unsteady, while 11% reported syncopal attacks. All of these were due to vertebral artery compression (Woods, 1978). Sessions et al. (2002) present the number of cases with TOS who have headaches that initiate in the occipital lobe, and then spread over the rest of the cranium, becoming global tension headaches. Although it is uncommon, the cephalalgia is hemicranial and can cause unilateral facial pain on the side of the TOS; these can become more painful than the upper extremity symptoms (Sessions et al., 2002).

Fields, Lemak, and Ben-Menachem (1986) identified several neurological effects due to TOS in a major-league baseball pitcher. His depth perception as well as his ability to transfer two-dimensional displays into three-dimensional displays was impaired. A neuro-ophthalmologic evaluation divulged no left visual field deficit, but during testing, the most frequent error the baseball pitcher made was the rotation of objects in space, which affected his ability to catch the balls returned on his left side by the catcher. When presented with a stimulus from both sides, he was unaware of the object in his left visual field. The neuro-ophthalmologic assessment also showed the presence of an incongruous upper left homonymous quadrantanopia, as well as acquired myopia secondary to ciliary spasm. Moreover, he also experienced weakness on the left side of his face (Fields et al., 1986).

The frustration involved with trying to obtain successful treatment may cause patients to lose motivation, and often there are deficits in their home, work, and social lives. More specifically, many patients reported difficulties styling their hair, driving, opening jars/bottles, and completing household chores such as vacuuming (Sessions et al., 2002).

DIAGNOSIS

Accurate diagnosis of TOS must include a history of the patient and physical examination (Urchel & Kourlis, 2007). Woods (1978) discusses the necessity of a psychological evaluation, because each TOS case requires legal attention that is often complicated by the fact that patients commonly suffered from financial losses due to disability (Woods, 1978). Many tests are used to diagnose TOS including EMG, nerve conduction velocity (NCV), and cervical spine and chest radiographic studies, such as MRI (Urchel & Kourlis, 2007). Radiographs of the cervical spine should be employed in all TOS patients (Ruckley, 1983). Urchel and Kourlis (2007) found that when the NCV moved down to less than 85 m/s of the median or ulnar nerves across the thoracic outlet, the patient had TOS. Such methods are essential when attempting to differentiate TOS from those presentations that may demonstrate some degree of clinical overlap including but not limited to brachial neuritis, carpal tunnel syndrome, cervical radiculopathy, peripheral neuropathy, reflex sympathetic dystrophy, and rotator cuff instability. Connective tissue diseases or infections may also be considered.

TREATMENT

Many TOS patients, especially those with an NCV surpassing 60 m/s, benefit from physical therapy; however, those with motor and vascular nerve difficulties cannot undergo physical therapy. Physical therapy serves to improve posture, strengthen the shoulder, loosen the muscles in the neck, and allow for space between the first rib and the clavicle. Patients may also need to modify their sleep and work habits, and lose weight (uchel). Woods (1978) treated his patients with TOS with medications, such as muscle relaxants, anti-inflammatory drugs, and ibuprofen. Almost one-fourth of his patients received physiotherapy, which proved beneficial in about 50% of the cases. In some of his patients, Woods also used transcutaneous electrostimulation, which temporarily

relived the pain for some of these patients (Woods, 1978).

Surgery might be necessary if patients have an NCV of less than 60 m/s (Urchel & Kourlis, 2007). Due to the possibility for severe complications, surgery should be carried out by a well-qualified and experienced surgeon (Ruckley, 1983). According to Urchel and Kourlis (2007), surgery first entails anterior scalenectomy, neurolysis of C7, C8, and T1 nerve roots and brachial plexus, first rib resection, and resection of the costoclavicular ligament. Patients with pseudo recurrences and real recurrences required a second procedure (Urchel & Kourlis, 2007).

Rachel Rock
Antonio E. Puente

Fields, W. S., Lemak, N. A., & Ben-Menachem, B. (1986). Thoracic outlet syndrome: Review and reference to stroke in a major league pitcher. *American Journal of Roentgenology, 146*(4), 809–814.

Ruckley, C. V. (1983). Thoracic outlet syndrome. *British Medical Journal, 287*(6390), 447–448.

Sessions, R. T., Ranavaya, M. I., & Brooks, C. N. (2002). The office diagnosis of thoracic outlet syndrome: A closer look. *Disability Medicine, 2*(4), 116–130.

Urchel, H. C., & Kourlis, H. (2007). Thoracic outlet syndrome: A 50-year experience at Baylor University Medical Center. *Baylor University Medical Center Proceedings, 20*(2), 125–135.

Woods, W. W. (1978). Thoracic outlet syndrome. *The Western Journal of Medicine, 128*(1), 9–12.

THYROTOXIC MYOPATHY

DESCRIPTION

Thyrotoxic myopathy, also referred to as hyperthyroid myopathy, is a neuromuscular disorder that develops when the thyroid produces an overabundance of thyroxine. The disorder occurs in the majority of patients who have hyperthyroidism, which is caused by either Graves' disease or a multinodular goiter. The incidence of myopathy among thyrotoxic patients can be as high as 82%. Common symptoms include muscle pain, fatigue, and exercise intolerance. In addition, there is a progressive weakness and wasting away of muscles, primarily those in the thighs and shoulders. The disease may progress to a point that suggests a motor system disease, especially if there is tremor and twitching during muscle contraction. Muscle weakness is predominantly proximal, which may be associated with respiratory problems and difficulty swallowing. Whereas thyrotoxicosis, the high metabolism syndrome resulting from elevations in thyroid hormone levels, is more prevalent in women, thyrotoxic myopathy is equally distributed between the sexes, which actually implies that men with high thyroid levels are more susceptible to the myopathy (Becker, 2001; Fleisher, 2005; Victor, Ropper, & Adams, 2002; Vinken, 1992).

NEUROPATHOLOGY/PATHOPHYSIOLOGY

Electromyograhy (EMG) displays abnormalities in proximal muscles. These anomalies are detected even when the patient is not experiencing relative weakness. Serum creatine kinase (CK) is usually normal, which indicates the scarcity of muscle fiber damage seen in the biopsy of the muscle. The main finding from the EMG is a nonselective muscle fiber atrophy. Motor nerve conduction studies are typical, but sensory amplitudes and conduction velocities may be reduced. Thyroxine impacts how striated muscle fibers contract, but has no impact on nerve fiber conduction or neuromuscular transmission. Therefore, in hyperthyroidism, the length of a muscle contraction is reduced, resulting in a lessening of muscle power and increased muscle fatigue (Becker, 2001; Victor, 2002).

NEUROPSYCHOLOGICAL/CLINICAL PRESENTATION

A person afflicted with thyrotoxic myopathy typically complains of weakness when rising from a low chair, climbing stairs, performing activities that require the arms to be raised above the head, or any activity that would require the movement of pelvic or shoulder muscles. Furthermore, the patient will experience pain and muscle stiffness in the extremities. Consequently, muscular atrophy is likely to be found upon clinical examination, particularly of the pectoral and pelvic girdle muscles (Vinken, 1992, 1998).

Thyrotoxic myopathy is sometimes distinguished into two categories: chronic and acute thyrotoxic myopathy. In chronic thyrotoxic myopathy, the clinical presentation is a slow, progressive weakness, and atrophy with weight loss. The degree of weakness is variable and can be severe. With chronic thyrotoxic myopathy, the weakness is mostly experienced in the pelvic and shoulder girdle muscles. Acute thyrotoxic myopathy has been described as more rarely seen. The patient here will present with profound muscle weakness that progresses rapidly within a few days. The patient may also suffer from respiratory insufficiency. Reflexes may be lessened or absent; however, sphincter functioning remains (Vinken, 1992, 1998).

DIAGNOSIS

Patients who are experiencing thyrotoxic myopathy will have an excess of thyroxine, and therefore have hyperthyroidism. A diagnosis of hyperthyroidism is performed by testing plasma thyroid stimulating hormone (TSH). Lower than normal levels of TSH are indicative of the disorder. The severity of hyperthyroidism is determined by measuring the levels of plasma-free thyroxine. In order to confirm thyrotoxic myopathy, a muscle biopsy can show atrophy of Types I and II fiber groups. While the EMG is usually normal, it may show short and polyphasic motor unit potentials in proximal muscles and creatine excretion will be elevated (Victor et al., 2002).

TREATMENT

Improvement of thyrotoxic myopathy requires treatment of the thyrotoxicosis or hyperthyroidism. Treatment of hyperthyroidism includes radioactive iodine, antithyroid drugs, or a thyroidectomy. Radioiodine is appropriate for patients who have reached normal thyroid hormone levels, who are over 40, who are unsuitable for surgery, or for those who have recurrent hyperthyroidism. The two antithyroid drugs most commonly used are propylthiouracil and methimazole. They work to prevent coupling of iodotyrosines in the thyroid gland. Antithyroid drugs are used as an ultimate treatment, or to prepare a patient for a thyroidectomy or treatment with radioiodine. The goal is to maintain a euthyroid state. Lastly, a thyroidectomy is preferred for patients who have a relatively large goiter, and for pregnant women and children (Doherty & Way, 2005; Fleisher, 2005; Victor et al., 2002).

Successful treatment of thyrotoxicosis usually results in improvement of the muscle weakness within a few months. Strength improves before muscle wasting begins to reverse. EMG changes and muscle weakness resolve gradually once a normal thyroid environment is reached. Full recovery may take several months. Propranolol may help alleviate muscle weakness (Vinken, 1998).

Kelly R. Pless
Charles Golden

Becker, K. L. (2001). *Principles and practice of endocrinology and metabolism.* Philadelphia: Lippincott Williams & Wilkins.

Doherty, G. M., & Way, L. M. (2005). *Current surgical diagnosis & treatment.* New York: McGraw-Hill Professional.

Fleisher, L. A. (2005). *Anesthesia and uncommon disease.* Philadelphia: Elsevier Health Sciences.

Victor, M., Ropper, A. H., & Adams, R. D. (2002). *Adam and Victor's manual of neurology.* New York: McGraw-Hill Professional.

Vinken, P. J. (1992). *Handbook of clinical neurology.* Philadelphia: Elsevier Health Sciences.

Vinken, P. J. (1998). *Systemic diseases: Handbook of clinical neurology series.* Philadelphia: Elsevier Health Sciences.

TODD'S PARALYSIS

DESCRIPTION

Robert Bentley Todd described postictal paralysis in his Lumleian Lectures that were given to the Royal College of Physicians in 1849. He termed it epileptic hemiplegia, which later became known as Todd paralysis (Koehler, Bruyn, & Pearce, 2000).

Todd's paralysis is a muscle weakness or paralysis that occurs in the postictal period following a seizure, often of the partial type. More rarely, it may follow a secondarily generalized seizure. In comparison, it is not known to follow absence seizures. The paralysis may be localized to the limbs affected by the seizure (Luders & Comair, 2000). As such, the weakness or paralysis may affect any muscle group but is rarely bilateral. Symptoms may last for minutes to days and duration is often in proportion to the length of the seizure (Adams & Victor, 276). Gallmetzer et al. (2004) reported that 13.4% of their sample of 328 seizure patients had postictal paralysis of mean duration 173.5 seconds and range 11 seconds to 22 minutes. Symptoms tend to last longer following focal status epilepticus but resolve over time (Luders & Comair, 2000). Todd's paralysis resolves on its own without treatment.

NEUROPATHOLOGY/PATHOPHYSIOLOGY

The cause of Todd's paralysis is unknown, although several theories have been posited. John Hughlings Jackson conceptualized it as an electrical exhaustion that follows the rapid and repetitive neuronal discharges of the seizure, which he credited as Todd and Robertson's hypothesis (Koehler et al., 2000). This may occur due to depletion of glucose in the neurons at the focal sight of the seizure (Popp, 233). It may also be a function of the excitotoxicity that occurs during the ictal or seizure period, or due to an excess or deprivation of oxygen or neurotransmitters (Luders & Comair, 2000).

Another theory states that neuronal inhibition of the motor centers continues to occur postictally after completion of the seizure (Gallmetzer et al., 2004). This theory was originally postulated by Gowers in 1881. This may occur due to inactivation of N-methyl-D-aspartic acid (NMDA) receptors that would restrict the opening of ion channels, thus prohibiting neural communication to complete a movement. The last hypothesis states that Todd's paralysis may be a cardiovascular phenomenon in which seizure activity causes vasomotor and metabolic changes such as arterial venous shunting, which restricts blood flow to a focal region of the brain for a short duration of time, or cerebral hyperperfusion, which increases blood flow (Yarnell, 1975).

Kimura, Sejima, Ozasa, and Yamaguchi (1998) presented two cases of focal seizures in children that resulted in Todd's paralysis. The authors utilized technetium-99m-HMPAO SPECT imaging to evaluate the patients' cerebral blood flow patterns following the seizure. Both cases showed contralateral cerebral hyperperfusion, or increased blood flow, within 36 hours of cessation of seizure activity, which continued after the paralysis had resolved and about 24 hours after cessation of seizure activity. MRI and EEG were normal and were thus seen as evidence against cerebral infarct. Furthermore, the authors concluded that increased cerebral blood flow did not seem to cause the Todd's paralysis since the paralysis resolved more rapidly.

Bergen, Rayman, and Heydemann (1992) reported two case studies of bilateral Todd's paralysis following focal seizure. Both patients had bilateral muscle weakness or paralysis of the arms and legs which lasted several minutes. The patients had flaccid muscle tone with unimpaired sensation of touch and pinprick. EEG and clinical observation showed that their seizures began in the supplementary motor cortex of the frontal lobe. They stated that this localization was further supported by the interconnection with the primary motor cortex, which would explain the more severe cases of transient paralysis.

Todd's paralysis occurs more often in patients with a tumor than in those with any other neurological condition that causes their seizures (Merritt, 1963). The condition is also associated with vascular lesions and arteriovenous malformations.

NEUROPSYCHOLOGICAL/CLINICAL PRESENTATION

Because the effects of Todd's paralysis rarely last more than 24 hours, neuropsychological testing would have to be performed during that brief period to find deficits of performance. Such impairments would be expected to include poor performance on motor tasks involving the affected side. Other neurological symptoms occur when the parietal, occipital, or frontal lobes are affected. Aphasia and other disturbances of speech, poor eye position, and disturbed vision may be disrupted and sensory changes and hallucinations have been reported. Decreased level of consciousness may follow the seizure and resolve rapidly (Mahadevan & Garmel, 2005).

DIAGNOSIS

Todd's paralysis most commonly follows unilateral motor seizure activity and less commonly follows generalized seizure. It is found most often in children and infants, although it can occur in adults. Symptoms last from minutes to hours, rarely for more than 24 hours (Niedermeyer & Lopes da Silva, 2004). Diagnosis is exclusionary and based upon history of seizure. When history is unknown, imaging techniques should be used to assess for head injury or stroke and drug levels should be analyzed to rule out withdrawal (Mahadevan & Garmel, 2005).

Because Todd's paralysis lateralizes the location of the seizure to the cerebral hemisphere contralateral to the muscle paralysis, it is useful for identification of the seizure focus. This measure is reliable even when the seizure activity spreads from the locus of onset throughout the cortex (Luders & Comair, 2000, p. 90).

Due to the short duration of symptoms, imaging may not be completed during every episode. This is supported by the fact that weakness or paralysis that occurs following a seizure does not guarantee that there is cortical bleeding or damage. However, when seizure and Todd's paralysis follows head trauma, patients should be evaluated for acute subdural hematoma because the trauma increases the risk of infarct (Anschel, 2006).

Imaging techniques have found various results from normal functioning to cerebral slowing. An EEG of the patient during an episode of Todd's paralysis may show marked slowing in the cerebral hemisphere contralateral to the side of motor weakness (Niedermeyer & Lopes da Silva, 2004). Gustavson, McIntyre, and Roberts (2003) presented a case study in which the patient's EEG during post-ictal paralysis showed higher amplitude and lower frequency activity on the contralateral side. The EEG may also be normal (Schwartzman, 2006). Von Kummer, Back, and Ay (2006) reported that they found no significant abnormalities on conventional MRI, MRA, DW1, or P1.

TREATMENT

Due to the short duration of symptoms, no treatment is warranted or conducted. The condition resolves on its own without intervention. The treatment and prognosis of the patient will depend upon his or her seizure activity. The presence of Todd's paralysis may increase the risk for recurrent seizures so patients should be carefully monitored (Mahadevan & Garmel, 2005).

Jessie L. Morrow
Charles Golden

Anschel, D. (2006). *Neurology* (6th ed.). New York: McGraw-Hill Professional.

Bergen, D. C., Rayman, L., & Heydemann, P. (1992). Bilateral Todd's Paralysis after focal seizures. *Epilepsia, 33*(6), 1101–1105.

Gallmetzer, P., Leutmezer, F., Serles, W., Assem-Hilger, E., Spatt, J., & Baumgartner, C. (2004). Postictal paresis in focal epilepsies—incidence, duration, and causes. A video-EEG monitoring study. *Neurology, 62*(12), 2160–2164.

Gustavson, A. R., McIntyre, B. B., & Roberts, H. W. (2003). Electrographic correlates of seizures with Todd's Paralysis. A case report. *Clinical Neurophysiology, 114*(2), 393.

Koehler, P. J., Bruyn, G. W., & Pearce, J. (2000). *Neurological eponyms.* New York: Oxford University Press.

Luders, H., & Comair, Y. G. (2000). *Epilepsy surgery.* Baltimore, MD: Lippincott Williams & Wilkins.

Mahadevan, S. V., & Garmel, G. M. (2005). *An introduction to clinical emergency medicine.* New York: Cambridge University Press.

Kimura, M., Sejima, H., Ozasa, H., Yamaguchi, S. (1998). Technetium-99m-HMPAO SPECT in patients with hemiconvulsions followed by Todd's paralysis. *Pediatric Radiology, 28*(2), 92–94.

Merritt, H. (1963). *Textbook of neurology.* London: Kimpton.

Niedermeyer, E., & Lopes da Silva, F. H. (2004). *Electroencephalography: Basic principles, clinical applications, and related fields.* Baltimore, MD: Lippincott Williams & Wilkins.

Schwartzman, R. J. (2006). *Differential diagnosis in neurology.* Fairfax, VA: IOS Press.

Von Kummer, R., Back, T., & Ay, H. (2006). *Magnetic resonance imaging in ischemic stroke.* New York: Birkhauser-Springer.

Yarnell, P. R. (1975). Todd's Paralysis: A cardiovascular phenomenon? *Stroke, 6,* 301–303.

TOURETTE'S SYNDROME AND OTHER TIC DISORDERS

DESCRIPTION

Tourette's syndrome disorder is named after Gilles de la Tourette, a late 19th century French neurologist. Although the term "Tourette's disorder" is used in the *Diagnostic and Statistical Manual* (fourth ed., text revision) (*DSM-IV-TR*; American Psychiatric Association [APA], 2000) and in the literature, it is more commonly referred to as Tourette's syndrome (TS). TS is a neurodevelopmental disorder characterized by the presence of multiple motor and vocal/phonic tics. Motor tics are rapid and repetitive movements that occur suddenly. They may be innocuous movements of any part of the body or, less frequently, obscene gestures referred to as copropraxia (Cavanna, Servo, Monaco, & Robertson, 2009). Vocal or phonic tics are rapid, meaningless sounds or noises. They can include sniffing, grunting, barking, and squeaking, or may be more complex and include syllables, words, or phrases (Leckman, Bloch, King, & Scahill, 2006). Although many researchers use the term "vocal," the term "phonic" tic is more often preferred, as the noises may not incorporate the individual's vocal cords (Jankovic & Mejia, 2006). The phonic tics may also be obscene in nature, referred to as coprolalia (Cavanna et al., 2009). The tics occur multiple times per day and individuals often report that the tics are preceded by an intense urge to move and/or make noise and are then followed by a sense of relief (Leckman et al., 2006).

The mean age of TS onset is approximately 6 years of age, although the copropraxic and coprolalic nature of the tics tends to emerge later, at about 14 years of age (Jankovic, 1997). Boys are more predisposed to tic disorders, at a rate of about 3.5:1.0 (Dure & DeWolfe, 2006). Other tic disorders include those that do not meet full diagnostic criteria for TS and include chronic multiple motor tic, or phonic, chronic single, transient, and nonspecific tic disorder (Tourette Syndrome Classification Study Group [TSCSG], 1993).

NEUROPATHOLOGY/PATHOPHYSIOLOGY

In Gilles de la Tourette's primary description of the disorder, he reported its familial nature (Abelson et al., 2005). Evidence from twin studies has indicated a genetic component (Price, Kidd, Cohen, Pauls, & Leckman, 1985), but the search for a clear genetic marker for the disorder has not been fruitful (O'Rourke, Scharf, Yu, & Pauls, 2009).

The role of the basal ganglia in TS was posited from observations that tic disorders may develop in individuals with lesions in this region (e.g., Pulst, Walshe, & Romer, 1983), and neuroimaging studies support this hypothesis (Peterson et al., 2003). Animal studies suggest that basal ganglia dysfunction leads to the disinhibition of excitatory neurons in the ventral thalamus, in turn leading to disinhibition of cortical motor areas (Gilbert, 2006). SPECT studies of TS generally indicate reduced blood flow in the basal ganglia and basal ganglia asymmetry (e.g., greater left-sided dysfunction; Butler, Stern, & Silbersweig, 2006). In persons with tic disorders, PET, fMRI, and SPECT studies provide convergent data that the basal ganglia, frontal cortex, midbrain, and paralimbic regions exhibit *abnormal* activity, whereas the motor cortex and supplemental motor area exhibit *increased* activity (Hampson, Tokoglu, King, Constable, & Leckman, 2009).

Clinical observations that dopamine antagonists decrease tics and dopamine agonists (e.g., Ritalin) elicit or increase tics suggest that persons with an abundance of D1 receptors may be at higher risk for the development of tic disorders (Gerfn et al., 1990).

NEUROPSYCHOLOGICAL/CLINICAL PRESENTATION

Beyond the presence of tics, there do not appear to be neuropsychological deficits specific to TS (Zinner & Coffey, 2009). In fact, one respected authority reports that persons with TS without comorbid psychopathology demonstrate higher psychometric intelligence than predicted (Denckla, 2006). Although individuals with TS may present with a reduction in fine motor dexterity (Bornstein, 1991), the primary effects of the tics on fine motor skills must be considered.

TS is often comorbid with other psychiatric disorders. Consequently, the neuropsychological deficit pattern tends to be consistent with comorbid disorders (Osmon & Smerz, 2005). TS is most often comorbid (about 60% of the time) with attention deficit hyperactivity disorder (ADHD; Denckla, 2006) and slightly less frequently (about 50% of the time) with obsessive-compulsive disorder (OCD; Hounie et al., 2006). In one large primary care clinic study (N = 3,500), only 8% of individuals with TS had *no* comorbid psychiatric diagnosis (Freeman et al., 2000). In addition to ADHD and OCD, TS is also often comorbid with depression, learning disorders, and conduct disorder (Zinner & Coffey, 2009).

DIAGNOSIS

The diagnosis of TS is based on observation (Cavanna et al., 2009), as suggested by the multidisciplinary TSCSG (1993). The criteria developed by the TSCSG (1993) included (1) multiple motor and one or more vocal/phonic tics present at some time during the course of the syndrome (though not necessarily concurrently); (2) tics occur multiple times per day for greater than 1 year; (3) onset occurs prior to age 21; (4) anatomic location, number, type, and severity of tics may change over time; (5) medical conditions do not account for the tics; and (6) the tics must be witnessed. The *DSM-IV-TR* (APA, 2000) modifies the TSCSG (1993) criteria by adding "[the tics] cause marked distress of significant impairment in social, occupation, or other important areas of functioning," age of onset prior to age 18, and the tics may not be absent for any longer than three consecutive months (p. 116). The tic disorder workgroup for the forthcoming *DSM-5* proposes removal of the criterion that tics may not be absent for longer than 3 months based on research evidence that a person with TS may experience periods of quiescence from tic movements, but that the tics ultimately recommence (APA, in press).

Persons may present with motor or vocal/phonic tics that do not meet criteria for TS (cf. TSCSG, 1993). For example, multiple motor tic or phonic tic disorder incorporates all the criteria for TS *except* the tics are *either* motor or vocal (not both). Single tic disorder incorporates all the criteria for TS *except* the tics are restricted to a *single* motor or vocal/phonic tic. Individuals with transient tic disorder may exhibit either single or multiple motor and/or vocal tics, but the tics are *not* present for longer than 12 consecutive months and must have begun more than 1 year ago. Persons diagnosed with nonspecific tic disorder exhibit tics but do not meet full criteria for TS or any of the other tic disorders.

Each of the criteria lists for TS and other tic disorders contain the criterion that the tics are not due to a general medical condition. Medical conditions that mimic features of TS include akathisia, chorea, dystonia, hyperekplexia, myoclonus, restless leg syndrome, rituals, and stereotypies (Jankovic & Mejia, 2006)

TREATMENT

Double-blind studies have demonstrated the effectiveness of pergolide (a dopamine agonist), clonidine (an alpha-2 adrenergic agonist), mecamylamine (a nonselective and noncompetitive antagonist of the nicotinic acetylcholine receptors), and tetrabenazine (a vesicular monoamine transporter inhibitor) in the control of tics, and clonidine has demonstrated effectiveness in combination with methylphenidate in the treatment of ADHD in children with tics without significantly increasing tics in a large multicenter, randomized, double-blind study (TSCSG, 2002). Compared with more recently developed medications (e.g., levetiracetam, an antiseizure medication), individuals prescribed clonidine exhibit a small but significant reduction in tic frequency (Hedderick, Morris, & Singer, 2009). Cannabis has also shown promise, although studies have not been randomized (Dure & DeWolfe, 2006).

Treatment of choice for ADHD is neurostimulant medication. Anecdotal information had suggested the use of methylphenidate in individuals with comorbid ADHD and TS may exacerbate the tics (Feinberg & Carroll, 1979). However, the results of one long-term longitudinal study suggested that relatively few persons experience increase in tics while taking methylphenidate (Gadow & Sverd, 2006), and the TSCSG (2002) study indicated an incidence of tics with methylphenidate use at 20%, and with placebo at 22% (the prevalence of tics with clonidine was 26%). When TS is comorbid with OCD, selective serotonin reuptake inhibitors (SSRIs) are the first-line approach (in particular, fluoxetine, fluvoxamine, sertraline, and paroxetine; Coffey et al., 2000). If SSRIs are not successful in controlling symptoms, the second-line approach is clomipramine (a non-SSRI similar to tricyclic antidepressants; Coffey et al., 2000).

Behavioral interventions for TS include relaxation training, biofeedback, massed negative practice, self-monitoring, and contingency management (Wilhelm et al., 2003; Woods, Himle, & Conelea, 2006). Available online is a 2-hour National Tourette's Syndrome Association (NTSA)-streamed video geared to professionals that provides instruction in the comprehensive behavioral intervention for tics approach for treating TS (NTSA, 2010, tsa-usa.org). In 2007, deep brain stimulation (DBS) was allowed as a humanitarian device exemption by the Food and Drug Administration for use with patients for whom pharmacologic interventions are not successful in treatment of their OCD. However, DBS use in TS is still under investigation with its use studied only in adults (Marks, Honeycutt, Acosta, & Reed, 2009).

Mary E. Haines
Melissa M. Swanson
Timothy F. Wynkoop

Abelson, J. F., Kwan, K. Y., O'Roak, B. J., Baek, D. Y., Stillman, A. A., Morgan, T. M., et al. (2005). Sequence variants in SLITRK1 are associated with Tourette's syndrome. *Science, 310,* 317–320.

T

American Psychiatric Association. (in press). *American psychiatric association: DSM-5 development*. Retrieved on March 30, 2010, from http://www.dsm5.org

American Psychiatric Association. (2000). *Diagnostic and statistical manual* (4th ed., text revision). Washington, DC: Author.

Bornstein, R. A. (1991). Neuropsychological performance in adults with Tourette's syndrome. *Psychiatry Research, 37,* 229–236.

Butler, T., Stern, E., & Silbersweig, D. (2006). Functional neuroimaging of Tourette syndrome: Advances and future directions. In J. T. Walkup, J. W. Mink, & P. J. Hollenbeck (Eds.), *Advances in neurology volume 99: Tourette syndrome* (pp. 115–129). Philadelphia: Lippincott Williams & Wilkins.

Cavanna, A., Servo, S., Monaco, F., & Robertson, M. (2009). The behavioral spectrum of Gilles de la Tourette syndrome. *Journal of Neuropsychiatry & Clinical Neurosciences, 21,* 13–23.

Coffey, B. J., Biederman, J., Smoller, J. W., Geller, D. A., Sarin, P., Schwartz, S., et al. (2000). Anxiety disorders and tic severity in juveniles with Tourette's disorder. *Journal of the American Academy of Child and Adolescent Psychiatry, 39,* 562–568.

Denckla, M. B. (2006). Attention deficit hyperactivity disorder: The childhood co-morbidity that most influences the disability burden in Tourette syndrome. In J. T. Walkup, J. W. Mink, & P. J. Hollenbeck (Eds.), *Advances in neurology volume 99: Tourette syndrome* (pp. 17–21). Philadelphia: Lippincott Williams & Wilkins.

Dure, L. S., & DeWolfe, J. (2006). Treatment of tics. In J. T. Walkup, J. W. Mink, & P. J. Hollenbeck (Eds.), *Advances in neurology volume 99: Tourette syndrome* (pp. 190–196). Philadelphia: Lippincott Williams & Wilkins.

Feinberg, M., & Carroll, B. J. (1979). Effects of dopamine agonists and antagonists in Tourette's disease. *Archives of General Psychiatry, 36,* 979–985.

Freeman, R. D., Fast, D. K., Burd, L., Kerbeshian, J., Robertson, M. M., & Sandor, P. (2000). An international perspective on Tourette's syndrome: Selected findings from 3,500 individuals in 22 countries. *Developmental Medicine and Child Neurology, 42,* 436–447.

Gadow, K. D., & Sverd, J. (2006). Attention deficit hyperactivity disorder, chronic tic disorder, and methylphenidate. In J. T. Walkup, J. W. Mink, & P. J. Hollenbeck (Eds.), *Advances in neurology volume 99: Tourette syndrome* (pp. 197–207). Philadelphia: Lippincott Williams & Wilkins.

Gerfn, C. R., Engber, T. M., Mahan, L. C., Susel, Z., Chase, T. N., Monsma, F. J., Jr., et al. (1990). D1 and D2 dopamine receptor-regulated gene expression of striatonigral and striatopallidal neurons. *Science, 250,* 1429–1432.

Gilbert, D. L. (2006). Motor cortex inhibitory function in Tourette syndrome, attention deficit disorder, and obsessive compulsive disorder: Studies using transcranial magnetic stimulation. In J. T. Walkup, J. W. Mink, & P. J. Hollenbeck (Eds.), *Advances in neurology volume 99: Tourette syndrome* (pp. 107–114). Philadelphia: Lippincott Williams & Wilkins.

Hampson, M., Tokoglu, F., King, R. A., Constable, R. T., & Leckman, J. F. (2009). Brain areas coactivating with motor cortex during chronic motor tics and intentional movements. *Biological Psychiatry, 65,* 594–599.

Hedderick, E. F., Morris, C. M., & Singer, H. S. (2009). Double-blind, crossover study of clonidine and levetiracetam in Tourette syndrome. *Pediatric Neurology, 40,* 420–425.

Hounie, A. G., Rosario-Campos, M. D., Diniz, J. B., Shavit, R. G., Ferrao, Y. A., Lopes, A. C., et al. (2006). Obsessive-compulsive disorder in Tourette syndrome. In J. T. Walkup, J. W. Mink, & P. J. Hollenbeck (Eds.), *Advances in neurology volume 99: Tourette syndrome* (pp. 22–38). Philadelphia: Lippincott Williams & Wilkins.

Jankovic, J. (1997). Phenomenology and classification of tics. In J. Jankovic (Ed.), *Neurologic clinics* (pp. 267–275). Philadelphia: W. H. Saunders Company.

Jankovic, J., & Mejia, N. I. (2006). Tics associated with other disorders. In J. T. Walkup, J. W. Mink, & P. J. Hollenbeck (Eds.), *Advances in neurology volume 99: Tourette syndrome* (pp. 61–68). Philadelphia: Lippincott Williams & Wilkins.

Leckman, J. F., Bloch, M. H., King, R. A., & Scahill, L. (2006). Phenomenology of tics and naturally history of tic disorders. In J. T. Walkup, J. W. Mink, & P. J. Hollenbeck (Eds.), *Advances in neurology volume 99: Tourette syndrome* (pp. 1–16), Philadelphia: Lippincott Williams & Wilkins.

Marks, W. A., Honeycutt, J., Acosta, F., & Reed, M. (2009). Deep brain stimulation for pediatric movement disorders. *Seminars in Pediatric Neurology, 16,* 90–98.

National Tourette Syndrome Association. (2010). *Comprehensive behavior intervention for tics (CBIT)*. Retrieved on April 16, 2010, from tsa-usa.org/Medical/medsci.html

O'Rourke, J. A., Scharf, J. M., Yu, D., & Pauls, D L. (2009). The genetics of Tourette syndrome: A review. *Journal of Psychosomatic Research, 67,* 533–545.

Osmon, D. C., & Smerz, J. M. (2005). Neuropsychological evaluation in the diagnosis and treatment of Tourette's syndrome. *Behavior Modification, 29,* 746–783.

Peterson, B. S., Thomas, P., Kane, M. J., Schahill, L., Zhang, H., Bronen, R., et al. (2003). Basal ganglia volumes in patients with Gilles de la Tourette syndrome. *Archives of General Psychiatry, 60,* 415–424.

Price, R. A., Kidd, K. K., Cohen D. J., Pauls, D. L., & Leckman, J. F. (1985). A twin study of Tourette syndrome. *Archives of General Psychiatry, 42,* 815–820.

Pulst, S. M. Walshe, T. M., & Romer, J. A. (1983). Carbon monoxide poisoning with features of Gilles de la Tourette's syndrome. *Archives of Neurology, 40*, 443–444.

Tourette Syndrome Classification Study Group. (1993). Definitions and classification of tic disorders. *Archives of Neurology, 50*, 1013–1016.

Tourette Syndrome Classification Study Group. (2002). Treatment of ADHD in children with tics: A randomized controlled trial. *Neurology, 58*, 527–536.

Woods, D. W., Himle, M. B., & C. A. Conelea (2006). Behavior therapy: Other interventions for tic disorders. In J. T. Walkup, J. W. Mink, & P. J. Hollenbeck (Eds.), *Advances in neurology volume 99: Tourette syndrome* (pp. 234–239), Philadelphia: Lippincott Williams & Wilkins.

Wilhelm, S., Deckersbach, T., Coffey, B. J., Bohne, A., Peterson, A. L., & Baer, L. (2003). Habit reversal versus supportive psychotherapy for Tourette's disorder: A randomized controlled trial. *American Journal of Psychiatry, 160*, 1175–1177.

Zinner, S., & Coffey, B. (2009). Developmental and behavioral disorders grown up: Tourette's disorder. *Journal of Developmental and Behavioral Pediatrics, 30*, 560–573.

TRANSIENT GLOBAL AMNESIA

DESCRIPTION

Transient global amnesia (TGA) is a disorder of unknown etiology typically occurring in adults between the ages of 34 and 92. Characteristic symptoms are sudden onset of both retrograde and anterograde amnesia lasting approximately 24–36 hours usually. Patients with this disorder tend to be confused and ask repetitive questions. TGA tends to occur only once in a patient's lifetime, although a review of the more recent literature indicates that as many as 16% of patients may have recurrences. Males have a slightly higher occurrence of TGA than do females, with a male-to-female ratio of 4:3. The incidence rate is uncertain. Precursors to the condition include coitus, cold baths, migraines, pain, and strong emotional episodes. The disorder tends to last from 4 to 8 hours but may last as long as 24 hours. TGA usually resolves itself gradually without medical intervention.

NEUROPATHOLOGY/PATHOPHYSIOLOGY

TGA's exact pathology is not yet conclusively understood. Many of the findings with recent literature have employed the use of a variety of neuroimaging technology including PET and diffusion-weighted MRI (DWI), which have indicated numerous brain regions that are affected in TGA (Strupp et al., 1998). PET and DWI research have suggested that areas of the brain specific to memory appear disrupted during the occurrence of a TGA. Theoretical proposals have suggested a potential role of medial temporal lobe seizure activity or a vascular etiology such as bilateral medial temporal lobe ischemia related to posterior cerebral artery (PCA) distribution (Love & Biller, 2007). Consistent with the latter vascular proposal, research using DWI techniques has pointed out the presence of tiny lesions in the hippocampus as well as diffuse lesions throughout other areas of the brain (Winbeck et al., 2005). Still the most commonly associated antecedent remains emotional distress (Miller, Petersen, Metter, Millikan, & Yanagihara, 1987). Owing to this, to date, the most accepted theory of TGA is that of a psychogenic basis, given the extent of neurological disruption presumed to be required to create such a complete cognitive, in particular amnestic, disruption.

NEUROPSYCHOLOGICAL/CLINICAL PRESENTATION

Although TGA patients are said to recover from their memory loss, neuropsychological results indicate that there may be a protracted deficit in verbal memory loss and impairment in verbal IQ scores (Pantoni et al., 2005). These results may occur even when patients return to their jobs and families with no subsequent complaints of neuropsychological difficulties. As suggested, the classic presentation of TGA is of a total amnesia (retrograde and anterograde), including loss of autobiographical memories (Quinette et al., 2006). Onset is sudden with complete resolution usually occurring within 24–36 hours. During the episode there are no sensory or motor deficits, visual disturbances, or brainstem abnormalities (Love & Biller, 2007). Upon resolution of symptoms, patients generally return to baseline and there is no recollection of the TGA period.

DIAGNOSIS

Generally TGA is diagnosed by the presence of the symptomology already outlined; however, other disorders must be ruled out. Differential diagnosis involves ruling out the following disorders: transient ischemic attacks (TIAs), epilepsy, psychogenic disturbance, encephalitis, trauma, tumors, migraine, alcohol

T

abuse, and hypoglycemia. Theories suggest that the disorder may have vascular causes or may be connected to migraines. TGA has also been said to be connected to allergic encephalopathy as a result of antitetanus serum; angiography; pituitary tumor; polycythemia; myxomatous degeneration of the mitral valve; and intoxication with digitalis, clioquinol, or diazepam. However, the most common link cited is of a psychogenic basis related to significant emotional stress (Miller et al., 1987). In differentially diagnosing TGA, it is important to recall that TGA patients do not have recognizable seizures and rarely display EEG abnormalities. Neuroimaging is generally unremarkable beyond features that may be seen in a fair portion of patients within this age range (e.g., small vessel ischemic changes). They are able to perform complex motor skills, and no neurologic signs or symptoms beyond memory loss and repetitive questioning are present. They tend to be oriented only to person.

TREATMENT

The symptoms of TGA resolve roughly within one day and therefore are not treated aggressively in an active sense. Rather, preventive measures (e.g., imaging and EEG) may be sought to determine if symptoms of TGA may be precursors or symptoms of further damage or the presence of other disorders. It is suggested that the patient and family be reassured and that invasive procedures be avoided. Those individuals with a history of migraines or at risk for cerebrovascular disorders should be closely monitored. Some physicians have found that prophylaxis with antiplatelet therapy is helpful when migraines are co-occurring with TGA.

At onset of TGA symptoms in a patient, it is important to reassure the patient and the patient's family. In addition, psychoeducational intervention by hospital personnel would be helpful in explaining what is known about the disorder and what the patient and family can expect after the disorder is resolved. In some cases, subsequent compensatory interventions may be advisable to assist the patient in adjusting to more chronic verbal memory or verbal IQ deficits. Typically, however, neither the patient nor the patient's family or coworkers report any subsequent deficit that impairs career functioning or interpersonal interactions. Thus, in general, patients would rarely require the services of a psychologist as a result of TGA.

Matthew Holcombe
Raymond S. Dean

Love, B. B., & Biller, J. (2007). Neurovascular system. In C. G. Goetz (Ed.), *Textbook of clinical neurology* (3rd ed.). Philadelphia, PA: W. B. Saunders Elsevier.

Miller, J. W., Petersen, R. C., Metter, E. J., Millikan, C. H., & Yanagihara, T. (1987). Transient global amnesia: Clinical characteristics and prognosis. *Neurology, 37*(5), 733–737.

Pantoni, L., Bertini, E., Lamassa, M., Pracucci, G., & Inzitari, D. (2005). Clinical features, risk factors, and prognosis in transient global amnesia: A follow-up study. *European Journal of Neurology, 12*(5), 350–356.

Quinette, P., Guillery-Girard, B., Dayan, J., de la Sayette, V., Marquis, S., Viader, F., et al. (2006). What does transient global amnesia really mean? Review of the literature and thorough study of 142 cases. *Brain, 129,* 1640–1658.

Strupp, M., Bruning, R., Wu, R. H., Deimling, M., Reiser, M., & Brandt, T. (1998). Diffusion-weighted MRI in transient global amnesia: Elevated signal intensity in the left mesial temporal lobe in 7 of 10 patients. *Annuals of Neurology, 43*(2), 164–170.

Winbeck, K., Etgen, T., von Einsiedel, H. G., Röttinger, M., & Sander, D. (2005). DWI in transient global amnesia and TIA: Proposal for an ischaemic origin of TGA. *Journal of Neurology Neurosurgery and Psychiatry, 76*(3), 438–441.

TRANSIENT ISCHEMIC ATTACKS

DESCRIPTION

Historically, transient ischemic attacks (TIAs) were defined as "a sudden onset of focal cerebral neurological dysfunction (e.g., hemiplegia) attributable to blood vessel disease which resolves in less than 24 hours" (Loring, 1999). Recently, the definition has been revised to "a transient episode of neurological dysfunction caused by focal brain, spinal cord, or retinal ischemia, without acute infarction" (Albers et al., 2002; Easton et al., 2009). Unilateral weakness, clumsiness, and/or heaviness are the most common initial symptoms of TIA. Other frequent presenting symptoms include unilateral sensory symptoms (numbness or tingling), dysphasic or dysarthric speech, and vision changes (partial vision loss, field cut, blurring or diminished vision). Multiple symptoms typically present simultaneously, gradually wear off over a few minutes, and are often accompanied by mild headache. Particularly in the elderly, misdiagnosis is believed to be common because patients may present with symptoms that are believed to be independently common in the elderly population including dizziness or vertigo, balance issues, falls, disorders of consciousness, or unawareness of deficits (Rancurel, 2005). On average, symptoms of a TIA last 10 minutes or less. Those that last longer than 1 hour are often evidenced as infarcts on today's more sensitive imaging technology, and therefore are not technically meeting the criteria for the definition and are better subsumed under the criteria for mild stroke.

TIAs and minor strokes comprise over half of all cerebrovascular events and are believed to imminently precede 20–30% of major disabling strokes (Pendlebury, Giles, & Rothwell, 2009; Rothwell & Warlow, 2005). Conversely, studies have shown that following a TIA, conversion to stroke appears to be at a rate of 10–15% at 3 months, with half occurring within 48 hours (Easton et al., 2009), much higher than previously thought. Because of the high conversion rate to full stroke, TIAs are considered a neurologic emergency that require immediate clinical and laboratory investigation targeted toward stabilizing the event and preventing acute infarction.

However, there is considerable variation in how patients with suspected TIA are managed in the acute phase. Some health care facilities provide immediate emergency inpatient care, whereas others recommend an outpatient clinical assessment. Recent guidelines recommend that hospitalization be considered for patients who experienced their first TIA within the past 48 hours (Johnston, Nguyen-Huynh, & Schwarz, 2006). Some of the advantages of in-hospital observation include improved ability to expedite workup and treatment and to facilitate the use of tissue plasminogen activator (tPA) in the event an acute stroke occurs (Nguyen-Huynh & Johnston, 2005). According to the guidelines, urgent (within 24–48 hours) assessment and evaluation are recommended for those not admitted to acute care.

Epidemiologically, varying criteria, lack of recognition, and lack of reporting make it difficult to estimate the incidence of TIA, but current estimates in the United States range from 200,000 to 500,000 per year with a population prevalence of approximately 5 million (Johnston, 2002). The prevalence of TIA in men is 2.7% for ages 65–69 and 3.6% for ages 75–79, compared with 1.6% for women aged 65–69 years and 4.1% for women aged 75–79 years (Price, Psaty, O'Leary, Burke, & Gardin, 1993). Notably, silent vascular infarct is also quite prevalent, with a 43% incidence rate above the age of 75 (Howard et al., 1998). Rates of TIA have been found to be higher in African Americans than in Caucasians (Kleindorfer et al., 2005) and appear to be higher during the week, perhaps because patients are less likely to seek medical attention on the weekend (Giles, Flossman, & Rothwell, 2006).

NEUROPATHOLOGY/PATHOPHYSIOLOGY

Although their mechanism is not fully understood, TIAs are often thought of as temporary strokes that usually reverse themselves. They are associated with hypertension and can involve any part of the vascular system.

Neuropathologic studies to date have shown that these transient attacks are usually linked to an atherosclerotic thrombosis. Clinically, it is important to separate attacks that last only a few minutes (up to 1 hour) and result in no permanent damage from those of longer duration, which are more likely embolic in nature.

Neuroimaging studies, such as diffusion- and perfusion-weighted MRI in particular, have had a positive influence on our understanding of the pathophysiology of TIA in recent years. MRI allows for confirmation of focal ischemia rather than another possible cause of a patient's deficit, improves accuracy of diagnosis of the vascular origin and cause of TIA, and examines the extent of previous cerebrovascular injury (Easton et al., 2009).

NEUROPSYCHOLOGICAL/CLINICAL PRESENTATION

Differential diagnosis of TIA includes a broad range of other possible etiologies that can produce transient neurological episodes including migraine, focal seizures, hypoglycemia, multiple sclerosis, benign paroxysmal positional vertigo, and psychological etiologies including panic attacks, dissociative disorders, and somatization. Even so, if the patient presents with stroke risk factors and transient deficits occur in a typical vascular pattern, TIA should be high on the list of probable diagnoses, and a formal diagnostic workup should be completed (Blumenfeld, 2002).

Although by definition TIAs do not result in permanent cognitive impairment by themselves, research has found that individuals with TIAs frequently do exhibit cognitive impairment upon further testing, suggesting that TIAs often reflect larger issues with vascular-related cognitive impairments. In a study of patients over the age of 60 years with hypertension, 12.3% showed cognitive impairment as measured by the Mini Mental State Examination and less than one-third of the patients had adequate blood pressure control (Vinyoles, De la Figuera, & Gonzalez-Segura, 2008). Other studies have found that about 50% of individuals with both carotid artery occlusion and TIAs have mild cognitive impairment, even though structural brain damage was not evident

T

(Bakker et al., 2003). Additionally, in a study of 2,105 patients who meet criteria for stroke, a large percentage (87%) were shown to exhibit cognitive syndromes compared with 36% of 309 TIA patients (Hoffmann, Schmitt, & Bromley, 2009).

Transient episodes of cognitive impairment, including aphasia and amnestic syndromes, often lead one to evaluation for TIAs, although epilepsy can be another precipitator. In patients who report symptoms often associated with TIAs, a history of transient weakness has been shown to be associated with memory impairments, although episodic numbness, loss of vision, inability to speak, and severe dizziness were not shown to be correlated with memory loss (Takahashi et al., 2009). Even patients who exhibit stroke risk factors in the absence of any identifiable vascular event appear to be at greater risk for exhibiting cognitive impairment later in life, particularly those with average or lower levels of cognitive functioning earlier in life (Elkins et al., 2004). Because many of these factors are modifiable, it again reinforces the need for primary prevention.

Although fatigue is more commonly reported post mild stroke, it is fairly frequent following TIA (56% vs. 29%) (Winward, Sackley, Metha, & Rothwell, 2009).

DIAGNOSIS

A number of tools have been devised for use in the acute identification of TIA or stroke including FAST (Face, Arm, Speech, Time test; Nor et al., 2004), LAPSS (Los-Angeles Pre-hospital Stroke Scale; Kidwell, Starkman, Eckstein, Weems, & Saver, 2000), CPSS (Cincinnati Pre-hospital Stroke Scale; Kothari, Pancioli, Liu, Brott, & Broderick, 1999), and ROSIER (Recognition of Stroke in the Emergency Room; Nor et al., 2005). Generally, these tools were designed to aid in the rapid differential diagnosis of stroke from other conditions in order to increase a patient's eligibility for thrombolysis within the first 3 hours following onset of a cerebrovascular event.

A history and physical examination is used to diagnose, prognosticate, and identify the potential cause of a TIA. Routine blood tests including complete blood count, serum electrolytes, creatinine, and fasting blood glucose and lipid levels are also recommended as part of the diagnostic workup (Johnston et al., 2006). Carotid imaging including carotid ultrasound, CT angiography, or MR angiography should be completed as soon as possible (within 24–48 hours) in patients with TIA who would be considered candidates for endarterectomy/stenting if a carotid stenosis were identified. ECG is recommended in all patients to diagnose atrial fibrillation and rule out other arrhythmias or acute myocardial ischemia (Elkins et al., 2002).

Brain imaging is frequently utilized during diagnostic evaluation in order to exclude stroke imitators such as tumors or subdural hematomas, to localize the site of the ischemia, and to differentiate between hemorrhagic and ischemic infarcts. Although CT and conventional MRI are the most commonly used methods of neuroimaging, recent studies have shown particular sensitivity for suspected TIA utilizing diffusion-weighted imaging (DWI) (Redgrave, Coutts, Schulz, Briley, & Rothwell, 2007; Redgrave, Schulz, Briley, Meagher, & Rothwell, 2007; Schulz, Briley, Meagher, Molyneux, & Rothwell, 2003, 2004). In addition to brain imaging, other techniques to image the vascular system may be utilized including catheter angiography, duplex sonography, perfusion studies with MR or CT, and transcranial Doppler sonography.

With the recent development of high-resolution DWI technology, many infarcts that would have been previously diagnosed as TIAs have been found to be associated with ischemic lesions that are not visible on conventional MR studies (Warach & Kidwell, 2004). Patients with new DWI abnormalities are 2–5 times more likely to have a stroke in the days following a TIA (Purroy et al., 2004). In individuals who present with TIA, silent brain infarcts and leucoaraiosis are frequent findings (Norrving, 2008), suggesting that the TIA is actually part of an overall profile of cerebrovascular events. Notably, evidence of a previous stroke is found in 20% of acute stroke patients utilizing CT scan, suggesting that the previous events were often clinically silent (Brainin, McShane, Steiner, Dachenhausen, & Seiser, 1995).

TREATMENT

The primary treatment for TIA is antiplatelet therapy. Other useful interventions include the administration of blood pressure–lowering medications, statins, or anticoagulation for atrial fibrillation. In addition, a TIA may be the first indicator that an endarterectomy is warranted and is the treatment of choice, if symptomatic carotid stenosis is identified. Studies suggest that through the use of these interventions, the risk of recurrent stroke could be reduced by 80–90% (Hackam & Spence, 2007). Because the goal of TIA management is prevention of a future stroke, efforts to control modifiable risk factors, such as diet, cholesterol, smoking, and physical activity level are critical.

With regard to secondary prevention, research efforts have focused on validating scales that utilize specific clinical factors in predicting risk of a subsequent stroke. The ABCD scale (age [A], blood pressure [B], clinical features [C], and duration of symptoms [D]) and ABCD(2) scale (all the previous with diabetes diagnosis [D]) were developed in an effort to predict risk of a subsequent stroke and as a method for triaging these patients (Asimos et al., 2009; Rothwell et al., 2005). Recent research has demonstrated the added value of MRI with the ABCD(2) tool in predicting recurrent stroke in those with a high score, showing a 90-day recurrent stroke risk of 32.1% versus 0.0% in those with a low score (Coutts et al., 2008).

Inpatient multidisciplinary stroke rehabilitation has been shown to significantly benefit outcomes following stroke (Langhorne & Duncan, 2001), but TIA seldom warrants inpatient rehabilitation services. Although rehabilitation efforts are generally reserved for those with more moderate to severe strokes, patients who present with TIA but experience impairments from cerebrovascular disease that have previously gone undetected may also benefit, particularly from experts trained in the diagnosis and rehabilitation of mild deficits. A recent study investigating the benefits of an individualized stroke care program for those with TIA or mild stroke found that providing follow-up occupational and neuropsychological screening 4–6 weeks after discharge, with therapy when appropriate, improved satisfaction at 6 months post event. Patients who were more satisfied were better able to perform activities of daily living (ADLs) and experienced a higher quality of life with less depressive symptoms reported (Arts, Kwa, & Dahmen, 2008).

Currently, a randomized controlled trial (CRAFTS trial) is underway that is investigating the application of the cardiac rehabilitation model following TIA (Lennon & Blake, 2009). The model focuses on lifestyle interventions and supervised aerobic activity to reduce modifiable risk factors and improve health-promoting behaviors. Outcomes will include measures of blood pressure, lipid profile, smoking and diabetic status, exercise, healthy eating, cardiovascular fitness, and health-related quality of life. It is hypothesized that similar to the benefits shown for recurrent cardiac event, this model will result in decreased risk for subsequent cerebrovascular event due to the similarity in modifiable risk factors.

Another concern following TIA is whether driving restriction is appropriate and necessary. Historically, countries that attempt to restrict driving privileges following TIA or minor stroke have had poor compliance (McCarron, Loftus, & McCarron, 2008). In spite of this, the recent research supporting a high conversion rate to full stroke after TIA provides further support for the enforcement of driving restrictions following TIA.

Lori S. Terryberry-Spohr
Amy J. Goldman

Albers, G. W., Caplan, L. R., Easton J. D., Fayad, P. B., Mohr, J. P., Saver, J. L., et al. (2002). Transient ischemic attack — proposal for a new definition. *The New England Journal of Medicine, 347*, 1713–1716.

Arts, M. L., Kwa, V. I., & Dahmen, R. (2008). High satisfaction with an individualized stroke care program after hospitalization of patients with a TIA or minor stroke: A pilot study. *Cerebrovascular Diseases, 25*(6), 566–571.

Asimos, A. W., Johnson, A. M., Rosamond, W. D., Price, M. F., Rose, K. M., Catellier, D, et al. (2010). A multi-center evaluation of the ABCD(2) score's accuracy for predicting early ischemic stroke in admitted patients with transient ischemic attack. *Annals of Emergency Medicine, 55*(2), 201–210.

Bakker, F. C., Klijn, C. J., Jennekens-Schinkel, A., van der Tweel, I., Tulleken, C. A., & Kappelle, L. J. (2003). Cognitive impairment in patients with carotid artery occlusion and ipsilateral transient ischemic attacks. *Journal of Neurology, 250*(11), 1340–1347.

Blumenfeld, H. (2002). *Neuroanatomy through clinical cases.* Sunderland, MA: Sinauer Associates.

Brainin, M., McShane, L. M., Steiner, M., Dachenhausen, A., & Seiser, A. (1995). Silent brain infarcts and transient ischemic attacks. A three-year study of first-ever ischemic stroke patients: The Klosterneuburg Stroke Data Bank. *Stroke, 26*(8), 1348–1352.

Coutts, S. B., Eliasziw, M., Hill, M. D., Scott, J. N., Subramaniam, S., Buchan, A. M., et al. (2008). An improved scoring system for identifying patients at high early risk of stroke and functional impairment after an acute transient ischemic attack or minor stroke. *International Journal of Stroke, 3*(1), 3–10.

Easton, J. D., Saver, J. L., Albers, G. W., Alberts, M. J., Chaturvedi, S., Feldmann, E., et al. (2009). Definition and evaluation of transient ischemic attack: A scientific statement for healthcare professionals from the American Heart Association/American Stroke Association Stroke Council; Council on Cardiovascular Surgery and Anesthesia; Council on Cardiovascular Radiology and Intervention; Council on Cardiovascular Nursing; and the Interdisciplinary Council on Peripheral Vascular Disease. The American Academy of Neurology affirms the value of this statement as an educational tool for neurologists. *Stroke, 40*(6), 2276–2293.

Elkins, J. S., O'Meara, E. S., Longstreth, W. T., Jr., Carlson, M. C., Manolio, T. A., & Johnston, S. C. (2004). Stroke risk factors and loss of high cognitive function. *Neurology, 63*(5), 793–799.

Elkins, J. S., Sidney, S., Gress, D. R., Go, A. S., Bernstein, A. L., & Johnston, S. C. (2002). Electrocardiographic findings predict short-term cardiac morbidity after transient ischemic attack. *Archives of Neurology, 59*(9), 1437–1441.

Giles, M. F., Flossman, E., & Rothwell, P. M. (2006). Patient behavior immediately after transient ischemic attack according to clinical characteristics, perception of the event, and predicted risk of stroke. *Stroke, 37*(5), 1254–1260.

Hackam, D. G., & Spence, J. D. (2007). Combining multiple approaches for the secondary prevention of vascular events after stroke: A quantitative modeling study. *Stroke, 38*(6), 1881–1885.

Hoffmann, M., Schmitt, F., & Bromley, E. (2009). Vascular cognitive syndromes: Relation to stroke etiology and topography. *Acta Neurologica Scandinavica, 120*(3), 161–169.

Howard, G., Wagenknecht, L. E., Cai, J., Cooper, L., Kraut, M. A., & Toole, J. F. (1998). Cigarette smoking and other risk factors for silent cerebral infarction in the general population. *Stroke, 29*(5), 913–917.

Johnston, S. C. (2002). Clinical practice. Transient ischemic attack. *The New England Journal of Medicine, 347*(21), 1687–1692.

Johnston, S. C., Nguyen-Huynh, M. N., & Schwarz, M. E., Fuller, K., Williams, C. E., Josephson, S. A., et al. (2006). National Stroke Association guidelines for the management of transient ischemic attacks. *Annals of Neurology, 60*, 301–313.

Kidwell, C. S., Starkman, S., Eckstein, M., Weems, K., & Saver, J. L. (2000). Identifying stroke in the field. Prospective validation of the Los Angeles prehospital stroke screen (LAPSS). *Stroke, 31*(1), 71–76.

Kleindorfer, D., Panagos, P., Pancioli, A., Khoury, J., Kissela, B., Woo, D., et al. (2005). Incidence and short-term prognosis of transient ischemic attack in a population-based study. *Stroke, 36*(4), 720–723.

Kothari, R. U., Pancioli, A., Liu, T., Brott, T., & Broderick, J. (1999). Cincinnati Prehospital Stroke Scale: Reproducibility and validity. *Annals of Emergency Medicine, 33*(4), 373–378.

Langhorne, P., & Duncan, P. (2001). Does the organization of postacute stroke care really matter? *Stroke, 32*(1), 268–274.

Lennon, O., & Blake, C. (2009). Cardiac rehabilitation adapted to transient ischaemic attack and stroke (CRAFTS): A randomized controlled trial. *BMC Neurology, 9*, 9.

Loring, D. W. (Ed.). (1999). *INS dictionary of neuropsychology*. New York: Oxford University Press.

McCarron, M. O., Loftus, A. M., & McCarron, P. (2008). Driving after a transient ischaemic attack or minor stroke. *Emergency Medicine Journal, 25*(6), 358–359.

Nguyen-Huynh, M. N., & Johnston, S. C. (2005). Is hospitalization after TIA cost-effective on the basis of treatment with tPA? *Neurology, 65*(11), 1799–1801.

Nor, A. M., Davis, J., Sen, B., Shipsey, D., Louw, S. J., Dyker, A. G., et al. (2005). The Recognition of Stroke in the Emergency Room (ROSIER) scale: Development and validation of a stroke recognition instrument. *Lancet Neurology, 4*(11), 727–734.

Nor, A. M., McAllister, C., Louw, S. J., Dyker, A. G., Davis, M., Jenkinson, D., et al. (2004). Agreement between ambulance paramedic- and physician-recorded neurological signs with Face Arm Speech Test (FAST) in acute stroke patients. *Stroke, 35*(6), 1355–1359.

Norrving, B. (2008). Leucoaraiosis and silent subcortical infarcts. *Revue Neurologique (Paris), 164*(10), 801–804.

Pendlebury, S. T., Giles, M. F., & Rothwell, P. M. (2009). *Transient ischemic attack and stroke.* New York: Cambridge University Press.

Price, T. R., Psaty, B., O'Leary, D., Burke, G., & Gardin, J. (1993). Assessment of cerebrovascular disease in the Cardiovascular Health Study. *Annals of Epidemiology, 3*(5), 504–507.

Purroy, F., Montaner, J., Rovira, A., Delgado, P., Quintana, M., & Alvarez-Sabin, J. (2004). Higher risk of further vascular events among transient ischemic attack patients with diffusion-weighted imaging acute ischemic lesions. *Stroke, 35*(10), 2313–2319.

Rancurel, G. (2005). [Transient ischemic attacks in the elderly: New definition and diagnostic difficulties]. *Psychol Neuropsychiatr Vieil, 3*(1), 17–26.

Redgrave, J. N., Coutts, S. B., Schulz, U. G., Briley, D., & Rothwell, P. M. (2007). Systematic review of associations between the presence of acute ischemic lesions on diffusion-weighted imaging and clinical predictors of early stroke risk after transient ischemic attack. *Stroke, 38*(5), 1482–1488.

Redgrave, J. N., Schulz, U. G., Briley, D., Meagher, T., & Rothwell, P. M. (2007). Presence of acute ischaemic lesions on diffusion-weighted imaging is associated with clinical predictors of early risk of stroke after transient ischaemic attack. *Cerebrovascular Diseases, 24*(1), 86–90.

Rothwell, P. M., & Warlow, C. P. (2005). Timing of TIAs preceding stroke: Time window for prevention is very short. *Neurology, 64*(5), 817–820.

Rothwell, P. M., Giles, M. F., Flossmann, E., Lovelock, C. E., Redgrave, J. N., Warlow, C. P., et al. (2005). A simple score (ABCD) to identify individuals at high early risk of stroke after transient ischaemic attack. *Lancet, 366*(9479), 29–36.

Schulz, U. G., Briley, D., Meagher, T., Molyneux, A., & Rothwell, P. M. (2003). Abnormalities on diffusion weighted magnetic resonance imaging performed several weeks after a minor stroke or transient ischaemic attack. *Journal of Neurology, Neurosurgery, and Psychiatry, 74*(6), 734–738.

Schulz, U. G., Briley, D., Meagher, T., Molyneux, A., & Rothwell, P. M. (2004). Diffusion-weighted MRI in 300 patients presenting late with subacute transient ischemic attack or minor stroke. *Stroke, 35*(11), 2459–2465.

Takahashi, P. Y., Dyrbye, L. N., Thomas, K. G., Cedeno, O. Q., North, F., Stroebel, R. J., et al. (2009). The association of transient ischemic attack symptoms with memory impairment among elderly participants of the Third US National Health and Nutrition Examination Survey. *Journal of Geriatric Psychiatry and Neurology, 22*(1), 46–51.

Vinyoles, E., De la Figuera, M., & Gonzalez-Segura, D. (2008). Cognitive function and blood pressure control in hypertensive patients over 60 years of age: COGNIPRES study. *Current Medical Research and Opinion, 24*(12), 3331–3339.

Warach, S., & Kidwell, C. S. (2004). The redefinition of TIA: The uses and limitations of DWI in acute ischemic cerebrovascular syndromes. *Neurology, 62*(3), 359–360.

Winward, C., Sackley, C., Metha, Z., & Rothwell, P. M. (2009). A population-based study of the prevalence of fatigue after transient ischemic attack and minor stroke. *Stroke, 40*(3), 757–761.

TRANSVERSE MYELITIS

DESCRIPTION

Transverse myelitis (TM) is a rare, neuroimmunological disorder related to focal spinal cord inflammation and neural injury. The end result of the process is varying degrees of motor, sensory and autonomic dysfunction (Bruna, Martinez-Yelamos, Martinez-Yelamos, Rubio, & Arbizu, 2006; Montalban, 2006). The acute presentation is divided based on the nature of the symptoms. Acute complete transverse myelitis (ACTM) is characterized by symmetrical and moderate to severe loss of function; acute partial transverse myelitis (APTM) presents in an asymmetrical manner with mild loss of spinal cord function (Ford, Tampieri, & Francis, 1992; Scott, Kassab, & Singh, 2005). Relapsing TM on the other hand, as the name suggests, demonstrates periods of active symptomology with periods of remission, or near remission in-between. When individuals with relapsing myelitis experience acute symptomatic periods, they often present as ACTM.

Epidemiology suggests an annual incidence of five people per million (Levin et al., 2009). The process may have its roots in a number of underlying pathological forces including multi focal central nervous system disease, direct injury to the spinal cord, a part of a systemic or autoimmune disease, or as an isolated, idiopathic entity (de Seze et al., 2001).

NEUROPATHOLOGY/PATHOPHYSIOLOGY

Acute transverse myelitis arises secondary to para-infectious inflammation of the spinal cord (Jeffery, Mandler, & Davis, 1993: Misra, Kalita, & Kumar, 1996). When it presents in a recurrent fashion, it has been more commonly noted as a symptom in relation to Lyme disease, herpes simplex virus infection, systemic lupus erythematosus, Sjörgen's syndrome, primary antiphospholipid syndrome, sarcoidosis, various forms of vasculitis, or an array of idiopathic inflammatory demyelinating disorders (IIDD). In these instances, CSF analysis may reveal mild pleocytosis, modest numbers of lymphocytes, elevated protein levels or oligoclonal bands (OCB) (Cordonnier et al., 2003; Montalban, 2006). However, idiopathic forms have also been noted and are believed to be related to an autoimmune process (Kim, 2003; Tippett, Fishman, & Panitch, 1991).

MRI often shows focal demyelination in the spinal cord involving all elements of the spinal cord on that transverse plane as opposed to unilateral involvement. When it only part of a cross section is affected, it is termed partial transverse myelitis. Further enhancement may be seen with gadolinium infusion. Similar demyelinating lesions may be observed in the cerebral hemispheres. This is usually seen when an intraparenchymal or perivascular cellular influx in the spinal cord actually results in the breakdown of the blood–brain barrier causing the variable demyelination and neuronal injury (Kerr & Ayetey, 2002).

Some cases of TM eventually expand into multiple sclerosis (MS) but is fairly rare, occurring in only 2% of cases within 5 years of symptom onset (Scott, Bhagavatula, Snyder, & Chieffe, 1998; Scott et al., 2005). In comparison, progression to Devic's disease (a.k.a. neuromyelitis optica) is more likely, occurring in more than 10% of cases of relapsing myelitis (Kim, 2003). It is noted that this is in regard to ACTM, whereas partial transverse myelitis has shown a greater frequency of progression to MS (Ford et al., 1992). Negative MRI at the onset of symptoms suggests a low risk for progression to MS (Morrissey et al., 1993).

NEUROPSYCHOLOGICAL/CLINICAL PRESENTATION

Clinically, TM is characterized by the emergence of paraparesis or paraplegia, ascending parasthesias, loss of deep sensibility in the feet, spincter dysfunc-tion, and bilateral Babinski (Ropper & Brown, 2005). The sensorimotor features may be symmetrical or asymmetrical and develop over the course of hours or days and often resolve over several days as well. Sensation is lost below the level of the lesion and radi-cular pain presents at a level even with the lesion. The motor symptoms eventually take on an upper-motor neuron paralysis appearance with hyper-reflexia and bilateral extensor plantar responses (Hammerstaad, 2007). Finally, autonomic dysfunction may also be observed including temperature dysregulation and vasomotor instability. Neurocognition is not com-monly associated with TM except when lesions are noted in cerebral cortex.

DIAGNOSIS

Neuroimaging with MRI of the spine and brain is essential to diagnosis with concentration being placed on the identification of aforementioned signs of demy-elination. While these lesions are hallmark of TM, it is not suggestive of definitive diagnosis (Polman et al., 2005; Wingerchuk, Lennon, Pittock, Lucchinetti, & Weinshenker, 2006). Such scans also allow for rule-out of cerebrovascular events as the basis of the clin-ical features. Additional workup should include CSF analysis making notation of pleocytosis, protein levels, and/or OCB. Workup should also consider those pre-sentations that TM may present in relation to including Lyme disease, herpes simplex virus infection, systemic lupus erythematosus, Sjörgen's syndrome, primary antiphospholipid syndrome, sarcoidosis, various forms of vasculitis, or an array of IIDD.

TREATMENT

Treatment for TM is not highly defined as there have been few clinical trials undertaken as most patients' symptoms remit spontaneously after several days past the peak of clinical features. High doses of corticoster-oids are commonly employed and can prove benefi-cial. These are most often used in idiopathic cases. For individuals who fail to respond to steroids, plasma-pharesis can be effective (Weinshenker et al., 1999).

When progression to MS is believed to be probable (i.e., asymmetric involvement of the spine in conjunc-tion with cerebral lesions), interferon beta-1a treatment has been found to delay the onset of MS (Jacobs et al., 2000). In those instances where progression to Devic's disease seems likely because of identification of neuro-myelitis optica antibodies, prophylactic immunosup-pression can be useful. Azathioprine, interferon-beta, and rituximab have all shown some efficacy

(Cree et al., 2007; Papeix, Deseze, Pierrot-Deseilligny, Tourbah, & Lebrun, 2005).

Chad A. Noggle
Michelle R. Pagoria

Agmon-Levin, N., Kivity, S., Szyper-Kravitz, M., & Shoe-nfeld, Y. (2009). Transverse myelitis and vaccines: A multi-analysis. *Lupus, 18*(13), 1198–1204.
Bruna, J., Martinez-Yelamos, S., Martinez-Yelamos, A., Rubio, F., & Arbizu, T. (2006). Idiopathic acute trans-verse myelitis: A clinical study and prognostic markers in 45 cases. *Multiple Sclerosis, 12,* 169–173.
Cordonnier, C., de Seze, J., Breteau, G., Ferriby, D., Michelin, E., Stojkovic, T., et al. (2003). Prospective study of patients presenting with acute partial transverse mye-lopathy. *Journal of Neurology, 250,* 1447–1452.
Cree, B. A. C., Lamb, S., Morgan, K., Chen, A., Waubant, E., & Genain, C. (2005). An open label study of the effects of rituximab in neuromyelitis optica. *Neurology, 64,* 1270–1272.
de Seze, J., Stojkovic, T., Breteau, G., Lucas, C., Michon-Pasturel, U., Gauvrit, J. Y. et al. (2001). Acute myelopa-thies: Clinical, laboratory and outcome profiles in 79 cases. *Brain, 124,* 1509–1521.
Ford, B., Tampieri, D., & Francis, G. (1992). Long-term follow-up of acute partial transverse Myelopathy. *Neurology, 42,* 250–252.
Hammerstaad, J. (2007). Strength and reflexes. In C. G. Goetz (Ed.), *Textbook of clinical neurology* (pp. 242–287). Phila-delphia, PA: Saunders Elsevier.
Jacobs, L. D., Beck, R. W., Simon, J. H., Kinkel, R. P., Brownscheidle, C. M., Murray, T. J., et al. (2000). Intra-muscular interferon beta-1a therapy initiated during a first demyelinating event in multiple sclerosis. *New England Journal of Medicine, 343,* 898–904.
Jeffery, D. R., Mandler, R. N., & Davis, L. E. (1993). Trans-verse myelitis: Retrospective analysis of 33 cases, with differentiation of cases associated with multiple sclero-sis and parainfectious events. *Archives of Neurology, 50,* 532–535.
Kerr, D. A., & Ayetey, H. (2002). Immunopathogenesis of acute transverse myelitis. *Current Opinion Neurology, 15,* 339–347.
Kim, K. K. (2003). Idiopathic recurrent transverse myelitis. *Archives of Neurology, 60,* 1290–1294.
Misra, U. K., Kalita, J., & Kumar, S. (1996). A clinical, MRI and neurophysiological study of acute transverse mye-litis. *Journal of the Neurological Sciences, 138,* 150–156.
Montalban, X. (2006). The importance of long-term data in multiple sclerosis. *Journal of Neurology, 253,* vi9–vi15.
Morrissey, S. P., Miller, D. H., Kendall, B. E., Kingsley, D. P., Kelly, M. A., Francis, D. A., et al. (1993). The significance of brain magnetic resonance imaging abnormalities at

presentation with clinically isolated syndromes suggestive of multiple sclerosis. *Brain, 116*, 135–146.

Papeix, C., Deseze, J., Pierrot-Deseilligny, C., Tourbah, A., & Lebrun, C. (2005). French therapeutic experience of Devic's disease: A retrospective study of 33 cases. *Neurology, 64*(Suppl. 1), A328.

Polman, C. H., Reingold, S. C., Edan, G., Filippi, M., Hartung, H. P., Kappos, L., et al. (2005). Diagnostic criteria for multiple sclerosis: 2005 revisions to the McDonald Criteria. *Annals of Neurology, 58*, 840–846.

Ropper, A. H., & Brown, R. H. (2005). *Adams and Victor's principles of neurology* (8th ed., pp. 529–545). New York: McGraw-Hill.

Scott, T. F., Bhagavatula, K., Snyder, P. J., & Chieffe, C. (1998). Transverse myelitis comparison with spinal cord presentations of multiple sclerosis. *Neurology, 50*, 429–433.

Scott, T. F., Kassab, S. L., & Singh, S. (2005). Acute partial transverse myelitis with normal cerebral magnetic resonance imaging: Transition rate to clinically definite multiple sclerosis. *Multiple Sclerosis, 11*, 373–377.

Tippet, D. S., Fishman, P. S., & Panitch, H. S. (1991). Relapsing transverse myelitis. *Neurology, 41*, 703–706.

Weinshenker, B. G., O'Brien, P. C., Petterson, T. M., Noseworthy, J. H., Lucchinetti, C. F., Dodick, D. W., et al. (1999). A randomized trial of plasma exchange in acute central nervous system inflammatory demyelinating disease. *Annals of Neurology, 46*, 878–886.

Wingerchuk, D. M., Lennon, V. A., Pittock, S. J., Lucchinetti, C. F., & Weinshenker, B. G. (2006). Revised diagnostic criteria for neuromyelitis optica. *Neurology, 66*, 1485–1489.

TRAUMATIC BRAIN INJURY

DESCRIPTION

Traumatic brain injury (TBI) refers to the "physiological disruption of brain functioning caused by an external force resulting in an acceleration/deceleration or a direct blow to the head" (Carroll, Cassidy, Holm, Kraus, & Coronado, 2004, p. 113). TBIs occur across a continuum of severity, ranging from a mild blow to the head, which results in brief disorientation but full recovery, to multiple crushing blows that lead to death. Of all TBIs, approximately 80% are mild in severity with the remaining being moderate to severe (10% each, respectively). Statistics from the Centers for Disease Control and Prevention (CDC, 2006) indicate that each year in the United States well over 1.5 million individuals sustain a TBI. The CDC (2006) estimated that over 2% of the U.S. population has some types of TBI-associated disability. Motor vehicle accidents are the most common cause for TBI in younger individuals, whereas in the elderly falls are most frequent. TBI is the leading cause of death in people under the age of 40 and males tend to sustain more severe brain injuries. TBI-related costs in the United States are estimated at approximately $60 billion dollars annually (Finkelstein, Corso, & Miller, 2006).

NEUROPATHOLOGY/PATHOPHYSIOLOGY

TBIs are broadly classified into two categories: open brain injuries and closed brain injuries. An open brain injury is where the intracranial cavity is breached by a foreign object, for example, a gunshot to the head. A closed brain injury occurs when there is a damage to the brain, but the skull remains intact. This would include acceleration/deceleration injuries, such as those commonly sustained in motor vehicle accidents. For both the open and the closed TBIs, a further distinction captures when and how the brain is damaged as follows: (a) primary damage and (b) secondary damage. Primary brain damage occurs directly from the forces resulting in, for example, focal lesions, mechanical compression, or diffuse tearing and shearing of brain tissues. Secondary damage refers to the brain damage that occurs in the hours or days after the impact, and includes damage caused by neurosurgical intervention, brain swelling, ischemia, brain infection, posttraumatic seizures, vasospasm, obstructive hydrocephalus, and hypoxia (Granacher, 2003). Secondary damage also includes metabolic and neurotransmitter changes associated with neuronal damage. In fact, research has captured TBI-related neurochemical and neurometabolic cascades that onset in the hours and days after the initial injury that leads to increased cell swelling and subsequent cell death (Bullock et al., 1998). As the individual's cerebral edema fluctuates, so does the level of consciousness, orientation, and agitation. Indeed, the length of loss of consciousness and disorientation provides important indicators for capturing TBI severity. In all, no unitary profile of TBI is seen. Rather, the resulting TBI symptom profile and recovery pattern are often variable and dependent upon the multifactorial interaction of pathology, severity, and environmental factors (Dykeman, 2003; Masson et al., 1996).

NEUROPSYCHOLOGICAL/CLINICAL PRESENTATION

Neuropsychological examinations are the accepted method for quantitatively determining the level of cognitive and emotional functioning after TBI. In the inpatient setting, neuropsychological consultation can assist the health care team to understand the interaction among the patient's physical, cognitive, and emotional symptoms. Neuropsychologists may also be called upon to comment on issues of capacity, readiness for discharge, and placement needs. As these severely brain-injured patients stabilize and recover from their injuries, they are usually better able to tolerate more comprehensive neuropsychological testing. Gauging whether the patient is putting forth adequate effort should be addressed and becomes crucial especially when the case involves legal issues. A comprehensive neuropsychological assessment typically assesses domains such as attention and concentration, memory and learning, language, visuospatial skills, executive functioning, and emotional functioning.

Mild TBI patients are infrequently hospitalized. However, neuropsychological testing can be requested in the early stages of recovery to assess the more subtle deficiencies that are present. Most mild TBI patients have a favorable recovery, but a minority continues to present with residual difficulties months or even years post accident. The *DSM-IV* (American Psychiatric Association [APA], 2000) specifies that if the TBI residuals persist beyond 3 months, then the diagnosis of a postconcussional disorder is warranted. A postconcussional disorder is typically composed of physical, emotional, and cognitive symptoms that occur subsequent to a TBI. According to *DSM-IV* (2000), the documented cognitive deficit should include deficits "in either attention (concentration, shifting focus of attention, performing simultaneous cognitive tasks) or memory (learning or recalling information)" (APA, p. 704). Other cognitive symptoms such as slowed motor movement, problems with executive functioning, and word finding difficulties may be prominent as well. Physical symptoms may include disordered sleep, headache, dizziness, and sensitivity to noise, medications, and light. Emotional symptoms include irritability, anxiety, depressive, affective lability, or other personality changes. Note that the diagnosis of the postconcussional disorder is most often used for milder forms of TBIs, whereas for very severe cases *DSM-IV* offers the diagnosis of dementia due to head trauma, with or without behavioral disturbances.

DIAGNOSIS

Introduced by a team of neurosurgeons in Scotland, the Glasgow Coma Scale (GCS) measures eye-opening, motor response, and verbal response and rates the severity of a TBI according to the patient's ability in each of these domains (Teasdale & Jeanette, 1974). The GCS, which ranges from 3 to 15, classifies TBI severity as mild (13–15), moderate (9–12), and severe (3–8). In general, the higher the GCS score, the better the prognosis. The GCS rating can be determined at the scene of the accident, and when indicated is repeated throughout the hospitalization, to determine the length of the coma or disorientation. It is important to note that the GCS score can be confounded by intoxication, pain, and medications. Although the GCS is the gold standard for triaging the more severe TBI patients, it often lacks the needed sensitivity for capturing mild TBIs (Marshall, 1989; Ruff, 2005; Stambrook, Moore, Lubusko, Peters, & Blumenschein, 1993). For example, if a patient receives a perfect score of 15 at admission to the emergency department, clinicians cannot rule out the likelihood of a mild TBI. Since the loss of consciousness associated with the mild TBI is usually brief, by the time health care providers arrive at the scene (if at all), the GCS will not retrospectively capture the patient's altered state. The most reliable diagnostic indicator for assessing a mild TBI is the patient's inability to store continues memories, and this inability to track ongoing events is called "posttraumatic amnesia."

In response to concerns that many mild TBIs were going undiagnosed, the American Congress of Rehabilitation Medicine in 1993 established a set of diagnostic criteria for mild TBI. Table 1 summarizes these guidelines for mild TBI, which also provide cutoffs for diagnosing more severe TBIs.

Recently, these guidelines have received further support by the World Health Organization

Table 1
DIAGNOSTIC CRITERIA FOR MILD TBI BY THE AMERICAN CONGRESS OF REHABILITATION MEDICINE SPECIAL INTEREST GROUP ON MILD TRAUMATIC BRAIN INJURY*

A traumatically induced physiological disruption of brain function, as manifested by *at least* one of the following:
- any loss of consciousness;
- any loss of memory for events immediately before or after the accident;
- any alteration in mental state at the time of the accident (e.g., feeling dazed, disoriented, or confused); and
- focal neurological deficit(s) that may or may not be transient;

But where the severity of the injury does not exceed the following:
- loss of consciousness of approximately 30 minutes or less;
- after 30 minutes, an initial Glasgow Coma Scale (GCS) score of 13–15; and
- posttraumatic amnesia not greater than 24 hours.

*Developed by the Mild Traumatic Brain Injury Committee of the Head Injury Interdisciplinary Special Interest Group (1993).

Neurotrauma Task Force on mild TBI (Carroll et al., 2004), and thus these guidelines are becoming the accepted standard for diagnosing mild TBI. Note that these diagnostic criteria do not depend upon neuroimaging. Indeed, many individuals with mild TBIs are never referred for neuroimaging. Thus, neuroimaging should not be used as the sole perimeter for determining the presence or absence of a mild TBI (Bazarian et al., 2005; Bigler, 2001; Iverson, Lovell, Smith, & Frazen, 2000; Ruff, Iverson, Barth, Bush, & Broshek, 2009).

TREATMENT

Poorer outcomes in individuals with TBIs have been associated with gender, age, repeated TBIs, premorbid psychopathology, structural intracranial injuries, increased stressors, and substance use (Edna & Cappelen, 1987; Hibbard et al., 2000; Iverson, 2006; Ponsford et al., 2000; Rapoport & Feinstein, 2000). An integrated understanding of the individual that is not limited to a specific discipline, but rather attempts to captures a patient-based perspective can help the clinicians to assess how synergistic symptom interactions can lead to poor outcomes (Ruff, 2005). To capture these interactions, it is essential for clinicians to also determine the individual's premorbid and comorbid functioning across the emotional, cognitive, and physical domains, as well as address the effects of the TBI on vocational, social, and recreational functioning in the individual's daily lives.

Given there is no unitary profile of TBI, treatment and intervention are symptom based. Physical deficits may be addressed within the context of physical and/or occupational therapy. In severe cases, where language is impacted, speech therapy may be used. Thorough neuropsychological assessment may prove priceless in identifying cognitive deficits upon which rehabilitation plans may be built. In conjunction with this, residuals that may interfere with an individual's return to school or work can be identified and addressed along, cognitive, behavioral, and physical lines. Emotional/psychiatric residuals may be addressed with psychotherapy and/or psychopharmacological intervention.

Christina Weyer Jamora
Ronald Ruff

American Psychiatric Association. (2000). *Diagnostic and statistical manual of mental disorders* (4th ed. TR). Washington, DC: Author.

Bazarian, J., McClung, J., Shah, M., Cheng, Y. T., Flesher, W., & Kraus, J. (2005). Mild traumatic brain injury in the United States, 1998–2000. *Brain Injury, 19*, 85–91.

Bigler, E. (2001). Quantitative magnetic resonance imaging in traumatic brain injury. *Journal of Head Trauma Rehabilitation, 16*, 117–134.

Bullock, R., Zauner, A., Woodward, J., Myseros, J., Choi, S., Ward, J., et al. (1989). Factors affecting excitatory amino acid release following severe human head injury. *Journal of Neurosurgery, 89*, 507–518.

Carroll, L., Cassidy, J., Holm, L., Kraus, J., & Coronado, V. G. (2004). Methodological issues and research recommendations for mild traumatic brain injury: The WHO Collaborating Centre Task Force on Mild Traumatic Brain Injury. *Journal of Rehabilitation Medicine, 43*, 113–125.

Centers for Disease Control and Prevention. (2006). *Traumatic brain injury in the United States: Emergency department visits, hospitalizations and deaths*. Retrieved July 31, 2007, from http://www.cdc.gov/ncipc/tbi/TBI_in_US_04/TBI_ED.htm

Dykeman, B. F. (2003). School-based intervention for treating social adjustment difficulties in children with traumatic brain injury. *Journal of Instructional Psychology, 30*(3), 225–230.

Edna, T., & Cappelen, J. (1987). Late post-concussional symptoms in traumatic head injury. An analysis of frequency and risk factors. *Acta Neurochirurgica, 86*, 12–17.

Finkelstein, E., Corso, P., & Miller, T. (2006). *The incidence and economic burden of injuries in the United States*. New York: Oxford University Press.

Granacher, R. (Ed.). (2003). The epidemiology and pathophysiology of traumatic brain injury. In *Traumatic brain injury: Methods for clinical assessment and forensic neuropsychiatric assessment* (pp. 1–24). Boca Raton, FL: CRC Press.

Hibbard, M., Bogdany, J., Uysal, S., Kepler, K., Silver, J., Gordon, W., et al. (2000). Axis II psychopathology in individuals with traumatic brain injury. *Brain Injury, 14*, 45–61.

Iverson, G. (2006). Complicated vs uncomplicated mild traumatic brain injury: Acute neuropsychological outcome. *Brain Injury, 20*, 1335–1344.

Iverson, G., Lovell, M., Smith, S., & Frazen, M. (2000). Prevalence of abnormal CT scans following mild traumatic brain injury. *Brain Injury, 14*, 1057–1061.

Marshall, L. (1989). A neurosurgeon's view of the epidemiology of minor and moderate head injury. In J. Hoff, T. Anderson, & T. Cole (Eds.), *Mild to moderate head injury* (pp. 29–34). Boston: Blackwell Scientific.

Masson, F., Salmi, L. R., Maurette, P., Dartigues, J. F., Vecsey, B., Garros, B., & Erny, P. (1996). Characteristics of head trauma in children: Epidemiology and a 5-year follow-up. *Archives de Pediatric, 3*, 651–660.

Ponsford, J., Willmont, C., Rothwell, A., Cameron, P., Kelly, A., Nelms, R., et al. (2000). Factors influencing outcome following mild traumatic brain injury in adults. *Journal of the International Neuropsychological Society, 6*, 568–579.

Rapoport, M., & Feinstein, A. (2000). Outcome following traumatic brain injury in the elderly: A critical review. *Brain Injury, 14*, 749–761.

Ruff, R. (2005). Two decades of advances in understanding of mild traumatic brain injury. *The Journal of Head Trauma Rehabilitation, 20*, 5–18.

Ruff, R., Iverson, G., Barth, J., Bush, S., & Broshek, D. (2009). Recommendations for diagnosing a mild traumatic brain injury. A National Academy of Neuropsychology position paper. *Archives of Clinical Neuropsychology, 24*, 3–10.

Stambrook, M., Moore, A., Lubusko, A., , Peters, L., & Blumenschein, S. (1993). Alternatives to the Glasgow Coma Scale as a quality of life predictor following traumatic brain injury. *Archives of Clinical Neuropsychology, 8*, 95–103.

Teasdale, G., & Jennett, B. (1974). Assessment of coma and impaired consciousness: A practical scale. *Lancet, 2*, 81–84.

TRIGEMINAL NEURALGIA

DESCRIPTION

Trigeminal neuralgia (TN), also known as "tic douloureux," is an uncommon disorder that typically presents as paroxysmal, brief, recurrent, unilateral facial pain (Sadosky, McDermott, Brandenburg, & Strauss, 2008). To date, two variants of the disorder have been identified: typical and atypical. Typical TN is thought to be caused by the compression of the fifth cranial nerve (trigeminal nerve), although the causes of atypical TN are unknown.

Prevalence estimates vary, largely due to the difficulty in diagnosis (Sadosky et al., 2008). However, the most recent epidemiological data suggest an incident rate ranging from 4.7 to 8.0 per 100,000 persons in the United States. TN is more likely to affect women than men (3.4:2.2). TN generally develops after the age of 50 and reaches a peak in the seventh decade of life, affecting about 1 in 1,000 persons aged 75 years and older. The disorder rarely occurs in children, although a small number of cases have been identified in children as young as 3 years of age (Bennetto, Patel, & Fuller, 2008).

NEUROPATHOLOGY/PATHOPHYSIOLOGY

Vascular compression of the trigeminal nerve root is the most common cause of TN (Edlich, Winters, Britt, & Long, 2006). Other causes include a primary demyelinating disorder or arteriovenous malformation, as well as cysts and tumors near the pons or medulla. An aberration of an artery or vein generally underlies vascular compression, which may in turn lead to irritative foci from the subsequent local demyelination. These foci may produce ectopic impulses resulting in the pain associated with TN.

NEUROPSYCHOLOGICAL/CLINICAL PRESENTATION

Pain is the essential feature of TN and is generally unilateral, although it may be bilateral (10% to 12%). Further, TN tends to wax and wane, with episodes lasting from a few seconds to several minutes (Sadosky et al., 2008). Attacks may occur several times a day, while remitting up to years before an episode reappears. Generally, the intensity and frequency of attacks increase over time (Carlson, 2007).

Neuropsychological studies were not located in the literature; however, some information regarding psychological factors associated with TN was found. Researchers have noted an increased rate of depression and anxiety in persons with chronic facial pain, as well as the presence of personality disorders (Kight, Gatchel, & Wesley, 1999; Korszun, Hinderstein, & Wong, 1996). Further, Curren et al. (1995) reported that 67% of chronic facial pain patients endorsed a history of sexual and/or physical abuse. In another study of 141 patients, 25% met criteria for posttraumatic stress disorder (Sherman et al., 2005).

DIAGNOSIS

TN pain is often initially misdiagnosed as a dental problem or mental health problem. Thus, it is not uncommon for individuals with TN to have seen several different professionals before TN is considered. The current diagnostic standards, according to the International Headache Society, include paroxysmal attacks of pain lasting from a fraction of a second to 2 minutes, which affect one or more divisions of the trigeminal nerve. Additionally, at minimum, the pain has one of the following characteristics: The pain is intense, sharp, superficial, or stabbing; it is precipitated from trigger areas or by trigger factors; attacks in the individual patient are stereotyped; no clinically evident neurologic deficit is present; and the pain is not attributed to another disorder (ICHD, 2004). More recently, Zebenholzer, Wöber, Vigl, Wessely, and Wöber-Bingöl (2006) have suggested that better diagnosis may result from altering the current diagnostic standard to a more liberal taxonomy to allow for individual variance.

Neuroimaging may be useful in accurate diagnosis, although the evidence is mixed. More recent research suggests that the routine use of imaging identifies structural causes of TN in 15% of the cases; thus, it is considered only potentially useful as a diagnostic tool (Gronseth et al., 2008).

TREATMENT

Treatment approaches include pharmacological, surgical, motor stimulation, and/or biobehavioral. For those persons without identified structural lesions, the initial treatment usually consists of carbamazepine, with nearly 70% of TN patients achieving significant relief from pain (Gronseth et al., 2008; He, Wu, & Zhou, 2006). The use of carbamazapine may have side effects that are intolerable to the patient (e.g., drowsiness, nausea and vomiting, and dizziness). Over time, patients may become resistant to carbamazepine as a monotherapy and need the addition of other agents (e.g., gabapentin) to optimize pain control.

Other anticonvulsant agents that have demonstrated efficacy in the management of TN include oxcarbazepine, gabapentin, lamotrigine, topiramate, and phenytoin. Additional pharmacological treatments include baclofen, benzodiazepines (e.g., clonazepam), opioids (e.g., methadone and morphine), and Botox injections.

Surgical interventions may provide relief for those whose pain is refractory to medication. Microvascular decompression is the most promising surgical option and involves the separation or removal of the offending vessel. Studies suggest that 64% of individuals achieved complete relief from pain 10 years postprocedure and remained pain free 20 years. Gamma knife radiosurgery has been effective for short-term relief from pain, although data are not as promising as that of vascular decompression (Linskey, Ratanatharathorn, & Peñagaricano, 2008; Tronnier, Rasche, Hamer, Kienle, & Kunze, 2001).

Biobehavioral treatment focuses on relaxation skills (progressive muscle, breathing) but also psychological factors that may be contributing to chronic pain, such as depression or PTSD (Carlson, 2007). These treatments have been shown to be effective for this patient group.

Jennifer Mariner
Jacqueline Remondet Wall

Bennetto, L., Patel, N. K., & Fuller, G. (2008). Trigeminal neuralgia and its management. *British Medical Journal, 334*(7586), 201–205.

Carlson, C. R. (2007). Psychological factors associated with orofacial pains. *Dental Clinics of North America, 51*, 145–160.

Curren, S. L., Sherman, J. J., Cunningham, L. C., Okeson, J. P., Reid, K. I., & Carlson, C. R. (1995). Physical and sexual abuse among orofacial pain patients: Linkages with pain and psychological distress. *Journal of Orofacial Pain, 10*, 141–150.

Edlich, R. F., Winters, K. L., Britt, L. D., & Long, W. B. (2006). Trigeminal neuralgia. *Journal of Long-Term Effects of Medical Implants, 16*(2), 185–192.

Gronseth, G., Cruccu, G., Alksne, J., Argoff, C., Brainin, M., Burchiel, K., et al. (2008). Practice parameter: The diagnostic evaluation and treatment of trigeminal neuralgia (an evidence-based review): Report of the Quality Standards Subcommittee of the American Academy of Neurology and the European Federation of Neurological Societies. *Neurology, 71*(15), 1183–1190.

He, L., Wu, B., & Zhou, M. (2006). Non-antiepileptic drugs for trigeminal neuralgia. *Cochrane Database of Systematic Reviews, 3*, 1–29.

International Headache Society. (2004). International Classification of Headache Disorders, 2nd edt. ICHD-II. *Cephalalgia* 2004; 24 (Suppl 1).

Kight, M., Gatchel, R. J., & Wesley, L. (1999). Temporomandibular disorders: Evidence for significant overlap with psychopathology. *Health Psychology, 18*, 177–182.

Korszun, A., Hinderstein, B., & Wong, M. (1996). Comorbidity of depression with chronic facial pain and temporomandibular disorders. *Oral Surgery, Oral Medicine, Oral Pathology, Oral Radiology, and Endodontology, 82*(5), 496–500.

Linskey, M. E., Ratanatharathorn, V., & Peñagaricano, J. (2008). A prospective cohort study of microvascular decompression and gamma knife surgery in patients with trigeminal neuralgia. *Journal of Neurosurgery, 109*(Suppl.), 160–172.

Sadosky, A., McDermott, A. M., Brandenburg, N. A., & Strauss, M. (2008). A review of the epidemiology of painful diabetic peripheral neuropathy, postherpetic neuralgia, and less commonly studied neuropathic pain conditions. *Pain Practice, 8*(1), 45–56.

Sherman, J. J., Carlson, C. R., Wilson, J. F., Okeson, J. P., & McCubbin, J. A. (2005). Post-traumatic stress disorder among patients with orofacial pain. *Journal of Orofacial Pain, 19*, 309–317.

Tronnier, V. M., Rasche, D., Hamer, J., Kienle, A. L., & Kunze, S. (2001). Treatment of idiopathic trigeminal neuralgia: Comparison of long-term outcome after radio frequency rhizotomy and microvascular decompression. *Neurosurgery, 48*(6), 1261–1268.

Zebenholzer, K., Wöber, C., Vigl, M., Wessely, P., & Wöber-Bingöl, Ç. (2006). Facial pain and the second edition of the international classification of headache disorders. *Headache, 46*, 259–263.

TROPICAL SPASTIC PARAPARESIS

DESCRIPTION

Tropical spastic paraparesis (TSP) is a chronic and progressive inflammatory disease primarily affecting the spinal cord (Osame et al., 1986). TSP was first described in the late 19th century (Strachan, 1897). Human T-cell lymphotropic virus type-I- (HTLV-I)-associated myelopathy (HAM) was later described in 1986 (Gessain et al., 1986; Osame et al., 1986; and it was shortly recognized that TSP and HAM are part of the same syndrome. HTLV-I is considered the likely cause of TSP/HAM (Carod-Artal, 2009). It is estimated that 20 million people are infected with HTLV-I throughout the world, and 0.3% to 4% will develop TSP/HAM (Carod-Artal, 2009). TSP is rarely diagnosed in the United States, but it occurs most often in southern Japan and the Caribbean basin (Osame et al., 1987), as well as West and Central Africa and some Latin American regions (Edlich, Arnette, & Williams, 2000). Those who contract the disease typically live in these endemic areas, have had sexual contact with infected individuals in the endemic areas, are intravenous drug users (IDU), or have had sexual contact with IDUs (Dixon et al., 1990; Kramer et al., 1995). Organ transplantation, blood transfusion, and breast-feeding have also been linked to transmission (Toro et al., 2002).

NEUROPATHOLOGY/PATHOPHYSISOLOGY

The pathophysiology of TSP/HAM also remains unclear. It has been suggested that the syndrome may be an autoimmune response from an HTLV reaction against CNS antigens (Levin et al., 2002). Some have further suggested that TSP/HAM may be similar to multiple sclerosis (MS), due to increased IgG and oligoclonal IgG in the cerebrospinal fluid (CSF), the preponderance of cases occurring in women, and the similar type of response pattern to MS-related treatments (Osame et al., 1987). Others have suggested that TSP/HAM is due to direct pathogenic action of the tax viral protein (Nagai & Jacobson, 2001; Orland, 2003). The pathology of TSP/HAM includes the spinal column, particularly at the thoracic level, with atrophy occurring around the lateral columns (Iwasaki, 1990). These lesions have been linked to perivascular and parenchymal lymphocytic infiltration (Umehara & Osame, 2003).

Brain lesions have been identified in some cases of TSP/HAM, but there is very little that is understood about the nature of the lesions, and how they may be related to spinal cord lesions (Moe et al., 2000). Yukitake et al. (2008) reviewed spinal cord MRIs of 38 patients with TSP/HAM. They found that patients who evidenced T2-hyperintensities evidenced severe paraparesis that rapidly progressed, which resulted in severe motor impairment. Kuroda et al. (1995) found that 30 of the 36 patients assessed demonstrated multiple white matter lesions on T2-weighted cranial MRI, with two fulfilling the criteria for MS. Puccioni-Sohler et al. (2007) found that the 17 patients assessed evidenced time-progressive and extensive multifocal white matter hyperintensities on T2-weighted images in the supra- and infratentorial areas of the brain. In addition, two patients had similar presentations in the spinal cord and gadolinium-enhancing brain lesions suggesting active disease (Puccioni-Sohler et al., 2007). Morgan et al. (2007) noted that white matter lesions are commonly observed on brain's MRI in HTLV-I carriers, but they do not help to discriminate those with TSP/HAM. Overall, there appears to be definite patterns of lesions on brain and spinal MRI; however, understanding the clinical correlates of these findings are where the study is needed.

NEUROPSYCHOLOGICAL/CLINICAL PRESENTATION

Patients can present with a variety of symptoms in TSP/HAM but those that may occur include widespread pyramidal signs, urinary urgency or incontinence, constipation, noncompressive paraparesis in the lower limbs, and subtle sensory changes (Araújo, Afonso, Schor, & Andrada-Serpa, 1993). Other changes may include disabling pain, which may occur in the lumbar region and radiate down the legs (Franzoi et al., 2005). In some cases, researchers assert that cognitive functioning is generally preserved in TSP/HAM (Orland, 2003). However, this is quite debatable in the literature, given that many cases of TSP/HAM appear to mimic MS. Thus, in addition to the noted abnormal neuroimaging results that have been in relation, the HTLV-I or TSP/HAM patients could lead one to presume that cognitive deficits also may be present. Nevertheless, these symptoms may be less likely to gain attention when detecting the disease process.

Silva, Mattos, Alfano, and Araujo (2003) found that HTLV-1 carrier groups and those with TSP/HAM exhibited a lower performance on neuropsychological testing when compared with controls. There were no observable differences between asymptomatic infected carriers and those with TSP/HAM. Observable changes included psychomotor slowing, deficits in alternate attention (mental flexibility), poor verbal and visual memory, including recognition, decreased verbal fluency, and diminished visuo-motor/construction skills. They pointed out that comorbid mood disorder was commonly observed in TSP/HAM, which could weaken this effect. They concluded that TSP/HAM as well as asymptomatic infection can be associated with mild cognitive deficits (Silva et al., 2002).

In a study of 43 patients, 31 of whom were women and diagnosed with TSP, it was found that at least 50% of the patients with TSP exhibited cognitive and affective impairment. Deficits were noted on the subtests of the WAIS, including digit span, digit symbol, object assembly, and picture arrangement. Deficits were also noted on the Benton Visual Retention Test. Overall, they found a positive relationship between cognitive and motor symptoms (Cartier & Gomez, 1999).

Overall, the research supports a subcortical type of disruption that can occur in cases of TSP/HAM. These findings are consistent with the type of profile that is commonly seen in MS as well as HIV infection.

DIAGNOSIS

In endemic areas of HTLV-I infection, differential diagnosis can be challenging for TSP/HAM and myelopathies of other etiologies as well as primary progressive MS (Puccioni-Sohler et al., 2007). Clear diagnostic criteria for TSP/HAM have yet to be established, which can also be especially complicating for mild cases of TSP/HAM (Orland, 2003). However, the World Health Organization has described certain characteristics of the condition. These may include diffuse hyperreflexia, clonus, leg weakness, loss of vibratory sense, and bladder dysfunction. In order to formally diagnose, confirmation of the presence of HTLV I or II virus of the antibodies must be detected in the CSF or peripheral blood (Orland et al., 2003). In the CSF, a diagnosis can be made using ELISA/western blot or by also using polymerase chain reaction in the CSF and the antibody index (AI) (Araújo, Leite, Lima, & Silva, 2009).

TREATMENT

Carod-Artal (2009) noted that many forms of treatment have been utilized in small open trials for TSP/HAM, but the efficacy has been limited to date. These treatments include plasma-exchange, intravenous immunoglobulins, corticosteroids, lamivudine, green-tea, danazol, pentoxifylline, lactobacillus-fermented milk, zidovudine, monoclonal antibodies (daclizumab), valproic acid, and interferon. Earlier

published studies note that similar to MS, corticosteroids and interferon — alpha or beta — have been successful in relieving some symptoms of TSP/HAM (Osame et al., 1987; Weiner & Hafler, 1988). In a systematic review of the effectiveness and safety of different interventions for treating HTLV-I and TSP/HAM, Uthman & Uthman (2007) found that high-dose human lymphobastoid interferon resulted in high efficacy with an acceptable degree of side effects. They concluded in their review that there was no significant benefit of using zidovudine plus lamivudine. They also noted that the data are limited because of small study sizes, short study durations, and some compromises noted in the designs (Uthman & Uthman, 2007).

Amy R. Steiner
Chad A. Noggle
Amanda Steiner

Araújo, A. C., Afonso, C. R., Schor, D., & Andrada-Serpa, M. J. (1993). Spastic paraparesis of obscure origin. A case-control study of HTLV-I positive and negative patients from Rio de Janerio, Brazil. *Journal of Neurological Science, 116*(16), 165–169.

Araújo, A. Q., Leite, A. C., Lima, M. A., & Silva, M. T. (2009). HTLV-1 and neurological conditions. When to suspect and when to order a diagnostic test for HTLV-1 infection? *Arquivos De Neuro-Psiquiatria* [serial on the Internet; cited 2009 Aug 27], *67*(1), 132–138. Retrieved from http://www.scielo.br/scielo.php?script=sci_arttext&pid=S0004-282X2009000100036&lng=en. doi: 10.1590/S0004-282X2009000100036.

Carod-Artal, F. J. (2009). Immunopathogenesis and treatment of myelopathy associated to the HTLV-I virus. *Revista De Neurologia, 48*(3), 147–155.

Cartier, L., & Gomaz, A. (1999). Subcortical dementia in HTLV-I tropical spastic paraparesis. Study of 43 cases. *Revista médica de Chile, 127*(4), 444–450.

Dixon, P. S., Bodner, A. J., Okihiro, M., Milbourne, A., Diwan, A., & Nakamura, J. M. (1990). Human T-lymphotropic virus type I (HTLV-I), and tropical spastic paraparesis or HTLV-I associated myelopathy in Hawaii. *Western Journal of Medicine, 152,* 261–267.

Edlich, R., Arnette, J., & Williams, F. (2000). Global epidemic of human T-cell lymphotropic virus type-I (HTLV-I). *Journal of Emergency Medicine, 18,* 109–119.

Franzoi, A.C., Araujo, A.Q.C. (2005). Disability profile of patients with HTLV-I-associated myelopathy/tropical spastic paraparesis using the Functional Independence Measure (FIM). *Spinal Cord*, 43, 236–240.

Gessain, A., Francis, H., Sonan, T., Sonan, T., Giordano, C. et al. (1986). HTLV-1 and Tropical Spastic Paraparesis in Africa. *The Lancet, 2* (8508), 698–698.

T

Iwasaki, Y. (1990). Pathology of chronic myelopathy associated with HTLV-I infections (HAM/TSP). *Journal of Neurological Science, 96,* 103–123.

Kramer, A., Maloney, E. M., Mogan O. S., Rodger-Johnson, P., Manns, A., Murphy, E. L., et al. (1995). Risk factors and cofactors for human T-cell lymphotropic virus type I (HTLV-I) associated meylopathy/tropical spastic paraparesis (HAM/TSP) in Jamaica. *American of Journal Epidemiology, 142,* 1212–1220.

Kuroda, Y., Matsui, M., Yukitake, M., Kurohara, K., Takashima, H. et. al. (1995). Assessment of MRI criteria for MS in Japanese MS and HAM/TSP. *Neurology, 45,* 30–33.

Levin, M. C., Lee, S. M., Kalume, F., Morcos, Y., Dohan, F. C., et al. (2002). Autoimmunity due to molecular mimicry as a cause of neurological disease. *Natural Medicine, 8,* 509–513.

Moe, M. A., Matsuoka, E., Moritoyo, T., Umehara, F., Suehara, M., Hokezu, Y., et al. (2000). Histopathological analysis of four autopsy cases of HTLV-I associated myelopathy/tropical spastic paraparesis: inflammatory changes occur simultaneously in the entire central nervous system. *Acta Neuropathologica, 100,* 245–252.

Morgan, D. J., Caskey, M. F., Abbehusen, C., Oliveira-Filho, J., Araujo, C., et al. (2007). Brain Magnetic resonance imaging white matter lesions are frequent in HTLV-1 carriers and do not discriminate from HAM/TSP. *AIDS Research and Human Retroviruses, 23*(12), 1499–1504.

Nagai, M., & Jacobson, S. (2001). Immunopathogenesis of human T cell lymphotropic virus type I-associated myelopathy. *Current Opinions in Neurology, 14,* 381–386.

Orland, J. R., Engstrom, J., Fridey, J., Sacher, R. A., Smith, J. W., et al. (2003). Prevalence and clinical features of HTLV neurologic disease in the HTLV outcomes study. *Neurology, 61,*1588–1594.

Osame, M., Usuku, K., Izumo, S., Ijichi, N., Amitani, H., Igata, A., et al. (1986). HTLV-I associated myelopathy, a new clinical entity *Lancet,* May 3; 1(8488):1031–1032.

Osame, M., Matsumoto, M., Usuku, K., Izumo, S., Ijichi, N., Amitani, H., et al. (1987). Chronic progressive myelopathy associated with elevated antibodies to human T-lymphotropic virus type I and adult T-cell leukemia like cells. *Annals of Neurology, 21,* 117–122.

Puccioni-Sohler, M., Yamano, Y., Rios, M., Carvalho, S. M. F., Vasconcelos, C. C. F., Papais-Alvarenga, R., et al. (2007). Differentiation of HAM/TSP from patients with multiple sclerosis infected with HTLV-I. *Neurology, 68,* 206–213.

Silva, M., Mattos, P., Alfano, A., & Araújo, A. (2003). Neuropsychological assessment in HTLV-1 infection: A comparative study among TSP.HAM, asymptomatic carriers, and healthy controls. *Journal of Neurosurgery Psychiatry, 74,* 1085–1089.

Strachan, H. (1897). On a form of multiple neuritis prevalent in the West Indies. *Practitioner (London), 59,* 477–484.

Umehara, F., & Osame, M. (2003). Histological analysis of HAM/TSP pathogenesis. In: K. Sugamura, T. Uchicyama, M. Masso, & M. Kannagi, (Eds.), *Two decades of adult T-cell leukemia and HTLV-I research.* Tokyo: Japan Scientific Societies Press.

Uthman, O. A., & Uthman, R. T. (2007). Interventions for the treatment of Human T-lymphotropic virus type-1-associated myelopathy: A systematic review of randomized controlled trials. *Neurology Asia, 12,* 81–87.

Weiner, H. L., & Hafler, D. A. (1988). Immunotherapy of multiple sclerosis. *Annals of Neurology, 23,* 211–222.

WHO (1989). Virus disease: Human T lymphotropic virus type I, HTLV-I. *The Weekly Epidemiological Record, 64,* 382–383.

Toro, C., Rodes, B., Aguilera, A., Caballero, E., Benito, R., Tuset, C., et al. (2002). Clinical Impact of HTLV-1 Infection in Spain: Implications for Public Health and Mandatory Screening. *Journal of Acquired Immune Deficiency Syndromes, 30*(3), 366–368.

Yukitake, M., Takase, Y., Nanri, Y., Kosugi, M., Eriguchi, M., Yakushiji, Y., et al. (2008). Incidence and clinical significances of human T-cell lymphotropic virus type I-associated myelopathy with T2 hyperintensity on spinal magnetic resonance images. *Internal Medicine, 47*(21), 1881–1886. [Epub 2008 Nov 4].

TROYER'S SYNDROME

DESCRIPTION

Troyer's syndrome is an autosomal recessive disorder that involves both developmental and degenerative processes. First identified in 1967, it is classified as a rare disease, which means that it impacts less than 200,000 individuals in the United States. The disease was first identified in the Amish, but recently has been identified in other populations. It is a complicated form of hereditary spastic paraplegia (HSP), a term used to describe a group of clinically heterogeneous neurodegenerative disorders in which the main feature is progressive lower limb spasticity. Being a complicated form of HSP, it differs from the pure form in that additional neurological signs such as mental retardation (MR), deafness, optic neuropathy, or extrapyramidal symptoms are present (Proukakis et al., 2004).

NEUROPATHOLOGY/PATHOPHYSIOLOGY

The complete pathogenic basis of Troyer's syndrome is unclear. However, the putative pathogenesis of

Troyer's syndrome is a mutation in the *SPG20* gene, which is responsible for encoding the protein spartin. Specifically, the 1110delA mutation in exon 4 appears to be the causal mutation in the *SPG20* gene (Patel et al., 2002). This gene is widespread throughout both adult and fetal tissue and mutation in *SPG20* invariably causing a complete loss protein spartin through either increased protein degradation or impaired translation (Bakowska, Wang, Xin, Sumner, & Blackstone, 2008), resulting in the manifestation of the Troyer's syndrome.

Radiological studies have noted that Troyer's syndrome may actually be a combination of brain abnormality and motor neuron disease (Auer-Grumbach et al., 1999). According to Proukakis et al. (2004), axonal degeneration of the corticospinal tracts, fasciculus gracilis, and the spinocerebellar tracts are common underlying pathology in Troyer's syndrome. Together, these make up the longest motor and sensory axons in the nervous system, and damage begins at the most distal portion near the neuromuscular junction, and works its way back to the cell soma.

Blood tests have been found normal in patients with Troyer's syndrome (Proukakis et al., 2004), however, electrophysiological studies by Auer-Grumbach et al. (1999) found motor nerve conduction to be below normal and compound motor action potentials to be markedly reduced, although sensory potentials and conduction were both in the normal range. Likely due to the degeneration in the aforementioned motor neurons, patients with Troyer's syndrome may display chronic denervation and loss of motor units in the lower extremities. Also likely due to the degeneration and chronic denervation, muscle fiber atrophy is possible.

MRI scans have repeatedly demonstrated deep white matter abnormalities in patients with Troyer's syndrome (Auer-Grumbach et al., 1999; Proukakis et al., 2004). Although there is no uniform pattern of signal change in Troyer's syndrome, there are some consistencies in the location of these hyperintensities as the temporoparietal periventricular white matter and posterior limbs of the internal capsule appear to be most highly implicated. There is also evidence of severe corpus callosum thinning throughout its entire length and a poorly defined cingulate gyrus, most notably in the frontal and posterior horns. Callosal changes appear to owe to a hypoplastic callosum rather than atrophy, due to the otherwise normal cerebral volume. This appears to implicate a fundamental cerebral developmental abnormality possibly due to impaired axonal growth or deficient myelination (Auer-Grumbach et al., 1999).

NEUROPSYCHOLOGICAL/CLINICAL PRESENTATION

The first presenting feature of Troyer's syndrome is a mild delay in reaching early milestones, specifically walking and talking, when compared to unaffected individuals (Proukakis et al., 2004). On average, patients with Troyer's syndrome will begin to walk at around 16 months of age, and talk at approximately 17 months. Throughout the later years, there is a slow deterioration of both, though a consistent timeline for this deterioration does not exist. The gait deterioration generally consists of a combination of spastic and ataxic features, a wide base, inward turned feet, and frequent reflexive plantar extension. Many of these patients are confined to a wheel chair by the 5th decade.

Because there is no distinct pattern of cerebral white matter disease, the specific cognitive deficits in Troyer's syndrome are inconsistent. However, in addition to a reduced IQ (Cross & McKusick, 1967), usually in the borderline range, generalized learning difficulties exist throughout the lifespan. There does not appear to be evidence of progressive cognitive decline. Cerebellar signs, which usually include dysdiadochokinesia (inability to make rapid hand movements), terminal dymetria (lack of coordination involving over- or under-shooting the intended position), choreoathetoid movements (continuous involuntary rapid, highly complex jerky movements), and dystonic limb posturinga, do, however, become more pronounced with age. Sensory exams are unremarkable with Troyer's syndrome patients as the disorder appears to be constricted to motor pathways. Speech difficulties are also often present, but correspond with dysarthric presentations, rather than damage to cortical speech areas. Emotional lability (e.g., inappropriate euphoria, depression, anger, and crying) is quite common in these patients, but not present in all cases.

DIAGNOSIS

Like many autosomal recessive disorders, prenatal diagnosis of at-risk pregnancies is possible for Troyer's syndrome. DNA analysis from fetal cells obtained by amniocentesis (amniotic fluid test) around 15–18 weeks of gestation or through chorionic villus sampling, which involves removal and examination of a small piece of placenta tissue, around 10–12 weeks of gestation. Prenatal diagnosis hinges on identification of a mutation in the *SPG20* gene, specifically, the 1110delA mutation in exon 4 (Patel et al., 2002).

If prenatal diagnosis of Troyer's syndrome is not conducted, genetic testing will likely occur within the 1st decade of life when clinical symptoms begin to appear. The pathognomonic clinical signs of Troyer's syndrome are spasticity in the lower limbs with hyper-reflexia and extensor plantar responses. Prior to this, delayed and dysarthric speech, combined with delayed, unsteady, and wide-based ambulation may be an early indicator of Troyer's syndrome. Genetic testing will be further warranted upon the presence of distal amyotrophy, choreoathetoid movements, and skeletal abnormalities. Specifically, patients with Troyer's syndrome appear to regularly have short stature, kyphoscoliosis (spinal curvature), and pes cavus (fixed plantar flexion). Finally, the previously mentioned cerebellar signs, learning difficulties, and emotional lability are also indicative of this disease. In conjunction with mutation in the *SPG20* gene, each of these clinical signs is diagnostic of Troyer's syndrome.

TREATMENT

Currently, there are no treatments available that will prevent or slow the progressive degeneration in Troyer's syndrome. The current best practice in the management of this disease consists of symptomatic therapy through antispasmodic drugs, physical therapy, and assistive devices to aid in walking. Physical therapy will not be able to combat the skeletal abnormalities or denervation in Troyer's syndrome, but may be able to help patients maintain and increase muscle strength and range of motion. Medicinal interventions, such as dantrolene or baclofen (orally or intrathecally) to reduce spasticity, zanaflex to treat muscle spasms, or benzodiazepines (i.e., diazepam and clonazepam), and botox injection as muscle relaxants may also be useful.

Finally, in patients with a much slower disease progression, lengthening the ankle plantar flexors through orthopedic surgery may be beneficial to reduce equine gait and extensor plantar flexion.

Daniel J. Heyanka
Charles Golden

Auer-Grumbach, M., Fazekas, F., Radner, H., Irmler, A., Strasser-Fuchs, S., & Hartung, H. P. (1999). Troyer syndrome: A combination of central brain abnormality and motor neuron disease? *Journal of Neurology, 246,* 556–561.

Bakowska, J. C., Wang, H., Xin, B., Sumber, C. J., & Blackstone, C. (2008). Lack of spartin protein in Troyer syndrome: A loss-of-function disease mechanism? *Archives of Neurology, 65,* 520–524.

Cross, H. E., & McKusick, V. A. (1967). The Troyer syndrome: A recessive form of spastic paraplegia with distal muscle wasting. *Archives of Neurology, 16,* 473–485.

Patel, H., Cross, H., Proukakis, C., Hershberger, R., Bork, P., & Ciccarelli, F. D., et al. (2002). SPG20 is mutated in Troyer syndrome, a hereditary spastic paraplegia. *Nature Genetics, 31,* 347–348.

Proukakis, C., Cross, H., Patel, H., Patton, M. A., Valentine, A., & Crosby, A. H. (2004). Troyer syndrome revisited: A clinical and radiological study of a complicated hereditary spastic paraplegia. *Journal of Neurology, 251,* 1105–1110.

TUBEROUS SCLEROSIS

DESCRIPTION

Tuberous sclerosis complex is an autosomal dominant neurocutaneous, multisystem disorder with a prevalence of 1 in 10,000 (Hunt & Lindenbaum, 1984). Although tuberous sclerosis is predominately reported as an inherited disorder, 60–70% of cases present secondary to spontaneous genetic mutations, most commonly related to anomalies of *TSC1* and *TSC2* genes that together produce hamartin and tuberin, respectively (Maria, Deidrick, Roach, & Gutmann, 2004; van Slegtenhorst et al., 1997). Although various systemic effects of the presentation can be seen, neurological involvement is common including mental retardation, higher incidence of autistic spectrum features, potential hydrocephalus, and seizures (e.g., infantile spasms). Treatment is usually focused on achieving good seizure control (Wong, 2006) and potential shunting if hydrocephalus presents. Surgical intervention may be employed for severe epileptiform activity and/or systemic issues such as kidney dysfunction. Medicinal intervention remains the most commonly used method of seizure control. Neuropsychological assessment is essential to identifying cognitive or behavioral deficits that are addressed as needed.

NEUROPATHOLOGY/PATHOPHYSIOLOGY

Tuberous sclerosis arises from mutations of *TSC1* and *TSC2* genes that are thought to be suppressor genes. The mutations lead to abnormalities in cell proliferation, differentiation, and migration that can affect the brain, heart, skin, retina, and kidneys (Ramesh, 2003).

These mutations arise spontaneously in more than 60% of cases.

Neurological features remain the most commonly seen sequelae of tuberous sclerosis. The neuropathology of the presentation corresponds with at least one supratentorial lesion characterized by the combined effects of cortical tubers and transmantle dysplasia, subcortical heterotopias, white-matter abnormalities, corpus callosum agenesis or dysplasia, and/or subependymal giant cell astrocytomas that can cause hydrocephalus and epileptogenic activity (van Slegtenhorst et al., 1997). The tubers that characterize the disorder are composed of poorly delineated mixtures of both neuronal and glial cell elements (Dabora et al., 2001). The cortical tubers and the abnormal tissue surrounding these formations serve as the basis of the seizures that present in conjunction with the disorder and are in many ways dependent upon the number, size, and location (Maeda, Tartaro, Matsuda, & Ishii, 1995). Periventricular and frontal regions may represent those areas with the highest prevalence of abnormalities such as ventricular enlargement in addition to supratentorial features previously discussed. Infratentorial brain lesions may also be seen but are far less common presenting in less than 5% of patients. These lesions include linear and gyriform cerebellar folia calcifications, cerebellar nodular white-matter calcifications, agenesis and hypoplasia of the cerebellar hemispheres and vermis, enlargement of the cerebellar hemispheres, and subependymal nodules and tubers in the brainstem and fourth ventricle (Maria et al., 2004).

NEUROPSYCHOLOGICAL/CLINICAL PRESENTATION

The clinical manifestations of tuberous sclerosis vary and include both neurological and physiological features. The type and amount of symptoms correspond with diagnosis. Definitive diagnosis is said to be concluded when two major or one major and two minor features present. If only one major symptom is seen in conjunction with only one minor symptom then diagnosis is said to be probable, whereas a possible diagnosis is noted when only one major feature is seen or two minor symptoms are seen (Maria et al., 2004). Major features include manifestations of the skin, other organs, and brain. Major skin presentations include facial angiofibromas, ungual fibroma, more than three hypomelanotic macules, and shagreen patch. Cardiac rhabdomyoma, lymphangioleiomyomatosis, and renal angiomyolipoma represent major symptoms that involve other organs. Finally, cortical tubers, subependymal nodules, and subependymal giant cell astrocytomas represent the major brain-based features. Minor symptoms include multiple randomly distributed pits in dental enamel, rectal polyps, bone cysts, cerebral white-matter migration abnormalities on brain imaging, gingival fibromas, nonrenal hamartomas, retinal achromic patches, confetti skin lesions, and multiple renal cysts (Maria et al., 2004).

Although central nervous system complications represent the most common sequelae, renal complications are the second most common cause of morbidity including kidney failure, angiomyolipomas, and polycystic kidney disease occurs in 5–8% of patients (Maria et al., 2004). Pulmonary distress may also be seen secondary to lung manifestations including lymphangioleiomyomatosis, multifocal cysts, and multifocal micronodular pneumocyte hyperplasia, which correspond with symptoms including cystic lung disease, dyspnea, cough, hemoptysis, recurrent pneumothoraces, lymphatic obstruction, and retroperitoneal and hilar adenopathy (Maria et al., 2004). Cardiac features may present as ventricular tachycardia and fibrillation, arrhythmia, bradycardia, and heart block (Maria et al., 2004).

Neurological degradation remains the most common feature of tuberous sclerosis. The disease is the leading cause of infantile spasms with a third of patients presenting with this type of seizure disorder although other seizure forms have also been noted (Maria et al., 2004). In fact, in upward of 90% of patients with tuberous sclerosis present with seizures. The presence of seizures is largely related to the manifestation of cognitive and/or behavioral deficits.

Mental retardation and other neuropsychological deficits, including attention and executive function impairments, present in approximately 45–57% of patients (Hunt & Shepherd, 1993; Jozwiak, Goodman, & Lamm, 1998; Shepherd & Stephenson, 1992; Shepherd, Houser, & Gomez, 1995). One of the more recent investigations demonstrated IQs falling below 70 in 44% of patients assessed (Joinson et al., 2003). Beyond mental retardation, autism or autistic-like behaviors have been noted in as high as 35% of patients; ADHD or ADHD-like symptoms have been noted in approximately 25% of patients; and aggression and destructiveness have been noted 48% of patients (Webb, Fryer, & Osborne, 1991; Webb, Thomson, & Osborne, 1991). Learning disabilities are also commonly seen.

DIAGNOSIS

As discussed previously, diagnosis is based on the type and the number of symptoms seen. Definitive diagnosis is said to be concluded when two major or one major and two minor features present. If only one major symptom is seen in conjunction with only one minor symptom then diagnosis is said to be probable, whereas a possible diagnosis is noted when only one major feature is seen or two minor symptoms are seen (Maria et al., 2004). Magnetic resonance imaging offers the most detailed view of the majority of brain lesions seen in tuberous sclerosis, although computed tomography scans can better display calcified areas (Maeda et al., 1995). EEG is essential given the high prevalence of seizures.

Genetic testing may also be employed but has been reported previously as only 80% accurate (Roach, Gomez, & Northrup, 1998). Dental examinations are also useful as 100% of people with tuberous sclerosis are said to present with dental pits and craters in permanent teeth and a majority have gingival fibromas.

Screening of behavioral and neurodevelopmental dysfunction has also been recommended by the National Institutes of Health at the time of diagnosis and at the start of a child's schooling and then at regular periods in time thereafter. Neuropsychological assessment is an essential component of these initial and follow-up evaluations.

TREATMENT

Treatment approaches are symptom based. For seizures that present in more than 90% of all patients with tuberous sclerosis, medication, vagus nerve stimulation, the ketogenic diet, and surgery have all been used (Maria et al., 2004). Medicinal intervention for seizures secondary to tuberous sclerosis is often different than medicinal control of seizures not associated with tuberous sclerosis. Research has demonstrated that children with tuberous sclerosis complex and epilepsy respond poorly to conventional antiseizure therapies (Maria et al., 2004). Rather, Vigabatrin, which is an irreversible 7-aminobutyric acid (GABA) transaminase inhibitor, is the preferred medicinal treatment for infantile. Surgical management of seizures in tuberous sclerosis is used rarely as there are often multiple bilateral lesions. Still, other research has suggested that reduction of lesion sites that correspond with seizure activity can reduce medicinal use and has been linked with improved development, behavior, and quality of life in some children (Romanelli, Najjar, Weiner, & Devinsky, 2002).

As noted previously, kidney complications are commonly seen in patients with tuberous sclerosis and are the second most common cause of morbidity.

Treatment can range from regular monitoring to partial or total nephrectomy. The presence of angiomyolipomas increases the risk of renal hemorrhage. In such instances, embolization may be used to prevent hemorrhage and reduce tumor size while maintaining kidney tissue that reduces the risk of dialysis need. Other physiological issues such as cardiac complaints are addressed through standard symptom management practices.

For cognitive and behavioral deficits, early intervention with speech-language, physical, and occupational therapies can prove essential. In children with problems in social interaction related to autism, which occurs at higher rates in tuberous sclerosis, behavioral modification can help remediate problem behaviors and improve functional skills (Wong, 2006). Oftentimes this treatment is also dependent upon aforementioned seizure treatment. Jambaqué, Chiron, Dumas, Mumford, and Dulac (2000) note that cognitive and behavioral difficulties in tuberous sclerosis complex can improve with reduction of seizure activity or structural lesions or therapeutic or medical interventions to treat specific disorders and that seizure control is associated with developmental gains. Problematic behaviors that may arise in relation to developmental delays, autism, and/or mental retardation can be addressed with psychotropic medications (Bruni et al., 1995; Romanelli et al., 2002).

Jacob M. Goings
Chad A. Noggle

Bruni, O., Cortesi, F., Giannotti, F., & Curatolo, P. (1995). Sleep disorders in tuberous sclerosis: A polysomnographic study. *Brain & Development, 17*(1), 52–56.

Dabora, S. L., Jozwiak, S., Franz, D. N., Roberts, P.S., Nieto, A., Chung, J., et al. (2001). Mutational analysis in a cohort of 224 tuberous sclerosis patients indicates increased severity of TSC2, compared with TSC1, disease in multiple organs. *American Journal of Human Genetics, 68*(1), 64–80.

Hunt, A., & Lindenbaum, R. H. (1984). Tuberous sclerosis: A new estimate of prevalence within the Oxford region. *Journal of Medical Genetics, 21*(4), 272–277.

Hunt, A., & Shepherd, C. (1993). A prevalence study of autism in tuberous sclerosis. *Journal of Autism and Developmental Disorders, 23*(2), 323–339.

Hunt, A., & Stores, G. (1994). Sleep disorder and epilepsy in children with tuberous sclerosis: A questionnaire-based study. *Developmental Medicine and Child Neurology, 36*(2), 108–115.

Jambaqué, I., Chiron, C., Dumas, C., Mumford, J., & Dulac, O. (2000). Mental and behavioural outcome of infantile epilepsy treated by vigabatrin in tuberous sclerosis patients. *Epilepsy Research, 38*(2–3), 151–160.

Joinson, C., O'Callaghan, F. J., Osborne, J. P., Martyn, C., Harris, T., & Bolton, P. F. (2003). Learning disability and epilepsy in an epidemiological sample of individuals with tuberous sclerosis complex. *Psychological Medicine, 33*(2), 335–344.

Jozwiak, S., Goodman, M., & Lamm, S. H. (1998). Poor mental development in patients with tuberous sclerosis complex: Clinical risk factors. *Archives of Neurology, 55*(3), 379–384.

Maeda, M., Tartaro, A., Matsuda, T., & Ishii, Y. (1995). Cortical and subcortical tubers in tuberous sclerosis and FLAIR sequence. *Journal of Computer Assisted Tomography, 19*(4), 660–661.

Maria, B. L., Deidrick, K. M., Roach, E. S., & Gutmann, D. H. (2004). Tuberous sclerosis complex: Pathogenesis, diagnosis, strategies, therapies, and future research directions. *Journal of Child Neurology, 19*(9), 632–642.

Ramesh, V. (2003, June). Aspects of tuberous sclerosis complex (TSC) protein function in the brain. *Biochemical Society Transactions, 31*(Pt 3), 579–583.

Roach, K. S., Gomez, M. R., & Northrup, H. (1998). Tuberous sclerosis complex consensus conference: Revised clinical diagnostic criteria. *Journal of Child Neurology, 13*(12), 624–628.

Romanelli, P., Najjar, S., Weiner, H. L., & Devinsky, O. (2002). Epilepsy surgery in tuberous sclerosis: Multistage procedures with bilateral or multilobar foci. *Journal of Child Neurology, 17*(9), 689–692.

Shepherd, C. W., Houser, O. W., & Gomez, M. R. (1995). MR findings in tuberous sclerosis complex and correlation with seizure development and mental impairment. *AJNR. American Journal of Neuroradiology, 16*(1), 149–155.

Shepherd, C. W., & Stephenson, J. B. (1992). Seizures and intellectual disability associated with tuberous sclerosis complex in the west of Scotland. *Developmental Medicine and Child Neurology, 34*(9), 766–774.

van Slegtenhorst, M., de Hoogt, R., Hermans, C., Nellist, M., Janssen, B., Verhoef, S., et al. (1997). Identification of the tuberous sclerosis gene TSC1 on chromosome 9q34. *Science (New York, N.Y.), 277*(5327), 805–808.

Webb, D. W., Fryer, A. E., & Osborne, J. P. (1991). On the incidence of fits and mental retardation in tuberous sclerosis. *Journal of Medical Genetics, 28*(6), 395–397.

Webb, D. W., Thomson, J. L. G., & Osborne, J. P. (1991). Cranial magnetic resonance imaging in patients with tuberous sclerosis and normal intellect. *Archives of Disease in Childhood, 66*(12), 1375–1377.

Wong, V. (2006). Study of the relationship between tuberous sclerosis complex and autistic disorder. *Journal of Child Neurology, 21*(3), 199–204.

TURNER'S SYNDROME

DESCRIPTION

Turner's syndrome (TS) is chromosomal disorder, arising in females, in which one of the X chromosomes is essentially absent. The presentation is thus represented as an XO combination as opposed to XX. The end result of this chromosomal defect is infertility in the affected female due to diminished estrogen levels and underdeveloped ovaries in combination with phenotypical traits of short stature, webbed neck, and cubitus valgus that is when the elbows are turned in slightly causing a wider carrying angle of the arms (Turner, 1938). TS presents in roughly 1 out of every 2,000 live female births (Saenger, 1996)

Functionally, hearing problems and ear defects may also be observed with the prior increasing with increasing age. Sensorineural hearing loss begins in adolescence and by age 40, hearing impairment is observed in more than 85% of women with TS (Hederstierna, Hultcrantz, & Rosenhall, 2008). Motor deficits and delays are also common, including hypotonia, delays in ambulation and coordination, and sensory-motor integration (Hagerman, 1999). In addition, neuropsychological deficits have been commonly reported. TS has been associated with a profile indicative of a nonverbal learning disability, including weak visuospatial skills compared with verbal and difficulties in mathematics (Mazzocco, 2009; Pennington et al., 1985). Attentional deficits, executive dysfunction, and working memory deficits have been reported, as has increased prevalence of attention deficit hyperactivity disorder (ADHD) (Bender, Linden, & Robinson, 1990; Russell et al., 2006). Both short-term and long-term memory deficits have also been reported in TS, including impaired visual memory (Ross et al., 2002). Increased risk of psychiatric presentations, such as anxiety and depression have also been reported (Cardoso et al., 2004)

Interventions and treatment vary and are multifaceted. Given that the presentation arises from a chromosomal defect there is no cure; rather, treatment seeks to reduce symptoms.

NEUROPATHOLOGY/PATHOPHYSIOLOGY

As previously discussed, TS is a chromosomal disorder, characterized by the essential absence of a second X chromosome in females, represented as XO in lieu of XX. More specifically, the most common

T

karyotype (49% of cases) is 45,X instead of 46,XX although others have been reported including those with mosaicism and structural defects of the second X (23%), 45,X/46,XX mosaicism (19%), and ill-defined structural defects of the second X not due to mosaicism (9%) (Birkebaek, Cruger, Hansen, Nielsen, & Bruun-Petersen, 2002).

Neuropathological alterations have been well researched in association with TS revealing structural and functional differences between these individuals and normal controls (Mullaney & Murphy, 2009). The summation of these studies has revealed abnormalities of the parietal lobe (Ross et al., 2002), thus explaining some of the most salient neurocognitive deficits best described as a nonverbal learning disability. Within this region reduced volume of both gray and white matter. Abnormalities have also been noted in the temporal lobe and limbic system, including the amygdala, hippocampus, and superior temporal gyrus, the cerebellum, and the midbrain (Kesler et al., 2003, 2004). Decreased white matter volume has been suggested on diffusion tensor imaging (DTI) in parieto-occipital and frontoparietal regions (Holzapfel, Barnea-Goraly, Eckert, Kesler, & Reiss, 2006). PET studies have reiterated anomalies in many of these areas, showing hypometabolism of glucose in parieto-occipital regions as well as medial temporal regions (Murphy et al., 1997). In fMRI studies, decreased functioning in the frontoparietal regions, including the inferior parietal lobe and dorsolateral prefrontal cortex, the caudate, and the left fusiform gyrus have been noted (Kesler et al., 2004; Skuse, 2005).

TS has also been associated with significantly higher concentrations of hippocampal Cho, and lower parietal N-acetylaspartate (NAA) (Mullaney & Murphy, 2009), which the authors cite as associated with healthy old age, thus suggesting TS, in some respects, neurochemically mimics aging. Specifically, the authors (i.e., Mullaney & Murphy, 2009) suggested TS anatomically was associated with (1) increased brain aging, (2) differences in neuronal membrane turnover and signal transduction that modify cell survival, and (3) reduced neuronal density/mitochondrial function in the parietal lobe.

In terms of the neuropathological and even functional features and deficits exhibited by individuals with TS, research has suggested a role of genetic imprinting outcomes (Skuse, 2000). In other words, outcomes may be related to which parent the defective X chromosome comes from or, the reverse, which parent provided the preserved X chromosome. Preservation of the paternal X chromosome (Xp) has been associated with better social adjustment, verbal skills, and executive functioning as well as better verbal

memory (Bishop et al., 2000); however, it has also been linked with poorer outcomes in visuo-spatial memory and functioning (Bishop et al., 2000). When it comes to neuroanatomical presentation, results are more mixed. Some have suggested a link between genomic imprinting and alterations of the brain, including bilateral temporal lobe white matter volume and midbrain gray matter volume (Cutter et al., 2006; Kesler et al., 2003), whereas others have failed to find any link between anatomical presentation and genomic imprinting (Good et al., 2003; Kesler et al., 2004).

NEUROPSYCHOLOGICAL/CLINICAL PRESENTATION

The clinical features of TS can be divided into physical, cognitive, and behavioral traits. Physically, as previously discussed, phenotypical traits of short stature, webbed neck, and cubitus valgus are hallmark of the presentation (Turner, 1938). The short stature observed presents secondary to a combination of mild growth retardation prenatally, slowed growth during infancy, delayed growth onset in childhood, and failed pubertal growth spurt (Taback et al., 1996). A broad chest, epicanthal folds, and low posterior hair line may be noted. Variability can be seen across these features based on the origin of the chromosomal defect. For example, some females will spontaneously enter puberty, but this is more commonly seen in relation to mosaicisms as opposed to the traditional 45,X karotype. Hearing loss is quite common, corresponding with a sensorineural origin. As previously noted, the superior temporal gyrus in the temporal lobes is often a site of volumetric reduction. Similarly, motor deficits are common, including developmental delays in walking, hypotonia, dyscoordination, and poor sensory-motor integration (Hagerman, 1999).

Cognitively, TS has been strongly linked with a profile indicative of nonverbal learning disability. That is, TS corresponds with significant deficits in performance IQ in comparison with verbal IQ (Temple & Carney, 1993). Despite this discrepancy, general IQ is often normal as verbal strengths often offer compensation for performance weaknesses. In some instances, TS has even been associated with hyperlexia and even normative strengths in linguistic knowledge and phonological processing (Murphy & Mazzocco, 2008). In comparison, response speed and oral/semantic fluency are areas of difficulty in TS (Mazzocco, 2001) but may be confounded by attention and executive defects.

In addition, neuropsychological deficits have been commonly reported. TS has been associated with a profile indicative of a nonverbal learning disability, including weak visuospatial skills compared with verbal and difficulties in mathematics (Mazzocco, 2009). Specific strengths in language have been reported in receptive vocabulary, phonemic processing, and lexical storage, whereas syntactic processing and semantic fluency tends to be impaired (Hong, Kent, & Kesler, 2009). As verbal tasks rely on spatial processes or higher level attention or executive functions, performance is impeded. For example, Inozemtseva, Matute, Zarabozo, and Ramírez-Dueñas (2002) found that individuals with TS exhibited impairments navigating maps when instructions were given verbally

Executive functioning and visuospatial processing represent those areas of greatest impairment in TS. Cognitive inflexibility may present (Buchanan, Pavlovic, & Rovet, 1998; Romans, Roeltgen, Kushner, & Ross, 1996). Attention and working memory deficits are also commonly reported (Russell et al., 2006). Consistent with these findings, Simon et al. (2008) found that on the WISC-IV and WISC-III, individuals with TS performed significantly worse than controls on both the POI and PRI. Finally, both short-term and long-term memory deficits have also been reported in TS, including impaired visual memory (Ross et al., 2002).

Increased risks of psychiatric, social, and adaptive difficulties have been associated with TS. As previously noted, increased risk of anxiety and depression has been associated with TS (Cardoso et al., 2004). However, this most often presents as increased self-report of anxiety, depression, low-self-esteem, and impaired social competence compared with same-aged peers (McCauley, Feuillan, Kushner, & Ross, 2001; Lagrou et al., 2006). In regard to social competence and functioning, both hearing loss and deficits in facial recognition have been identified as mediators (Bergamaschi et al., 2008).

Finally, in regard to academic performance, as noted, mathematics tends to be an area of relative weakness for individuals, potentially requiring special education services. In comparison, reading tends to be a relative strength, presenting as hyperlexia.

DIAGNOSIS

Definitive diagnosis of TS is accomplished through genetic testing. Oftentimes it is indicated upon noticing the phenotypical traits associated with the presentation, but not confirmed until such analysis is completed. MRI and functional imaging may be completed, but are not necessary for diagnosis. Rather, neuropsychological assessment is more essential as it provides a means by which neurocognitive strengths and weaknesses are identified and appropriate interventions may be designed. Audiology evaluations are highly recommended given the high prevalence of sensorineural hearing loss. Motor development assessment should also be carried out.

TREATMENT

There is no cure for TS given it is a chromosomal defect. Treatment and intervention is thus directed at addressing symptoms and features of the presentation. Again, treatments fall across physical, cognitive, and behavioral lines.

Physically, treatment has sought to address both the short stature and pubertal absence experienced with TS as well as potential hearing loss. Historically, growth hormone has been used to offset the short stature exhibited in TS. As described previously, delay or slowness in growth has been reported across much of infancy, childhood, and adolescence. However, results have been mixed, with increases being reported as ranging from minimal growth (less than 5 cm) to as much as 17 cm (van Pareren et al., 2003). Indications vary in terms of when treatment should be started. Some have suggested that it can be started as early as 2 years of age, whereas others suggest growth itself is the determining factor with treatment starting once individuals drop below the fifth percentile of the normal female growth curve (Ismail et al., 2010). Hormone replacement therapy with estrogen is used to initiate puberty and to counteract gonadal dysgenesis. Still yet, as many as 30% of females enter puberty spontaneously (Birgit et al., 2009; Modi, Sane, & Bhartiya, 2003).

Cognitively, variable reports of effectiveness have been reported for psychostimulants in offsetting deficits in attention, processing speed, and features of ADHD (Hagerman, 1999). However, risk is increased with these agents if cardiac defects are present, thus cardiological consultation is often needed first to determine safety. Interestingly, estrogen therapy has also been correlated with improvements in cognition. Ross et al. (1998) found that estrogen led to improvements in motor skills. Special education services are often required to address deficits in mathematics. Oxandrolone, an oral androgen, has shown some utility in improving mathematics deficits in TS when used over a 4-year period (Ross et al., 2009).

Chad A. Noggle

Bender, B., Linden, M., & Robinson, A. (1990). SCA: In search of developmental patterns. In D. Berch & B. Bender

(Eds.), *Sex chromosome abnormalities and human behavior: Psychological studies, AAAS Selected Symposium*. Boulder, CO: Westview Press.

Bergamaschi, R., Bergonzoni, C., Mazzanti, L., Scarano, E., Mencarelli, F., Messina, F., et al. (2008). Hearing loss in Turner syndrome: Results of a multicentric study. *Journal of Endocrinological Investigation, 31*, 779–783.

Birgit, B., Julius, H., Carsten, R., Maryam, S., Gabriel, F., Victoria, K., et al. (2009). Fertility preservation in girls with Turner syndrome: Prognostic signs of the presence of ovarian follicles. *The Journal of Clinical Endocrinology & Metabolism, 94*, 74–80.

Birkebaek, N. H., Cruger, D., Hansen, J., Nielsen, J., & Bruun-Petersen, G. (2002). Fertility and pregnancy outcome in Danish women with Turner syndrome. *Clinical Genetics, 61*(1), 35–39.

Bishop, D. V., Canning, E., Elgar, K., Morris, E., Jacobs, P. A., & Skuse, D. H. (2000). Distinctive patterns of memory function in subgroups of females with Turner syndrome: Evidence for imprinted loci on the X-chromosome affecting neurodevelopment. *Neuropsychologia, 38*, 712–721.

Buchanan, L., Pavlovic, J., & Rovet, J. (1998). The contribution of visuospatial working memory to impairments in facial processing and arithmetic in Turner syndrome. *Brain Cognition, 37*, 72–75.

Cardoso, G., Daly, R., Haq, N. A., Hanton, L., Rubinow, D. R., Bondy, C. A., et al. (2004). Current and lifetime psychiatric illness in women with Turner syndrome. *Gynecological Endocrinology, 19*(6), 313–319.

Cutter, W. J., Daly, E. M., Robertson, D. M., Chitnis, X. A., van Amelsvoort, T. A., Simmons, A., et al. (2006). Influence of X chromosome and hormones on human brain development: A magnetic resonance imaging and proton magnetic resonance spectroscopy study of turner syndrome. *Biological Psychiatry, 59*, 273–283.

Good, C. D., Lawrence, K., Thomas, N. S., Price, C. J., Ashburner, J., Friston, K. J., et al. (2003). Dosage-sensitive X-linked locus influences the development of the amygdala and orbitofrontal cortex, and fear recognition in humans. *Brain, 126*, 2431–2446.

Hagerman, R. J. (1999). *Neurodevelopment disorders: Diagnosis and treatment*. New York: Oxford University Press.

Hederstierna, C., Hultcrantz, M., & Rosenhall, U. (2008). Estrogen and hearing from a clinical point of view; characteristics of auditory function in women with Turner syndrome. *Hearing Research, 252*, 3–8. December 6 (Epub ahead of print).

Holzapfel, M., Barnea-Goraly, N., Eckert, M. A., Kesler, S. R., & Reiss, A. L. (2006). Selective alterations of white matter associated with visuospatial and sensorimotor dysfunction in Turner syndrome. *Journal of Neuroscience, 26*, 7007–7013.

Hong, D., Kent, J. S., & Kesler, S. (2009). Cognitive profile of turner syndrome. *Developmental Disabilities Research Reviews, 15*, 270–278.

Hovatta, O. (1999). Pregnancies in women with Turner's syndrome. *Annals of Medicine, 31*, 106–110.

Inozemtseva, O., Matute, E., Zarabozo, D., & Ramírez-Dueñas, L. (2002). Syntactic processing in Turner's syndrome. *Journal of Child Neurology, 17*, 668–672.

Ismail, N. A., Eldin Metwaly, N. S., El-Moguy, F. A., Hafez, M. H., Abd El Dayem, S. M., & Farid, T. M., (2010). Bone age is the best predictor of growth response to recombinant human growth hormone in Turner's syndrome. *Indian Journal of Human Genetics, 16*(3), 119–126.

Kesler, S. R., Blasey, C. M., Brown, W. E., Yankowitz, J., Zeng, S. M., Bender, B. G., et al. (2003). Effects of Xmonosomy and X-linked imprinting on superior temporal gyrus morphology in Turner syndrome. *Biological Psychiatry, 54*, 636–646.

Kesler, S. R., Garrett, A., Bender, B., Yankowitz, J., Zeng, S. M., & Reiss, A. L. (2004). Amygdala and hippocampal volumes in Turner syndrome: A high-resolution MRI study of X-monosomy. *Neuropsychologia, 42*, 1971–1978.

Lagrou, K., Froidecoeur, C., Verlinde, F., Craen, M., De Schepper, J., François, I., et al. (2006). Pyschosocial functioning, self-perception and body image and their auxologic correlates in growth hormone and oestrogen-treated young adult women with Turner syndrome. *Hormone Research, 66*, 277–284.

Mazzocco, M. M. M. (2001). Math learning disability and math LD subtypes: Evidence from studies of Turner syndrome, fragile X syndrome, and neurofibromatosis type 1. *Journal of Learning Disabilities, 34*(6), 520–533.

Mazzocco, M. M. M. (2009). Mathematical learning disability in girls with Turner syndrome: A challenge to defining MLD and its subtypes. *Developmental Disabilities Research Reviews, 15*, 35–44.

McCauley, E., Feuillan, P., Kushner, H., & Ross, J. L. (2001). Psychosocial development in adolescents with Turner syndrome. *Journal of Developmental and Behavioral Pediatrics, 22*, 360–365.

Modi, D., Sane, S., & Bhartiya, D. (2003). Accelerated germ cell apoptosis in sex chromosome aneuploid fetal human gonads. *Molecular Human Reproduction, 9*, 219.

Mullaney, R., & Murphy, D. (2009). Turner syndrome: Neuroimaging findings: Structural and functional. *Developmental Disabilities Research Reviews, 15*, 279–283.

Murphy, D. G. M., Mentis, M. J., Pietrini, P., Grady, C., Daly, E., Haxby, J. V., et al. (1997). A PET study of Turner's syndrome: Effects of sex steroids and the X chromosome on brain. *Biological Psychiatry, 41*, 285–298.

Murphy, M. M., & Mazzocco, M. M. M. (2008). Rote numeric skills may mask underlying mathematical disabilities in girls with fragile X syndrome. *Developmental Neuropsychology, 33*, 345–364.

Pennington, B., Heaton, R., Karzmark, P., Pendleton, M. G., Lehman, R., & Shucard, D. W. (1985). The neuropsychological phenotype in Turner syndrome. *Cortex, 21,* 391–404.

Romans, S. M., Roeltgen, D. P., Kushner, H., & Ross, J. L. (1996). Executive function in females with Turner syndrome. *Archives of Clinical Neuropsychology, 11,* 442.

Ross, J. L., Mazzocco, M. M., Krushner, H., Kowal, K., Cutler, G. B., Jr., & Roeltgen, D. (2009). Effects of treatment with oxandrolone for 4 years in the frequency of severe arithmetic learning disabilities in girls with turner syndrome. *The Journal of Pediatrics, 155*(5), 714–720.

Ross, J. L., Roeltgen, D., Feuillan, P., Kushner, H., & Cutler, G. B., Jr. (1998). Effects of estrogen on nonverbal processing speed and motor function in girls with Turner syndrome. *The Journal of Clinical Endocrinology and Metabolism, 83*(9), 3198–3204.

Ross, J. L., Stefanatos, G. A., Kushner, H., Zinn, A., Bondy, C., & Roeltgen, D. (2002). Persistent cognitive deficits in adult women with Turner syndrome. *Neurology, 58,* 218–225.

Russell, H. F., Wallis, D., Mazzocco, M., Moshang, T., Zackai, E., Zinn, A., et al. (2006). Increased prevalence of ADHD in Turner syndrome with no evidence of imprinting effects. *Journal of Pediatrics Psychology, 31*(9), 945–955.

Saenger, P. (1996). Turner's syndrome. *The New England Journal of Medicine, 335,* 1749–1754.

Simon, T. J., Takarae, Y., DeBoer, T., McDonald-McGinn, D. M., Zackai, E. H., Ross, J. L., et al. (2008). Overlapping numerical cognition impairments in children with chromosome 22q11.2 deletion or Turner syndromes. *Neuropsychologia, 46,* 82–94.

Skuse, D. H. (2000). Imprinting, the X-chromosome, and the male brain: Explaining sex differences in the liability to autism. *Pediatric Research, 47,* 9–16.

Skuse, D. H. (2005). X-linked genes and mental functioning. *Human Molecular Genetics, 14,* R27–R32.

Taback, S. P., Collu, R., Deal, C. L., Guyda, H. J., Salisbury, S., & Dean, H. J. (1996). Does growth-hormone supplementation affect adult height in Turner's syndrome? *Lancet, 348,* 25–27.

Temple, C. M., & Carney, R. A. (1993). Intellectual functioning of children with Turner syndrome: A comparison of behavioural phenotypes. *Developmental Medicine & Child Neurology, 35,* 691–698.

Temple, C. M., & Carney, R. (1996). Reading skills in children with Turner's syndrome: An analysis of hyperlexia. *Cortex, 32,* 335–345.

Turner, H. H. (1938). A syndrome of infantilism, congenital webbed neck and cubitus valgus. *Endocrinology, 23,* 556–574.

T

VASCULITIS

DESCRIPTION

The term "vasculitis" is derived from the Latin word *vasculum* meaning vessel and *itis*, which means inflammation. Although the exact mechanisms of the condition are unknown, it is primarily characterized by an inflammation in the veins, arteries, or capillaries. Many diseases exist — over 30 — that are characterized by vasculitis as the primary symptom including, but not limited to Kawasaki's disease, Behcet's disease, polyarteritis nodosa, Wegener's granulomatosis, cryoglobulinemia, Takayasu's arteritis, Churg–Strauss syndrome, giant cell arteritis (temporal arteritis), and Henoch–Schonlein's purpura (Watts & Scott, 2009). Other conditions maintain vasculitis as a secondary or atypical symptom (i.e., infection, cancer, etc.).

Prevalence rates vary based on the specific subtype of vasculitis. For example, in the United States, the prevalence for giant cell arteritis in the elderly is approximately 20 per 100,000, 4–15 per 100,000 for Kawasaki's disease, 6 per 100,000 for allergic angiitis, 3 per 100,000 for Wegener's granulomatosis, 3 per 100,000 for polyarteritis nodosa, and 1 per 100,000 for Takayasu's arteritis (Khasnis & Langford, 2009). It is estimated that 100,000 individuals are hospitalized each year in the United States for vasculitis, and may or may not exhibit differences based on race, gender, or age (i.e., giant cell arteritis that tends to occur in those over 50s in Caucasian women and Kawasaki's disease that tends to occur in children) (Khasnis & Langford, 2009).

Prognosis of vasculitis depends upon the organ systems involved and the number of sites affected in the body with systemic vasculitis often leading to debilitating conditions (i.e., stroke, myocardial infarction, blindness, or end stage renal disease) and, at times, fatality (Perez et al., 2004).

NEUROPATHOLOGY/PATHOPHYSIOLOGY

The pathophysiology of vasculitis is largely unknown; however, generalities of the disease process can be mentioned. As the blood vessels become inflamed, they may narrow and eventually close or stretch and weaken, eventually bursting (aneurysm) (Khasnis & Langford, 2009). Although the exact etiology or risk factors of the disease are unknown for the majority of vasculitis subtypes, it is proposed that inflammation is secondary to abnormal immune response where blood vessels are targeted (Perez et al., 2004).

Those variants of vasculitis with unknown etiology are referred to as primary vasculitides, whereas the variants where an identified disease is the etiology are referred to as secondary vasculitides (Merkel, Choi, & Niles, 2002). In regard to secondary vasculitides, individuals present with abnormal proteins in their blood, cryoglobulinemia, most commonly seen in individuals with a hepatitis C virus infection or in those with hepatitis B virus infection who develop polyarteritis nodosa (Watts & Scott, 2009). Autoimmune disorders, such as rheumatoid arthritis, lupus erythematosus, and Sjögren's syndrome, may also result in inflammation, and even allergic reactions to medication may result in vasculitis (Merkel, Choi, & Niles, 2002).

NEUROPSYCHOLOGICAL/CLINICAL PRESENTATION

Vasculitis may present in many ways given the plethora of variants and distinctive involvement in organ systems. General symptoms for vasculitis may include fever, swelling, headache, and weight loss (Khasnis & Langford, 2009). If the skin system is involved, then palpable pupura and livedo reticularis may be evident (Xu, Esparza, Anadkat, Crone, & Brasington, 2009). When muscles and joints are involved, then myalgia, arthralgia, or arthritis may be observed (Watts & Scott, 2009). Cardiovascular system involvement may result in hypertension, gangrene, or myocardial infarction (Mukhtyar, Brogan, & Luqmani, 2009). Respiratory system involvement may evince lung infiltrates, bloody cough, or nose bleeds (Watts & Scott, 2009). Gastrointestinal system involvement often results in abdominal pain, perforations, or bloody stool (Morgan & Savage, 2005). Renal system involvement often exhibits glomerulonephritis (Samarkos, Loizou, Vaiopoulos, & Davies, 2005).

Vasculitis may also involve the nervous system resulting in the following common symptoms: confusion, forgetfulness, stroke, or mononeuritis multiplex (Khasnis & Langford, 2009). Given the blood vessel perfusion of the brain, cognitive impairments may likely be diffuse, with impairments being either transient or persisting.

DIAGNOSIS

There are more than 30 types of vasculitis that have been named from the primary author who initially identified the condition, the clinical setting where it occurs, the size of the blood vessel involved, or features from the biopsy. Differential diagnosis may be difficult to ascertain because vasculitis resembles many other medical disorders. Common differential diagnoses include: infection, drug toxicity or poisoning, coagulopathy, malignancy, atrial myxoma, multiple cholesterol emboli, congenital collagen disorders, or fibromuscular dysplasia (Khasnis & Langford, 2009).

Common tests to elucidate the presence of vasculitis include blood tests, imaging, urinalysis, or biopsy. Specific blood tests may analyze erythrocyte sedimentation rate, C-reactive protein, platelets, white blood cell count, antineutrophyl cytoplasmic antibodies, rheumatoid factor, or antinuclear antibody (Eleftheriou & Brogan, 2009). Imaging may be performed through ultrasound, CT, MRI, or angiogram (Perez et al., 2004). Urine samples may be analyzed to rule out infection or renal involvement. Finally, biopsy is considered the most conclusive test for differential diagnosis (Perez et al., 2004).

TREATMENT

In general, vasculitis is considered a rare condition, which requires specialized medical care. Consistent with the variability in diagnosis noted above and the plethora of subtypes of vasculitis, treatment and outcome tend to be complex. Some individuals with vasculitis may experience minor symptoms and full recovery without treatment (i.e., Henoch–Schonlein's purpura), whereas other cases may be terminal, or even if successfully treated may recur (i.e., giant cell arteritis, Wegener's granulomatosis, and Takayasu's arteritis), thereby requiring chronic monitoring and treatment (Merkel, Choi, & Niles, 2002). To further complicate matters, pharmaceutical treatments can be toxic resulting in permanent sequelae in the blood vessel.

Although, medication tends to be the primary intervention utilized for vasculitis with common prescriptions being in the order of increasing severity: nonsteriodal anti-inflamatory drugs (i.e., aspirin and ibuprofen), corticosteroids (i.e., prednisone or methylprednisolone), or — for particularly intractable vasculitis — cytotoxic drugs (i.e., azathioprine or cyclophosphamide) (Eleftheriou & Brogan, 2009; Khasnis & Langford, 2009). Response to medication and disease progression is monitored with routine blood tests, and follow-up with the treating physician is recommended.

Javan Horwitz
Natalie Horwitz
Chad A. Noggle

Eleftheriou, D., & Brogan, P. A. (2009). Vasculitis in children. *Best Practice & Research Clinical Rheumatology, 23*(3), 309–323.

Khasnis, A., & Langford, C. A. (2009). Update on vasculitis. *The Journal of Allergy and Clinical Immunology, 123*(6), 1226–1236.

Merkel, P. A., Choi, H. K., & Niles, J. L. (2002). Evaluation and treatment of vasculitis in the critically ill patient. *Critical Care Clinics, 18*(2), 321–344.

Morgan, M., & Savage, C. (2005). Vasculitis in the gastrointestinal tract. *Best Practice & Research Clinical Gastroenterology, 19*(2), 215–233.

Mukhtyar, C., Brogan, P., & Luqmani, R. (2009). Cardiovascular involvement in primary systemic vasculitis. *Best Practice & Research Clinical Rheumatology, 23*(3), 419–428.

Perez, V. L., Chavala, S. H., Ahmed, M., Chu, D., Zafirakis, P., Baltatzis, S., et al. (2004). Ocular manifestations and concepts of systemic vasculitides. *Survey of Ophthalmology, 49*(4), 399–418.

Samarkos, M., Loizou, S., Vaiopoulos, G., & Davies, K. (2005). The clinical spectrum of primary renal vasculitis. *Seminars in Arthritis and Rheumatism, 35*(2), 95–111.

Watts, R. A., & Scott, D. G. (2009). Recent developments in the classification and assessment of vasculitis. *Best Practice & Research Clinical Rheumatology, 23*(3), 429–443.

Xu, L. Y., Esparza, E. M., Anadkat, M. J., Crone, K. G., & Brasington, R. D. (2009). Cutaneous manifestations of vasculitis. *Seminars in Arthritis and Rheumatism, 38*(5), 348–360.

VON ECONOMO DISEASE

DESCRIPTION

von Economo disease (VED), commonly known as encephalitis lethargica, was pandemic from 1917 to

1926 with affected individuals suffering both acute and chronic symptoms. Originally thought to be related to influenza, there is presently no definitive identifiable etiology and current estimates of the prevalence of VED have not been established. Originally, mortality rates were between 20% and 40%, with survivors developing parkinsonian features and dyskinesias. However, at the present time, the prognosis of VED is highly variable depending upon accompanying complications and disorders (Dale et al., 2003). Common features of VED may include diplopia, lethargy, mutism, facial and cranial nerve palsies, motor disturbances, dyskinesias, and other parkinsonian features.

NEUROPATHOLOGY/PATHOPHYSIOLOGY

The etiology of the original VED epidemic remains a mystery, and the present form of the disease may be entirely different today than the disease originally explained by von Economo (Dale, Webster, & Gill, 2007). Because the original acute form of VED disappeared following the 1920s, a direct study of the disease is not possible. Epidemiological studies of the brain samples from the 1917 epidemic have failed to associate VED with influenza. However, some believe that the samples may have been contaminated or influenced by a myriad of impending factors that may have eliminated any trace evidence of viral encephalitis, if present (McCall, Vilensky, Gilman, & Taubenberger, 2008). Rather than finding evidence of influenza RNA, some studies have found the presence of intrathecal oligoclonal bands and elevated protein suggesting neurotropic viral encephalitis as an unlikely etiology (Dale et al., 2003).

Postencephalitic individuals may present similar neuropathology as individuals with idiopathic Parkinson's disease such as dopaminergic denervation in the caudate nuclei and putamen (Caparros-Lefebvre et al., 1998). Furthermore, some individuals with VED display bilateral abnormalities in the substantia nigra, increased signal in the tegmentum and basal ganglia, and lesions to the right striatum during MRI (Dale et al., 2003; Verschueren & Crols, 2001). Although imaging has found deep gray matter lesions in individuals with VED, many have normal MRI scans. The present form of VED may be subsequent to postinfectious autoimmunity in deep gray matter. Individuals with VED have been found to have significantly more autoantibodies that were reactive toward basal ganglia antigens than normal individuals, which results in movement and psychiatric disorders (Dale et al., 2003).

NEUROPSYCHOLOGICAL/CLINICAL PRESENTATION

Visuoconstructional abilities may be impaired as measured by Rey's figure copy and recall measure. Individuals with VED may present with executive and cognitive impairment, and impairment on measures of concept formation, mental flexibility, verbal abstraction, nonverbal recall and recognition, and verbal associate learning (Dewar & Wilson, 2005). Postencephalitic individuals who have been diagnosed with VED are at a higher risk of developing obsessive-compulsive disorder, depression, or other psychiatric disorders (Caparros-Lefebvre, et al., 1998; Dale et al., 2003; Dale et al., 2007). Individuals may experience diplopia, lethargy, mutism, facial and cranial nerve palsies, motor disturbances, hyperesthesia, dyskinesias (e.g., distonia, stereotypes, motor tics, facial grimacing, chorea, or facial grimacing), and/or other common parkinsonian features such as bradykinesia with postural instability, tremor, or rigidity (Dale et al., 2003; Taylor, 1921). Differentiation between postencephalitic parkinsonian and idiopathic Parkinson's disease may be made in part based upon age of onset. VED-related parkinsonian features may manifest as early as childhood, whereas the mean age of onset for idiopathic Parkinson's disease is approximately 59 years (Li et al., 2003). Sleep disorders are also common including hypersomnolence, insomnia, and sleep inversion (Dale et al., 2003; Ocular palsies in encephalitis lethargica, 1924). Individuals may experience additional symptoms associated with intracranial pathology. In a study by Dale et al. (2003), over half of individuals contracted pharyngitis preceding onset of VED.

DIAGNOSIS

Raghav et al. (2007) suggest that diagnosis can be made based on clinical features, laboratory investigation, exclusion of other disorders, and circumstantial evidence. Specific manifestations of VED that aid in diagnosis include the characteristic parkinsonian signs, which are very common. In fact, many individuals with VED may actually meet the diagnostic criteria for Parkinson's syndrome (Dale et al., 2003). As noted previously, in contrast to idiopathic Parkinson's disease, parkinsonian symptoms may develop at an early age. Such features may include, but are not limited to, bradykinesia, resting tremor, or rigidity. Dyskinesias as well as sleep disturbances including hypersomnolence, sleep inversion, and insomnia are of diagnostic utility as they occur frequently in

uv

individuals with VED. Additional symptomology of diagnostic utility include lethargy, oculogyric crisis, cranial nerve palsies, and diplopia. To make a correct diagnosis, Raghav and colleagues identified clinical features from the original epidemic disease, such as acute encephalitis associated with symptoms from basal ganglia dysfunction, neuropsychiatric signs, respiratory problems, and oculogyric posturing as a comparison for making a present diagnosis.

Due to the fact that almost half of the individuals with VED have normal MRIs, the MRI may be used to differentiate between VED and other neuropathological conditions. Although neuropsychological test data exist for VED, due to the lack of replication in the literature it is recommended that the aforementioned neuropsychological signs be used as supplement additional data and independently. Deep gray matter lesions may help identify underlying neuropathology typical of VED. The presence of intrathecal oligoclonal bands and elevated protein may also be useful in making a diagnosis (Dale et al., 2003).

TREATMENT

Treatment for VED is largely symptomatic in nature, and treatment outcomes are mixed. However, some individuals with VED have experienced full recovery following electroconvulsive therapy, which may be due to the treatment's effect on underlying dopaminergic activity (Delkeva & Husain, 1995). Individuals with VED oftentimes are very reactive to L-dopa, experiencing many side effects. Hypersensitive dopamine receptors may be responsible for the development of dyskinesias during L-dopa treatment. Foster and Hoffer (2003) suggest that accompanying an L-dopa treatment with an antioxidant supplement may reduce oxidative stress, and prolong the benefits of the medication in comparison to subsequent side effects. McAuley, Shahmanesh, and Swash (1999) treated a patient with trials of apomorphine infusion followed by oral L-dopa without the individual experiencing additional dyskinetic problems. Lorazepam may also be useful in improving behavioral agitation that sometimes accompanies VED (Dale et al., 2007). However, full recovery from VED is likely to occur only in a minority of individuals (Dale et al., 2003).

Cognitive rehabilitation may be useful for individuals with memory or executive impairment. Compensatory strategies aimed at managing memory impairment such as the use of memory diaries or other memory aids, restructuring the individual's environment, or providing a problem-solving template may allow an affected individual to improve memory functioning (Dewar & Wilson, 2005).

Anthony P. Odland
Charles Golden

Caparros-Lefebvre, D., Cabaret, M., Godefroy, M., Seinling, M., Rémy, P., Samson, Y., et al. (1998). PET study and neuropsychological assessment of a long-lasting postencephalitic parkinsonism. *Journal of Neural Transmission, 105,* 489–495.

Dale, R. C., Church, A. J., Surtees, R. A., Lees, A. J., Adcock, J. E., Harding, B., et al. (2003). Encephalitis lethargica syndrome: 20 new cases and evidence of basal ganglia autoimmunity. *Brain, 127*(1), 21–33.

Dale, R. C., Webster, R., & Gill, D. (2007). Contemporary encephalitis lethargica presenting with agitated catatonia, stereotypy, and dystonia-parkinsonism. *Movement Disorders, 22*(15), 2281–2284.

Delkeva, K. B., & Husain, M. M. (1995). Sporadic encephalitis lethargica: A case treated successfully with ECT. *The Journal of Neuropsychiatry and Clinical Neurosciences, 7,* 237–239.

Dewar, B. K., & Wilson, B. A. (2005). Cognitive recovery from encephalitis lethargica. *Brain Injury, 19*(14), 1285–1291.

Foster, H. D., & Hoffer, A. (2004). The two faces of L-DOPA: Benefits and adverse side effects in the treatment of encephalitis lethargica, Parkinson's disease, multiple sclerosis and amyotrophic lateral sclerosis. *Medical Hypotheses, 62,* 177–181.

Li, Y. J., Oliveira, S. A., Xu, P., Martin, E. R., Stenger, J. E., Scherzer, C. R., et al. (2003). Glutathione S-transferase omega-1 modifies age-at-onset of Alzheimer disease and Parkinson disease. *Human Molecular Genetics, 12*(24), 3259–3267.

McAuley, J., Shahmanesh, M., & Swash, M. (1999). Dopaminergic therapy in acute encephalitis lethargica. *European Journal of Neurology, 6*(2), 235–237.

McCall, S., Vilensky, J. A., Gilman, S., & Taubenberger, J. K. (2008). The relationship between encephalitis lethargica and influenza: A critical analysis. *Journal of Neurovirology, 14,* 177–185.

Ocular palsies in encephalitis lethargica. (1924). *British Journal of Ophthalmology, 8,* 421.

Raghav, S., Seneviratne, J., McKelvie, P. A., Chapman, C., Talman, P. S., & Kempster, P. A. (2007). Sporadic encephalitis lethargica. *Journal of Clinical Neuroscience, 14,* 696–700.

Taylor, J. (1921). Some cases of encephalitis lethargica. *The British Journal of Ophthalmology,* 1–4.

Verschueren, H., & Crols, R. (2001). Bilateral substantia nigra lesions on magnetic resonance imaging in a patient with encephalitis lethargica. *Journal of Neurology, Neurosurgery and Psychiatry, 71*(2), 275.

uv

VON HIPPEL–LINDAU SYNDROME

DESCRIPTION

von Hippel–Lindau syndrome (VHL) is so named for the two researchers most linked with its discovery and delineation as a syndrome. Eugene von Hippel originally discovered hemangioblastomas (benign tumors that are cystic in nature that occur throughout the central nervous system [CNS]) involving the retina. Twenty years later, Arvid Lindau made the connection between retinal, cerebral, and visceral hemangioblastomas (Morantz & Walsh, 1993). The *VHL* gene is a tumor suppressor gene commonly found in different areas throughout the body.

As a result, tumors commonly occur in many different sites throughout the body. In the brain, hemangioblastomas occupy space and compress the fourth ventricle. The initial effects can be ataxia of gate or ataxia of one side of the body. Other signs might include increased intracranial pressure, retinal angioma, or hepatic and pancreatic cysts. The last two symptoms are normally verified through imaging such as MRI or CT and will be further discussed in association with VHL. VHL is a genetic syndrome that can be traced through familial descent in approximately 75% of cases (Morantz & Walsh, 1993).

Through genetic mapping it has been determined that VHL is a problem with the third chromosomal arm. This relatively common (compared with other genetic disorders) autosomal disorder has been estimated to occur in 1 in 35,000 individuals (Greenburg & Cheung, 2005). In many cases, this syndrome presents later in life, but is not isolated to later life. The syndrome presents in different ways and there are a variety of ways to diagnose the disorder.

NEUROPATHOLOGY/PATHOPHYSIOLOGY

Diagnosis needs to take into account two different variations when attempting to understand the clinical presentation. The first type of presentation occurs in those who have no familial history of VHL. These patients have the simplex version and are completely diagnosed based on their symptom presentation. This should include at least two of the following: retinal hemangioblastomas, multicystic renal disease, renal cell carcinoma, pheochromocytoma, pancreatic cysts, epididymal cysts, cerebellar hemangioblastomas, and/or hemangioblastomas of other CNS locations (e.g., cortex, brainstem, spinal cord) (Morantz & Walsh, 1993). In the familial version of the syndrome,

the patient only needs to have one of the above-mentioned symptoms and a family member with VHL or gene coding for the disorder. The most common method of diagnosis is through the identification of retinal hemangioblastomas, which occur in a majority of the cases. Presentation of the retinal hemangioblastomas can begin without symptoms but in most cases retinal detachment occurs.

Common techniques for establishing the criterion mentioned above involve the use of CT and MRI scans. These types of scans have the ability to view CNS tumors, pheochromocytomas (tumor of the adrenal glands or extra chromaffin cells), and endolymphatic tumors (tumors of the endolymphatic sac inside the ear). Both T-1 and T-2 MRIs are used. The use of ultrasound is also warranted in cases of epididymis and broad ligament or for kidney screening.

Other methods used include radioiodine-labeled MIBG, PET, and urinary catecholamine metabolites. Genetic testing has also been used in order to confirm diagnosis by looking for the factors associated with familial version and for prenatal testing. Genetic testing has been advised for all individuals who are thought to have VHL (Rasmussen et al., 2006).

NEUROPSYCHOLOGICAL/CLINICAL PRESENTATION

The effects of VHL on neuropsychological assessment have not been formally analyzed due to the semi-rare nature of the disorder. The neurological symptoms associated with VHL occur from the CNS pathology that occurs in concert with the syndrome. VHL has CNS pathology within the cerebellum. Although many of the tumors occur in the CNS, the location and the pressure that they exert cause both peripheral and central symptoms. The location of any tumors in the spinal cord must also be taken into account when looking at the physical symptoms of the syndrome.

The cerebellum is associated with coordinated movement; tumors here usually lead to some type of ataxic movement. Neurological signs associated with VHL include various manifestations of ataxia as well as slurred speech and nystagmus. Consequently, these symptoms would be expected to affect the results of neuropsychological testing that require motor movements or visual motor skills. If the ataxia occurs on one side of the body, symptoms of lateralized motor problems can be generated. Furthermore, slurred speech could interfere with any verbal tests, especially those involving expressive speech and verbal fluency. If nystagmus is present, it could be difficult for the person to complete subtests that require any type of fine vision. In cases where hydrocephalus

uv

develops, there can be diffuse and global changes in cognitive abilities. Within this context, confusional states, feeling cloudy, and memory impairment are all possible symptoms. Agitation and vomiting can also occur, as well as personality change.

DIAGNOSIS

As mentioned, the syndrome requires one or two symptoms depending upon the familial status. The patient's symptoms must include one or two of the following: retinal hemangioblastomas, multicystic renal disease, renal cell carcinoma, pheochromocytoma, pancreatic cysts, epididymal cysts, cerebellar hemangioblastomas, and/or hemangioblastomas of other CNS locations (Morantz & Walsh, 1993). This presentation should be confirmed through either MRI and/or CT in order to better understand the symptom presentation. Furthermore, the confirmation should include genetic testing because it is highly reliable and could also help to take preventative measures in the future for the individual and their family. EEG and ultrasound can also help because of their diagnostic abilities. Ultrasound is an efficacious diagnostic tool as it permits the viewing of the kidneys for different pathologies associated with the disorder. In comparison, EEG will sometimes have nonspecific slowing of the wave patterns that may serve to demonstrate a pathological course. As a hallmark of the disorder, it is important to also note when attempting to diagnose VHL that cysts occur in the viscera of most people and therefore cannot be the sole diagnosing feature.

The ability to differentially diagnose this disorder from other similar disorders is apparent. The complexity of the symptoms and the pervasive nature of the VHL tumor suppressor gene make the non-CNS-affected sites look similar to other disorders. Hay, Haywood, Levin, and Sondheimer (2000) noted that there are a wide variety of lethal disorders in children, which can present similar to VHL. However, the likelihood of a person developing VHL before 15 is low. Given the diagnostic complexity surrounding the disorder, in the more complex cases of VHL, it is important to use genetic testing to verify the disorder.

Another important marker associated with the disorder is the lack of cutaneous abnormalities. Although the disorder is listed under the cutaneous class of disorders it has no cutaneous abnormalities. The absence of such symptoms allows VHL to be separated from other disorders like Birt–Hogg–Dubé (BHD) syndrome and hereditary leiomyomatosis, as well as renal cell cancer (HLRCC), a disorder that overlaps with VHL but will be accompanied by cutaneous malformations.

TREATMENT

Treatment of VHL begins with preventative measures and scans. If an individual has a family history of the disorder it is extremely important to get scanned continually for the different types of hemangioblastomas mentioned above. As mentioned above, the preventative genetic testing allows for knowledge regarding an individual who may develop VHL. Along with the scanning techniques, eye examinations should be conducted because of the high likelihood of retinal hemangioblastomas. These can be treated through surgical intervention or laser removal. These detection methods can help identify the signs of the disorder prior to the physical and psychological symptoms occurring. In the case of cerebral hemangioblastomas the utmost caution must be taken, as symptoms may not develop due to their commonly benign nature. If these symptoms are observed, surgical intervention may be warranted.

David M. Scarisbrick
Charles Golden

Greenburg, A., & Cheung, A. K. (2005). *Primer on kidney diseases*. Elsevier Health Sciences.

Hay, W. W., Haywood, A. R., Levin, M. J., & Sondheimer, J. M. (2000). *Current pediatric diagnosis & treatment*. McGraw-Hill Professional.

Morantz, R. A., & Walsh, J. W. (1993). *Brain tumors: A comprehensive text*. Informa Health Care.

Rasmussen, A., Nava-Salazar, S., Yescas, P., Alonso, E., Revuelta, R., Ortiz, I., et al. (2006). Von Hippel-Lindau disease germline mutations in Mexican patients with cerebellar hemangioblastoma. *Journal of Neurosurgery, 104*, 389–394.

W

WALLENBERG'S SYNDROME

DESCRIPTION

Wallenberg's syndrome (also known as lateral medullary syndrome) is one of the most commonly recognized conditions resulting from brainstem infarction (Rigueiro-Veloso, Pego-Reigosa, Brañas-Fernández, Martínez-Vázquez, & Cortés-Laíño, 1997). The condition also commonly involves the posterior cerebellar regions, and therefore is also often characterized as posterior inferior cerebellar artery syndrome. The condition is caused by infarction of the brainstem involving the dorsolateral medulla (Ross, Biller, Adams, & Dunn, 1986), and onset is often progressive, typically occurring after the age of 40, and one study identified a predominance of middle-aged men (age range 30–78 years) among patients presenting with Wallenberg's syndrome (Rigueiro-Veloso et al., 1997). A variety of cerebrovascular risk factors, including hypertension, hypercholesterolemia, and diabetes are often present prior to the cerebrovascular event resulting in Wallenberg's syndrome, and arterial hypertension is known to be the primary risk factor (52%; Rigueiro-Veloso et al., 1997).

Despite the higher prevalence of Wallenberg's syndrome due to cerebrovascular accident, cases of symptom emergence resulting from brain tumor have also been reported (Hanyu, Yoneda, Katsunuma, Miki, & Miwa, 1990). Clinical outcome is often favorable, although death secondary to either respiratory or cardiac failure has been previously described but is uncommon (Hanyu at al., 1990; Rigueiro-Veloso et al., 1997). Additional lesions within the cerebellum are possible, as noted above, resulting in a similar pattern of clinical symptoms. However, further complications including acute hydrocephalus resulting from brainstem compression are also common with this combined syndrome type (Ross et al., 1986).

NEUROPATHOLOGY/PATHOPHYSIOLOGY

Wallenberg's syndrome results from infarction within the arterial supply of the medulla. More specifically, the condition results from vertebral artery occlusion and infarction of the lateral medulla posterior to the inferior olivary nucleus (Nowak & Topka, 2006). Posterior cerebellar infarction is also common. Consequently, the neuropsychiatric and neurocognitive sequelae of Wallenberg's syndrome appears to be attributable to corticocerebellar circuits connecting the ventral posterior cerebellum to associative (parietal) and paralimbic cortical areas (Exner, Weniger, & Irle, 2004).

NEUROPSYCHOLOGICAL/CLINICAL PRESENTATION

Wallenberg's syndrome manifests in a collection of symptoms including vertigo and dizziness (91%), cerebellar gait ataxia (88%), dysphagia (61%), dysphonia (55%), Horner's syndrome (73%), and sensory abnormalities including facial (85%) and hemibody (94%) sensory changes (Kim, Lee, Suh, & Lee, 1994; Zhang, Liu, Wan, & Zheng, 2008). Approximately 25% of patients presenting with lateral medullary infarction also later develop central poststroke pain (Kim, 2007).

Although investigation fails to suggest a significant role of the medulla in cognitive processing, research has demonstrated the importance of the cerebellum for higher-order cognitive processing, to which deficits in reasoning, executive function, and memory may be attributed. As such, the cognitive symptoms may reach sufficient severity to warrant a diagnosis of dementia (Chafetz, Friedman, Kevorkian, & Levy, 1996). Previous work has also documented a particularly specialized role of the posterior cerebellum in both cognitive and affective processing (Schmahmann & Sherman, 1998; cerebellar cognitive affective syndrome); in contrast, individuals with lesions in the superior or anterior cerebellar regions tend to remain cognitively and behaviorally unaffected. However, infarction of the posterior inferior cerebellar artery results in deficits noted in the areas of executive functioning, visuospatial ability, memory function, and neuropsychiatric/personality changes including affective blunting.

More recent work (Exner et al., 2004) has demonstrated a similar pattern of memory impairment, with visuospatial, working, and episodic memories preferentially impaired in combination with emotional withdrawal noted in subjects with focal posterior cerebellar lesions (i.e., individuals with lesions in the posterior inferior cerebellar artery territory). This effect appears to be specific to the posterior cerebellar regions, as similar findings were not demonstrated for lesions within the superior cerebellar artery. Lesion size was not responsible for these cognitive findings, and, in fact, subjects with superior cerebellar lesions were virtually identical to control subjects in both cognitive and affective functioning.

DIAGNOSIS

The diagnosis of Wallenberg's syndrome is done by clinical observation (i.e., signs) as well as the patient's report of physical symptoms, although clinical confirmation using neuroradiological methods are often employed for diagnostic support.

CT imaging appears to be insufficient for the evaluation of medullary lesions, although MRI has been found to be a more useful method for correlating neuropathological diagnosis with clinical symptoms (Ross et al., 1986).

One prior report (Ross et al., 1986) indicated the presence of medullary infarction using MRI, but not CT, in four patients with clinical diagnosis of Wallenberg's syndrome. Axial-plane MRI results also revealed cerebellar infarction of three of the four patients without CT or clinical evidence of cerebellar infarction. This latter finding was particularly revealing, as symptoms associated with coexisting cerebellar lesions often mimic medulla infarction, which may obscure clinical diagnosis and prognostic implications as the secondary lesion may provoke serious and life-threatening complications.

A second prior MRI study (Kim et al., 1994) found that symptoms of nausea and vomiting as well as Horner's sign were common regardless of the lesion location. Rostral medullary lesions were often associated with presence of facial paresis, severe dysphagia, and hoarseness, although caudal lateral medullary lesions were observed in the presence of notable vertigo, nystagmus, and gait ataxia. Ventromedially extending lesions often correlated with contralateral facial sensory change. The investigators concluded that rostrocaudal and dorsoventral MRI findings allows foranato micro-clinical correlations in the evaluation of lateral medullary stroke syndrome patients.

A final study (Rigueiro-Veloso et al., 1997) that employed a larger sample revealed positive MRI findings for 22 of the 23 subjects studied.

More advanced neuroimaging methods, including diffusion-weighted imaging, have been used to image patients presenting with Wallenberg's lateral medullary syndrome. In one recent study (Kitis, Calli, Yunten, Kocaman, & Sirin, 2004), 13 patients presenting in acute or subacute clinical stages underwent diffusion-weighed imaging and results indicated posterolateral medullary localization (positive scan) for 12 of the 13 subjects who underwent imaging. The false-negative result occurred in a patient imaged 10 hr following the onset of symptoms. Clinical observation of imaging results indicated improved detection of normal versus infarcted regions for the high b-value images when compared with the apparent diffusion coefficient map. Researchers concluded that diffusion-weighted neuroimaging is an effective method for examining patients presenting with signs and symptoms of Wallenger's syndrome, although disease detection for patients within the hyperacute stage of the syndrome remains unclear.

TREATMENT

In regard to treatment, compensatory strategies for improving cognitive impairment resulting from cerebellar dysfunction have been attempted. Memory strategies might include the use of external memory devices, such as electronic organizers, whereas rehabilitative strategies for higher cognitive functions such as executive functioning may include implementing increased daily/activity structure. For cases in which new learning is impaired, behaviorally based forms of rehabilitation relying upon development of newly conditioned associations may be warranted (Chafetz et al., 1996).

Treatment for noncognitive functional deficits has also been attempted. In particular, bulbar pain (dysesthesia on the opposite side of the body) caused by lateral medullary infarct may be attenuated with stimulation therapy. In one study (Katayama, Tsubokawa, & Yamamoto, 1994), four subjects underwent thalamic stimulation and three underwent motor cortex stimulation. Although pain control was not obtained by thalamic stimulation, two of the three subjects treated with motor cortex stimulation reported satisfactory pain control. Researchers concluded that motor cortex stimulation was significantly more useful than thalamic stimulation for controlling deafferentation pain secondary to lesion of the central nervous system.

Jessica Foley
Charles Golden

Chafetz, M. D., Friedman, A. L., Kevorkian, C. G., & Levy, J. K. (1996). The cerebellum and cognitive function: Implications for rehabilitation. *Archives of Physical Medicine Rehabilitation, 77*, 1303–1308.

Exner, C., Weniger, G., & Irle, E. (2004). Cerebellar lesions in the PICA but not SCA territory impair cognition. *Neurology, 63*, 2132–2135.

Hanyu, H., Yoneda, Y., Katsunuma, H., Miki, T., & Miwa, T. (1990). Wallenberg's syndrome caused by a brain tumor—a case report and literature review. *Rinsho Shinkeigaku, 30*, 324–326

Katayama, Y., Tsubokawa, T., & Yamamoto, T. (1994). Chronic motor cortex stimulation for central deafferentation pain: Experience with bulbar pain secondary to Wallenberg syndrome. *Stereotactic and Functional Neurosurgery, 62*, 295–299.

Kim, J. S. (2007). Medial medullary infarct aggravates central poststroke pain caused by previous lateral medullary infarct. *European Neurology, 58*, 41–43.

Kim, J. S., Lee, J. H., Suh, D. C., & Lee, M. C. (1994). Spectrum of lateral medullary syndrome. Correlation between clinical findings and magnetic resonance imaging in 33 subjects. *Stroke, 25*, 1405–1410.

Kitis, O., Calli, C., Yunten, N., Kocaman, A., Sirin, H. (2004). Wallenberg's lateral medullary syndrome: Diffusion-weighted imaging findings. *Acta Radiologica, 45*(1), 78–84.

Nowak, D. A., & Topka, H. R. (2006). The clinical variability of Wallenberg's syndrome: The anatomical correlate of ipsilateral axial lateropulsion. *Neurology, 53*, 507–511.

Rigueiro-Veloso, M. T., Pego-Reigosa, R., Brañas-Fernández, F., Martínez-Vázquez, F., & Cortés-Laíño, J. A. (1997). Wallenberg syndrome: A review of 25 cases. *Revista de Neurologia, 59*, 211–215.

Ross, M. A., Biller, J., Adams, H. P., & Dunn, V. (1986). Magnetic resonance imaging in Wallenberg's lateral medullary syndrome. *Stroke, 17*, 542–545.

Schmahmann, J. D., Sherman, J. C. (1998). The cerebellar cognitive affective syndrome. *Brain, 121*, 561–579.

Zhang, S. Q., Liu, M. Y., Wan, B., & Zheng, H. M. (2008). Contralateral body half hypalgesia in a patient with lateral medullary infarction: Atypical Wallenberg syndrome. *European Neurology, 59*, 211–215.

WEGENER'S GRANULOMATOSIS

DESCRIPTION

Wegener's granulomatosis is a form of vasculitis, a disorder characterized by inflammation of the blood vessel(s), involving either the arteries or the veins. The inflammation, necrosis, and vasculitis in Wegener's granulomatosis most frequently targets the upper (sinuses, nose, and trachea) and lower respiratory tracts (lungs) and the kidneys. Other organs that can be affected include the eyes, skin, or peripheral nerves. Along with inflamed blood vessels, Wegener's granulomatosis also forms granulomas around the blood vessels that can destroy normal tissue.

Granuloma is a collection of inflammatory tissue, often a small nodular aggregation of inflammatory cells or a collection of macrophages resembling epithelial cells. Wegener's granulomatosis is part of a large group of vasculitic syndromes. This group presents with an abnormal type of circulating antibody, antineutrophil cytoplasmic antibodies (ANCAs), and affect small- to medium-sized blood vessels. Wegener's usually occurs in middle age, but is found in people of all ages. This disease is typically not often found in children, but there have been some cases.

Wegener's granulomatosis is found within both sexes, but is slightly more prevalent in men. The cause of Wegener's is unknown, but appears to be due to an inflammation-causing event that triggers an abnormal reaction from the immune system. This combination of events may ultimately lead to vasculitis, inflamed and constricted blood vessels, and tissue masses.

NEUROPATHOLOGY/PATHOPHYSIOLOGY

The traditional tissue abnormality associated with Wegener's granulomatosis is inflammation with granuloma formation against a nonspecific inflammatory background. It has been determined that the ANCAs are responsible for the inflammation in Wegener's. The ANCAs found in the disease are those that react with proteinase 3, an enzyme prevalent in granulocytes. This particular type of ANCA is distinguished as cANCA, where "c" indicates cytoplasmic. In Wegener's, the lungs are sometimes afflicted with inflammation of the alveoli.

Necrotizing granulomatosis can develop and may initially appear as small pus-filled abscesses or necrosis of irregularly shaped areas. Inflammation of the arterial walls may occur (arteritis) and may include small and medium vessels, both arteries and veins. Inflammation of these arteries has been both chronic and acute. Scarring of the vasculature can be permanent. The kidneys are typically affected by lesions causing necrotizing glomerulonephritis in Wegener's. Necrotizing glomerulonephritis is a form of kidney disease that causes damage to the inner structures of the kidney (glomeruli) that help filter waste and fluid from the blood. Inflammation in the kidneys can be seen around the glomeruli or the small renal arteries.

Neurological involvement is quite common in Wegener's; however, pathologic reports of neurological involvement are not as prevalent. Some available studies have determined that about one half of patients with Wegener's manifested neurologic involvement prior to beginning treatment with cyclophosphamide. A large series study of the neurological involvement in Wegener's was completed by Nishino, Rubino, DeRemee, Swanson, and Parisi (1993). In their series of 324 patients, most were affected by peripheral or cranial neuropathies. In these neuropathies, cranial nerves II, VI, and VII are most commonly affected by injury compression or extension of the disease. Tissue ischemia may also occur due to the direct effects of inflammation. Overall nervous system involvement in the series included peripheral neuropathy, cranial neuropathy, mononeuritis multiplex, external ophthalmoplegia, seizures, cerebritis, and stroke syndromes. On rare occasions, neurological disorders such as myopathy, aseptic meningitis, and diabetes insipidus have been noted. MRI studies have shown increased dural enhancement in patients with signs of meningeal inflammation.

NEUROPSYCHOLOGICAL/CLINICAL PRESENTATION

Wegener's granulomatosis presents with upper and lower respiratory tract symptoms including sinusitis, nasal ulceration, coughing up blood, and uncomfortable breathing. There may also be hearing loss due to auditory tube dysfunction, sensorineural hearing loss, ulcerations in the mouth, pseudotumors of the eyes, scleritis, conjunctivitis, and subglottic stenosis of the trachea. Renal involvement may be present but is much less common than respiratory tract symptoms. Symptoms related to kidneys include a rapidly necrotizing glomerulonephritis that leads to chronic renal failure. This manifests itself through excess proteins in the urine (proteinuria), blood in the urine (hematuria), and renal insufficiency. Fever, weight loss, and anorexia may be present in the systemic version of the disease. Neurological presentations are variable and focus on the impact of Wegener's on the central nervous system. These presentations include seizures, altered cognition, stroke syndromes, and focal motor and sensory complaints. They may involve chronic, acute, or a stepwise deterioration of tissue inflammation and scarring. This may also be seen in peripheral nerve syndromes and cranial neuropathies related to the disease. Presentation of headaches may be a sign of Wegener's due to parenchymal and meningeal inflammation.

DIAGNOSIS

Initial signs of Wegener's granulomatosis are variable and diagnosis may be delayed due to the nonspecific nature of the symptoms. Wegener's is a suspected diagnosis when there is a presentation including upper respiratory tract symptoms such as chronic sinusitis and/or nasal ulceration, or lower respiratory tract symptoms including coughing up blood (hemoptysis), uncomfortable breathing (dyspnea), or cough. Determination of ANCAs can aid in diagnosis, but positive ANCAs are not conclusive to diagnosis and negative ANCAs are not enough to dismiss the diagnosis. In order to determine ANCAs related to Wegener's, cytoplasmic staining is used. If the ANCAs react with proteinase 3 in neutrophils, they are typically associated with Wegener's. If a patient presents with renal failure or skin vasculitis, these would be the most obvious organs to biopsy. On a rare occasion, a lung biopsy may be needed. A biopsy will show leukocytoclastic vasculitis and clumps of typically arranged white blood cells. Many biopsies, however, are nonspecific and provide too little information for diagnosis.

Criteria for diagnosis include a granulomatous inflammation involving the respiratory tract and a vasculitis of small- to medium-sized vessels. In addition, there must be nasal or oral inflammation (ulcers or nasal discharge), abnormal chest X-ray with nodules, infiltrates or cavities, urinary sediment, and granulomatous inflammation. Differential diagnosis for this disorder is extensive. Other forms of vasculitis can present with very similar symptoms and the antibodies can be positive after certain drug usage. Some differentials include sarcoidosis and neuropathy, complex partial seizures, cerebellar hemorrhage, diabetic neuropathy, multiple sclerosis, cerebellar aneurysms, amyotrophic lateral sclerosis, and acute disseminated encephalomyelitis. Other problems that may need to be differentiated include lymphoma, neurosyphilis, lymphomatoid granulomatosis, carotid disease, and stroke.

TREATMENT

Before medication regimens were determined, Wegener's was uniformly fatal. However, Wegener's granulomatosis is now typically treated with various medication regimens using immunosuppressants with a much better prognosis. Most often, a combination of steroids and antimetabolites (i.e., cyclophosphamide, azathioprine, or methotrexate) may prove useful in treating Wegener's. Antimetabolites inhibit cell growth and proliferation and have some immunosuppressant qualities to them. Cyclophosphamide is now the usual drug for bringing about remission. Cyclophosphamide is administered through pulse IV as the standard administration due to the toxicity of the oral version of the medication.

Azathioprine is used as initial therapy if the patient is unable to tolerate cyclophosphamide; however, it is usually used as maintenance therapy. Cyclophosphamide is an alkylating agent with potential toxicity to bone marrow, liver, and bladder. Azathioprine is an agent that inhibits DNA, RNA, and protein synthesis and antagonizes purine metabolism. This drug may also decrease autoimmune activity by decreasing the spreading of the immune cells in the body.

If the disease is in the severe stages, plasmapheresis may be beneficial. This involves removal, treatment, and return of (components of) blood plasma from blood circulation. Due to the possible side effects of the drugs, doctors may prescribe additional drugs to help prevent the side effects from occurring. These drugs include ones such as trimethoprim/ sulfamethoxazole (Bactrim or Septra) to prevent infection of the lungs, bisphosphonates (Fosamax) to prevent osteoporosis associated with prednisone and other steroids, and folic acid (vitamin B) to prevent sores and other depletion of folate in the body. Finally, surgery may be needed if there has been organ failure as a result of Wegener's granulomatosis (i.e., kidney transplant to restore proper renal function).

Erin L. Tireman
Charles Golden

Wernicke–Korsakoff Syndrome

DESCRIPTION

Carl Wernicke in 1881 was the first to describe a triad of symptoms observed in three patients including a rapid progression of weakness of eye muscles, abnormal gait, and changes of mood, a syndrome now known as Wernicke's encephalopathy (WE). Shortly thereafter, S. S. Korsakoff (1887) published of a series of articles that described an amnesic syndrome, now commonly referred to as Korsakoff syndrome (KS) (both cited in Victor, Adams, & Collins, 1989). In a subsequent 1889 article, Korsakoff described symptoms of peripheral nerve damage starting with paralysis beginning in the lower extremities then continuing to the arms, trunk, bladder, and diaphragm as well as psychic symptoms including irritability, confusion, and disturbances of memory, particularly recent memories (cited in Victor & Yakovlev, 1955). It has become evident that WE and

KS are two aspects of the same disease process but manifested at different points along a continuum of severity and chronicity. A majority of alcoholic patients who survive acute WE develop KS; however, nonalcoholic WE rarely develops into Korsakoff psychosis. The mortality rate of WE is 17–20%, and 85% of survivors develop KS (Victor et al., 1989).

WE commonly occurs in chronic alcoholics but has also been documented in adults following bariatric surgery, gastrointestinal (GI) carcinoma, HIV/ AIDS, and any disease in which nutrient absorption is compromised. Wernicke–Korsakoff syndrome (WKS) has also been documented in pediatric patients with cancer, GI diseases, food allergy, and malnutrition (Vasconcelos et al., 1999).

NEUROPATHOLOGY/PATHOPHYSIOLOGY

In the 1930s, it was established that animals deprived of vitamin B_1, thiamine, developed "biochemical lesions" similar to those seen in WE and KS (Peters, 1936). Further studies have confirmed that WE and Korsakoff amnesia are the result of chronic thiamine deficiency. Thiamine is absorbed by the GI tract, and it is possible that chronic alcohol consumption may lead to impairments in the absorption of thiamine. The body stores enough thiamine to last 4–6 weeks after which time symptoms of WE may be seen. Thiamine crosses the blood–brain barrier via active and passive transport. Active transport of thiamine occurs at approximately the same rate at which thiamine is used by the brain ($0.3 \ \mu g/h/g$) (Cook, Hallwood, & Thomson, 1998).

Two thiamine-dependent enzymes, α-ketoglutarate (αKGDH) and transketolase (TK), have been implicated in symptoms and lesions of WKS. A reduction in thiamine leads to a subsequent reduction in αKGDH, a rate-limiting enzyme of the citric acid cycle involved in glucose metabolism. In addition, reduction of αKGDH may be responsible for increased lactate in the brain, which may play an important role in the formation of biochemical lesions that are characteristic of WKS (Butterworth, 1989, 1995, 2003; Hazell & Butterworth, 2009). It has also been suggested that αKGDH is associated with increased nitric oxide production that has also been implicated in neuronal damage. TK is a second thiamine-dependent enzyme believed to be involved in symptoms of WKS. TK is involved in the synthesis of components that are essential for the reduction of nicotinamide adenine dinucleotide phosphate (NADPH). Important cellular functions are lost with the reduction of TK (Butterworth, 1995). In one study, investigators found that in rats treated with pyrithiamine, a

W

thiamine antagonist, 36% showed a reduction in alpha-ketoglutarate dehydrogenase and abbreviated (α-KGDH) and up to 69% showed a reduction in TK. The animals were then treated with thiamine at which time KGDH activity returned to normal, but TK activity remained 30% lower. The authors suggested that KGDH may be responsible for reversible symptoms and functional lesions by impaling ACh synthesis but that TK is responsible for more permanent lesions (Gibson, Ksiezak-Reding, Sheu, Mykytyn, & Blass, 1984).

Glutamatergic neurotransmission has also been implicated in WKS. Alcohol acts as an N-methyl-D-aspartic acid receptor antagonist disallowing stimulation of the receptor via calcium influx (Tsai, Gastfriend, & Coyle, 1995). Butterworth (2003) suggested that the best current explanation for this degeneration is a down-regulation of glutamate transporters leading to an increase in radical oxygen and nitrous oxide.

Wernicke reported autopsy findings showing lesions of the gray matter around the third and fourth ventricles as well as the cerebral aqueduct. Research using MRI shows that WKS is associated with lesions of the diencephalon, particularly the periventricular area of the third ventricle (Zuccoli et al., 2007), the medial thalamus, the periaqueductal region of the midbrain, the mamillary bodies, and the caudate nuclei (Zhong, Jin, & Fei, 2005). Neuroimaging studies have found reduction in the volume of mamillary bodies and thalamus (Reed et al., 2003). Other research has indicated cerebellar atrophy in approximately 26.8% of patients with WKS (Torvik & Torp, 1986). Lesions of the cerebellar vermis found in WKS may be responsible for ataxic symptoms (Zuccoli et al., 2007). In another study of patients with WE, the medial mamillary nucleus showed the greatest neuronal loss, but severe losses in the medial dorsal nucleus were also found. In addition, the authors found damage to the anterior principal nucleus and concluded that damage to this area is a requirement for amnesia to develop (Harding, Halliday, Caine, & Kril, 2000). Another study showed that increased signals or enhancement of the paramedian thalamus or the mamillary bodies on MRIs of patients with WE were associated with significantly worse outcome, with three of four patients developing KS even after thiamine treatment (Weidauer, Nichtweiss, Lanfermann, & Zanella, 2003).

Reed et al. (2003) examined fluorodeoxyglucose-positron emission tomography (FDG-PET) scans from Korsakoff patients compared with controls and found significant white matter hypermetabolism, specifically in the frontotemporal lobes, which they suggested may be due to inflammatory process or subsequent glial proliferation. In addition, they found hypometabolism of the retrosplenial and medial temporal regions with no atrophy in medial temporal volume, suggesting that changes in the metabolism of this region are not solely due to atrophy of the tissue. Finally, they found hypometabolism in the cortical tissue of the frontotemporal lobe that was directly related to atrophy in that area in one-third of the patients they examined.

NEUROPSYCHOLOGICAL/CLINICAL PRESENTATION

Crowe and El Hadj (2002) investigated the effects of thiamine deficiency coupled with alcohol exposure in chicks and found permanent and irreversible memory dysfunction that remained even following subsequent thiamine treatment. In a study with rats, animals exposed to thiamine deficiency and alcohol did not meet criteria for a learning task. The authors conclude that this suggests a synergistic effect of alcohol and thiamine deficiency (Ciccia & Langlais, 2000).

Wechsler Adult Intelligence Scale (WAIS-III) and Wechsler Memory Scale (WMS-III) scores from 10 participants diagnosed with KS indicated that intelligence quotients remain relatively intact (PIQ = 92.2; VIQ = 94.5; PSI = 88.2) as do working memory scores (97.8); however, the mean general memory score was 57.8 with a range from 45 to 66 and auditory immediate memory scores averaged 73.1. Results suggest that attention and working memory remain relatively intact, but patients with WKS suffer severe deficits in encoding and storage of information (Psychological Corporation, 1997). Another study found that patients with alcoholic KS had deficits in long-term memory and some executive functions including verbal fluency and working memory but that cognitive abilities remained stable over 2 years. Jacobson and Lishman (1987) examined performance of 38 Korsakoff patients on memory and intelligence tests and found that 63% demonstrated marked deficits in memory with small decline of intellectual functioning; 22% showed only mild impairments in memory and IQ scores; and 11% demonstrated marked deficits in both memory and intelligence scores.

DIAGNOSIS

WE has classically been recognized by the triad of symptoms first described by Wernicke in 1881: opthalmoplegia, ataxia, and a global confusional state. However, more recent literature has recognized that relying on this full triad of symptoms as the diagnostic marker leads to misdiagnosis of up to 80% of cases (Butterworth, 2003). In one study, researchers found that only 10% of patients presented with all three symptoms. A literature review revealed that disorientation is the most common symptom observed in up to 82% of this population, poor memory in 30%, ataxia presented in 23%, and nystagmus or ophthalmoplegia presented in 29% of cases (Harper, Giles, & Finaly-Jones, 1986).

In 1997, Caine, Halliday, Kril, and Harper operationalized the criteria for WKS stating that, in order for WE to be diagnosed, at least two of four criteria must be met: dietary deficiencies, eye signs, cerebellar signs, or memory impairment. They also concluded that for WKS to be diagnosed, patients must fulfill the criteria for WE, and have documented evidence of amnesia or disorientation in the absence of an acute confusional state. Using these criteria, they found that patients with WE shared a progressive course of deterioration with a maximum survival of 3 years; however, patients with WKS lived longer.

Differential diagnosis between WKS and Alzheimer's disease may be made in several ways. One way is that patients with WKS do not have plaques as seen in Alzheimer patients. Also, the operational criteria aforementioned enable clinicians to diagnose WKS with high sensitivity and specificity. Finally, lesions of the areas surrounding the third and fourth ventricles are characteristic of WKS.

TREATMENT

Administration of vitamin B_1 has been effective in reversing some of the symptoms of WKS. However, oral administration may not be sufficient because chronic alcohol consumption reduces thiamine transport in the GI tract. Oral and parenteral thiamine are not equally available to the brain, and it is recommended that thiamine be delivered via IM or IV for the treatment of WKS (Tanev, Roether, & Yang, 2009). Thiamine has been effective at not only ameliorating some of the symptoms of Wernick–Korsakoff syndrome, but has also demonstrated effective reduction of lesions (Zhong et al., 2005).

In one patient who developed symptoms of WE after bariatric surgery, oral thiamine was not effective in preventing an acute episode of WE from occurring. It is recommended that thiamine be delivered either intramuscularly or intravenously for 6 weeks postsurgery (Loh et al., 2004). One method of prevention proven relatively effective in some countries is the enrichment of thiamine into staple foods such as bread flour (Harper & Matsumoto, 2005).

Mandi Musso
Alyse Barker
William Drew Gouvier

Butterworth, R. F. (1989). Effects of thiamine deficiency on brain metabolism: Implications for the pathogenesis of the Wernicke-Korsakoff syndrome. *Alcohol & Alcoholism, 24*(4), 271–279.

Butterworth, R. F. (1995). Pathophysiology of alcoholic brain damage: Synergistic effects of ethanol, thiamine deficiency and alcoholic liver disease. *Metabolic Brain Disease, 10*(1), 1–8.

Butterworth, R. F. (2003). Thiamine deficiency and brain disorders. *Nutrition Research Reviews, 16*, 277–283.

Caine, D., Halliday, G. M., Kril, J. J., & Harper, C. G. (1997). Operational criteria for the classification of chronic alcoholics: Identification of Wernicke's encephalopathy. *Journal of Neurology, Neurosurgery, and Psychiatry, 62*(1), 51–60.

Ciccia, R. M., & Langlais, P. J. (2000). An examination of the synergistic interaction of ethanol and thiamine deficiency in the development of neurological signs and long-term cognitive and memory impairments. *Alcoholism: Clinical and Experimental Research, 24*(5), 622–634.

Cook, C. C. H., Hallwood, P. M., & Thomson, A. D. (1998). B vitamin deficiency and neuropsychiatric syndromes in alcohol misuse. *Alcohol & Alcoholism, 33*(4), 317–336.

Crowe, S. F., & El Hadj, D. (2002). Phenytoin ameliorates the memory deficit induced in the young chick by ethanol toxicity in association with thiamine deficiency. *Pharmacology Biochemistry and Behavior, 71*(1–2), 215–222.

Gibson, G. E., Ksiezak-Reding, H., Sheu, K. R., Mykytyn, V., & Blass, J. P. (1984). Correlation of enzymatic, metabolic, and behavioral deficits in thiamin deficiency and its reversal. *Neurochemical Research, 9*(6), 803–814.

Harding, A., Halliday, G., Caine, D., & Kril, J. (2000). Degeneration of anterior thalamic nuclei differentiates alcoholics with amnesia. *Brain, 123*, 141–154.

Harper, C. G., Giles, M., & Finaly-Jones, R. (1986). Clinical signs in the Wernicke-Korsakoff complex: A retrospective analysis of 131 cases diagnosed at necropsy. *Journal of Neurology, Neurosurgery, and Psychiatry, 49*, 341–345.

Harper, C., & Matsumoto, I. (2005). Ethanol and brain damage. *Current Opinion in Pharmacology, 5*, 73–78.

Hazell, A. S., & Butterworth, R. F. (2009). Udpate of cell damage mechanisms in thiamine deficiency: Focus on oxidative stress, excitotoxicity and inflammation. *Alcohol & Alcoholism, 44*(2), 141–147.

Jacobson, R. R., & Lishman, W. A. (1987). Selective memory loss and global intellectual deficits in alcoholic Korsakoff's syndrome. *Psychological Medicine, 17*(3), 649–655.

Loh, Y., Watson, W. D., Verma, A., Chang, S. T., Stocker, D. J., & Labutta, R. J. (2004). Acute Wernicke's encephalopathy following bariatric surgery: Clinical course and MRI correlation. *Obesity Surgery, 14*, 129–132.

Peters, R. A. (1936). The biochemical lesion in vitamin B1 deficiency. Application of modern biochemical analysis in its diagnosis. *Lancet, 1*, 1161–1164.

W

Psychological Corporation. (1997). *Wechsler Adult Intelligence Scale-third edition and Wechsler Memory Scale-third edition technical manual*. San Antonio, TX: Author.

Reed, L. J., Lasserson, D., Marsden, P., Stanhope, N., Stevens, T., Bello, F., et al. (2003). FDG-PET findings in the Wernicke-Korsakoff syndrome. *Cortex, 39*, 1027–1045.

Tanev, K. S., Roether, M., & Yang, C. (2009). Alcohol dementia and thermal dysregulation: A case report and review of the literature. *American Journal of Alzheimer's Disease and Other Dementias, 23*(6), 563–570.

Torvik, A., & Torp, S. (1986). The prevalence of alcoholic cerebellar atrophy: A morphometric and histological study of an autopsy material. *Journal of the neurological science, 75*(1), 43–51.

Tsai, G., Gastfriend, D. R., & Coyle, J. T. (1995). The glutamatergic basis of human alcoholism. *The American Journal of Psychiatry, 152*(3), 332–340.

Vasconcelos, M. M., Silva, K. P., Vidal, G., Silva, A. F., Domingues, R. C., & Berditchevsky, C. R. (1999). Early diagnosis of pediatric Wernicke's encephalopathy. *Pediatric Neurology, 20*(4), 289–294.

Victor, M., Adams, R. D., & Collins, G. H. (1989) *The Wernicke-Korsakoff syndrome and related neurologic disorders due to alcoholism and malnutrition* (2nd ed.). Philadelphia, PA: F. A. Davis.

Victor, M., & Yakovlev, P. (1955). S. S. Korsakoff's psychic disorder in conjunction with peripheral neuritis: A translation of Korsakoff's original article with brief comments on the author and his contribution to clinical medicine. *Neurology, 5*, 394–406.

Weidauer, S., Nichtweiss, M., Lanfermann, H., & Zanella, F. E. (2003). Wernicke encephalopathy: MR findings and clinical presentation. *European Radiology, 13*, 1001–1009.

Wernicke, C. (1881). Die acute haemorrhagische polioencephalitis superior. In *Lehrbuch der Gehirn Krankheiten Fr Aerzte und studirende* (Vol. 2, pp. 229–242). Kassle, Germany: Theodor Fischer.

Zhong, C., Jin, L., & Fei, G. (2005). MR imaging of nonalcoholic Wernicke encephalopathy: A follow-up study. *American Journal of Neuroradiology, 26*, 2301–2305.

Zuccoli, G., Gallucci, M., Capellades, J., Regnicolo, L., Tumiati, B., Cabada Giadas, T., et al. (2007). Wernicke encephalopathy: MR findings at clinical presentation in twenty-six alcoholic and nonalcoholic patients. *American Journal of Neuroradiology, 28*, 1328–1331.

WEST'S SYNDROME

DESCRIPTION

West's syndrome (WS), often referred to as infantile spasms, is a severe epileptic disease arising in infancy, characterized by spasms and hypsarrhythmia on EEG (Akiyama et al., 2005; Asano et al., 2005). In reality, WS is a variant of infantile spasms. The presentation was first described by West in 1841 when he observed a case that he described as a peculiar form of infantile convulsions. The average prevalence is 0.25 per 1,000 children. To date, classification of the core clinical features of WS has been described. The spasms are very brief and usually occur in a series or cluster. The motor involvement is often asymmetric and presents in conjunction with diverted or other pathological eye movements, facial grimaces, or motionless, blank stares (Donat & Wright, 1991; Gaily, Shewmon, Chugani, & Curran, 1995, 1999; Kellaway, Hrachovy, Frost, & Zion, 1979; Watanabe, Toshiko, Tamiko, Kousaburo, & Norihide, 1994). EMG demonstrates a typical diamond-like pattern with a pattern of rapid increasing/decreasing muscle contraction. Over time, psychomotor regression is seen. Symptoms first onset within the first year of life, but cases have been described with a latent onset later in childhood.

WS is divided into three groups: symptomatic, cryptogenic and idiopathic (Baselli et al., 1987). The groups are so defined by their etiological roots. When WS arises from identified brain damage it is referred to as symptomatic. Cryptogenic WS is believed to be secondary to brain damage, but the latter has yet to be or is not definitively related to brain damage. Finally, cases are defined as idiopathic when no suggested cause is established and there are no markers of a possible link to brain damage.

From a prognosis standpoint, outcomes are mixed. Although spasms dissipate over time with development and maturation, cognitive deficits may persist that stem from the seizure activity and their resulting insults that themselves increase risk of future epileptic disorders (Chugani, 2002). Still yet, some children, particularly those with an idiopathic etiology, may demonstrate remission of seizures in combination with preservation of cognitive deficits (Drury, Beydoun, Garofalo, & Henry, 1995; Dulac et al., 1994). Adrenocorticotropic hormone (ACTH), vigabatrin, and corticosteroids are usually the first line of treatment; however, the presentation can often remain refractory to treatment and these agents often fail to alter outcome (Camfield, Camfield, Lortie, & Darwish, 2003; Chugani & Chugani, 1999).

NEUROPATHOLOGY/PATHOPHYSIOLOGY

WS is characterized by spasms and hypsarrhythmia on EEG (Asano et al., 2005; Avanzini, Panzica, & Franceschetti, 2002). Although hypsarrhythmia is the most commonly noted feature on EEG, asymmetric or hypersynchronous presentations, and the presence of consistent epileptic foci may be noted instead (Drury et al., 1995; Panzica-Hrachovy, Frost, & Kellaway, 1984; Hrachovy & Frost, 2006). Seizures and spasms present in the same ictal sequence, suggesting a common pathophysiological substrate. Ictal discharge commonly arises cortically, with focal origin, and presents with an asymmetric EEG pattern involving rhythmic bursts of fast activity preceding symmetric and asymmetric spasms (Avanzini et al., 2002; Panzica et al., 1999). Focal or diffuse, low- amplitude fast rhythms have also been reported on ictal EEG in association with symptomatic and cryptogenic WS (Asano et al., 2005; Kang et al., 2006; Kobayashi et al., 2004). The occurrence of diffuse, low-amplitude rhythms has suggested the potential of concurrent subcortical activity that some have suggested arises from the brainstem (Fusco & Vigevano, 1993; Vigevano, Fusco, & Pachatz, 2001).

Although focal cortical origins may be seen, they are not necessarily tied to specific cortical malformations (Avanzini et al., 2002; Kobayashi et al., 2004; Panzica and Chugani, 1999). For example, Chugani and Chugani (1999) demonstrated that while MRI and CT scans in patients with idiopathic WS remained unremarkable, PET revealed focal cortical abnormalities related to glucose utilization. Following resection of the identified tissue, microscopic analysis revealed subtle malformations and dysplastic cortical lesioning.

Anatomically, WS has been associated with diffuse atrophy and delayed myelination. Relative prevalence of lesions arising in the right hemisphere versus the left and in the temporal and/or occipital lobes as opposed to frontal have been reported (Hamano et al., 2000; Koo & Hwang, 1996). Hypometabolism and hypoperfusion in parieto-occipito-temporal areas have been noted on PET and SPECT scans. The corpus callosum may appear thinner than normal. Functional imaging has suggested basal ganglion and brainstem involvement secondary to cortical recruitment (Chugani, 2002; Chugani & Chugani, 1999; Mori et al., 2007; Munakata et al., 2004).

In the case of symptomatic WS, in which the presentation arises from neurological disturbance, multiple disorders have been associated with the manifestation of WS, including perinatal hypoxia, viral encephalitis, bacterial meningitis, head injury, vascular disorders, cortical dysplasias, and tuberous sclerosis, among others.

NEUROPSYCHOLOGICAL/CLINICAL PRESENTATION

As previously described, WS is a severe epileptic syndrome arising in infancy and marked by brief,

clustered, asymmetric spasms often seen with additional abnormalities of eye movements, facial grimaces, and/or blank stares (Donat & Wright, 1991; Gaily et al., 1995, 1999; Kellaway et al., 1979; Watanabe et al., 1994). Severe EEG derangement (i.e., hypsarrhythmia) is also seen. These spasms may manifest as forward head nodding, jackknife bowing when sitting (bending over forward from the waist when sitting), and rigid extension of the neck, torso, or extremities among others.

Neuropsychological and developmental issues are quite common in association with WS. Over time, following onset of the aforementioned spasms and hypsarrhythmia, psychomotor regression and mental deterioration are noted. However, prior to this, there may be soft signs of impairment. Guzzetta, Frisone, Ricci, Randò, and Guzzetta (2002) noted that as early as 3 months of age and preceding the onset of spasms, the median DQ on Griffiths' scales in WS infants was borderline. Following onset of spasms, a general deterioration of cognition was observed, particularly in language competencies. At the time of a 2-year follow-up only minor improvements had been noted. Truly, cognitive impairment seems to occur in the majority of patients, yet variability is seen across patients and even within patients. In infancy, visual impairments have been commonly reported (Guzzetta, Crisafulli, & Isaya Crinò, 1993; Jambaquè, Chiron, Dulac, Raynaud, & Syrota, 1993). Within this domain, visual inattention, decreased acuity, ocular motility, decreased eye contact, and impaired visual scanning skills have all been reported (Brooks, Simpson, Leer, Robertson, & Archer, 2002; Castano, Lyons, Jan, & Connolly, 2000; Guzzetta et al., 2002; Randó et al., 2004). Auditory functioning is also commonly affected, having been correlated previously with decreased brainstem auditory evoked potential (Kaga, Marsh, & Fukuyama, 1982).

Long-term outcomes in cognition suggest deficits present in approximately 80% of individuals (Riikonen, 2001; Trevathan, Murphy, & Yeargin-Allsopp, 1999). Deficits in memory, attention, and learning have all been reported, even in the presence of preserved or normal intelligence (Gaily et al., 1999). Neurological regression in infancy has also included hypotonia, loss of head control and reaching ability, lack of responsiveness, poor smiling, and decrease of alertness (Guzzetta et al., 1993). Deficits in eye-hand coordination are often below age expectations (Randó et al., 2005).

Behavioral disorders have been reported at higher rates in WS (Riikonen & Amnell, 1981; Thronton & Pampiglione, 1979). Among these presentations, increased risk of autism and autistic features has been noted in the literature (Guzzetta et al., 1993; Jambaqué et al., 1993).

From a prognosis and long-term outcome standpoint, idiopathic WS is associated with the most favorable outcomes. Furthermore, outcomes related to cryptogenic WS are more favorable than in symptomatic WS (Hamano, Tanaka, Mochizuki, Sugiyama, & Eto, 2003; Hamano et al., 2006; Ito et al., 2002; Koo, Hwang, & Logan, 1993; Nabbout, 2001; Yanagaki et al., 1999). Still, long-term deficits have been associated with all variants as discussed above; symptomatic and cryptogenic variants being associated with the greatest deficits. Across all variants, only 16% of patients on average exhibit normal development and over 40% present with neurological deficits with mental retardation being among the most common long-term outcomes; moderate to severe deficits being observed in more than half of patients with cryptogenic or symptomatic forms (Hamano et al., 2003; Ito et al., 2002; Koo et al., 1993). In some cases, the long-term outcomes were related to the timing of treatment initiation, with earlier intervention and seizure management being associated with better outcomes (Koo et al., 1993). When no treatment is received, 75% to 96% of patients present with mental retardation (Jeavons & Bower, 1964).

Increased mortality rates have been reported in conjunction with WS, with an average of around 12% including heightened susceptibility to infections that can be serious and even fatal during ACTH treatment (Riikonen, 1993, 1995).

DIAGNOSIS

Diagnosis of WS is multifaceted, involving a combination of imaging, EEG, and clinical evaluation and history taking. Regarding the latter, a thorough history is necessary including detailed description of the symptoms and their onset. An MRI is critical as it can identify underlying neurological defects. When no such anomalies are identified, yet EEG and history are suggestive of WS, diagnosis is still made and classified as idiopathic or cryptogenic. PET can be quite valuable in the diagnosis of WS, as it permits detection of functional cortical abnormalities as well as indentifying small lesions not clearly identifiable on CT or MRI. SPECT can also be used in the instance that PET even though it is inferior in comparison with PET.

An EEG is essential to the diagnostic workup of WS. As noted, WS presents with EEG patterns characterized by spasms and hypsarrhythmia (Asano et al., 2005; Avanzini et al., 2002). Asymmetric or hypersynchronous presentations, and the presence of consistent epileptic foci may be noted as may ictal discharge commonly arising cortically, with focal origin, and presenting with an asymmetric EEG pattern involving rhythmic bursts of fast activity preceding symmetric and asymmetric spasms (Avanzini et al., 2002; Drury et al., 1995; Panzica-Hrachovy et al., 1984; Hrachovy & Frost, 2006; Panzica et al., 1999). Again, focal or diffuse low amplitude fast rhythms have been associated with ictal EEG in symptomatic and cryptogenic WS (Asano et al., 2005; Kang et al., 2006; Kobayashi et al., 2004). Video-monitored EEG can aid in better evaluating the seizure characteristics.

Neuropsychological evaluation should be sought to document the nature and extent of any neurocognitive deficits as they present in most cases. This is essential to treatment as well in terms of setting up proper educational plans for children as services are often needed.

Physical and occupational therapy evaluations may also be sought to document potential psychomotor deficits. Optometry examination should be requested given the high prevalence of visual deficits. Consultation with a neuro-ophthamologist may be required. Auditory examinations are also recommended as such deficits present in higher frequency.

TREATMENT

Medicinal treatment is the most common approach to treatment. ACTH, vigabatrin, prednisolone, and tetracosactide have all shown some efficacy in acute treatment (Camfield et al., 2003; Chugani & Chugani, 1999; Lux et al., 2004). They have demonstrated utility in diminishing seizure activity acutely in a short span of time; however, prolonged use is concerning due to significant side effects. For example, vigabatrin can cause loss or reduction of peripheral vision. Anti-epileptic drugs may also be useful, but are discussed less. These include topiramate, valproic acidm felbamate, and lamotrigine. Neurosurgical intervention may be considered if individuals are refractory to medicinal treatment.

Beyond medicinal intervention, patients may be aided by a ketogenic diet. Physical and occupational therapy may be needed as individuals present with psychomotor regression early in the disorder do not fully resolve always. Special education services will likely be needed in more than 80% of cases. Necessity of services and type of services required should be based off of assessment findings.

Chad A. Noggle

W

Akiyama, T., Otsubo, H., Ochi, A., Ishiguro, T., Kadokura, G., Ramachandrannair, R., et al. (2005). Focal cortical high-frequency oscillations trigger epileptic spasms: Confirmation by digital video subdural EEG. *Clinical Neurophysiology, 116*, 2819–2825.

Asano, E., Juhasz, C., Shah, A., Muzik, O., Chugani, D. C., Shah, J., et al. (2005) Origin and propagation of epileptic spasms delineated on electrocorticography. *Epilepsia, 46*, 1086–1097.

Avanzini, G., Panzica, F., & Franceschetti, S. (2002). Brain maturational aspects relevant to pathophysiology of infantile spasms. *International Review Neurobiology, 49*, 353–365.

Baselli, G., Cerutti, S., Civardi, S., Lombardi, F., Malliani, A., Merri, M., et al. (1987). Heart rate variability signal processing: A quantitative approach as an aid to diagnosis in cardiovascular pathologies. *International Journal of Biomedical Computing, 20*, 51–70.

Brooks, B. P., Simpson, J. L., Leer, S. M., Robertson, P. L., & Archer, S. M. (2002). Infantile spasms as a cause of acquired perinatal visual loss. *Journal of American Association for Pediatric Ophthalmology and Strabismus, 6*, 385–388.

Camfield, P., Camfield, C., Lortie, A., & Darwish, H. (2003). Infantile spasms in remission may reemerge as intractable epileptic spasms. *Epilepsia, 44*, 1592–1595.

Castano, G., Lyons, C. J., Jan, J. E., & Connolly, M. (2000). Cortical visual impairment in children with infantile spasms. *Journal of American Association for Pediatric Ophthalmology and Strabismus, 4*, 175–178.

Chugani, H. T. (2002). Pathophysiology of infantile spasms. *Advances in Experimental Medicine and Biology, 497*, 111–121.

Chugani, H. T., & Chugani, D. C. (1999). Basic mechanisms of childhood epilepsies: Studies with positron emission tomography. *Advances in Neurology, 79*, 883–891.

Donat, J. F., & Wright, F. S. (1991). Unusual variants of infantile spasms. *Journal of Child Neurology, 6*, 313–318.

Drury, I., Beydoun, A., Garofalo, E. A., & Henry, T. R. (1995). Asymmetric hypsarrhythmia: Clinical electroencephalographic and radiological findings. *Epilepsia, 36*, 41–47.

Dulac, O., Chiron, C., Robain, O., Plouin, P., Jambaque, I., & Pinard, J. M. (1994). Infantile spasms: A pathophysiological hypothesis. *Seminars in Pediatric Neurology, 1*, 83–89.

Fusco, L., & Vigevano, F. (1993). ICTAL clinical electroencephalographic findings of spasms in West syndrome. *Epilepsia, 34*, 671–678.

Gaily, E., Appelqvist, K., Kantola-Sorsa, E., Liukkonen, E., Kyyrönen, P., Sarpola, M., et al. (1999). Cognitive deficits after cryptogenic infantile spasms with benign seizure evolution. *Developmental Medicine & Child Neurology, 41*, 660–664.

Gaily, E. K., Shewmon, D. A., Chugani, H. T., & Curran, J. G. (1995). Asymmetric and asynchronous infantile spasms. *Epilepsia, 36*, 873–882.

Guzzetta, F., Crisafulli, A., & Isaya Crinò, M. (1993). Cognitive assessment of infants with West syndrome: how useful is it for diagnosis and prognosis? *Developmental Medicine & Child Neurology, 35*, 379–387.

Guzzetta, F., Frisone, M. F., Ricci, D., Randò, T., & Guzzetta, A. (2002). Development of visual attention in West syndrome. *Epilepsia, 43*, 757–763.

Hamano, S., Tanaka, M., Kawasaki, S., Nara, T., Horita, H., Eto, Y., et al. (2000). Regional specificity of localized cortical lesions in West syndrome. *Pediatric Neurology, 23*, 219.

Hamano, S., Tanaka, M., Mochizuki, M., Sugiyama, N., & Eto, Y. (2003). Long-term follow-up study of West syndrome: differences of outcome among symptomatic etiologies. *Journal of Pediatrics, 143*, 231–235.

Hamano, S., Yamashita, S., Tanaka, M., Yoshinari, S., Motoyuki, M., & Eto, Y. (2006) Therapeutic efficacy and adverse effects of ACTH therapy in West syndrome: Differences in dosage of ACTH, onset of age and etiology. *Journal of Pediatrics, 148*, 485–488.

Hrachovy, R. A., & Frost, J. D. (2006). The EEG in selected generalized studies. *Journal of Clinical Neurophysiology, 23*, 312–332.

Ito, M., Aiba, H., Hashimoto, K., Kuroki, S., Tomiwa, K., Okuno, T., et al. (2002). Low-dose ACTH therapy for West syndrome: initial effects and long-term outcome. *Neurology, 58*, 110–114.

Jambaqué, I., Chiron, C., Dulac, O., Raynaud, C., & Syrota, P. (1993). Visual inattention inWest syndrome: A neuropsychological and neurofunctional imaging study. *Epilepsia, 34*, 692–700.

Jeavons, P. M., & Bower, B. D. (1964). Infantile spasms, a review of the literature and a study of 112 cases. In *Clinics in developmental medicine* (Vol. 82, pp. 8–25). London: Heineman.

Kaga, K., Marsh, R. R., & Fukuyama, Y. (1982). Auditory brainstem responses in infantile spasms. *International Journal of Pediatrics Otorhinolaryngology, 4*, 57–67.

Kang, H. C., Hwang, Y. S., Park, J. C., Cho, W. H., Kim, S. H., Kim, H. D., et al. (2006). Clinical and electroencephalographic features of infantile spasms associated with malformations of cortical development. *Pediatric Neurosurgery, 42*, 20–27.

Kellaway, P., Hrachovy, R. A., Frost, J. D., Jr., & Zion, T. (1979). Precise characterization and quantification of infantile spasms. *Annals of Neurology, 6*, 214–218.

Kobayashi, K., Oka, M., Akiyama, T., Inoue, T., Abiru, K., Ogino, T., et al. (2004). Very fast rhythmic activity on scalp EEG associated with epileptic spasms. *Epilepsia, 45*, 488–496.

Koo, B., & Hwang, P. (1996). Localization of focal cortical lesions influences age of onset of infantile spasms. *Epilepsia, 37,* 1068.

Koo, B., Hwang, P. A., & Logan, W. J. (1992). Infantile spasms: Outcome and prognostic factors of cryptogenic and symptomatic groups. *Neurology, 43,* 2322–2327.

Koo, B., Hwang, P. A., & Logan, W. J. (1993). Infantile spasms: Outcome and prognostic factors of cryptogenic and symptomatic groups. *Neurology, 43,* 2322–2327.

Lux, A. L., Edwards, S. W., Hancock, E., Johnson, A. L., Kennedy, C. R., Newton, R. W., et al. (2004). The United Kingdom Infantile Spasms Study comparing vigabatrin with prednisolone or tetracosactide at 14 days: A multicentre, randomised controlled trial. *Lancet, 364,* 1773–1778.

Mori, K., Toda, Y., Hashimoto, T., Miyazaki, M., Saijo, T., Ito, H., et al. (2007). Patients withWest syndrome whose ICTAL SPECT showed focal cortical hyperperfusion. *Brain Development, 29,* 202–209.

Munakata, M., Haginoya, K., Ishitobi, M., Sakamoto, O., Sato, I., Kitamura, T., et al. (2004). Dynamic cortical activity during spasms in three patients with West syndrome: a multichannel near-infrared spectroscopic topography study. *Epilepsia, 45,* 1248–1257.

Nabbout, R. (2001). A risk-benefit assessment of treatments for infantile spasms. *Drug Safety, 24,* 813–828.

Panzica, F., Franceschetti, S., Binelli, S., Canafoglia, L., Granata, T., & Avanzini, G. (1999). Spectral properties of EEG fast activity ICTAL discharges associated with infantile spasms. *Clinical Neurophysiology, 110,* 593–603.

Panzica-Hrachovy, R. A., Frost, J. D., & Kellaway, P. (1984). Hypsarrhythmia: Variations on the theme. *Epilepsia, 25,* 317–325.

Randó, T., Bancale, A., Baranello, G., Bini, M., De Belvis, A. G., Epifanio, R., et al. (2004). Visual function in infants withWest syndrome: Correlation with EEG patterns. *Epilepsia, 45,* 781–786.

Randó, T., Baranello, G., Ricci, D., Guzzetta, A., Tinelli, F., Biagioni, E., et al. (2005). Cognitive competence at the onset of West syndrome: correlation with EEG patterns and visual function. *Developmental Medicine and Child Neurology, 47,* 760–765.

Riikonen, R. (1993). Infantile spasms: Infectious disorders. *Neuropediatrics, 24,* 274.

Riikonen, R. (1995). In O. Dulac, H. T. Chugani, & B. Dalla Bernardina (Eds.), *Infantile spasms and West syndrome* (pp. 216–225). London: W.B. Saunders.

Riikonen, R. (2001). Long-term outcome of patients with West syndrome. *Brain Development, 21,* 683–687.

Riikonen, R., & Amnell, G. (1981). Psychiatric disorders in children with earlier infantile spasms. *Developmental Medicine & Child Neurology, 23,* 747–760.

Thornton, E., & Pampiglione, G. (1979). Psychiatric disorders following infantile spasms. *Lancet 1*(8129), 1297.

Trevathan, E., Murphy, C. C., & Yeargin-Allsopp, M. (1999). The descriptive epidemiology of infantile spasms among Atlanta children. *Epilepsia, 40,* 748–751.

Vigevano, F., Fusco, L., & Pachatz, C. (2001). Neurophysiology of spasms. *Brain Development, 23,* 467–472.

Yanagaki, S., Oguni, H., Hayashi, K., Imai, K., Funatuka, M., Tanaka, T., et al. (1999). A comparative study of high-dose and low-dose ACTH therapy for West syndrome. *Brain and Development, 21,* 461–467.

Watanabe, K., Toshiko, H., Tamiko, N., Kousaburo, A., & Norihide, M. (1994). Focal spasms in clusters, focal delayed myelination, and hypsarrhythmia: Unusual variant of West Syndrome. *Pediatric Neurology, 11,* 47–49.

WHIPLASH

DESCRIPTION

Whiplash, a term coined in 1928 by Crowe, constitutes soft-tissue damage to the neck following abrupt flexion or extension often secondary to an automobile accident, sports injury, fall, or assault, typically resulting in neck pain and other assorted symptoms (Crowe, 1964). Motor vehicle accidents as low as 3.6 mph (8.0 km/hr) have been shown to result in whiplash symptoms (Howard, Bowles, Guzman, & Krenrich, 1998). Due to the complex and confusing symptoms, including no overt evidence of injury and longer periods of disabling symptoms than expected, this syndrome has been debated, criticized, and debunked for over a century (Scaer, 2001). During the 19th and early 20th centuries, this seemingly unusual presentation of symptoms was considered by some practitioners to be a result of psychiatric compensation. However, following research demonstrating pendular effects showing forces 3–4 times greater on the head and neck than those exerted on the body, the medical community has come to recognize this collection of symptoms, which appears to be similar among patients, as a legitimate medical condition (Howard et al., 1998).

NEUROPATHOLOGY/PATHOPHYSIOLOGY

Tissues often damaged in such an injury include intervertebral joints, disks, ligaments, cervical muscles, and nerves. Velocity-related injuries can result in minor traumatic brain injury with postconcussion symptoms. The shearing of axons during this event may result in some of the cognitive, somatic, or psychological conditions described below (Rodriguez, Barr, & Burns, 2004).

NEUROPSYCHOLOGICAL/CLINICAL PRESENTATION

The primary symptom of whiplash typically includes neck pain, which tends to be focal and spreads to contralateral areas. Additionally, neck stiffness, injuries to the muscles in the face and neck (i.e., myofacial injuries), and shoulder and/or back pain are other common musculoskeletal symptoms. With regard to sensory functions, paresthesias consisting of burning or prickling sensations may occur. Neurologic symptoms typically include headaches and dizziness (Rodriguez et al., 2004).

Additional less common symptoms may occur. Infrequent neurologic symptoms may include vertigo, balance problems, fainting, or blurred vision. Neurocognitive dysfunctions may occur and typically includes memory loss and/or concentration impairment secondary to axonal shearing similar to that found in traumatic brain injury. Neurocognitive testing of Grade 3 whiplash (see classification system below) will typically reveal impairments in memory and concentration, with other neurocognitive domains generally remaining intact (Randanov & Dvorak, 1996). Psychiatric disturbances may include nervousness, irritability, sleep disturbances, fatigue, or depression (Randanov & Dvorak, 1996). In general, psychological symptoms appear to be significantly exacerbated by disability and restriction from previous work and leisure activities.

Conditions that exacerbate whiplash include being young and involved in contact sports, wearing a seatbelt with a shoulder restraint (which prevents other injuries), poor posture, poor head restraints, being female (likely due to less developed neck muscles), and congenital or acquired narrowing of the cervical spinal canal (Lankester, Garneti, Gargan, & Bannister, 2006). High risk factors include age 65 or greater, paresthesia in extremities, and a "dangerous mechanism of injury," which is defined as "a fall from a height of greater than 1 meter or 3.28 feet, an axial load to the head, motor vehicle collision of greater than 100 km/hr (45.45 mph) with rollover or ejection, collision involving a motorized recreational vehicle, or a bicycle collision" (Lankester et al., 2006). Low risk factors include rear-end collisions, maintaining ambulation, remaining seated rather than prone, delayed onset of neck pain, and absence of midline cervical spine tenderness (Randanov & Dvorak, 1996).

DIAGNOSIS

No independent imaging, physiological, or psychological study provides specific diagnostic criteria. X-Rays, CT or MRI, and EMG are often utilized to rule out injuries, but generally provide little information resulting in normal readings. Recent preliminary and follow-up neuroradiology studies have provided evidence of fatty infiltrates in the cervical extensor muscles, which may allow for a strong MRI diagnostic test in the future (Elliott et al., 2005). A comprehensive clinical interview and neurobehavioral evaluation examining the neurocognitive and sensorimotor domains will help a practitioner identify the pattern of impairments commonly found with whiplash. Whiplash symptoms or whiplash-associated disorders are graded on a scale of 0–4 based on the severity of symptoms: Grade 0 means no complaints of physical signs; Grade 1 indicates neck complaints but no physical signs; Grade 2 indicates neck complaints and musculoskeletal signs; Grade 3 indicates neck complaints and neurological signs; and Grade 4 indicates neck complaints and fracture or dislocation (Verhagen, Scholten-Peeters, de Bie, & Bierma-Zeinstra, 2004).

Differential diagnosis of acute neck pain and stiffness include spinal fracture, cervical disc herniation, subarachnoid hemorrhage, meningitis, myocardial infarction, cervical spondylosis, and brain and bone tumors (Rodriguez et al., 2004).

TREATMENT

Treatment for whiplash includes pain medications, nonsteroidal anti-inflammatory drugs, antidepressants, muscle relaxants, and a cervical collar (Verhagen et al., 2004). The latter is often worn for 2–3 weeks, but recent research has shown that extended use of a cervical collar may actually prolong the recovery time (Rodriguez et al., 2004). Range of motion exercises, physical therapy, and cervical traction may also be prescribed and tend to result in rehabilitation (Rodriguez et al., 2004). Supplemental heat application may relieve muscle tension.

In general, the prognosis for individuals with whiplash is varied, based on the nature of the injury, but generally good with neck and head pain clearing within a few days to weeks (Rodriguez et al., 2004). Typical recovery often follows a slower than expected and unpredictable course compared to other muscle injuries. Researchers have found that the factors that showed significant association with poor outcome on both physical and psychological outcome scales were pre-injury back pain, high frequency of physician attendance, evidence of pre-injury depression or anxiety symptoms, front position in the vehicle, and pain radiating away from the neck after injury (Lankester et al., 2006). Although the majority of patients (70% to 80%) recover completely within 3–6 months post-injury, some may experience chronic neck pain and headaches for several years with periods of worsening symptoms (Scaer, 2001).

Javan Horwitz
Natalie Horwitz
Chad A. Noggle

Crowe, H. (1964). A new diagnostic sign in neck injuries. *California Medicine, 100*, 12–13.

Elliott, J., Galloway, G., Jull, G., Noteboom, J., Centeno, C., & Gibbon, W. (2005). Magnetic resonance imaging analysis of the upper cervical spine extensor musculature in an asymptomatic cohort: An index of fat within muscle. *Clinical Radiology, 60*(3), 355–363.

Howard, R., Bowles, A., Guzman, H., & Krenrich, S. (1998). Head, neck, and mandible dynamics generated by "whiplash." *Accident; Analysis and Prevention, 30*(4), 525–534.

Lankester, B., Garneti, N., Gargan, M., & Bannister, G. (2006). Factors predicting outcome after whiplash injury in subjects pursuing litigation. *European Spine Journal, 15*(6), 902–907.

Randanov, B., & Dvorak, J. (1996). Spine update. Impaired cognitive functioning after whiplash injury of the cervical spine. *Spine, 21*(3), 392–397.

Rodriguez, A., Barr, K., & Burns, S. (2004). Whiplash: Pathophysiology, diagnosis, treatment, and prognosis. *Muscle Nerve, 29*(6), 768–781.

Scaer, J. (2001). *The body bears the burden: Trauma, dissociation, and disease* (pp. 23–53). New York: The Haworth Medical Press.

Verhagen, A., Scholten-Peeters, G., van Wijngaarden, S., de Bie, R., & Bierma-Zeinstra, S. (2004). Conservative treatments for whiplash. *Cochrane Database of Systematic Reviews, 1*, CD003338.

WHIPPLE'S DISEASE

DESCRIPTION

Whipple's disease, also referred to as intestinal lipodystrophy, is a rare, chronic, and infectious disease that can affect multiple systems. However, the disease primarily affects the intestinal tract. The disease is caused by an infection of a rod-shaped bacterium, *Tropheryma whippelii*, and possibly a genetic anomaly in the host. Common symptoms include abdominal pain, diarrhea, fever, weight loss, and malabsorption in the small intestines. Malabsorption may affect the heart, brain, lungs, joints, and eyes. There is pathological evidence of central nervous system (CNS) involvement in most cases, although only 10% of cases present with neurological symptoms. Such symptoms may include progressive dementia, personality changes, ophthalmoplegia, seizures, and hemiparesis. This is almost exclusively a disease of middle-aged, Caucasian males.

NEUROPATHOLOGY/PATHOPHYSIOLOGY

The infecting organism, *T. whippelii*, is a rod-shaped bacterium. *T. whippelii* is a common soil and water saprophyte, and those who are infected frequently work at building sites or farms (Anderson, Dalton, & Davies, 1999; McPhee, Tierney, & Papadakis, 2006).

T. whippelii is a gram-positive actinomycete that thrives in the phagosomes of the macrophages that aid the digestive tract. The macrophages swell from the infection, and, in turn, block drainage from the lymph nodes and the spaces where the macrophages accumulate. The result is malabsorption and excess fat in the bowels. The vacuoles within the macrophages can be detected with a periodic acid–Schiff (PAS) stain if they do contain the pathogen (Burmester, Pezzutto, Ulrichs, & Aicher, 2003).

When an endoscopy is performed on the affected person, the duodenal mucosa will likely have thickened mucosal folds and will have a scattered granular covering of yellowish plaques. Biopsy of the discolored areas will be most helpful in diagnosis. If the biopsy has no discolorations, the person may have been infected mildly. Intestinal villi may be normal or club shaped, which causes distension of the lamina propria, with the characteristic foamy macrophages. A PAS stain will show many positive inclusions that distend the cytoplasm of the macrophages as well. The PAS-positive bacilli and macrophages are most evident at the tips of the villi; however, the entire mucosa may be involved. Mesenteric lymph nodes that are infected will be enlarged and contain many of the macrophages. In addition, there are rare cases where biopsies of organs not involved with the intestines will be positive for the macrophages (Chandrasoma, 1998).

As previously noted, involvement of the CNS is seen in the majority of cases of Whipple's disease. This is usually seen in the early course of the disease, but is also recognized as the most common site of involvement for recurrence (Suzer, Demirkan, Tahta, Coskun, & Cetin). Suzer et al. (1999), in their review of the literature identified cases of Whipple's disease in which CNS involvement was seen as the primary presentation, which is rare. Synthesis of these reports identified primary neurological involvement of the cortical gray matter (including temporal parietal and

W

occipital regions), diencephalon (including both the thalamus and hypothalamus), putamen, leptomeninges, pons, midbrain, and both the supratentorial, and infratentorial white matter.

NEUROPSYCHOLOGICAL/CLINICAL PRESENTATION

The symptoms of Whipple's disease can be considerably variable and nonspecific; therefore, it is often the case that a diagnosis is not reached until later stages of the disease. The disease most often presents as a wasting illness with fever, inflamed and painful joints, skin darkening, and diarrhea. Swollen lymph glands are also common. When the small intestine is involved, steatorrhea, or fatty liver, is likely. Other common symptoms include severe weight loss, sluggishness, chronic diarrhea, and malabsorption. Ninety percent of patients will be anemic.

Other systems that may be involved include the central nervous, cardiovascular, and respiratory systems. Ten percent of patients will experience neurological difficulties including dementia, seizures, weakness on only one side of the body (hemiparesis), and paralysis of the eyes (ophthalmoparesis). The involvement of the central nervous system is often indicative of long-term morbidity. Chest discomfort, chronic cough, and shortness of breath (dyspnea) are prevalent in most cases. These respiratory symptoms may be confused for sarcoidosis (Anderson et al., 1999; Miskovitz, 2005).

DIAGNOSIS

The organism primarily affects the small bowel and therefore, a definitive diagnosis is obtained with a biopsy of the distal duodenum. This biopsy will differentiate Whipple's disease from other disorders that cause malabsorption. Positive biopsies will show increased numbers of histiocytes within the lamina propria. The cytoplasm will be relatively foamy, and there will be clear intracytoplasmic inclusion. Tissues that have been affected by Whipple's disease will have PAS-positive granules within the macrophages. The bacilli can sometimes be seen using electron microscopy. When the central nervous system is involved, collections of PAS-positve cells can be found in the brain and spinal cord. It is definitively diagnosed by PCR (polymerase chain reaction) amplification for *T. whipplei* from a bowel biopsy, brain biopsy, or other appropriate specimen. The bacteria is a gram-positive actinomycete (Anderson et al., 1999; McPhee et al., 2006

Examining *T. whippelii* DNA from a biopsy sample using PCR is the best method of confirming a diagnosis of Whipple's disease. The PCR will be positive in mucosal areas that have not shown to be positive histologically. PCR testing of cerebrospinal fluid is recommended in all patients to detect neurological involvement. Neurological relapse is a common cause of treatment failure (Chandrasoma, 1998).

The biopsy also helps distinguish Whipple's disease from other disorders that cause malabsorption and that have a similar clinical presentation. These include celiac disease, AIDS patients who have intestinal infection, sarcoidosis, Reiter's syndrome, systemic vasculitides, intestinal lymphoma, and subacute infective endocarditis (McPhee et al., 2006).

TREATMENT

Left untreated, Whipple's disease will progress and be fatal usually within 1 year. The goal of treatment is to prevent this progression. Treatment with antibiotics is mandatory for successful recovery, and dramatic clinical improvement is evident within several weeks. Relapse is possible, and therefore prolonged antibiotic treatment for at least 1 year is important. For those in an advanced disease state, recommended treatment includes 2 weeks of intravenous ceftriaxone, followed with trimethoprim-sulfamethoxazole taken twice daily for 1 year. Some patients may be resistant or allergic to sulfonamides in which case treatment with doxycycline and hydroxychloroquine may be effective. After the first year of treatment, patients should have duodenal biopsies obtained to ensure no recurrence of the disease (McPhee et al., 2006).

For patients who do exhibit recurrence, a cyclic course, rather than a continuous course of antibiotics should be used to avoid antibiotic resistance. Interventions should also aim to reduce fever, correct malabsorption and malnutrition, correct anemia, and replenish fluids and electrolytes. (Escott-Stump, 2007; McPhee et al., 2006).

Kelly R. Pless
Charles Golden

Anderson, S. H. C., Dalton, H. R., & Davies, G., (1999). *Key topics in gastroenterology*. New York: Informa Health Care.

Burmester, G. R., Pezzutto, A., Ulrichs, T., & Aicher, A. (2003). *Color atlas of immunology*. New York: Thieme.

Chandrasoma, P. (1998). *Gastrointestinal pathology*. New York: McGraw-Hill Professional.

Escott-Stump, S. (2008). *Nutrition and diagnosis-related care*. Philadelphia: Lippincott Williams & Wilkins.

McPhee, S. J., Tierney, L. M., & Papadakis, M. A. (2006). *Current medical diagnosis and treatment.* New York: McGraw-Hill Professional.

Miskovitz, P. F. (2005). *The doctor's guide to gastrointestinal health: Preventing and treating acid reflux, ulcers, irritable bowel syndrome, diverticulitis, celiac disease, colon cancer, pancreatitis, cirrhosis, hernias and more.* New Jersey: John Wiley and Sons.

Suzer, T., Demirkan, N., Tahta, K., Coskun, E., & Cetin, B. (1999). Whipple's disease confined to the central nervous system: Case report and review of the literature. *Scandinavian Journal of Infectious Disease, 31,* 411–414.

WILLIAMS' SYNDROME

DESCRIPTION

Williams' syndrome (WS) is a genetic disorder caused by the deletion of approximately 25 genes on chromosome 7q11.23 (Donnai & Karmiloff-Smith, 2000). The genotype corresponds with a mixed phenotypical pattern of physical, cognitive, and behavioral features. Physically, distinct facial appearance, cardiovascular disease, connective tissue abnormalities, and growth deficiency are noted (Mervis & Morris, 2007). Cognitively, the syndrome is often characterized by mild to moderate mental retardation with hallmark impairments in spatial cognition and motor skill learning in the presence of relatively spared language functioning (Brock, 2007; Mayer-Lindenberg, Mervis, & Berman, 2006). Socially, WS has been linked with atypical social features categorized as hypersociability (Doyle, Bellugi, Korenberg, & Graham, 2004).

WS presents with a relative prevalence between 1 in 7,500 and 1 in 20,000 (Strømme, Bjørnstad, & Ramstad, 2002). Because it is genetically based, there is no cure. Treatment is symptom based and primarily focused on addressing cognitive and behavioral sequelae. However, as physical symptoms arise (e.g., cardiovascular issues) they must also be addressed as they can have a direct impact on mortality.

NEUROPATHOLOGY/PATHOPHYSIOLOGY

Although genetically based, corresponding with an approximate deletion of 25 genes on chromosome 7q11.23, the clinical profile has more defined pathological foundations. Cognitive and behavioral profiles have been associated with specific neurological abnormalities. Broadly, individuals with WS present with reduced global brain volume (Meyer-Lindenberg et al., 2005). Focal anomalies have also been described and have been linked with the behavioral picture of WS. Particular attention has been paid to the dorsal stream and parietal regions as well as the amygdala.

WS has been linked to impeded development of the dorsal visual stream and parietal regions. These regions present structurally with reduced gray matter and sulci depth as well as reduced functional activation (Chiang et al., 2007; Meyer-Lindeneberg, et al., 2004; Van Essenet al., 2006). In comparison, ventral stream regions seem relatively normal. Meyer-Lindenberg et al. (2004) demonstrated this by comparing dorsal and ventral streams via fMRI of individuals with WS and IQ-matched controls. WS was associated with decreased parietal activation bilaterally in comparison with controls as well as decreased gray matter volume in the intraparietal sulci. Similarly, previous literature also indicated dorsal stream regions while demonstrating preservation of ventral stream regions owing to functional profiles of impaired visuospatial processing in the presence of preserved functions such as motion perception and object identification (Jordan, Reiss, Hoffman, & Landau, 2002; Landau, Hoffman, & Kurz, 2006; Paul, Stiles, Passarotti, Bavar, & Bellugi, 2002; Tager-Flusberg, Plesa-Skwerer, Faja, & Joseph, et al., 2003). Consequently, structural anomalies in parietal regions have also led to the interest in mathematical functioning in WS that is discussed in the following.

Abnormalities in the amygdala of individuals with WS has also been commonly reported and been linked to the hypersociable behavior exhibited (Jawaid, Schmolck, & Schulz, 2008). Research has demonstrated abnormalities both in the structure and size, but more importantly the nature of amygdala activation in individuals with WS (Plesa-Skwerer et al. 2009; Reiss et al., 2004). Reiss et al. (2004) suggested localized hyperactivity of particular nerve clusters in the amygdala when viewing facial expressions in comparison with controls. In comparison, Plesa-Skwerer et al. (2009) demonstrated hypoarousal of autonomic responses in individuals with WS when watching facial expressions compared with normal controls. These discrepancies may suggest that the strength of connection between the amygdale and autonomic nervous system (ANS) in individuals with WS may be weaker owing to the amygdala's tendency to by hyperactive yet correspond with reduced autonomic responsiveness.

Others have suggested that amygdala dysfunction in WS is compounded by their behavioral actions. Specifically, although normal developing children and adults learn to occasionally avert their gaze in social settings to reduce cognitive load (Doherty-Sneddon, Bruce, Bonner, Longbotham, & Doyle, 2002), individuals with WS often do not do this. Maintaining direct eye gaze illicits a physiological response of arousal as the autonomic nervous system is activated by the amygdala (Andreassi, 2000). Normal functioning children and adults avert their gaze to reduce heightened physiological arousal caused by prolonged mutual gaze (Field, 1981). It may be the case that the hyperactivity of the amygdala in WS corresponds with their hypersociability, which itself is reinforced by a lack of gaze aversion that is only possible because their reduced ANS activation prevents them from reaching a point of arousal that would otherwise become uncomfortable. Porter, Coltheart, and Langdon (2007) suggestion of frontal lobe disinhibition may also explain some of this presentation although this proposal is still being evaluated. This latter dysfunction may well explain the higher prevalence of attention-deficit/hyperactivity disorder (ADHD) in WS, however.

NEUROPSYCHOLOGICAL/CLINICAL PRESENTATION

The clinical presentation of WS spans physical, cognitive, and behavioral domains. Physically, WS is characterized by fairly distinct facial dysmorphic features. Individuals commonly present with a constellation of a sunken nasal bridge, small papebral fissures (i.e., eye slits), epicathal fold, eye puffiness, long upper lip owning to a wide mouth in comparison with ears, prominent lower lip, small widely spaced teeth (observable in toddlerhood and through childhood), and a small chin (Bellugi, Lichtenberger, Jones, Lai, & St. George, 2001). In addition, their eyes are blue, they have short stature, and commonly present with cardiovascular defects in which supravalvar aortic stenosis is the most frequently seen. From a cognitive and behavioral standpoint, in many respects, one could conceptualize WS as the polar opposite of autism as verbal skills are spared while visuospatial domains are severely impaired and individuals are hypersocial with overly fixed eye contact. Even toddlers with WS show intense looking behavior toward faces (Mervis et al., 2003).

Cognitively, individuals with WS most commonly present with mild to moderate mental retardation although low-average to average intellectual ability can be seen in some individuals. Severe mental retardation may also be seen in small percentage of individuals. Beyond this more global impairment of cognition, WS is associated with a fairly distinct profile (in comparison with the predicted capabilities) of severe visuospatial impairments, mostly construction, and mathematic disabilities in the presence of relatively spared language functioning. Verbal short-term memory is also spared (Bellugi et al., 2001; Mervis et al., 2000). Of interest, as individuals age, some of their deficits increase. In a longitudinal study of individuals with WS, Jarrold, Baddeley, and Hewes (1998) found that verbal and spatial abilities develop in a divergent way, and the difference between the two abilities increases with age in these subjects.

Behaviorally, WS presents with a distinct personality profile that is hallmark of the presentation itself. Individuals often demonstrate overfriendliness, gregariousness, and high levels of empathy, with an undercurrent of anxiety (Klein-Tasman & Mervis, 2003). In addition, high comorbidity rates have been suggested between WS and various psychiatric manifestations including ADHD, specific phobia, and generalized anxiety disorder beginning in early adolescence (Leyfer, Woodruff-Borden, Klein-Tasman, Fricke, & Mervis, 2006). Furthermore, although irritability and low frustration tolerance has been reported in association with WS (Gosch & Pankau, 1997), oppositional and conduct behaviors are rare (Gosch & Pankau, 1994).

DIAGNOSIS

Diagnostic consideration often starts in infancy or early childhood in response to noted facial abnormalities that often include a sunken nasal bridge, small papebral fissures (i.e., eye slits), epicathal fold, eye puffiness, long upper lip owing to a wide mouth in comparison with ears, prominent lower lip, small widely spaced teeth (observable in toddlerhood and through childhood), and a small chin. Eyes are blue with a starry pattern. Genetic testing may then be requested with definitive diagnosis determined through identification of the aforementioned profile of 25 deletions on chromosome 7q11.23. Neuropsychological evaluation remains essential in determining the cognitive and behavioral profile of individuals, with particular attention placed on visuospatial and mathematic domains. Cardiovascular evaluation is recommended given the high prevalence of such issues, particularly supravalvar aortic stenosis. The same is true of connective tissue abnormalities and growth deficiencies whose identification does not aid in the diagnosis of WS but should be evaluated for once WS is diagnosed.

TREATMENT

Treatment is symptom-based and begins with thorough evaluation of the patient's neuropsychological profile. As suggested, particular attention in assessment should be placed on visuospatial domains and mathematics as well as other domains with a high parietal loading/dependence. Still, as global impairment in the form of mild to moderate mental retardation is seen at higher than average rates, comprehensive evaluation is necessary. Special education services can be utilized with some success to address mathematic difficulties. Depending upon the particular nature of their deficits in this domain, individualized recommendations are necessary.

Applied behavior analysis is recommended at the outset to better determine the nature of the individuals behavioral profile so that specific recommendations can be made. Medicinal interventions have been employed with some success depending upon the severity of the behavioral symptoms.

Chad A. Noggle
Amy R. Steiner

Andreassi, J. L. (2000). *Psychophysiology: Human behaviour and physiological response* (4th ed). Mahwah, NJ: Lawrence Erlbaum Associates.

Bellugi, U., Lichtenberger, L., Jones, W., Lai, Z., & St George, M. (2001). The neurocognitive profile of Williams syndrome: A complex pattern of strengths and weaknesses. In U. Bellugi & M. St. George (Eds.), *Journey from cognition to brain to gene: Perspectives from Williams syndrome* (pp. 1–41). Cambridge, MA: The MIT Press.

Bellugi, U., Wang, P., & Jernigan, T. (1994). Williams syndrome: An unusual neuropsychological profile. In S. Broman & J. Grafman (Eds.), Atypical cognitive deficits in developmental disorders: Implications for brain function. Hillsdale, NJ: Lawrence Erlbaum Associates.

Brock, J. (2007). Language abilities in Williams syndrome: A critical review. *Development and Psychopathology, 19*, 97–127.

Chiang, M. C., Reiss, A. L., Lee, A. D., Bellugi, U., Galaburda, A. M., Korenberg, J. R., et al. (2007). 3D pattern of brain abnormalities in Williams syndrome visualized using tensor-based morphometry. *NeuroImage, 36*, 1096–1109.

Doherty-Sneddon, G., Bruce, V., Bonner, L., Longbotham, S., & Doyle, C. (2002). Development of gaze aversion as disengagement from visual information. *Developmental Psychology, 38*, 438–445.

Donnai, D., & Karmiloff-Smith, A. (2000). Williams syndrome: From genotype through to the cognitive phenotype. *American Journal of Medical Genetics: Seminars in Medical Genetics, 97*(2), 164–171.

Doyle, T. F., Bellugi, U., Korenberg, J. R., & Graham, J. (2004). "Everybody in the world is my friend" hypersociability in young children with Williams syndrome. *American Journal of Medical Genetics Part A, 124A*(3), 263–273.

Field, T. (1981). Infant gaze aversion and heart rate during face-to-face interactions. *Infant Behaviour and Development, 4*, 307–315.

Gosch, A., & Pankau, R. (1994). Social-emotional and behavioral-adjustment in children with Williams-Beuren syndrome. *American Journal of Medical Genetics, 53*(4), 335–339.

Gosch, A., & Pankau, R. (1997). Personality characteristics and behavior problems in individuals of different ages with Williams syndrome. *Developmental Medicine & Child Neurology, 39*(8), 527–533.

Jarrold, C., Baddeley, A. D., & Hewes, A. K. (1998).Verbal and nonverbal abilities in the Williams syndrome phenotype: Evidence for diverging developmental trajectories. *Journal of Child Psychology & Psychiatry & Allied Disciplines, 39*, 511–523.

Jawaid, A. Schmolck, H., & Schulz, P. E. (2008). Hypersociability in Williams syndrome: A role for the amygdala? *Cognitive Neuropsychiatry, 13*(4), 338–342.

Jordan, H., Reiss, J. E., Hoffman, J. E., & Landau, B. (2002). Intact perception of biological motion in the face of profound spatial deficits: Williams syndrome. *Psychological Science, 13*, 162–167.

Klein-Tasman, B. P., & Mervis, C. B. (2003). Distinctive personality characteristics of 8-, 9-, and 10-year-old children with Williams syndrome. *Developmental Neuropsychology, 23*, 271–292.

Landau, B., Hoffman, J. E., & Kurz, N. (2006). Object recognition with severe spatial deficits in Williams syndrome: Sparing and breakdown. *Cognition, 100*, 483–510.

Leyfer, O. T., Woodruff-Borden, J., Klein-Tasman, B. P., Fricke, J. S., & Mervis, C. B. (2006). Prevalence of psychiatric disorders in 4–16-year-olds withWilliams syndrome. *American Journal of Medical Genetics Part B, 141B*, 615–622.

Mayer-Lindenberg, A., Mervis, C. B., & Berman, K. F. (2006). Neural mechanism in Williams syndrome: A unique window to genetic influences on cognition and behaviour. *Nature Reviews Neuroscience, 7*, 380–393.

Mervis, C. B., & Morris, C. A. (2007). Williams syndrome. In M. M. M. Mazzocco & J. L. Ross (Eds.), Neurogenetic developmental disorders: Variation of manifestation in childhood (pp. 199–262). Cambridge, MA: The MIT Press.

Mervis, C. B., Morris, C. A., Klein, T., Bonita, P., Bertrand, J., Kwitny, S., et al. (2003). Attentional characteristics of infants and toddlers with Williams syndrome during triadic interactions. *Developmental Neuropsychology, 23*, 243–268.

Mervis, C. B., Robinson, B. F., Bertrand, J., Morris, C. A., Klein-Tasman, B. P., & Armstrong, S. C. (2000). The Williams Syndrome Cognitive Profile. *Brain and Cognition, 44*, 604–628.

Meyer-Lindenberg, A., Kohn, P., Mervis, C. B., Kippenhan, J. S., Olsen, R. K., Morris, C. A., et al. (2004). Neural basis of genetically determined visuospatial construction deficit in Williams syndrome. *Neuron, 43,* 623–631.

Meyer-Lindenberg, A, Mervis, C. B., Sarpal, D., Koch, P., Steele, S., Kohn, P., et al. (2005). Functional, structural, and metabolic abnormalities of the hippocampal formation in Williams syndrome. *The Journal of Clinical Investigation, 115,* 1888–1895.

Paul, B. M., Stiles, J., Passarotti, A., Bavar, N., & Bellugi, U. (2002). Face and place processing in Williams syndrome: Evidence for a dorsal-ventral dissociation. *Neuroreport, 13,* 1115–1119.

Plesa Skwerer, D., Borum, L., Verbalis, A., Schofield, C., Crawford, N., Ciciolla, L. & Tager-Flusberg, H. (2009). Autonomic responses to dynamic displays of facial expressions in adolescents and adults with Williams syndrome. *Social Cognitive and Affective Neuroscience, 4*(1), 93–100.

Porter, M. A., Coltheart, M., & Langdon, R. (2007). The neuropsychological basis of hypersociability in Williams and down syndrome. *Neuropsychologia, 45,* 2839–2849.

Reiss, A. L., Eckert, M. A., Rose, F. E., Karchemskiy, A., Kesler, S., Chang, M., et al. (2004). An experiment of nature: Brain anatomy parallels cognition and behavior in Williams syndrome. *Journal of Neuroscience, 24,* 5009–5015.

Strømme, P., Bjørnstad, P. G., & Ramstad, K. (2002). Prevalence estimation of Williams syndrome. *Journal of Child Neurology, 17,* 269–271.

Tager-Flusberg, H., Plesa-Skwerer, D., Faja, S., & Joseph, R. M. (2003). People with Williams syndrome process faces holistically. *Cognition, 89,* 11–24.

Van Essen, D. C., Dierker, D., Snyder, A. Z., Raichle, M. E., Reiss, A. L., & Korenberg, J. (2006). Symmetry of cortical folding abnormalities in Williams syndrome revealed by surface-based analyses. *Journal of Neuroscience, 26,* 5470–5483.

WILSON'S DISEASE

DESCRIPTION

Wilson's disease (WD) is a rare (1 in 30,000–100,000 worldwide), autosomal recessively inherited deficiency of copper metabolism. The result is excessive deposits of copper in the liver, brain, and other organs. WD is often categorized as *neurologic* or *liver* depending upon presenting symptoms, and as *juvenile* or *adult* depending upon the age at onset. It is named after S. A. K. Wilson, a neurologist who described the syndrome as "hepatolenticular degeneration" in the early 20th century (Wilson, 1912).

NEUROPATHOLOGY/PATHOPHYSIOLOGY

When foods rich in copper are ingested (e.g., liver, shellfish, nuts), copper is absorbed in the small intestine, bound to circulating proteins, with excess copper deposited in the liver for out-processing via the bile (de Bie, Muller, Wijmenga, & Klomp, 2007). Copper as a trace mineral assists in the transfer of electrons and is necessary for healthy bones, nerves, and skin. Too little copper (hypocupremia) may result in anemia, bone lesions, kinky hair syndrome, and so forth (Cordano, 1978). In WD excessive amounts of copper can begin to accumulate in the liver as early as birth, with onset of observed symptoms as early as 5 (juvenile-onset type), but more typically as the patient approaches middle age (adult-onset type). Juvenile onset is associated with a more virulent course than is adult-onset WD (Mendez & Cummings, 2003). Age of observable symptom onset in the literature ranges from younger than 2 into the 70s (Roberts & Schilsky, 2008).

Concentrations of copper in WD become excessive first in the liver and then in the brain, eyes, kidneys, and joints (Ala, Walker, Ashkan, Dooley, & Schilsky, 2007; Roberts & Schilsky, 2008). Symptoms can include signs of liver damage including cirrhosis (e.g., abdominal pain, jaundice, anemia, vomiting blood, ascites, lower extremity edema, enlarged spleen), neurological involvement (e.g., "wing-beating" tremor, unsteady gait, muscle spasms and/or stiffness, dysarthria, drooling), endocrine problems (e.g., hypoparathyroidism), cardiac (e.g., cardiomyopathy, arrhythmias), corneal (Kayser-Fleischer's rings — copper deposited in the cornea, typically first observed during slit-lamp eye exam), renal problems (including renal stones), and osteoporosis. Psychosis as well as behavior and personality changes have been documented (e.g., mood swings and affective disorders, agitation; Shanmugiah et al., 2008), including confusion, forgetfulness, and aggression and paranoid-driven violence (Dening & Berrios, 1989; Wynkoop, 1994). In fact, psychiatric symptoms are the first manifestation in 20% to 24% of WD cases (Dening & Berrios, 1989; Shanmugiah et al., 2008). Left untreated, liver failure via cirrhosis or fulminating hepatitis can be debilitating and/or fatal (Scheinberg & Sternlieb, 1984). However, early detection and treatment can lead to a fairly normal life.

The genetic mutation for WD is found on chromosome 13 and affects a protein (ATP7B) that assists in the transport of copper in bile and also in the

W

bloodstream via the incorporation of copper into ceruloplasmin. Essentially, both parents have to carry the mutated gene and have a 1-in-4 chance of having a child with the disease with each pregnancy. One in 90 persons carry the genetic mutation. WD's autosomal recessive pattern of inheritance places carrier families and some consanguineous groups at higher risk and results in equal incidence across sexes. The presence of the APOE-3 genotype is believed to contribute to delayed onset of symptoms in WD for reasons that are unclear (Mendez & Cummings, 2003). The neurologic form of adult-onset WD has also been known as Westphal–Strumpell's pseudosclerosis.

In neurologic WD, the areas of the brain believed to be most susceptible to copper deposition are the globus pallidus and putamen (lenticular formation; de Bie et al., 2007). Abnormalities of these structures are observed on CT (Medalia, Isaacs-Glaberman, & Scheinberg, 1988), and the basal ganglia are known to be more sensitive to copper than the thalamus (via MR spectroscopy; Tarnacka, Szeszkowski, Golebiowski, & Czlonkowska, 2009). SPECT has implicated dysfunction in a variety of brain regions including superior frontal, prefrontal, parietal, occipital, select temporal gyri, caudate, and putamen (Piga et al., 2008). Cortical and subcortical regions have been implicated. MRI is the standard of neuroimaging care for WD patients with neurological symptoms at present (Roberts & Schilsky, 2008).

NEUROPSYCHOLOGICAL/CLINICAL PRESENTATION

There is no clear pattern of neurocognitive test results in WD. Some of the factors responsible for this include variability in copper deposition in the brain, age at onset, degree of liver involvement (e.g., hepatic encephalopathy), presence of psychiatric symptoms, and severity of the patient's neurocognitive decline when tested. As above, in addition to the lenticular formation, a variety of cerebral regions may be affected in any given patient and across patients (Piga et al., 2008). Counterintuitively, there may not be a direct linear relationship between level of copper toxicity and neurocognitive deficits (Rathbun, 1996).

Decline in general psychometric intelligence, problematic concentration, slowed mentation, apathy, forgetfulness, and problems with abstraction, concept formation, mental flexibility, arithmetic, and spatial orientation have been observed in different patients at different times during the course and treatment of WD (cf. Mendez & Cummings, 2003; Szutkowska-Hoser, Seniow, Czlonkowska, & Laudanski, 2005).

DIAGNOSIS

In all likelihood, WD will not be initially diagnosed by the neuropsychologist. However, WD's neurologic and/or behavioral symptoms often result in referral to characterize neurocognitive functioning. If not already diagnosed, but suspected by the neuropsychologist, a gastroenterology consultation is prudent. A neurology consultation may also be appropriate, given that the patient will likely be experiencing neurological symptoms by virtue of having been referred to neuropsychology. Suspicion of WD is the first step in its diagnosis. Patients with liver disease who are members of consanguineous groups and/or those with biological relatives who have been diagnosed with WD or who have died of undiagnosed liver failure should be suspected.

Diagnostic tests include urine copper, serum copper, serum ceruloplasmin, slit-lamp examination (for Kayser–Fleischer's rings, which occur in 66% of WD cases; Merle, Schaefer, Ferenci, & Stremmel, 2007), liver copper needle biopsy, radio copper ceruloplasmin incorporation test, and DNA analysis of linked markers (Mendez & Cummings, 2003). Not all tests need to be conducted, and diagnostic recommendations have been promulgated (e.g., Roberts & Schilsky, 2008). Regarding genetic testing, the Wilson's Disease Association (WDA) suggests that all siblings and children of WD patients and other relatives with symptoms or lab tests suggestive of liver or neurological disorder be tested genetically for WD (a description of various genetic tests for WD is provided at the WDA Web site).

TREATMENT

The goal of treatment is to eliminate excess copper (acute intervention) and then to prevent excessive reaccumulation (maintenance therapy; Mendez & Cummings, 2003). Chelating agents (e.g., trientine, penicillamine) are most effective at rapidly reducing the amount of stored copper, whereas preventing further absorption of copper in the stomach and small intestine (via zinc acetate) is a second-line therapy for those who cannot tolerate chelation therapy. Copper reducing therapy is required for life in addition to minimizing dietary intake of copper (e.g., avoiding water containing more that 100 mcg of copper per liter; avoiding supplements containing copper; avoiding chocolate, nuts, liver, shellfish, bran, etc.). Liver transplantation as a cure for WD is rarely used (typically in instances of fulminant liver failure or in which the patient does not respond to other therapies) because of the risks involved. The neuropsychologist can provide the patient and family support in addition to serial assessments as needed.

Timothy F. Wynkoop

Ala, A., Walker, A. P., Ashkan, K., Dooley, J. S., & Schilsky, M. L. (2007). Wilson's disease. *Lancet, 369*, 397–408.

Cordano, A. (1978). Copper deficiency in clinical medicine. In K. M. Hambidge & B. L. Nichols (Eds.), *Zinc and copper in clinical medicine* (pp. 119–122). New York: Spectrum.

de Bie, P., Muller, P., Wijmenga, C., & Klomp, L. W. (2007). Molecular pathogenesis of Wilson and Menkes disease: Correlation of mutations with molecular defects and disease phenotypes. *Journal of Medical Genetics, 44*, 673–688.

Dening, T. R., & Berrios, G. E. (1989). Wilson's disease: Psychiatric symptoms in 195 cases. *Archives of General Psychiatry, 46*, 1126–1134.

Medalia, A., Isaacs-Glaberman, K., & Scheinberg, I. H. (1988). Neuropsychological impairment in Wilson's disease. *Archives of Neurology, 45*, 502–504.

Mendez, M. F., & Cummings, J. L. (2003). *Dementia: A clinical approach*. Philadelphia: Butterworth/Heinemann.

Merle, U., Schaefer, M., Ferenci, P., & Stremmel, W. (2007). Clinical presentation, diagnosis and long-term outcome of Wilson's disease: a cohort study. *Gut, 56*, 115–120.

Piga, M., Murru, A., Satta, L., Serra, A., Sias, A., Loi, G., et al. (2008). Brain MRI and SPECT in the diagnosis of early neurological involvement in Wilson's disease. *European Journal of Nuclear Medicine and Molecular Imaging, 35*, 716–724.

Rathbun, J. K. (1996). Neuropsychological aspects of Wilson's disease. *International Journal of Neuroscience, 85*, 221–229.

Roberts, E. A., & Schilsky, M. L. (2008). Diagnosis and treatment of Wilson's disease: An update. *Hepatology, 47*, 2089–2111.

Scheinberg, I. H., & Sternlieb, I. (1984). Wilson's disease. In L. H. Smith (Ed.), *Major problems in internal medicine* (Vol. 23). Philadelphia: W. B. Saunders.

Shanmugiah, A., Sinha, S., Taly, A. B., Prashanth, L. K., Tomar, M., Arunodaya, G. R., et al. (2008). Psychiatric manifestations in Wilson's disease: A cross-sectional analysis. *Journal of Neuropsychiatry and Clinical Neurosciences, 20*, 81–85.

Szutkowska-Hoser, J., Seniow, J., Czlonkowska, A., & Laudanski, K. (2005). Cognitive functioning and life activity in patients with hepatic form of Wilson's disease. *Polish Psychological Bulletin, 36*, 234–238.

Tarnacka, B., Szeszkowski, W., Golebiowski, M., & Czlonkowska, A. (2009). Metabolic changes in 37 newly diagnosed Wilson's disease patients assessed by magnetic resonance spectroscopy. *Parkinsonism & Related Disorders, 15*, 582–586.

Wilson, S. A. K. (1912). Progressive lenticular degeneration: A familial nervous disease associated with cirrhosis of the liver. *Brain, 34*, 295–509.

Wynkoop, T. F. (1994). Psychiatric symptomatology and type of treatment in Wilson's disease: A retrospective case analysis. *Advances in Medical Psychotherapy, 7*, 181–190.

Online Resources

Wilson's Disease Association (WDA; http://www.wilsonsdisease.org) provides a wide variety of educational materials for patients, families, and medical professionals in pdf format, as well as advocacy updates (go to Patients → WDA Publications).

National Institutes of Health's National Institute of Neurological Disease and Stroke provides the NINDS Wilson's Disease Information Page (http://www.ninds.nih.gov/disorders/wilsons/wilsons.htm). The "Additional resources from MEDLINEplus" link offers additional links and a wealth of information to share with patients and their families.

WOLMAN'S DISEASE

DESCRIPTION

Wolman's disease is a rare autosomal recessive lysosomal storage disease due to a lysosomal lipase deficiency (Uniyal, Colaco, Bharath, Pradhan, & Murthy, 1995) that results in a toxic accumulation of triglycerides and cholesterol esters throughout major organs. Though effecting less than 200,000 people in the United States, it is a fatal disorder in which most of the patients die during the first year of life (Ben-Haroush, Yogev, Levit, Hod, & Kaplan, 2003). Infants will initially present with failure to thrive, persistent vomiting, and abdominal distension (Hoeg, Demosky, Pescovitz, & Brewer, 1984). As the disease progresses, the symptoms worsen and additional symptoms appear including anemia, hypotonia, inanition, and hepatosplenomegaly (enlargement of the liver and spleen).

NEUROPATHOLOGY/PATHOPHYSIOLOGY

A malfunction of chromosome 10, in which the acid lipase enzyme is located, is the putative causal factor of Wolman's disease (Uniyal et al., 1995). The paucity of the acid lipase enzyme results in the accumulation of cholesterol esters and triglycerides at a toxic level, causing death in the first year. The pathognomonic pathophysiological aspects of Wolman's disease include bilateral adrenal gland enlargement and calcification (Hill, Hoeg, Dwyer, Vucich, & Doppman, 1983), vacuolated lymphocytes, hepatosplenomegaly, and foam cells within the patient's bone marrow, which owe to accumulation of cholesterol esters and are dangerous as build-up may cause atherosclerosis (Uniyal et al., 1995).

The adrenal calcification is primarily confined to the outer edges of the glands, and though they enlarge, the glands retain natural shape. This calcification results in adrenocortical insufficiency, and is similar in process to that found in a milder form of acid lipase deficiency, cholesteryl ester storage disease (CESD), but is more devastating to the patient with Wolman's disease. An increase in the adrenal cortex is the causal factor of the gland enlargement, and CT scans are the most sensitive neuroradiological modality for identifying this pathognomonic characteristic.

Another essentially pathognomonic sign of Wolman's disease is hepatosplenomegaly, an enlargement of the spleen and liver. According to Crocker, Vawter, Neuhauser, and Rosowsky (1965), the cholesterol levels in the liver are 15–20 times higher than that seen in normal infants and 4–5 times higher than normal in the spleen. This due to the lack of degradation of triglycerides and cholesterol esters from acid lipase enzyme deficiency. In addition to enlargement, the liver loses density (Hill et al., 1983) due to vacuolation of the hepatic parenchymal cells (Uniyal et al., 1995). Interestingly, fibroblast cultures of the skin from patients with Wolman's disease show increased lipid and cholesterol levels, thus lending further support for deficient triglyceride and cholesterol degradation (Kyriakides, Filippone, Paul, Grattan, & Balint, 1970). Density loss, coupled with gross enlargement due to lipid deposits, contribute to the subsequent liver failure.

NEUROPSYCHOLOGICAL/CLINICAL PRESENTATION

Assessing for neurocognitive impairments is not feasible as the disease is fatal in infancy without treatment (Stein et al., 2007). Patients show failure to thrive syndrome, which is one of the diagnostic phenotypes of the disorder. This lack of growth results in muscular deficiencies that cause hypotonia and motor delays. In late-onset Wolman's disease, the muscle tone may initially develop, though there will be deterioration.

The enlargement and calcification of the adrenal glands result in adrenocortical insufficiency. This leads to the hypotonia, nausea, vomiting, and gastrointestinal difficulties. Though the adrenal medulla maintains its shape, it is reduced in size (Ozmen et al., 1992) due to gland expansion and calcification that results in a reduction in the release of epinephrine and norepinephrine as hormones into the blood stream.

DIAGNOSIS

A diagnosis of Wolman's disease first requires an examination of patient symptomatology. The essential symptom presentation is failure to thrive, vomiting, diarrhea, anemia, hypotonia (low muscle tone), and abdominal distension due to an enlarged liver and spleen. In the presence of these symptoms, there are two definitive pathognomonic signs of Wolman's disease: bilateral adrenal gland enlargement and calcification and dermal fibroblast cultures that demonstrate deficient acid esterase activity (Wolman, 1995) with a substantial elevation in cholesterol levels compared with normals (Kyriakides et al., 1970). Other diagnostic signs of Wolman's disease are hepatosplenomegaly with diminished liver density as identified through a CT scan (Ozmen et al., 1992), vacuolated lymphocytes, and foam cells in bone marrow (Uniyal et al., 1995).

Research has also demonstrated the ability for a prenatal diagnosis of Wolman's disease in at-risk pregnancies (Coates, Cortner, Mennuti, Wheeler, & Kaback, 1978; Patrick, Willcox, Stephens, & Kenyon, 1976; van Diggelen et al., 1988). Patrick et al. (1976) found severe deficiency of acid esterase activity in cultured amniotic fluid cells (amniocentesis) in the 15th week of pregnancy, suggesting a diagnosis of Wolman's disease. Van Diggelen et al. (1988) supported the ability to diagnose Wolman's disease in the first trimester by identifying acid lipase deficiency in the chorionic villi. Finally, Coates et al. (1978) identified deficient acid lipase.

The primary differential diagnosis of Wolman's disease is its milder version, CESD, which does not lead to early death. CESD presents with deficient acid esterase-lipase activity that is less severe (Wolman, 1995). CESD patients are generally asymptomatic in childhood and are eventually diagnosed due to less severe hepatomegaly (Hoeg et al., 1984). The pathognomonic sign of Wolman's disease is rarely present (Hill et al., 1983; Ozmen et al., 1992). CESD patients have higher lysosomal acid lipase activity (Ozmen et al., 1992) and the lipid deposition is more widespread.

TREATMENT

Wolman (1995) posited that the disease process may be slowed by avoiding the introduction of nontransportable and noncatabolizable lipids to the infant from breast milk or formula containing lipid esters. Though effective in slowing the process, reducing lipid intake is unsuccessful in curing the disease. Recent research has suggested that it may indeed be remedied through umbilical cord blood (UCB) transplantation from an unrelated donor, an optimal source of stem cells (Stein et al., 2007). These authors reported successfully restoring acid lipase levels through UCB transplantation at 3 months, with cells engrafting within a few weeks and complete platelet transfusion independence in just over 2 months. Normal levels of acid lipase were identified 7 weeks after UCB transplantation. A follow-up MRI at 18 months noted age-appropriate myelinization 6 months later (Stein et al., 2007). Four years after UCB transplantation, the patient no longer suffered from hepatosplenomegaly, was growing at the normal rate, and motor and intellectual achievements were age appropriate.

Hematopoietic cell transplantation (HCT), the transplantation of blood cells derived from bone marrow, has also been found effective in the treatment of Wolman's disease (Tolar et al., 2008). Tolar et al. (2008) reported that this method was successful in preventing hepatic failure in Wolman's disease patients, and improves hepatosplenomegaly, and sometimes adrenal function. The authors reported mild to moderate psychomotor developmental delay in one of the patients treated with HCT, but were unable to determine whether the neurocognitive deficits owed to treatment or other medical problems. The patients treated by these authors at an earlier age displayed age-appropriate neurodevelopment.

Both HCT and UCB transplantations are best implemented in the first few months of life, and decreasing lipid intake enhances treatment efficacy. Long-term survival rates, and neurocognitive or medical sequelae are not available as both Stein et al. (2007) and Tolar et al. reported these therapies as some of the first known successes, with the eldest surviving patients under the age of 5 at study completion.

Daniel J. Heyanka
Charles Golden

Ben-Haroush, A., Yogev, Y., Levit, O., Hod, M., & Kaplan, B. (2003). Isolated fetal ascites caused by Wolman disease. *Ultrasound in Obstetrics and Gynecology, 21,* 297–298.

Coates, P. M., Cortner, J. A., Mennuti, M. T., Wheeler, J. E., & Kaback, M. M. (1978). Prenatal diagnosis of Wolman disease. *American Journal of Medical Genetics, 2,* 397–407.

Crocker, A. C., Vawter, G. F., Neuhauser, E. B. D., & Rosowsky, A. (1965). Wolman's disease: Three new patients with a recently described lipidosis. *Pediatrics, 35,* 627–640.

Hill, S. C., Hoeg, J. M., Dwyer, A. J., Vucich, J. J., & Doppman, J. L. (1983). CT findings in acid lipase deficiency: Wolman disease and cholesteryl ester storage disease. *Journal of Computer Assisted Tomography, 7,* 815–818.

Hoeg, J. M., Demosky, S. J., Jr., Pescovitz, O. H., & Brewer, H. B., Jr. (1984). Cholesteryl ester storage disease and Wolman disease: Phenotypic variants of lysosomal acid cholesteryl ester hydrolase deficiency. *American Journal of Human Genetics, 36,* 1190–1203.

Kyriakides, E. C., Filippone, N., Paul, B., Grattan, W., & Balint, J. A. (1970). Lipid studies in Wolman's disease. *Pediatrics, 46,* 431–436.

Ozmen, M. N., Aygiin, N., Kilic, I., Kuran, L., Yalcin, B., & Besim, A. (1992). Wolman's disease: Ultrasonographic and computed tomographic findings. *Pediatric Radiology, 22,* 541–542.

Patrick, A. D., Willcox, P., Stephens, R., & Kenyon, V. G. (1976). Prenatal diagnosis of Wolman's disease. *Journal of Medical Genetics, 13,* 49–51.

Stein, J., Garty, B. Z., Dror, Y., Fenig, E., Zeigler, M., & Yaniv, I. (2007). Successful treatment of Wolman disease by unrelated umbilical cord blood transplantation. *European Journal of Pediatrics, 166,* 663–666.

Tolar, J., Petryk, A., Khan, K., Bjoraker, K. J., Jessurun, J., & Dolan, M., et al. (2008). Long-term metabolic, endocrine, and neuropsychological outcome of hematopoietic cell transplantation for Wolman disease. *Bone Marrow Transplant.* [EPub ahead of print].

Uniyal, K. J., Colaco, M. P., Bharath, N. S., Pradhan, M. R., & Murthy, A. K. (1995). *Indian Pediatrics, 32,* 232–235.

Van Diggelen, O. P., Von Kuskull, H., Ammala, P., Vredeveldt, G. T. M., Janse, H. C., & Kleijer, W. J. (1988). First trimester diagnosis of Wolman's disease. *Prenatal Diagnosis, 8,* 661–663.

Wolman, M. (1995). Wolman disease and its treatment. *Clinical Pediatrics, 34,* 207–212.

ZELLWEGER'S SYNDROME

DESCRIPTION

Zellweger's syndrome is a progressive developmental metabolic disease attributable to deficient biogenesis of peroxisomes and resulting in a generalized loss of peroxisomal functions (Poll-The et al., 2004). The condition manifests in a distinctive dysmorphic phenotype despite a highly variable range of severity levels (Weller, Rosewich, & Gärtner, 2008). All peroxisomal biogenesis disorders are associated with similar clinical, biochemical, pathological, and genetic findings (Folz & Trobe, 1991; Poll-The et al., 2004). Zellweger's syndrome is part of a group of three peroxisomal disorders, resulting in defective biogenesis of the peroxisome; others included within this category are neonatal adrenoleukodystrophy and infantile Refsum disease (Folz & Trobe, 1991)—all syndromes are collectively known as Zellweger's spectrum.

Zellweger's syndrome constitutes the most severe variant of the three peroxisomal biogenesis disorders and has been found to be associated with seizures, infantile hypotonia, and death within the first year (Folz & Trobe, 1991), although a significant subset of patients live beyond the age of 4. When it does occur, death is most often attributable to the consequences of respiratory dysfunction, dehydration, renal or liver failure, and gastrointestinal hemorrhage. There is a 77% probability that a nonprogressive child living past the age of 1 will continue to live to school age (Poll-The et al., 2004).

NEUROPATHOLOGY/PATHOPHYSIOLOGY

The peroximal biogenesis disorders reflect malformation syndromes resulting from metabolic error and highlight the important role that biochemical pathways play in human development. Zellweger's spectrum disorders are caused by the inability to import peroxisomal matrix proteins into peroxisomes, which are targeted to peroxisomes by one of two different peroxisome targeting signals (i.e., PTS1 and PTS2). The failure to form peroxisomes, as is the case in

these conditions, leads to impairment of many peroxisomal functions including the formation of poly-unsaturated Zellweger's syndrome, and prior investigation has revealed MRI to be particularly useful for this purpose (Barkovich & Peck 1997; Barth et al., 2001, 2004; van der Knaap & Valk, 1991). More recently, Weller et al. (2008) evaluated 18 patients presenting with Zellweger's syndrome using conventional MRI and documented a variety of abnormal findings, including an atypical gyration pattern, delayed myelination leukoencephalopathy, and brain atrophy. Polymicrogyria and pachygyria were more common in patients presenting with a more severe variant of the condition, whereas abnormal gyration appears to be more frequent in the milder conditions. Leukoencephalopathy was also found to increase with age in longer-surviving patients.

One study of six cases of Zellweger's syndrome revealed polymicrogyria in both cerebral and cerebellar cortices, neuronal heterotopia in the cerebral white matter, and dysplasia of the inferior olivary nucleus and subependymal cyst (Takashima et al., 1992). Diffuse dysmyelination and neuronal migratory dysfunction also occur in this condition: Although diffuse dysmyelination is likely related to abnormal development of oligodendrocytes, migration dysfunction is due to abnormal endothelial cells or radial glial cells (Takashima et al., 1992). Neurodevelopmentally, neuronal migratory processes are strikingly abnormal, and there are areas of polymicrogyria, Purkinje cell heterotopic and olivary nucleus abnormalities (Steinberg et al., 2006).

Molecularly, 21 of 31 patients in a relatively recent investigation showed mutations in the PEX1 gene, and the most common mutations included the G843D (c.2528G → A; improved outcome and milder phenotype) missense mutation, and the c.2097insT frameshift mutation (severe phenotype). Intermediate severity is shown in patients heterozygous for G843D/c.2097insT (Poll-The et al., 2004).

NEUROPSYCHOLOGICAL/CLINICAL PRESENTATION

A recent investigation conducted on 31 patients (aged 1.2–24 years) with biochemically confirmed peroxisome biogenesis disorders presenting with prolonged survival revealed overlapping cognitive and motor dysfunction, retinopathy, sensorineural hearing impairment, eye abnormalities, craniofacial abnormalities, and hepatic involvement. Postnatal growth failure was present among many subjects, and hyperoxaluria was found in 10 subjects. Despite notable cognitive and motor deficits, a range of severity was revealed. In particular, speech ranged from nonverbal communication to grammatically correct speech and comprehensive reading, and motor skills ranged from supported sitting to normal gait (Poll-The et al., 2004).

For peroxisome biogenesis disordered patients surviving past age 4, early developmental skills (e.g., unsupported sitting, intentional hand use, unsupported walking, hearing, and purposeful vocalization) were attained by greater than 75% of the individuals studied. Unsupported sitting occurred between 9 and 30 months of age and unsupported walking occurred between 14 and 66 months of age. In contrast, more advanced developmental milestones such as grammatical language (21%) and reading (4%) were seen only in a minority of subjects. Seizures have been observed in 23% of cases, with an average seizure onset between 0 and 2.7 years of age; presentations may vary considerably and include automatisms, myoclonic, atonic, tonic–clonic, and infantile spasms. All subjects studied exhibited severe visual disturbance, which ranged from total blindness originating at birth to corrected vision with prescription glasses; common symptoms included refractive anomalies, strabismus, nystagmus, retinopathy, cataracts, optic nerve atrophy, corneal clouding, glaucoma, and failure to achieve pursuit eye movements. All 31 patients in the study demonstrated hearing impairment. Liver, spleen, and kidney dysfunction were also common.

Finally, peroxisome biogenesis disorder has been associated with facial dysmorphic features, including high forehead, epicanthic folds, and abnormal and attached ear lobules (Poll-The et al., 2004; Steinberg et al., 2006).

DIAGNOSIS

Diagnosis of Zellweger's syndrome is determined by clinical presentation and the biochemical evaluation of peroxisomal metabolites, and is confirmed based upon mutation detection in 1 out of 12 genes coding for proteins involved in the biogenesis of peroxisomes. Biochemical studies are performed in the blood and urine to screen for the peroxisome biogenesis disorders. DNA testing is also possible (Steinberg et al., 2006).

However, in some cases, clinical symptoms are less readily detectable and MRI may prove useful in diagnostic confirmation. Positive MRI findings include abnormal gyration patterns including polymicrogyria and pachygyria, leukoencephalopathy, germinolytic cysts, and heterotopias (Weller et al., 2008).

TREATMENT

The myriad of biochemical abnormalities resulting from peroxisome assembly failure, as detailed above, lead to significant developmental disturbances that present at birth and progress further postnatally. Therapeutic approaches for Zellweger's syndrome are primarily supportive in nature as effective treatments for attenuating the primary effects of the condition remain to be discovered (Poll-The et al., 2004). Currently available treatments are intended to target seizure disorder, liver dysfunction, sensory abnormalities (e.g., hearing via external aids), ophthalmologic conditions, and other related developmental dysfunction, as described above (Steinberg et al., 2006).

Cognitive and motor treatments have not yet been investigated for individuals diagnosed with Zellweger's syndrome. For milder cases of individuals surviving until school age, treatments may involve participation in schools targeting developmentally disabled students, as well as educational plans aimed at increasing accommodation to cognitive and sensory difficulties (Poll-The et al., 2004).

Jessica Foley
Charles Golden

Barkovich, A. J., & Peck, W. W. (1997). MR of Zellweger syndrome. *AJNR American Journal of Neuroradiology, 18*, 1163–1170.

Barth, P. G., Gootjes, J., Bode, H., Vreken, P., Majoie, C. B., & Wanders, R. J. (2001). Late onset white matter disease in peroxisome biogenesis disorder. *Neurology, 57*, 1949–1955.

Barth, P. G., Majoie, C. B. L. M., Gootjes, J., Wanders, R. J. A., Waterham, H. R., van der Knaap, M. S., et al. (2004). Neuroimaging of peroxisome biogenesis disorders (Zellweger spectrum) with prolonged survival. *Neurology, 62*, 439–444.

Folz, S. J., & Trobe, J. D. (1991). The peroxisome and the eye. *Survey of Ophthalmology, 35*, 353–368.

Poll-The, B. T., Gootjes, J., Duran, M., De Klerk, J. B., Wenniger-Prick, L. J., Admiraal R. J., et al. (2004). Peroxisome biogenesis disorders with prolonged survival: Phenotypic expression in a cohort of 31 patients.

American Journal of Medical Genetics. Part A, 126A, 333–338.

Steinberg, S. J., Dodt, G., Raymond, G. V., Braverman, N. E., Moser, A. B., & Moser H. W. (2006). Peroxisome biogenesis disorders. *Biochimica et Biophysica Acta, 1763,* 1733–1748.

Takashima, S., Houdou, S., Kamei, J., Hasegawa, M., Mito, T., Suzuki, Y., et al. (1992). Neuropathology of peroxisomal disorders: Zellweger syndrome and neonatal adrenoleukodystrophy. *No To Hattatsu. Brain and Development, 24,* 186–193.

van der Knaap, M. S., & Valk, J. (1991). The MR spectrum of peroxisomal disorders. *Neuroradiology, 33,* 30–37.

Weller, S., Rosewich, H., & Gärtner, J. (2008). Cerebral MRI as a valuable diagnostic tool in Zellweger spectrum patients. *Journal of Inherited Metabolic Disease.* [Epub ahead of print].

XYZ

INDEX